AF393370

PROGRESS IN ALZHEIMER'S AND PARKINSON'S DISEASES

ADVANCES IN BEHAVIORAL BIOLOGY

Recent Volumes in This Series

Volume 37   KINDLING 4
Edited by Juhn A. Wada

Volume 38A   BASIC, CLINICAL, AND THERAPEUTIC ASPECTS OF ALZHEIMER'S AND PARKIN-
SON'S DISEASES, Volume 1
Edited by Toshiharu Nagatsu, Abraham Fisher, and Mitsuo Yoshida

Volume 38B   BASIC, CLINICAL, AND THERAPEUTIC ASPECTS OF ALZHEIMER'S AND PARKIN-
SON'S DISEASES, Volume 2
Edited by Toshiharu Nagatsu, Abraham Fisher, and Mitsuo Yoshida

Volume 39   THE BASAL GANGLIA III
Edited by Giorgio Bernardi, Malcolm B. Carpenter, Gaetano Di Chiara, Micaela Morelli,
and Paolo Stanzione

Volume 40   TREATMENT OF DEMENTIAS: A New Generation of Progress
Edited by Edwin M. Meyer, James W. Simpkins, Jyunji Yamamoto,
and Fulton T. Crews

Volume 41   THE BASAL GANGLIA IV: New Ideas and Data on Structure and Function
Edited by Gérard Percheron, John S. McKenzie, and Jean Féger

Volume 42   CALLOSAL AGENESIS: A Natural Split Brain?
Edited by Maryse Lassonde and Malcolm A. Jeeves

Volume 43   NEUROTRANSMITTERS IN THE HUMAN BRAIN
Edited by David J. Tracey, George Paxinos, and Jonathan Stone

Volume 44   ALZHEIMER'S AND PARKINSON'S DISEASES: Recent Developments
Edited by Israel Hanin, Mitsuo Yoshida, and Abraham Fisher

Volume 45   EPILEPSY AND THE CORPUS CALLOSUM 2
Edited by Alexander G. Reeves and David W. Roberts

Volume 46   BIOLOGY AND PHYSIOLOGY OF THE BLOOD–BRAIN BARRIER: Transport, Cellular
Interactions, and Brain Pathologies
Edited by Pierre-Olivier Couraud and Daniel Scherman

Volume 47   THE BASAL GANGLIA V
Edited by Chihiro Ohye, Minoru Kimura, and John S. McKenzie

Volume 48   KINDLING 5
Edited by Michael E. Corcoran and Solomon L. Moshé

Volume 49   PROGRESS IN ALZHEIMER'S AND PARKINSON'S DISEASES
Edited by Abraham Fisher, Israel Hanin, and Mitsuo Yoshida

PROGRESS IN ALZHEIMER'S AND PARKINSON'S DISEASES

Edited by

Abraham Fisher
Israel Institute for Biological Research
Ness Ziona, Israel

Israel Hanin
Loyola University of Chicago
Maywood, Illinois

and

Mitsuo Yoshida
Jichi Medical School
Tochigi, Japan

Volume I

SPRINGER SCIENCE+BUSINESS MEDIA, LLC

Library of Congress Cataloging-in-Publication Data

Progress in Alzheimer's and Parkinson's diseases / edited by Abraham
  Fisher, Israel Hanin, and Mitsuo Yoshida.
        p.   cm. -- (Advances in behavioral biology ; v. 49)
    "Proceedings of the Fourth International Conference on Progress in
  Alzheimer's and Parkinson's Diseases, held May 18-23, 1997, in
  Eilat, Israel"--T.p. verso.
    This Conference was also the 41st in the series of annual OHOLO
  Conferences sponsored by the Israel Institute for Biological
  Research, and conducted under the auspices of the Alzheimer's
  Association's Ronald and Nancy Reagan Research Institute.
    Includes bibliographical references and index.
    ISBN 978-1-4613-7435-0   ISBN 978-1-4615-5337-3 (eBook)
    DOI 10.1007/978-1-4615-5337-3
      1. Alzheimer's disease--Congresses.   2. Parkinson's disease-
  -Congresses.   I. Fisher, Abraham. II. Hanin, Israel.
  III. Yoshida, Mitsuo, 1933-   . IV. Makhon le-mehkar biyologi be
  -Yisra 'el.   V. Ronald and Nancy Reagan Research Institute.
  VI. International Conference on Progress in Alzheimer's and
  Parkinson's Diseases (4th : 1997 : Eilat, Israel) VII. OHOLO
  Conference (41st : 1997 : Eilat, Israel) VIII. Series.
      [DNLM: 1. Alzheimer Disease--congresses.   2. Parkinson Disease-
  -co.   W3AD215 v.49 1998]
  RC523.P763 1998
  616.8'31--dc21
  DNLM/DLC
  for Library of Congress   98-26174
                                                         CIP

Proceedings of the Fourth International Conference on Progress in Alzheimer's and Parkinson's
Diseases, held May 18-23, 1997, in Eilat, Israel

ISBN 978-1-4613-7435-0

© 1998 Springer Science+Business Media New York
Originally published by Plenum Press,New York in 1998
Softcover reprint of the hardcover 1st edition 1998
http://www.plenum.com

10 9 8 7 6 5 4 3 2 1

PREFACE

This book represents the fourth in a series of international conferences related to Alzheimer's (AD) and Parkinson's (PD) diseases. The first one took place in Eilat, Israel in 1985; the second in Kyoto, Japan, in 1989; and the third in Chicago, IL, USA in 1993. This book incorporates the proceedings of the Fourth International Conference on Progress in Alzheimer's and Parkinson's Diseases, held in Eilat, Israel, on May 18–23, 1997. This Conference was the 41st in the series of annual OHOLO Conferences sponsored by the Israel Institute for Biological Research (IIBR). It was also conducted under the auspices of the Alzheimer's Association Ronald and Nancy Reagan Research Institute, USA.

The Conference was attended by 550 participants from 28 countries, representing a broad spectrum of research interests; and included a well-balanced representation from academia, clinical institutions and pharmaceutical industry. The four-and-one-half day meeting served as an excellent medium for surveying the current preclinical and clinical developments in AD, PD, and other related disorders. The scientific program was divided into 24 oral sessions and daily poster sessions. The conference culminated in a round table discussion. There were 122 talks and 161 posters. This book incorporates a combination of both.

Many people and organizations were instrumental in the success of this multidisciplinary international conference and the scientific quality of this book. We thank the members of the Scientific Advisory Board, the Local Advisory Committee, and Prof. Y. Mitzuno from Japan, for their constructive input and their excellent service as chairpersons and speakers in the conference. We would like to acknowledge the backup of IIBR, and in particular Dr. A. Shafferman, the Director of IIBR for contributing his moral support for this endeavor. Mr. G. Rivlin and Ms. D. Dreman and their devoted team from Kenes are to be commended for the excellent organization of this Conference. Also thanks to Ms. Dalia Wallach for her dedicated secretarial support for the conference. In particular, we would like to acknowledge the supreme effort of Ms. Corrine Arthur for reformatting and reprinting most of the chapters in these proceedings.

The conference would not have been as successful as it turned out to be without the financial support of a number of important contributors. These are listed on the following pages in a special acknowledgment section.

Finally, the measure of a conference is dependent upon the participants themselves. The diverse international community was well represented at this meeting. It is hoped that this conference provided the medium for friendly and active exchange among all the participants, and that it contributed to the development of new collaborative efforts for the future.

Abraham Fisher
Israel Hanin
Mitsuo Yoshida

ACKNOWLEDGMENTS

The Organizing Committee wishes to express its gratitude to the following, who through their generosity and support have helped to make this Conference possible:

Sponsors

Alzheimer's Association Ronald and Nancy Reagan Research Institute, USA
Applied Genetics, USA
Bayer A.G., Germany
Hoechst Marion Roussel Inc., USA
MitoKor, USA
Neuroscience and Aging Institute of Loyola University Chicago, Stritch School of Medicine, USA
Novartis Pharma A.G., USA
Snow Brand Milk Products Co. Ltd., Japan

Contributors

Amgen Inc., USA
Astra Arcus AB, Sweden
Banyu Pharmaceutical Company, Japan
Bayer Corp., USA
Bristol-Myers Squibb Co., USA
Boehringer Ingelheim, Germany
Boehringer Ingelheim, Japan
California Peptide Research Inc., USA
Cephalon, Inc., USA
Eisai America, Inc., USA
El Al Israel Airlines
Eli Lilly, Japan
Fujimoto Pharmaceutical Company, Japan
GlaxoWellcome, UK
Guilford Pharmaceuticals, USA
Kissei Pharmaceutical Company, Japan
Medtronic, Inc., USA
Merck Sharpe & Dohme Research Labs, UK

Merck & Co., Inc., USA
Merck KGaA., Germany
Ministry of Tourism, Israel
National Parkinson Foundation, USA
Nihon Med-Physics Co. Ltd., Japan
Novartis Pharma, Japan
Pharmacia, Italy
Pfizer, Inc., USA
Roche, Japan
Rhone-Poulenc Rorer S.A., France
Schering, Japan
Servier, France
SmithKline Beecham, USA
SmithKline Beecham, Japan
Sumitomo Pharmaceutical Company, Japan
Synthelabo, France
Tokyo Fujisawa Pharmaceutical Company, Japan
UCB SA, Belgium
The Upjohn Company, USA
Warner Lambert Parke-Davis Pharmaceuticals Research, USA
Zeneca Pharmaceuticals Group, USA

Local Organizing Committee

Amos D. Korczyn, M.D.
Ichilov Hospital, Tel-Aviv

Danny M. Michaelson, Ph.D.
Tel-Aviv University, Tel-Aviv

Menachem Segal, Ph.D.
The Weizmann Institute, Rehovot

Hermona Soreq, Ph.D.
The Hebrew University of Jerusalem, Jerusalem

Scientific Advisory Board

Yves Agid, M.D.
Laboratoire de Medecine Experimentale
INSERM U289, Paris, France

David Bowen, Ph.D.
University of London
London, United Kingdom

Peter Davies, Ph.D.
Albert Einstein College of Medicine
Bronx, New York, USA

Ezio Giacobini, M.D., Ph.D.
Institutions Universitaires de Geriatrie de Geneve
Switzerland

Paul Greengard, Ph.D.
The Rockefeller University
New York, New York, USA

Kazuo Hasegawa, M.D.
St. Marianna University
Kawasaki, Japan

Franz Hefti, Ph.D.
Merck Research Laboratories
Essex, United Kingdom

Ichiro Kanazawa, M.D.
University of Tokyo
Tokyo, Japan

Zaven S. Khachaturian, Ph.D.
Ronald and Nancy Reagan Research Institute
Alzheimer Association
Potomac, MD, USA

Irwin J. Kopin, M.D.
NINDS, NIH
Bethesda, Maryland, USA

Toshiharu Nagatsu, M.D.
Fujita Health University
Aichi, Japan

Agneta Nordberg, Ph.D.
Karolinska Institutet
Huddinge University Hospital, Sweden

Elaine K. Perry, Ph.D.
MRC Medical Research Council
Newcastle General Hospital, United Kingdom

Paavo J. Riekkinen, Sr., M.D.
University of Kuopio
Kuopio, Finland

Dennis J. Selkoe, M.D.
Brigham and Women's Hospital
Boston, Massachusetts, USA

CONTENTS

Pathology in Alzheimer's Disease: General

1. The Pathogenesis of Alzheimer's Disease 1
   Robert D. Terry

2. Molecular and Cellular Abnormalities of Tau in Early Alzheimer's Disease 7
   Peter Davies, Charles Weaver, and Gregory A. Jicha

Apolipoprotein E

3. ApoE and Memory in Alzheimer's Disease 13
   Hilkka S. Soininen and Paavo J. Riekkinen, Sr.

4. Divergent Metabolism of Apolipoproteins E3 and E4 by Cells 17
   Robert E. Pitas, Zhong-Sheng Ji, Lubica Supekova, and Robert W. Mahley

5. APP, ApoE, and Presenilin Transgenics: Toward a Genetic Model of Alzheimer's
   Disease 25
   L. Pradier, C. Czech, L. Mercken, S. Moussaoui, M. Reibaud, P. Delaère, and
   G. Tremp

6. Differential Susceptibility of Human Apolipoprotein E Isoforms to Oxidation
   and Consequences on Their Interaction with Phospholipids 31
   Corinne Jolivalt, Brigitte Leininger-Muller, Philippe Bertrand, and
   Gérard Siest

7. The Apolipoprotein E ε4 Allele: Association with Alzheimer's Disease and
   Depression in Elderly Patients 39
   A. S. Rigaud, L. Traykov, L. Caputo, J. de Rotrou, F. Moulin, R. Couderc,
   M. L. Seux, M. B. Perol, A. Le Divenah, F. Latour, P. Bouchacourt,
   F. Boller, and F. Forette

Apoptosis; Oxidative Stress; Amyloids, Inflammation, and Other Defects

8. Apoptosis in Alzheimer's Disease: Inductive Agents and Antioxidant Protective
   Factors 45
   Carl W. Cotman and Christian J. Pike

9. Membrane Constituencies and Receptor Subtype Contribute to Age-Related Increases in Vulnerability to Oxidative Stress: Implications for Neurodegenerative Disease 53
   J. A. Joseph, N. Denisova, D. Fisher, I. Cantuti-Castelvetri, and S. Erat

10. Mitochondrial Dysfunction and Alzheimer's Disease 59
    Soumitra S. Ghosh, Scott Miller, Corinna Herrnstadt, Eoin Fahy, Leslie A. Shinobu, Douglas Galasko, Leon J. Thal, M. Flint Beal, Neil Howell, W. Davis Parker, Jr., and Robert E. Davis

11. Mitochondrial Dysfunction in Parkinson's Disease: Potential Applications for Cybrid Modeling of the Disease 67
    Russell H. Swerdlow, Janice K. Parks, Scott W. Miller, John N. Davis II, Patricia A. Trimmer, Jeremy B. Tuttle, James P. Bennett, G. Frederick Wooten, Robert E. Davis, and W. Davis Parker

12. Neuronal Oxidative Stress Is a Common Feature of Alzheimer's and Parkinson's Diseases 77
    George Perry and Mark A. Smith

13. Common Mechanisms in Cell Cycle and Cell Death 81
    D. Uberti, M. Belloni, C. Rizzini, A. Fontanini, L. Piccioni, M. Grilli, P. F. Spano, and M. Memo

14. Intracerebroventricular Administration of Beta-Amyloid Peptide (25–35) Induces Oxidative Stress and Neurodegeneration in Rat Brain 89
    Natalia V. Gulyaeva, Ilya V. Victorov, Mikhail Yu. Stepanichev, Mikhail V. Onufriev, Olga S. Mitrokhina, Yulia V. Moiseeva, and Natalia A. Lazareva

15. Molecular Characterization of the Neuroprotective Activity of Salicylates 99
    M. Grilli, M. Pizzi, F. Goffi, M. Benarese, G. M. Gerardi, M. Memo, and P. F. Spano

16. N-Methyl(R)Salsolinol: A Neurotoxin Candidate to Induce Parkinson's Disease Causes Apoptosis in Dopamine Cells 105
    Wakako Maruyama and Makoto Naoi

17. Age-Related Na,K-ATPase mRNA Expression and Alzheimer's Disease 113
    George J. Siegel, Neelima B. Chauhan, and John M. Lee

18. HB-GAM a Novel Amyloid Associated Protein Is Present in Prion Related Disorders and Other Cerebral Amyloidoses 121
    Maciej M. Lalowski, Marc Baumann, Heikki Rauvala, Blas Frangione, and Thomas Wisniewski

19. Regulation of APP Metabolism by Protein Phosphorylation 133
    J. D. Buxbaum, A. Ikin, Y. Luo, J. Naslund, S. Sabo, B. Vincent, T. Watanabe, and P. Greengard

20. Identification of Peptides Binding to Presenilin 1 by Screening of Random
   Peptide Display Libraries   141
   Alexander Schwarzman, Maria Tsiper, Michael Vitek,
   Peter St. George-Hyslop, and Dmitry Goldgaber

21. Matrix-Metalloproteinases (MMPS) in Astroglial Cells: Modulation by TNF-α
   and Interacting Cytokines   149
   Nitza Lahat, Sarah Shapiro, Michael Inspector, Reuben Reich,
   Rosa Gershtein, and Ariel Miller

22. Polyamines and Related Compounds in Nerve Cell Death and Survival: An
   Overview   159
   Gad M. Gilad, Varda H. Gilad, Tatiana Prohorov, and Jose M. Rabey

23. Haloperidol Induces Neurotoxicity in Mouse Embryo Brain Tissue: Evidence
   for Oxidative Damage Mechanism, and Implication for Tardive Dyskinesia   163
   I. Gil-Ad, D. Offen, B. Shtaif, R. Galili-Mosberg, and A. Weizman

24. Direct Evidence that Lactate Is an Obligatory Aerobic Energy Substrate for
   Functional Recovery Posthypoxia in Vitro   171
   Avital Schurr, Ralphiel S. Payne, James J. Miller, and Benjamin M. Rigor

25. Comparative Study of Antioxidants' Action on Membrane-Bound
   Acetylcholinesterase (AChE) of Blood Erythrocytes and Brain
   Synaptosomes   177
   Faina I. Braginskaya, Elena M. Molochkina, Olga M. Zorina,
   Irina B. Ozerova, and Elena B. Burlakova

26. Ultra-Low Doses of Antioxidant and Acetylcholine Modify the Lipid Phase and
   Kinetic Properties of Acetylcholinesterase in Murine Brain Membranes . .   183
   E. M. Molochkina, I. B. Ozerova, and E. B. Burlakova

Amyloid Aggregation

27. Amyloid-β Hypothesis of Alzheimer's Disease   187
   Mark S. Shearman

28. Discovery and Characterization of Peptidoorganic Inhibitors of Amyloid
   β-Peptide Polymerization   191
   Mark A. Findeis and Susan M. Molineaux

29. Anthracyclines and Amyloidosis   197
   C. Post, F. Tagliavini, R. A. Mc Arthur, F. Della Vedova, M. Gerna,
   T. Bandiera, M. Varasi, A. Molinari, and J. Lansen

30. The Amino Terminus of the β-Amyloid Peptide Contains an Essential Epitope
   for Maintaining Its Solubility   205
   Beka Solomon, Eilat Hanan, Rela Koppel, Dan Frankel, Ilana Ophir, and
   Dale Schenck

31. Animal Models of Amyloid Aggregation and Deposition 213
Robert Kisilevsky

Tau in Alzheimer's Disease

32. The Conformations of Tau Protein and Its Aggregation into Alzheimer Paired
Helical Filaments 223
Eckhard Mandelkow, Peter Friedhoff, Jacek Biernat, and
Eva-Maria Mandelkow

33. Role of Neurofibrillary Degeneration in Alzheimer's Disease 235
Inge Grundke-Iqbal and Khalid Iqbal

34. Cytoskeletal Protein Gene Expression after Neuronal Injury Recapitulates
Developmental Patterns: Implications for Tau Protein in Alzheimer's
Disease 241
Nancy A. Muma and Christopher B. Chambers

35. Hyperphosphorylation of Tau in Apolipoprotein E-Deficient Mice 251
Idit Genis and Daniel M. Michaelson

36. Aβ Induces Cell Death in PC12 Cells and Tau-Transfected Cho Cells, but Only
Tau Phosphorylation in PC12 Cells 257
Lone Fjord-Larsen, Jens D. Mikkelsen, and Ole F. Olesen

**Alzheimer's Disease/Parkinson's Disease and Related Disorders:
Clinical and Etiological Aspects**

37. Different Cognitive Profiles on Memory Tests in Parkinson's Disease and
Alzheimer's Disease 265
Ricardo F. Allegri, Paula Harris, and Raúl L. Arizaga

38. Neuropsychological Subtypes and Rate of Progression in Alzheimer's Disease   271
C. Piccini, D. Campani, M. Piccininni, G. Manfredi, L. Amaducci, and
L. Bracco

39. Brain Banking in Aging and Dementia Research—the Amsterdam Experience   277
R. Ravid, D. F. Swaab, W. Kamphorst, and A. Salehi

40. Insulin, Insulin Receptors, and Igf-I Receptors in Post-Mortem Human Brain in
Alzheimer's Disease 287
F. Frölich, D. Blum-Degen, S. Hoyer, H. Beckmann, and P. Riederer

41. Demonstration of Aluminum in the Brain of Patients with Alzheimer's Disease   293
Sakae Yumoto, Shigeo Kakimi, Hideki Matsushima, Akira Ishikawa, and
Yoshikazu Homma

42. Lipid Composition of Different Brain Regions in Patients with Alzheimer's
Disease and Multi-Infarct Dementia 301
D. Řípová, V. Němcová, C. Höschl, E. Fales, E. Majer, and A. Strunecká

43. Verbal and Motor Memory in Alzheimer's Disease: Release from Proactive
    Inhibition 309
    Joseph Harris, Malcolm Dick, Veronica Sandoval, Daniel Gallegos,
    Sean Lozano, Sergio Rangel, and Mary-Louise Kean

44. Cognitive and Non-Cognitive Symptoms in Senile Dementia 317
    A. Sellers, L. Pérez, C. Carrera, J. C. Bustos, J. M. Caamaño, B. Rodríguez,
    R. Mouzo, P. Pérez, J. I. Lao, K. Beyer, X. A. Álvarez, and R. Cacabelos

45. Dementia Associated Sleep Disorders 323
    A. Sellers, L. Pérez, B. Rodríguez, V. M. Pichel, J. M. Caamaño, M. Laredo,
    M. Alcaraz, X. A. Álvarez, and R. Cacabelos

46. Freezing Phenomenon, the Fifth Cardinal Sign of Parkinsonism 329
    Nir Giladi and Stanley Fahn

47. Cognitive Impairment in Patients with Parkinsonism 337
    C. N. Homann, K. Suppan, K. Polmin, R. Schmidt, E. Floh, S. Horner, and
    E. Ott

48. Cognitive Impairment without Dementia in Parkinson's Disease 343
    Abraham Lieberman

49. Neuroleptic Malignant Syndrome and Dementia with Lewy Bodies:
    A Case Study 351
    Howard Feldman, Kevin Solomons, Tom Cooney, and Thomas G. Beach

50. Case Report on a Generalized Epilepsy in a Patient Suffering from Parkinson's
    Disease 359
    Emanuel Kogan, Irma Schöll, and Alexandra E. Henneberg

51. Pathophysiology of Hereditary Progressive Dystonia with Marked Diurnal
    Fluctuation—Its Characteristics in Contrast to Other Dopa-Responsive
    Disorders 363
    Masaya Segawa and Yoshiko Nomura

52. Effects of Progressive Neurological Disease on Interpersonal Relations between
    Patients and Family Members 371
    L. L. Sprinzeles

53. Cognitive Deficits in Alzheimer's Disease, Parkinson's Disease, and
    Huntington's Chorea 377
    Elka Stefanova, Vladimir Kostic, Gordana Ocic, and Ljubomir Ziropadja

54. Recall of Ytzhak Rabin's Assassination by Demented People 385
    T. A. Treves, S. Klimowitzky, R. Verchovsky, and A. D. Korczyn

55. Study of Dementia in China 389
    Xianhao Xu, Hong Guo, Bin Qin, Hua Zhang, Xiangyu Zeng, Dantao Peng,
    Xiuyun Wang, Hong Sun, Shiguang Wen, Yun Jiang, Baolin Li,
    Fengzhen Pang, and Hong Wang

Parkinson's Disease: Etiology, Genetics, Treatment

56. Genetic Aspects of Parkinson's Disease 393
Yoshikuni Mizuno, Hiroto Matsumine, Nobutaka Hattori,
Satoe Matsubayashi, Tomonori Kobayashi, Asako Yoritaka, and Mei Wang

57. A Chromosome 6q-Linked Parkinsonism 401
Hiroto Matsumine, Masaaki Saito, Atsushi Ishikawa, Yasuhiro Yamamura,
Shoji Tsuji, and Yoshikuni Mizuno

58. Cytokines in Parkinson's Disease 407
Toshiharu Nagatsu and Makio Mogi

59. N-Methyl(R)Salsolinol and (R)Salsolinol N-Methyltransferase as Possible
Pathogenic Factors in Parkinson's Disease 413
Makoto Naoi and Wakako Maruyama

60. Antioxidant and Cytoprotective Properties of Apomorphine 421
Michael Gassen, Aviva Gross, and Moussa B. H. Youdim

61. Toxicity of 1BnTIQ, Endogenous Amine in the Brain, in Mesencephalic Slice
Culture 429
Yaichiro Kotake, Masaki Sakurai, Ichiro Kanazawa, Shigeru Ohta

62. Dopaminergic Responsiveness of Hypokinesia but Not of Rigidity and Tremor
Is Reduced in Fluctuating Parkinson's Disease 435
Jan Roth, Evžen Růžička, Irena Svobodová, Robert Jech, and Petr Mečíř

63. Motor Fluctuation and Levodopa Absorption 439
Miho Murata and Ichiro Kanazawa

Cholinergic Strategies in Alzheimer's and Parkinson's Disease

64. The Rationale for Development of Cholinergic Therapies in AD 445
Albert Enz and Paul T. Francis

65. Dementia with Lewy Bodies: A New Avenue for Research into Neurobiological
Mechanisms of Consciousness? 451
Robert H. Perry, Matthew Walker, and Elaine K. Perry

66. Nicotinic Receptors as a New Target for Treatment of Alzheimer's Disease 463
Agneta Nordberg, Anne-Lie Svensson, Ulrika Warpman, Linda Bud,
Amelia Marutle, Hui Miao, Olga Gorbounova, Ivan Bednar,
Ewa Hellström-Lindahl, and Xiao Zhang

67. S 12024-2, a Cognitive Enhancer, Interacts with Nicotinic Neurotransmission .. 469
Jean M. Lépagnol, Philippe Morain, Jean-Yves A. Thomas, Murielle Méen,
Marianne Rodriguez, and Pierre J. Lestage

68. Lewy Body Influence on Tacrine Efficacy 477
Florence Lebert, Lydie Souliez, Florence Pasquier, and Henri Petit

69. Tacrine Treatment in Parkinson's Disease Dementia 481
    A. E. Werber, S. Perlov, B. Mildorf, and J. M. Rabey

Alzheimer's Disease: Muscarinic Treatment and Therapy — β-Amyloids

70. APP Localization and Trafficking in the Central Nervous System 487
    J. D. Buxbaum, A. Ikin, Y. Luo, J. Naslund, S. Sabo, B. Vincent, T. Watanabe,
    and P. Greengard

71. The Cholinergic but Not the Serotonergic Phenotype of a New Neuronal Cell
    Line Is Sensitive to β-Amyloid-Induced Toxicity 495
    Ole F. Olesen, Lone Fjord-Larsen, and Jens D. Mikkelsen

72. The Molecular Basis Underlying the Discrete Activation of Signal Transduction
    Pathways by Selective Muscarinic Agonists: Relevance to Treatment of
    Alzheimer's Disease 503
    E. Heldman, Z. Pittel, R. Haring, N. Eshhar, R. Levy, Z. Vogel, D. Marciano,
    Y. Kloog, and A. Fisher

73. Muscarinic Modulation of β-Amyloid Precursor Protein (βAPP) Processing in
    Vitro and in Vivo 509
    Zipora Pittel, Nomi Eshhar, Eliahu Heldman, Michal Sapir, Rachel Haring,
    Moshe Kushnir, and Abraham Fisher

74. M1 Muscarinic Agonists: From Treatment toward Delaying Progression of
    Alzheimer's Disease 515
    Abraham Fisher, Rachel Haring, Zipora Pittel, Nomi Eshhar, Yishai Karton,
    Rachel Brandeis, Haim Meshulam, Daniella Marciano, and
    Eliahu Heldman

Cholinesterase Inhibitors for Treatment of Alzheimer's Disease

75. Crystallographic Studies on Complexes of Acetylcholinesterase with the Natural
    Cholinesterase Inhibitors Fasciculin and Huperzine A 523
    Israel Silman, Michal Harel, Mia Raves, and Joel L. Sussman

76. What Can Be Learned from the Use of HuAChE Mutants for Evaluation of
    Potential Alzheimer's Drugs 531
    Avigdor Shafferman, Arie Ordentlich, Naomi Ariel, Dov Barak,
    Chanoch Kronman, Tamar Bino, Moshe Leitner, Dino Marcus, Arie Lazar,
    and Baruch Velan

77. Cholinesterases in Neurogenesis: Pharmacological and Transfection Studies of
    the Reaggregating Chick Retina 541
    Paul G. Layer, Andrea Robitzki, Alexandra Mack, and Elmar Willbold

78. The Non-Catalytic Role and Complex Management of Acetylcholinesterase in
    the Mammalian Brain Call for RNA-Based Therapies 551
    Hermona Soreq and Shlomo Seidman

79. Antisense Oligodeoxynucleotide Dependent Suppression of
    Acetylcholinesterase Expression Reduces Process Extension from Primary
    Mammalian Neurons   557
    Mirta Grifman, Dalia Ginzberg, and Hermona Soreq

80. Tacrine Reduces the Secretion of Soluble Amyloid Beta-Peptides in a
    Neuroblastoma Cell Line   563
    Debomoy K. Lahiri and Martin R. Farlow

81. Cholinesterase Inhibitors for Alzheimer's Disease Therapy: Do They Work? . . .   571
    Ezio Giacobini

82. The Preclinical Pharmacology of Metrifonate, a Long-Acting and Well Tolerated
    Cholinesterase Inhibitor for Alzheimer Therapy   579
    Bernard H. Schmidt, Volker C. Hinz, and F. Josef van der Staay

83. Increase in Cerebral Blood Flow and Glucose Utilization in Beneficial Effect of
    a Cholinesterase Inhibitor, ENA713, in Alzheimer's Disease   587
    Marta Weinstock

84. Quaternary-Lipophilic Carbamates with Blood Brain Barrier Permeability as
    Potential Drugs for Memory Impairment Associated with Cholinergic
    Deficiency   595
    Gabriel Amitai, Eliezer Rachaman, Rachel Adani, Ishai Rabinovitz,
    Rachel Brandeis, and Eliahu Heldman

85. Characterization of C-10 Substituted Analogues of Huperzine A as Inhibitors of
    Cholinesterases   601
    Ashima Saxena, Alan P. Kozikowski, Shaomeng Wang, Giuseppe Campiani,
    Qingjie Ding, and B. P. Doctor

Neurotrophic Factor Therapy: Neuroprotection, Neurotransplantation, and Other Treatment Strategies

86. Functional Effects of GDNF on Dopamine Neurons in Animal Models of
    Parkinson's Disease   607
    Alexander F. Hoffman, Meleik A. Hebert, Barry J. Hoffer, Zhiming Zhang,
    Wayne A. Cass, Don M. Gash, and Greg A. Gerhardt

87. Development and Uses of Small Molecule Ligands of TrkA Receptors   615
    Lynne LeSauteur, Natalia Beglova, Kalle Gehring, and H. Uri Saragovi

88. Molecular Cloning, Transient Expression, and Neurotrophic Effect for DA
    Neurons of Human Brain Derived Neurotrophic Factor   627
    Wang Jia-Zheng, Chen Qian, Yu Yun-Kai, and Fan Ming

89. Preventive Treatment of Alzheimer's Disease: Peptide-Mediated Neuroprotection   635
    Illana Gozes, Ariane Davidson, Michal Bachar, Amos Bardea, Orly Perl,
    Sara Rubinraut, Mati Fridkin, Eliezer Giladi, and Douglas E. Brenneman

90. Clinical Aspects of Neurotransplantation of Embryonal Brain Tissue: Long Term
   Results 643
   Miron Šramka, Július Rattaj, and Martin Novotný

91. Gene Therapy of a Rodent Model of Parkinson's Disease Using
   Adeno-Associated Virus (AAV) Vectors 647
   Dong-Sheng Fan, Matsuo Ogawa, Ken-ichi Fujimoto, Kunihiko Ikeguchi,
   Yoji Ogasawara, Masashi Urabe, Akihiro Kume, Masatoyo Nishizawa,
   Imaharu Nakano, Mitsuo Yoshida, Hiroshi Ichinose, Toshiharu Nagatsu,
   Gary J. Kurtzman, and Keiya Ozawa

92. S 17092-1, a New Post-Proline Cleaving Enzyme Inhibitor: Memory Enhancing
   Effects and Substance P Neuromodulatory Activity 653
   Pierre Lestage, Cécile Lebrun, Fabrice Iop, Anne Hugot, Nathalie Rogez,
   Philippe Grève, Dominique Favale, Marie-Hélène Gandon,
   Odile Raimbault, and Jean Lépagnol

Animal Models in Alzheimer's and Parkinson's Diseases

93. Age Dependence of Muscarinic Plasticity in the Rat Hippocampus 661
   J. M. Auerbach and M. Segal

94. Models of Cholinergic Degeneration: AF64A and 192-IgG-Saporin 667
   Thomas J. Walsh

95. Molecular Mechanisms of AF64A Toxicity in the Cholinergic Neuron 675
   Israel Hanin

96. The AF64A Model of Cholinergic Hypofunction: Role of Nitric Oxide in
   AF64A-Mediated Neurodegeneration 681
   M. Lautenschlager, A. Arnswald, D. Freyer, J. R. Weber, and H. Hörtnagl

97. Effect of AF64A/NGF Treatment on ChAT mRNA Expression in the
   Septo-Hippocampal Pathway and Striatum 687
   Qing I. Fan, Christopher A. Willson, and Israel Hanin

98. Induction, Secretion, and Pharmacological Regulation of β-APP in Animal
   Model Systems 695
   V. Haroutunian, S. A. Ahlers, N. Greig, and W. C. Wallace

99. Anapsos Improves Learning and Memory in Rats with βA(1-28) Deposits into
   the Hippocampus 699
   Antón Alvarez, José Javier Miguel-Hidalgo, Lucía Fernández-Novoa,
   Joaquín Díaz, José Miguel Sempere, and Ramón Cacabelos

100. *In Vivo* Neurotoxicity of β-Amyloid 1-40 in the Rat Hippocampus 705
   José Javier Miguel-Hidalgo, Antón Álvarez, and Ramón Cacabelos

101. Impairments of Cholinergic But Not of Nigrostriatal Dopaminergic Projections
   in Apolipoprotein E Deficient Mice 711
   Shira Chapman and Daniel M. Michaelson

102. Interval Hypoxic Training Prevents Oxidative Stress in Striatum and Locomotor
Disturbances in a Rat Model of Parkinsonism 717
Natalia V. Gulyaeva, Mikhail Yu. Stepanichev, Mikhail V. Onufriev,
Ilya V. Sergeev, Olga S. Mitrokhina, Yulia V. Moiseeva, and
Elena N. Tkatchouk

103. An α_2-Adrenoceptor Agonist, Clonidine, Disrupts Attentional Performance 725
Pekka Jäkälä, Kosti Kejonen, Matti Vanhanen, Esa Koivisto, and
Paavo Riekkinen, Jr.

Diagnostic Tools in Alzheimer's and Parkinson's Diseases

104. Functional Neuroimaging Reveals Decline from Premorbid Functioning in AD   733
Isak Prohovnik

105. Novel Phenyltropanes: Affinity to Monoamine Transporters in Rat Forebrain ... 739
John L. Neumeyer, Ross J. Baldessarini, Nora S. Kula, and Gilles Tamagnan

106. APP Isoforms in Platelets: A Peripheral Marker of Alzheimer's Disease 747
M. Di Luca, A. Padovani, L. Pastorino, A. Bianchetti, J. Perez, S. Govoni,
L. A. Vignolo, G. L. Lenzi, M. Trabucchi, and F. Cattabeni

107. Neuropsychological and Positron Emission Tomographic Comparisons of
Alzheimer's, Multi-Infarct, and Parkinson's Disease Dementias 751
Daphne Alroy Harris, Rowena Gomez, Gerardo Bedolla, Edward Lee,
Ingrid Ochoa, Bond Ren, Susan Vasquez, and Joseph Harris

108. $\alpha1$-Antichymotrypsin and Apolipoprotein E Polymorphism in Alzheimer's
Disease 757
Akira Ueki, Mieko Otsuka, Yoshio Namba, Takeshi Ishii, and Kazuhiko Ikeda

109. Influence of the APOE Genoptype on Serum ApoE Levels in Alzheimer's
Disease Patients 765
L. Corzo, L. Fernández-Novoa, R. Zas, K. Beyer, J. I. Lao, X. A. Alvarez,
and R. Cacabelos

110. Development of a Specific Diagnostic Test for Measurement of β-Amyloid
(1-42) [βA_4(1-42)] in CSF 773
H. Vanderstichele, K. Blennow, N. D'Heuvaert, M.-A. Buyse, A. Wallin,
N. Andreasen, P. Seubert, A. Van de Voorde, and E. Vanmechelen

111. Indices of Oxidative Stress in the Peripheral Blood of *de Novo* Patients with
Parkinson's Disease 779
Tihomir V. Ilic, Marina Jovanovic, Aco Jovicic, and Mirjana Tomovic

112. Acylphosphatase Levels in Alzheimer's Disease Cultured Skin Fibroblasts 787
S. Latorraca, C. Cecchi, A. Pieri, G. Liguri, L. Amaducci, and S. Sorbi

113. Centromeric Disturbances Affecting All Chromosomes of Cultured
Lymphocytes Obtained from Alzheimer's Disease Patients 793
José Ignacio Lao Villadóniga, Katrin Beyer, and Ramón Cacabelos

114. APOE Genotype-Related Blood Pressure in Senile Dementia 799
Ricardo Mouzo, X. Antón Alvarez , V. Manuel Pichel, Angeles Sellers,
Jose M. Caamaño, Marta Laredo, Katrin Beyer, Jose I. Lao, Paula Perez,
Margarita Alcaraz, M. Carmen Rúa, Lola Corzo, Lucía Fernández-Novoa,
René Fernández, and Ramón Cacabelos

115. Apolipoprotein E (Apo E) Phenotype in Alzheimer's Disease, Vascular Dementia
and Parkinson's Disease with and without Dementia in Northern Ireland . . 805
Cathal J. Foy, Anthony P. Passmore, Djamil M. Vahidassr, Ian S. Young,
Michael Smye, and John T. Lawson

116. Changes in Cerebral Blood Flow Associated with Disease Staging and APOE
Genotyping in Patients with Senile Dementia 811
V. M. Pichel, J. M. Caamaño, A. Sellers, R. Mouzo, X. A. Alvarez, P. Pérez,
M. Laredo, and R. Cacabelos

117. Apolipoprotein E ε4 Allele Does Not Influence the Development of Dementia in
Parkinsonian Patients 817
D. Paleacu, R. Inzelberg, J. Chapman, E. Orlov, A. Asherov, and A. D. Korczyn

118. A Simple Procedure of Immunochemical Detection of Amyloid β Proteins Using
Milligram Amounts of Brain Tissues of Patients with Alzheimer's Disease 823
B. Kaplan, B. Martin, S. Yakar, M. Pras, T. Wisniewski, J. Ghiso,
B. Frangione, and G. Gallo

Developments in Treatment Strategies in Alzheimer's Disease

119. Bridging Studies in Alzheimer's Disease: Finding the Optimal Dose for Efficacy
Studies 829
Neal R. Cutler and John J. Sramek

120. How Can We Improve the Drug Development Process in Alzheimer's Disease? 833
C. Brazell and T. H. Corn

121. Trial to Prevent Neurodegeneration in Persons Genetically Predisposed to
Alzheimer's Disease 841
Natalia Ponomareva, Vitaly Fokin, and Natalia Selesneva

122. Delaying Endpoints in Alzheimer's Disease and Mild Cognitive Impairment . . . 847
Leon J. Thal

123. Current Neurotransmitter Strategies in AD Drug Development 851
Paul T. Francis, J. Tracy Alder, Kate L. Cole, Kirsten E. Heslop,
Stephen L. Minger, and Maria J. Ramirez

124. Harmonization of Drug Approval Guidelines in Alzheimer's and Parkinson's
Diseases 861
Rachelle Smith Doody, Michael Davidson, Ira Shoulson, and
Peter Whitehouse

Index 867

PROGRESS IN ALZHEIMER'S AND PARKINSON'S DISEASES

THE PATHOGENESIS OF ALZHEIMER'S DISEASE

Robert D. Terry

Departments of Neurosciences and Pathology
University of California, San Diego
9500 Gilman Drive
La Jolla, California 92093-0624

The great majority of Alzheimer investigators seems to be convinced that the deposition of β-amyloid lies at the heart of the pathogenetic problem. More than 2,500 papers have been published in the last 15 years concerning this Alzheimer amyloid (Aβ), and that is more publications than on almost any other protein. While we know an enormous amount of detail about this amyloid—its origin, anabolism, catabolism, configuration, *in vitro* function, etc., there remains a number of reasons why its primary, causal significance in Alzheimer disease must be regarded with some skepticism.

For example, the beta amyloid which is characteristic of Alzheimer disease (AD) is not specific to that disorder, but has been found in such remote and diverse situations as human congenital cerebral vascular anomalies and rat gracile nucleus (Ichihara et al., 1995). Many studies have shown that there is no correlation between the clinical severity of the cortical symptoms and the quantity of cortical amyloid (Arriagada et al., 1992). Only two reports disagree. One is quite old and has been much disputed on the basis of its statistical methods (Blessed et al., 1968). The other involves the entorhinal cortex (Cummings et al., 1995) where amyloid containing plaques are a minor epiphenomenon relative to neurofibrillary tangles. Particularly significant in regard to this failure of correlation is the point that pharmacologic reduction or prevention of amyloid might have only a minimal effect on the clinical severity of the disease unless the therapy has other, more primary physiologic effects.

To advance arguments against amyloid as a primary factor, one might also point out that Aβ can be present in large quantities in the normal, nondemented elderly brain. Neocortical tangles are not to be found or are very rare in such situations, but numerous neuritic plaques containing beta amyloid are quite common in patients whose cognition is apparently normal. This also indicates that the presence of Aβ does not induce the formation of neurofibrillary tangles. Diffuse plaques are frequent in both normal elderly and in demented Alzheimer patients. If one examines these diffuse plaques which lack filamentous amyloid for the presence of synapse markers, one finds that the apparent concentra-

Progress in Alzheimer's and Parkinson's Diseases
edited by Fisher *et al.*, Plenum Press, New York, 1998.

tion of presynaptic elements is normal in the area of the unformed, diffusely deposited Aβ (Masliah et al., 1990). So this kind of amyloid is not toxic to synapses.

The toxicity of amyloid is well documented *in vitro* (Yankner, 1989), but proof is lacking *in vivo,* where it is to be seen that inoculation of fibrillar amyloid into the brain does not result in toxic changes, but only in trauma, such as one might see with any inert material. If amyloid contains a soluble toxic component, we would expect there to be a gradient of observable damage to the brain parenchyma extending from the nidus of amyloid deposition. In fact, however, such a gradient is not present. The diminished concentration of synapses typical of AD is quite uniform from the edge of one plaque to the edge of another.

It is said that in Down's syndrome, amyloid is deposited very early in life (Burger et al., 1973). One wonders whether this is indeed the case in Alzheimer disease. Electron microscopic examination of human brains (Terry et al., 1970), as well as these of nonhuman primates (Wisniewski et al., 1973) and dogs (Wisniewski et al., 1970) reveals that dystrophic neurites appear prior to the deposition of the amyloid and certainly in its topographic absence. This might also be the case in Down's, but preceding dystrophy has not been sought there.

In regard to instances of APP mutations, it must be pointed out that in the human such mutations of chromosome 21 account for only about one-tenth of one percent (0.1%) of the Alzheimer population. Mutations on chromosomes 14 and 1 are more common but do not directly or exclusively effect the metabolism or the synthesis of amyloid. In the Athena mouse, where amyloid deposition is present in well formed plaques (Games et al., 1995), this phenomenon actually follows loss of synapses and diminished GAP43 (Masliah, personal communication).

Now, there is no doubt that Aβ is present in every case of Alzheimer disease, for without it the diagnosis is untenable. The Aβ is thus a totally consistent marker of AD, but that alone does not prove it to be a primary causal factor. For example, fever is an almost constant sign of infection, but it does not cause the infection, and treating the fever alone will not change the progress of the disease. The phlogiston theory has disappeared in the face of contrary evidence concerning etiology and pathogenesis.

So, how is it that amyloid has so captured the attention of the research community? Glenner very importantly isolated Aβ from Alzheimer meningeal vessels in the mid-1980s, and reported it to be a specific small peptide (Glenner et al., 1984). That period of scientific development involved especially technology of protein chemistry, and Aβ was an ideal subject. First, it had to do with a major human disease as had been shown, and second, the technology for its study was readily available, and so was the peptide itself. Dozens of laboratories were attracted and became involved. Had the same peptide been discovered 10–20 years earlier, very little could have been done with it, and attention might have been turned elsewhere.

The leading theory concerning amyloid-dominant pathogenesis of AD has it that amyloid precursor protein (APP) is synthesized in many cells, but most importantly in the cell body of neurons from which it is transported by rapid axoplasmic flow (Price et al., 1994)) to the presynaptic terminals where the Aβ itself is released to damage the synaptic terminal either from within the cell or from the extracellular space. It is the last part of that sequence which is problematic. It has been stated that the formed element of amyloid, that is the filament, is the toxic part, at least *in vitro* (Pike et al., 1991); but formed filaments are not to be found at the synapse by electron microscopic study of the tissue. Synapses are being lost throughout the neuropil without visible amyloid filaments. If it is soluble amyloid which is doing the damage, then this is contrary to the major *in vitro* evidence, as well as being contrary to the findings concerning the diffuse plaque (vide supra) in tissue.

No, despite it popularity, the amyloid hypothesis seems to be inadequate. But there are several other possibilities as to the cause of Alzheimer disease; as for example, oxidative stress (Beal, 1994), calcium homeostasis (Mattson et al., 1992), even infections (Itzhak et al., 1997). The one which came up early and still holds my own attention has to do with the neuronal cytoskeleton. We noticed in the early electron microscopic studies 35 years ago, that in brain biopsies from Alzheimer patients, there was a paucity of microtubules in the cortical neurons especially obvious in those cells with tangles. We suggested in 1967 (Suzuki et al.) that the dystrophic terminals in the plaques and in the neuropil could be the result of inadequate substrate coming from the remote cell bodies due to deficient axoplasmic flow, that function being dependent on the microtubules. The latter structures are essential for bi-directional linear movement in axons, where material flows at different rates, thanks to certain motor proteins acting along the cytoskeleton.

More recently, it has been shown that hyperphosphorylation of tau protein destabilized microtubules and that this hyperphosphorylation is prominent in neurofibrillary tangles (Goedert, 1993). But the number of tangles in the neocortex is not at all great enough to account for the much larger loss of neuronal cell bodies (Gomez-Isla et al., 1977). Therefore, there must be other causes of neuronal death, and there might well be other forms of cytoskeletal abnormalities leading to the diminished axoplasmic flow. In this regard, it has very recently been shown that the actin gene is up-regulated in cells expressing amyloid precursor protein (Ramakrishna et al., 1997).

Destabilization of the microtubules leads to dispersion of the Golgi apparatus (Stieber et al., 1996) which would result in abnormal Golgi functions. Since these must include post translational effects on amyloid precursor protein (APP), this dispersion might ultimately result in excessive production of amyloid that we see in Alzheimer disease. It is interesting the presenilin 1 and 2 from chromosomes 14 and 1 are both Golgi (Kovacs et al., 1996) or endoplasmic reticulum (Walter et al., 1996) proteins, and may have similar disruptive functions in their mutated forms.

The markedly diminished axoplasmic flow should certainly cause the loss of synapses, since they are dependent on substrate coming from the perikaryon. Degenerative synapses elicit activation of the microglia (McGeer et al., 1994) which then secrete cytokines adding to the destruction. Synaptic loss is greater than neuronal loss and, therefore, probably comes first. Furthermore, synapse concentrations are the best correlate of cognitive function in AD (Terry et al., 1991).

The loss of terminal axons, again due to diminished axoplasmic flow, would lead to diminished return of trophic factors to the cell bodies since these factors come from the target areas and are returned to the cell body by means of retrograde axoplasmic flow. Diminution of trophic factors available to the cells causes apoptosis, and it has been shown that apoptotic cells secrete amyloid. The neurons disappear by way of apoptosis, which is a quite rapid process and is therefore rarely found *in situ* in the histologic study of the brain. Finally, the deficiency of synapses results in transmitters not being available to receptors. Thus, cerebral functions are disconnected, and dementia is the result (Terry, 1996).

The appended (Terry, 1996) chart (Figure 1) shows a possible mechanism which envelopes all the known changes regarding the histologic lesions and the transmitter chemistry. It might be regarded as a sort of final common pathway into which the several causal genes, as well as the risk gene (apoE) feed. It is to be noted that amyloid appears as a bi-product of the Golgi abnormalities and of the dystrophic neurites, but that it does not contribute significantly to the dementia. Microglia, as stated above, are activated by degeneration of the synapses, but their cytokine secretions once activated add to the damage. The death by apoptosis of neuronal cell bodies is the result of a failure of neurotrophic substance, which

Pathogenesis of Alzheimer Disease

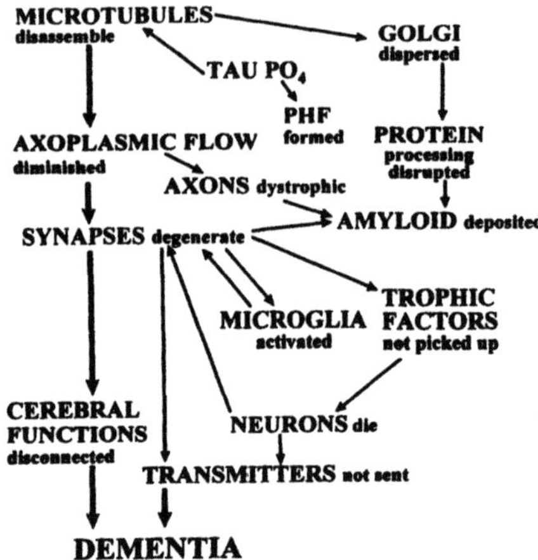

Figure 1. Pathogenesis of Alzheimer's Disease.

is due to the loss of synapses and the loss of retrograde axoplasmic flow associated with cytoskeletal deficiency.

REFERENCES

Arriagada, P.V., Grouden, J.H., Hedley-White, E.T., and Hyman, B.T., 1992, Neurofibrillary tangles but not senile plaques parallel duration and severity of Alzheimer disease. *Neurology.* 42:631–639.

Beal, M.F., 1994, Energy, oxidative damage, and Alzheimer's disease: Clues to the underlying puzzle. *Neurobiol. Aging.* 15(suppl 2):171–174.

Blessed, G., Tomlinson, B.E., and Roth, M., 1968, The association between quantitative measures of dementia and of senile changes in the cerebral grey matter of elderly subjects. *Br. J.Psychiat.* 114:797–811.

Burger, P.C., and Vogel, F.S., 1973, The development of the pathologic changes of Alzheimer's disease and senile dementia in patients with Down's syndrome. *Am. J. Path.* 73:457–476.

Cummings, B.J., and Cotman, C.W., 1995, Image analysis of beta-amyloid load in Alzheimer's disease and relation to dementia severity. *Lancet.* 346:1524–1528.

Games, D., Adams, D., Alessandrini, R., Barbour, R., Berthelette, P., Blackwell, C., Carr, T., Clemens, J., Donaldson, T., Gillespie, F., Guido, T., Hagopian, S., Johnson-Wood, K., Khan, K., Lee, M., Leibowitz, P., Lieberburg, I., Little, S., Masliah, E., McConlogue, L., Montoya-Zavala, M., Mucke, L., Paganini, L., Penniman, E., Power, M., Schenk, D., Seubert, P., Snyder, B., Soriano, F., Tan, H., Vitale, J., Wadsworth, S., Wolozin, B., and Zhao, J., 1995, Alzheimer-type neuropathology in transgenic mice overexpressing V717Fβ-amyloid precursor protein. *Nature.* 373:523–527.

Glenner, G.G., and Wong, C.W., 1984, Alzheimer's disease and Down's syndrome: sharing of a unique cerebrovascular amyloid fibril protein. *Biochem. Biophys. Res. Comm.* 122:1131–1135.

Goedert, M., 1993, Tau protein and the neurofibrillary pathology of Alzheimer's disease. *Trends Neurosci.* 16:460–465.

Gomez-Isla., T., Hollister, R., West, H., Miu, S., Growdon, J.H., Petersen, R.C. Parisi, J.E., and Hyman, B.T., 1997, Neuronal loss correlates with but exceeds neurofibrillary tangles in Alzheimer's disease. *Ann. Neurol.* 41:17–24.

Ichihara, N., Wu, J., Chui, D.H., Yamazaki, K., Wakabayashi, T., and Kibuchi, T., 1995, Axonal degeneration promotes abnormal accumulation of amyloid beta protein ascending gracile tract of gracile axonal dystropy (GAO) mouse. *Brain Res.* 695:173–178.

Itzhaki, R., Lin., W.R., Shang, D. et al., 1997, Herpes simplex versus type 1 in brain and risk of Alzheimer disease. *Lancet.* 349:241–244.

Kovacs, D.M., Fausett, H.J., Page, K.J., Kim, T.W., Moir, R.D., Merriam, D.E., Hollister, R.D., Hallmark, O.G., Mancini, R., Felsenstein, K.M. et al., 1996, Alzheimer-associated presenilin 1 and 2: neuronal expression in brain and localization to intracellular membranes in mammalian cells. *Nat. Med.* 2:224–229.

Masliah, E., Terry, R.D., Mallory, M., Alford., M., and Hansen, L.A., 1990, Diffuse plaques do not accentuate synapse loss in Alzheimer disease. *Am. J. Pathol.* 137:1293–1297.

Mattson, M.P., Cheng, B., Davis, D., Bryant, K., Lieberberg, I., and Rydel, R.E., 1992, β-amyloid peptides destabilize calcium homeostasis and render human cortical neurons vulnerable to excitotoxicity. *J. Neurosci.* 12:376–389.

McGeer, P.L., Walker, D.G., Akiyama, H. et al., 1994, Involvement of microglia in Alzheimer's disease. *Neuropathol. Appl. Neurobiol.* 20:191–192.

Pike, C.J., Walencewicz, A.J., Glabe, C.G., and Cotman, C.W., 1991, *In vitro* aging of β-amyloid causes peptide aggregation and neurotoxicity. *Brain Res.* 563:311–314.

Price, D.L., and Sisodia, S.S., 1994, Cellular and molecular biology of Alzheimer's disease and animal models. *Ann. Rev. Med.* 45:435–446.

Ramakrishna, N., Smedman, M., Ramakruskna, V., and Gillam, B., 1997, Upregulation of actin gene expression in cells expressing exogenous β-amyloid precursor protein. *Biochem. Biophys. Res. Commun.* 231:615–618.

Stieber, A., Mourelatos, Z., and Gonatas, N.K., 1996, In Alzheimer's disease the Golgi apparatus of a population of neurons without neurofibrillary tangles is fragmented and atrophic, *Amer. J. Path.* 148:415–426.

Suzuki, K., and Terry, R.D., 1967, Fine structural localization of acid phosphatase in senile plaques in Alzheimer's presenile dementia, *Acta Neuropathol.* 8:276–284.

Terry, R.D., 1996, The pathogenesis of Alzheimer disease: an alternative to the amyloid hypothesis, *J. Neuropathol. Exper. Neurol.* 55:1023–1025.

Terry, R.D., Masliah, E., Salmon, D.P., Butters, N., DeTeresa, R., Hill, R., Hansen, L.A., Katzman, R., 1991, Physical basis of cognitive alterations in Alzheimer disease: Synapse loss is the major correlate of cognitive impairment, *Ann. Neurol.* 30:572–580.

Terry, R.D., and Wisniewski, H.M., 1970, The Ultrastructure of the Neurofibrillary Tangle and the Senile Plaque. In: *CIBA Foundation Symposium on Alzheimer's Disease and Related Conditions.* Wolstenholme, G.E.W., and O'Connor, M., eds., J. & A. Churchill, London pp. 145–168.

Walter, J., Capell, A., Grunberg, J., Pesold, B., Schindzielorz, A., Prior, R., Podlisny, M., Fraser, P., Hyslop, P.S., Selkoe, D.J. et al. 1996, the Alzheimer's disease-associated presenilin are differentially phosphorylated proteins located predominately within the endoplasmic reticulum, *Mol. Med.* 2:673–691.

Wisniewski, H.M., Ghetti, B., and Terry, R.D., 1973, Neuritic (senile) plaques and filamentous changes in aged rhesus monkeys, *J. Neuropathol. Exper. Neurol.* 32:566–584.

Wisniewski, H.M., Johnson, A.B., Raine, C.S., Kay, W.J., and Terry, R.D., 1970, Senile plaques and cerebral amyloidosis in aged dogs. A histochemical and ultrastructural study, *Lab. Invest.* 23:287–296.

Yankner, B.A., Dawes, L.R., Fisher et al., 1989, Neurotoxicity of a fragment of the amyloid precursor associated with Alzheimer's disease, *Science.* 245:417–420.

2

MOLECULAR AND CELLULAR ABNORMALITIES OF TAU IN EARLY ALZHEIMER'S DISEASE

Peter Davies, Charles Weaver, and Gregory A. Jicha

Departments of Pathology and Neuroscience
Albert Einstein College of Medicine
1300 Morris Park Avenue
Bronx, New York 10461

INTRODUCTION

The formation of neurofibrillary tangles in patients with Alzheimer's Disease is probably the end result of a number of biochemical processes which take place in specific neuronal populations. The Braak's and their colleagues (Braak and Braak, 1991; Braak, Braak and Bohl, 1993) have provided a very useful staging system which has been extensively used to attempt to work out the temporal sequence of biochemical events. This scheme defines the stage of disease essentially through definition of the brain regions containing neurofibrillary pathology within neurons. The transentorhinal cortex appears to be the first area in which these abnormalities are found, with subsequent "spread" to the hippocampal formation and then to association cortex. For the work described in this report, Braak staging was used to identify cases of Alzheimer's Disease very early in the course of the illness.

A new series of monoclonal antibodies has been developed to examine the early biochemical changes taking place in neurons in the brains of patients with Alzheimer's Disease. Antibodies were produced by immunization of mice with proteins prepared by immunoaffinity chromatography using an IgG1 class switch variant of Alz-50 (Wolozin et al., 1986; Vincent and Davies, 1992) These new antibodies define two distinct abnormalities that distinguish tau in the normal brain from what has been called PHF-tau. These antibodies have been used in both biochemical and immunocytochemical studies, especially of the hippocampus of early Alzheimer's Disease cases. The results outlined here suggest that the earliest detectable abnormalities of tau occur in the perikarya of entorhinal cortex and hippocampal neurons, before the formation of neurofibrillary tangles and indeed before formation of paired helical filaments. In early Alzheimer's Disease (AD) cases, this

Progress in Alzheimer's and Parkinson's Diseases
edited by Fisher *et al.*, Plenum Press, New York, 1998.

abnormal tau is very prominently localized to the perikarya and proximal portions of both basal and apical dendrites of hippocampal pyramidal cells, rather than in the axons of these neurons.

Antibodies Sensitive to Tau Conformation

The MCI and Alz-50 antibodies both appear to define a conformational change that tau undergoes in early AD. Neither antibody reacts with recombinant tau or with tau prepared from the normal human or animal brain if solution assays such as ELISA or immunoprecipitation are used. They both react well with tau from Alzheimer's Disease brain tissue in these assays, and with all forms of tau after treatment with SDS/ beta mercaptoethanol and immobilization on nitrocellulose. Using recombinant tau and assaying antibody reactivity by immunoblotting, we have shown that both antibodies require two widely separated tau sequences for reactivity (Jicha et al., 1997). There is an essential N-terminal sequence, limited to the first 15 amino acids reported previously (Goedert et al., 1991) and which requires Phe8 (Ksiezak-Reding et al., 1995) and the two glutamates at positions 7 and 9 (the numbering system used refers to the 441 amino acid form of tau). The second required sequence is in the region 312 to 342, which includes the third microtubule binding domain (MTBD). Neither the first nor the second MTBD can substitute for the third, despite suggestions to the contrary (Carmel et al., 1996). The simplest interpretation of this data is that tau from the AD brain is folded such that the N-terminus is in close association with the third MTBD (see Figure 1), and that this conformation does not occur at significant levels in the normal brain. Other interpretations are possible, including a variety of models in which the presence of the third MTBD leads to "exposure" of the N-terminus. These seem difficult to reconcile with the existing models of tau structure, which indicate essentially a random coil structure in solution (Schweers et al., 1994). Further work is in progress, but it seems clear that both MCI and Alz-50 binding requires a conformational modification of tau that is associated with AD, in that tau from normal brain in solution is simply not reactive with these antibodies.

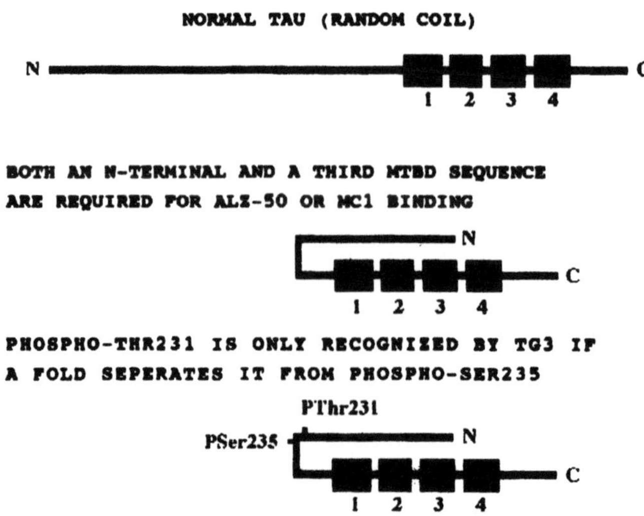

Figure 1. A simple model of how tau might be folded in the Alzheimer brain.

Antibodies Recognizing Phosphoepitopes

The second group of antibodies used recognize phosphorylated epitopes on tau that are associated with the formation of paired helical filaments (see for example, Hasegawa et al., 1992). There is considerable confusion in the literature concerning the "abnormality" of some of these phosphorylations. Immunoblot studies of biopsy-derived human brain tissues show that tau is phosphorylated at more sites than can be detected in autopsy derived normal brain tissues (e.g., serines 235 and 396) (Greenberg et al., 1992; Matsuo et al., 1994). However, it is also clear that these phosphoepitopes are much more stable in autopsy AD brain tissue than in normal, and that this difference in stability results from the nature of the phosphorylated tau, rather than from a difference in protein phosphatase activity (Vincent and Davies, 1990; and unpublished data). When present in PHF, all the phosphoepitopes we have examined are considerably more resistant to the action of alkaline phosphatase than are the same phosphoepitopes on recombinant tau. It also seems to be the case that the extent of phosphorylation at any given site is higher in the tau from autopsy AD brain than it is in tau from biopsied normal brain.

One monoclonal antibody, designated TG3 (Dickson et al., 1995; Vincent Rosado and Davies, 1996), that specifically recognizes a phosphorylation of threonine 231 of tau also appears to be sensitive to the conformation of the phosphorylated tau. Threonine 231 appears to be phosphorylated at low levels in the normal (biopsy) brain, although the epitope is not usually detectable in normal autopsy brain (Goedart et al., 1994; Matsuo et al., 1994). Phosphorylation of serine 235 appears to follow the same pattern. However, when both sites are phosphorylated, normal tau is not reactive with TG3, although tau from the AD brain, also phosphorylated at both sites, is strongly reactive. These results argue for a conformational difference between normal tau phosphorylated at these two sites and similarly phosphorylated AD derived tau. Recent work in collaboration with Otvos and Hoffmann (Jicha et al., submitted 1997) has been able to find support for this idea in studies of TG3 reactivity with a diphosphopeptide, phosphothreonine 231 – phosphoserine 235, which is only TG3 reactive under certain solvent conditions which stabilize a beta turn in the peptide molecule. This work provides further support for the notion that tau in the AD brain is quite different in conformation than that in the normal brain (see Figure 1).

Immunocytochemistry

Investigations are ongoing in an attempt to answer the important and obvious question of which comes first in Alzheimer's Disease, the conformational change in tau or the accumulation of phosphoaminoacids. These studies are greatly facilitated by the fact that both MC1 and TG3 appear by immunocytochemistry of routine autopsy tissues fixed in formalin to be very specifically reactive with neurons undergoing the neurofibrillary degeneration of Alzheimer's Disease (both antibodies also demonstrate the same specificity in paraffin embedded tissue, which allows studies of archival material). Detailed immunocytochemical studies of early AD cases have been conducted with the two types of antibodies described in brief above. Light and electron microscope single and double labeling studies have been conducted on a series of cases which fit into the Braak staging scheme as Stage 1 and 2 cases, in which neurofibrillary pathology is largely confined to the entorhinal cortex and hippocampus. In these cases both MCI and TG3 reveal hippocampal pyramidal cell staining that has never been found in brain tissue from young normal individuals. This staining is particularly intense in the perikarya of CA1 and sometimes CA2 neurons, where there often appears to be a perinuclear intensification of the staining. Immunoreactivity extends into both the basal and apical dendrites, fading out some 200-300 nanometers from the cell body. Electron microscopy reveals that in most cases the staining is cytoplasmic, and is not associated with filaments of any type. Staining is also occasionally observed in pyramidal cells of CA4 and to a surprising extent in both cell bodies and dendrites of dentate granule neurons. Again, in these early AD cases, most of the staining is cytoplasmic rather than filamentous.

Hippocampal CA1 neurons in a relatively small number of cases (11) have been examined with double labeling at the EM level, to attempt to determine if there are neurons which do not contain paired helical filaments that are positive for either TG3 or MC 1 (but not both). To date, it appears that MC1 labeling of such cells is quite frequently found in the absence of TG3 staining, implying that the conformational change in tau precedes the accumulation of phosphoepitopes. It is noteworthy that it is very rare to find evidence for phosphorylation at serine 235 or serine 396 in the hippocampal pyramidal cells of these cases, implying that these phosphoepitopes accumulate fairly late in the process of filament formation and degeneration.

CONCLUSION

This work raises many questions about the nature of the neurodegenerative process in AD. At the very earliest stages, neurons that do not appear to be abnormal by morphologic criteria have accumulations of a highly abnormal tau in the somatodendritic compartment. Does the tau accumulate because it is abnormal in conformation and sometimes highly phosphorylated, thus preventing axonal localization? Does the tau accumulate in cell bodies and dendrites because of some failure in axonal transport and then become abnormally folded and phosphorylated? The new generations of monoclonal antibodies seem to allow studies of molecular events taking place in the earliest stages of AD, although they do not allow us to define the relative importance of the biochemical changes they detect. Two quite different interpretations are possible. In the first, the abnormalities of tau are critical to the state of the microtubule system of the neuron, and degeneration proceeds because of lack of functional tau. In the second, the changes in tau conformation and phosphorylation state are simply results of derangement of neuronal biochemistry, and serve as markers for the degenerative process without having any direct consequences for the cell. Cell and molecular biological studies will be needed to address these intriguing questions.

ACKNOWLEDGMENTS

The authors' work is supported by NIMH grant MH38623 and NIA grant 06803.

REFERENCES

Braak, H., and Braak, E., 1991, Neuropathologic staging of Alzheimer-related changes. *Acta Neuropath.* 82:239–259.

Braak, H., Braak E., and Bohl, J., 1993, Staging of Alzheimer-related cortical destruction. *Eur. Neurol.* 33:403–408.

Carmel, G., Mager, E.M., Binder, L.I., and Kuret, J., 1996, The structural basis of monoclonal antibody Alz-50's selectivity for Alzheimer's disease pathology. *J. Biol. Chem.* 271:32789–32795.

Dickson, D.W., Crystal, H.A., Bevona, C., Honer, W.H., Vincent, I.J., and Davies, P., 1995, Correlations of synaptic and pathologic markers with cognition of the elderly. *Neurobiol Aging* 16:285–298.

Goedert, M., Spillantini, M.G., and Jakes, R., 1991, Localization of the Alz-50 epitope in recombinant human microtubule-associated protein tau. *Neurosci. Lett.* 126:149–154.

Goedert, M., Jakes, R., Crowther, R.A., Cohen, P., Vanmechelen, E., Vandermeeren, M. and Cras, P., 1994, Epitope mapping of monoclonal antibodies to the paired helical filaments of Alzheimer's disease: identification of phosphorylation sites in tau protein. *Biochem J.* 301:871–7.

Greenberg, S.G., Davies, P., Schein, J.D., and Binder, L.I., 1992, Hydrofluoric acid-treated tau-PHF proteins display the same biochemical properties as normal tau. *J. Biol. Chem.* 267:564 - 569.

Hasegawa, M., Morishima-Kawashima, M., Takio, K., Suzuki, M., Titani, K., and Ihara, Y., 1992, Protein sequence and mass spectrometric analyses of tau in the Alzheimer's disease brain. *J. Biol. Chem.* 267: 17047–17054.

Jicha, G.A., Bowser, R., Kazam, I.G., and Davies, P., 1997, Alz-50 and MC-1, a new monoclonal antibody raised to paired helical filaments, recognize conformational epitopes on recombinant tau. *J. Neurosci Res.* 48:128–132.

Jicha, G.A., Lane, E.,Vincent, I.J., Otvos, L., Hoffmann, R., and Davies, P., 1997, A conformation and phosphorylation dependent antibody recognizing the paired helical filaments of Alzheimer's Disease. Submitted.

Ksiezak-Reding, H., Leibowitz, R.L., Bowser, R. , and Davies, P., 1995, Binding of Alz50 depends on Phe8 in tau synthetic peptides and varies between native and denatured tau proteins. *Brain Res.* 697:63–75.

Matsuo, E.S., Shin, R.W., Billingsley, M.L., Van Devoorde, A., O'Connor, M., Trojanowski, J.Q., and Lee, V.M., 1994, Biopsy-derived adult human brain tau is phosphorylated at many of the same sites as Alzheimer's disease paired helical filament tau. *Neuron.* 13: 989–1002.

Schweers, O., Schonbrunn-Hanebeck, E., Marx, A., and Mandelkow, E., 1994, Structural studies of tau protein and Alzheimer paired helical filaments show no evidence for beta structure. *J. Biol. Chem.* 269: 24290–24297.

Vincent, I.J. and Davies, P., 1990, Phosphorylation characteristics of the A68 protein in Alzheimer's Disease. *Brain Res.* 531:127–135.

Vincent, I.J., and Davies, P., 1992, A protein kinase associated with the paired helical filaments in Alzheimer's Disease. *Proc. Natl. Acad. Sci.* 89:2878–2882.

Vincent, I.J., Rosado, M. and Davies, P., 1996, Mitotic mechanisms in Alzheimer's Disease? *J. Cell. Biol.* 132:413–425.

Wolozin, B.L., Pruchnicki, A., Dickson, D.W., and Davies, P. , 1986, A neuronal antigen in the brains of patients with Alzheimer's disease. *Science* 232:648–650.

3

ApoE AND MEMORY IN ALZHEIMER'S DISEASE

Hilkka S. Soininen[1] and Paavo J. Riekkinen, Sr.[2]

[1]Department of Neuroscience and Neurology
Kuopio University and University Hospital
[2]AIVirtanen Institute
Kuopio, Finland

INTRODUCTION

The role of apolipoprotein E (ApoE) allele ε4 as a risk factor for AD is generally agreed (Strittmatter and Roses, 1995). ApoE can be detected by immunohistochemistry in senile plaques, neurofibrillary tangles, and cerebrovascular amyloid, the major neuro-pathologic changes in AD brain. ApoE contributes to the transport of cholesterol and other lipids, and it is also involved in the growth and regeneration of nerves during development or following injury (Poirier, 1994). ApoE isoforms also differ in their binding properties to amyloid β-protein (Aβ) and tau protein suggesting that ApoE might be involved in the pathogenesis of AD (Strittmatter and Roses, 1995). ApoE ε4 allele is associated with earlier age of onset of AD, increased accumulation of β amyloid (Aβ) in AD brains (Schmechel et al., 1993; Rebeck et al., 1993) and even brains of elderly nondemented subjects (Polvikoski et al., 1995), increased counts of neurofibrillary tangles (Nagy et al., 1995), and decreased plastic response (Arendt et al., 1997). Moreover, recent data have indicated that the degree of the cholinergic deficit in AD brains is related to the number of ε4 alleles (Poirier, 1994; Soininen et al., 1995).

Loss of memory is often the first symptom of AD accompanied later by impairment in visuospatial, executive, and verbal functions. Many studies have shown that reduction of the hippocampal volume measured on magnetic resonance imaging (MRI) scans is a sensitive and early indicator of AD. Hippocampal atrophy also correlates with degree of memory impairment in tests assessing delayed recall (Lehtovirta et al., 1995).

Recent data have suggested that the presence of the ApoE ε4 allele may significantly enhance the magnitude of hippocampal atrophy. The ε4 allele seems also to be associated with severe memory impairment in AD and is related to impaired learning ability even in the nondemented elderly. Therefore, ApoE ε4 allele may to be a significant contributor to memory impairment in the elderly population.

Progress in Alzheimer's and Parkinson's Diseases
edited by Fisher *et al.*, Plenum Press, New York, 1998.

HIPPOCAMPAL VOLUMES AND MEMORY ARE AFFECTED BY ApoE ε4 ALLELE

A study evaluating the deficits in cognitive performance in AD patients showed that the only difference in the cognitive profile of AD patients related to the number of ApoE ε4 alleles, was more severe memory impairment (Lehtovirta et al., 1995 and 1996). AD patients carrying the ε4 allele also showed more severe hippocampal damage than AD patients without ε4. The patients were in the early stage of the disease, and patients with 2, 1, or 0 ApoE ε4 alleles were comparable in global severity of dementia assessed by rating scales. The AD ε44 subjects displayed the most pronounced volume loss, they had significantly smaller volumes of the right hippocampus (−54% of control) than all the other study groups. The AD ε44 patients also had the lowest scores in delayed memory tests, and differed from ε33 AD patients in delayed recognition of learned words.

Nondemented elderly carrying ε4 were also reported to have minor hippocampal changes (Soininen et al., 1995), namely a decrease in hippocampal asymmetry that is detected in normal controls.

Data from a population based study supported these findings and suggested that ApoE ε2 might be protective for learning and memory functions whereas ε4 seemed to be deleterious (Helkala et al., 1995). This study of 916 nondemented subjects showed that the individuals with 22 or 23 phenotype had better learning ability that than those carrying an ε4 allele. The groups did not differ in Mini-Mental Status scores or performance in psychometric tests assessing other cognitive domains. Three years later, 632 subjects participated in a follow-up screening, and the subjects with ε22 or ε23 had maintained their verbal learning performance, whereas learning ability of subjects with other ApoE phenotypes deteriorated (Helkala et al., 1996).

CHOLINERGIC DEFICIT AND ApoE GENOTYPE

Depletion of choline acetyltransferase (ChAT) in the neocortex and hippocampus and degeneration of the cholinergic neurons in the nucleus basalis of Meynert are the most consistent neurochemical changes in AD brain. A post-mortem study indicated that AD patients carrying the ε4 allele have a more severe cholinergic deficit (−72% of control) in the frontal cortex than the AD patients without the ε4 allele (−48% of control) (Soininen et al., 1995). The ChAT deficit was most pronounced for the AD patients with the ε44 genotype. These data are in line with a report of a decrease of ChAT proportional to the number of ε4 alleles in the post mortem temporal cortex and hippocampus of AD patients (Poirier, 1994). Moreover, decreased number of nicotine binding sites and decreased neuronal density in the nucleus basalis have been reported to associate with the ApoE ε4 in AD brain (Poirier et al., 1995). Interestingly, AD patients carrying ε4 have shown a decreased response to tacrine, an acetylcholinesterase inhibitor. Moreover, another study reported increased activity of acetylcholinesterase, an enzyme degrading acetylcholine, in the CSF of AD patients carrying ε4 (Soininen et al., 1995). These findings may have implication for drug treatment of AD patients with cholinomimetics. At the moment, in many drug trials the ApoE genotype will be determined and its effect to the drug response will be analyzed.

TEMPORAL LOBE STRUCTURES ARE VULNERABLE TO ApoE ε4

Both in AD patients and in nondemented elderly subjects, memory functions and medial temporal lobe structures such as the hippocampus, seem to be particularly susceptible to adverse effects of the ApoE ε4 allele. In contrast, ε2 might be protective; elderly subjects with ε2 maintain their learning ability (Helkala et al., 1996). Bondi and coworkers (1995) also showed that episodic memory changes were associated with the ApoE ε4 allele in nondemented older adults. Another study in normal older twins showed lower cognitive performance in subjects carrying the ApoE ε4 allele (Reed et al., 1994). The ApoE ε4 allele has been reported to be a strong predictor of development of AD in memory impaired individuals (Petersen et al., 1995). Moreover, many studies have documented earlier in age of onset in AD patients carrying 2 ε4 alleles. This kind of data propose that ε4 carriers among the elderly suffering from memory impairment may be a group that is at high risk for dementia and outline a possible target group for preventive procedures if these become available in the future.

How ApoE exerts its action AD, is not known yet. However, new data about its possible mechanisms of action have rapidly accumulated. ApoE isoforms differ in binding to Aβ and tau (Strittmatter and Roses, 1995), and ApoE is involved in regeneration and synaptogenesis following injury. ApoE-deficient mice have also shown reduced synaptic density and diminished regenerative capacity following hippocampal lesions (Mashliah et al., 1995). Moreover, *in vitro* studies have indicated that ApoE3 enhances while ApoE4 inhibits neurite outgrowth in neuronal cell cultures (Nathan et al., 1994). Because transport of cholesterol and other lipoproteins plays a crucial role in synaptogenesis, it is possible that AD patients differing in ApoE phenotype also differ in their capacities for plastic response and synaptogenesis. Finally, the ε4 allele is related to severe cholinergic deficit in the frontal cortex (Soininen et al., 1995), temporal cortex and hippocampus (Poirier, 1994). ApoE may be of major importance for the cholinergic system which is partly dependent of phospholipid metabolism in neurons (Wurtman, 1992). In concert with results from AD patients, ApoE knocked out mice were reported to have cholinergic depletion in the frontal cortex and hippocampus and also impairments in working memory but not in reference memory (Gordon et al. 1995).

To sum up, increasing evidence is accumulating that the ApoE ε4 may be harmful, particularly, for memory functions. The ApoE ε4 allele is associated with severe hippocampal damage and memory impairment in AD. In contrast, the ApoE ε2 seems to be protective for memory functions in the elderly. ApoE ε4 is also associated with severe cholinergic deficit in AD that may imply a reduced response to cholinomimetics as has been found concerning tacrine.

REFERENCES

Arendt, T., Schindler, C., Bruckner, M.K., Eschrich, K., Bigl, V., Zedlick, D., and Markova, L., 1997, Plastic neuronal remodeling is impaired in patients with Alzheimer's disease carrying apolipoprotein ε4 allele, *J. Neurosci.* 17:516.

Bondi, M.W., Salmon, D.P., Monsch, A.U., Galasko, D., Butters, N., Klauber, M.R., Thal, L.J. and Saitoh, T., 1995, Episodic memory changes are associated with APOE-ε4 allele in nondemented older adults, *Neurology* 45:2203–2206.

Gordon, I., Grauer, E., Genis, I., Sehayek, E. and Michaelson, D.M., 1995, Memory deficits and cholinergic impairments in apolipoprotein E-deficient mice, *Neurosci. Lett.* 199:1–4.

Helkala, E.L., Koivisto, K., Hänninen, T., Vanhanen, M., Kervinen, K., Kuusisto, J., Mykkänen, L., Kesäniemi, Y.A., Laakso, M. and Riekkinen, P.Sr., 1995, The association of apolipoprotein E with memory: a population based study, *Neurosci. Lett.* 1991:141–144.

Helkala, E.L., Koivisto, K., Hänninen, T., Vanhanen, M., Kervinen, K., Kuusisto, J., Mykkänen, L., Kesäniemi, Y.A., Laakso, M. and Riekkinen, P.Sr., 1996, Memory functions in human subjects with different apolipoprotein E phenotypes during a 3-year population-based follow-up study, *Neurosci. Lett.* 204:177–180.

Lehtovirta, M., Laakso, M.P., Soininen, H., Mannermaa, A., Helkala, E.-L., Partanen, K., Ryynänen, M., Vainio, P., Hartikainen, P. and Riekkinen, P.J. Sr., 1995, Volumes of hippocampus, amygdala, and frontal lobe in Alzheimer patients with different apolipoprotein E genotypes, *Neuroscience* 67:65–72.

Lehtövirta, M., Soininen, H., Helisalmi, S., Mannermaa, A., Helkala, E.-L., Hartikainen, P., Hänninen, T., Ryynänen, M. and Riekkinen P.J., 1996, Clinical and neuropsychological characteristics in familial and sporadic Alzheimer's disease: relation to apolipoprotein E polymorphism, *Neurology* 46:413–419.

Masliah, E., Mallory, M., Alford, M., Ge, N. and Mucke, L., 1995, Abnormal synaptic regeneration in hAPP695 transgenic and apoE knockout mice. In: *Research Advances in Alzheimer's Disease and Related Disorders,*. Iqbal, K., Mortimer, J.A, Winblad, B., Wisniewski ,H.M., eds,Wiley, New York, pp.405–414.

Nagy, Z., Esiri, M.M., Jobst, K.A., Johnston, C., Litchfield, S., Sim, E. and Smith, A.D., 1995, Influence of the apolipoprotein E genotype on amyloid deposition and neurofibrillary tangle formation in Alzheimer's disease, *Neuroscience* 69:757–761.

Nathan, B.P., Bellosta, S., Sanan, D.A., Weisgraber, K.H., Mahley, R.W. and Pitas, R.E., 1994, Differential effects of apolipoproteins E3 and E4 on neuronal growth in vitro, *Science* 264:850–852.

Petersen, R.D., Smith, G.E., Ivnik, R.J., Tangalos, E.G., Schaid, D.J., Thibodeau, S.N., Kokmen, E., Waring, S.C. and Kurland, L.T., 1995, Apolipoprotein E status as a predictor of the development of Alzheimer's disease in memory-impaired individuals, *JAMA* 273:1274–1278.

Poirier, J., Delisle, M.C., Quirion, R., Aubert, I., Farlow, M., Lahiri, D., Hui, S., Bertrand, P., Nalbantoglu, J., Gilfix, B.M. et al., 1995, Apolipoprotein E4 allele as a predictor of cholinergic deficits and treatment outcome in Alzheimer's disease, *Proc. Natl. Acad. Sci. USA* 92:12260–12264.

Poirier, J., 1994, Apolipoprotein E in animal models of CNS injury and Alzheimer's disease, *Trends Neurosci.* 17:525–530.

Polvikoski, T., Sulkava, R., Haltia, M., Kainulainen, K., Vuorio, A., Verkkoniemi, A., Niinistö, L., Halonen, P. and Kontula, K., 1995, Apolipoprotein E, dementia, and cortical deposition of β-amyloid protein, *New. Engl. J. Med.* 333:1242–1247.

Rebeck, G.W., Reiter, J.S., Strickland, D.K. and Hyman, B.T., 1993, Apolipoprotein E in sporadic Alzheimer's disease: allelic variation and receptor interactions, *Neuron* 11:575–580.

Reed, T., Carmelli, D., Swan, G.E., Breitner, J.C., Welsh, K.A., Jarvik, G.P., Deeb, S. and Auwerx, J., 1994, Lower cognitive performance in normal older adult male twins carrying the apolipoprotein E epsilon 4 allele, *Arch. Neurol.* 51:1189–1192.

Schmechel, D.E., Saunders, A.M., Strittmatter, W.J., Crain, B.J., Hulette, C.M., Joo, S.H., Pericak-Vance, M.A., Goldgaber, D. and Roses, A., 1993, Increased amyloid β-peptide deposition as a consequence of apolipoprotein E genotype in late-onset Alzheimer's disease, *Proc Natl Acad Sci USA* 90:9649–9653.

Soininen, H., Kosunen, O., Helisalmi, S., Mannermaa, A., Paljärvi, L., Talasniemi, S., Ryynänen, M. and Riekkinen, P.J. Sr., 1995, A severe loss of choline acetyltransferase in the frontal cortex of patients carrying apolipoprotein E ε 4 allele, *Neurosci. Lett.* 187:79–82.

Soininen, H., Lehtovirta, M., Helisalmi, S., Linnaranta, K., Heinonen, O., Riekkinen, P. Sr., 1995, Increased acetylcholinesterase activity in the CSF of Alzheimer patients carrying apolipoprotein ε4 allele, *NeuroReport* 6:2518–2520.

Soininen, H., Partanen, K., Pitkänen, A., Hallikainen, M., Hänninen, T., Helisalmi, S., Ryynänen, M., Koivisto, K., Riekkinen, P. Sr., 1995, Decreased hippocampal volume asymmetry on MRI scans in nondemented elderly subjects carrying apolipoprotein E ε 4 allele, *Neurology* 45:391–392.

Soininen, H.S. and Riekkinen, P.J. Sr., 1996, Apolipoprotein E, memory and Alzheimer's disease. *Trends Neurosci.* 19:224–228.

Strittmatter, W.J. and Roses, A.D., 1995, Apolipoprotein E and Alzheimer disease, *Proc. Natl. Acad. Sci. USA* 92:4725–4727.

Wurtman, R.J., 1992, Choline metabolism as a basis for the selective vulnerability of cholinergic neurons, *Trends Neurosci.* 15:117–122.

4

DIVERGENT METABOLISM OF APOLIPOPROTEINS E3 AND E4 BY CELLS[*]

Robert E. Pitas,[1,2] Zhong-Sheng Ji,[1] Lubica Supekova,[1] and
Robert W. Mahley[1,2,3]

[1]Gladstone Institute of Cardiovascular Disease
P.O. Box 419100
San Francisco, California 94141-9100
The Cardiovascular Research Institute and
[2]The Department of Pathology
[3]The Department of Medicine
University of California
San Francisco, California 94141-9100

INTRODUCTION

Apolipoprotein (apo-) E is a 299-amino acid, 34-kDa protein that is synthesized and secreted by hepatocytes, macrophages, and astrocytes. It is a component of both plasma and cerebrospinal fluid lipoproteins (Borghini et al., 1995; Mahley, 1988; Pitas, 1997; Pitas et al., 1987). As a component of lipoproteins, apo-E is a ligand for several members of the low density lipoprotein (LDL) receptor gene family, including the LDL receptor itself and the LDL receptor-related protein (LRP) (Krieger and Herz, 1994; Mahley, 1988; Pitas et al., 1979). Apo-E occurs in three common forms that are products of different alleles at the same gene locus (Zannis and Breslow, 1981). The proteins apo-E2, apo-E3, and apo-E4 differ by single amino acid changes at amino acids 112 and 158 (Mahley, 1988). Apo-E2 has cysteine at both positions, apo-E4 has arginine at both positions, and apo-E3 has cysteine at position 112 and arginine at 158 (Mahley, 1988; Weisgraber, 1994). These amino acid substitutions have a profound impact on the metabolic properties of the proteins and their association with disease. Of particular interest is the observation that the apo-E4 allele is overrepresented in subjects with late-onset Alzheimer's disease (AD) and furthermore that subjects who carry the apo-E4 allele develop AD at an earlier age than

[*] This research was funded in part by NIA Grant AG13619 and NHLBI Program Project Grant HL41633 from the National Institutes of Health. Additional funding was obtained from a Cambridge Neuroscience/Gladstone collaborative research agreement.

Progress in Alzheimer's and Parkinson's Diseases
edited by Fisher *et al.*, Plenum Press, New York, 1998.

those with the apo-E3 allele (Corder et al., 1993; Mayeux et al., 1993; Poirier et al., 1993; Saunders et al., 1993). Apo-E4 is therefore a major risk factor for the development of late-onset AD.

In our initial attempts to determine how apo-E4 might contribute to AD, we examined the effect of apo-E-enriched lipoproteins on the outgrowth of neurites from neurons in culture. In primary cultures of dorsal root ganglion neurons (Nathan et al., 1994) and a murine neuroblastoma cell line (Neuro-2a) (Nathan et al., 1995), incubation with apo-E3-enriched lipoproteins stimulated neurite outgrowth, whereas incubation with apo-E4-enriched lipoproteins inhibited neurite outgrowth. Free apo-E, which is not a ligand for lipoprotein receptors, had no effect. Similar results were observed in Neuro-2a cells stably transfected to secrete either apo-E3 or apo-E4 (Bellosta et al., 1995). Cerebrospinal fluid lipoproteins or β-VLDL (cholesterol-rich plasma very low density lipoproteins) stimulated neurite outgrowth from cells expressing apo-E3 and inhibited outgrowth from cells expressing apo-E4. Several lines of evidence demonstrate that the effect of the apo-E3- and apo-E4-enriched lipoproteins on neurite outgrowth is mediated after interaction with the LRP (Bellosta et al., 1995; Holtzman et al., 1995).

The differential effects of apo-E3 and apo-E4 on neurite outgrowth were associated with differential effects on the cytoskeleton (i.e., microtubules are disrupted in apo-E4-treated but not in apo-E3-treated cells) and with the differential accumulation of apo-E3 and apo-E4 in cells (Nathan et al., 1995). Immunocytochemical detection of apo-E in Neuro-2a cells demonstrated greater accumulation of apo-E in the cell body and neurites in cells incubated for 48 hr with apo-E3-enriched lipoproteins than in cells incubated with apo-E4-enriched lipoproteins. These results were confirmed by studies with iodinated apo-E. This differential accumulation of apo-E3 and apo-E4 in neurons is somewhat surprising because apo-E3 and apo-E4 stimulate LRP-mediated uptake of lipoprotein-derived cholesterol to a similar extent in non-neuronal cells (Kowal et al., 1990).

The goals of the current study were to determine the reason for the differential accumulation of apo-E3 and apo-E4 in neurons and to determine if the differential accumulation occurs in other cell types as well (Ji et al., 1997).

METHODS

To examine the metabolism of apo-E-enriched β-VLDL by cells and to determine the mechanism for the differential accumulation of apo-E3 and apo-E4, two types of experiments were performed. In one set of studies, the metabolism of the apo-E-enriched β-VLDL particles was examined by using either iodinated β-VLDL or β-VLDL labeled with the fluorescent molecule 1,1 dioctadecyl-3,3,3′,3′-tetra-methylindocarbocyanine (DiI) to follow the metabolism of the major protein component of the lipoprotein, apo-B, or the lipid moieties of the particles, respectively. In the other set of studies, apo-E metabolism was assessed directly using three different techniques: immunofluorescence detection of cellular apo-E, western blotting of cellular apo-E, and by examining the metabolism of β-VLDL enriched with iodinated apo-E.

In the various studies, the cells were incubated at 37°C or, where indicated, at 18°C with β-VLDL alone or with β-VLDL enriched with apo-E3 or apo-E4. The apo-E3 or apo-E4 were preincubated with the β-VLDL for 1 hr at 37°C before addition to the cells. The cells were then assayed for cell association or internalization of ligand. Cell association includes both bound and internalized material, whereas internalization was assayed after the release of surface-bound ligand with suramin.

RESULTS

In experiments performed with iodinated β-VLDL, apo-E3 and apo-E4 increased the cell association of β-VLDL with Neuro-2a cells to a similar extent, as compared with the cell association of β-VLDL alone. Similar results were observed with the DiI-labeled β-VLDL, where the internalization of the fluorescently labeled lipoproteins was quantitated. Both apo-E4 and apo-E3 stimulated the uptake of DiI-labeled β-VLDL to a comparable extent. Incubation of cells with apo-E3- and E4-enriched β-VLDL also resulted in similar increases in the cholesterol content of the cells. These results, which are consistent with data previously obtained in fibroblasts, demonstrate that apo-E3 and apo-E4 mediate the delivery of an equivalent number of lipoprotein particles to neurons. When the uptake of apo-E by the cells was assessed more directly, different results were obtained.

Cells were incubated with apo-E-enriched β-VLDL for various periods of time, and cell-associated immunoreactive apo-E was quantitated by confocal microscopy in 60 cells at each time point. Starting at the earliest time point measured (2 hr) and continuing through 48 hr, apo-E3 accumulated to a greater extent than apo-E4. Western blot analysis of cell extracts confirmed the differential cell association of apo-E3 and apo-E4; the greater accumulation of apo-E3 was noted at 1 hr, the earliest time point measured and continued through 36 hr. The apo-E was intact and migrated at the same position as purified apo-E. We next performed studies in which Neuro-2a cells and human fibroblasts were incubated with β-VLDL enriched with iodinated apo-E. Neuro-2a cells internalized twice as much apo-E3 as apo-E4 (Fig. 1). Similar results were obtained in fibroblasts.

Subsequent experiments to determine the mechanism for the differential accumulation were performed with fibroblasts because they adhere better in the cell culture experiments than neurons and because mutant fibroblasts are available as tools to help dissect the pathways responsible for the differential accumulation. To determine if preferential degradation of apo-E4 accounted for the difference in accumulation, the internalization of iodinated apo-E-enriched β-VLDL was examined in fibroblasts treated with chloroquine to block lysosomal degradation or maintained at 18°C, a temperature at which lipoprotein internalization occurs but degradation does not. In these studies, apo-E3 also accumulated in the cells to a greater extent than apo-E4, demonstrating that the differential accumulation was not secondary to lysosomal degradation. Similar results were obtained with Neuro-2a cells.

Figure 1. Cell association of ^{125}I-apo-E-enriched β-VLDL with Neuro-2a cells. Neuro-2a cells were grown to ~100% confluence, washed twice with serum-free medium, and incubated overnight. They were then incubated with either ^{125}I-apo-E3-enriched β-VLDL or ^{125}I-apo-E4-enriched β-VLDL at 37°C for 2 hr. The ^{125}I-apo-E (7.5 μg/ml) and β-VLDL (5 μg protein/ml) were mixed and incubated for 1 hr at 37°C before addition to the cells. The cells were washed five times on ice with 0.1M phosphate-buffered saline (PBS) containing 0.2% bovine serum albumin and once with 0.1M PBS and then dissolved in 0.1N NaOH. The ^{125}I-apo-E cell association was measured by gamma counting and cellular protein determined.

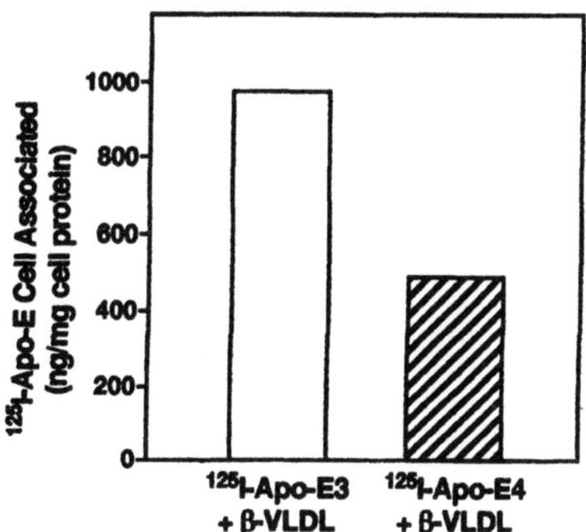

Next we examined the importance of the LDL receptor, the LRP, and heparan sulfate proteoglycans (HSPG) in the differential accumulation of apo-E3 and apo-E4. To study the role of the LDL receptor, we used normal human fibroblasts, which express the LDL receptor, and human fibroblasts from patients with familial hypercholesterolemia, which do not express LDL receptors. The differential accumulation of apo-E3 and apo-E4 occurred in both types of fibroblasts, demonstrating that the LDL receptor is not involved. Heparinase totally blocked the differential accumulation, suggesting that the effect is mediated either by the HSPG–LRP complex or by cell-surface HSPG. To distinguish between these possibilities, we used murine fibroblasts (obtained from J. Herz) that were either heterozygous for LRP expression or lacked LRP expression. Again, the differential accumulation was observed in both types of fibroblasts, demonstrating that the LRP is not required for the effect. To examine the role of HSPG directly, we performed a similar experiment in wild-type Chinese hamster ovary (CHO) cells and in CHO cells deficient in either HSPG expression or in expression of all proteoglycans (obtained from J.D. Esko) (Fig. 2). The differential accumulation of apo-E3 and apo-E4 was observed in the wild-type cells but not in the HSPG-deficient cells, clearly demonstrating that HSPG are required for this process.

Proteoglycans can associate with cell membranes either by phospholipid anchors or by transmembrane spanning of their core proteins (Bernfield et al., 1992; Yanagishita, 1992). These proteoglycans undergo different rates of cellular processing (Yanagishita, 1992). The glycero-phosphatidylinositol (GPI)–anchored proteoglycans undergo fast endosome-to-lysosome transport, resulting in lysosomal degradation within 30 min after internalization. In contrast, the core protein–anchored proteoglycans undergo slow endosome-to-lysosome transport, resulting in delayed processing of up to 4 hr. Retention of apo-E by the cells would be consistent with use of the slow pathway for degradation and would suggest that the differential accumulation of apo-E3 and apo-E4 in the cells is not due to internalization of apo-E with GPI-anchored proteoglycans.

To test this hypothesis, we examined the effect of specific phospholipase C on the cell association of iodinated apo-E-enriched β-VLDL with fibroblasts. Treatment with

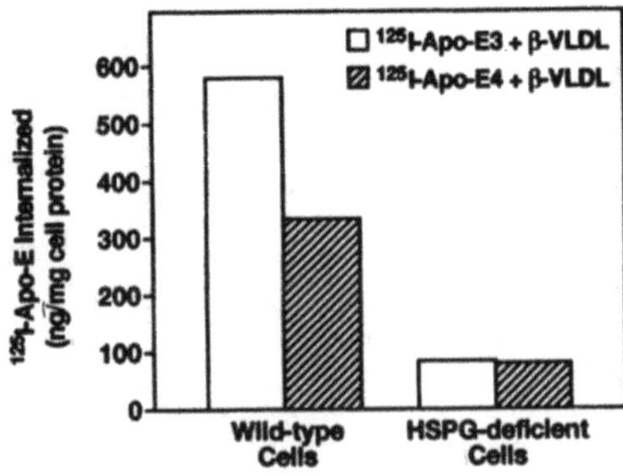

Figure 2. Internalization of ^{125}I-apo-E-enriched β-VLDL by wild-type and mutant CHO cells. Wild-type and HSPG-deficient CHO cells were grown to ~100% confluence in F12 medium containing 7.5% fetal bovine serum, washed twice with serum-free F12 medium, and incubated with either ^{125}I-apo-E3-enriched β-VLDL or ^{125}I-apo-E4-enriched β-VLDL at 37°C for 2 hr. The ^{125}I-apo-E and β-VLDL (7.5 µg/ml and 5 ug protein/ml, respectively) were mixed and incubated together at 37°C for 1 hr before use. After incubation, the cells were washed twice on ice with Dulbecco's modified Eagle's medium–Hepes. The cells were then incubated with 10 mM suramin at 4°C for 30 min, washed with 0.1M PBS, and dissolved in 0.1 N NaOH. The radioactivity and protein concentration of the cells were determined.

phospholipase C, which removes GPI-anchored HSPG, did not affect the differential accumulation of apo-E3 and apo-E4 in the cells, demonstrating that GPI-anchored HSPG are not involved.

DISCUSSION

These studies demonstrate that the differential cellular accumulation of apo-E3 and apo-E4 from apo-E-enriched β-VLDL occurs in fibroblasts as well as in neurons, that the LDL receptor and the LRP are not responsible for the differential accumulation, and that cell-surface HSPG are required for the differential accumulation of apo-E3 and apo-E4. Whereas the accumulation of apo-E in the cells clearly requires HSPG, the mechanism for the differential accumulation of apo-E3 and apo-E4 remains to be determined. The differential accumulation could result from a different affinity of apo-E3- or apo-E4-enriched lipoproteins for a specific HSPG, with apo-E3 having a higher affinity and hence greater uptake leading to a higher intracellular concentration. Alternatively, there could be a different intracellular fate for the HSPG-bound apo-E. Apo-E3 may be sequestered and retained, whereas apo-E4 might undergo retroendocytosis and loss from the cell, resulting in a lower intracellular accumulation. At present there are no data to differentiate these possibilities. In addition the current studies do not rule out the possibility that an as yet unidentified co-receptor functions together with the HSPG in the accumulation of apo-E in cells.

The cellular compartment where apo-E is retained has not been determined; however, certain studies suggest that apo-E can occur in the cytoplasm of neurons (Han et al., 1994; Han et al., 1994). If so, apo-E might be available to interact with cytoplasmic components that could affect the cytoskeleton and neurite outgrowth. *In vitro* studies have shown that apo-E3, but not apo-E4, interacts with the microtubule-associated proteins tau and MAP2c (Huang et al., 1994; Huang et al., 1995; Strittmatter et al., 1994), and it has been postulated that apo-E3 may bind to tau in cells, preventing overphosphorylation and neurofibrillary tangle formation (Roses, 1994; Strittmatter et al., 1994). This hypothesis has not been tested, but there is evidence suggesting that apo-E3, but not apo-E4, may in fact interact with tau *in vivo*. Lovestone et al. recently showed that the intracellular distribution of apo-E3 and apo-E4 differs in COS cells transfected to express tau (Lovestone et al., 1996). When the cells were incubated with cerebrospinal fluid lipoproteins, the site of intracellular apo-E was dependent upon the apo-E genotype. Apo-E4 was sequestered in vesicles, whereas apo-E3 was observed diffusely in the cells, and was colocalized with tau, suggesting that apo-E might be present in the cytoplasm. In future studies, it will be important to identify the intracellular compartments where apo-E3 and apo-E4 reside and to determine definitively whether intracellular apo-E4 contributes to the microtubule disruption and inhibition of neurite outgrowth observed *in vitro* (Bellosta et al., 1995; Nathan et al., 1994; Nathan et al., 1995) and to the pathogenesis of AD.

REFERENCES

Bellosta, S., Nathan, B. P., Orth, M., Dong, L.-M., Mahley, R. W., and Pitas, R. E. (1995). Stable expression and secretion of apolipoproteins E3 and E4 in mouse neuroblastoma cells produces differential effects on neurite outgrowth. J. Biol. Chem. *270*, 27063–27071.

Bernfield, M., Kokenyesi, R., Kato, M., Hinkes, M. T., Spring, J., Gallo, R. L., and Lose, E. J. (1992). Biology of the syndecans: A family of transmembrane heparan sulfate proteoglycans. Annu. Rev. Cell Biol. *8*, 365–393.

Borghini, I., Barja, F., Pometta, D., and James, R. W. (1995). Characterization of subpopulations of lipoprotein particles isolated from human cerebrospinal fluid. Biochim. Biophys. Acta *1255*, 192–200.

Corder, E. H., Saunders, A. M., Strittmatter, W. J., Schmechel, D. E., Gaskell, P. C., Small, G. W., Roses, A. D., Haines, J. L., and Pericak-Vance, M. A. (1993). Gene dose of apolipoprotein E type 4 allele and the risk of Alzheimer's disease in late onset families. Science *261*, 921–923.

Han, S.-H., Einstein, G., Weisgraber, K. H., Strittmatter, W. J., Saunders, A. M., Pericak-Vance, M., Roses, A. D., and Schmechel, D. E. (1994). Apolipoprotein E is localized to the cytoplasm of human cortical neurons: A light and electron microscopic study. J. Neuropathol. Exp. Neurol. *53*, 535–544.

Han, S.-H., Hulette, C., Saunders, A. M., Einstein, G., Pericak-Vance, M., Strittmatter, W. J., Roses, A. D., and Schmechel, D. E. (1994). Apolipoprotein E is present in hippocampal neurons without neurofibrillary tangles in Alzheimer's disease and in age-matched controls. Exp. Neurol. *128*, 13–26.

Holtzman, D. M., Pitas, R. E., Kilbridge, J., Nathan, B., Mahley, R. W., Bu, G., and Schwartz, A. L. (1995). Low density lipoprotein receptor-related protein mediates apolipoprotein E-dependent neurite outgrowth in a central nervous system-derived neuronal cell line. Proc. Natl. Acad. Sci. USA *92*, 9480–9484.

Huang, D. Y., Goedert, M., Jakes, R., Weisgraber, K. H., Garner, C. C., Saunders, A. M., Pericak-Vance, M. A., Schmechel, D. E., Roses, A. D., and Strittmatter, W. J. (1994). Isoform-specific interactions of apolipoprotein E with the microtubule-associated protein MAP2c: Implications for Alzheimer's disease. Neurosci. Lett. *182*, 55–58.

Huang, D. Y., Weisgraber, K. H., Goedert, M., Saunders, A. M., Roses, A. D., and Strittmatter, W. J. (1995). ApoE3 binding to tau tandem repeat I is abolished by tau serine$_{262}$ phosphorylation. Neurosci. Lett. *192*, 209–212.

Ji, Z.-S., Mahley, R. W., Supekova, L., and Pitas, R. E. (1997). Differential accumulation of apolipoproteins E3 and E4 by cells is mediated by cell-surface heparan sulfate proteoglycans. Abstract submitted for the 27th Annual Meeting of the Society for Neuroscience, to be held in New Orleans, October 25–30, 1997

Kowal, R. C., Herz, J., Weisgraber, K. H., Mahley, R. W., Brown, M. S., and Goldstein, J. L. (1990). Opposing effects of apolipoproteins E and C on lipoprotein binding to low density lipoprotein receptor-related protein. J. Biol. Chem. *265*, 10771–10779.

Krieger, M. and Herz, J. (1994). Structures and functions of multiligand lipoprotein receptors: Macrophage scavenger receptors and LDL receptor-related protein (LRP). Annu. Rev. Biochem. *63*, 601–637.

Lovestone, S., Anderton, B. H., Hartley, K., Jensen, T. G., and Jorgensen, A. L. (1996). The intracellular fate of apolipoprotein E is tau dependent and apoe allele-specific. Neuroreport *7*, 1005–1008.

Mahley, R. W. (1988). Apolipoprotein E: Cholesterol transport protein with expanding role in cell biology. Science *240*, 622–630.

Mayeux, R., Stern, Y., Ottman, R., Tatemichi, T. K., Tang, M.-X., Maestre, G., Ngai, C., Tycko, B., and Ginsberg, H. (1993). The apolipoprotein ε4 allele in patients with Alzheimer's disease. Ann. Neurol. *34*, 752–754.

Nathan, B. P., Bellosta, S., Sanan, D. A., Weisgraber, K. H., Mahley, R. W., and Pitas, R. E. (1994). Differential effects of apolipoproteins E3 and E4 on neuronal growth in vitro. Science *264*, 850–852.

Nathan, B. P., Chang, K.-C., Bellosta, S., Brisch, E., Ge, N., Mahley, R. W., and Pitas, R. E. (1995). The inhibitory effect of apolipoprotein E4 on neurite outgrowth is associated with microtubule depolymerization. J. Biol. Chem. *270*, 19791–19799.

Pitas, R. E. (1997). Cerebrospinal fluid lipoproteins, lipoprotein receptors, and neurite outgrowth. Nutr. Metab. Cardiovasc. Dis. In press.

Pitas, R. E., Boyles, J. K., Lee, S. H., Hui, D., and Weisgraber, K. H. (1987). Lipoproteins and their receptors in the central nervous system. Characterization of the lipoproteins in cerebrospinal fluid and identification of apolipoprotein B,E(LDL) receptors in the brain. J. Biol. Chem. *262*, 14352–14360.

Pitas, R. E., Innerarity, T. L., Arnold, K. S., and Mahley, R. W. (1979). Rate and equilibrium constants for binding of apo-E HDL$_c$ (a cholesterol-induced lipoprotein) and low density lipoproteins to human fibroblasts: Evidence for multiple receptor binding of apo-E HDL$_c$. Proc. Natl. Acad. Sci. USA *76*, 2311–2315.

Poirier, J., Davignon, J., Bouthillier, D., Kogan, S., Bertrand, P., and Gauthier, S. (1993). Apolipoprotein E polymorphism and Alzheimer's disease. Lancet *342*, 697–699.

Roses, A. D. (1994). Apolipoprotein E affects the rate of Alzheimer disease expression: β-amyloid burden is a secondary consequence dependent on APOE genotype and duration of disease. J. Neuropathol. Exp. Neurol. *53*, 429–437.

Saunders, A. M., Strittmatter, W. J., Schmechel, D., St George-Hyslop, P. H., Pericak-Vance, M. A., Joo, S. H., Rosi, B. L., Gusella, J. F., Crapper-MacLachlan, D. R., Alberts, M. J., Hulette, C., Crain, B., Goldgaber, D., and Roses, A. D. (1993). Association of apolipoprotein E allele ε4 with late-onset familial and sporadic Alzheimer's disease. Neurology *43*, 1467–1472.

Strittmatter, W. J., Saunders, A. M., Goedert, M., Weisgraber, K. H., Dong, L.-M., Jakes, R., Huang, D. Y., Pericak-Vance, M., Schmechel, D., and Roses, A. D. (1994). Isoform-specific interactions of apolipoprotein E with microtubule-associated protein tau: Implications for Alzheimer disease. Proc. Natl. Acad. Sci. USA *91,* 11183–11186.

Weisgraber, K. H. (1994). Apolipoprotein E: Structure–function relationships. Adv. Protein Chem. *45,* 249–302.

Yanagishita, M. (1992). Glycosylphosphatidylinositol-anchored and core protein-intercalated heparan sulfate proteoglycans in rat ovarian granulosa cells have distinct secretory, endocytotic, and intracellular degradative pathways. J. Biol. Chem. *267,* 9505–9511.

Zannis, V. I. and Breslow, J. L. (1981). Human very low density lipoprotein apolipoprotein E isoprotein polymorphism is explained by genetic variation and posttranslational modification. Biochemistry *20,* 1033–1041.

5

APP, ApoE, AND PRESENILIN TRANSGENICS

Toward a Genetic Model of Alzheimer's Disease

L. Pradier, C. Czech, L. Mercken, S. Moussaoui, M. Reibaud, P. Delaère, and
G. Tremp

Rhône-Poulenc Rorer
Centre de Recherches de Vitry-Alfortville
94400 Vitry, France

INTRODUCTION

Both environmental and genetic factors are involved in Alzheimer's Disease (AD) aetiology. Mutations in the amyloid precursor protein (APP) and in presenilin PS1 and PS2 genes cause early-onset forms of the disease while the apolipoprotein ApoEε4 allele is a risk factor for AD (reviewed in Selkoe, 1996; Hardy, 1997). Environmental factors such as trauma and inflammation have also been implicated in the pathology but the overall mechanism of the disease is poorly understood, hampering the development of therapeutic treatments. An animal model of the disease would be of great interest to both unravel the pathophysiological mechanism *in vivo* and to provide a model for testing of therapeutic approaches. Recently, large overexpression of mutated forms of APP in two transgenic mouse models has been shown to lead to amyloid plaque formation and behavioral deficits (Games et al., 1995; Hsiao et al., 1996). However, mutations in APP and PS's proteins have also been recently shown to contribute to a similar pathological process, the increase in production of the long form of Aβ (Aβ1–42, Selkoe, 1996, Duff e$Xal., 1996; Borchelt et al., 1996), possibly through a direct physical interaction (Weidemann et al, 1997). Therefore, rather than large overexpression, transgenic models based on a combination of the known genetic factors expressed at more physiological levels could potentially lead to a more suitable model of the disease. Towards that goal, we have generated several human mutant APP, and PS's transgenic rodent lines and combined them by breeding both together and with ApoE-KO animals.

APP TRANSGENICS

Several mutant and truncated forms of APP have been expressed in transgenic mice under the control of a modified HMG-CoA reductase promoter. Of special interest is the

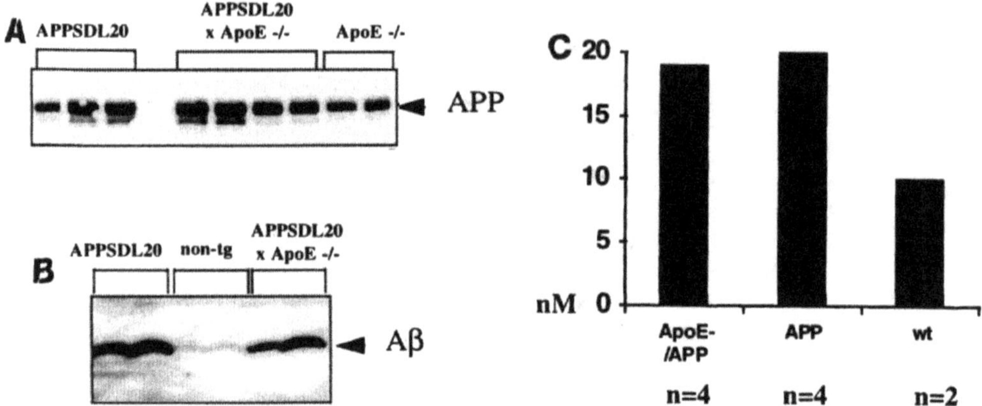

Figure 1. Expression and processing of APP in the brain of APPSDL20 and ApoE–/– mice. Brain homogenates were analyzed by western blot for (A) total APP expression using the 22C11 antibody, (B) Aβ production after immunoprecipitation with a polyclonal Aβ antibody. (C) Aβ levels were quantified by RIA using the Peninsula laboratory kit as directed.

mutant APP line bearing three mutations (Swedish, Dutch and London) on the same human APP 695 cDNA (line APPSDL20, Czech et al., 1997). The expression levels of the transgene are moderate with total APP representing 1.3–1.5 times APP levels in litter-mate controls (Fig.1A), starting early in embryogenesis. The expression of hAPP was demonstrated by immunohistochemistry to be essentially neuronal with a broad distribution in the brain. Aβ peptide and APP amyloidogenic C-terminal fragments could be clearly detected in these animals (Fig. 1B, lane APPSDL20), but without formation of amyloid plaques even at 12–16 months of age (Czech et al., 1997).

To analyze behavioral performances in the Morris water maze, the APPSDL20 line was transferred onto a C57Bl6 genetic background by 3 rounds of backcrossing with C57Bl6 mice. This genetic background is the most suitable for the water maze analysis. At both 3 and 12 months of age, the transgenic animals displayed learning capacities identical to litter mate controls both in the acquisition (7-day training) and in the retention (probe test with platform removed) phases (M.R., in preparation). In the probe test, treatments with amnesic agents, scopolamine (1 mg/kg i.p., 1h before test) or MK801 (0.125 mg/kg i.p., 1h before test), induced a total loss of retention in control animals. However, transgenic animals were totally insensitive to these treatments, preferentially spending time in the correct quadrant (where the platform was previously located) with no difference as compared to untreated transgenic or control animals (Fig. 2). Interestingly, the APPSDL20 were also less sensitive to systemic injections of lethal doses of NMDA (data not shown). Since APPSDL20 display lesser sensitivity to both NMDA antagonist and agonist, it is conceivable that the NMDA component of the glutamatergic pathways has been selectively decreased during embryogenesis. These observations can be linked to the known increased sensitivity to NMDA of neurons treated with low doses of Aβ (Mattson and Rydel, 1992) since the APPSDL20 animals produce Aβ early in embryogenesis. Additionally, a similar decreased sensitivity to NMDA agents has recently been reported in another APP transgenic model (Moechards et al., 1996) displaying apoptosis in the CNS.

The behavioral phenotype of the APPSDL20 is somewhat counterintuitive since a straight loss of mnesis capacities would have been expected. However, Aβ-induced glutamate toxicity occuring early on in embryogenesis could lead to compensatory mechanisms

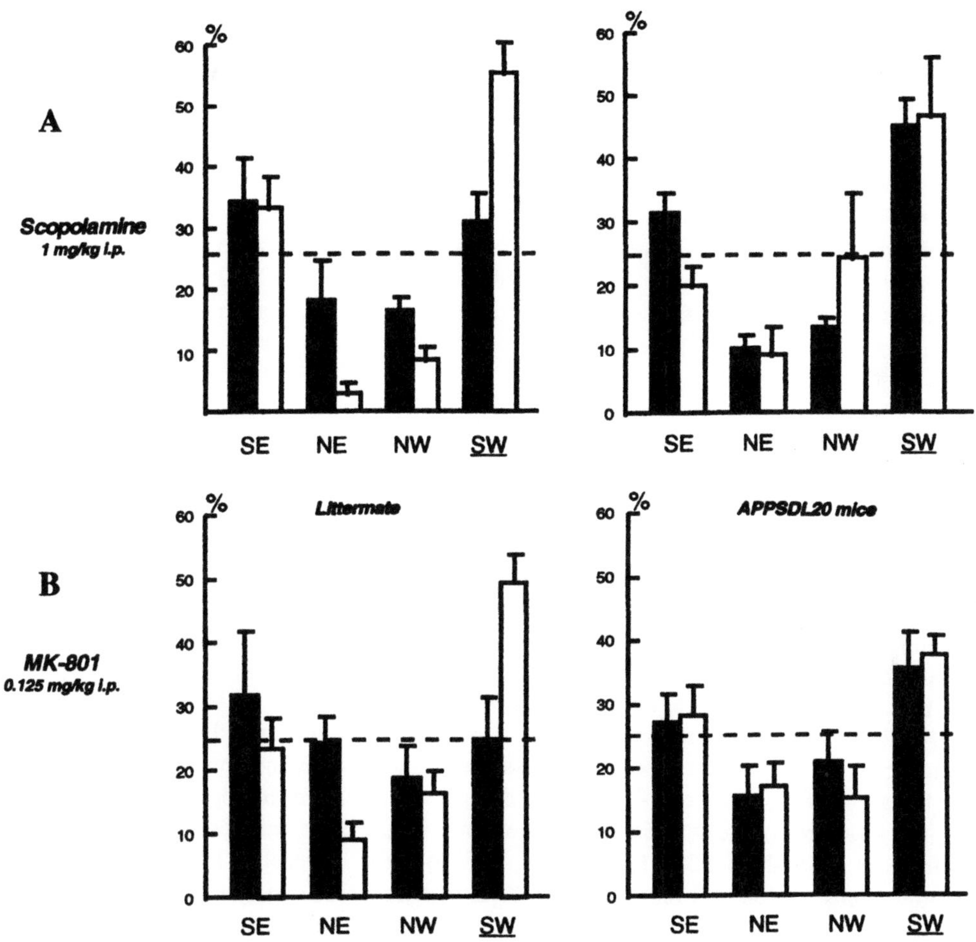

Figure 2. Decreased sensitivity to amnesic treatments in APPSDL20 mice. After 7 days of training, mice (n = 6) were subjected to a probe test. The platform was removed from its former SW location and the percentage of time spent in each quadrant was measured. Mice were treated (closed bars) or not (open bars) one hour before test. Note the sharp decrease of time spent in the SW quadrant for treated litter mate controls but not the treated APPSDL20 mice.

leading to replacement by non-NMDA type of receptors and normal behavior and we are currently testing this hypothesis.

Although the APPSDL20 mice do not present an obvious AD-like pathology, they provide us with a valuable tool to measure Aβ levels *in vivo* (and APP processing in general) and present a slight behavioral deficit which might reflect some aspects of Aβ toxicity in vivo.

APP AND ApoE-KO DOUBLE TRANSGENICS

The molecular mechanism underlying the ApoE4 involvement in AD pathology has not been elucidated yet although an increase in Aβ load in ε4 carrier would suggest an interaction with Aβ production. Some authors have demonstrated that ApoE levels in the brain of ε4 carriers are decreased, suggesting a loss of function (Poirier, 1994), whereas a gain of function for ApoE4 is also conceivable. To test the loss of function hypothesis, we transferred the APPSDL20 transgenics on an ApoE-KO genetic background by breeding and analyzed APP processing and Aβ production. At 6 month of age, the double transgenics showed neither modification of APP nor elevation of Aβ levels both in Western blot analysis (Fig. 1b) and by RIA assay (Fig. 1c). This result would indicate that ApoE does not participate in the clearance mechanism or homeostasis of Aβ in the rodent brain unless compensatory mechanisms have been elicited in the ApoE-KO. Our results would rather point towards a gain of function of ApoE4 and human ApoE4 transgenic mice would be of great interest.

PRESENILIN TRANSGENICS

In accordance with our overall strategy of combining the different genetic factors of AD, wild-type PS1 transgenic mice and rats and mutated PS1 mice have also been generated. Different lines have been studied displaying various levels of expression in the brain. In vivo, PS1 is essentially present as a 30 kD N-terminal (Fig. 3, lane: non transgenic) and 19–20 kDa C-terminal proteolytic fragments as previously described (Thinakaran et al., 1996). On high resolution SDS-PAGE, the N-ter fragment migrate as a doublet. A similar cleavage occurs for the transgenic human PS1 with, however, slightly different molecular weights which makes it possible to distinguish between transgenic and endogenous mouse PS1 (data not shown). In the low expressing transgenic lines only fragments of hPS1 can be detected whereas in the high expressing transgenic lines (approximately 5 times endogeneous levels), the full length PS1 protein is detectable at around 44 kDa (Fig. 3, from left to right increasing levels of expression with appearance of the full length PS1 with high expression) suggesting that PS1 cleavage processes are saturated. A similar processing of PS1 and its saturation was also observed in our different lines of PS1 wt transgenic rats. The FAD mutation M146 L does not seem to affect this proteolytic cleavage neither qualitatively nor quantitatively (data not shown). Transgenic PS1 protein is detectable in various brain regions like cortex, cerebellum, striatum, and hippocampus. No pathology has been detected in 12-month-old animals.

To study the effects of PS1 overexpression on human APP processing, we crossed one transgenic mouse line expressing high amounts of PS1wt and of PS1M146L with the APPSDL20 mice. Since the same promoter has been used for the two types of transgenics, it is probable that the same neurones will express both transgenes simultaneously in the double transgenics. Processing of PS1 is not modified in double transgenic mice (Fig. 3, lane 5). Conversely, the hAPP and the APP C-terminal fragment (12 kDa) levels in the double transgenic are comparable to APPSDL 20 mice alone. Regarding total Aβ levels, we have observed a high interindividual variability in double transgenics with both wt and mutant PS1 which was not apparent in the parental APPSDL20 line. We are currently testing a larger set of animals at different ages for total Aβ as well as more specific Aβ1–40 and Aβ1–42 levels as selective increase of the latter has been shown with mutant PS1 (Duff et al., 1996; Borchelt et al., 1996). Pathological and behavioral characterization of these lines, especially of aged animals, is under progress. In parallel, PS2 wt and mutant transgenic animals are under analysis.

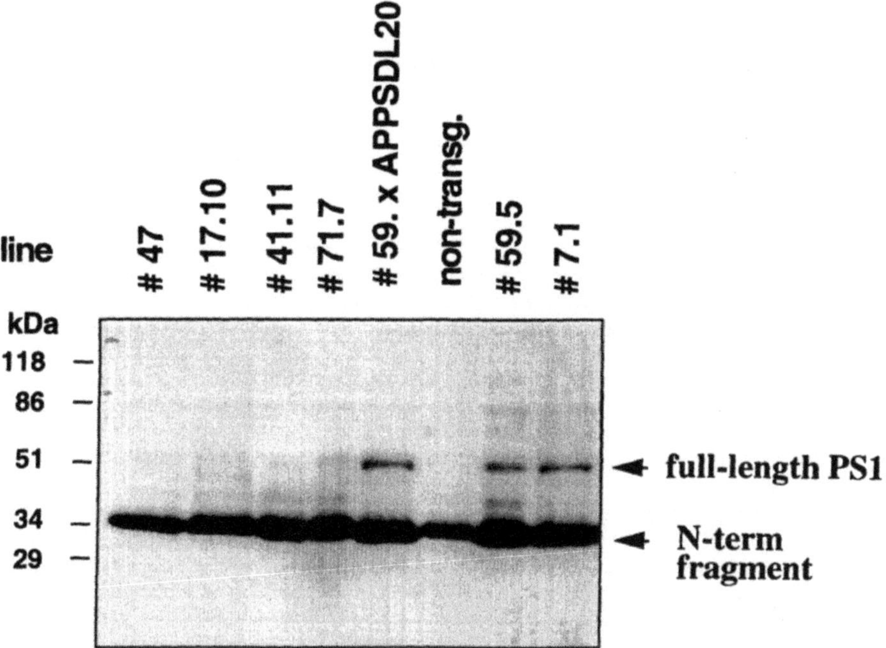

Figure 3. Expression levels of PS1 in transgenic mice. Brain homogenates of several lines PS1 transgenic mice were analyzed in Western blot using an antibody (93/23, generous gift from C. Masters) directed against the N-term of PS1.

CONCLUSION

We have generated transgenic animals for most of the different genetic factors of AD. By breeding, combination of these factors at levels which individually do not induce a pathology, could potentially lead to new animal models of AD. Such models would offer the opportunity to reanalyze each of the mono-transgenics to detect some of the early signs of the pathology and to unravel the functional interactions between the different factors. Additional external stress factors like trauma or lesions could further contribute to the development of an AD-like pathology. The development of such animal models of AD would provide key elements for the understanding of the pathophysiological mechanisms and the development of new therapeutic approaches.

ACKNOWLEDGMENTS

We are grateful to Drs. Colin Masters (Melbourne) and Akihiko Takashima (Tokyo) for providing us with PS1 antibodies.

REFERENCES

Borchelt, D.R., Thinakaran, G., Eckman, C., Lee, M.K., Davenport, F., Ratovitsky, T., Prada, C.-M., Kim, G., Seekins, S., Yager, D., Slunt, H.H., Wang, R., Seeger, M., Levey, A.I., Gandy, S.E., Copeland, N.G., Jenkins, N., Price, D.L., Younkin, S.G. and S. Sisodia, 1996, Familial Alzheimer's disease-linked presenilin 1 variants elevate Aβ1–42/1–40 ratio in vitro and in vivo. *Neuron* 17:005–1013.

Czech, C., Delaère, P., Macq, A.-F., Reibaud, M., Dreisler, S., Touchet, N. , Schombert, B., Mazadier, M., Mercken, L., Theisen, M., Pradier, L., Octave, J.-N., Beyreuther, K. and G. Tremp, 1997, Proteolytical processing of mutated human amyloid precursor protein in transgenic mice. *Mol. Brain Res.* 47:108–116

Duff, K., Eckman, C., Zehr, C., Yu, X., Prada, C.-M., Perez-tur, J., Hutton, M., Buee, L; Harigaya, Y., Yager, D., Morgan, D., Gordon, M.N., Holcomb, L., Refolo, L., Zenk, B., Hardy, J. and S. Younkin, 1996, Increased amyloid-β42(43) in brains of mice expressing mutant presenilin1. *Nature* 383:710–713.

Games, D., Adams, D., Alessandrini, R., Barbour, R., Berthelette, P., Blackwell, C., Carr, T., Clemens, J., Donaldson, T., Gillespie, F. et al., 1995, Alzheimer-type neuropathology in transgenic mice overexpressing V717F beta-amyloid precursor protein, *Nature* 373:523–527.

Hardy, J., 1997, Amyloid, the presenilins and Alzheimer's disease. *Trends in Neurosci.* 20 154–159.

Hsiao, K., Chapman, P., Nilsen, S., Eckman, C., Harigaya, Y., Younkin, S., Yang, F. and G. Cole, 1996, Correlative memory deficits, Aβ elevation and amyloid plaques in transgenic mice. *Science* 274:99–102.

Mattson, M.P. and Rydel, R.E., 1992, β-amyloid precursor protein and Alzheimer's disease: the peptide plot thickens. *Neurobiol. Aging* 13:617–621.

Moechars, D., Lorent, K., De Strooper, B., Dewachter, I. and Van Leuven, F., 1996, Expression in brain of amyloid precursor protein mutated in the α-secretase site causes disturbed behavior, neuronal degeneration and premature death in transgenic mice. *EMBO J.* 15:1265–1274.

Poirier, J., 1994, Apolipoprotein E in animal models of CNS injury and in Alzheimer's disease. *Trends in Neurosci.* 17: 525–530.

Selkoe, D.J., 1996, Amyloid β-protein and the genetics of Alzheimer's disease. *J. Biol. Chem.* 271: 18295–18298.

Thinakaran, G., Borchelt, D.R., Lee, M.K., Slunt, H.H., Spitzer, L., Kim, G., Ratovitsky, T., Davenport, F., Nordstedt, C., Seeger, M., Hardy, J., Levey, A.I., Gandy, S.E., Jenkins, N.A., Copeland, N.G., Price, D.L. and S. Sisodia ,1996, Endoproteolysis of presenilin1 and accumulation of processed derivatives in vivo. *Neuron* 17:181–190.

Weidemann, A., Paliga, K., Dürrwang, U., Czech, C., Evin, G., Masters, C.L. and Beyreuther, K., 1997, Formation of stable complexes between the two Alzheimer's disease gene products: presenilin-2 and β-amyloid precursor protein, *Nature Med.* 3:328–332.

6

DIFFERENTIAL SUSCEPTIBILITY OF HUMAN APOLIPOPROTEIN E ISOFORMS TO OXIDATION AND CONSEQUENCES ON THEIR INTERACTION WITH PHOSPHOLIPIDS

Corinne Jolivalt, Brigitte Leininger-Muller, Philippe Bertrand, and
Gérard Siest

Centre du Médicament
University Henri Pioncaré Nancy I
30 rue Lionnois, 54000 Nancy, France

INTRODUCTION

According to current hypotheses, neurodegenerative pathologies could be due to an increase of free radicals production in the brain and/or to a deficit in protective enzymatic mechanisms, physiologically lower in the brain than in the liver (Minn et al.,1991). In fact, cerebral oxidative processes seem to increase in normal aging, and even more in pathological aging such as Alzheimer's disease (AD) (Volicer et al., 1990, Mattson, 1995, Smith et al., 1995). AD is also accompanied by a loss of brain cholesterol and phospholipids (PL) (Wurtman, 1992). Among the protein accumulating in the brain amyloid deposits characteristic of this disease, amyloid-β (Aβ) and apolipoprotein E (apo E) are largely studied. The Apo E gene presents a polymorphism defining the 3 major isoforms E2, E3, E4. The $\varepsilon4$ allele has widely been shown to be a risk factor, while $\varepsilon2$ allele seems to be a protective factor, for AD (reviewed by Siest et al., 1995). The major function described for apo E is the transport and the redistribution of cholesterol and PL among cells. In addition, apo E plays a central role in nerve regeneration (Mahley, 1988) and synaptic plasticity (Poirier, 1994). Apo E is a major apolipoprotein present in the brain and can constitute a potential target to oxidation in the brain, as is the case for the major circulating apolipoprotein apo B (Lecomte et al., 1993). Oxidation of apo E could impair its function, thus contributing to biological features of pathological cerebral aging, as an early neuronal density decrease (Gomez-Isla et al., 1996).

Moreover, the increase of the $\varepsilon4$ allele frequency in AD points to the question of the differential implication of the 3 apo E isoforms. While apo E could be a pathological chaperone favoring the fibrillogenesis of Aβ (Wisniewski et al., 1992), the oxidation of apo E was proposed to favor the interaction between apo E and Aβ (Strittmatter et al., 1993). The aim of this work was to study the oxidation of the 3 apo E isoforms in presence of free radicals or chloramines produced by the action of neutrophils-secreted myeloperoxidase (MPO), an oxidative enzyme also present in the brain (Jolivalt et al., 1996). Furthermore, most studies to date were performed with lipid-free apo E while most of the physiologically relevant apo E is complexed to lipids as to form high density lipoproteins (HDL)-like particles in cerebrospinal fluid. We thus examined the consequences of apo E oxidation on its interaction with PL, and compared PL-free and PL-bound apo E oxidation.

MATERIALS AND METHODS

The 3 isoforms of recombinant human apo E (E2, E3, E4) cDNAs were cloned in modified pARHS-2 and produced in *E. Coli* BL21(DE3) as a fusion protein of about 44 kDa. This 44 kDa apo E results from the fusion of apo E and a peptide containing a polyhistidine sequence, which allows the recombinant proteins to be purified by single-step affinity chromatography on nickel gel (Barbier et al., 1997).

In vitro oxidation assays with MPO, isolated from polymorphonuclear neutrophils, were performed as previously described (Jolivalt et al., 1996), with slight modifications of pH adapted to the formation of apo E/PL discoidal complexes. Chloramines were formed by the reaction of MPO in 55 mM phosphate buffer (pH 4.5), 100 mM NaCl and 10 mM leucine with different concentrations of H_2O_2 (0;1.25; 4; 5.75; 7.6 mM). Then, native apo E was oxidized by these chloramines at physiological pH (pH 7.4). Proteins were submitted to SDS-PAGE in non-reducing conditions and tranferred to PVDF (Millipore) membranes.

The protein carbonyl content was measured by forming labelled protein hydrazone derivatives using 2,4-dinitrophenyl hydrazine (DNPH) (Keller et al., 1993). The dinitrophenyl moities formed on apo E were revealed by enhanced chemiluminescence (ECL, Pierce) after blot incubation with rabbit anti-DNP antibodies (Sigma) followed by incubation with HRP-labelled anti-rabbit antibodies (Sigma). After stripping, western blots were incubated with monoclonal anti-apo E antibodies (kind gift from Dr. Y. Marcel, Canada) followed by incubation with secondary anti-mouse antibodies labelled with HRP (Sigma), and then revealed by ECL.

Discoidal complexes were made by a detergent reconstitution method adapted from Jonas (1984). The PL, dipalmitoyl phosphatidylcholine (DPPC), was dispersed in sodium cholate and incubated with apo E in a 3/1 (w/w) ratio of PL/protein. The spontaneously formed apo E/PL discs were isolated from cholate by adsorption on Bio Beads (Biorad). Lipoproteic complexes were separated from free apo E and PL by gel filtration, and concentrated by centrifugation on Centriplus 100 (Amicon). DPPC complexes formed were detected at 280 nm. Apo E and DPPC contents of the resulting protein/PL complexes were estimated, respectively, by absorbance measurement at 280 nm and by PL measurement using a colorimetric assay (Boehringer Mannheim).

RESULTS

The oxidation based on MPO activity was initially established at pH 4.5, the optimal pH of the enzyme in neutrophils (Jolivalt et al., 1996). We then slighty modified experi-

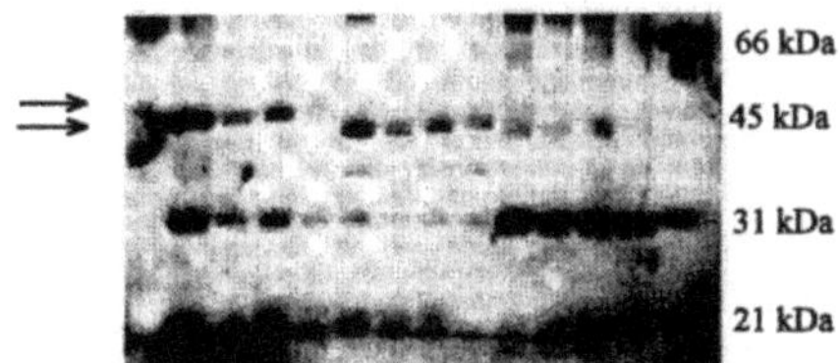

Figure 1. Immunoblotting analysis of the 3 isoforms of apo E after oxidation at pH 7.4, using anti-DNP antibodies. Line 1: apo E4; line 2: apo E4 +MPO; line 3: apo E4 + MPO + 0.025 mM H_2O_2; line 4: apo E4 + MPO +.5 mM H_2O_2; line 5: apo E3; line 6: apo E3 +MPO; line 7: apo E3 + MPO + 0.025 mM H_2O_2; line 8: apo E3 + MPO + 0.5 mM H_2O_2; line 9: apo E2; line 10: apo E2 +MPO; line 11: apo E2 + MPO + 0.025 mM H_2O_2; line 12: apo E2 + MPO + 0.5 mM H_2O_2; line 13: molecular weight ladder. Arrows indicate specific apo E material.

mental conditions to allow protein oxidation at pH 7.4 by using the formation of chloramines (Zcliczynski et al., 1993). At pH 4.5, SDS-PAGE analysis revealed that the apo E-specific band migrated with a higher apparent molecular weight (MW) with simultaneous formation of high molecular weight polymerization products (60 kDa and higher) (not shown). At pH 7.4, the apo E-specific band mainly exhibited a shift in MW (Figure 1). These shifts were visualized for the 3 apo E isoforms, and are differential according to the apo E isoforms. The difference observed between the main apo E band before and after oxidation is more important for apo E4 than apo E3 than apo E2 (Table 1).

The capacity of apo E isoforms to interact with DPPC was evaluated through the elution profiles of apo E/DPPC complexes. Material eluted in fractions 2 to 10 represent apo E/DPPC complexes, while fractions eluting after fraction 10 correspond to free apo E (Figure 2). All 3 native apo E isoforms form heterogeneous complexes with similar efficiency (about 65%). In contrast, oxidized apo E isoforms exhibit a differential decrease in their ability to interact with DPPC. Actually, yields of oxidized apo E complexed to DPPC are 0, 17 and 33% for apo E4, apo E3 and apo E2 complexes, respectively.

Thus, oxidation of apo E makes the protein greatly lose its ability to interact with PL. Such decrease in apo E interaction with PL led us to check for apo E oxidative profile by oxidizing apo E/PL complexes. Figure 3 illustrates that oxidation of apo E in DPPC discs gives rise to apo E alterations different from those observed with lipid-free apo E.

Table 1. Apparent molecular weight of the major band of the 3 isoforms of apo E after oxidation at pH 7.4

	Major apo E band (kDa)	MW shift (%)
E4	46	
ox 0.025 mM	47.3	+ 2.8
ox 0.5 mM	49.1	+ 6.7
E3	44.7	
ox 0.025 mM	45.7	+ 2.2
ox 0.5 mM	46.2	+ 3.3
E2	45.2	
ox 0.025 mM	45.2	+ 0
ox 0.5 mM	45.7	+ 1.1

These values are obtained by scanning autoradiogram shown in Figure 1, using a Biomax software (Kodak). Similar results were obtained when comparing apo E isoforms oxidized at pH 4.5.

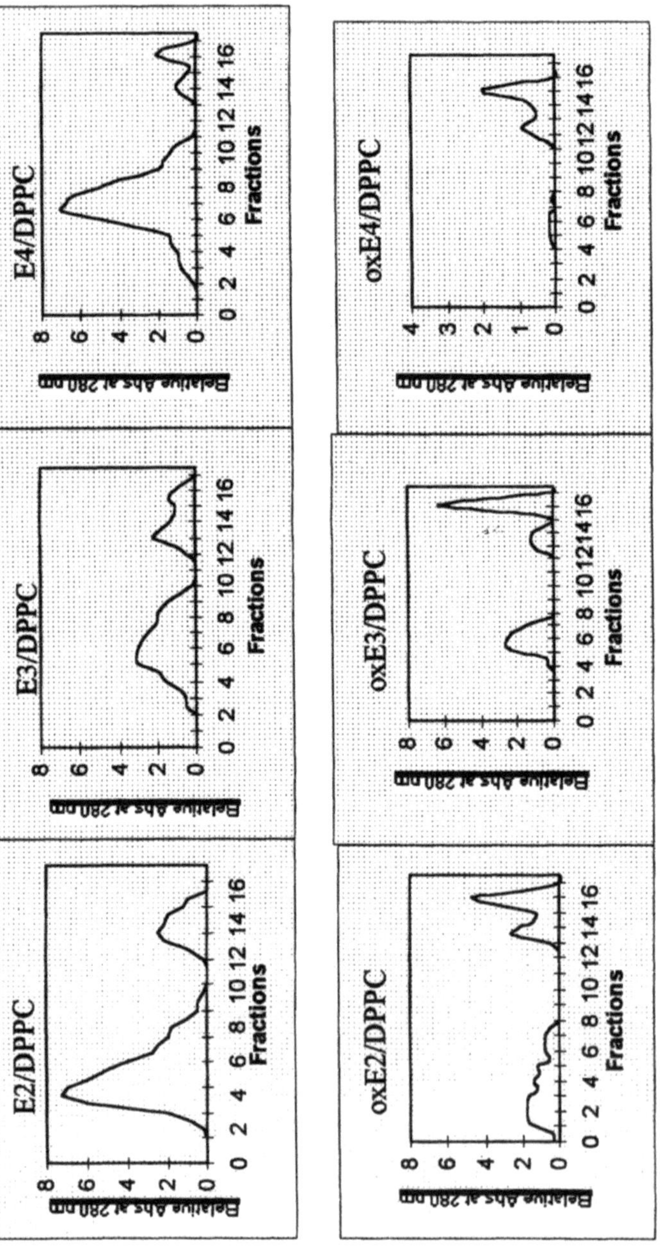

Figure 2. Elution profiles of apo E and oxidized apo E complexes on gel filtration. Apo E/DPPC complexes were separated from free apo E by gel filtration on Sephacryl HR300. The flow rate was 30 ml/h and 1.5 ml fractions were collected.

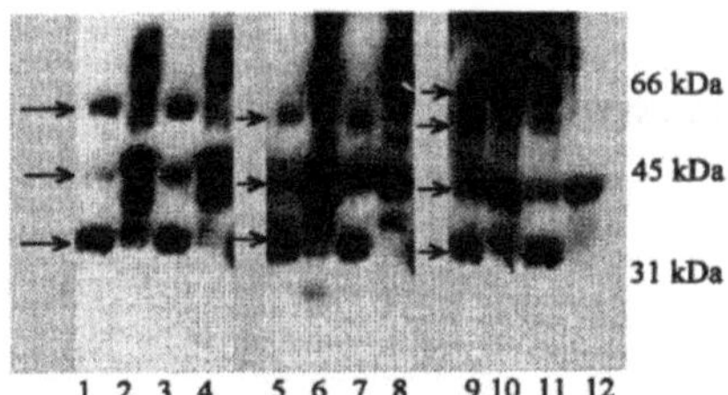

Figure 3. Immunoblotting analysis of oxidized lipid-bound apo E isoforms, after oxidation at pH 7.4, using anti-apo E antibodies. Line 1: apo E4/DPPC + MPO + 0.025 mM H_2O_2; line 2: apo E4 +MPO + 0.025 mM H_2O_2; line 3: apo E4/DPPC + MPO + 0.5 mM H_2O_2; line 4: apo E4 + MPO +0.5 mM H_2O_2; line 5: apo E3/DPPC + MPO + 0.025 mM H_2O_2; line 6: apo E3 + MPO + 0.025 mM H_2O_2; line 7: apo E3/DPPC + MPO + 0.5 mM H_2O_2; line 8: apo E3 + MPO + 0.5 mM H_2O_2; line 9: apo E2/DPPC + MPO + 0.025 mM H_2O_2; line 10: apo E2 + MPO + 0.025 mM H_2O_2; line 11: apo E2/DPPC + MPO + 0.5 mM H_2O_2; line 12: apo E2 + MPO + 0.5 mM H_2O_2. Numbers on the right indicate position of molecular weight. Arrows indicate specific apo E material.

Namely, the apo E band is shifted in both cases towards higher MW, but oxidation of apoE/PL results in the appearance of bands at about 30 and 60 kDa, while oxidation of native apo E results in the appearance of a high MW smear probably reflecting aggregated material. In addition, most of the initial apo E specific band (see Figure 1) is lightly revealed to the benefit of both the ≈30 and ≈60 kDa bands, and the patterns resulting from oxidation of apo E2 in DPPC discs is different from those observed for apo E3 and E4. No bands of MW below 30 kDa were observed.

DISCUSSION

Apo E4 is associated with AD (Siest et al., 1995). Moreover, oxidative process are increased in AD whose apo E could be a target (Montine et al., 1996). The apo E allele specificity linked to pathological aging points to the differential susceptibility of apo E to oxidation. Indeed, apo E4 is more oxidized than apo E3, itself more than apo E2. This differential oxidation is characterized by a differential mobility in SDS-PAGE. Oxidation may modify amino acid residues, which in turn modify the function and/or the protein structure. The amino acid residues the more susceptible to oxidation are cystein, methionine, tryptophane, proline, lysine, histidine, tyrosine, in a decreasing order. As shown by Anantharamaiah et al. (1988) through a combination of reverse-phase high performance liquid chromatography (RP-HPLC) and cyanogen bromide cleavage, oxidation of apo AI methionine alters the secondary structure of the protein. By RP-HPLC, we confirmed the apo E structural modification by the decrease of the retention time of apo E after oxidation (data not shown). Moreover, Heinecke et al. (1993) showed crosslinking of protein after oxidation by MPO, through formation of bityrosine. Oxidative modification of apo E can lead to polymerization products at pH 4.5, a condition of oxidation stronger than at pH 7.4 (Jolivalt et al., 1996). The difference between the 3 apo E isoforms could be due to a difference in their structure, by differentially exposing oxidable amino acids residues. It is known that discrete amino acid residues may mediate isoform-specific conformational changes which alter apo E interaction with lipids and receptors (Weisgraber, 1994, Dong et al., 1996). Furthermore, the differential susceptibility of apo E isoforms to oxidation may be related to their primary structure as they differ in their cysteine content: cysteine residues may act as antioxidants, and apo E4 is Arg112-Arg158, apo E3 is Arg112-

Cys158, and apo E2 is Cys112-Cys158. In addition, methionine residues were recently proposed to also act as internal antioxidants in proteins (Levine et al., 1996). Depending on the exposure of the methionine residues (8 in apo E), we might expect a differential capacity of apo E isoforms to resist to reactive species attack. Cyanogen bromide cleavage experiments are in progress to precise the impact of methionine residues in apo E oxydation. Such properties could correlate with the differential antioxidant properties of apo E isoforms (Miyata et al., 1996).

It is likely that oxidation linked modifications in apo E conformation alters its capacity to interact with PL and other components. To test this hypothesis, we prepared complexes of oxidized apo E and DPPC for the 3 apo E isoforms. Oxidation of apo E before its incorporation in DPPC discs leads to the decrease of its binding to PL. This results are in agreement with those obtained by Anantharamaiah et al. (1988), showing that apo AI affinity for DMPC is reduced after oxidation. In addition, the 3 apo E isoforms show a differential decrease in their interaction with DPPC after oxidation. More the apo E isoform is susceptible to oxidation, greater is its loss in DPPC binding ability after oxidation. Indeed, oxidized apo E4 becomes unable to form apo E/DPPC complexes after oxidation.

Furthermore, we obtained preliminary evidence showing that oxidation of apo E isoforms does not modify their effect on Aβ fibrillogenesis (data not shown). Other functional implications of apo E oxidation must be sought at the level of the antioxidant properties of apo E. Apo E decreases Aβ neurotoxicity in an isoform-dependent manner (Miyata et al., 1996), presumably by counterbalancing Aβ-generated reactive species (Miyata et al., 1996, Behl et al., 1994). Apo E isoforms active as antioxidants are thus logically targets of reactive species, with apo E4 presenting the greater susceptibility to oxidation, and the lowest antioxidant ability. Taken altogether, these observations reinforce the link between apo E4 and AD, and could correlate with the loss of brain PL in AD, due to the loss of the PL recycling activity of apo E4, and with the increased levels of crosslinking of apo E with products of lipid peroxydation in apo E4-AD brains (Miyata et al., 1996).

Apo E inclusion in DPPC discs modifies its conformation, which could lead to expose oxidation-susceptible amino acid residues in a pattern distinct than those exposed in lipid-free apo E. Effectively, apo E included in DPPC discs is differently altered by oxidation than lipid-free apo E. Oxidation at pH 7.4 was usually not accompanied by the appearance of aggregated material of high MW. This phenomenon was consistently observed at pH 4.5 (Jolivalt et al., 1996), and was minor in some experiments at pH 7.4 (Figure 3). Although we can not exclude that the aggregated material is secondary to the initial fragmentation of apo E, the evidence for the generation of apo E fragments upon oxidation is clearly illustrated by the oxidation pattern of DPPC-bound apo E. Most importantly, these results indicate that PL-bound apo E is more prone to fragmentation upon oxidation, with apo E2 generating additional bands as compared with the two other isoforms (Figure 2). The precise identity of the 30 and 60 kDa bands observed after oxidation of apo E/DPPC complexes remains to be elucidated. As we could not detect any apo E fragments with a size below 30 kDa, whether using monoclonal (Figure 3) or polyclonal (data not shown) antibodies, we speculate that the 30 kDa band might correspond to the N-terminal domain of apo E, while the 60 kDa band might correspond to the aggregated C-terminal domain of the protein. If true, such fragmentation pattern of physiological apo E-containing lipoproteins might be relevant of the neuropathology of AD, since C-terminal fragments were detected in senile plaques (Castano et al., 1995), and N-terminal fragments of the protein were shown to exhibit isoform-specific neurotoxicity (Marques et al., 1996).

CONCLUSION

The differential susceptibility to oxidation of the 3 apo E isoforms and its consequence on the ability of apo E to bind PL could explain at least part of apo E implication in AD. The apo E association with PL seems to be determinant, not only for binding to lipoproteins receptors and further PL recycling, but also for the generation of specific apo E fragments. Studies are required to further precise the link between apo E and oxidation on the one hand, and apo E- and Aβ-related neurotoxicity on the other hand.

ACKNOWLEDGMENT

This study was supported by a grant from Ipsen Foundation (Paris), PIR (Pôle Interuniversitaire Régionale, Recherche biologique médicale et santé) and the Région Lorraine. We thank A. Dergunov (Russia) for helpful discussion.

REFERENCES

Anantharamaiah, G.M., Hughes, T.A., Iqbal, M., Gawish, A., Neame, P.J., Medley, M.F., Segrest , J.P., 1988, Effect of oxidation on the properties of apolipoproteins AI and AII. *J. Lip. Res.* 29:309–318.

Barbier, A., Visvikis, A., Mathieu, F., Diez, L., Havekes, L., Siest, G., Characterization of three human apolipoprotein E isoforms (E2, E3 and E4) expressed in *Escherichia coli*.Eur. J. *Clin. Chem. Clin. Biochem.*, in press.

Behl, C., Davis, J.B., Lesley, R., Schubert, D., 1994, Hydrogen peroxyde mediates amyloid beta protein toxicity. *Cell,* 77:817–827.

Castano, E.M., Prelli, F., Wisniewski, T., Golabek, A., Kumar, R.A., Soto, C., Frangione, B., 1995, Fibrillegenesis in Alzheimer's disease of amyloid β peptides and apolipoprotein E. *Biochem. J.* 306:599–604.

Dong, L.-M., Parkin, S., Trakhanov, S.D., Rupp, B., Simmons, T., Arnold, K.S., Newhouse, Y.M., Innerarity, T.L., Weisgraber, K.H., 1996, Novel mechanism for defective receptor binding of apolipoprotein E2 in type III hyperlipoproteinemia. *Nature Struct. Biol.* 3:718–722.

Gomez-Isla, T., Price, J.L., McKeel, Jr., D.W., Morris, J.C., Growdon, J.H., Hyman, B.T., 1996, Profound loss of layer II entorhinal cortex neurons occurs in very mild Alzheimer's disease. *J. Neurosci.* 16:4491–4500.

Heinecke, J.W., Li, W., Francis, G.A., Golstein, J.A., 1993, Tyrosyl radical generated by myeloperoxidase catalyzes the oxidative cross-linking of proteins. *J. Clin. Invest.* 91:2866–2872.

Jolivalt, C., Leininger-Muller, B., Drozdz, R., Naskalski, J.W., Siest, G., 1996, Apolipoprotein E is highly susceptible to oxidation by myeloperoxidase, an enzyme present in the brain. *Neurosci. Lett.* 210:61–64

Jonas, A., 1984, A review of plasma apolipoprotein A-I interaction with phosphatidylcholines. *Exp. Lung Res.* 6:255–70.

Keller, R.J., Halmes, N.C., Hinson, J.A., Pumford, N.R., 1993, Immunochemical detection of oxidized proteins. *Chem. Res. Toxicol.* 6:430–33

Lecomte, E., Artur,Y., Chancerelle, Y., Herbeth, B., Galteau, M.-M., Jeandel, C., Siest, G., 1993, Malondialdehyde adducts to, and fragmentation of, apolipoprotein B from human plasma. *Clin. Chim. Acta* 218:39–46.

Levine, R.L., Mosoni, L., Berlett, B.S., Stadtman, E.R., 1996, Methionine residues as endogenous antioxidants in proteins. *Proc. Natl. Acad. Sci. (USA)* 93:15036–15040.

Mahley, R.W.,.1988, Apolipoprotein E : cholesterol transport protein with expanding role in cell biology. *Science* 240:622–630.

Marques, M., Tolar, M., Harmony, J.A.K., Crutcher, K.A., 1996, A thrombin cleavage fragment of apolipoprotein E exhibits isoform-specific neurotoxicity. *Neuroreport* 7:2529–2532.

Mattson, M.P., 1995, Free radical and disruption of neuronal ion homeostasis in AD: A role for amyloid β-peptide ? *Neurobiol. Aging,* 16:679–682.

Minn, A., Ghersi-Egea, J.-F., Perrin, R., Leininger, B., Siest, G., 1991, Drug metabolizing enzymes in the brain and cerebral microvessels. *Brain Res. Rev.* 16:65–82.

Miyata, M., Smith, J.D., 1996, Apolipoprotein E allele-specific antioxidant activity and effects on cytotoxicity by oxidative insults and β-amyloid peptides. *Nature Genet.* 14:55–61.

Montine,T.J., Huang, D.Y., Valentine, W.M., Amarnath, V., Saunders, A., Weisgraber, K.H., Graham, D.G., Strittmatter, W.J., 1996, Crosslinking of apolipoprotein E by products of lipid peroxidation. *J. Neuropathol. Exp. Neurol.* 55:202–210.

Montine, K.S., Olson, S.J., Amarnath, V., Whetsell, W.O., Graham, D.G., Montine, T.J., 1997, Immunohistochemical detection of 4-hydroxy-2-nonenal adducts in Alzheimer's disease is associated with inheritance of apo E4. *Am. J. Pathol.* 150:437–443.

Poirier, J., 1994, Apolipoprotein E in animal models of brain injury and in Alzheimer's disease. *Trends Neurosci.* 12:525–530.

Siest, G., Pillot, T., Régis-Bailly, A., Leininger-Muller, B., Steinmetz, J., Galteau, M.-M., Visvikis, S., 1995, Apolipoprotein E: An important gene and protein to follow in laboratory medicine. *Clin. Chem.* 41:1068–1086.

Smith, M.A., Sayre, L.M., Monnier, V.M., Perry, G., 1995, Radical AGEing in Alzheimer's disease. *Trends Neurosci.* 18:172–176.

Strittmatter, W.J., Saunders, A., Schmechel, D., Pericakvance, M., Englhild, J., Salvesen, O.S., Roses, A.D., 1993, Apolipoprotein E: High affinity binding β-amyloid and increased frequency of type 4 allele in late onset Alzheimer's disease. *Proc. Natl. Acad. Sci. (USA)* 90:1977–1981.

Volicer, L., Crino, P.B., 1990, Involvement of free radicals in dementia of the Alzheimer type: A hypothesis. *Neurobiol. Aging* 11:567–571.

Weisgraber, K.H., 1994, Apolipoprotein E: structure-function relationships. *Adv. Prot.Chem.* 45:249–302.

Wisniewski, T., Frangione, B., 1992, Apolipoprotein E: a pathological chaperone protein in patients with cerebral and systemic amyloid. *Neurosci. Lett.* 135:235–238.

Wurtman, R.J., 1992, Choline metabolism as a basis for the selective vulnerability of cholinergic neurons. *Trends Neurosci.* 15:117–122.

Zcliczynski, J.M., Stelmaszynska, T., Domanski, J., Ostrowski, W., 1971, Chloramines as intermediates of oxidation reaction of amino acids by myeloperoxidase. *Bioch. Biophys.Acta* 235:419–424.

7

THE APOLIPOPROTEIN E ε4 ALLELE

Association with Alzheimer's Disease and Depression in Elderly Patients

A. S. Rigaud,[1] L. Traykov,[2] L. Caputo,[2] J. de Rotrou,[1] F. Moulin,[1]
R. Couderc,[3] M. L. Seux,[1] M. B. Perol,[1] A. Le Divenah,[1] F. Latour,[1]
P. Bouchacourt,[1] F. Boller,[2] and F. Forette[1]

[1]Hôpital Broca
CHU Cochin Port-Royal
Université René Descartes, Paris V
54/56 rue Pascal, 75013 Paris, France
[2]INSERM Unité 324
[3]Hôpital Tenon
Paris, France

INTRODUCTION

The overlap between symptoms of depression and dementia in elderly patients has been well established. Depressed elderly patients often complain of poor memory. They may develop cognitive dysfunction which in some cases may be severe enough to meet the criteria for dementia. Some authors have suggested that depression in the elderly increases the risk of dementia. Alternatively, depression may be an early manifestation of dementia (Davanand et al., 1996).

A major task in this field is to identify distinct biologic features which could serve as markers and help to provide information about the underlying pathology. Recently, a great deal of interest has been generated in the status of the apolipoprotein E gene (ApoE) as a risk factor for Alzheimer's disease (AD). It appears that the ε4 allele is over-represented in patients with familial or sporadic AD relative to control subjects (Corder et al., 1993; Saunders et al., 1993). To gain insight into the relationship between depression and AD in late life, we compared the distribution of ApoE phenotypes and of ApoE allele frequencies in depression and in AD, in a sample of community dwelling elderly patients.

Progress in Alzheimer's and Parkinson's Diseases
edited by Fisher *et al.*, Plenum Press, New York, 1998.

PATIENTS AND METHODS

The study included 87 consecutively admitted outpatients attending a memory clinic in Paris. We selected patients who were 60 years or older and met the DSMIIIR criteria for either a current major depressive episode or dementia (APA, 1987). Demented patients had to fulfil the NINCDS/ARDRA criteria for AD (Mckhann et al., 1984). We excluded patients suffering from either AD with depressive symptoms or depression with severe cognitive impairment.

Cognitive status was evaluated by the Mini Mental Test (MMSE) (Folstein et al., 1975) and a battery of neuropsychologic screening tests known as the Cognitive Efficiency Profile (CEP) which has been shown to detect early impairment of cognitive functions (De Rotrou et al., 1991). Psychiatric diagnoses and previous history of depression were derived from the results of semi-structured inpatient evaluation supplemented by information from family members (usually the patient's spouse or child) or another caregiver. The intensity of depression was assessed by the Geriatric Depression Scale (GDS) (Yesavage and Brink, 1983) and a self-administered questionnaire for the self-evaluation of depressive symptoms in elderly patients (QD2A) (Pichot et al., 1984).

Patients underwent a complete physical and neurologic examination, laboratory tests (including blood count, creatinine, electrolytes, thyroid hormones, vitamin B12 and folates and TPHA assay). All the demented patients had brain computed tomography. Apolipoprotein E phenotyping was performed by an agarose isoelectric focusing immunoblot method (Bailleul et al., 1993). As this method has been used in large population studies, population estimates of APOE allele frequencies based on this method are available. ApoE typing was performed blindly in relation to clinical diagnosis.

We compared patients with AD or depression to aged-matched controls from a previous French study (Brousseau et al., 1994.). Characteristics and mean test scores of patients with AD and depression were compared by Student's t test. ApoE phenotype distributions and ApoE allele frequencies were respectively compared by Fisher's exact test and the chi square test.

RESULTS

AD was diagnosed in 53 patients, and depression in 34 (Table 1). The two groups did not differ significantly as regards age. Thirty-nine out of 53 patients in the AD group were women, and 19 out of 34 in the depressed group.

Cognitive functions were significantly more impaired in AD than in depressed patients as shown by MMSE (19 ± 5 versus 29 ± 1), and by CEP (25 ± 12 versus 73.1 ± 11.3, $p < 0.001$). The respective evaluations of depressive symptoms by a psychiatrist and a neuropsychologist were in close agreement. The severity of depressive symptoms was greater in depressed than in AD patients, as shown by GDS (16 ± 5 versus 7 ± 5), and by QD2R (8 ± 3 versus 4 ± 3, $p < 0.001$).

As shown in Table 2, there was no significant difference between the distribution of ApoE phenotypes in depressed and AD patients, but their distribution in each group differed significantly from that of the controls ($p = 0.005$ for depression and $p < 0.0001$ for AD).

ApoE $\varepsilon2$ allele frequency was significantly lower in AD patients than controls ($p = 0.0047$). ApoE $\varepsilon4$ allele frequencies in AD and depression were nearly four times higher than in the controls but were not significantly different from each other (Table 3).

Table 1. Characteristics of patients with
Alzheimer's disease (AD) and depression

	Subjects	Sex (F/M)	Age (mean ± SD)
Controls	38	33/5	80 ± 8.2
AD	53	39/14	79 ± 8
Depression	34	26/8	73.1 ± 7

Data for controls were derived from the French study by Brousseau *et al.* (1994).

DISCUSSION

The results of this study confirm previous reports of increased ApoE ε4 frequency and decreased ApoE ε2 allele frequency in AD patients compared to control subjects (Corder et al., 1993; Saunders et al., 1993). However, our principal findings suggest an association between the presence of the ApoE ε4 allele and the major depression that occurs late in life. A spurious increase in ApoE ε4 allele frequency in the subjects with depression, due to mistaken diagnosis, i.e. that they were suffering from AD with depression rather than primary major depression, seems unlikely, because we used a highly sensitive battery of neuropsychologic tests in a careful attempt to exclude from this study patients suffering from AD with depressive symptoms.

Several authors have proposed that depression late in life is a heterogeneous condition in which organic factors play a key role. Thus, an increasing number of changes in white brain matter were detected by both computerized tomography and magnetic resonance imaging in elderly patients with depression suggesting the importance of vascular factors in this pathology (Greenwald et al., 1996; Lesser et al., 1996; O'Brien et al., 1996). Some authors recently proposed that the particular form of vascular depression should be individualized (Alexopoulos et al., 1997; Krishnan et al., 1997). However, other neuroimagery and biochemical studies in elderly depressive subjects with cognitive impairment showed alterations in brain regional volume (Pearlson et al., 1989) and in platelet monoamine oxidase-specific activity (Alexopoulos et al., 1987) similar to those found in patients with AD. In follow-up studies, a substantial number of depressed elderly patients presenting with either mild cognitive impairment or disability were found to de-

Table 2. Comparative distributions of ApoE phenotypes in patients
with Alzheimer's disease (AD) or depression versus controls

Phenotype frequencies	Controls (n = 38)	AD (n = 53)	Depression (n = 34)
ε2/ε2	0.025	0	0
ε2/ε3	0.21	0.05	0.09
ε3/ε3	0.66	0.49	0.53
ε3/ε4	0.08	0.4	0.35
ε4/ε4	0	0.05	0.03
ε4/ε2	0.025	0	0

Controls vs AD: p < 0.0001*
AD vs Depression: NS
Controls vs Depression: p = 0.005*

Data for controls were derived from the French study by Brousseau *et al.* (1994).
*Fisher's exact test. NS = not significant.

Table 3. Comparison of ApoE allele frequencies in patients with
Alzheimer's disease (AD) or depression versus controls

Allele frequencies	Controls (n = 76)	AD (n = 106)	Depression (n = 68)
ε2	0.15	0.03	0.04
		p = 0.0047*	
ε3	0.8	0.72	0.75
ε4	0.05	0.25	0.21
		p = 0.0003*	
		p = 0.02*	

Data for controls were derived from the French study by Brousseau *et al.* (1994). *Chi square test.

velop primary dementia (Alexopoulos et al., 1997; Kivela et al., 1994; Reding et al., 1985). Furthermore, in community-residing elderly subjects without dementia, Davanand et al. (1996) showed that the presence of a depressed mood was associated with a moderate risk of dementia, which on follow-up was mostly proved to be AD. The present study lends support to this hypothesis.

An association between the ε4 allele and major depression in late life has already been shown by Krishnan et al. (1996). However, these authors did not compare the frequency of the ApoE ε4 in depressed and AD patients as we did in the present work. Zubenko et al. (1996) found that apoE ε4 allele frequency increased in depressed patients with psychotic symptoms but was not increased either in patients with cognitive impairment or in their depressed group. The depressed patients described by these authors were of the same age as ours (73 ± 8 and 73 ± 7 respectively), but unlike ours, included inpatients with severe major depression, mostly accompanied by psychotic features and previous depressive episodes. The patients in the present series were communitky-living and were undergoing a milder depressive episode—in most cases their first—than Zubenko et al.'s patients. One possible explanation for the divergent results of Zubenko's study and ours may be the difference between the depressed groups in each study and consequently the probable difference in the underlying pathology.

It is thus tempting to postulate that AD may be the underlying condition in a group of late-onset depressed patients such as the one considered here. Such late-onset depressive subjects may be in an early stage of some form of dementia that cannot be diagnosed at first, but manifests itself later. Although the trend was not significant, the mean age of our depressed subjects tended to be lower than that of the AD patients. Alternatively, we cannot rule out the hypothesis that the ApoE ε4 allele is a risk factor for AD in elderly subjects with depression. A prospective study in which those patients presenting with both depression and ApoE ε4 are followed up should help to clarify this issue.

REFERENCES

Alexopoulos, G.S., Young, R.C., Liberman, K.W., and Shamoian, C.A., 1987, Platelet MAO activity in geriatric patients with depression and dementia. *Am. J. Psychiatry* 144:1480–1483.

Alexopoulos, G.S., Meyers, B.S., Young, R.C., Mattis, S., and Kakuma, T., 1993, The course of geriatric depression with reversible dementia: a controlled study. *Am. J. Psychiatry* 150:1693–1699.

Alexopoulos, G.S., Meyers, B.S., Young, R.C., Kakuma, T., Silbersweig, D., and Charlson, M., 1997, Clinically defined vascular depression. *Am. J. Psychiatry* 154:562–565.

American Psychiatric Association Diagnostic and Statistical Manual of Mental Disorders, 1987, (third edition-revised, DSM IIIR), APA ed, Washington D.C.

Bailleul, S., Couderc, R., Landais, V., Lefèvre, G., Raichvarg, D., Etienne, J., 1993, Direct Phenotyping of human apolipoprotein E in plasma:Application to population frequency distribution in Paris (France). *Hum. Hered.* 43:159–165.

Brousseau, T., Legrain, S., Berr, C., Gourlet, V., Vidal, O., and Amouyel, P., 1994, Confirmation of the ε4 allele of the apolipoprotein E gene as a risk factor for late-onset Alzheimer's disease. *Neurology* 44: 342–344.

Corder, E.H., Saunders, A.M., Strittmatter, W.J., Schmechel, D.E., Gaskell, P.C., Small, G.W., Roses, A.D., and Pericak-Vance, M.A., 1993, Gene dose of apolipoprotein E Type 4 allele and the risk of Alzheimer's disease in late onset families. *Science* 261:921–923.

Davanand, D.P., Sano, M., Tang, M.X., Taylor, S., Gurland, B.J., Wilder, D., Stern, Y., Mayeux, R., 1996, Depressed mood and the incidence of Alzheimer's disease in the elderly living in the community. *Arch. Gen. Psychiatry* 53:175–182.

De Rotrou, J., Forette, F., Hervy, M.P., Tortra, D., Fermanian, J., Boudou, M.R., and Boller, F., 1991, The cognitive efficiency profile:description and validation in patients with Alzheimer disease. *Int. J. Geriatr. Psychiatr.* 6:501–509.

Folstein, M.F., Folstein, S.E., McHugh, P.R., 1975, "Mini-Mental Test". A practical method for grading the cognitive state of patients for the clinician. *J. Psychiatr. Res.* 12:189–198.

Greenwald, B.S., Kramer-Ginsberg, E., Krishnan, K.R.R., Ashtari, M., Aupperle, P.M., Patel, M., 1996, MRI Signal Hyperintensities in Geriatric Depression. *Am. J. Psychiatry* 153:1212–1215.

Kivela, S.L., Kongäs-Saviaro, P., Kesti, E., Pahkala, K., Laippala, P., 1994, Five-year prognosis for depression in old age. *Int. Psychogeriatr.* 6(1):69–78.

Krishnan, K.R.R., Tupler, L.A., Ritchie, J.C., McDonald, W.M., Knight, D.L., Nemeroff, C.B., Caroll, BJ., 1996, Apolipoprotein E-e4 frequency in Geriatric Depression. *Biol Psychiatry* 40:69–71

Krishnan, K.R.R., Hays, J.C., and Blazer, D.G., 1997, MRI-defined vascular depression. *Am. J. Psychiatry 154:497–501.*

Lesser, I.M., Boone, K.B., Mehringer, C.M., Wolh, M.A., Miller, B.L., and Berman, NG., 1996, Cognition and White Matter Hyperintensities in Older Depressed Patients. *Am. J. Psychiatry* 153:1280–1287.

Mckhann, G., Drachman, D., Folstein, M., Katzman, R., Price, D., Stadlan, E.M., 1984, Clinical diagnosis of Alzheimer's disease: Report of the NINCDS-ADRDA work group under the auspices of Department of Health and Human Services Task Force on Alzheimer disease. *Neurology* 34:939–944.

O'Brien, J., Desmond, P., Ames, D., Schweitzer, I., Harrigan, S., Tress, B. A., 1996, Magnetic Resonance Imaging Study of White Matter Lesions in Depression and Alzheimer's disease. *Brit.J. Psychiatr.* 168:477–485.

Pearlson, G.D., Rabins, P.V., Kims, W.S., Speedie, L.J., Moberg, P.J., Burns, A., Bascom, M.J., 1989, Structural brain CT changes and cognitive deficits in elderly depressives with and without reversible dementia. *Psychol. Med.* 19:573–584.

Pichot, P., Boyer, P., Pull, C.B., Rein, W., Simon, M., Thibault,A., 1984, Un questionnaire d'auto-évaluation de la symptomatologie dépressive, le questionnaire QD2II, forme abrégée QD2A. *Rev. Psychol. Appl.* 34(4):323–340.

Reding, M., Haycox, J., and Blass, J., 1985, Depression in Patients Referred to a Dementia Clinic. A Three-Year Prospective Study. *Neurology* 42:894–896.

Saunders, A.M., Strittmatter, W.J., Schmechel, D.E., Hyslop, P.H.S., Pericak-Vance, M.A., Joo, S.H., Rosi, B.L., Gusella, J.F., Crapper-McLachlan, D.R., Alberts, M.J., Hulette, C., Crain, B., Goldgaber, D., and Roses, A.D., 1993, Association of apolipoprotein E allele ε4 with late-onset familial and sporadic Alzheimer's disease. *Neurology* 43:1467–1472.

Yesavage, J., Brink, T.L., 1983, Development and validation of a Geriatric Depression Screening Scale: a preliminary report. *J Psychiatr. Res.* 17:37–49.

Zubenko, G.S., Henderson, R., Stiffler, J.S., Stabler, S., Rosen, J., and Kaplan, B.B., 1996, Association of the APOE ε4 Allele with Clinical Subtypes of Late Life Depression. *Biol. Psychiatry* 40:1008–1016.

8

APOPTOSIS IN ALZHEIMER'S DISEASE

Inductive Agents and Antioxidant Protective Factors

Carl W. Cotman and Christian J. Pike

Institute for Brain Aging and Dementia
University of California Irvine
Irvine, California 92697-4540

INTRODUCTION

It is a common premise that the irreversible loss of brain function in AD is due to the disruption of synapses and the loss of neurons that make those synapses. Accordingly, identification of the mechanisms causing circuit disruption and neuronal loss is critical to understanding and interrupting the progression of AD pathology.

Recent evidence suggests that neuronal loss in AD may be caused at least in part by apoptotic mechanisms. While apoptosis is a normal process that is known to occur during the developmental elimination of excess neurons, it may be reinitiated pathologically during aging by certain stimuli causing the loss of significant numbers of neurons and leading to dementia. Indeed, as discussed in this chapter, increasing evidence supports the hypothesis that apoptosis is a mechanism that contributes to neuronal death in AD.

Our approach for experimentally evaluating this theory has been to use cell culture to identify possible mechanisms and markers of neuronal apoptosis, then examine postmortem AD brain tissues for the presence or absence of similar events. In this chapter, we will briefly summarize evidence demonstrating that cultured neurons are induced to undergo apoptosis when subjected to many of the conditions that develop in the AD brain, suggesting that apoptosis may be a cell death mechanism for at least some neurons in AD. Second, we will describe new data on the relative effectiveness of various antioxidants for their ability to protect neurons from various inducers of neuronal apoptosis. These data are particularly relevant in view of recent data showing that vitamin E appears to slow the progression of the disease. The unexpected finding is that on primary neurons a variety of antioxidants are ineffective against β-amyloid induced apoptosis but are effective against induction by hydrogen peroxide, tertiary butyl hydroperoxide and iron.

Progress in Alzheimer's and Parkinson's Diseases
edited by Fisher *et al.*, Plenum Press, New York, 1998.

β-Amyloid Initiates Apoptosis in Cultured Primary Neurons

In the aging and AD brain, β-amyloid accumulates in the extracellular space as small deposits and larger senile plaques. Based on the observation that neurites surrounding β-amyloid deposits show sprouting and degenerative responses, we proposed that this peptide is not metabolically inert as was initially believed, but rather possesses biological activity. We discovered that β-amyloid stimulates a transient growth of neuronal processes, and then, as it self-assembles into small aggregates and β-sheet structures, it acquires an ability to activate degenerative mechanisms (Cotman et al., 1995; Cotman et al., 1996; Yankner, 1996) that culminate in cell death via apoptotic mechanisms (Loo et al., 1993; Watt et al., 1994). This observation has been confirmed by many laboratories (Forloni et al., 1993; Copani et al., 1995; Geschwind and Huber, 1995; Paradis et al., 1996).

β-Amyloid induces classic properties of apoptosis, including membrane blebbing, cell shrinkage, DNA damage, the generation of nuclear apoptotic bodies and a DNA ladder. Consistent with other neuronal apoptosis paradigms (Estus et al., 1994; Ham et al., 1995) apoptosis induced by β-amyloid involves an early and sustained elevation in the immediate early gene product c-Jun within vulnerable, but not resistant neurons (Anderson et al., 1995). Similarly, in the AD brain we have observed DNA damage, cell shrinkage, nuclear apoptotic bodies and increases in c-Jun levels within degenerating neurons (Cotman et al., 1995; Anderson et al., 1994).

Many Inducers of Apoptosis Accumulate in the AD Brain

Apoptosis can be induced in most neurons by a variety of stimuli many of which are present in the AD brain (Table 1). As discussed above, β-amyloid can initiate apoptosis and this inducer accumulates in proximity to neurons and neuronal processes. In parallel with characteristic AD pathology, β-amyloid induces the formation of dystrophic-like neurite morphology in cultured neurons (Pike et al., 1992). Also, oxidative insults readily initiate neuronal apoptosis (Whittemore et al., 1994; Ratan et al., 1994) and oxidative damage is known to occur in the aging and AD brain (Behl, 1995; Beal, 1995; Smith et al., 1995). Similarly, reductions in glucose metabolism have been suggested to contribute to

Table 1. Many inducers of apoptosis correspond to conditions present in the AD brain

Stimuli/Inducers of Apoptosis	AD Conditions
β-amyloid	Accumulation of β-amyloid
Reactive oxygen species	Increased oxidative damage
Elevated intracellular calcium	Abnormalities in calcium homeostasis
Low neurotrophic support	BDNF deficiency, defect in connectivity and retrograde transport
Low energy	Reduced metabolism (vascular angiopathy prevalent) proposed but not established
Excitotoxins (e.g., Glutamate)	Presence of lipid peroxidation products
4-hydroxynoneal (HNE) oxidants	Combinations of the above conditions increases with disease progression
Combinations of conditions (e.g., β-amyloid, oxidation)	
Genetic Risk Factors	**AD Conditions**
PS1, PS2	Familial AD
APP	Familial AD

neurodegeneration in AD (McGeer et al., 1995; Hoyer, 1993; Behl et al., 1993; Beal et al., 1993; Finch et al., 1997), and β-amyloid has been shown to exacerbate neurodegeneration in cultured neurons when glucose levels are reduced (Copani et al., 1991). Multicomponent insults may accumulate and drive neurons toward their apoptotic threshold. Furthermore, the recently described presenilin genes appear to make cells more vulnerable to apoptotic inducers.

Inhibition of Oxidative Neuronal Loss by Antioxidants

To evaluate the potential contribution of oxidative stress to Aβ neurotoxicity vs. other apoptosis inducers, the effective doses of antioxidants were first determined for defined oxidative insults and then tested for protective effects against Aβ. Three classic, widely utilized oxidative insults were chosen for study: iron, hydrogen peroxide (H_2O_2) and tert-butyl hydroperoxide (tBOOH). As shown in Figure 1, each oxidant induced dose-dependent neuronal loss over the 18–24 h experimental period. Cell injury mediated by H_2O_2 and tBOOH typically was visible within a few hours after treatment and appeared complete within approximately 12 hours. In contrast, cell damage caused by iron generally was not noticeable for at least 12 hours, but rapidly progressed thereafter. Using these data, a single concentration of each oxidant was chosen that would generate levels of oxidative stress sufficient to induce robust cell death (70–100%).

Next, several antioxidant agents were evaluated to determine the maximally effective dose to protect against oxidative insults. The tested antioxidants included two free-radical scavengers propyl gallate and Trolox, a water-soluble analog of vitamin E, and the lipid peroxidation inhibitor probucol, since several groups have reported Aβ-induced lipid peroxidation and suggested this event as a primary site of Aβ's oxidative actions (Butterfield et al., 1994; Mark et al., 1997).

Dose-response neuroprotection curves for each of these antioxidants were generated using iron as the oxidative insult. As shown in Figure 2, all of the antioxidants were extremely effective against iron-mediated toxicity, providing at least 80% protection. Based upon these data, maximally protective doses of these antioxidants were established for further study: 1 mM Trolox, 5 μM propyl gallate, and 10 μM probucol. These optimized antioxidant doses also were assessed for protection against both H_2O_2 and tBOOH. Similar to their inhibition of iron-mediated toxicity, the free radical scavengers Trolox and propyl gallate significantly reduced cell death induced by H_2O_2 and tBOOH. However, the lipid

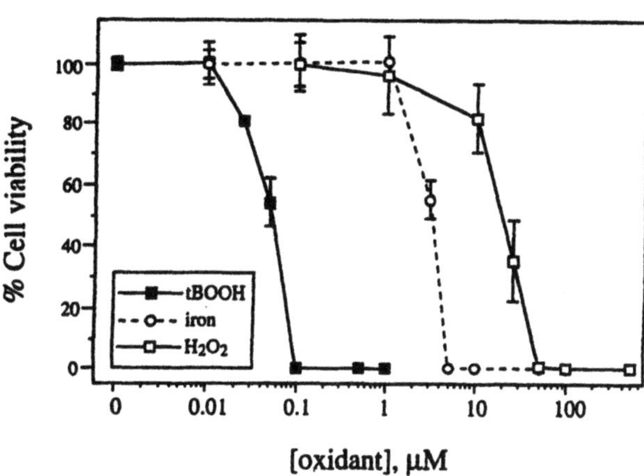

Figure 1. Oxidative stress induced by tert-butyl hydroperoxide (tBOOH; ■) iron (O), hydrogen peroxide (H_2O_2; □), and tBOOH results in dose-dependent toxicity in cultured hippocampal neurons. From these curves, toxic doses of each agent were established for further study: 7 μM iron, 25 μM H_2O 100 nM tBOOH.

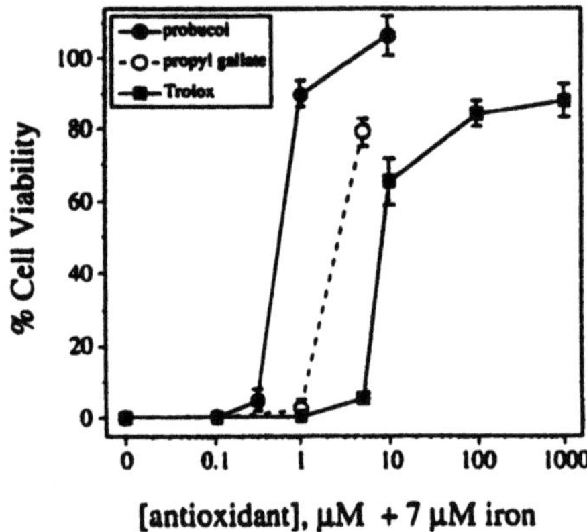

Figure 2. Iron-induced toxicity was inhibited by the antioxidants propyl gallate (open circles), probucol (filled circles), and Trolox (filled boxes, dashed line).

peroxidation inhibitor probucol was ineffective against these insults. These data suggest that antioxidants differ significantly in their ability to protect neurons even against primarily oxidative type insults.

Antioxidants Do Not Inhibit Aβ Toxicity

After establishing the efficacy of several antioxidant agents in inhibiting oxidative cell death, their effectiveness against aggregated Aβ peptides was examined. The experimental design paralleled that used for the oxidative insults: cultures were preloaded with antioxidants, pre-aggregated Aβ peptides were added at an established toxic concentration (25 μM) and cell viability was quantified 24 h later. In contrast to the robust protection antioxidants afforded to classic oxidative insults, the tested antioxidants did not significantly reduce neurotoxicity mediated by Aβ1-42 (Fig. 3).

Induction of Lipid Peroxidation by Iron and Aβ

The data presented above fail to support a classic oxidative mechanism of Aβ toxicity but do not directly address whether Aβ induces oxidative stress. Several investigators who have observed attenuation of Aβ-toxicity by antioxidants also reported that Aβ caused a sig-

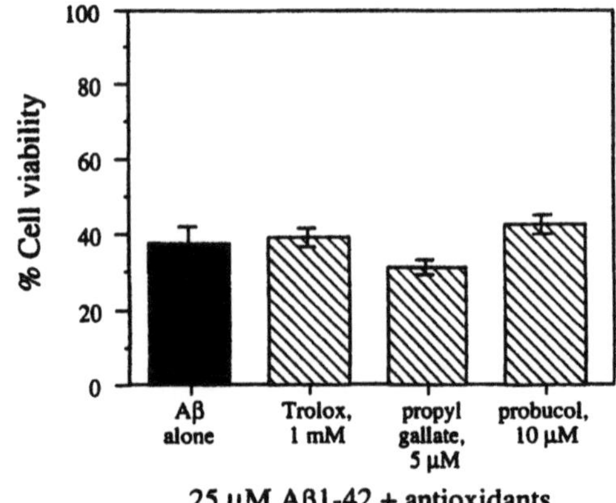

Figure 3. Antioxidants did not provide significant protection against toxicity induced by Aβ1-42.

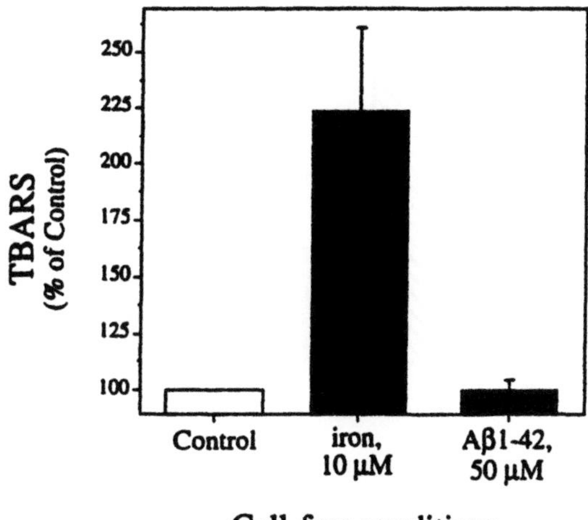

Figure 4. Iron, but not Aβ, induced lipid peroxidation in neuronal membranes in a cell free system.

nificant increase in lipid peroxidation (Butterfield et al., 1994; Mark et al., 1997). Lipid peroxidation is an attractive candidate for Aβ-induced oxidative damage since Aβ readily associates with lipid components in membranes and synthetic bilayers and appears to induce cell death subsequent to membrane interactions. Accordingly, levels of lipid peroxidation products were quantified using a TBARS assay. Initial experiments examined lipid peroxidation in a cell-free, neuronal lysate system to evaluate the possibility that Aβ may act as a direct peptide radical. As shown in Figure 4, iron caused a large increase in TBARS whereas Aβ had no significant effect on TBARS in this cell-free paradigm.

To evaluate the possibility that Aβ indirectly induces lipid peroxidation following neuronal interaction, TBARS were measured in neuronal cultures treated for various times (0–24 h) with iron or Aβ. Toxic doses of iron rapidly caused a mild but significant increase in TBARS that increased to approximately 200% of control values after 16–24 h. Aβ peptide also induced a mild increase in lipid peroxidation with significant values appearing within one hour of treatment. However, unlike the robust TBARS values observed with iron, Aβ levels were typically only 30–50% above control values.

Notably, induction of TBARS by both iron and Aβ occurred well before cell death, which suggests possible contributions of lipid peroxidation to the degenerative mechanism(s) of these insults. To evaluate this possibility, we examined how an inhibitor of lipid peroxidation affected TBARS values and cell viability. Pretreatment of cultures with the antioxidant probucol (10 μM) significantly inhibited the induction of lipid peroxidation by both iron and Aβ. This probucol-mediated reduction in TBARS was paralleled by significant neuroprotection against iron but not Aβ (Fig. 5).

Oxidative Stress Potentiates Aβ-Mediated Neurotoxicity

The data presented above show that although Aβ toxicity is not inhibited by a variety of antioxidants it is associated with increased TBARS, an indication of oxidative stress. This finding suggests a possible degenerative synergism between Aβ and oxidative stress whereby neurons under oxidative challenge may exhibit significantly enhanced sensitivity to Aβ. To begin evaluation of this possibility, we compared the neurotoxicity of Aβ in the presence and absence of a 24 h pretreatment with subtoxic doses (1–3 μM) of iron.

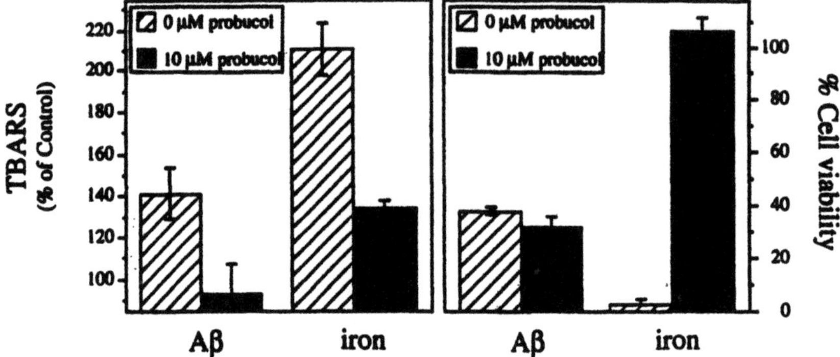

Figure 5. In cultured neurons, both iron and Aβ induced significant lipid peroxidation that was inhibited by probucol (left panel). However, probocol protected against iron but not Aβ induced neuronal apoptosis (right panel). Thus some insults that drive neurons into apoptosis are relatively resistant to most antioxidants.

We observed that the toxicity of Aβ over a complete dose-response range was significantly increased by iron. Notably, the combination of otherwise non-toxic levels of Aβ (1 μM) and iron caused significant neuronal loss.

CONCLUSION

Increasing evidence suggests that a proportion of neurons in the AD brain may degenerate by apoptotic mechansims. Neurons show many of the molecular and morphological signatures of apoptosis and many of the conditions which accumulate in the AD brain are inducers of apoptosis. In the studies discussed in this chapter it is clear that antioxidants can protect neurons in culture from some but not all insults. In particular, relatively classic inducers of oxidation readily induce apoptosis as expected and the neurons are protected by antioxidants though some are more effective than others. In contrast, Aβ induced apoptosis occurs in the presence of antioxidant doses that protect against such oxidative inducers as hydrogen peroxide and iron. We suggest that the primary mechanism driving Aβ apoptosis is not oxidative damage to the cell but rather some other mechanism. That is, select antioxidants reduced Aβ induced lipid peroxidation but did not reduce neuronal degeneration. One alternative mechanism we have previously suggested is that Aβ may cause cross-linking of cell surface receptors and thereby induce activation induced cell death in neurons in a manner analogous to Fas induced apoptosis.

The AD brain contains many conditions which can induce apoptosis and these can act together to be additive or synergistic. Indeed, the concentration of Aβ necessary to induce apoptosis was reduced in the presence of subthreshold doses of iron. Thus it would be predicted that antioxidants would act to reduce the toxicity of Aβ in the presence of some other insults but not eliminate it. While the actual site of action of Vitamin E in AD is unknown it may be that it affords some protection to neurons affected later in the disease by inhibiting the accumulation of adverse conditions that can promote entry into a cycle of terminal apoptosis.

REFERENCES

Anderson, A.J., Cummings, B.J., and. Cotman, C.W., 1994, Increased immunoreactivity for Jun- and Fos-related proteins in Alzheimer's disease: association with pathology. *Exp. Neurol.* 125:2286–295.

Anderson, A.J., Pike, C.J., and. Cotman, C.W., 1995, Differential induction of immediate early gene proteins in cultured neurons by beta-amyloid (Aβ): association of c-jun with Aβ-induced apoptosis. *J. Neurochem.* 65:1487–1498.

Beal, M.F., 1995. Aging, energy, and oxidative stress in neurodegenerative diseases. *Ann. Neurol.* 38(3): 357–366.

Beal, M.F., Hyman, B.T., and. Koroshetz, W., 1993, Do deficits in mitochendrial energy metabolism underlie the pathology of neurodegenerative diseases? *TINS* 16(4):178–184.

Behl, C., Hovey, L., Krajewski, S., Schubert, D., and. Reed, J.C., 1993, BCL-2 prevents killing of neuronal cells by glutamate but not by amyloid beta protein. *Biochem. Biophys. Res. Commun.* 197(2): 949–956.

Behl, M.F., 1995, Aging, energy, and oxidative stress in neurodegenerative diseases. *Ann. Neurol.* 38:357–366.

Butterfield, D.A., Hensley, K., Harris, M., Mattson, M., and Carney, J., 1994, â-Amyloid peptide free radical fragments initiate synaptosomal lipoperoxidation in a sequence-specific fashion: implications to Alzheimer's disease. *Biochem. Biophys. Res. Commun.* 200(2):710–715.

Copani, A., Koh, J.-Y., and. Cotman, C.W, 1991, β-Amyloid increases neuronal susceptibility to injury by glucose deprivation [see comments]. *NeuroReport* 2(12):763–765.

Copani, A., Bruno, V., Gattalglia, G., Leanza, G., Pellitteri, R., Russo, A., Stanzani, S., and Nicholletti, F., 1995, Activation of metabotropic glutamate receptors protects cultured neurons against apoptosis induced by beta-amyloid peptide.*Mol. Pharmacol.* 47(5):890–897.

Cotman, C.W., and Anderson, A.J., 1995, A potential role for apoptosis in neurodegeneration and Alzheimer's disease. *Mol. Neurobiol.* 10(1):19–45.

Cotman, C.W., and Su, J.H., 1996, Mechanisms of neuronal death in Alzheimer's disease. *Brain Pathol.6:*493–506.

Estus, S., Zaks, W., Freeman, R.S., Gruda M., Bravo, R., and Johnson, E.M., Jr., 1994, Altered gene expression in neurons during programmed cell death: identification of c-jun as necessary for neuronal apoptosis. *J. Cell. Biol.* 127(6):1717–1727.

Finch, C.E., and. Cohen, D.M., 1997, Aging, metabolism, and Alzheimer disease: review and hypotheses. *Exp. Neuro.* 143(1): 82–102.

Forloni, G., Chiesa, R., Angeretti, N., and Smiroldo, S., 1993, Apoptosis mediated neurotoxicity induced by chronic application of beta amyloid fragment 25–35. *Neuroreport* 4(5): 523–526.

Geschwind, M., and Huber, G., 1995, Apoptotic cell death induced by beta-amyloid 1–42 peptide is cell type dependent. *J. Neurochem.* 65(1):292–300.

Ham, J., Babij, C., Whitfield, J., Pfarr, C.M., Lallenmand, D., Yaniv, M., and Rubin,L.L., 1995, A c-Jun dominant negative mutant protects sympathetic neurons against programmed cell death. *Neuron* 14(5):927–939.

Hoyer, S., 1993, Abnormalities in brain glucose utilization and its impact on cellular and molecular mechanisms in sporadic dementia of Alzheimer type. *Ann. NY Acad. Sci.* 695:77–80.

Loo, D.T., Copani, A.G., Pike, C.J., Whittemore, E.R., Walencewicz, A.J., and Cotman, C.W., 1993, Apoptosis is induced by beta-amyloid in cultured central nervous system neurons. *Proc. Natl. Acad. Sci.* USA, 90(17): 7951–7955.

Mark, R.J., Lovell, M.A., Markesbury, W.R., Uchida, K., and. Mattson, M.P., 1997, A role for 4-hydroxynonenal,an aldehydic product of lipid peroxidation, in disruption of ion homeostasis and neuronal death induced by amyloid beta-peptide. *J. Neurochem.* 68(1):255–264.

McGeer, P.L., Kamo, H., Harrop, R., Li, K.K., Tuokko, H., McGeer, E.G., Adam, M.J., Ammann, W., Beattie,B.L., and Calne, D.B., 1986, Positron emission tomography in patients with clinically diagnosed Alzheimer's disease. *Can. Med. Assoc. J.* 134(6): 597–607.

Paradis, E., Douillard, H., Koutroumanis, M., Goodyer, C., and LeBlanc, A., 1996, Amyloid beta peptide of Alzheimer's disease downregulates Bcl-2 and upregulates bax expression in human neurons. *J.Neurosci.* 16(23): 7533–7539.

Pike, C.J., Cummings, B.J., and Cotman, C.W., 1992, β-amyloid induces neuritic dystrophy in vitro similarities with Alzheimer pathology. *Neuroreport* 3:769–772.

Ratan, R.R., Murphy, T.H., and Baraban, J.M., 1994, Oxidative stress induces apoptosis in embryonic cortical neurons. *J. Neurochem.* 62(1):376–379.

Smith, M.A., Sayre, L.M., Monnier, V.M., and. Perry, G., 1995, Radical AGEing in Alzheimer's disease. *Trends Neurosci.* 1995. 18(4):172–6.

Watt, J.A., Pike, C.J., Walencewicz-Wasserman, A.J., and Cotman, C.W., 1994, Ultrastructural analysis of β-amyloid-induced apoptosis in cultured hippocampal neurons. *Brain Res.* 661:147–156.

Whittemore, E.R., Loo, D.T., and Cotman, C.W., 1994, Exposure to hydrogen peroxide induces cell death via apoptosis in cultured rat cortical neurons. *NeuroReport* 5(13):585–1588.

Yankner, B.A., 1996. Mechanisms of neuronal degeneration in Alzheimer's disease. *Neuron* 16(5): 921–932

9

MEMBRANE CONSTITUENCIES AND RECEPTOR SUBTYPE CONTRIBUTE TO AGE-RELATED INCREASES IN VULNERABILITY TO OXIDATIVE STRESS

Implications for Neurodegenerative Disease

J. A. Joseph, N. Denisova, D. Fisher, I. Cantuti-Castelvetri, and S. Erat

USDA Human Nutrition Research Center on Aging
Tufts University
Boston, Massachusetts 02111

INTRODUCTION

Since the populations of many countries are increasing in age, with all the attendant age-related functional alterations increasing in frequency, delineation of the mechanism(s) involved in neurodegeneration and neuronal dysfunction, especially in diseases that increase in incidence as a function of age, has become extremely important. This is particularly true in the case of neuronal dysfunction and associated behavioral changes (i.e., decrements in memory and motor behavior functions). It should be noted here that these changes can occur even in the absence of specific age-related neurodegenerative diseases. Unfortunately, very little is known about the mechanisms involved in these age-related declines in memory and motor functions, and attempts to reverse or retard their decline have been, with very few exceptions, singularly unsuccessful. However there is a great deal of evidence which suggests the involvement of oxidative stress (OS) in these declines.

OXIDATIVE STRESS

OS is defined as an imbalance between oxidants and antioxidants in favor of the former, resulting in oxidative damage to molecules such as lipids, DNA, and proteins. As is well known (e.g., see Halliwell and Gutteridge, 1989; Halliwell, 1994; Yu 1994; for reviews), this insult can arise from both extra metabolic (e.g., pollution, radiation, toxins,

Progress in Alzheimer's and Parkinson's Diseases
edited by Fisher *et al.*, Plenum Press, New York, 1998.

etc.) and metabolic sources. Concerning the latter of these, among the most significant biological sources of free radicals are those that lead to O_2 derived superoxide ($O_2^{\cdot-}$) from electron transport associated with mitochondrial membranes. In this case the conversion of oxygen to water requires electron transfer. Among the products formed by these reactions are the: hydroperoxyl radical ($HO_2^{\cdot}$), hydrogen peroxide (H_2O_2) and the hydroxyl radical ($\cdot OH$), which is potentially the most damaging pro-oxidant in cellular systems. Other cellular sources of free radical generation are those of microsomal and nuclear membranes. Fortunately, during normal functioning, cells contain a number of antioxidant defenses that remove excess superoxides and H_2O_2. These include superoxide dismutase (SOD), catalase and various peroxidases. In addition, there are low molecular mass antioxidants such as glutathione, vitamin E and ascorbic acid. Since organisms do not scavenge free radicals with 100% efficiency, the repair of oxidative damage in DNA, proteins and lipids is extremely important. Thus, a wide variety of enzymes, proteases and chain-breaking antioxidants exist to aid in this repair (see reviews by Halliwell, 1994; Yu, 1994). In both aging and age-related neurodegenerative disease there appear to deficits in both protection and repair mechanisms to offeset the deleterious OS effects that lead to increased vulnerability to continued free radical insult.

NEURODEGENERATION, AGING, AND BEHAVIOR

As can be seen from the brief description above, there are numerous free radicals that can be generated by a variety of systems with associated protection systems. In aging, however, there may be decreases in the efficacy of these scavenging systems that are associated with an increasing inability to cope with OS that occurs throughout the life-span. After life-long free-radical insult on an organ, which already shows increased vulnerability to OS, functional deficits are observed. Indeed, one of the primary efforts in aging research is to investigate putative changes in these repair processes, as well as in the antioxidant defenses. In this regard, there is a great deal of evidence suggesting that oxidation is a primary factor in cellular aging (e.g., Harman, 1981; Halliwell, 1994; Shigenaga et al., 1994). However, there is less evidence demonstrating a role for OS in normal aging, especially in the brain. In fact, it is only recently that this is beginning to be specified with respect to the nervous system. The brain may show greater vulnerability to the effects of OS than other extraneuronal sites, since it is relatively deficient in free radical protection, and utilizes high amounts of oxygen (Olanow, 1992). Moreover, there is increasing evidence to suggest that OS may contribute to the declines seen in age-related neurodegenerative diseases (e.g., Youdim et al., 1994; Alzheimer's Disease, Benzi and Moretti, 1995; Choi-Miura and Oda, 1996; Jenner, 1996; Simonian and Coyle, 1996; Parkinson's Disease, Jenner, 1996; Jenner and Olanow, 1996; Ebadi et al., 1996). Research also indicates that several indices of antioxidant protection appear to be reduced in aging. As examples: a) The ratio of oxidized to total glutathione in the reduced form (GSH) increased as a function of age in several brain areas including: hippocampus, cortex and striatum (Zhang et al., 1993); b) Higher levels of α-tocopherol were observed in older age groups, possibly indicating an attempt to respond to age-related increases in OS (Zhang et al., 1993); and c) Significant lipofuscin accumulation with bcl-2 increases and membrane lipid peroxidation have been observed as a function of age (Yu, 1994) in lipofuscin-containing vacuoles of neurons, glia and vascular cells (Migheli et al., 1994).

However, there have been few studies directed toward demonstrating age-related increases in sensitivity to OS on neuronal parameters that are known to change with age. In this regard, we have developed two such tests (oxotremorine-enhancment of K^+-evoked dopamine release from striatal slices and carbachol-stimulated GTPase activity) which are age- and OS-sensitive (Joseph et al., 1996). These tests were utilized to examined the nature of the rather ubiquitous loss in sensitivity expressed by muscarinic receptors as a function of age in the striatum. The findings, thus far, have indicated that: a) Oxotremorine (oxo) enhancement of dopamine (DA) release (K^+-ERDA) (in superfused striata) shows significant declines with aging; b) K^+-ERDA deficits are exacerbated by OS in an age-dependent manner; c) These changes were associated with significant deficits in motor function on several tests. Several subsequent studies have shown that these deficits are primarily the result of deficits in signal transduction, since carbachol-stimulation of GTPase activity (an indicator of receptor-G protein coupling/uncoupling) was also found to be reduced with aging and OS (Yamagami et al., 1992; Joseph et al., 1996).

Thus, if these age-related changes in signal transduction are the result of OS and if OS vulnerability increases as a function of age, then it is extremely important to delineate the mechanisms involved in these alterations.. Recent ongoing work from our laboratory has suggested that in addition to the putative decreases in antioxidant protection that are cited above, vulnerability increases also may be the result of increases in membrane lipids, particularly sphingomyelin and may be dependent to a large extent on the composition of the receptor population in a particular brain area.

MEMBRANE LIPIDS AND OXIDATIVE STRESS

It has been shown in numerous experiments that alterations cell membrane lipid constituencies in aging can increase rigidity and lead to decreased signal transduction, and cell loss. These include significant age-related increases in membrane cholesterol (Viand, et al., 1991; Cho et al., 1995; Lope et al., 1995) and sphingomyelin (Giusto et al., 1992) and/or lipid peroxidation (Yu et al., 1992; Cho et al., 1995). Since previous findings indicate that among, its other effects, OS increases membrane rigidity, it was hypothesized that in aging OS impinges upon membranes that are already exhibiting increases in rigidity and therefore, there may be an enhancement of the effects of OS. Moreover, it has been shown that one common effect of OS appears to be to induce a deficit in Ca^{2+} homeostasis that may lead to cell death (e.g., see McCord 1987; Lee et al., 1991; Cheng et al., 1994) and that there are elevations of intracellular Ca^{2+} in normal aging (e.g., Landfield and Eldridge, 1994) and age-related neurodegenerative diseases (e.g. see Pagliusi et al., 1994). From these and other studies it has been suggested that a direct, initial free radical insult which increases the intracellular calcium ($[Ca^{2+}]_I$) and decreases Ca^{2+} extrusion may lead to the indirect generation of additional pro-oxidants. Thus, in aging and age-related neurodegenerative diseases, OS appears to impinge upon systems that are already compromised in their ability to regulate Ca^{2+} flux.

In order to examine in relative isolation the interaction of membrane lipids and OS on specific indices of Ca^{2+} flux, PC-12 cells were assessed. Cells were incubated in maintenance media (RPMI-1640 with 2 mM glutamine, 10% horse serum and 5% fetal bovine serum (FBS) and 120 U/ml penicillin/streptomycin). These media were removed and replaced with the same media with or without 300 μM H_2O_2 and further incubated at 37°C for 30 minutes. Cells were then washed 3 times with the maintenance media, incubated in RPMI-1640 with 1% FBS and 2 μM Fura-2 AM (45 minutes), followed by Kreb's-Ringers-Hepes (KRH) Buffer (30 min) to allow hydrolyzation of the Fura-2 AM and then held on ice for up to 2 hours. A coverslip with treated PC-12 cells was then inserted into a

Leiden cover slip dish (37°C) that was mounted on the stage of an Olympus IMT-2 inverted fluorescent microscope

For each test, a group of 5 to 15 representative cells was selected. Near simultaneous images of the cells at 510 nm emission and either 340 or 380 excitation wavelengths were captured (Compix, Inc.). The interval between capture ranged from 2.4 to 3.5 seconds. After approximately 60 seconds, the cells were depolarized by the addition of 0.1 ml of 300 mM KCl (for a final concentration of 30 mM), and image capture continued for an additional 15 minutes.

Pixel-by-pixel comparisons of the captured images were made, and a ratio of Ca^{2+}-bound fura (340 nm excitation) to unbound fura (380 nm excitation) was generated for each pair of images. Three parameters of Ca^{2+} flux were examined using fluorescence imaging: *baseline*, pre-KCl Ca^{2+} levels), *depolarization* (expressed as % of Ca^{2+} increase) (to 30 mM KCl), and *recovery* ($[Ca^{2+}]_I$ extrusion). Results showed that baseline Ca^{2+} levels were significantly increased by H_2O_2 treatment (e.g., 300 μM, 200%), while the rise in free intracellular Ca^{2+} following KCl stimulation (i.e., peak) was decreased (e.g., 300 μM, 50%) and Ca^{2+} recovery time following depolarization was significantly decreased and led eventually to cell death 24 hrs after H_2O_2 (Live/Dead Eukolight Kit, Molecular Probes) (Joseph et al., 1997).

In a subsequent study attempts were made to determine if these response patterns would be altered further after modification of membrane lipid composition induced by incubating the PC-12 cells (All lipid or lipid metabolite [see below] incubations were carried out for 1h at 37°C prior to H_2O_2 treatment). with 660 μM cholesterol (CHL) in the presence or absence of 500 μM sphingomyelin (SPM). Following incubation, the membrane levels of CHL or SPM were similar to those seen in aging.

While neither CHL nor SPH had synergistic effects with H_2O_2 on baseline, SPH significantly decreased recovery in the presence or absence of H_2O_2 by 50% and significantly increased level of conjugated dienes by 750%. These effects were not seen with CHL pretreatment. The results indicated that membrane sphingomyelin could be a critical factor in determining OS vulnerability and Ca^{2+} translocation in membranes. This may be especially important in aging where there is increased membrane SPH and significant loss of calcium homeostasis (Densiova et al., 1997).

In additional experiments, attempts were made to determine the particular metabolite of SPM that might be contributing to the increased effectiveness of H_2O_2 on recovery. In these studies, membrane SPM was depleted by incubating the PC-12 cells in either 100 mU/ml *Staphylococcus aureus* sphingomyelinase(Sase) or 2 mM L-Cycloserine (L-CS) 500 μM SPH and incubated in H_2O_2 or incubation medium alone and Ca^{2+} recovery examined. Results showed that endogenously induced depletion of SPH by L-CS significantly increased the ability of the cells to recover. With Sase pretreatment increases in the vulnerability to H_2O_2 were observed that were similar to those seen with SPM incubation. These findings indicated that a metabolite of SPM was involved in these increases in OS vulnerability, since L-CS primarily antagonized the synthesis of SPM and thus, decreased membrane SPM metabolite levels.

Subsequent evaluations in which the cells were incubated in SPM metabolites C2-ceramide (Cer, 100 μM) or 1 μM sphingosine-1-phosphate (S-1-P, 1 μM) indicated that Cer had no effect on the H_2O_2-decreases in recovery, while S-P-1P significantly increased the vulnerability of cells to H_2O_2-induced decreases in recovery. The nature of this effect is not clear. It seems there are at least two different SPM pools (plasma membrane and new-synthesized in *cis-medial* Golgi stacks). Both pools affect Ca^{2+} homeostasis but only the newly-synthesized SPH was able to significantly decrease cells vulnerability to OS.

Therefore, these findings do indicate that one factor that is important in determining OS vulnerabilty is membrane lipid content and that age-related increases in membrane SPM content may be extremely critical in this regard.

MUSCARINIC RECEPTOR SUBTYPES

In addition to lipid modifications, a second factor that might be important in determining OS vulnerability in aging may involve qualitative/quantitative differences in receptor subtypes in various neuronal populations. For example, it has been known for many years that there are region-specific variations in brain aging and some areas show more deleterious effects than others (e.g., striatum). Therefore, if OS is involved in inducing these changes, selective regional vulnerability to OS may reflect the qualitative make-up of the receptor populations. To this end we exposed COS-7 cells transfected with one of five muscarinic receptor subtypes (M_1-M_5 AChR) to low concentrations of H_2O_2 (0, 300 or 500 μM for 30 minutes in growth medium) or DA (1 mM for 4 hrs) and examined intracellular Ca^{2+} levels prior to and following 500 μM oxotremorine (to induce depolarization) (oxo), as well as cell death following OS exposure.

Following H_2O_2 exposure the number of cells showing oxo-induced depolarization and Ca^{2+} recovery varied as a function of transfected mAChR subtype. The percent of cells showing the greatest decreases in responding (depolarizing) to oxo were those transfected with the M_1 (300 or 500 μM H_2O_2, 30%) and M_2 (45%) subtypes while $M_{3,\ 4}$, and $_5$ cells showed no significant decreases in responding with H_2O_2. However with respect to recovery, $M_{1,\ 2}$, or M_4-transfected cells showed the greatest decreases following H_2O_2 (50–100%) or DA (25–50%). Recovery in M_3- and M_5-transfected DA- or H_2O_2-exposed cells was not significantly decreased. Similar patterns in were observed in subsequent examinations of the degree of alterations in cell viability (Live/Dead Eukolight kit) in cells transfected with M_1 or M_3 at 4 hrs and 24 hrs post DA treatment to these seen for Ca^{2+} recovery. Analysis of the degree of cell death by apoptosis following DA exposure (Apo-Tag Kit) indicated that it was about 10% of the 40% cell death in M_1-transfected cells. No cell death was observed in M_3-transfected, DA- exposed cells. Thus, it may be that receptor differences in OS vulnerability may determine, in-part, regional susceptibility to cell death. For example, it has been shown in the striatum that: a) M_1 receptor protein is expressed in 78% of the neurons; b) M_2 receptors may be the predominant muscarinic receptor; c) M_4 receptors were localized to 44% of striatal cells (Hersch et al., 1994); and d) there are high concentrations of DA (which form a variety of OS-based toxic products e.g., Ben-Shachar et al., 1995; Hastings and Zigmond, 1994). Thus the profound age-related changes in the striatum may be reflective of the interactions between DA and specific populations of OS vulnerable receptors. We are examining these possibilities. However, it should be clear that in age-related neurodegenerative diseases (AD and PD) there are even greater decreases in the ability to respond to OS superimposed upon a nervous system that is already showing increased sensitivity to free radical insult.

REFERENCES

Benzi, G. and Moretti, A., 1995, Are reactive oxygen species involved in Alzheimer's Disease? *Neurobiol. Aging* 16:661.

Ben-Shachar, D., Zuk, R., and Glinka,, Y., 1995, Dopamine neurotoxicity: Inhibition of mitochondrial respiration, *J. Neurochem.* 64:718.

Cheng Y., Wixom P., James-Kracke M. R., and Sun A. Y., 1994, Effects of extracellular ATP on Fe²⁺- induced cytotoxicity in PC-12 cells, *J. Neurochem.* 66:895.

Cho, E. M., Jackson, C., and Yu, B. P., 1995, Lipid peroxidation contributes to age-related membrane rigidity, *Free Radic. Biol. Med.* 18:977.

Choi-Miura, N. H ., and Oda, T., 1996, Relationship between multifunctional protein "clusterin" and Alzheimer disease. *Neurobiol. Aging* 17:717.

Denisova, N. A.., Strain, J. G., and Joseph, J. A., 1997, Oxidant injure in PC-12 cells: A possible model of calcium "dysregualtion in aging" II. Interactions with membrane lipids, *J. Neurochem.*, in press.

Ebadi, M., Srinivasan, S. K., and Baxi, M. D., 1996, Oxidative stress and antioxidant therapy in Parkinson's disease, *Prog. in Neurobiol.* 48:1.

Giusto N., Roque M., Iiincheta M. E., and de Boschero M.G., 1992, Effect of aging on the content, composition and synthesis of sphingomyelin in the central nervous system, *Lipids* 27:835.

Halliwell, B., 1994, Free radicals and antioxidants: A personal view, *Nutr. Rev.* 52:253.

Halliwell, B. and Gutteridge J. M.C., 1989, *Free Radic. Biol. Med.* Oxford, England Clarendon Press.

Harman, D., 1981, The aging process, *PNAS USA* 78:7124.

Hastings, T. G. and Zigmond, M. J., 1994, Identification of catechol- protein conjugates in neostriatal slices incubated with [³H] dopamine: Impact of ascorbic acid and glutathione, *J. Neurochem.*63:1126.

Hersch, S. M., Guteknust, C. A., Rees, H. D., Heilman, C. J., and Levey, A. I., 1994, Distribution of m1-m4 muscarinic receptor proteins in the rat striatum: light and electron microscopic immunocytochemistry using subtype-specific antibodies. *J. Neurosci.* 14:3351.

Jenner, P., 1996, Oxidative stress in Parkinson's disease and other neurodegenerative disorders, *Pathol. Biol.* 44:57.

Jenner, P. and Olanow, C. W., 1996, Oxidative stress and the pathogenesis of Parkinson's disease, *Neurol.* 47 (Suppl 3):S161.

Joseph, J. A., Strain, J., and Jimenez, N. D., 1997, Oxidant injure in PC-12 cells: A possible model of calcium "dysregualtion in aging" I. Selectivity of antioxidant protection, *J. Neurochem.*, in press.

Joseph, J. A., Villalobos-Molina, R., Denisova, N., Erat, S., Cutler, R., Strain, J., 1996, Age differences in sensitivity to H_2O_2 or NO-induced reductions in K⁺ - evoked dopamine release from superfused striatal slices: Reversals by PBN or Trolox, *Free Radic. Biol. Med.* 20:821.

Landfield P. W. and Eldridge J. C., 1994, The glucocorticoid hypothesis of age-related hippocampal neurodegeneration: Role of dysregulated intraneuronal calcium, *Ann. N. Y. Acad. Sci.* 746:308.

Lee K. S., Frank S., Vanderklish P., Arai A., and Lynch G., 1991, Inhibition of proteolysis protects hippocampal neurons from ischemia, *PNAS USA* 88:7233.

Lope, G. H., Ilincheta de Boschero, M. G., Castagnet, P. I., and Gusto, N. M., 1995, Age-associated changes in the content and fatty acid composition of brain glycerophospholipids, *Comp. Biochem. Physiol. Part B, Biochem. Molec. Biol.*112:331.

McCord J. M., 1987, Oxygen-derived radicals: A link between reperfusion injury and inflammation, *Fed. Proc.* 46:2402.

Migheli, A., Cavalla, P., Piva, R., Giordana, M. T., and Schiffer, D., 1994, Bcl-2 protein expression in aged brain and neurodegenerative diseases, *Neurorep.* 5:1906.

Olanow, C. W., 1992, An introduction to the free radical hypothesis in Parkinson's disease, *Ann. Neurol.* 32:S2.

Pagliusi ,S. R., Gerrard, P., Abdallah, M., Talabot D., and Catisicas ,S., 1994, Age-related changes in expression of AMPA-selective glutamate receptor subunits: is calcium-permeability altered in hippocampal neurons? *Neuroscience* 61:429–433.

Shigenaga, M. K., Hagen, T. M., and Ames, B.N. 1994. Oxidative damage and mitochondrial decay in aging, *PNAS USA* 91:10771.

Simonian, N. A. and Coyle, J. T., 1996, Oxidative stress in neurodegenerative diseases., *Ann. Rev. Pharmacol. Tox.* 36:83.

Viand, P., Cervato, G., Fioilli, A., and Cestaro, B., 1991, Age-related differences in synaptosomal peroxidative damage and membrane properties, *J. Neurochem.* 56:253.

Yamagami, K., Joseph, J. A., and Roth, G. S., 1992, Decrement of muscarinic receptor-stimulated low K_m GTPase activity in striata and hippocampus from aged rat, *Brain Res.* 576:327.

Yu, B. P., Suescun, E. A. and Yang, S. Y., 1992, Effect of age-related lipid peroxidation on membrane fluidity and phospholipase A2: modulation by dietary restriction, *Mech. Ageing Dev.* 65:17.

Youdim, M. B. H., Lavie, L., and Riederer, P., 1994, Oxygen free radicals and neurodegeneration in Parkinson's disease: A role for nitric oxide, *Ann. New York Acad. Sci.* 738:64.

Yu, B.P., 1994, Cellular defenses against damage from reactive oxygen species, *Physiol. Rev.*76:139.

Zhang, J.R. Andrus, P.K., and Hall, E.D., 1993, Age-related regional changes in hydroxyl radical stress and antioxidants in gerbil brain, *J. Neurochem.* 61:1640.

10

MITOCHONDRIAL DYSFUNCTION AND ALZHEIMER'S DISEASE

Soumitra S. Ghosh,[1] Scott Miller,[1] Corinna Herrnstadt,[1] Eoin Fahy,[1]
Leslie A. Shinobu,[2] Douglas Galasko,[3] Leon J. Thal,[3] M. Flint Beal,[2]
Neil Howell,[4] W. Davis Parker, Jr.,[5] and Robert E. Davis[1]

[1]MitoKor
San Diego, California
[2]Massachusetts General Hospital
Boston, Massachusetts
[3]University of California at San Diego
La Jolla, California
[4]University of Texas Medical Branch
Galveston, Texas
[5]University of Virginia
Charlottesville, Virginia

INTRODUCTION

Alzheimer's disease (AD) is a progressive neurodegenerative disease that culminates in selective neuronal loss in discrete regions of the brain. AD is genetically heterogeneous and is best characterized as a syndrome with a common but variable pathologic sequela. Rare familial forms of AD follow conventional patterns of autosomal dominant Mendelian inheritance (St. George-Hyslop et al., 1990; Schellenberg et al., 1992; Levy-Lahad et al., 1995a,b), occur earlier in life and account for less than 5% of all AD cases. The vast majority of AD cases (approximately 95%) appear late in life after the age of 60, without clearly discernible chromosomal linkages. However, first-degree relatives of affected probands are at higher risk for AD than the general population (Silverman et al., 1994a,b) and lack of a family history is a negative risk factor for AD (Payami et al., 1994). Further, the risk of AD increases when a maternal relative is afflicted with AD (Duara et al., 1993; Edland et al., 1996). Sporadic inheritance with familial association, maternal transmission, and variable phenotypic expression are hallmarks of mitochondrial genetic disease (Johns, 1995; Luft, 1994). These features typify the mode of genetic presentation of late-onset AD in the population.

Progress in Alzheimer's and Parkinson's Diseases
edited by Fisher *et al.*, Plenum Press, New York, 1998.

We have proposed that a significant proportion of AD cases is associated with oxidative stress that arises from a primary and focal enzymatic defect in cytochrome *c* oxidase (CO), the terminal complex of the mitochondrial electron transport chain (ETC) (Davis, et al, 1997; Swerdlow et al., 1997). We have examined the functional consequences of mitochondrial dysfunction associated with AD through the analysis of cytoplasmic cellular hybrid (cybrid) systems. AD cybrids have been generated by fusing platelets from AD donors with ρ^o cell lines lacking endogenous mitochondrial DNA (mtDNA). We have shown that cybrids transformed with mitochondria from sporadic AD donors exhibit a specific decrease of cytochrome *c* oxidase activity, increased production of reactive oxygen species (ROS) and altered calcium homeostasis.

MITOCHONDRIAL DYSFUNCTION AS A CENTRAL ETIOLOGIC EVENT IN AD

Mounting evidence suggests that the AD is associated with focal defects in energy metabolism with accompanying increases in oxidative stress. Positron emission tomography studies have reported regionally specific deficits in energy metabolism in AD brains (Kuhl et al., 1985; Haxby et al., 1990, Azari et al., 1993). Functional magnetic resonance spectroscopy studies indicate decreased production of ATP in AD brain as inferred from elevated inorganic phosphate to phosphocreatine ratios (Pettegrew et al., 1994; Pettigrew et al., 1995). AD pathology shows prominent signs of oxidative injury, implicating ROS in neuronal degeneration. AD brains at autopsy show increased levels of DNA, protein and lipid oxidation (Palmer & Burns, 1994; Pappolla et al., 1992; Jeandel et al., 1989; Balazs & Leon, 1994; Mecocci et al., 1994, Smith et al., 1996). Neurofibrillary tangles also appear to be prominent sites of protein oxidation (Schweers et al., 1995). In addition, the activity of critical antioxidant enzymes, particularly catalase, are reduced (Gsell et al., 1995) suggesting that the AD brain is vulnerable to increased ROS production.

Several lines of evidence place mitochondrial dysfunction at the center of AD pathology. Cell death in AD is presumed to be apoptotic because signs of programmed cell death (PCD) have been observed (Smale et al., 1995; Cotman & Anderson, 1995). It is likely that apoptotic cell death of neurons in the AD brain occurs as a consequence of mitochondrial dysfunction. Evidence suggests that alterations of mitochondrial function occurs early in the PCD pathway (Kroemer et al., 1995). In several cell types, including neurons, sequential reduction of the mitochondrial membrane potential ($\Delta\Psi$m) and generation of ROS precede nuclear DNA degradation (Zamzami et al., 1995a,b). Mitochondria release cytochrome *c* in apoptotic cells that triggers activation of caspases and DNA fragmentation (Liu et al., 1996). Importantly, the Bcl-2 family of anti-apoptosis gene products are located within the outer mitochondrial membrane (Monaghan et al., 1992) and overexpression of Bcl-2 prevents cells from undergoing apoptosis in response to a variey of stimuli (Reed, 1994). Recent studies show that Bcl-2 prevents the apoptotic process by inhibiting the release of cytochrome *c* from mitochondria (Yang et al., 1997, Kluck et al., 1997). To the extent that apoptotic cell death is a prominent feature of neuronal loss in AD, mitochondrial dysfunction may be critical to the progression of this disease.

Excitotoxic neuronal death is associated with inadequate mitochondrial ATP synthesis. This can lead to partial neuronal depolarization, followed by activation of NMDA receptors by ambient glutamate concentrations (Beal, 1992). Overstimulation of NMDA receptors, in turn, triggers massive calcium influx into the cell. Since the mitochondrion is the critical cellular organelle for maintaining calcium homeostasis (Harrington et al., 1996), its dysfunction can lead the induction of glutamate neurotoxicity (Schinder et al., 1996).

The clearest link implicating mitochondrial dysfunction with the bioenergetic defects and oxidative stress in AD is the observation of specific defects in the catalytic activity of CO in platelets from AD patients and in AD brain at autopsy (Parker et al. 1990; Kish et al., 1992; Parker et al., 1994; Parker et al., 1994; Mutisya et al., 1994; Chagnon et al., 1995; Parker & Parks, 1995). The activities of other components of the ETC are normal in AD brain and platelets. Importantly, these findings differ from those demonstrating a complex I dysfunction in Parkinson's disease brain and platelets (Schapira et al. 1992; Krige et al., 1992). These data indicate that the CO defect associated with AD is disease specific, and that it is not simply a non-specific consequence of neurodegeneration, postmortem change or aging. A pronounced catalytic impairment of CO would be expected to result in bioenergetic failure and increased ROS production that could contribute to neurodegeneration.

AD CYBRID CELLS: AN *IN VITRO* MODEL OF AD MITOCHONDRIAL DYSFUNCTION

The indication of an anatomically generalized expression of the CO defect as seen in both neuronal and non-neuronal AD tissues was suggestive of alterations in DNA. The functional implication of this observation was probed by fusion of platelets from donor individuals into SY5Y neuroblastoma cells that were depleted of endogenous mtDNA, but not nuclear DNA (essentially mtDNA knockout cells). Exogenous mtDNA along with other cytoplasmic contents were introduced into ρ^0 SY5Y cells by polyethylene glycol-mediated fusion of platelets derived from blood of AD patients and cognitively normal, age-matched controls (Miller, et. al., 1996). This procedure creates cybrids where the mitochondrial DNA (mtDNA) from the donor is expressed in the nuclear and cellular environment of the host ρ^0 cell. Cybrids derived from normal age-matched controls (control cybrids) displayed the normal aerobic phenotype with complex I and CO activities that were equivalent to the parental cell lines. In contrast, cybrids derived from AD individuals generally had reduced CO activity whereas complex I activity remained normal (Figure 1). Since the nuclear environments in the AD and control cybrid cell lines are identical, the CO defect in the AD cybrids must arise from the mitochondrial DNA transfer from AD donors. In addition, AD cybrids displayed increased basal cytosolic calcium concentration and impaired intracellular calcium homeostasis (Sheehan et al., 1997).

A CO defect should lead to increased leakage of electrons from the ETC that can subsequently react with molecular oxygen to generate ROS. As anticipated, the fluorescent probe, dichlorofluorescin diacetate (DCF-DA), detected significantly elevated production of ROS in AD cybrids as compared to control cybrids (Figure 2). In response to increased oxidative stress, significant induction of radical scavenging enzymes such as glutathione reductase and glutathione peroxidase is seen in SH-SY5Y AD cybrids as compared to control cybrids (Miller and Davis, unpublished results). Upregulation of Cu/Zn superoxide dismutatase (SOD) and Mn SOD in Ntera2/D1 (NT2) AD cybrids has been observed as a compensatory response to increased ROS (Swerdlow et al., 1997). AD cybrids also show increased vulnerability to apoptosis in response to a variety of stimuli (Dykens and Davis, unpublished results).

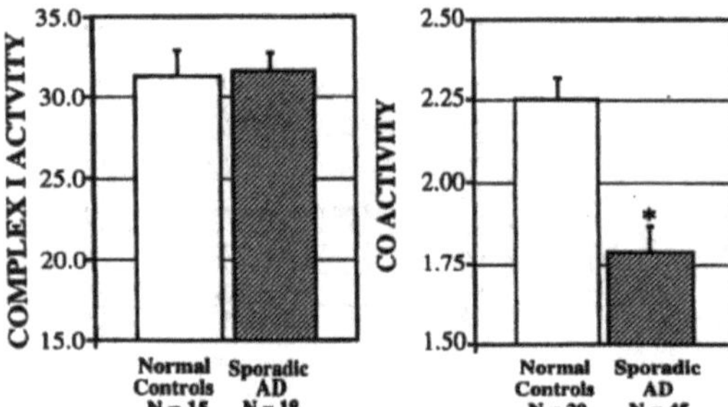

Figure 1. Characterization of complex I and IV activity of AD and control cybrids. Complex I and CO activity were assayed in isolated cells as described previously and expressed as rate for complex I (nmol.min^{-1}.mg^{-1}) and relative rate for CO (min^{-1}.mg^{-1}). (Miller et al., 1996). CO activity was significantly decreased in AD cybrids relative to control cybrids. The group means were significantly different (p = 0.00005). In contrast, complex I activity, another complex encoded in part by the mitochondrial genome, was not different in a subset of AD and normal control cybrids.

INCREASED RATIOS OF NUCLEAR PSEUDOGENE DNA/mtDNA CORRELATE WITH AD

CO is a thirteen polypeptide multimeric complex and three of its subunits (COI, COII & COIII) are encoded by mtDNA. The lack of nuclear genetic associations in most AD cases and a transferable CO defect into AD cybrids prompted us to search for AD-associated mutations in the mitochondrial genes. White buffy coat fraction of blood was isolated from AD patients, cognitively normal age matched controls, patients with non-insulin diabetes mellitus (NIDDM) and neurological controls. The cells were lysed by a boiling procedure to release the DNA. Clonal sequence analysis revealed a unique DNA sequence that carried a linked set of specific point mutations in the CO1 and CO2 genes. This DNA was found to be over-represented in a majority of AD patients (Davis et al., 1997). We originally suggested that these polymorphisms were disease related. Subsequent work (Hirano et al., 1997; Wallace et al., 1997) established these polymorphisms to be present in a nuclear pseudogene. We have characterized the pseudogene as a 5.8 kb fragment that is largely in frame with mitochondrial nucleotide positions 3911–9755 (Herrnstadt et al., 1998). The sequence is found with flanking non-mitochondrial sequences and is absent in immunopurified mitochondria from SH-SY5Y and blood cells. Since these polymorphisms are apparently not expressed, it is unlikely to account for decreases in CO activity in AD cybrids. The etiology and genetics of this focal CO defect therefore requires further investigation.

Nonetheless, the association of AD with increased levels of pseudogene DNA in relation to wild type mtDNA is significant and has diagnostic potential. A competitive

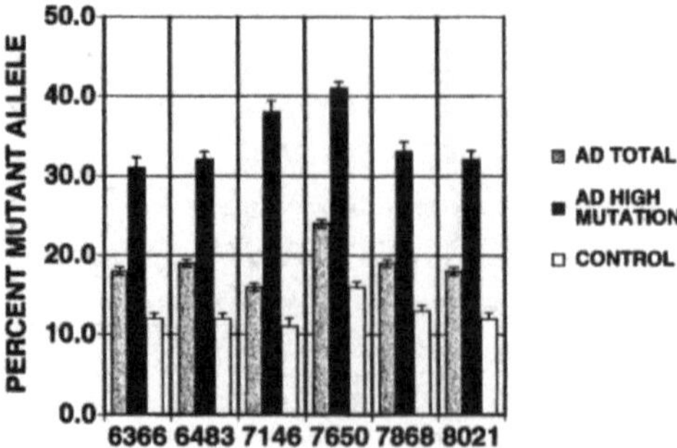

Figure 2. Intracellular generation of reactive oxygen species in AD and control cybrids. ROS was measured by the DCF-DA assay in a subset of the normal control and AD cybrids. Each bar represents the group mean percent change from the level of DCF fluorescence of parental SH-SY5Y cells (relative mean fluorescence/cell number). AD cybrids produced significantly more reactive oxygen species than control cybrids (p = 0.0007).

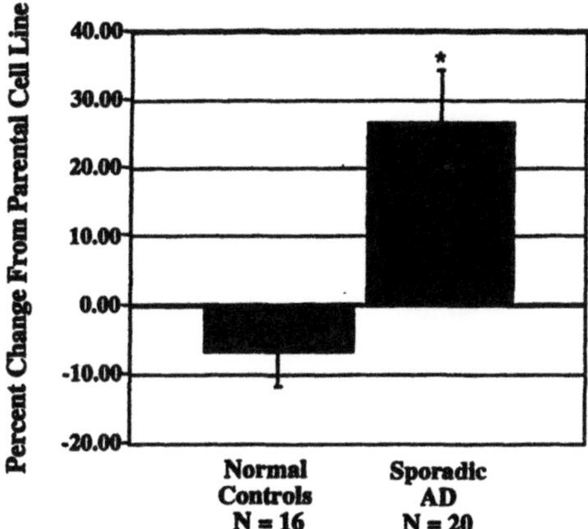

Figure 3. Nuclear pseudogene DNA/mtDNA ratios for AD patients and controls. Six nucleotide positions that distinguish the nuclear pseudogene from mtDNA were monitored by a quantitative primer extension assay. Each bar represents the group mean percentage of the polymorphic base in the nuclear pseudogene relative to the wild-type mtDNA base. Error bars represent the SEM for each group. AD total group represents 660 AD cases, and controls (N = 124) comprised cognitively normal, age matched individuals, neurologic controls and patients with NIDDM. The AD high ratio group (Å20% of all AD cases) represents those AD cases whose pseudogene DNA/mtDNA ratios exceeded those of any control case. At each site, AD cases had significantly higher levels of the mean pseudogene DNA/mtDNA ratio than controls as determined by independent t tests (p < 0.001).

primer extension assay on approximately 800 AD patients and controls revealed that the pseudogene appears at low levels in most controls, but the pseudogene to mtDNA ratio was elevated in most AD cases. Approximately 20% of AD cases can be detected with absolute specificity based on their high pseudogene to mtDNA ratios, whereas Å60% of suspected AD cases against 20% of controls can be identified at an intermediate pseudogene to mtDNA ratio threshold. The appearance of elevated pseudogene to mtDNA ratios is relatively disease specific. Elevated pseudogene to mtDNA ratios were not observed in patients with NIDDM or in neurologic controls.

Mitochondrial DNA in AD blood cells must be altered for the above disease association to hold. Preliminary evidence suggests that these changes are due to inefficient extraction of mtDNA from AD blood tissue when using heat lysis. It is likely, but not proven, that the mtDNA in AD patients is associated with membrane lipids or proteins, which is consistent with other evidence for mtDNA alterations in AD.

DISCUSSION

While a clear molecular link has yet to be established, our studies provide strong evidence that AD cybrids prepared from two different host cell lines (SY5Y and Ntera2/D1) recapitulate important features of the AD phenotype: metabolic dysfunction, focal decreases in cytochrome c oxidase activity, and increased generation of reactive oxygen species with attendant display of oxidative markers. In addition, AD cybrids show perturbations in calcium homeostasis, induction of antioxidant enzyme defense systems, and pronounced susceptibility to apoptotic stimuli. The finding that the cytochrome c oxidase defect can be transferred from AD platelets to cybrid cell lines supports the evidence that mitochondrial abnormalities are present in AD blood cells.

REFERENCES

Azari N.P.; Pettigrew K.D., Schapiro M.B., Haxby J.V., Grady C.L., Pietrini P., Salerno J.A., Heston L.L., Rapoport S.I., and Horwitz B. 1993, Early detection of Alzheimer's disease: a statistical approach using positron emission tomography. *J Cereb. Blood Flow Metab.* 13: 438–447.

Balazs, L., and Leon, M. 1994, Evidence of an oxidative challenge in the Alzheimer's brain. *Neurochem. Res.* 19: 1131–1137.

Beal, M.F. 1992, Does impairment in energy metabolism result in excitotoxic neuronal death in neurodegenerative illness. *Ann. Neurol.* 31: 119–130.

Chagnon, P., Betard, C., Robitaille, Y., Cholette, A., and Gauvreau, D. 1995, Distribution of brain cytochrome oxidase activity in various neurodegenerative diseases. *NeuroReport* 6: 711–715.

Cohen, J.J. 1993, Apoptosis. *Immunol. Today* 14: 126–130.

Cotman, C.W., and Anderson, A.J. 1995, A potential role for apoptosis in neurodegeneration and Alzheimer's disease. *Mol. Neurobiol.* 10: 19–45.

Davis, R.E., Miller, S., Herrnstadt, C., Ghosh, S.S., Fahy, E., Shinobu, L.E., Galasko, D., Thal, L.J., Beal, M.F., Howell, N., and Parker Jr, W.D. 1997, Mutations in mitochondrial cytochrome *c* oxidase genes segregate with late-onset Alzheimer disease *Proc. Natl. Acad. Sci. USA* 94:4526–4531.

Duara, R., Lopez-Alberola, R.F., Barker, W.W., Loewenstein, D.A., Zatinsky, M., Eisdorfer, C.E., and Weinberg, G.B. 1993, A comparison of familial and sporadic Alzheimer's disease. *Neurol.* 43:1377–1384.

Edland, S.D., Silverman, J., Peskind, E.R., Tsaung, D., Wijsman, E., and Morris, J.C. 1996, Increased risk of dementia in mothers of Alzheimers disease cases: Evidence for maternal inheritance. *Neurol.* 47:254–256.

Gsell, W., Conrad, R., Hickethier, M., Sofic, E., Frolich, L., Wichart, I., Jellinger, K., Moll, G., Ransmayr, G., Beckmann, H., and Riederer, P. (1995). Decreased catalase activity but unchanged superoxide dismutase activity in brains of patients with dementia of Alzheimer type. *J. Neurochem.* 64:1216–1223.

Haxby, J.V., Grady, C.L., Koss, E., Horwitz, B., Heston, L., Schapiro, M., Friedland, R.P., and Rapoport, S.I 1990, Longitudinal study of cerebral metabolic asymmetries and associated neuropsychological patterns in early dementia of the Alzheimer type. *Arch. Neurol.* 47:753–760.

Harrington, J., Park, Y.B., Babcock, D.F., and Hille, B. 1996, Dominant role of mitochondria in clearance of large Ca^{2+} loads from rat adrenal chromaffin cells. *Neuron* 16:219–228.

Herrnstadt, C., Clevenger, W., Ghosh, S.S., Anderson, C., Fahy, E., Miller, S., Thal, L.J., Beal, M.F., Howell, N. and Davis, R.E. A unique mitochondrial DNA-like sequence in the human nuclear genome: characterization of an ancient mtDNA fossil. (submitted for publication)

Hirano, M., Shtilbans, A., Mayeux, R., Davidson, M.C., DiMauro, S., Knowles, J.A. and Schon, E.A. 1997, Apparent mtDNA heteroplasmy in Alzheimer's disease patients and in normals due to PCR amplification of nucleus-embedded pseudogenes. *Proc. Natl. Acad. Sci. USA* 94:14894–14899.

Jeandel, C., Nicolas, M.B., Dubois, F., Nabet-Belleville, F., Penin, F., and Cuny, G. 1989, Lipid peroxidation and free radical scavengers in Alzheimer's disease. *Gerontology* 35:275–282.

Johns, D.R. (1995). Mitochondrial DNA and disease. *New Eng. J. Med.* 333:638–644.

Kish, S.J., Bergeron, C., Rajput, A., Dozic, S., Mastrogiacomo, F., Chang, L.J., Wilson, J.M., DiStefano, L.M., and Nobrega, J.N. 1992, Brain cytochrome oxidase in Alzheimer's disease. *J. Neurochem.* 59: 776–779.

Kluck, R.M., Bossy-Wetzel, E., Green, D.R., and Newmeyer, D.D. 1997, The release of cytochrome *c* from mitochondria: a primary site for Bcl-2 regulation of apoptosis. *Science,* 275:1132–1136.

Krige, D., Carroll, M.T., Cooper, J.M., Marsden, C.D. and Schapira, A.H.V. 1992, Platelet mitochondrial function in Parkinson's disease. *Ann. Neurol.* 32:782–788.

Kroemer, G, Petit, P., Zamzami, N., Vayssiere, J.-L., and Mignotte, B. 1995, The biochemistry of programmed cell death. *FASEB* 9:1277–1287.

Kuhl, D.E., Metter, E.J., and Riege, W.H. 1985, Patterns of cerebral glucose utilization in depression, multiple infarct dementia, and Alzheimer's disease. *Res. Publ. Assoc. Nerv. Ment. Dis.* 63: 211–226.

Levy-Lahad, E., Wasco, W., Poorkaj, P., Romano, D.M., Oshima, J., Pettingell, W.H., Yu, C., Jondro, P.D., Schmidt, S.D., Wang, K., Crowley, A.C., Fu, YH., Guenette, S.Y., Galas, D., Nemens, E., Wijsman, E.M., Bird, T.D., Schellenberg, G.D., and Tanzi, R.E. 1995a, Candidate gene for the chromosome 1 familial Alzheimer's disease locus. *Science* 269, 973–977.

Levy-Lahad, E., Wijsman, E.M., Nemens, E., Anderson, L., Goddard, K.A.B., Weber, J.L., Bird, T.D., and Schellenberg, G.D. 1995b, A familial Alzheimer's disease locus on chromosome 1. *Science* 269:970–973.

Liu, X., Kim, C.N., Yang, J., Jemmerson, R., and Wang, X. 1996, Induction of apoptotic program in cell-free extracts: requirement for dATP and cytochrome *c*. *Cell* 86:147–57.

Luft, R. 1994, The Development of Mitochondrial Medicine. *Proc. Natl. Acad. Sci. USA* 91:8731–8738.

Mecocci, P., MacGarvey, U., and Beal, M.F. 1994, Oxidative damage to mitochondrial DNA is increased in Alzheimer's disease. *Ann. Neurol.* 36:747–751.

Miller, S.M, Trimmer, P.A., Parker, W.D. and Davis, R.E. 1996, Creation and characterization of mitochondrial DNA depleted cell lines with 'neuronal-like' properties. *J. Neurochem.* 67:1897–1907.

Monaghan, P., Robertson,.D., Amos, T.A.S., Dyer, M.J.S., Mason. D.Y., and Greaves, M.F., 1992, Ultrastructural localization of the Bcl-2 protein. *J. Histochem. Cytochem.* 40:1819–1825.

Mutisya, E.M., Bowling, A.C., and Beal, M.F. 1994, Cortical cytochrome oxidase activity is reduced in Alzheimer's disease. *J. Neurochem.* 63:2179–84.

Palmer, A.M., and Burns, M.A. 1994, Selective increase in lipid peroxidation in the inferior temporal cortex in Alzheimer's disease. *Brain Res.* 645:338–342.

Pappolla, M.A., Omar, R.A., Kim, K.S., and Robakis, N.K. 1992, Immunohistochemical evidence of antioxidant stress in Alzheimer's disease. *Am. J. Pathol.* 140: 621–628.

Parker, W.D., Filley, C.M., and Parks, J.K. 1990, Cytochrome oxidase deficiency in Alzheimers disease. *Neurol.* 40:1320–1303.

Parker Jr., W.D. Mahr, N.J., and Filley, C.M. 1994, Reduced platelet cytochrome oxidase activity in Alzheimers disease. *Neurol.* 44:1086–1090.

Parker Jr., W.D., Parks, J.K, Filley, C.M., and Kleinschmidt-DeMasters, B.K. (1994). Electron transport defects in Alzheimers disease brain. *Neurol.* 44: 1090–1096.

Parker Jr., W.D., and Parks, J.K. (1995). Cytochrome *c* oxidase in Alzheimer's disease brain: Purification and characterization. *Neurol.* 45:482–486.

Payami, H., Montee, K., and Kaye, J. 1994, Evidence for familial factors that protect against dementia and outweigh the effect of increasing age. *Am. J. Hum. Genet.* 54:650–657.

Pettegrew, J.W., Klunk, W.E., Panchalingam, K., Kanfer, J.N., and McClure, R.J. 1994, Alterations of cerebral metabolism in probable Alzheimer's disease. *Neurobiol. of Aging* 15:117–132.

Pettegrew, J.W., Klunk, W.E., Kanal, E., Panchalingam, K., and McClure, R.J. 1995, Changes in brain membrane phospholipid and high-energy phosphate metabolism precede dementia. *Neurobiol. of Aging* 16: 973–975.

Reed, J.C. 1994, *J. Cell Biol.* 124, 1–6.

Schapira, A.H., Mann, V.M., Cooper, J.M., Krige, D., Jenner, P.J. and Marsden, P.J. 1992, Mitochondrial function in Parkinson's disease. *Ann. Neurol.* 32:S116-S124

Schellenberg, G.D., Bird, T.D., Wijsman, E.M., Orr, H.T., Anderson, L., Nemens, E., White, J.A., Bonnycastle, L., Weber, J.L., Alonos, M.E., Potter, H., Heston, L.L., and Martin, G.M. 1992, Genetic linkage evidence for a familial Alzheimer's disease locus on chromosome 14. *Science* 258:668–671.

Schinder, A.F., Olson, E.C., Spitzer, N.C. and Montal, M. 1996, Mitochondrial Dysfunction is a primary event in glutamate toxicity. *J. Neurosci.* 16:6125–6133

Schweers, O., Mandelkow, E.-M., Biernat, J., and Mandelkow, E. 1995, Oxidation of cysteine-322 in the repeat domain of microtubule-associated protein tau controls the in vitro assembly of paired helical filaments. *Proc Natl Acad Sci USA* 92:8463–8467.

Sheehan, J. P., Swerdlow, R. H., Miller, S. W., Davis, R. E., Parks, J. K., Parker, W. D., and Tuttle, J. B. 1997, Calcium homeostasis and reactive oxygen species production in cells transformed by mitochondria from individuals with sporadic Alzheimer's disease. *J. Neurosci.* 17:4612–4622.

Silverman, J.M., Li, G., Zaccario, M.L., Smith, C.J., Schmeidler, J., Mohs, R.C., and Davis, K.L. (1994a). Patterns of Risk in First-Degree Relatives of Patients with Alzheimer's disease. *Arch. Gen. Psychiat.* 51: 577–586.

Silverman, J.M., Raiford, K., Edland, S., Fillenbaum, G., Morris, J.C., Clark, C.M., Kukull, W., and Heyman, A. (1994b). The Consortium to Establish a Registry for Alzheimer's Disease (CERAD). Part VI. Family history assessment: A multicenter study of first-degree relatives of Alzheimer's disease probands and nondemented spouse controls. *Neurol.* 44:1253–1259.

Smale, G., Nichols, N.R., Brady, D.R., Finch, C.E., and Horton Jr., W.E. 1995, Evidence for apoptotic cell death in Alzheimer's disease. *Exptl. Neurol.* 133:225–230.

Smith, M.A., Perry, G., Richey, P.L., Sayre, L.M., Anderson, V.M., Beal, M.F., and Kowall, N. 1996, Oxidative damage in Alzheimer's Disease. *Nature* 382:120–121.

St George-Hyslop, P.H. Haines, J.L., Farrer, L.A., Van Broeckhoven, C., Goate, A., Crapper McLachlan, D.R., Orr, H., Bruni, A.C., Sorbi, S., Rainero, I., Foncin, J.-F., Pollen, D., Cantu, J.-M., Tupler, R., Voskresenskaya, N., Mayeux, R., Growdon, J., Fried, V.A., Myers, R.H., Nee, L., Backhovens, H., Martin, J.-J., Rosser, M., Owen, M.J., Mullan, M., Percy, M.E., Karlinsky, H., Rich, S., Heston, L., Montesi, M., Mortilla, M., Nacmias, N., Gusella, J.F., Hardy, J.A., and other members of the FAD Collaborative Study group. 1990, Genetic linkage studies suggest that Alzheimer's disease is not a single homogeneous disorder. *Nature* 347:194–197.

Swerdlow, R.H., Parks, J.K., Cassarino, B.S., Maguire, D.J., Maguire, R.S., Bennett, J.P., Davis, R.E. and Parker Jr., W.D. 1997, Cybrids in Alzheimer's disease: a cellular model of the disease? *Neurol.* 49:918–925.

Wallace, D.C., Stugard, C., Murdock, D., Schurr, T. and Brown, M.D. 1997, Ancient mtDNA sequences in the human nuclear genome: a potential source of errors in identifying pathogenic mutations. *Proc. Natl. Acad. Sci. USA* 94:14900–14905.

Yang, J., Liu, X., Bhalla, K., Kim, C.N., Ibrado, A.M., Cai, J., Peng, T.-I., Jones, D.P. and Wang, X. 1997, Prevention of apoptosis by Bcl-2: release of cytochrome *c* from mitochondria blocked. *Science* 275:1129–1132.

Zamzami, N., Marchetti, P., Castedo, M., Decaudin, D., Macho, A., Hirsch, T., Susin, S., Petit, P., Mignotte, B., and Kroemer, G. 1995a, Sequential reduction of mitochondrial transfembrane potential and generation of reactive oxygen species in early programmed cell death. *J. Exp. Med.* 182:367–377.

Zamzami, N., Marchetti, P., Castedo, M., Zanin, C., Vayssiere, JL., Petit, P.X., and Kroemer, G. 1995b, Reduction in mitochondrial potential constitutes an early irreversible step of programmed lymphocyte death in vivo. *J. Exp. Med.* 181:1661–1672.

11

MITOCHONDRIAL DYSFUNCTION IN PARKINSON'S DISEASE

Potential Applications for Cybrid Modeling of the Disease

Russell H. Swerdlow,[1] Janice K. Parks,[1] Scott W. Miller,[2] John N. Davis II,[1] Patricia A. Trimmer,[1] Jeremy B. Tuttle,[1] James P. Bennett,[1] G. Frederick Wooten,[1] Robert E. Davis,[2] and W. Davis Parker[1]

[1]Center for the Study of Neurodegenerative Diseases and
Department of Neurology, Box 394
University of Virginia Health Sciences Center
Charlottesville, Virginia 22908
[2]MitoKor
11494 Sorrento Valley Rd.
San Diego, California 92121

INTRODUCTION

In 1983, Langston et al. determined that a recreational opiate contaminant, *N*-methyl-4-phenyl-1,2,3,6-tetrahydropyridine (MPTP), was responsible for an epidemic of parkinsonism in a group of California drug addicts (Langston et al., 1983). Two years later, Nicklas and Heikkila showed that 1-methyl-4-phenyl pyridinium (MPP+), a pyridine metabolite of MPTP, inhibited the mitochondrial electron transport chain (ETC) enzyme NADH:ubiquinone oxidoreductase (complex I) (Nicklas and Heikkila, 1985). Relevance of this finding to those with idiopathic Parkinson's disease (PD) was established in 1989, when several groups announced Parkinson's disease patients also manifested complex I abnormalities (Parker et al., 1989; Schapira et al., 1989; Mizuno et al., 1989).

Distribution of Complex I Dysfunction in PD

The tissue distribution of complex I dysfunction in PD patients was initially controversial. Schapira et al. proposed that PD complex I dysfunction was limited to substantia nigra (Schapira et al., 1990), even though Parker et al. observed a complex I defect in enriched mitochondria from PD platelets (Parker et al., 1989). Support for a nigra-limited complex I defect was provided by the London group (Mann et al., 1992), who studied PD patient complex I activity in crude platelet homogenates rather than enriched platelet mitochondria and did not find a defect. Additional support for a nigra-limited defect came from the study of Schapira et al. who assayed complex I activity in multiple regions of PD brain but only found a relative (to control brain) defect in substantia nigra (Schapira et al., 1990). Assays in this brain study also used crude tissue homogenates instead of enriched mitochondria.

The study of Krige et al. underscored the technical shortcomings of assaying ETC activities in crude homogenates. When the London group again assayed complex I activity in PD platelet mitochondria, this time using an enriched mitochondrial fraction, a complex I defect was detected. Multiple studies from multiple laboratories now confirm the finding of Parker et al. that complex I is defective in PD platelet mitochondria (Krige et al., 1992; Yoshino et al., 1992; Benecke et al., 1993; Haas et al., 1995). Unfortunately, no standardized method for assaying PD platelet complex I activity has emerged, and negative PD platelet complex I studies using different methods continue to enter the literature (Blake et al., 1997). These studies do not refute the positive studies because methodology is not comparable. Potential pitfalls encountered in our experience include the use of decylubiquinone (DB) as a coenzyme Q analog instead of Q1 and the addition of bovine serum albumin to the spectrophotometric assay, which minimize differences between PD and control complex I activities clearly present when measured by other methods. Failure to detect PD platelet complex I dysfunction in these studies appears more consistent with methodological complications than the lack of a complex I defect in mitochondria from this tissue.

Methodologic issues also complicate the question of whether complex I dysfunction is present in PD muscle. Multiple studies demonstrate the presence of complex I dysfunction in this tissue in PD patients (Bindoff et al., 1991; Shoffner et al., 1991; Nakagawa-Hattori et al., 1992; Cardellach et al., 1993; Blin et al., 1994). Some studies failed to find a complex I defect in this tissue, but as in the platelet literature, methodology in these negative studies was unique to these studies or else not described in adequate detail to allow for comparison and so do not refute the positive studies (Mann et al., 1992; Anderson et al., 1993; DiDonato et al., 1993). Finally, there is the study of Mytilineau et al. demonstrating complex I dysfunction in fibroblasts from PD patients (Mytelineau et al., 1994) and the study of Barroso et al. (Barroso et al., 1993) reporting a complex I defect in PD lymphocytes. Overall, data support the presence of complex I dysfunction in multiple tissues of PD patients, and complex I dysfunction in PD most likely represents a systemic defect. The presence of complex I dysfunction in non-degenerating tissues indicates this observed enzymatic defect is unlikely to be occurring as a consequence of tissue degeneration. Taken with the observation that toxic complex I inhibition by MPP+ causes a clinical and pathological PD-like syndrome (Langston et al., 1983; Forno et al., 1986), a primary role for complex I dysfunction in PD is envisioned.

Mitochondrial DNA in Parkinson's Disease

A potential role for mutation of mitochondrial DNA (mtDNA) in the PD complex I defect was initially proposed by Parker and co-investigators (1989). Mitochondrial DNA codes for seven of the 41 known subunits of complex I. Furthermore, mtDNA, like most idiopathic PD, does not follow the rules of Mendelian inheritance. Mutation of mtDNA leading to complex I dysfunction is thus consistent with the epidemiology of PD.

Initial studies of mtDNA mutation in PD concentrated on the search for large scale deletions, particularly the so-called "common deletion". An early report from Ikebe et al.

found the proportion of mtDNA genomes containing the common deletion to be increased in PD brain relative to control brain (Ikebe et al., 1990). Subsequent studies suggested that this deletion was not quantifiably different between PD and control brains and therefore both this deletion and other deletions of significant size were not likely to account for the complex I defect of PD (Schapira et al., 1990; Lestienne et al., 1990; Lestienne et al., 1991; Mann et al., 1992; Sandy et al., 1993; DiDonato et al., 1993).

Shoffner et al. used a restriction fragment length polymorphism strategy to screen for mtDNA mutations in PD and Alzheimer's disease (AD) subjects. Despite the fact that less than 10% of the mitochondrial genome was surveyed, a missense point mutation in a tRNA gene (tRNA^{Gln}, nucleotide pair 4336) was found to exist in higher amounts in a group of AD/PD patients than in control patients (Shoffner et al., 1993). More recently, Ikebe et al. sequenced mtDNA complex I genes in five PD patients and found point mutations in all five (Ikebe et al., 1995).

Swerdlow et al. used cytoplasmic hybrids (cybrids) to screen for mtDNA mutation in sporadic PD subjects (Swerdlow et al., 1996). Briefly, a human neuroblastoma cell line was depleted of endogenous mtDNA to form ñ⁰ cells. Mitochondria (and hence mtDNA) from PD subjects was then transferred to these ñ⁰ cells to form unique cybrid cell lines that express the transferred mitochondrial genes. Control cybrid lines were also created using mtDNA from age-matched control subjects. This system allows for controlling of nuclear genetic and environmental input between PD and control subjects because nuclear DNA is clonal (the same) between cybrid lines and all cybrid lines are handled identically. At the genetic level cybrids differ only in that their mtDNA is derived from different individuals. Therefore, phenotypic/biochemical differences observed between cell lines is most consistent with differences in mtDNA.

Twenty four PD cybrid lines and 28 control cybrid lines were created and complex I activity was assayed spectrophotometrically. Complex I activity was decreased in the PD cybrid group relative to the control cybrid group (Figure 1). This finding is most consistent with abberation of PD mtDNA, since transfer of complex I dysfunction to this system was associated with transfer of mtDNA from PD subjects. Complex IV activity was not significantly decreased, suggesting the genetic defect was restricted to one or a combination of the seven complex I encoding genes of mtDNA.

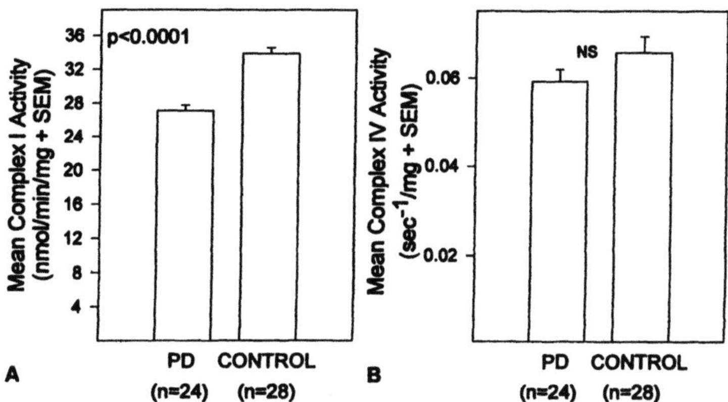

Figure 1. A complex I defect transfers to cybrid cell lines with mtDNA from PD subjects (A). Complex IV activities in PD cybrids are not significantly reduced (B).

Cybrids in PD: A Potential Model for the Disease?

The magnitude of the catalytic defect observed in our PD cybrids was small. Compared to control cybrids, PD cybrid complex I activity was reduced by only 20%. This is comparable to the magnitude of the complex I defect observed in some studies showing complex I dysfunction in non-nigral tissues of PD subjects (Krige et al., 1992; Yoshino et al., 1992; Cardellach et al., 1993; Haas et al., 1995). It is possible that the magnitude of the complex I defect in PD platelets is not as great as that of brain, a post mitotic tissue in which defective mtDNA may accumulate over time. Regardless, the PD cybrid complex I defect does confer substantial functional consequences to the cybrid cells that express it.

Mitochondria are important sites of free radical generation, ETC dysfunction is associated with increased free radical production, and evidence of oxidative stress is observed in PD patients (Dexter et al., 1994; Sanchez-Ramos et al., 1994). We hypothesized that the apparent mtDNA-determined complex I defect could act as a free radical generator. To test this, we incubated control and PD cybrid lines with 2′,7′-dichlorodihydroflourescein diacetate (DCFDA), a dye which flouresces in the presence of reactive oxygen species (ROS). As a group, DCFDA flourescence was higher in the PD cybrid group, indicating the PD mtDNA-encoded complex I product acted as a genetically determined free radical generator (Figure 2). Increased ROS production thus represents an important gain-of-function consequence of the complex I PD defect, at least in our cybrid system. This increase was observed despite the presence of a significant increase in free radical scavenging enzymes in PD cybrids (glutathione reductase and peroxidase; total, Mn-dependent, and Cu/Zn dependent superoxide dismutase; and catalase), thereby recapitulating to some extent oxidative pathology in PD patients (Martilla et al., 1988; Saggu et al., 1989; Kalra et al., 1992; Damier et al., 1993).

PD cybrids also exhibit impaired calcium homeostasis (Sheehan et al., 1997). Mitochondria, together with endoplasmic reticulum and plasma membrane transporters, play an important role in cellular calcium buffering. In neurons, mitochondria appear to help regulate even mild to moderate cytosolic calcium fluctuations (Werth and Thayer, 1994). We incubated PD and control cybrids in the presence of fura-2, a dye which flouresces in the

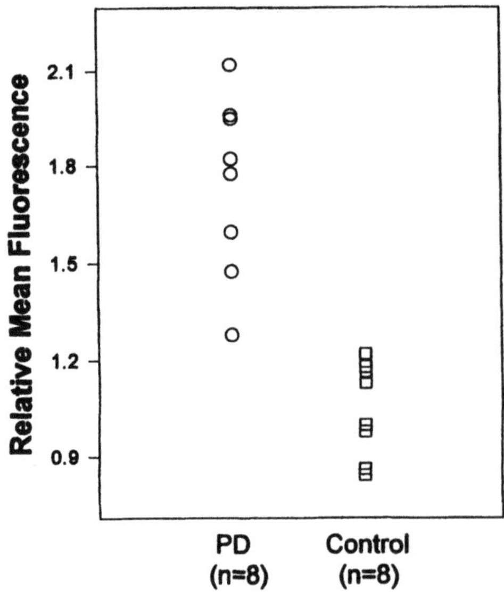

Figure 2. As shown by DCFDA fluorescence, ROS generation is increased in PD cybrids. Fluorescence shown is relative to that of native SH-SY5Y neuroblastoma cells.

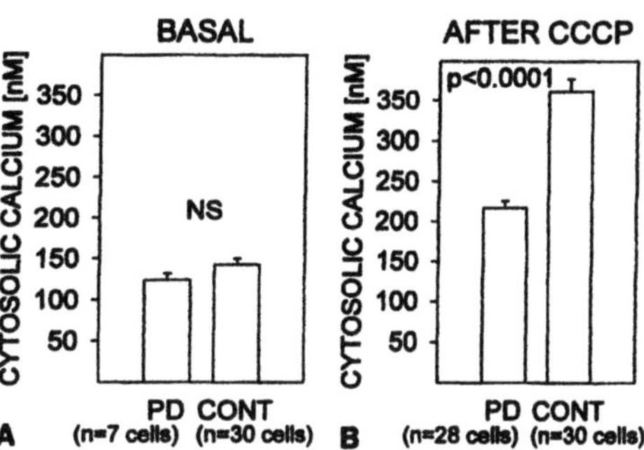

Figure 3. In the basal state, cytosolic calcium concentrations are equivalent between PD and control cybrids as shown by fura-2 imaging (A). However, the same experiment performed following CCCP exposure reveals that mitochondrial calcium sequestration in this basal state is reduced in PD cybrids, since following CCCP exposure PD cybrid cytosolic calcium increased less than control cybrid cytosolic calcium (B).

presence of cytosolic calcium. Basal cytosolic calcium levels were equivalent in the non-manipulated state. Following exposure to the ETC uncoupler carbonyl cyanide m-chlorophenylhydrazone (CCCP), which eliminates the mitochondrial membrane potential and causes efflux of sequestered matrix calcium, cytosolic calcium was higher in the control cybrid lines. This indicates that PD mitochondrial calcium sequestration was diminished, presumably as a consequence of the mtDNA-determined complex I defect in these cells (Figure 3).

In addition to alterations of basal cytosolic calcium homeostasis, dynamic calcium handling was impaired in PD cybrids. Cybrids were exposed to carbachol, a cholinergic agonist which binds to acetylcholine receptors and causes an IP3 mediated calcium signalling transient. The generated cytosolic calcium "spike" is removed via transport of calcium to other compartments. In PD cybrids, elimination of cytosolic calcium was diminished following carbachol exposure. We determined that this was due to decreased mitochondrial calcium buffering. The mtDNA-determined PD complex I defect therefore effects the ability of cells to respond to neurotransmitter induced, receptor mediated calcium signalling transients. Since impairments of calcium signalling can play a role in programmed cell death (Nicotera and Orrenius, 1992: Hartley et al., 1993; Oshimi and Miyazaki, 1995), we believe this is another pathway by which a primary bioenergetic defect (complex I dysfunction) contributes to neurodegeneration in PD.

The genetically determined complex I defect observed in our PD cybrids also conferred increased susceptibility to the toxin MPP+. PD and control cybrid lines were exposed to MPP+ at varying concentrations and durations. Resultant cybrid cell death was consistently higher in the PD cybrids compared to control cybrids. This indicates that toxins may still play an important role in the development of PD, especially in persons carrying the specific complex I defect seen in our PD cybrids. A genetic-toxin interaction such as this one may explain why some persons exposed to a given toxin at a particular concentration and for a particular duration develop PD whereas others exposed to the same toxin under similar conditions do not.

Mitochondrial ultrastructure was also altered in PD cybrids. Electron microscopy studies revealed that PD cybrid mean mitochondrial size was larger than that of control cybrids. Therefore, even though the magnitude of the complex I defect was small in PD cybrids, mitochondria were adversely effected by the genetically determined complex I defect as shown by a number of physiologic and anatomic measures. The relevance of complex I catalytic dysfunction to PD neurodegeneration, even if it is as small in brain *in vivo* as it is in our PD cybrids, should not be underestimated. The functional consequences resulting from this abnormal enzyme, even when the catalytic defect is small, are substantial. There is precedence for this phenomenon. Transgenic mice expressing the G37R superoxide dismutase (SOD) mutation develop ALS pathology, despite the fact that their SOD catalytic activity is normal (Wong et al., 1995). We propose that even if complex I catalytic activity in a PD patient is comparable to activity in non-PD subjects, the enzyme may not necessarily be normal and may still contribute to neurodegeneration in that person.

To further consider the relationship of defect magnitude to disease relevance, it is important to note that individual cybrid line mtDNA subclones were not selected for analysis in these experiments. The advantage of treating all subclones generated within a given line as part of an overall cybrid line population is that it helps avoid subclone selection bias while still addressing the question of whether mtDNA defects are or are not transferred from a given mtDNA donor. This strategy does not, however, address the potential mtDNA heteroplasmic variation that may exist from cell to cell. Some cells within a cybrid line may indeed carry a substantial complex I catalytic defect that is not readily apparent when the complex I activities from all the cells of a line are averaged. This phenomenon requires consideration since the distribution of complex I dysfunction between individual PD neurons *in vivo* is unknown. If a population of neurons crippled by severe complex I dysfunction were assayed together with neurons exhibiting little-to-absent dysfunction, only a mild to moderate defect would be apparent. Under such circumstances it would be a mistake to declare the observed defect irrelevant because of its overall low magnitude.

Origin of Complex I mtDNA Mutation(s)

The mutation rate of mtDNA is higher than that of nuclear DNA (Linnane et al., 1989). The proximity of mtDNA to a site of free radical generation could also contribute to somatic mutation/degradation of the genome. It is possible that mtDNA is degraded or mutated as a consequence or epiphenomenon of an independent primary PD pathophysiologic process, and that the mitochondrial pathophysiology observed in our cybrid system is simply an effect of the disease and not a cause. We think that this explanation is unlikely. The use of platelets instead of brain as mtDNA donors in the aforementioned experiments makes tissue degeneration an unlikely causative factor in our cybrid system. The finding that activity of cytochrome c oxidase, another ETC enzyme with mtDNA encoded subunits, was not significantly depressed in PD cybrids is not consistent with random degradation of the mitochondrial genome. As was already discussed, PD mtDNA does not appear to carry large scale deletions. The most likely mutation(s) responsible for the PD complex I defect are therefore point mutation(s) in one or a combination of the seven ND genes of mtDNA.

PD epidemiology further argues that the cybrid-implied mtDNA mutation(s) are not somatic. A recent study by Wooten et al. found a maternal inheritance bias in PD when probands with both an affected sibling and parent were considered (Wooten et al., 1997). This strategy screens for PD cohorts that are not large enough to demonstrate clear Mendelian inheritance patterns, yet are not truly "sporadic" and appear to have a genetic etiology. In this study, the likelihood that the proband's affected parent was the mother was greater than what should have been observed by chance. This is consistent with the presence of a maternally transmitted genetic factor (mtDNA). Somatic mtDNA mutations cannot account for this observation.

We studied a family in which PD is present in multiple family members over three generations (Wooten et al., 1997). While the pedigree does not rule out the presence of a Mendelian genetic factor, it is notable that in each generation the disease is passed through maternal lines. We prepared cybrids from 15 members of this family encompassing two generations. Eight cybrids were constructed using mitochondrial genes from family members descended through female lineages and seven cybrid lines were constructed using mitochondrial genes from family members descended through male lineages. Complex I activity in the maternal descendents was significantly lower than that of the paternal descendents, suggesting the presence of non-somatic, inherited mutation of mtDNA. Although the techniques used are different from those employed in linkage studies of Mendelian genes in human disease, the end result is the same—localization of a genetic defect to a particular stretch of DNA (in this case mtDNA).

SUMMARY

We propose that the PD complex I defect is systemic and that in sporadic PD it arises from mutation of mtDNA. We further propose that this genetic ETC defect results from inherited rather than somatic mutation of the mitochondrial genome. This genetically determined bioenergetic defect is responsible for both loss-of-function and gain-of-function consequences that are relevant to neurodegenerative pathophysiology. Epidemiologic studies suggest an etiologic role for mtDNA mutation in sporadic PD. The cybrid strategy appears useful for studying PD pathophysiology. However, definitive validation of the results of cybrid methodology in PD basic research will result only upon demonstration of actual specific mtDNA sequence alterations in PD patients, and after drugs ameliorating mitochondrially-related pathophysiology in cybrids are shown to benefit persons with the disease.

REFERENCES

Anderson J.J., Bravi D., Ferrari R., Davis T.L., Baronti F., Chase T.N., Dagani F., 1993, No evidence for altered muscle mitochondrial function in Parkinson's disease. *J. Neurol. Neurosurg. Psych.* 56:477–480.

Barroso N., Campos Y., Huertas R., Esteban J., Molina J.A., Alonso A., Gutierrezrivas E., Arenas J., 1993, Respiratory chain enzyme activities in lymphocytes from untreated patients with Parkinson disease. *Clin. Chem.* 39:667–669.

Benecke R., Strumper P. Weiss H., 1993, Electron transfer complexes I and IV of platelets are abnormal in Parkinson's disease but normal in Parkinson-plus syndromes. *Brain* 116:1451–1455.

Bindoff L.A., Birch-Machin M.A., Cartlidge N.E., Parker W.D. Jr., Turnbull D.M., 1991, Respiratory chain abnormalities in skeletal muscle from patients with Parkinson's disease. *J. Neurol. Sci.* 104:203–208.

Blin O., Desnuelle C., Rascol O., Borg M., Peyro Saint Paul H., Azulay J.P., Bille F., Figarella D., Coulom F., Pellissier J.F., Montastruc J.L., Chatel M., Serratrice G., 1994, Mitochondrial respiratory failure in skeletal muscle from patients with Parkinson's disease and multiple system atrophy. *J. Neurol. Sci.* 125:95–101.

Blake C.I., Spitz E., Leehey M., Hoffer B.J., Boyson S.J., 1997, Platelet mitochondrial respiratory chain function in Parkinson's disease. *Mov. Dis.* 12:3–8.

Cardellach F., Marti M.J., Fernandez-Sola J., Marin C., Hoek J.B., Tolosa E., Urbano-Marquez A., 1993, Mitochondrial respiratory chain activity in skeletal muscle from patients with Parkinson's disease. *Neurology* 43:2258–2262.

Damier P., Hirsch E.C., Zhang P., Agid Y., Javoy-Agid F., 1993, Glutathione peroxidase, glial cells and Parkinson's disease. *Neuroscience* 52:1–6.

Dexter D.T., Holley A. E., Flitter W.D., Slater T.F., Wells F.R., Daniel S.E., Lees A.J., Jenner P., Marsden C.D., 1994, Increased levels of lipid hydroperoxides in the Parkinsonian substantia nigra: an HPLC and ESR study. *Mov. Dis.* 9:92–97.

DiDonato S., Zeviani M., Giovannini P., Savarese N., Rimoldi M., Mariotti C., Girotti F., Caraceni T., 1993, Respiratory chain and mitochondrial DNA in muscle and brain in Parkinson's disease patients. *Neurology* 43:2262–2268.

Forno L.S., Langston J.W., DeLanney, Irwin I., Ricuarte G.A., 1986, Locus ceruleus lesions and eosinophilic inclusions in MPTP-treated monkeys. *Ann. Neurol.* 20:449–455.

Haas R.H., Nasirian F., Nakano K., Ward D., Pay M., Hill R., Shults C.W., 1995, Low platelet mitochondrial complex I and complex II/III activity in early untreated Parkinson's disease. *Ann. Neurol.* 37:714–722.

Hartley D.M., Kurth M.C., Bjerkness L., Weiss J.H., Choi D.W., 1993, Glutamate receptor-induced $^{45}Ca^{2+}$ accumulation in cortical cell culture correlates with subsequent neuronal degeneration. *J. Neurosci.* 13:1993–2000.

Ikebe S.I., Tanaka M., Ohno K., Sato W., Hattori K., Kondo T., Mizuno Y., Ozawa T, 1990, Increase of deleted mitochondrial DNA in the striatum in Parkinson's disease and sensescence. *Biochem. Biophys. Res. Comm.* 170:1044–1048.

Ikebe S.I., Tanaka M., Ozawa T., 1995, Point mutations of mitochondrial genome in Parkinson's disease. *Mol. Brain Res.* 28:281–295.

Kalra J., Rajput A.H., Mantha S.V., Prasad K., 1992, Serum antioxidant enzyme activity in Parkinson's disease. *Mol. Cell. Biochem.* 110:165–168.

Krige D., Carrol M.T., Cooper J.M., Marsden C.D., Schapira A.H.V., 1992, Platelet mitochondrial function in Parkinson's disease. The Royal Kings and Queens Parkinson Disease Research Group. *Ann. Neurol.* 32:782–788.

Langston J.W., Ballard P.A., Tetrud J.W., Irwin I., 1983, Chronic parkinsonism in humans due to a product of meperidine-analog synthesis. *Science* 219:979–980.

Lestienne P., Nelson J., Riederer P., Jellinger K., Reichmann H., 1990, Normal mitochondrial genome in brain from patients with Parkinson's disease and complex I defect. *J. Neurochem.* 55:1810–1812.

Lestienne P., Nelson I., Reiderer P., Reichmann H., Jellinger K., 1991, Mitochondrial DNA in postmortem brain from patients with Parkinson's disease. *J. Neurochem.* 56:1819.

Linnane A.W., Marzuki S., Ozawa T., Tanaka M., 1990, Mitochondrial DNA mutations as an important contributor to aging and degenerative diseases. *Lancet* 1(8639):642–645.

Mann V.M., Cooper J.M., Krige D., Daniel S.E., Schapira A.H., Marsden C.D., 1992, Brain, skeletal muscle and platelet homogenate mitochondrial function in Parkinson's disease. *Brain* 115:333–342.

Mann V.M., Cooper J.M., Schapira A.H.V., 1992, Quantitation of a mitochondrial DNA deletion in Parkinson's disease. *FEBS* 299:218–222.

Mizuno Y., Ohta S., Tanaka M., Takamiya S., Suzuki K., Sato T., Oya H., Ozawa T., Kagawa Y., 1989, Deficiencies in complex I subunits of the respiratory chain in Parkinson's disease. *Biochem. Biophys. Res. Commun.* 163:1450–1455.

Mytilineou C., Werner P., Molinari S., Di Roco A., Cohen G., Yahr M.D., 1994, Impaired oxidative decarboxylation of pyruvate in fibroblasts from patients with Parkinson's disease. *J. Neural. Transm.* 8:223–228.

Martilla R.J., Lorentz H., Rinne U.K., 1988, Oxygen toxicity protecting enzymes in Parkinson's disease. Increase of superoxide dismutase-like activity in the substantia nigra and basal nucleus. *J. Neurol. Sci.* 86:321–331.

Nakagawa-Hattori Y., Yoshino H., Kondo T., Mizuno Y., Horai S., 1992, Is Parkinson's disease a mitochondrial disorder? *J. Neurol. Sci.* 107:22–33.

Nicklas W.J., Heikkila R.E., 1985, Inhibition of NADH-linked oxidation in brain mitochondria by 1-methyl-4-phenylpyridine, a metabolite of the neurotoxin, 1-methyl-4-phenyl-1,2,3,6-tetrahydropyridine. *Life Sci.* 36:2503–2508.

Nicotera P. and Orrenius S., 1992, Calcium and death. *Ann. N.Y. Acad. Sci.* 648:17–27.

Oshimi Y. and Miyazaki S., 1995, Fas antigen-mediated DNA fragmentation and apoptotic morphologic changes are regulated by elevated cytosolic Ca^{2+} level. *J. Immunol.* 154:599–609.

Parker W.D., Boyson S.J., Parks J.K., 1989, Electron transport chain abnormalities in idiopathicParkinson's disease. *Ann. Neurol.* 26:719–723.

Saggu H., Cooksey J., Dexter D., Wells F.R., Lees A., Jenner P., Marsden C.D., 1989, A selective increase in particulate superoxide dismutase activity in parkinsonian substantia nigra. *J. Neurochem.* 53:692–697.

Sanchez-Ramos J.R., Overvik E., Ames B.N., 1994, A marker of oxyradical-mediated DNA damage (8-hydroxy-2'deoxyguanosine) is increased in nigro-striatum of Parkinson's disease brain. *Neurodegeneration* 3:197–204.

Sandy M.S., Langston J.W., Smith M.T., Di Monte D.A., 1993, PCR analysis of platelet mt DNA: Lack of specific changes in Parkinson's disease. *Mov. Dis.* 8:74–82.

Schapira A.H.V., Cooper J.M., Dexter D., Jenner P., Clark J.B., Marsden C.D., 1989, Mitochondrial complex I deficiency in Parkinson's disease. *Lancet* i: 1289.

Schapira A.H.V., Mann V.M., Cooper J.M., Dexter D., Daniel S.E., Jenner P., Clark J.B., Marsden C.D., 1990, Anatomic and disease specificity of NADH CoQ$_1$ Reductase (Complex I) deficiency in Parkinson's disease. *J. Neurochem.* 55:2142–2145.

Schapira A.H.V., Cooper J.M., Dexter D.,Clark J.B., Jenner P., Marsden C.D., 1990, Mitochondrial complex I deficiency in Parkinson's disease. *J. Neurochem.* 54: 823–827.

Schapira A.H.V., Holt I.J., Sweeney M., Harding A.E., Jenner P., Marsden C.D., 1990, Mitochondrial DNA analysis in Parkinson's disease. *Mov. Dis.* 5 294–297.

Sheehan J.P., Swerdlow R.H., Parker W.D., Miller S.W., Davis R.E., Tuttle J.B., 1997, Altered calcium homeostasis in cells transformed by mitochondria from individuals with Parkinson's disease. *J. Neurochem.* 68:1221–1233.

Shoffner J.M., Watts R.L., Juncos J.L., Torroni A., Wallace D.C., 1991, Mitochondrial oxidative phosphorylation defects in Parkinson's disease. *Ann. Neurol.* 30:332–339.

Shoffner J.M., Brown M.D., Torroni A., Lott M.T., Cabell M.F., Mirra S.S., Beal M.F., Yang C.C., Gearing M., Salvo R., Watts R.L., Juncos J.L., Hansen L.A., Crain B. J., Fayad M., Reckord C.L., Wallace D.C., 1993, Mitochondrial DNA variants observed in Alzheimer disease and Parkinson disease patients. *Genomics* 17:171–184.

Swerdlow R.H., Parks J.K., Miller S.W., Tuttle J.B., Trimmer P.A., Sheehan J.P., Bennett J.P., Davis R.E., Parker W.D., 1996, Origin and functional consequences of the complex I defect in Parkinson's disease. *Ann. Neurol.* 40:663–671.

Werth J.L. and Thayer S.A., 1994, Mitochondria buffer physiological calcium loads in cultured rat dorsal ganglion neurons. *J. Neurosci.* 14:348–356.

Wong P.C., Pardo C.A., Borchelt D.R., Lee M.K., Copeland N.G., Jenkins N.A., Sisodia S.S., Cleveland D.W., Price D.L., 1995, An adverse property of familial ALS-linked SOD1 mutation causes motor neuron disease characterized by vacuolar degeneration of mitochondria. *Neuron* 14:1105–1116.

Wooten G.F., Currie L.J., Bennett J.P., Harrison M.B., Trugman J.M., Parker W.D. Jr., 1997, Maternal inheritance in Parkinson's disease. *Ann. Neurol.* 41:265–268.

Wooten G.F., Currie L.J., Bennett J.P., Trugman J.M., Harrison M.B., 1997, Maternal inheritance in two large kindreds with Parkinson's disease. *Neurology* 48:A333.

Yoshino H., Nakagawa-Hattori Y., Kondo T., Mizuno Y., 1992, Mitochondrial complex I and II activities of lymphocytes and platelets in Parkinson's disease. *J. Neural. Transm.* 41:27–34.

12

NEURONAL OXIDATIVE STRESS IS A COMMON FEATURE OF ALZHEIMER'S AND PARKINSON'S DISEASES

George Perry and Mark A. Smith

Institute of Pathology
Case Western Reserve University
2085 Adelbert Road, Cleveland, Ohio 44106

INTRODUCTION

One of the most striking features of the intraneuronal inclusions of Alzheimer (AD) and Parkinson (PD) diseases is that, although they are derived from the neuronal cytoskeleton, they are fundamentally altered. Among these alterations is their insolubility in denaturants (Selkoe et al., 1982; Galloway et al., 1992) and it is our contention that the elucidation of the posttranslational modifications responsible for insolubilization will provide a fundamental insight into the cytopathology of AD and PD.

ROLE OF POSTTRANSLATIONAL MODIFICATION IN INSOLUBILITY

Extensive phosphorylation of τ protein (Grundke-Iqbal et al., 1986) and neurofilaments (Sternberger and Sternberger, 1983) found in neuronal inclusions provided a putative link between insolubilization and abnormalities in kinases (Trojanowski et al., 1993). Unfortunately, the role of increased phosphorylation and insolubilization is complex. First, the phosphorylation of cytoskeletal proteins found in inclusions is not abnormal but rather part of the normal pattern of axonal metabolism (Sternberger and Sternberger, 1983; Goedert et al., 1993; Matsuo et al., 1994). Therefore, terms such as "hyper-" or "aberrant" phosphorylation which imply a nonphysiological process are misleading. Instead, the phosphorylation associated with the inclusions in AD and PD is quite similar, if not identical, to that found normally and differs only in location, occurring in the cell body rather than in the axon (Sternberger et al., 1985). Further, phosphorylation of τ protein is not an absolute requirement for its incorporation into the inclusion since non-phosphorylated τ is also present in NFT (Bondareff et al., 1995). Finally, NFT insolubility persists even following complete dephosphorylation (Smith et al., 1996a). Therefore, overall, these findings suggest that the relationship between phosphorylation and NFT formation is indirect, i.e., phosphorylation acts to free τ protein from its role in stabilizing microtubules and to instead promote τ protein self-assembly into the abnormal filaments of NFT. Indeed, it is likely that phosphorylation may be the molecular switch controlling pathological versus physiological interaction.

While NFT and Lewy bodies are insoluble in chaotropes and denaturants, they are soluble at high pH (Smith et al., 1996a) as well as in amines (Perry and Smith, unpublished observations). These solubility properties are consistent with well known oxidative cross-linking from aldol condensation of carbonyl adducts. Protein-based carbonyls arise from at least three sources; reducing sugars, lipid peroxidation products and direct oxidation, and all three are associated with NFT and Lewy bodies (Smith et al., 1994a, 1996b; Castellani et al., 1996; Sayre et al., 1997). Glycation, the most established oxidative posttranslational modifications of proteins in aging (Cerami et al., 1987), perhaps better known as the Maillard reaction, is the adduction of reducing sugars to free amines and, while glycation was first known from the food industry as being responsible for spoilage of canned food, more recent studies show that glycation, *in vivo*, can be rapid and dynamic. Indeed, while the reaction between glucose and the amines of lysine residues is slow and of little consequence, save increased insolubility, in contrast, *in vivo* far more reactive sugars are involved. Further, the subsequent transition metal-catalyzed oxidations, in addition to creating free radicals, also leads to the formation of advanced glycation end products (AGEs). Pentosidine and pyrraline, two well characterized AGE products, have been found in NFT, senile plaques and Lewy bodies (Smith et al., 1994a; Castellani et al., 1996).

NEURONS ARE THE TARGET OF OXIDATIVE STRESS

The chemistry of lipid peroxide adduction to proteins is analogous to glycation since the most reactive products are, as reducing sugars, carbonyl-containing intermediates. Subsequent rearrangement leads to stable advanced lipid-peroxidation endproducts, some of which are identical to products of AGEs (Baynes et al., 1991). Significantly, increased lipid peroxidation is a sensitive and direct index of oxidative damage since polyunsaturated lipids are the most oxidation-susceptible class of macromolecules found in cells. Further, while the carbonyl-containing and other intermediates of lipid peroxidation are short-lived, the resultant advanced products are not only stable, but through extensive crosslinking, can also inhibit proteolysis (Friguet et al., 1994). The most well studied lipid adducts are those between proteins and malondialdehyde (MDA) or hydroxynonenal (HNE). While MDA is the dominant product of lipid peroxidation, HNE is the most reactive with proteins (Esterbauer et al., 1991), and adducts of both MDA and HNE are found in AD (Yan et al., 1994; Montine et al., 1997; Sayre et al., 1997). Of note, instead of being confined to NFT, the neuronal cytoplasm in regions affected by NFT in AD also shows increased HNE adduction compared to controls (Sayre et al., 1997). This latter finding not only indicates that increased lipid peroxidation is independent of NFT formation but further suggests that AD is associated with a global increase in neuronal oxidative stress.

Two other assessments of oxidative damage also show global increases in neuronal oxidative stress. First, peroxynitrite-mediated damage, evidenced by nitrotyrosine, has essentially the same distribution as HNE-adducts (Smith et al., 1997a). Second, analysis of free carbonyls, resulting from direct oxidation as well as adduction by lipid and sugars, also shows an identical pattern of neuronal involvement. In sum, these findings support a widespread increase in oxidative stress in neurons in the CNS of AD.

ANTIOXIDANT RESPONSE

As a result of oxidative stress, cells upregulate antioxidant defenses. In one such case, inducible heme oxygenase-1 (HO-1) catalyzes the first step in the conversion of heme to bilirubin, producing an antioxidant from a prooxidant. In AD and PD, HO-1 is associated with the cytoskeletal abnormalities leading to inclusion formation (Smith et al., 1994b; Castellani et al., 1996), however, in the case of AD, it exactly overlaps the distribution of intraneuronal τ protein accumulation, even that preceding NFT (Smith and Perry, unpublished findings). Therefore HO-1 induction does not appear to be simply a response to increased oxidative stress but, rather, to oxidative damage extensive enough to involve cytoskeletal proteins. This apparent correlation may even be direct since *in vitro* studies with neuroblastoma cells demonstrate that AGE-modified τ can increase oxidative stress (Yan et al., 1994, 1995).

While HO-1 activation increases the antioxidant bilirubin, its additional products, CO and free iron, may have damaging effects. Iron catalyzes the formation of hydroxyl radicals that are essential to both advanced glycation and lipid peroxidation endproducts. Understanding whether HO-1 is a source of excess free iron associated with NFT in AD (Smith et al., 1997b) is critical to understanding whether the brain's response to chronic oxidative damage actually exacerbates the problem.

SUMMARY

In just three years, results from a number of laboratories have implicated oxidative stress in the pathogenesis of AD. One of the most important unresolved issues is whether the production of free radicals is a result of the pathology or serves to initiate pathological damage. The importance of resolving these and other issues is all the clearer from recent clinical and epidemiological findings showing that antioxidants slow down or delay the onset of Alzheimer disease. Therefore, efforts to understand and reduce oxidative stress may have direct therapeutic value in both assisting patients and in solving the complex pathogenesis of AD.

ACKNOWLEDGMENTS

This work was supported through grants from the National Institutes of Health (AG09287) and the American Health Assistance Foundation (AHAF). M.A.S. is a Daland fellow of the American Philosophical Society.

REFERENCES

Baynes, J.W., 1991, Role of oxidative stress in development of complications in diabetes, *Diabetes* 40:405–412.

Bondareff, W., Harrington, C.R., Wischik, C.M., Hauser, D.L., and Roth, M., 1995, Absence of abnormal hyperphosphorylation of tau in intracellular tangles in Alzheimer's disease, *J. Neuropathol. Exp. Neurol.* 54:657–663.

Castellani, R., Smith, M.A., Richey, P.L., and Perry, G., 1996, Glycoxidation and oxidative stress in Parkinson disease and diffuse Lewy body disease, *Brain Res.* 737:195–200.

Cerami, A., Vlassara, H., and Brownlee, M., 1987, Glucose and aging, *Sci. Amer.* 256:90–96.

Esterbauer, H., Schaur, R. J., and Zollner, H., 1991, Chemistry and biochemistry of 4-hydroxynonenal, malonaldehyde and related aldehydes, *Free Radic. Biol. Med.* 11:81–128.

Friguet, B., Stadtman, E.R., and Szweda, L.I., 1994, Modification of glucose-6-phosphate dehydrogenase by 4-hydroxy-2-nonenal. Formation of cross-linked protein that inhibits the multicatalytic protease, *J. Biol. Chem.* 269:21639–21643.

Galloway, P.G., Mulvihill, P., and Perry, G., 1992, Filaments of Lewy bodies contain insoluble cytoskeletal elements, *Am. J. Pathol.* 140:809–822.

Goedert, M., Jakes, R., Crowther, R.A., Six, J., Lubke, U., Vandermeeren, M., Cras, P., Trojanowski, J.Q., and Lee, V.M., 1993, The abnormal phosphorylation of tau protein at Ser-202 in Alzheimer disease recapitulates phosphorylation during development, *Proc. Natl. Acad. Sci. USA* 90:5066–5070.

Grundke-Iqbal, I., Iqbal, K., Tung, Y.C., Quinlan, M., Wisniewski, H.M., and Binder, L.I., 1986, Abnormal phosphorylation of the microtubule-associated protein τ (tau) in Alzheimer cytoskeletal pathology, *Proc. Natl. Acad. Sci. USA* 83:4913–4917.

Matsuo, E.S., Shin, R.W., Billingsley, M.L., Van deVoorde, A., O'Connor, M., Trojanowski, J.Q., and Lee, V.M., 1994, Biopsy-derived adult human brain tau is phosphorylated at many of the same sites as Alzheimer's disease paired helical filament tau, *Neuron* 13:989–1002.

Montine, K.S., Olson, S.J., Amarnath, V., Whetsell, W.O. Jr., Graham, D.G., and Montine, T.J., 1997, Immunohistochemical detection of 4-hydroxy-2-nonenal adducts in Alzheimer's disease is associated with inheritance of APOE4, *Am. J. Pathol.* 150:437–443.

Sayre, L.M., Zelasko, D.A., Harris, P.L.R., Perry, G., Salomon, R.G., and Smith, M.A., 1997, 4-Hydroxynonenal-derived advanced lipid peroxidation end products are increased in Alzheimer's disease, *J. Neurochem.* 68:2092–2097.

Selkoe, D.J., Ihara, Y., and Salazar, F.J., 1982, Alzheimer's disease: insolubility of partially purified paired helical filaments in sodium dodecyl sulfate and urea, *Science* 215:1243–1245.

Smith, M.A., Taneda, S., Richey, P.L., Miyata, S., Yan, S.-D., Stern, D., Sayre, L.M., Monnier, V.M., and Perry, G., 1994a, Advanced Maillard reaction end products are associated with Alzheimer disease pathology, *Proc. Natl. Acad. Sci. USA* 91:5710–5714.

Smith, M.A., Kutty, R.K., Richey, P.L., Yan, S.-D., Stern, D., Chader, G.J., Wiggert, B., Petersen, R.B., and Perry, G., 1994b, Heme oxygenase-1 is associated with the neurofibrillary pathology of Alzheimer's disease, *Am. J. Pathol.* 145:42–47.

Smith, M.A., Siedlak, S.L., Richey, P.L., Nagaraj, R.H., Elhammer, A., and Perry, G., 1996a, Quantitative solubilization and analysis of insoluble paired helical filaments from Alzheimer disease, *Brain Res.* 717:99–108.

Smith, M.A., Perry, G., Richey, P.L., Sayre, L.M., Anderson, V.E., Beal, M.F., and Kowall, N., 1996b, Oxidative damage in Alzheimer's, *Nature* 382:120–121.

Smith, M.A., Harris, P.L.R., Sayre, L.M., Beckman, J.S., and Perry, G., 1997a, Widespread peroxynitrite-mediated damage in Alzheimer's disease, *J. Neurosci.* 17:2653–2657.

Smith, M.A., Harris, P.L.R., Sayre, L.M., and Perry, G., 1997b, Iron accumulation in Alzheimer disease is a source of redox-generated free radicals, *Proc. Natl. Acad. Sci. USA*, in press.

Sternberger, L.A. and Sternberger, N.H., 1983, Monoclonal antibodies distinguish phosphorylated and nonphosphorylated forms of neurofilaments *in situ.*, *Proc. Natl. Acad. Sci. USA* 80:6126–6130.

Sternberger, N.H., Sternberger, L.A., and Ulrich, J., 1985, Aberrant neurofilament phosphorylation in Alzheimer disease, *Proc. Natl. Acad. Sci. USA* 82:4274–4276.

Trojanowski, J.Q., Schmidt, M.L., Shin, R.-W., Bramblett, G.T., Goedert, M., and Lee, V.M.-Y., 1993, PHF-tau (A68): From pathological marker to potential mediator of neuronal dysfunction and degeneration in Alzheimer's disease, *Clin. Neurosci.* 1:184–191.

Yan, S.-D., Chen, X., Schmidt, A.-M., Brett, J., Godman, G., Zou, Y.-S., Scott, C.W., Caputo, C., Frappier, T., Smith, M.A., Perry, G., Yen, S.-H., and Stern, D., 1994, Glycated tau protein in Alzheimer disease: a mechanism for induction of oxidant stress, *Proc. Natl. Acad. Sci. USA* 91:7787–7791.

Yan, S.D., Yan, S.F., Chen, X., Fu, J., Chen, M., Kuppusamy, P., Smith, M.A., Perry, G., Godman, G.C., Nawroth, P., Zweier, J.L., and Stern, D., 1995, Non-enzymatically glycated tau in Alzheimer's disease induces neuronal oxidant stress resulting in cytokine gene expression and release of amyloid ß-peptide, *Nature Med.* 1:693–699.

13

COMMON MECHANISMS IN CELL CYCLE AND CELL DEATH

D. Uberti, M. Belloni, C. Rizzini, A. Fontanini, L. Piccioni, M. Grilli,
P. F. Spano, and M. Memo

Division of Pharmacology
Department of Biomedical Sciences and Biotechnologies
School of Medicine
University of Brescia
Brescia, Italy

INTRODUCTION

The central core of the hypothesis underlying the present chapter is that terminally differentiated cells like neurons that have irreversibly exited the cell cycle have acquired programmed cell death (apoptosis) as an alternative effector pathway. This pathway may be activated in response to molecular events that lead to transformation of dividing stem cell populations. For example, alterations of those genes that can cause transformation in dividing cell populations, can cause apoptosis of terminally differentiated neurons. Up to now, it is quite evident that apoptosis is an important component in many progressive and acute neurodegenerative diseases. The extracellular signals as well as the intracellular mechanisms inducing and regulating apoptosis (or different types of apoptosis) of neuronal cells are still a matter of investigation.

The present chapter will review some recent data obtained in our laboratory with the aim both to identify and to characterize the mechanism of action of cytosolic and nuclear proteins known to be involved in cell cycle regulation as well as in promoting degeneration and apoptosis of neurons. Since their established role in regulating cell cycle of peripheral and/or tumor cells, two molecules have to be taken into consideration: p53 and MSH2. These proteins are apparently linked one to each other by consecutive transcriptional activation, thus suggesting the existence of an intracellular pathway responsible for the induction and progression of neuronal apoptosis. Identification of such mechanisms could be relevant for understanding the apoptosis associated with various neurodegenerative diseases, as well as for developing novel strategies of pharmacological intervention.

Progress in Alzheimer's and Parkinson's Diseases
edited by Fisher *et al.*, Plenum Press, New York, 1998.

THE TUMOR SUPPRESSOR PROTEIN p53 IN THE CNS

The tumor suppressor protein p53 is a cell cycle checkpoint protein that contributes to the preservation of genetic stability. Upon certain conditions, including physical or chemical DNA damage, p53 gene expression can be activated to either arrest cell cycle progression in the late G1 phase, thus allowing the DNA to be repaired before its replication, or induce apoptosis (Lane, 1992). Due to its role, p53 has been defined as a "safeguard against tumorigenesis". Indeed, in tumor cells lacking functional p53, the above described pathways are not functional, resulting in inefficient DNA repair and the emergence of genetically unstable cells (Vogelstain and Kinzier, 1992). More recently, it was found that p53 may also play a role in cell differentiation (Eizenberg et al., 1996).

The mechanism(s) by which p53 can induce cell cycle arrest and/or apoptosis is still largely unknown. Development of transgenic mice deficient for p53 has recently gained further insight on the functional role of p53 (Donehover et al., 1992). Interestingly, mice homozygous for p53 null allele appear normal. Thus, at least from these data and with the awareness of the intrinsic limitation of the experimental model, p53 function appears to be dispensable in many apoptotic processes that occur physiologically during the entire lifespan in a large variety of organs and systems. However, p53 deficient mice are prone to the spontaneous development of a variety of neoplasms by 6 months of age, suggesting that the lack of the p53 gene predisposes the animal to neoplastic diseases, although it is not obligatory for tumorigenesis. Interestingly, normal development and high risk of tumor are found in family members with dominantly inherited Li-Fraumeni syndrome and this syndrome has been associated with germ line p53 mutation (Srivastava et al., 1990).

Nevertheless, p53 appears to play an important role in promoting apoptosis and this function could have relevant implications for brain function. Indeed, apoptosis of neurons is observed physiologically during development and aging. Furthermore, apoptosis has been associated, at least in part, with neurodegeneration detectable in various neurological diseases, including Huntington's (Portera-Cailliau et al., 1995) and Alzheimer's diseases (Duguid et al., 1989).

A series of recent papers have mainly contributed to unravel the role of p53 during a neurodegenerative process (Li et al., 1994; Sakhi et al., 1994; Xiang et al., 1996). In particular, systemic injection of kainic acid, a potent excitotoxin that produces seizures associated with a defined pattern of neuronal cell loss, induced p53 expression in neurons exhibiting morphological evidence of damage (Sakhi et al., 1994). More recently, Morrison et al., (1996) found that systemic injection of kainic acid to p53 gene deficient mice did not induce neuronal cell death. A further indirect although intriguing link between excitotoxicity and p53 has been provided by Didier et al., (1996) who showed accumulation of single-strand DNA damage as an early event in excitotoxicity. This particular DNA damage is indeed capable of inducing p53 expression (Jayaraman and Prives, 1995; Lee et al., 1995).

We studied the role of p53 in cultured, genetically unmodified neurons, namely rat cerebellar granule cells, during development *in vitro* and in response to neurotoxicity induced by excitatoxins. Primary cultures of cerebellar granule cells offer not only a morphologically defined system for studying transsynaptic regulation of neuronal gene expression, but also provide the opportunity to analyze the precise temporal sequence of molecular events following stimulation of specific glutamate receptor subtypes. Advantages of this experimental model also include the possibility to study the function of a given gene product using the oligonucleotide antisense technology, thus avoiding redundancy on compensation that may occur in transgenic animal models.

We found that primary cultures of rat cerebellar granule cells, although definitely post-mitotic and terminally differentiated, express the tumor suppressor phosphoprotein p53 (Uberti et al., 1997). In particular, granule cells both expressed significant levels of p53 mRNA and positively reacted to an anti-p53 antibody, from the first day of culturing. During neuron differentation, p53 mRNA content did not significantly change, at least up to 12 days in vitro, while p53 immunoreactivity increased gradually. p53 expression appeared to be further modulable, being upregulated after stimulation of glutamate ionotropic receptors by glutamate or kainate. Although qualitatively similar, p53 induction by glutamate and kainate differed in terms of intensity and time-course. The glutamate-induced increase of p53 immunoreactivity appeared within 30 min after the treatment and lasted for at least 2 h. Kainate-induced increase of p53 immunoreactivity was delayed, becoming apparent within 2 h and lasting for at least 8 h. As shown by the electrophoretic mobility shift analysis, both glutamate and kainate induced increases of p53 DNA binding activity. Blockade of p53 induction by a specific p53 antisense oligonucleotide resulted in a partial reduction of excitotoxicity with a complete inhibition of the excitatory aminoacids-induced apoptosis. Our data suggest that stimulation of ionotropic glutamate receptors in neurons results in a p53-dependent apoptosis.

DNA DAMAGE REPAIR SYSTEM(S) IN THE CNS

DNA repair is one of the most essential system for mantaining the inherited nucleotide sequence of genomic DNA over time. In eukaryotic cells, damaged DNA can be repaired by the activation of different pathways which involve nucleotide or base excision, and pair mismatch recognition. Previous studies have demonstrated the presence in brain cells of different factors involved in DNA repair processes (Walker and Bachelard, 1988; Dragunow, 1995; Ono et al., 1995). Up to now, very little is known about the mismatch DNA repair systems in neurons (Brooks et al., 1996). It is still unclear whether or not they are expressed, functioning, and modulable and, maybe more important, if there is any reason for them to be expressed in postmitotic cells like neurons. In this regard, it should be noted that repair of non-replicating DNA would be expected to be particularly important in neurons, because neurons are among the longest-living cells in the body. There are at least three different events which may induce mismatched nucleotides in DNA: i) genetic recombination; ii) misincorporation of nucleotides during DNA replication; and iii) physical damage. Since neurons are definitely postmitotic cells thus unable to replicate, only the latter possibility can be taken into consideration as a possible inducer of DNA mispair. Indeed, physical damage induced by water, oxygen, ultraviolet light, ionizing irradiation, or drugs, to DNA can give rise to mismatched bases (Friedberg, 1985).

Mismatched nucleotides produced by these mechanisms are known to be recognized and repaired by specific enzyme systems. The MutHLS mismatch repair pathway has been originally identified as one of the major repair systems in *E. Coli* (see Modrich 1994 as review). DNA mismatch recognition in human cells is thought to be mediated by a series of components, homologs of MutHLS, that have been named MSH2, MSH3, MSH6, MLH1 and PMS2 (Kunkel, 1995). In response to a DNA mismatch proliferating cells arrest at various checkpoints (Wiebauer and Jiricny, 1990; Modrich, 1994; Habraken et al., 1996; Acharya et al., 1996). The arrest in G1 phase, possibly mediated by p53 activation, gives the cells time to repair critical damage before DNA replication occurs, thereby avoiding the propagation of genetic lesions to progeny cells. In theory, these functions can be applied only partially to neurons. In fact, terminally differentiated neurons do not reenter the cell cycle, and they cannot be transformed. However, DNA damage can be developed in neuron both in physiological and pathological conditions and this may represent the functional basis for the expression of such systems (Robbins, 1985; Anderson et al., 1996; Evans et al., 1996).

We first studied the distribution of MSH2 in rat brain by immunohistochemical analysis. A heterogeneous level of expression was observed in the different brain areas (Belloni et al., 1997). Immunoreactivity was found in the pyramidal neurons of the hippocampus and in the granular cells of the dentate gyrus. The staining was observed in all the fields of the hippocampus and in the dentate gyrus, without appreciable changes in intensity. The immunoreactivity was specifically localized in the nucleus. According to the localization of the positive cells the expression of the protein is generally restricted to the neurons. High levels of expression were observed in the entorhinal cortex and in the fronto-parietal cortex. Positive cells were also observed in the substantia nigra and in the cerebellum (granular cells and Purkinje cells).

We then investigated the possible correlation between activation of DNA mismatch repair system and cell death in rat brain neurons both *in vivo* and *in vitro* (Belloni et al., 1997). Excitotoxicity was chosen as the experimental paradigm to induce cell death. In recent years dysfunction of the ionotropic glutamate-activated neurotransmitter receptors, which are the principal providers of fast neurotrasmission in mammalian brain, has been extensively implicated in neurodegeneration since excessive or persistent activation of these receptors results in neuronal death. Brain damage through excitotoxicity has been closely associated to acute conditions like stroke, trauma, ischaemia, hypoglycemia, but also to epilepsy and ALS. In addition a contribution of excitotoxicity to chronic and progressive neuropathologies like Alzheimer's and Parkinson's diseases has also been suggested (Lipton 1994). Interestingly, DNA damage has been found to be deeply involved in many of these diseases, including ischaemia and Alzheimer's Disease (Robbins et al., 1985; Mazzarello et al., 1992; Boerrigter et al., 1992; Liu et al., 1996).

Systemic administration of kainic acid induces various behavioural alterations and a typical pattern of neuropathology, with cell death in specific brain areas. The pyramidal neurons of the fields CA1 and CA3 of the hippocampus appear to be the most vulnerable. In our study, rats were treated intraperitoneally with kainic acid at the dose of 10 or 15 mg/kg body weight and their brains examined after a survival period of 8 h. We found a marked increase in MSH2 immunoreactivity in the hippocampal neurons. The effect was particularly in the CA1 and CA3 fields and specific, since no changes in immunoreactivity were detected in other hippocampal fields and brain areas. The overexpression was induced also by the lowest dose, which did not result in a significant cell loss.

TRANSCRIPTIONAL CASCADE LEADING TO CELL DEATH

There is an emerging consensus that glutamate, through the activation of specific glutamate receptor subtypes, activates a series of genes whose products trigger long-term phenotypic changes in neurons. Nevertheless, the relative functional contribution of the individual gene products in processing the glutamate signal to induce neuronal death is still unknown. Stimulation of NMDA-sensitive glutamate receptor subtypes that are present in primary cultures of cerebellar granule cells results in the induction of a number of transcription factors, including the NFκB/rel transcription factor family (Kaltschmidt et al., 1994; Guerrini et al., 1995; Grilli et al., 1996a). We recently showed that blockade of glutamate-induction of NFκB by salicylate results in a complete prevention of glutamate-induced cell death (Grilli et al., 1996b, Grilli and Memo, 1997). Since p53 is one of the target genes of NFκB (Wu and Lozano, 1994), it may be inferred that glutamate, possibly by increasing intracellular calcium concentration, may activate a restricted number of transcription factors, including NFκB, which in turn amplify the signal by recruiting other genes to dictate a long-lasting transcriptional program. At present, the p53 target genes triggered by glutamate receptor stimulation are largely unknown. Studies in normally or abnormally proliferating cells have shown that several genes are indeed transcriptionally regulated by p53, most of them regulating cell cycle arrest and DNA repair (Kastan et al., 1992; El-Diery et al., 1993; Barak et al., 1993; Miyashita et al., 1994). One of the genes involved in recognizing and repairing mismatch DNA lesions, and transcriptionally activated by p53 (Scherer et al., 1996), is the MSH2 gene (Palombo et al., 1994). In this regards, we found that cerebellar granule cells contain MSH2 protein and that its expression is up-regulated by glutamate injury (Belloni et al., 1997). It may be inferred that a number of cytosolic and nuclear proteins, known to be involved in cell cycle regulation, are indeed relevant contributors in promoting degeneration and apoptosis of neurons. Among the others, since their established role is in regulating cell cycle of peripheral and/or tumor cells, are p53 and MSH2. These proteins are apparently linked one with another by consecutive transcriptional activation, possibly triggered by glutamate-induced NF-κB induction. This cascade of transcription factor recruitment suggests the existence of an intracellular pathway responsible for the induction and progression of neuronal apoptosis. The understanding of this diverging cascade of nuclear events may unravels novel targets for pharmacological intervention for those neurological diseases in which necrosis and apoptosis play a differential role.

REFERENCES

Acharya, S., Wilson, T., Gradia, S., Kane, M.F., Guerrette, S., Marsischky, G.T., Kolodner, R., and Fishel, R., 1996, hMSH2 forms specific mispair-binding complexes with hMSH3 and hMSH6. *Proc. Natl. Acad. Sci. U.S.A.* 93:13629–13634.

Anderson, A.J., Su, J.H., and Cotman, C.W., 1996, DNA damage and apoptosis in Alzheimer's disease: colocalization with c-Jun immunoreactivity, relationship to brain area, and effect of postmortem delay. *J. Neurosci.* 16(5):1710–1719.

Barak, Y., Juven, T., Haffine, R. and Oren, M., 1993, *mdm2* expression is induced by wild-type p53 activity. *EMBO J.* 12:461–468.

Belloni, M., Uberti, D., Rizzini, C., Spano, P.F., and Memo. M., 1997, Expression of the DNA mismatch repair protein MSH2 in rat brain and primary neurons: induction by excitatory aminoacids. (Submitted for publication).

Boerrigter, M.E.T.I., Wei, J.Y., and Vijg, J., 1992, DNA repair and Alzheimer's disease. *J Gerontol.* 47(6):B177-B184.

Brooks, P.J., Marietta, C., and Goldman, D., 1996, DNA mismatch repair and DNA methylation in adult brain neurons. *J. Neurosci.* 16(3):939–945.

Didier, M., Bursztajn, S., Adamec, E., Passani, L., Nixon, RA., Coyle, JT., Wei, JY., and Berman, SA., 1996, DNA strand breaks induced by sustained glutamate excitatotoxicity in primary neuronal cultures. *J. Neurosci.* 16:2238–2250.

Donehover, L.A., Harvey, M., Slagle, B.L., McArthur, M.J., Montgomery Jr, C.A., Butel, J.S. and Bradley, A., 1992, Mice deficient for p53 are developmentally normal but susceptible to spontaneous tumours. *Nature* 356:215–221.

Dragunow, M., 1995, Ref-1 expression in adult mammalian neurons and astrocytes. *Neurosci. Lett.* 191:189–192.

Duguid, J.R., Bohmot, C.W., Liu, N., and Tourtellotte, W.W., 1989, Changes in brain gene expression shared by scrapie and Alzheimer's disease. *Proc. Natl. Acad. Sci. U.S.A.* 86:7260–7264.

Eizenberg, O., Faber-Elman, A., Gottlier, E., Oren, M., Rotter, V., and Schwartz, M., 1996, p53 plays a regulatory role in differentiation and apoptosis of central nervous system-associated cells. *Mol. Cell Biol.* 16:5178–5185.

El-Deiry, W.S., Tokino, T., Veculescu, V.E., Levy, D.B., Parsons, R., Trent, J.M., Lin, D., Mercer, W.E., Kinzler, K.W., and Vogelstein, B., 1993, WAF1, a potent mediator of p53 tumor suppression. *Cell.* 75:817–825.

Enokido, Y., Araki, T., Tanaka, K., and Hatanaka, H., 1996, Involvement of p53 in DNA strand break-induced apoptosis in postmitotic CNS neurons. *Eur. J. Neurosci.* 8:1812–1821.

Evans, D.A.P., Burbach, J.P.H., Swaab, D.F., and van Leeuwen, F.W., 1996, Mutant vasopressin precursors in the human hypothalamus: evidence for neuronal somatic mutations in man. *Neuroscience.* 71(4):1025–1030.

Friedberg, E.C., 1985, DNA repair. Freeman, W.H., New York.

Grilli, M., Goffi, F., Memo, M., and Spano, P.F., 1996a, Interleukin-1β and glutamate activate the NF-κB/Rel binding site from the regulatory region of the amyloid precursor protein gene in primary neuronal cultures. *J. Biol. Chem.* 271:15002–15007.

Grilli, M., Pizzi, M., Memo, M., and Spano, P.F., 1996b, A novel property for aspirin and sodium salicylate: neuroprotection through blockade of NF-κB activation. *Science.* 274:983–1985.

Grilli, M., and Memo, M., 1997, Transcriptional pharmacology of neurodegenerative disorders: novel venue towards neuroprotection against excitotoxicity? *Mol.Psychiatry* 2:192–195.

Guerrini, L., Blasi, F., and Denis-Donini, S., 1995, Synaptic activation of NF-κB by glutamate in cerebellar granule neurons in vitro. *Proc. Natl. Acad. Sci. USA* 92: 9077–9081.

Habraken, Y., Sung, P., Prakash, L., and Prakash, S., 1996, Binding of insertion/deletion DNA mismatches by the heterodimer of yeast mismatch repair proteins MSH2 and MSH3. *Curr. Biol.* 6(9):1185–1187.

Jayaraman, JL., and Prives, C., 1995, Activation of p53 sequence-specific DNA binding by short single strand of DNA requires the p53 C-terminus. *Cell.* 81:1021–1029.

Kaltschmidt, C., Kaltschmidt, B. Neumann, H., Wekerle, H., and Baeuerle, P. A., 1994, Constitutive NFkB activity in neurons. *Mol. Cell. Biol.* 14:3981–3992.

Kastan, M.B., Zhan, Q., El-Deiry, W.S., Carrier, F., Jacks, T., Walsh. W.V., Plunkett, B.S., Vogelstein, B., and Forance, A.J., 1992, A mammalian cell cycle check point pathway utilizing p53 and GADD45 is defective in ataxia-teleangectasia. *Cell.* 71:587–597.

Kolodner, R.D., 1995, Mismatch repair: mechanisms and relationship to cancer susceptibility. *Trends in Biochem. Sci.* 20:397–401.

Kunkel, T.A., 1995, The intricacies of eukaryotic spell-checking. *Curr. Biol.* 5(10):1091–1094.

Lane, D.P., 1992, Cancer. p53, guardian of the genome. *Nature* 358:15–16.

Lee, S., Elenbaas, B., Levine, A., and Griffith, J., 1995, p53 and its 14 kDa C-terminus domain recognize primary DNA damage in the form of insertion/deletion mismatches. *Cell.* 81:1013–1020.

Li, Y., Chopp, M., Zhang, ZG., Zaloga, C., Neiwenhuis, L., and Gautam, S., 1994, p53-immunoreactive protein and p53 mRNA expression after transient middle cerebral artery occlusion in rats. *Stroke* 25:849–855.

Lipton, S.A., and Rosemberg, P.A., 1994, Excitatory aminoacids as a final common pathway for neurologic disorders. *N. Engl. J. Med.* 330(9):613–622.

Liu, P.K., Hsu, C.Y., Dizdaroglu, M., Floyd, R.A., Kow,Y.W., Karakaya, A., Rabow, L.E., and Cui, J-K., 1996, Damage, repair, and mutagenesis in nuclear genes after mouse forebrain ischemia-reperfusion. *J. Neurosci.* 16(21):6795–6806.

Mazzarello, P., Poloni, M., Spadari, S., and Focher, F., 1992, DNA repair mechanism in neurological diseases: facts and hypotheses. *J. Neurol. Sci.* 112:4–14.

Myashita, T., Karjewska, S., Krajewska, M., Wang, H.C., Lin, H.K., Liebermann, D.A., Hoffman, B., and Reed, J.C., 1994, Tumor suppressor p53 is a regulator of bcl-2 and bax gene expression in vitro and in vivo. *Oncogene.* 9:1799–1805.

Modrich, P., 1991, Mechanisms and biological effects of mismatch repair. *Ann. Rev. Genet.* 25:229–253.

Morrison, R.S., Wenzel, H.J., Kinoshita, Y., Robbins, C.A., Donehower, L.A., and Schwartzkroin, P.A., 1996, Loss of the p53 tumor suppressor gene protects neurons from kainate-induced cell death. *J. Neurosci.* 16:1337–1345.

Ono, Y., Watanabe, M., Inoue, Y., Ohmoto, T., Akiyama, K., Tsutsui, K., and Seki, S., 1995, Developmental expression of APEX nuclease, a multifunctional DNA repair enzyme, in mouse brains. *Dev. Brain. Res.* 86:1–6.

Palombo, F., Hughes, M., Jiricny, J., Truong, O., and Hsuan, J., 1994, Mismatch repair and cancer.*Nature (Lon.)* 367:417–418.

Pellegata, N.S., Antoniono, R.J., Redpath, J.L., and Stanbridge, E.J., 1996, DNA damage and p53-mediated cell cycle arrest: a reevaluation. *Proc. Natl. Acad. Sci. U.S.A.* 93:15209–15214.

Portera-Cailliau, C., Hedreen, J.C., Price, D.L., and Koliatsos, V.E., 1995, Evidence of apoptotic cell death in Huntington diseases and an excitotoxic animal model. *J. Neurosci.* 15:3775–3787.

Robbins, J.H., Otsuka, F., Tarone, R.E., Polinsky, R.J., Brumback, R.A., Nee, L.E., 1985, Parkinson's disease and Alzheimer's disease: hypersensitivity to X rays in cultured cell lines. *J. Neurol. Neurosurg. Psychiatry* 48: 916–923.

Sakhi, S., Bruce, A., Sun, N., Tocco, G., Baudry, M., and Schreiber, SS., 1994, p53 induction is associated with neuronal damage in the central nervous system. *Proc. Natl. Acad. Sci. USA.* 89:12028–12032.

Scherer, S., Welter, C., Zang, KD., and Dooley S., 1996, Specific in vitro binding of p53 to the promoter region of the human mismatch repair hMSH2. *Biochem. Biophys. Res. Commun.* 221:722–728.

Srivastava, S., Zou, Z., Pirollo, K., Blattner, W., and Chang, E.H., 1990, Germ-line transmission of a mutated p53 gene in a cancer-prone family with Li-Fraumeni syndrome. *Nature* 348:747–749.

Uberti, D., Belloni, M., Grilli, M., Spano, P.F., and Memo. M., 1997, Induction of tumour suppressor phosphoprotein p53 in the apoptosis of cultured rat cerebellar neurons triggered by excitatory aminoacids. *Eur. J. Neurosci.*, in press.

Walker A.P., and Bachelard H.S., 1988, Studies on DNA damage and repair in the mammalian brain. *J. Neurochem.* 51:1394–1399.

Wiebauer, K., and Jirikny, J., 1990, Mismatch-specific thymine DNA glycosylase and DNA polymerase beta mediate the correction of G-T mispairs in nuclear extracts from human cells. *Proc. Natl. Acad. Sci. U.S.A.* 87:5842–5845.

Wu, H., and Lozano, G., 1994, NF-κB activation of p53. A potential mechanism for suppressing cell growth in response to stress. *J. Biol. Chem.* 269:20067–20074.

Xiang, H., Hochman, D.W., Saya, H., Fujiwara, T., Schwartzkroin, P.A., and Morrison, R.S., 1996, Evidence for p53-mediated modulation of neuronal viability. *J. Neurosci.* 16:6753–6765.

14

INTRACEREBROVENTRICULAR ADMINISTRATION OF BETA-AMYLOID PEPTIDE (25–35) INDUCES OXIDATIVE STRESS AND NEURODEGENERATION IN RAT BRAIN

Natalia V. Gulyaeva,[1] Ilya V. Victorov,[2] Mikhail Yu. Stepanichev,[1] Mikhail V. Onufriev,[1] Olga S. Mitrokhina,[1] Yulia V. Moiseeva,[1] and Natalia A. Lazareva[1]

[1]Institute of Higher Nervous Activity and Neurophysiology
Russian Academy of Sciences
5A Butlerov Street
Moscow 117865, Russia
[2]Brain Research Institute Russian Academy of Medical Sciences
5, Pereulok Obukha
Moscow 103064, Russia

INTRODUCTION

The cytotoxic action of beta-amyloid has been considered to be the primary determinant of the neurodegeneration observed in Alzheimer's disease. Many aspects of the molecular mechanisms associated with neurotoxic activity of beta-amyloid are being investigated using the synthetic peptide—the active fragment of beta amyloid protein containing residues from 25 to 35 of the parent compound [beta (25–35)].

Beta (25–35) is highly lipophilic and inserts into the membrane hydrocarbon core. Following the intercalation of beta (25–35) to this location in the membrane, the protein fragment may interact with regulatory membrane proteins (Mason et al., 1996). Neurotoxicity of beta-amyloid in vitro is dependent upon its spontaneous adoption of an aggregated structure, significant levels of beta (25–35) aggregation being always associated with significant neurotoxicity (Pike et al., 1995).

Beta (25–35) displays direct cytotoxicity to neurons. Chronic exposure of neuronal cultures to the peptide induces neuronal death by apoptosis (Forloni et al., 1993; Forloni et al., 1996). There are data suggesting that beta (25–35) induces apoptotic cell death through the protein kinase A-mediated pathway (Ueda et al., 1996) and through the modifications in the control of calcium homeostasis (Scorziello et al., 1996). Chen et al. (1996) demonstrated that beta (25–35) produced a cavitational lesion in rat hippocampus and also reduced tyrosine hydroxylase and glutamate immunoreactivities in locus coeruleus as well as choline acetyltransferase immunoreactivity in medial septum. Singh et al. (1995) revealed the stimulation of phospholipases A, C and D activities of LA-N-2 cells by beta (25–35).

Beta (25–35) increased the membrane permeability of brain neurons, resulting in a destabilized intracellular homeostasis leading to neuronal death (Furukawa et al., 1994). Not only membrane permeability of inorganic ions such as Ca^{2+}, Na^+ and K^+ increased, but also that of organic molecules. Therefore, the brain neuron membrane was suggested to lose its integrity in the presence of beta (25–35) that resulted in neuronal death (Oyama et al., 1995). Using nerve growth factor-treated PC12 cells, Joseph and Han (1992) noted that beta (25–35) caused a specific and dose-dependent increase in intracellular Ca^{2+} due to an influx of extracellular Ca^{2+}. Beta (25–35) potentiated the Ca^{2+}-dependent release of excitatory amino acids from depolarized hippocampal slices (Arias et al., 1995) and enhanced excitatory activity in glutamatergic synaptic networks, causing excitatory potentials and Ca^{2+}influx, property probably contributing to the toxicity of beta (25–35) (Brorson et al., 1995).

There is evidence that oxidative damage plays a causative role in Alzheimer's disease and amyloid beta protein toxicity (see Gulyaeva and Erin, 1995 and Richardson et al., 1996, for review). Zhou et al. (1996) showed that both the disruption of Ca^{2+} homeostasis and the reduction of cell viability produced by beta-amyloid in PC12 cells are mediated by free radical-based processes. The neurotoxic effects of of beta (25–35) and its effects on cytosolic free Ca^{2+} were blocked by the antioxidant lazaroid U-83836E and by vitamin E. The hydrophilic antioxidant ascorbic acid and the lipophilic antioxidant 2-mercaptoethanol both protected significantly against beta (25–35) neurotoxicity in cultured rat hippocampal neurons (Prehn et al., 1996, Zhou and Kumar, 1996). Harris et al. revealed that beta (25–35) significantly inhibited L-glutamate uptake in rat hippocampal astrocyte cultures and this inhibition was prevented by the antioxidant Trolox. Decreases in astrocyte function, in particular L-glutamate uptake, may contribute to neuronal degeneration, these results leading to a revised excitotoxicity/free radical hypothesis of beta amyloid toxicity involving astrocytes.

Iron is frequently a potent facilitator of free radical production due to its ability to mediate the conversion of H_2O_2 to hydroxyl radicals via the Fenton reaction or by virtue of hypervalent iron compounds. Schubert et al. (1995) showed that iron facilitated beta amyloid toxicity to cultured cells. Beta (25–35) stimulated release of NO in a neuronal cell line, this phenomenon contributing to understanding the molecular basis of amyloid-induced oxidative stress (Hu and el-Fakahany, 1993).

There are only few studies on the effects of beta (25–35) administrated to animals. Beta (25–35) could impair short-term memory when infused in the rat: a significant amnesia in the social recognition test was observed after intraseptal injection of of beta (25–35) (Terranova et al., 1996). Maurice et al. (1996) showed potent amnestic ability of aggregated beta (25–35), injected intracerebroventricularly, in mice. They also revealed beta (25–35)-induced neurodegeneration and beta-amyloid deposits in rat brain areas. Delobette et al. (1997) demonstrated that aggregated beta (25–35) was a better inducer of amnesia in rats as compared with soluble beta (25–35).

Herein, we report on the neurodegeneration and oxidative stress in rats after intracerebroventricular injection of beta (25–35).

METHODS

Animals

Male Wistar rats (n = 63), weighing 230–290 g at the beginning of the experiment, were housed five per cage and maintained on a natural light/dark cycle. Food and water were provided ad libitum. Rats were randomly divided into two groups: sham-operated and beta (25–35)-treated.

Stereotaxic Surgery

Animals under ketamine anesthesia (150 mg/kg) (Calipsol, Gedeon Richter, Hungary) were positioned in a stereotaxic instrument and a midline sagittal incision was made in the scalp. Holes were drilled in the skull over the lateral ventricles using the following coordinates: 0.8 mm posterior to bregma; 1.5 mm lateral to the sagittal suture; 3.8 mm beneath the surface of the brain. Either artificial CSF or 7.5 nmol of beta (25–35) (RBI) aggregated according to Maurice et al. (1996) was injected at a rate of 1 µl/min into each cerebral ventricle.

Behavioral Tests

Twenty seven rats (13 sham-operated and 14 with beta (25–35) administration) were used in behavioral experiments. Spatial working memory performance was assessed 16 days after the surgery by recording spontaneous alternation behavior in a Y-maze (Sarter et al., 1988). Twenty days after the surgery, long-term memory was examined using the step-through type of the passive avoidance task (Bures et al., 1983). The "open field" test (Kelley, 1993) was carried out on the 9 and 28 days after the surgery. The following parameters were evaluated during 5 min: latency of movement start, horizontal and vertical locomotor activity, number of entries to the center of the lighted area, grooming, defecation number, freezing time.

Tissue Preparation

The animals were killed by decapitation 1, 3, 5, and 30 days after the surgery (n = 6 in each group). Brain was immediately taken out and washed in isotonic NaCl solution. Neocortex, hippocampus and cerebellum were isolated. Brain tissue was handled as described by Gulyaeva et al. (1994).

Evaluation of Free Radical-Mediated Processes

2-Thiobarbituric acid (TBA) reactive substances were detected using spectrophotometric method according to Kagan et al. (1979). The analysis of H_2O_2 - induced luminol-dependent chemiluminescence (total light emission) was used for watching free radical generation (Gulyaeva et al., 1994). Superoxide scavenging/generating activity (SSGA)was determined according to method described by Gulyaeva et al. (1989) based on the spectrophotometric assay of superoxide dismutase elaborated by Nishikimi et al. (1972). The method makes it possible to evaluate the steady state between superoxide generation and superoxide scavenging in brain tissue revealing the prevalence of either process. If superoxide scavenging is higher than superoxide generation, the metod can assess the net superoxide scavenging activity (SSGA is positive), if superoxide generation is higher, SSGA is negative. Protein concentration was determined by using the method of Bradford (1976).

Histology

Thirty days after the surgery brains of sham-operated and beta (25–35)-treated rats were fixed by intracardial perfusion with 10% neutral formalin prepared on phosphate buffer. Dissected brains were postfixed in the same fixing solution during 4 days and then were embedden in paraffin. frontal serial paraffin sections (12 μm) mounted on gelatinized slides were deparaffinized and stained with Nissl (cresyl fast violet), haematoxylin-eosin and vanadium acid fuchsin-toluidin blue. The latter method selectively reveals necrotic neurons as red cells and chromatophylic neurons as blue (Victorov and Barskov, 1993). Congo red (Putchler et al., 1962) and thioflavin S (Francis, 1990) staining were used for identification of beta-amyloid deposites. As a positive control, paraffin sections of postmortal brain (frontal cortex) from a patient with clinical diagnosis of Alzheimer's disease were stained in parallel in each experiment. Sections from each brain were also silver impregnated for neurofibrilary tangles and neuritic plaques (Reusche, 1991).

Materials

All chemicals were from Sigma, unless otherwise stated.

Data Analysis

The results are expressed as mean ± S. E. M. Statistical analysis of the data was performed using Mann-Whitney criterion.

RESULTS

Behavior

The i.c.v. administration of aggregated beta (25–35) resulted in a significant decrease in alternation behavior. Though the total number of alternation during the 8-min session did not differ in sham-operated group (15.3 ± 1.7) and beta (25–35)-treated rats (13.7 ± 1.5), the percent alternation significantly decreased (76.9 ± 3.1 and 62.6 ± 2.4%, respectively, p = 0.02).

In step-through passive avoidance test, latencies did not differ in sham-operated and beta (25–35 group) initially (10.5 ± 3.1 s and 9.8 ± 0.7 s), 1 day after the training session (143.3 ± 8.0 and 144.4 ± 33.2 s) and 7 days after the session (128.9 ± 31.9 and 145.0 ± 34.7, respectively).

No difference in the «open field» test indices were revealed 9 and 28 days after the surgery (data not shown), with the exception of horizontal locomotor activity which was significantly lower (p = 0.03) in beta (25–35) group (42.6 ± 6.3 squares crossed/5 min) than in sham-operated group (64.2 ± 6.8 squares) 28 days after beta (25–35) administration.

Free Radical-Mediated Processes

Beta (25–35) administration induced a generalized, slowly developing oxidative stress in the brain: most expressed accumulation of TBA-reactive substances (Table 1) and increase of superoxide generation (Table 2) were revealed 30 days after the surgery. However, the time course of free radical-mediated processes was region-specific. E.g., free radical generation increased in cerebellum 5 days after the surgery and in cerebral cortex—30 days after the surgery (Table 3).

Table 1. TBA-reactive substances (OD/mg protein) in
rat brain after i.c.v. injection of aggregated beta (25–35)

Days	Groups	Cerebral cortex	Hippocampus	Cerebellum
			Brain structure	
1	Sham	0.21 ± 0.02	0.24 ± 0.02	0.18 ± 0.01
	Beta (25–35)	0.20 ± 0.02	0.23 ± 0.01	0.19 ± 0.01
3	Sham	0.18 ± 0.01	0.19 ± 0.02	0.26 ± 0.09
	Beta (25–35)	0.22 ± 0.03	$0.27 \pm 0.02**$	0.18 ± 0.04
5	Sham	0.14 ± 0.01	0.21 ± 0.02	0.17 ± 0.02
	Beta (25–35)	$0.21 \pm 0.03**$	$0.27 \pm 0.01**$	0.16 ± 0.02
30	Sham	0.19 ± 0.01	0.21 ± 0.02	0.19 ± 0.01
	Beta (25–35)	$0.37 \pm 0.06***$	$0.28 \pm 0.03**$	$0.24 \pm 0.01***$

$**P < 0.05$; $***P < 0.02$ sham-operated vs. beta (25–35).

Table 2. Superoxide scavenging/generating activity (arbitrary units)
in rat brain after i.c.v. injection of aggregated beta (25–35)

Days	Groups	Cerebral cortex	Hippocampus	Cerebellum
			Brain structure	
1	Sham	-10.7 ± 1.4	0.2 ± 2.0	-12.9 ± 2.2
	Beta (25–35)	-9.3 ± 3.7	-0.6 ± 2.9	$-2.9 \pm 2.1***$
3	Sham	-5.8 ± 3.11	-2.4 ± 3.5	-4.9 ± 3.4
	Beta (25–35)	$-16.4 \pm 4.0*$	-1.2 ± 4.7	-6.9 ± 2.4
5	Sham	-10.1 ± 2.0	-4.3 ± 2.8	-5.4 ± 0.9
	Beta (25–35)	-10.9 ± 5.1	-4.1 ± 2.2	-2.5 ± 5.6
30	Sham	4.2 ± 1.9	1.3 ± 2.4	-1.8 ± 0.4
	Beta (25–35)	$-5.7 \pm 0.6***$	$-7.4 \pm 2.7*$	$-5.4 \pm 1.4*$

$*P < 0.08$; $**P < 0.05$; $***P < 0.02$ sham-operated vs. beta (25–35).

Table 3. Free radical generation (arbitrary units) in rat brain
after i.c.v. injection of aggregated beta (25–35)

Days	Groups	Cerebral cortex	Hippocampus	Cerebellum
			Brain structure	
1	Sham	488.2 ± 49.0	178.7 ± 6.3	442.3 ± 37.7
	Beta (25–35)	496.1 ± 34.6	$158.1 \pm 2.9**$	404.4 ± 32.7
3	Sham	469.6 ± 27.2	175.2 ± 10.0	414.1 ± 22.6
	Beta (25–35)	509.3 ± 43.7	171.4 ± 3.2	408.6 ± 29.4
5	Sham	508.0 ± 27.1	174.3 ± 8.2	367.2 ± 5.9
	Beta (25–35)	469.2 ± 46.1	169.1 ± 6.1	$431.4 \pm 19.7**$
30	Sham	514.9 ± 30.2	174.5 ± 6.5	544.0 ± 39.9
	Beta (25–35)	$648.7 \pm 36.1**$	176.0 ± 5.3	506.3 ± 52.3

$**P < 0.05$; $***P < 0.02$ sham-operated vs. beta (25–35).

Histology

In all animals bilateral symmetric neuronal degeneration was observed in anterior cingulate and posterior cingulate (retrosplenial) cortex and primary olfactory cortex. In neocortex, single and grouped degenerating neurons were found in fronto-parietal motor and somatosensory areas of neocortex. In neocortex, degenerated neurons often formed vertical columns and were localized near radial arterioles. In hippocampal region, neuronal degeneration was most expressed in enthorinal cortex and CA3 field of Ammon's horn, however, degenerating neurons were observed also in CA1 field and fascia dentata. Single degenerating neurons were found in septum, caudato-putamen and amygdala (Figs 1 and 2).

No traces of amyloid depositions or signs of neurofibrillary neuronal degeneration and neuritic plaques were found in cortical and subcortical structures of all rat brains studied.

DISCUSSION

Maurice et al. (1996) attempted to induce a potential Alzheimer's-type amnesia in mice after direct i.c.v. administration of aggregated beta (25–35). Pretraining administration of aggregated beta (25–35) induced dose-dependent decreases in both alternation behaviour and step-down type passive avoidance. Treatment of animals with cholinergic agents: cholinesterase inhibitor tacrine and the nicotinic receptor agonist (–)-nicotine resulted in a dose-dependent abrogation of the beta (25–35)-induced decreases in alternation behaviour and passive avoidance and also reversed the beta (25–35)-induced impairment of place learning and retention in the water-maze. Histological examination indicated a moderate cell loss within the frontoparietal cortex and the hippocampal formation of mice treated with aged beta (25–35). Examination of Congo red-stained sections in the same animals demonstrated the presence of amyloid deposits throughout these brain areas. These results confirmed that the deposition of beta-amyloid peptide in the brain is in some way related to impairment of learning and cholinergic degeneration.

In the present study we demonstrated that i.c.v. administration of aggregated beta (25–35) to Wistar rats (15 nmol/rat) resulted in the impairment of spontaneous alternation performance (spatial working memory performance) in a Y-maze. However, there were no differences between rats treated with beta (25–35) and sham operated rats in the performance of a step-through passive avoidance task. Thus, beta (25–35) induced impairments of working memory without any effect on long-term memory. The spontaneous locomotor activity in the «open field» test decreased, this decrease being evident 28 days after beta (25–35) administration.

Pathohistological staining revealed numerous degenerated neurones in cingulate cortex, neocortex and hippocampus of rats treated with beta (25–35). However, no reliable data indicating beta-amyloid deposits were obtained. Takashima et al. (1995) reported about in vitro accumulation of amyloid precursor protein derivatives in the cytoplasm of neurons induced by beta (25–35), and Maurice et al. (1996) revealed amyloid deposits in mouse brain after i.c.v. administration of beta (25–35). The absence of beta-amyloid deposits in the rat model may be related to differences in beta-amyloid metabolism in mouse and rat brain. It also can't be excluded that amyloid deposition after beta(25–35) administration takes more time in rats and one month is not enough for this process or that higher doses of beta (25–35) can induce amyloidogenesis in rat brain.

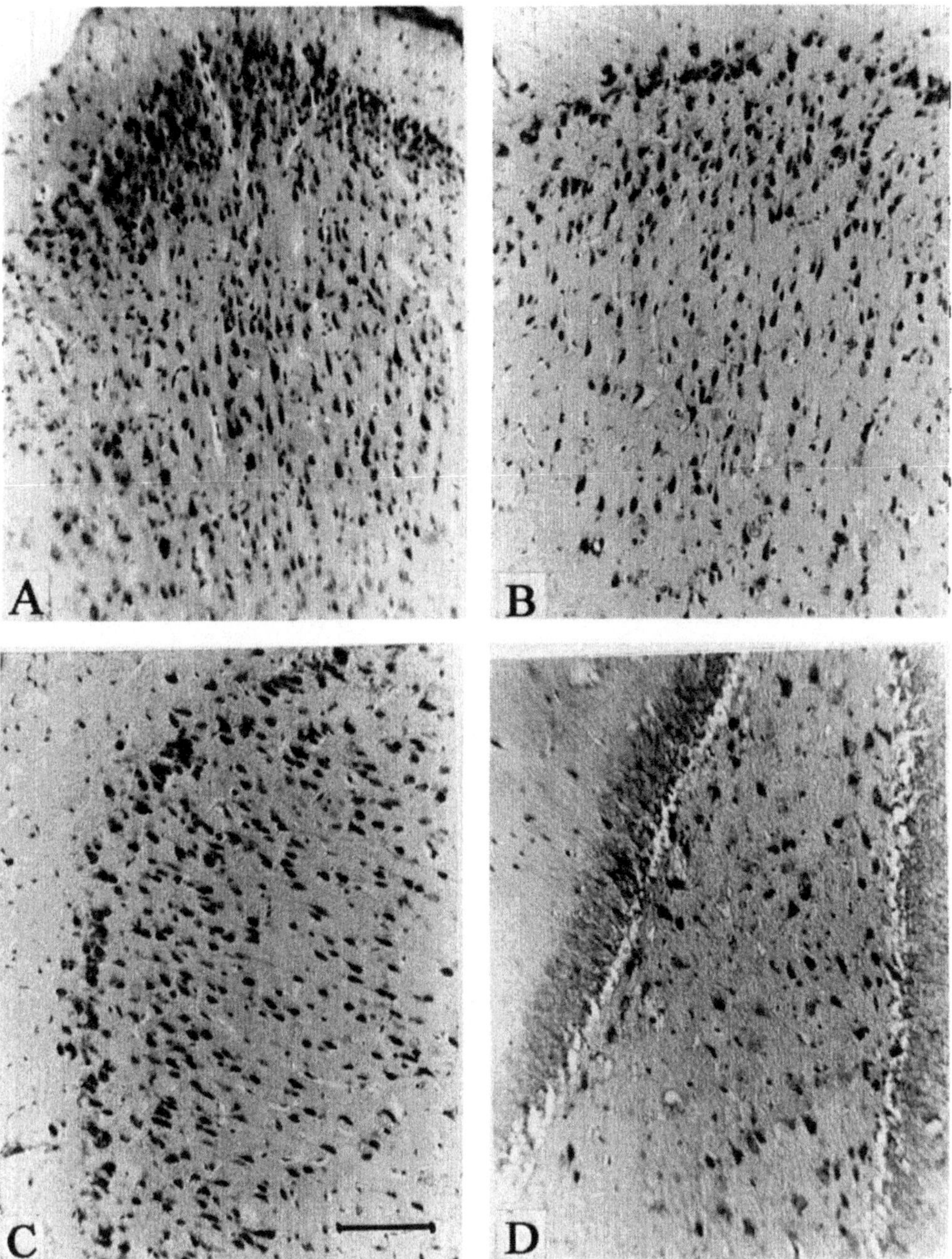

Figure 1. Neuronal degeneration in allocortex and hippocampal region. A) Retrosplenial granular cortex; B) Primary olfactory cortex; C) enthorinal cortex; D) CA3 field of Ammon's horn and Fascia dentata. Vanadium acid fuchsin - Toluidin blue staining. Bar: 100 μm.

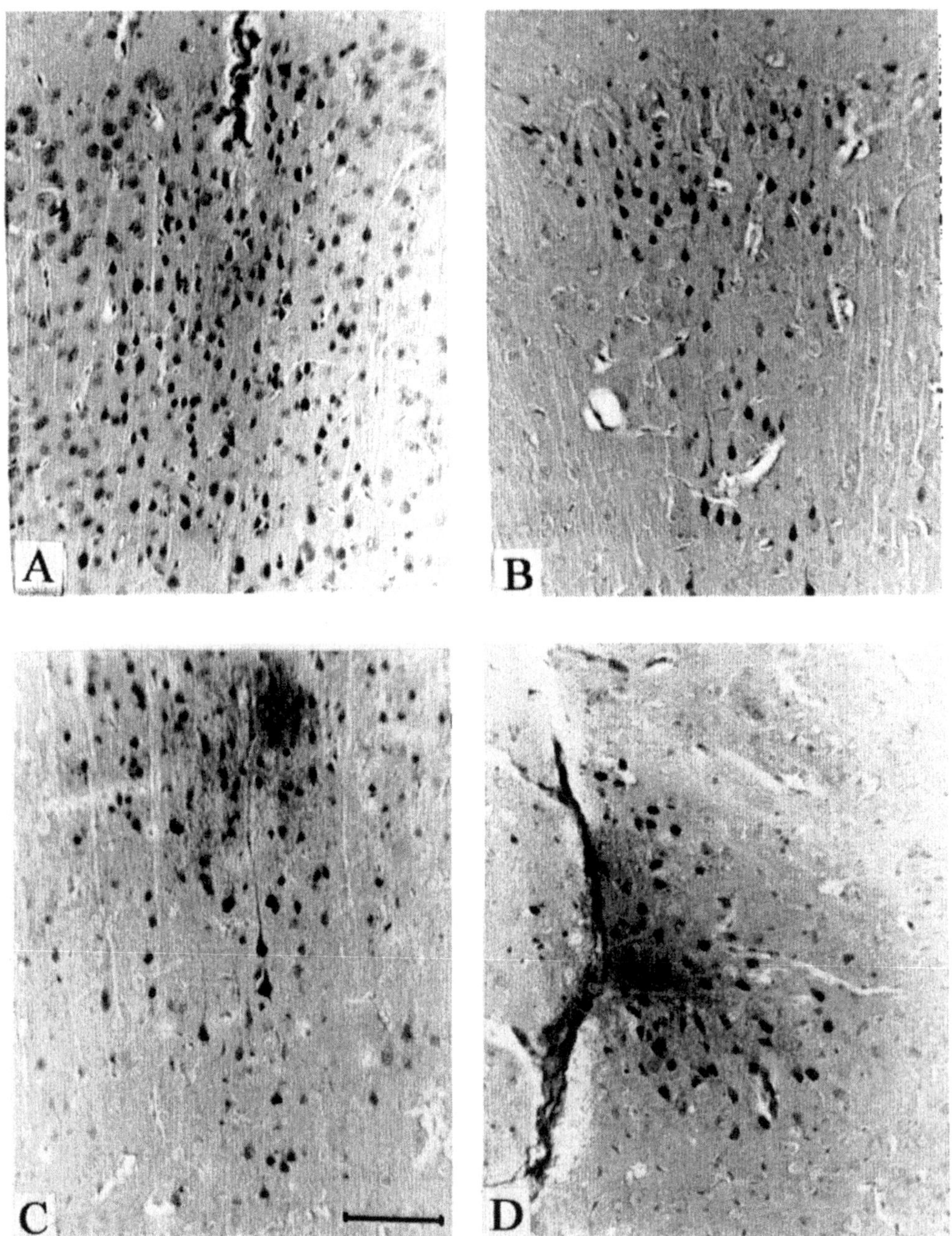

Figure 2. Neuronal degeneration in neocortex. A) Fronto-parietal somato-sensory cortex; B,C) Fronto-parietal motor cortex; D) perivasal localization of degenerating neurons. Vanadium acid fuchsin - Toluidin blue staining. Bar: 100 μm.

Signs of beta (25–35)-induced oxidative stress were evident in all brain regions studied. One month after the surgery, manifestations of oxidative stress (TBA-reactive substances accumulation and increased superoxide generation) were most striking: However, the time course of different indices of free radical-mediated processes was dependent on the region. It should be noted that along with increases in free radical generation, compensatory changes in hippocampus and cerebellum (decrease of free radical generation) could be seen.

The results of the present study confirm that beta (25–35) induces Alzheimer's type amnesia, neurodegeneration and oxidative stress in rat brain and suggest that oxidative stress and neurodegeneration are in some way related to impairment of learning in rats after beta (25–35) administration.

ACKNOWLEDGMENT

The authors are grateful to Dr. Tangui Maurice for valuable suggestions regarding the experiment.

REFERENCES

Arias, C., Arrieta, I., and Tapia, R., 1995, Beta-Amyloid peptide fragment 25–35 potentiates the calcium-dependent release of excitatory amino acids from depolarized hippocampal slices, *J. Neurosci. Res.* 41:561–566.

Bradford, M. M., 1976, A rapid and sensitive method for the quantitation of microgram quantities of protein using the principle of protein-dye binding, *Anal. Biochem.* 72:248–254.

Brorson, J. R., Bindokas, V. P., Iwama, T., Marcuccilli, C. J., Chisholm, J. C., and Miller, R. J., 1995, The Ca2+ influx induced by beta-amyloid peptide 25–35 in cultured hippocampal neurons results from network excitation, *J. Neurobiol.* 26:325–338.

Bures, J., Buresova, O., and Huston, J. P., 1983, *Techniques and Basic Experiments for the Study of Brain and Behavior*, Elsevier, Amsterdam, N. Y., *pp.* 117.-132.

Chen, S. Y., Harding, J. W., and Barnes, C. D., 1996, Neuropathology of synthetic beta-amyloid peptide analogs in vivo. *Brain. Res.* 715:44–51.

Delobette, S., Privat, A, and Maurice, T., 1997, In vitro aggregation facilitates beta-amyloid peptide-(25–35)-induced amnesia in the rat, *Eur. J. Pharmacol,* in press.

Forloni, G., Chiesa, R., Smiroldo, S., Verga, L., Salmona, M., Tagliavini, F., and Angeretti, N., 1993, Apoptosis mediated neurotoxicity induced by chronic application of beta amyloid fragment 25–35, *Neuroreport* 4:523–535.

Forloni, G., Bugiani, O., Tagliavini, F., and Salmona, M., 1996, Apoptosis-mediated neurotoxicity induced by beta-amyloid and PrP fragments. *Mol. Chem. Neuropathol.* 28:163–170.

Francis, R., 1990, Amyloid. In: *Theory and practice of histological techniques.* Bankroff, T.D., Stavens, A., eds., 3rd edition, Edinburg. Churchill Livingstone, pp. 110–132.

Furukawa, K., Oyama, Y., Chikahisa, L., Hatakeyama, Y., and Akaike, N., 1994, Flow cytometric analysis on cytotoxic action of amyloid beta protein fragment 25–35 on brain neurons dissociated from the rats, *Brain Res.* 662:259–262.

Gulyaeva, N. V., Levshina, I. P., and Obidin, A. B., 1989, Indices of free radical-mediated oxidation of lipids and antiradical protection of the brain: Neurochemical correlates of development of the general adaptation syndrome, *Neurosci. Behav. Physiol.* 19:376–381.

Gulyaeva, N. V., Onufriev, M. V., and Stepanichev, M. Yu., 1994, NO synthase and free radical generation in old rats: Correlations with individual behavior, *NeuroReport.* 6:94–96.

Gulyaeva, N. V., and Erin, A. N.,1995, The role of free radical processes in development of neurodegenerative diseases, Neurochemistry (*Neurokhimija, Rus.)* 12:3–15.

Harris, M. E., Wang, Y., Pedigo, N. W., Jr., Hensley, K., Butterfield, D. A., and Carney, J. M. ,1996, Amyloid beta peptide (25–35) inhibits Na+-dependent glutamate uptake in rat hippocampal astrocyte cultures, *J. Neurochem.* 67: 277–284.

Hu, J., and el-Fakahany, E. E., 1993, Beta-Amyloid 25–35 activates nitric oxide synthase in a neuronal clone, *Neuroreport* 4:760–762.

Joseph, R., and Han, E., 1992, Amyloid beta-protein fragment 25–35 causes activation of cytoplasmic calcium in neurons, *Biochem. Biophys. Res. Commun.* 184: 1441–1147.

Kagan, V. E., Prilipko, L. L., Savov, V. M., Pisarev, V. A., Eluashvili, I. A., Kozlov Yu. P., 1979, Participation of free active forms of oxygen in enzymatic peroxidation of lipids in biomembranes, *Biochemistry (Biokhimija)* 44:379–385.

Kelley, A. E.,1993, Locomotor activity and exploration, In: *Behavioral Neuroscience. V. 2. A Practical Approach*, Sahgal A., ed., IRL Press. Oxford et al., pp. 1–24.

Maurice, T., Lockhart, B. P., and Privat, A., 1996, Amnesia induced in mice by centrally administered beta-amyloid peptides involves cholinergic dysfunction. *Brain Res.* 706: 181–193.

Mason, R. P., Estermyer, J. D., Kelly, J. F., Mason, P. E., 1996, Alzheimer's disease amyloid beta peptide 25–35 is localized in the membrane hydrocarbon core: x-ray diffraction analysis. *Biochem. Biophys. Res. Commun.* 222:78–82.

Nishikimi, N., Rao, A., and Yagi, K., 1972, The occurence of the superoxide anion in the reaction of reduced phenazine methosulfate and molecular oxygen, *Biochem. Biophys. Res. Comm.* 46:849–855.

Oyama, Y., Chikahisa, L., Ueha, T., Hatakeyama, Y., and Kokubun, T., 1995, Change in membrane permeability induced by amyloid beta-protein fragment 25–35 in brain neurons dissociated from rats. *Jpn. J. Pharmacol.* 68:77–83.

Pike, C. J., Walencewicz-Wasserman, A. J., Kosmoski, J., Cribbs, D. H., Glabe, C. G., and Cotman, C. W., 1995, Structure-activity analyses of beta-amyloid peptides: contributions of the beta 25–35 region to aggregation and neurotoxicity, *J. Neurochem.* 64:253–261.

Prehn, J. H., Bindokas, V. P., Jordan, J., Galindo, M. F., Ghadge, G. D., Roos, R. P., Boise, L. H., Thompson, C. B., Krajewski, S., Reed, J. C., and Miller, R. J., 1996, Protective effect of transforming growth factor-beta 1 on beta-amyloid neurotoxicity in rat hippocampal neurons, *Mol. Pharmacol.* 49:319–328.

Putchler, H., Sweat, F., and Levine, M., 1962, On the binding of Congo red by amyloid, *J. Histochem. Cytochem.* 10:355–374.

Reusche, E., 1991, Silver staining of senile plaque and neurfibrillary tangles in paraffin sections. A simple and effective method. *Path.. Res. Pract.* 187:1045–1057.

Richardson, J. S., Sarter, M., Bodewitz, G., and Stephens, D., 1988, Attenuation of the scopolamine-induced impairment of spontaneous alternation behaviour by antagonist but not inversed agonist and agonist β-carbolines, *Psychopharmacology*, 94:491–497.

Scorziello, A., Meucci, O., Florio T., Fattore M., Forloni G., Salmona M., and Schettini G., 1996, beta 25–35 alters calcium homeostasis and induces neurotoxicity in cerebellar granule cells, *J. Neurochem.* 66:1995–2002.

Schubert, D., and Chevion, M., 1995, The role of iron in beta amyloid toxicity, *Biochem. Biophys. Res. Commun.* 216:702–707.

Singh, I. N., McCartney, D. G., and Kanfer, J. N., 1995, Amyloid beta protein (25–35) stimulation of phospholipases A, C and D activities of LA-N-2 cells. *FEBS Lett.* 365:125–128.

Takashima, A., Yamaguchi, H., Noguchi, K., Michel, G., Ishiguro, K., Sato, K., Hoshino, T., Hoshi, M., and Imahori, K., 1995, Amyloid beta peptide induces cytoplasmic accumulation of amyloid protein precursor via tau protein kinase I/glycogen synthase kinase-3 beta in rat hippocampal neurons. *Neurosci. Lett.* 198:83–86.

Terranova, J. P., Kan, J. P., Storme, J. J., Perreaut, P., Le Fur, G., and Soubrie, P., 1996, Administration of amyloid beta-peptides in the rat medial septum causes memory deficits: reversal by SR 57746A, a non-peptide neurotrophic compound, *Neurosci. Lett.* 213:79–83.

Victorov, I. V, and Barskov, I. V., 1993, Method of ischemic neurons staining in the brain and spinal cord, *Pathol. Physiol. Experim. Therapy* 2:53–55.

Ueda, K,. Yagami, T., Kageyama, H., and Kawasaki, K., 1996, Protein kinase inhibitor attenuates apoptotic cell death induced by amyloid beta protein in culture of the rat cerebral cortex, *Neurosci. Lett.* 203:175–178.

Zhou, Y., Gopalakrishnan, and V., Richardson, J. S., 1996, Actions of neurotoxic beta-amyloid on calcium homeostasis and viability of PC12 cells are blocked by antioxidants but not by calcium channel antagonists, *J. Neurochem.* 67:1419–1426.

Zhou, Y., and Kumar, U., 1996, Free radicals in the neurotoxic actions of beta-amyloid, *Ann. N. Y. Acad. Sci.* 777:362–365.

15

MOLECULAR CHARACTERIZATION OF THE NEUROPROTECTIVE ACTIVITY OF SALICYLATES

M. Grilli, M. Pizzi, F. Goffi, M. Benarese, G. M. Gerardi, M. Memo, and P. F. Spano

Division of Pharmacology
Department of Biomedical Sciences and Biotechnologies
School of Medicine
University of Brescia
Brescia, Italy

INTRODUCTION

The idea that inflammatory processes contribute to the pathology of neurodegenerative diseases and in particular of Alzheimer's disease (AD), has been supported by epidemiological and clinical studies. Multiple retrospective epidemiological analyses indicate that patients receiving anti-inflammatory drugs or suffering from conditions in which such drugs are routinely used, have a decreased risk of developing AD (see McGeer and McGeer, 1995, as review). In a preliminary double-blind clinical trial, the non steroidal anti-inflammatory drug (NSAID) indomethacin has proven to reduce progression of cognitive decline in AD patients (Rogers et al., 1993). Obviously, more comprehensive clinical trials need to be carried out, but the future of anti-inflammatory therapy in AD holds great promise.

Among NSAIDs, aspirin is still one of the most widely prescribed compounds to treat inflammation (Insel, 1996). More recently, other previously unappreciated beneficial effects of prophylactic doses of acetyl salicyclic acid (ASA), including reduced risk of heart disease, transient ischemic attacks and decreased incidence of breast, colon and lung cancer have been demonstrated, as evidence of the peculiarly wide spectrum of action of this drug.

Here we provide further evidence for such a pleiotropic therapeutic value of ASA. In particular we demonstrate for ASA and its metabolite sodium salicyclate (NaSal) a novel effect, which could potentially synergize with their strict anti-inflammatory properties to ameliorate neurodegenerative states. At concentrations which are compatible with plasma levels maintained during chronic inflammatory therapeutic regimens (i.e. arthritis) (Insel,

Progress in Alzheimer's and Parkinson's Diseases
edited by Fisher *et al.*, Plenum Press, New York, 1998.

1996), the drugs potently counteract neurotoxicity elicited by the excitatory amino acid glutamate (Grilli et al., 1996).

SALICYLATES AND EXCITOTOXICITY

Glutamate is the most abundant excitatory neurotransmitter in the brain; however, under certain undefined conditions, it may become a potent excitotoxin whose contribution to the neurodegeneration associated with acute and chronic neurodegenerative diseases is widely recognized (Lipton and Rosenberg, 1995). Several models of neurons in culture have been extensively used to unravel the molecular events triggered by glutamate and leading to cell death as well as to develop a variety of pharmacological compounds able to counteract excitotoxicity. Among them, there is the primary culture of rat cerebellar granule cells, where a brief pulse of glutamate, through activation of the NMDA-type of glutamate receptor, induces cell death (Gallo et al., 1982). In the present study, ASA and NaSal were added to the culture medium 5 min before and during a 50 µM glutamate pulse, a concentration which is able to reduce cell survival by 70–80%. Cell viability after a glutamate pulse, applied in the absence or presence of the antiinflammatory drugs was evaluated 24 h later and expressed as percentage of neuroprotection. The range of concentration for the tested drugs was accurately chosen to correlate with the plasma concentrations for optimal antiinflammatory effects in patients with rheumathic diseases (Table 1) (Insel, 1996). A dose-dependent protection against glutamate-induced neurotoxicity was observed in the presence of both drugs (Grilli et al., 1996). For ASA the calculated EC_{50} value was 1.7 mM, with maximal effect (equivalent to 90% protection) exerted at 3 mM. The concentration of NaSal giving 50% of protection was about 5 mM, while maximal response (87% protection) was observed at 10 mM. Indomethacin, an effective antiinflammatory drug, was tested under the same experimental conditions. Unlike salicylates, at doses compatible with the plasma levels during drug chronic treatment (1–20 µM), indomethacin was unable to prevent glutamate-evoked cell death (Table 1).

Neuroprotection was also evaluated in a different experimental model involving slices of 8 day-old rat hippocampus (Garthwaite and Garthwaite, 1989). This experimental setting offers several advantages compared to primary cultures of neurons which make it more predictive for an *in vivo* effect of these drugs. First of all, the hippocampus contains neurons which are most vulnerable to excitotoxic damage, namely pyramidal and granular cells; additionally, the *ex vivo* preparation represents a heterogenous population of neurons which have been differentiated *in vivo*. In agreement with previous findings (Pizzi et al., 1996a), stimulation of the NMDA receptor subtype by application of the selective agonist

Table 1. Correlation between plasma levels maintained during chronic anti-inflammatory therapy and neuroprotective effects of the tested drugs

Agent	Plasma levels during chronic antiinflammatory therapy in humans[a]	Tested doses[b]	Neuroprotection in hippocampal slices (EC50)[b]	Neuroprotection in primary neurons (EC50)[b]	Inhibition of glutamate-induced NF-κB activation
Aspirin	1–3 mM	1–3 mM	< 3 mM	1.7 mM	+
NaSalicylate	1–3 mM	2–10 mM	< 2 mM	5 mM	−
Indomethacin	1–20 µM	1–20 µM	ND	NS	+

ND, not determined; NS, not significant.
[a]Data from Insel, 1996; [b]data from Grilli et al., 1996.

(30 μM, for 30 min), specifically induced a characteristic cell injury. Most of the pyramidal neurons of CA1, CA3 and granule cells of dentate gyrus (DG) became acutely necrotic: they exhibited highly swollen cytoplasm containing large vacuoles, nuclear shrinkage and focal clumping of chromatin. We found that application of ASA preserved hippocampal cell viability from the NMDA-mediated injury. The effect of ASA was evaluated at concentrations ranging from 1 to 10 mM. ASA did not modify cell viability at 1 mM concentration, while at 3 mM specifically the drug produced a significant neuroprotection in the CA3 region. Higher concentration of ASA elicited almost complete prevention of the NMDA effect even in CA1 and DG, besides CA3. Per se, the drug did not modify neuron viability. Interestingly, compared to what was observed in primary culture of rat cerebellar granule cells, as low as 2 mM NaSal was sufficient to efficiently counteract NMDA-mediated toxicity in hippocampal slices.

SALICYLATES AND GLUTAMATE-REGULATED CALCIUM HOMEOSTASIS

In an attempt to dissect the molecular mechanisms by which salicylates protect against glutamate-induced neurotoxicity, we first evaluated the possibility that these drugs might counteract glutamate-evoked cell death by diminishing the NMDA-mediated calcium entry. The hypothesis was tested in primary cultures of rat cerebellar granule cells by measuring $[Ca^{2+}]_i$ at the single cell level using microfluorimetry technology (Pizzi et al., 1996b). Application of glutamate in the absence of external Mg^{2+} caused a rapid increase of $[Ca^{2+}]_i$ followed by a sustained plateau, principally due to the NMDA receptor subtype activation. ASA, applied at the neuroprotective concentrations (1–3 mM) 2 min before glutamate exposure, induced a low transient increase of $[Ca^{2+}]_i$ but it did not modify cell responsiveness to the following glutamate response. Similarly, NaSal at neuroprotective concentrations ranging from 2 to 10 mM, produced a transient $[Ca^{2+}]_i$ elevation without altering glutamate response. These results strongly excluded a possible negative modulatory effect of both ASA and NaSal on the NMDA receptor efficiency and suggested their interference with intracellular molecular targets further downstream from glutamate receptor activation in the cascade of events triggering excitotoxicity. In this regard, salicylates appear distinguishable from most of the drugs endowed with neuroprotective properties. Moreover, the data indicate that, in contrast to what it is usually believed, neuroprotection can also occur independently of mechanisms controlling $[Ca^{2+}]_i$ homeostasis.

SALICYLATES AND NF-κB TRANSCRIPTION FACTORS

Despite their wide use in several clinical settings, the mechanisms underlying the anti-inflammatory properties of aspirin-like drugs have not been completely established. Drug effectiveness has been mainly ascribed to ability to prevent prostaglandin (PG) and thromboxane (TX) production by inhibiting the Prostaglandin Endoperoxide H Synthase (PGHS) enzyme (Insel, 1996). Nevertheless, some inconsistences within this hypothesis make the mechanism of action of these drugs still a matter of debate. For instance, salycilic acid lacks inhibitory activity on PGHS (Amin et al., 1995); moreover, doses of drugs needed to treat chronic inflammatory diseases are consistently higher than those required to inhibit PGs synthesis (Insel, 1996). The recent finding that, at plasma concentrations maintained during treatment of chronic inflammatory diseases, ASA and NaSal inhibit the activation of NF-κB transcription factors (Kopp and Gosh, 1994), has provided an additional explanatory mechanism for the anti-inflammatory properties of these drugs. The NF-κB/Rel family of transcription factors is indeed widely implicated in controlling expression of a large number of genes crucially involved in immune and inflammatory function (Grilli et al., 1993). Recently our and other groups (Kaltschmidt et al., 1994; Grilli et al., 1995; Guerrini et al. 1995; Grilli et al., 1996a) have demonstrated the presence of NF-κB/Rel proteins in primary neurons and in several brain areas. The functional significance of these proteins is still not completely understood but since certain subsets of neurons appear to contain constitutively active DNA-binding activity, it seems likely that they may participate in normal brain function. On the other hand, NF-κB/Rel proteins may be hypothesized as well as crucial third messengers in pathological brain states. In fact: i) in neurons, the NF-κB activity can be further modulated by signals like cytokines and glutamate, which are commonly involved in neurodegenerative processes (Guerrini et al., 1995; Kaltschmidt et al., 1995; Grilli et al., 1996a); ii) among the genes under the control of NF-κB molecules there is the amyloid precursor protein gene, whose involvement in the neuropathology associated with Alzheimer's disease is well established (Grilli et al., 1995; 1996a); iii) Yan and colleagues (1995) have shown a specific activation of NF-κB in brains of AD patients, and in particular in neuron subsets which show signs of degeneration, i.e tau accumulation.

As previously demonstrated, administration of glutamate to primary cultures of rat cerebellar granule cells, under the appropriate experimental conditions which elicit cell death via NMDA-receptor activation, results in a significant upregulation of NF-κB nuclear activity (Grilli et al. 1996; 1996a). In the present study, cells were exposed to a neurotoxic dose of glutamate (50 μM, 15 min pulse) in the absence or presence of ASA (1, 3 mM) and NaSal (3, 10 mM). Nuclear extracts were prepared 1 h after stimulation. We found that both drugs inhibited glutamate-induced increase of NF-κB activity in a dose-dependent manner (Grilli et al., 1996). Parallel experiments of cell viability, performed at later times (24 h), revealed a strict correlation between doses of anti-inflammatory drugs which are neuroprotective and blockade of induction of NF-κB. The salicylate effect on NF-κB/Rel proteins was specific. In fact, neuroprotective concentrations of ASA and Na-Sal failed to modify, under the same conditions, the glutamate-mediated nuclear induction of transcriptional complex AP1 (Curran and Franza, 1988).

CONCLUSION

In this report we demonstrate that, at concentrations compatible with plasma levels reached during treatment of chronic inflammatory states, ASA prevents glutamate-induced neurotoxicity. The neuroprotective effect does not appear to correlate with the anti-inflammatory properties of this compound since: 1) indomethacin was inactive; ii) in our experimental settings, aspirin is equi- or more potent than its metabolite salicylic acid; iii) preliminary studies of structure-activity relationship indicate in derivatives of benzoic acid the simplest core molecules that still retain neuroprotective ability (unpublished results).

The molecular target for ASA and sodium salicylate to exert neuroprotection appears to be localized downstream from the glutamate receptor. Along the cascade of events triggered by stimulation of the NMDA receptor the compounds are able to counteract glutamate-mediated induction of NF-κB activity. A strict correlation was observed between doses of the drugs able to prevent cell death and to block induction of the nuclear activity. The effect was specific, since under the same conditions, glutamate-mediated induction of AP-1 was unaffected.

The impact of the novel pharmacological property of salicylates in clinical use and in particular in acute and chronic neurodegenerative disorders, has still to be evaluated but it could be of great relevance. Our results offer a novel contribution to the emerging theme of anti-inflammatory therapy in AD, since they suggest an additional unexpected effect of salicylates which could beneficially counteract neurodegenerative states. These molecules would appear to possess a wider pharmacological spectrum compared to other NSAID. In view of their dual and distinct ability of acting not merely as anti-inflammatory compounds but also directly as antidegenerative molecules, we would predict a potential high benefit from the employment of aspirin-like drugs in neurodegenerative processes.

REFERENCES

Amin, A. R., Vyas, P., Attur, M., Leszczynska-Piziak, J., Patel, I.R., Weissmann, G., and Abramson, S.B., 1995, The mode of action of aspirin-like drugs: effect on inducible nitric oxide synthase, *Proc. Natl. Acad. Sci USA* 92:7926–7930.

Curran, T., and Franza, B.R., 1988, Fos and Jun: the AP-1 connection, *Cell.* 55:395–397.

Gallo, V., Ciotti, M.T., Coletti, F., Aloisi, F., and Levi, G., 1982, Selective release of glutamate from rat cerebellar granule cells differentiating in culture, *Proc. Natl. Acad. Sci.* USA.79:7919–7923.

Garthwaite, G., and Garthwaite, J., 1989, Differential dependence on calcium of N-methyl-D-aspartate and kainate neurotoxicity in young rat hippocampal slices, *Neurosci. Lett.* 97:316–321.

Grilli, M., Chiu, J-S., and Lenardo, M.J., 1993, NF-KB and Rel: participants in a multiform transciptional regulatory system, *Int. Rev. Cytol.* 143:1–62.

Grilli, M., Ribola, M., Alberici, A., Valerio, A., Memo, M., and Spano, P.F., 1995, Identification and characterization of a kB/Rel binding site in the regulatory region of the Amyloid Precursor Protein gene, *J. Biol. Chem.* 270:26774–26777.

Grilli, M., Pizzi, M., Memo, M., and Spano, P.F., 1996, Neuroprotection by aspirin and sodium salicylate through blockade of NF-B activation, *Science* 274:1383–1385.

Grilli, M., Goffi, F., Memo, M., and Spano, P.F., 1996a, Interleukin-1β and glutamate activate the NF-kB/Rel binding site from the regulatory region of the Amyloid Precursor Protein gene in primary neuronal cultures, *J. Biol. Chem.* 271:15002–15007.

Guerrini, L., Blasi, F., and Denis-Donini, S., 1995, Synaptic activation of NF-êB by glutamate in cerebellar granule neurons in vitro, *Proc. Natl. Acad. Sci.* USA 92:9077–9081.

Insel, P., 1996, in Goodman and Gilman's The Pharmacological Basis of Therapeutics, (McGraw-Hill, New York), pp. 617–657.

Kaltschmidt, C., Kaltschmidt, B., Neumann, H., Wekerle, H., and Baeuerle, P.A., 1994, Constitutive NFkB activity in neurons, *Mol. Cell. Biol.* 14:3981–3992.

Kaltschmidt, C., Kaltschmidt, B., and Baeuerle, P.A., 1995, Stimulation of ionotropic glutamate receptors activates transcription factor NF-kB in primary neurons, *Proc. Natl. Acad. Sci.* USA 92:9618.

Kopp, E., and Ghosh, S., 1994, Inhibition of NF-kB activity by sodium salicylate and aspirin, *Science* 265:956–959.

Lipton, S.A., and Rosenberg, P.A., 1995, Excitatory aminoacids as a final common pathway for neurological disorders, *New Engl. J. Med.* 330:613–622.

McGeer P.L., and McGeer E.G., 1995, The inflammatory response system of brain: implications for therapy of Alzheimer and other neurodegenerative diseases. *Brain Res. Rev.* 21:195–218.

Pizzi, M., Consolandi, O., Memo, M., and Spano, P.F., 1996a, Activation of multiple metabotropic glutamate receptor subtypes prevents NMDA-induced excitotoxicity in rat hippocampal slices. *Eur. J. Neurosci.* 8:1516–1521.

Pizzi, M., Galli, P., Consolandi, O., Arrighi, V., Memo, M., and Spano, P.F., 1996b, Metabotropic and ionotropic transducers of glutamate signal inversely control cytoplasmic Ca^{2+} concentration and excitotoxicity in cultured cerebellar granule cells: pivotal role of protein kinase C. *Mol. Pharmacol.* 49:586–594.

Rogers, J, Kirby, L.C., Hempelman, S.R., Berry, D.L., McGeer, P.L., Kaszniak, A.W., Zalinski, J., Cofield, M., Mansukhani, L., Willson, P., and Kogan, F., 1993, Clinical trial of indomethacin in Alzheimer's disease. *Neurology.* 43:1609–1611.

Yan, S.D., Yan, S.F., Chen, X., Fu, J., Chen, M., Kuppusamy, P., Smith, S.M., Perry, G., Godman, G.C., Nawroth, P., Zweier, J.L., and Stern, D., 1995, Non-enzymatically glycated tau in Alzheimer's disease induces oxidant stress resulting in cytokine gene expression and release of amyloid β-peptide. *Nature Med..* 1:693–699.

16

N-METHYL(R)SALSOLINOL: A NEUROTOXIN CANDIDATE TO INDUCE PARKINSON'S DISEASE CAUSES APOPTOSIS IN DOPAMINE CELLS

Wakako Maruyama[1] and Makoto Naoi[2]

[1]Laboratory of Biochemistry and Metabolism
Department of Basic Gerontology
National Institute for Longevity Sciences
Obu 474, Japan
[2]Department of Biosciences
Nagoya Institute of Technology
Gokiso-cho, Showa-ku
Nagoya 466, Japan

INTRODUCTION

Recently, it has been indicated that apoptosis is a type of cell death in the neurodegenerative disorders, such as Parkinson's disease (PD) and Alzheimer's disease. In PD, the apoptotic features were detected in the dopamine neurons of the substantia nigra by the terminal deoxylnucteotidyl transferase-mediated nick end labeling (TUNEL) method (Mochizuki et al., 1996) and also by electromicroscopic study (Anglade et al., 1997). However, the detailed mechanism to induce apoptosis has not been well clarified.

The discovery of 1-methyl-4-phenyl-1,2,3,6-tetrahydropyridine (MPTP), which elicits parkinsonism in humans, supports a hypothesis that a neurotoxin synthesized and accumulated in the dopamine neurons might induce PD. Among neurotoxin candidates, 1(R), 2(N)-dimethyl-1,2,3,4-tetrahydroisoquinoline [N-methyl(R)salsolinol, NM(R)Sal] is one of the most probable ones (Naoi et al., 1997). After injection of NM(R)Sal in the striatum, the rat showed behavioral changes, such as hypokinesia, rigidity of the tail and rhythmical twitch of the limbs. By histo-pathological study dopamine neurons were found to be selectively depleted in the substantia nigra without necrotic tissue reaction, which might indicate that NM(R)Sal induces apoptosis (Naoi et al., 1996).

In this paper, the mechanism of the cell death was examined using human dopaminergic neuroblastoma SH-SY5Y cells, which were differentiated with retinoic acid. DNA

Progress in Alzheimer's and Parkinson's Diseases
edited by Fisher *et al.*, Plenum Press, New York, 1998.

damage caused by NM(R)Sal and related compounds was quantitatively analyzed by use of a single cell gel electrophoresis (comet) assay (Ostling and Johanson, 1984; Singh et al., 1988). NM(R)Sal was found to induce apoptosis in the cells. The involvement of oxidative stress to apoptotic cell death and factors to protect the death process will be discussed in relation to the pathogenesis of PD.

MATERIALS AND METHODS

The (R)- and (S)enantiomers of 1-methyl-6,7-dihydroxy-1,2,3,4-tetrahydroisoquinoline (salsolinol, Sal) and NMSal were synthesized according to Teitel et al. (1972). 1,2-Dimethyl-6,7-dihydroxyisoquinolinium ion ($DMDHIQ^+$) was synthesized by the method of Bembenek et al. (1990). Cycloheximide, retinoic acid and superoxide dismutase were purchased from Sigma (St. Louis, MO); catalase, 4′,6-diamidino-2-phenylindole (DAPI), agarose (low melting-temperature), reduced glutathione (GSH) and other reagents were from Nacalai Tesque (Kyoto, Japan). *In situ* apoptosis detection kit was obtained from Takara Biomedicals (Kyoto, Japan) for the TUNEL method (Gavrieli et al., 1992).

SH-SY5Y cells were cultured in the abscence or presence of 10 μM retinoic acid for 3 days, and after the morphological change and arrest of the proliferation were confirmed in the cells treated with retinoic acid, they were used for the comet assay. SH-SY5Y cells were dissociated with trypsin, gathered, washed with Cosmedium-serum solution, then washed twice with phosphate-buffered saline (PBS). The cells were then suspended in 500 μl (a total volume) of the Krebs-Ringer solution and incubated with NM(R)Sal and other isoquinotines at 37°C. Then, the cells were centrifuged, washed with PBS, and DNA damage was assessed by the comet assay. The cells (5×10^4 cells) were suspended in 100 μl of PBS free from calcium and magnesium, 20 μl of which was mixed with 14 μl of 1% low-melting agarose in PBS. The mixture (100 μl) was applied on a microscope slide, and allowed to stand at 4°C for 10 min. The slide was subjected to alkaline lysis at 4°C for 1 hour in 10 mM Tris buffer, pH 10.0, containing 2.5 M NaCl, 100 mM EDTA, 1% sarcosine and 1% Triton X-100, to which dimethyl sulfoxide (DMSO) was added to 10% just before use. The slides were equilibrated with an alkaline electrophoresis buffer, 300 mM NaOH solution containing 1 mM EDTA 2Na, at 4°C for 20 min. Electrophoresis was carried out with 25 V and 300 mA at 4°C for 20 min. After neutralization with 0.4 M Tris-HCl buffer, pH 7.5, DNA was stained with DAPI solution (1 μg/ml). The comet image was observed through a video camera attached to a fluorescence microscope at 200 time magnification. Two hundred images were randomly selected and their length (the nucleus plus migrated DNA tail) was measured on the screen.

The effects of antioxidants and other compounds were examined. The cells were incubated at 37°C for 20 min in a total volume of 500 μl with GSH (100 μM, final concentration), catalase (0.5 mg), superoxide dismutase (2000 units), deprenyl (20 μM) or semicarbazide (100 μM), or 60 min with cycloheximide (5 μM). Then, NM(R)Sal (0.5 mM) was added and the effects were examined after a 3 hour incubation. The effects of the antioxidants were examined also in the cells differentiated by the retinoic acid. The cells were pre-incubated with mannitol (10 mM), N-acetylcysteine (500 μM), n-propyl gallate (5 μM), tocopherol (250 μM), Tris (10 mM) and butylated hydroxyanisole (20 μM), and then NM(R)Sal (0.2 mM) was added and incubated for 3 hours.

Morphological detection of apoptosis was performed by staining differentiated SH-SY5Y cells treated with NM(R)Sal after stained by the TUNEL method and with hematoxylin-eosin (H-E) solution. The cells were incubated with NM(R)Sal at 37°C for 3 hours as in the case of the comet assay. Control and NM(R)Sal-treated cells were resuspended in PBS and applied on a slide glass, dried immediately by cool air, stained using H-E and the TUNEL method according to the manufacture's instructions, and viewed by a light microscopy. After H-E stain, the cytoarchitectural characteristic of apoptosis was assessed by cell shrinkage, condensation of nuclear chromatin, formation of membrane blebs and apoptotic bodies.

RESULTS

One mM of NM(R)Sal induced DNA damage in almost all cells (Fig. 1), whereas in the cells incubated without isoquinotines or with (R)- and (S)Sal and DMDHIQ$^+$, DNA damage was negligible. The distance from the comet head to the tip of the tail was determined as the comet length and the cells with the length longer than 45 μm was assessed as positive for DNA damage.

The nature of DNA damage by NM(R)Sal was investigated by morphological observation. After incubation with NM(R)Sal, some of the cells showed morphological features specific for apoptosis; condensation of chromatin materials and also "apoptotic" bodies. The specific immuno-cytochemical TUNEL method was applied to detect 3'-OH ends of increased small nucleosomal units. Positive staining was detected in the cells incubated with NM(R)Sal.

A protein synthesis inhibitor, cycloheximide, prevented DNA damage induced by 0.5 mM NM(R)Sal, as shown in Table 1. Pre-incubation of the cells with 5 μM cycloheximide reduced occurrence of the DNA damage. Allowing for the fact that cycloheximide itself induced some DNA damage, it can be seen that pre-treatment with cycloheximide prevented the DNA damage essentially completely.

Table 2 summarizes the effects of 1 mM NM(R)Sal and its related compounds on the tail length of the cells. Only (R)- and (S)-enantiomers of NMSal induced significant DNA damage, but the effect of NM(R)Sal was much profound than NM(S)Sal. The effect of both enantiomers of NMSal was further compared with different concentrations. The rate of induced DNA damage was dependent on the concentration (p < 0.01) for both the enantiomers and the effect of NM(R)Sal was about 20 times greater than the (S)-enantiomer.

The differentiation of the cells by retinoic acid clearly increased the sensitivity to the neurotoxicity by NM(R)Sal. As shown in Fig. 2, in the differentiated cells apoptosis was observed with NM(R)Sal at much lower concentrations than the cells without treatment.

The effects of anti-oxidants and anti-oxidative enzymes were examined. With 0.5 mM NM(R)Sal about 18% cells showed the typical comet image of DNA damage. Pretreatment with catalase, GSH, deprenyl or semicarbazide protected the cells from the DNA damage. On the other hand, superoxide dismutase did not prevent the DNA damage induced by NM(R)Sal, and the number of cells with DNA damage was not different from the cells incubated with NM(R)Sal alone. The cells treated with retinoic acid were pre-incubated with anti-oxidants, and the effect of 0.2 mM of NM(R)Sal was examined. Mannitol, N-acetylcysteine, n-propyl gallate, Trisand butylated hydroxyanisole reduced DNA damage, but tocopherol did not.

DISCUSSION

Apoptosis is an active process of cell death observed during development, but recently postmitotic cells such as neurons were found to apoptose. Apoptosis can be initi-

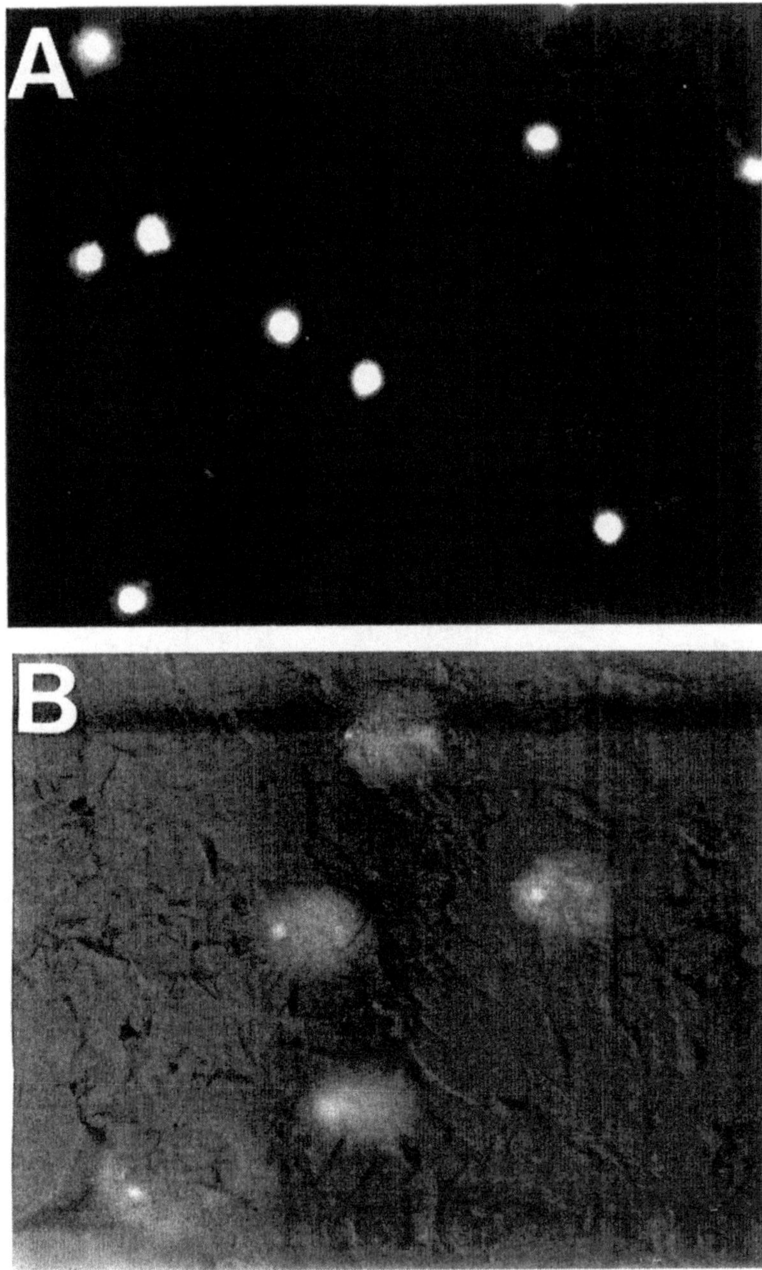

Figure 1. Fluorescence photomicrographs of SH-SY5Y cells. Cells were incubated without (A) or with (B) 1 mM of N-methyl(R)salsolinol for 3 hours and subjected to the comet assay, as described in Materials and Methods.

ated by various stimuli such as oxidative stress and ATP depletion (Hartley et al., 1994, Wolvetang et al., 1994) and a neurotoxin 1-methyl-4-phenylpyridinium ion (MPP$^+$) was reported to induce apoptosis (Dipasquale et al., 1991, Mutoh et al., 1994). In this article endogenous dopaminergic neurotoxin NM(R)Sal was found to induce DNA damage in

Table 1. Effect of cycloheximide on DNA damage induced by N-methyl(R)salsolinol

SH-SY5Y cells treated with	% of DNA damaged cells
Control	1.30 ± 0.65
Cycloheximide (5 µM)	15.34 ± 6.90
N-methyl(R)salsolinol (0.5 mM)	28.13 ± 3.72
Cycloheximide + N-methyl(R)salsolinol	6.40 ± 4.20*

SH-SY5Y cells were pre-treated with 5 µM of cycloheximide for 1 hour and then, 0.5 mM of N-methyl(R)salsolinol was added in the cell suspension and incubated further for 3 hours. The cells with the comet length greater than 40 µm were determined as DNA damaged cells. Percentage of DNA damaged cells was compared with cells without treatment (control), cells treated with cycloheximide alone or N-methyl(R)salsolinol alone. Each value represents the mean ± SD of 3 independent experiments. *p < 0.05 compared to cells treated with N-methyl(R)salsolinol alone by ANOVA.

Table 2. Effect of dopamine-derived isoquinolines on SH-SY5Y cells

SH-SY5Y cells incubated with	Comet length (µm)
Control	11.00 ± 1.00
(R)Salsolinol	10.45 ± 2.21
(S)Salsolinol	9.92 ± 1.60
N-methyl(R)salsolinol	57.24 ± 5.08*
N-methyl(S)salsolinol	12.60 ± 4.53**
DMDHIQ+	10.44 ± 1.47

SH-SY5Y cells were treated with 1 mM of each isoquinolines for 3 hours as described in Materials and Methods. The comet length was measured on a TV screen attached to a fluorescence microscope. Each value represents the mean ± SD of comet length of 100 cells. *p < 0.01, **p< 0.05 compared to control by analysis of variance (ANOVA).

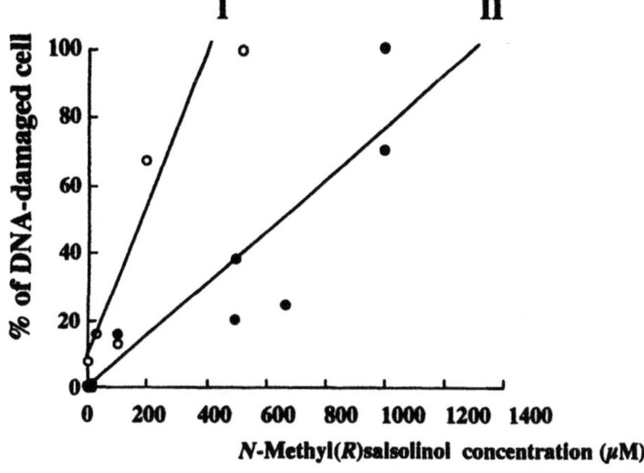

Figure 2. The effect of N-methyl(R)salsolinol on SH-SY5Y cells cultured with (I, open circle) and without (II, filled circle) retinoic acid. SH-SY5Y cells were cultured with 10 µM of retinoic acid for 3 days prior to the experiment. Then, the cells were suspended in Krebs-Ringer solution and treated with various concentration of N-methyl(R)salsolinol for 3 hours. The cells with comet length greater than 40 µm were assessed to be positive for DNA damage. Each circle represents the mean of 2 independent experiments.

dopaminergic neuroblastoma cells. An inhibitor of protein synthesis, cycloheximide, protected the cells from the damage, indicating that active intracellular process was involved in the mechanism. In addition, the morphological study confirmed DNA damage was apoptosis. This is the first report to demonstrate apoptosis induced by an endogenous neurotoxin. The (R)-enantiomer of NMSal was found to be more potent to induce DNA damage than the (S)-enantiomer. It indicates that some intracellular molecules may distinguish the enantiomeric characteristics of NMSal and initiate the death process. NM(R)Sal was found to produce hydroxyl radical *in vivo and in vitro* and DMDHIQ$^+$ simultaneously (Maruyama et al., 1995a,b). Catalase and other radical scavengers, GSH, semicarbazide, mannitol, N-acetylcysteine, n-propyl gallate and Tris protected the cell from DNA damage. It suggests the radical generation may account for apoptosis induced by NM(R)Sal.

The mechanism of the protective effect of deprenyl should not be ascribed to its inhibition of type B monoamine oxidase (MAO-B), because SH-SY5Y cells do not have MAO-B activity (Maruyama et al., 1997b). Recently there are reports supporting that the neuroprotective action of deprenyl cannot be simply ascribed to MAO-B inhibition, but that deprenyl can modulate the transcription of genes involved in apoptotic process (Tatton et al., 1996).

The analysis of human brains showed that there exist only (R)-enantiomer of Sal and NMSal. In addition, (R)Sal distributed in whole brain regions examined, whereas NM(R)Sal occurred in the substantia nigra and the caudate-putamen, and DMDHIQ$^+$ was detectable only in the substantia nigra (Maruyama et al., 1997a). NM(R)Sal might be synthesized and accumulated in dopamine neurons of the nigro-striatal system and oxidized and accumulated in the substantia nigra. Increased activity of a (R)Sal N-methyltransferase in the PD lymphocyte (Naoi et al., this book) and probably in the brain might result in an increase of NM(R)Sal, as already shown in the cerebrospinal fluid of untreated Parkinsonian patients (Maruyama et al., 1996). The result here indicates NM(R)Sal might induce apoptosis in dopamine neurons of the substantia nigra and subsequently PD after long term of accumulation.

ACKNOWLEDGMENTS

This work was supported by a Grant-In-Aid for Scientific Research on Priority Area, and (C) from a Ministry of Education, Science and Culture, Japan.

REFERENCES

Anglade, P., Vyas, S., Javoy-Agid, F., Herrero, M.T., Michel, P.P., Marquez, J., Mouratt-Prigent, A., Ruberg, M., Hirsh, E.C. and Agid, Y., 1997, Apoptosis and autophagy in nigral neurons of patients with Parkinson's disease. *Histol. Histopathol.* 12:25–31.

Bembenek, M.E., Abell, C.W., Chrisey, L.A., Rowadowska, M.D., Gesser, W. and Brossi, A., 1990, Inhibition of monoamine oxidase A and B by simple isoquinoline alkaloids: racemic and optically active 1,2,3,4-tetrahydro, 3,4-dihydro, and fully aromatic isoquinolines. *J. Med. Cliem.* 33:147–152.

Dipasquale, B., Marini, A.M. and Youle, R.J., 1991, Apoptosis and DNA degradation induced by 1-methyl-4-phenylpyridinium in neurons. *Biochem. Biophys. Res. Commun.* 181:1442–1448.

Hartley, A., Stone, J.M., Heronm, C., Cooper, J.M. and Shapira, A.H.V., 1994, Complex I inhibitors induce dose-dependent apoptosis in PC12 cells: Relevance to Parkinson's disease. *J. Neurochem.* 63:1987–1990.

Maruyama, W., Dostert, P., Matsubara, K. and Naoi, M., 1995a, N-Methyl(R)salsolinol produces hydroxyl radicals: Involvement to neurotoxicity. *Free Radic. Biol. Med.* 19:67–75.

Maruyama, W., Dostert, P. and Naoi, M., 1995b, Dopamine-derived 1-methyl-6,7-dihydroxyisoquinolines as hydroxyl radical promoters and scavengers in the rat brain: *in vivo* and *in vitro* studies. *J. Neurochem.* 64:2635–2743.

Maruyama, W., Abe, T., Tohgi, H., Dostert, P. and Naoi, M., 1996, A dopaminergic neurotoxin, (R)-N-methylsalsolinol, increases in parkinsonian CSF. *Ann. Neurol.* 40:119–122.

Maruyama, W., Sobue, G., Matsubara, K., Hashizume, Y., Dostert, P. and Naoi, M., 1997a, A dopaminergic neurotoxin, 1(R), 2(N)-dimethyl-6,7-dihydroxy-1,2,3,4-tetrahydroisoquinoline, and its oxidation product, 1,2(N)-dimethyl-6,7-dihydroxyisoquinolinium ion, accumulate in the nigro-striatal system in the human brain. *Neurosci. Lett.* 223:61–64.

Maruyama, W., Naoi, M., Kasamatsu, T., Hashizume, Y., Takahashi, T., Kohda, K. and Dostert, P., 1997b, An endogenous dopaminergic neurotoxin, N-methyl(R) salsolinol, induces DNA dwnage in human dopaminergic neuroblastoma SH-SY5Y cells. *J. Neurochem.*, in press.

Mochizuki, H., Goto, G., Mori, H. and Mizuno, Y., 1996, Histochemical detection of apoptosis in Parkinson's disease. *J. Neurol. Sci.* 137:120–123.

Mutoh, T., Tokuda, A., Marini, A.M. and Fujiki, N., 1994, 1-Methyl-4-phenylpyridinium kills differentiated PC12 cells with a concomitant change in protein phosphorylation. *Brain Res.* 661:51–55.

Naoi, M., Maruyama, W., Dostert, P., Hashizume, Y., Nakahara, D., Takahashi, T. and Ota, M., 1996, Dopamine-derived endogenous 1(R), 2(N)-dimethyl-6,7-dihydroxy-1,2,3,4-tetrahydroisoquinoline, N-methyl-(R)-salsolinol, induced parkinsonism in rat: Biochemical, pathological and behavioral studies. *Brain Res.* 709:285–295.

Naoi, M., Maruyama, W., Dostert, P. and Hashizume, Y., 1997, N-Methyl-(R)salsolinol as a dopaminergic neurotoxin: From an animal model to an early marker of Parkinson's disease. *J. Neural Transm.* [Suppl 50]:89–105.

Ostling, 0. and Johanson, K.J., 1984, Microelectrophoretic study of radiation-induced DNA damage in individual mammalian cells. *Biochem. Biophys. Res. Commun.* 123:291–298.

Teitel, S., O'Brien, J. and Brossi, A., 1972, Alkaloids in mammalian tissues. 2. Synthesis of (+) and (-)-1-substituted-6,7-dihydroxy-1,2,3,4-tetrahydroisoquinolines. *J. Med. Chem.* 15:845–846.

Tatton, W.G. and Chalmers-Redman, R.M.E., 1996, Modulation of gene expression rather than monoamine oxidase inhibition: (–)-Deprenyl-related compounds in controlling neurodegeneration. *Neurology* 47 [Suppl 3]:S171–183.

Wolvetang, E.J., Johnson, K.L., Knauer, K., Ralph, S.J. and Linnane, A.W., 1994, Mitochondrial respiratory chain inhibitors induce apoptosis. *FEBS Lett.* 339:40–44.

17

AGE-RELATED Na,K-ATPase mRNA EXPRESSION AND ALZHEIMER'S DISEASE

George J. Siegel,[1,2] Neelima B. Chauhan,[1] and John M. Lee[3]

[1]Molecular and Cellular Neuroscience Laboratory
Neurology Service
Edward Hines Jr. Veterans Affairs Hospital
Hines, Illinois
[2]Departments of Neurology and Molecular and Cellular Biochemistry
[3]Departments of Pathology and Pharmacology and Experimental Therapeutics
Loyola University Chicago
Stritch School of Medicine
Maywood, Illinois

INTRODUCTION

The pathogenesis of Alzheimer's disease (AD) is believed to involve multiple factors including known and unknown genetic as well as acquired influences (Selkoe, 1994). The known genetic mutations involve the amyloid precursor protein (APP), trisomy 21 in Down's syndrome, presenilin 1 and presenilin 2 (Selkoe, 1994; Hardy, 1997). However, in more than 90% of AD patients, the disease is sporadic with onset in late adulthood although the probability of developing AD is increased by the presence of the ε4 allele of apolipoprotein E (Corder et al., 1993). While all the inherited and sporadic cases of AD are believed to involve abnormal processing and deposition of fibrillar amyloid (Aβ) peptides derived from APP (Selkoe, 1994; Hardy, 1997), there are many indications that Aβ peptide processing is not the only critical factor in AD dementia, and that other factors may interact with Aβ peptide to potentiate the toxicity.

It is notable that in all of the sporadic, familial and congenital (trisomy 21) forms of AD, the incidence of dementia increases with advancing age. In trisomy 21, the incidence of AD type of dementia and behavioral changes increases with increasing age after 40, the mean age of onset being 56 years (Zigman et al., 1996; Visser et al., 1997), although the histopathology characteristic of AD begins earlier and is almost uniform over 35 years (Del Bo et al., 1997). These data suggest the existence of general factors in normal aging that potentiate AD or AD type of dementia. Such age-related factors may be: (1) effects accumulated over time from the environment or from endogenous metabolic processes, such as reactive oxygen species; or (2) effects of postadult differentiation of gene expression with age, which is manifested as cell-specific changes in expression of selective genes with advancing age after reproductive years. (Chauhan and Siegel, 1996). While presumably not subject to evolutionary pressure, these changes in gene regulation may or may not be desirable to the organism living past the reproductive phase. Candidates for this type of gene, the regulation of which might potentiate AD pathogenesis, would be those (a) that show changes in normal aging and (b) that show greater than normal changes correlated with the earliest pathologic events in AD.

Although there have been numerous studies of gene expression in AD brains compared to age-matched controls, there have been very few comparisons of expression in normal aged to young human subjects. The only available data for changes in expression in both normal aging human brain and in AD indicate increases in mRNA for glial fibrillary acidic protein (GFAP) (Nichols et al., 1993) and glial S-100 (Sheng et al., 1996), decreases in mRNA for calbindin-28K (Iacopino and Christakos, 1990), and alterations in the proportions among the three mRNA constructs for APP (Oyama et al., 1993; Tanaka et al., 1993).

On the other hand, studies of rat brain have shown age-related, cell-specific differentiation of Na,K-ATPase catalytic (α) subunit isoform expression. The mRNA for the α3 or neuron-specific catalytic subunit isoform of Na,K-ATPase is reduced 3 to 4-fold in neurons while the α1-isoform mRNA, which is found in glia and in some neurons, is increased 7 to 8-fold in regions of aged rat brain (Chauhan and Siegel, 1996, 1997a, 1997b). Na,K-ATPase is the enzyme responsible for the major portion of brain energy expenditure and the Na^+ gradients critical to many nerve functions (Albers et al., 1994). Age-related differentiation of this enzyme, if it occurs also in humans, might be a candidate for potentiation of neurodegeneration. Therefore, we analyzed cell-specific Na,K-ATPase α1- and α3-isoform mRNAs by in situ hybridization in the superior frontal cortex of five cases of AD and five cases of nondemented control males between 69 and 84 years and three cases of young control males between 35 and 46 years of age.

METHODS

Cases were selected from the Loyola University/Hines VAH Brain Bank. Severity of AD was graded according to CERAD criteria.Total cellular RNA was extracted from isopentane-frozen samples, electrophoretically separated on denaturing gels, transferred to GeneScreen membranes, and hybridized with ^{32}P-labeled human β-actin cRNA. Only cases with excellent preservation of 18S and 28S ribosomal RNA bands and consistent labeling with the β-actin probe were studied. In situ hybridization was performed on 10% buffered formalin-fixed, 5μm-thick Paraplast sections with the use of [^{35}S]CTP-riboprobes. Cloned rat α-isoform cDNAs, provided by Dr. Robert Levenson (Yale University) and by Dr. Jerry Lingrel (University of Cincinnati College of Medicine) were used to prepare subclones containing portions of α1- and α3-subunit cDNAs. Preparation of riboprobes and procedures for in situ hybridization and quantitative image analysis with the BioQuant OS/2 System were carried out as described previously (Chauhan and Siegel, 1996). Total grain densities for α1- and α3-mRNAs were counted under dark-field illumination in five cortical columns separated by ~1.0–1.2 cm in each of two adjacent sections. Each column of 180μm-width was divided into 4 depths orthogonal to the pial surface between the pia and the white matter. For each case, 10 measurements per depth were obtained. In addition, within depth 4, grain-clusters over individual pyramidal neuron were counted. Ten pyramidal neurons within depth 4 of each column, in 3 columns per section and 6 columns per case, totaling 60 pyramidal neurons per case were analyzed. Diffuse and neuritic plaques were counted in the same regions on adjacent sections stained with the Bielschowsky silver method. Data were statistically analyzed by two-way ANOVA for testing variations in $\alpha1$- and $\alpha3$-mRNA-densities within total neuropil of (1) different cortical depths, and (2) different groups; and one-way ANOVA for comparing mean $\alpha3$-mRNA density over pyramidal neurons within different groups. $\alpha1$- and $\alpha3$-mRNA densities can not be compared to each other since the actual amount of radioactivity bound per molecule is not known. Ratios for the different regions and isoforms are the means based on 3 cases of young normal, and 5 cases each of the aged normal and AD.

RESULTS

Grains representing $\alpha1$-mRNA were distributed diffusely through the cortex. Density measurements showed that the mean $\alpha1$-mRNA per unit area of neuropil was slightly increased by 10% in the deepest layer of the normal aged relative to young brains but this value did not reach significance. In AD brains, however, the $\alpha1$-mRNA density was increased significantly by 13–18% in all the layers relative to both the normal aged ($p < 0.003$) and young ($p < 0.003$) brains.

On the other hand, grains representing $\alpha3$-mRNA were localized in clusters over pyramidal neurons. In addition, there was an even distribution of $\alpha3$-mRNA as fine grains throughout the dendritic neuropil, presumably in neuronal extensions (although electron microscopy would be required to distinguish these from glial processes), in all the cortical layers of normal young and aged brains (Fig. 1). No amyloid plaques were seen in the normal aged brain (Fig. 2). When clusters of grains over individual neurons in depth 4 were counted, it was found that the mean $\alpha3$-mRNA content per neuron was decreased by 14% in the normal aged group ($p < 0.01$) and by 44% in the AD group relative to young brains ($p < 0.001$). Density measurements of total $\alpha3$-mRNA in the neuropil were significantly decreased by 31–38% in all cortical layers of the AD brains relative to the normal aged (compare Figs. 1 and 3) and young controls ($p < 0.0001$). However, $\alpha3$-mRNA grain density in the neuropil was not significantly different between the normal aged and normal young groups. AD brains showed marked reductions in $\alpha3$-mRNA content per neuron (Fig. 3) and accumulation of amyloid plaques in adjacent sections (Fig. 4).

Sections of cerebellar vermis from the same cases were carried through the same procedures with the frontal cortex sections. There were no significant differences with respect to $\alpha1$- or $\alpha3$-mRNA densities in granular, Purkinje cell or molecular layers among the three groups of subjects ($p = 0.2$). These data together with the facts that the $\alpha1$- and $\alpha3$-mRNA densities change in opposite directions in the cortex prove that the differences observed in frontal cortex between young, normal aged and AD groups cannot be ascribed to artifacts of tissue shrinkage or fixation, differential postmortem preservation of $\alpha1$- and $\alpha3$-mRNAs, agonal conditions, or handling of tissues or sections. Moreover, since not even a tendency for small differences in the vermis was observed, the significant changes, albeit small, observed in the pyramidal neuron perikarya of the normal aged frontal cortex relative to the young are considered of probable biological significance with respect to aging. However, data are needed from more cases at various ages and with other types of neurodegeneration.

In order to test a correlation of changes in mRNA density with neuropathologic characteristics of AD, the cortical burdens of diffuse and of neuritic/core plaques were

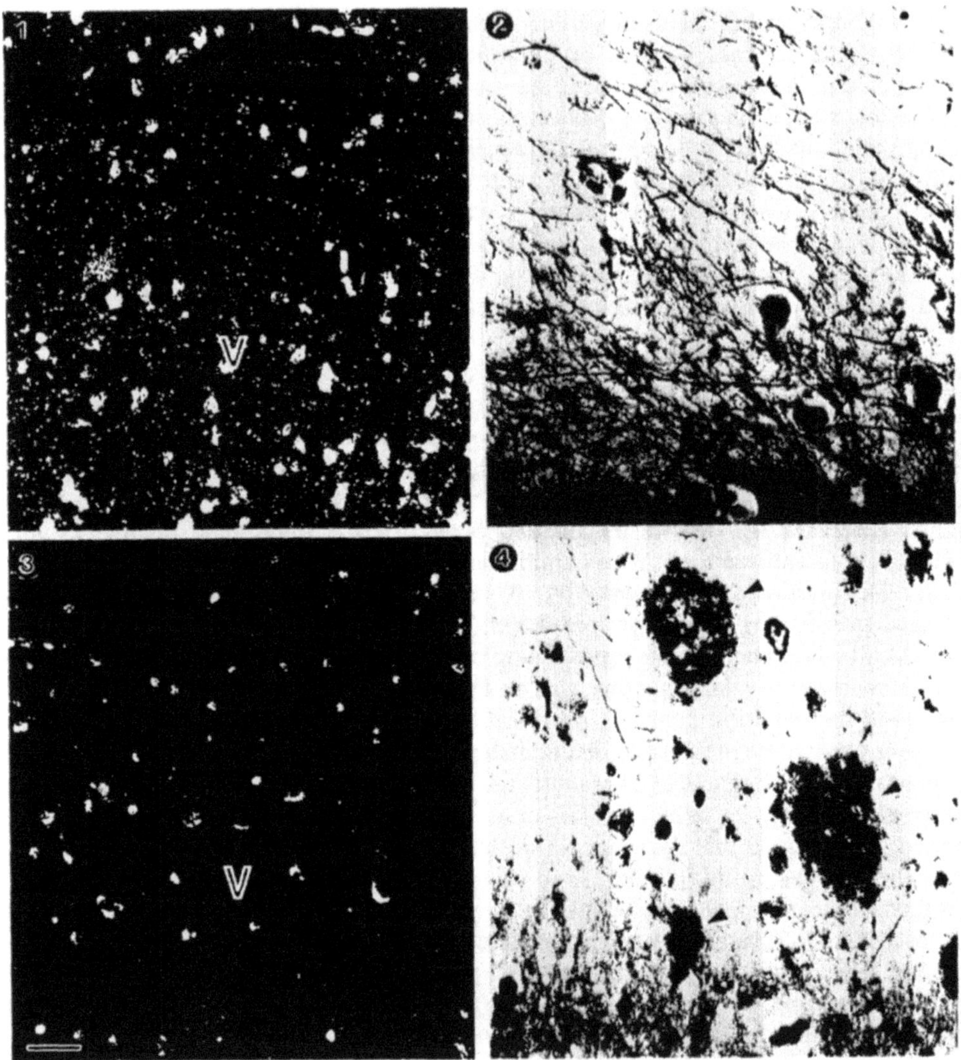

Figure 1-4. *In situ* distribution of Na,K-ATPase α3-mRNA (Figs. 1 and 3) and modified Bielschowsky silver stain (Figs. 2 and 4) in layer V of the superior frontal cortex from a 78 year-old male control brain (Figs. 1 and 2) and 83 year-old male Alzheimer's disease (AD) brain (Figs. 3 and 4). The control brain shows abundant distribution of α3-mRNA in the neuropil and pyramidal neurons (Fig. 1) and absence of plaques in the adjacent section (Fig. 2). The AD brain shows marked reduction in α3-mRNA (Fig. 3) and accumulation of amyloid plaques (arrowheads) in the adjacent section (Fig. 4). Scale bar = 25 μm.

plotted versus the densities of α1-mRNA and of α3-mRNA in each cortical depth for each case of AD. Linear regression analysis suggests an inverse correlation of the diffuse plaque counts with total neuropil α3-mRNA density in depths 1, 3 and 4 from case to case (r values: 0.806, 0.805, 0.753; p values: 0.099, 0.1, 0.142). However, given the small N of five, additional cases are needed to establish statistical significance. There was no obvious correlation of α3-mRNA with neuritic plaque counts nor of α1-mRNA with either diffuse or neuritic plaques.

DISCUSSION

This study shows that the normal aged group exhibits small but significant declines of α3-mRNA in the deep cortical neuronal perikarya, but not in the neuropil, relative to young controls, while the AD group is subject to 3-fold greater (44%) perikaryal reductions than in the normal aged group and significant 31–38% decreases in the neuropil of all the cortical layers as well. These data taken together indicate that declines of α3-mRNA in neuronal perikarya begin in normal aging, independently of AD, and are accelerated in AD. In AD, the declines in perikaryal α3-mRNA are exaggerated and are accompanied by further declines of total α3-mRNA in perikarya as well as in cell extensions in the neuropil. The declines in α3-mRNA are in contrast to the significant increases (13–18%) of total α1-mRNA in neuropil. The increased α1-mRNA is probably related to glial hypertrophy or activation as evidenced by increases in GFAP (Nichols et al., 1993) and S-100 mRNAs (Sheng et al., 1996). This is not to say that such changes occur only in AD, since other types of neurodegenerations have not yet been studied in this way. Also, it should be kept in mind that these data represent steady-state levels of mRNA and that information regarding turnover of either the mRNA or proteins is lacking.

If diffuse plaques represent one of the earliest forms of Aβ deposition and Aβ is critical to the pathogenesis (Cummings et al., 1996), then their inverse correlation with α3-mRNA density in the neuropil in individual cases suggests that the decline in α3-mRNA begins early in the disease, certainly before neuronal dystrophic changes or neuritic plaques, and that the acceleration of declines relative to the normal aged group is also an intrinsic part of the disease progression. The questions are: which is the cause and which the effect, or is it a vicious cycle? Although these data clearly show that declines in α3-mRNA do not depend on AD histopathology since they begin in normal aging, we do not know what is the earliest age at which an AD-specific process actually begins.

Mattson and colleagues have found that β-amyloid peptides inhibit Na,K-ATPase prior to producing cytotoxicity, Ca^{++} influx and cell death in cell cultures (Mark, et al., 1995). Exposure of cultured cells to ouabain, the specific inhibitor of Na,K-ATPase, also produces cytotoxic effects similar to those of the β-amyloid peptides (Mark et al., 1995). In addition, inhibition of Na,K-ATPase potentiates glutamate excitotoxicity (Brines and Robbins, 1992).

It is plausible to hypothesize that reductions in the capacity to upregulate neuron-specific Na,K-ATPase in vivo, such as may result from decreased mRNA levels in normal aging, would either predispose to or potentiate any pathologic process that produces inhibition of the enzyme. According to this hypothesis, age-related declines in neuronal expression of catalytic subunit would be synergistic with Aβ inhibition of Na,K-ATPase in the pathogenic process, which would lead to further cell toxicity and exaggerated reductions of α3-mRNA in a vicious cycle. It is possible, moreover, that Aβ itself, which activates tyrosine phosphorylation in cell cultures (Luo et al, 1996), produces intracellular signaling effects that lead to synergistic reductions in Na,K-ATPase mRNA levels. The elements of this hypothesis can be tested better in cell cultures and transgenic mouse models of AD than in humans.

CONCLUSIONS

These observations do not mean that reduced Na,K-ATPase mRNA is the cause of AD but that (1) these changes in Na,K-ATPase gene regulation occur with normal aging and that (2) these changes are exaggerated in neurons prior to any obvious dystrophic cell changes early in the course of AD. Postadult differentiation of Na,K-ATPase isoform expression may be a normal age-dependent factor that potentiates AD. Elucidation of normal age-related differentiation of gene expression and the possible impact of such changes on the cell toxicity of AD-specific factors such as amyloid and neurofibrillary tangles may open new avenues for interventions to delay or ameliorate the AD disease as well as for studying the neurobiology of normal aging.

ACKNOWLEDGMENTS

This work was supported in part by the Chicago Association for Research, Education and Science, Hines Veterans Affairs Hospital and the Bane Charitable Trust, Loyola University Chicago. The authors acknowledge the assistance provided by Phyllis Anderson and Gerda Kirshner, Medical Media Service, Hines Veterans Affairs Hospital and the technical support of Debra Magnuson, Department of Pathology, Loyola University Medical Center.

REFERENCES

Albers, R.W., Siegel, G.J.and Stahl, W.L., 1994, Membrane Transport, in *Basic Neurochemistry: Molecular, Cellular and Medical Aspects*, 5th edit., Siegel, G.J., et al., eds., Raven Press, New York, pp. 49–74.

Brines,M.L. and Robbins, R.J., 1992, Inhibition of α2/ α3 sodium pump isoform potentiates glutamate neurotoxicity. *Brain Res.* 591:94–102.

Chauhan, N.B. and Siegel, G.J., 1996, In situ analysis of Na,K-ATPase α1- and α3-isoform mRNAs in aging rat hippocampus. *J. Neurochem.* 66 (4):1742–1751.

Chauhan, N.B. and Siegel, G.J., 1997a, Differential expression of Na,K-ATPase α-isoform mRNAs in aging rat cerebellum. *J. Neurosci. Res.* 47 (3): 287–299.

Chauhan, N.B. and Siegel, G.J., 1997b, Na,K-ATPase: Increases in α1-messenger RNA and decreases in α3-messenger RNA levels in aging rat cerebral cortex. *Neuroscience* 78:7–11.

Corder, E.H.,Saunders, A.M., Strittmatter, W.J., et al.. 1993, Gene dose of apolipoprotein E type 4 allele and the risk of Alzheimer's disease in late onset families. *Science* 261:921–923.

Cummings, B.J., Satou, T., Head, E., et al., 1996, Diffuse plaques contain C-terminal A-beta(42) and not A-beta(40). Evidence from cats and dogs. *Neurobiol. Aging* 17 (4):653–659.

Del Bo, R., Comi, G.P., Bresolin, N., et al., 1997, The apolipoprotein E epsilon 4 allele causes a faster decline of cognitive performances in Down's syndrome subjects. *J. Neurol. Sci. 145* (1):87–91.

Hardy, J., 1997, Amyloid, the presenilins and Alzheimer's disease. *Trend Neurosci.* 20:154–159.

Iacopino, A.M. and Christakos, S., 1990, Specific reduction of calcium-binding protein (28-kilodalton calbindin-D) gene expression in aging and neurodegenerative diseases. *Proc Natl. Acad. Sci. U.S.A.* 87 (11): 4078–4082.

Lou, Y., Sunderland,T. and Wolozin, B., 1996, Physiologic levels of â-amyloid activate phosphatidylinositol 3 -kinase with the involvement of tyrosine phosphorylation. *J. Neurochem.* 67:978–987

Mark, R.J., Hensley, K., Butterfield, D.A. and Mattson, M.P., 1995, Amyloid â-peptide impairs ion-motive ATPase activities: Evidence for a role in loss of Ca^{++} homeostasis and cell death. *J. Neurosci.* 15 (9):6239–6249.

Nichols, N.R., Day, J.R., Laping, N.J., et al., 1993, GFAP mRNA increases with age in rat and human brain. *Neurobiol. Aging* 14 (5): 421–429.

Oyama, F., Shimada, H., Oyama, R., et al., 1993, Beta-amyloid protein precursor and tau mRNA levels versus beta-amyloid plaque and neurofibrillary tangles in the aged human brain. *J. Neurochem.* 60 (5):1658–1664.

Selkoe, D.J., 1994, Normal and abnormal biology of the β-amyloid precursor protein. *Ann. Rev. Neurosci.* 17: 489–517.

Sheng, J.G., Mrak, R.E., Rovnaghi, C.R., et al., 1996, Human brain S 100 beta and S 100 beta mRNA expression increases with age: Pathogenic implications for Alzheimer's disease. *Neurobiol. Aging* 17 (3):359–363.

Tanaka, S., Nakamura, S., Kimura, J., et al., 1993, Age-related change in the proportion of amyloid precursor protein mRNAs in the gray matter of cerebral cortex. *Neurosci. Lett.* 163 (1):19–21.

Visser, F.E., Aldenkamp, A.P., van Huffelein, A.C., et al., 1997, Prospective study of the prevalence of Alzheimer-type dementia in institutionalized individuals with Down's syndrome. *Am. J. Ment. Retard.* 101 (:4): 400–412.
Zigman, W.B., Schupf, N., Sersen E., et al., 1996, Prevalence of dementia in adults with and without Down syndrome. *Am. J. Ment. Retard.* 100 (4): 403–412.

18

HB-GAM, A NOVEL AMYLOID ASSOCIATED PROTEIN, IS PRESENT IN PRION RELATED DISORDERS AND OTHER CEREBRAL AMYLOIDOSES

Maciej M. Lalowski,[1,2] Marc Baumann,[4] Heikki Rauvala,[5] Blas Frangione,[2] and Thomas Wisniewski[3]

[1]Polish Academy of Science, Medical Research Centre
Department of Cellular Signalling
5 Pawinskiego Street, 2-106 Warsaw, Poland
[2]Department of Pathology and
[3]Department of Neurology
New York University Medical Center
550 First Avenue, New York, New York 10016
[4]Institute of Biomedicine
Department of Medical Chemistry, P.O. Box 8
University of Helsinki
FIN-00014, Finland
[5]Laboratory of Molecular Neurobiology
Institute of Biotechnology, P.O. Box 45
University of Helsinki
FIN-00014, Helsinki, Finland

INTRODUCTION

The amyloidoses form a collection of diseases sharing several common properties including the deposition of a protein, which has a soluble precursor, as a fibril with a predominantly β-pleated secondary structure. There are over 16 biochemically distinct forms of amyloid (Ghiso et al., 1994). Each of these amyloid deposits are associated with a group of amyloid associated proteins. The progressive deposition of amyloid β peptide (Aβ) occurs as part of Alzheimer's disease (AD), Down's Syndrome (DS), Hereditary Cerebral Hemorrhage with Amyloidosis-Dutch Type (HCHWA-D) and with aging. A feature of all Gerstman-Sträussler-Scheinker (GSS) and about 10% of Creutzfeld Jakob disease (CJD) cases is the presence of PrP amyloid plaques. British amyloidosis is a cerebral

Progress in Alzheimer's and Parkinson's Diseases
edited by Fisher *et al.*, Plenum Press, New York, 1998.

amyloidosis characterized by deposition of cerebral amyloid in the forms of congiophilic angiopathy and parenchymal amyloid plaques, which are not yet biochemically fully characterized (Plant et al., 1990; Baumann et al., 1996). Meningocerebrovascular amyloidosis-Hungarian type (AHun) is a cerebral amyloidosis caused by a novel transthyrethin mutation at codon 18 where Asp is replaced by Gly (D18G) in a Hungarian kindred (Vidal et al., 1996). To date several proteins have been found to be associated with both cerebral and systemic amyloid deposits including: apolipoproteins E, J and A1, amyloid P-component and proteoglycans (Ghiso et al., 1994), while other proteins, such as β_1-antichymotrypsin and presenilin-1 are more closely associated with AD amyloid deposits (Abraham et al., 1988; 27). Although the precise role of these molecules is not known, it was suggested that some may act to promote or stabilize a β-sheet structure (Wisniewski et al., 1992; Ma et al., 1994). Alternatively the binding of some of these proteins may be related to the known hydrophobic and "sticky" nature of amyloid deposits. HB-GAM-heparin binding growth associated molecule, or pleiotrophin is a novel 18 Kda novel type of developmentally regulated cytokine, initially identified as a mitogen for fibroblasts and neurite outgrowth-promoting factor (Li et al., 1990; Rauvala, 1989; Merenmies et al., 1991; Raulo et al., 1992). Several studies showed the expression of HB-GAM in a variety of tissues including the central nervous system (CNS), according to a temporal and spatial pattern during development (Li et al., 1990; Rauvala, 1989; Hampton et al., 1992). While HB-GAM is downregulated in non-brain tissues, in the brain it persists beyond neonatal stages (Li et al., 1990; Rauvala, 1989). As shown by *in vitro* assays it exhibits neurite outgrowth-promoting activities activities due to substrate bound- proteins (Li et al., 1990; Rauvala, 1989; Hampton et al., 1992). Additionally HB-GAM forms extracellular tracts along growing neurites in tissue, suggesting a role in formation of neural connections (Rauvala et al., 1994). It is also known that HB-GAM binds to syndecan-3/N-syndecan, one of the HSPG's (heparan sulfate proteoglycans) and 6B4-proteoglycan/phosphacan, one of the ChSPG's (chondroitin sulfate proteoglycans) with high affinity (Li et al., 1990; Rauvala 1989; Merenmies et al., 1991; Raulo et al., 1992; Hampton et al., 1992; Maeda et al., 1996). Previously we have identified HB-GAM as a component of both diffuse (preamyloid) and neuritic plaques, as well as in the amyloid laden vessels in cerebral amyloidoses of Alzheimer's disease and Down's syndrome (Wisniewski et al., 1996). It was suggested that HB-GAM is one of the cofactors associated with cerebral plaques of Aβ and acts as a marker of neuronal injury (Wisniewski et al., 1996). Here we explore the role played by HB-GAM in other cerebral and systemic amyloidoses, as well its interactions with amyloid peptides *in vitro*.

MATERIALS AND METHODS

Immunohistochemistry

Paraffin embedded, formalin fixed 6 μm brain tissue sections were obtained from autopsy material from three cases of CJD, one with GSS syndrome, 3 cases with HCHWA-D, one with ABri, one case of novel meningocerebrovascular amyloidosis of Hungarian type, 3 cases of light chain deposition and one case of gelsolin related amyloidosis. The tissue sections were stained with Congo Red and Thoflavin S for the presence of amyloid. The adjacent sections were stained with affinity purified rabbit polyclonal antibodies against recombinant protein HB-GAM (HB-GAM rec.) (2 μg/ml) (Merenmies et al., 1991) and against the N-terminus of HB-GAM rec. (2 βg/ml) (Rauvala, 1989), monoclonal anti-apolipoprotein E (apoE) (1:300) (Biodesign Int., Kennenbunk, ME), monoclonal anti-α-chain of apolipoprotein J (apo J) (1:100) (a kind gift from Dr.Nam-Ho-Choi Miura), monoclonal anti-heparan sulfate proteoglycan (HSPG) (a kind gift from Dr.R.N. Kalaria). As positive controls 4G8, monoclonal anti-Aβ17–24 (1:500) (Senetec, Plc.), monoclonal anti-prion protein 3F4 (Senetec.Plc.), polyclonal anti-British amyloid (Baumann et al., 1996) and polyclonal anti-TTR (Pras et al., 1983) were used. Systemic sections were stained with anti-amyloid A (Dako), polyclonal anti-gelsolin-related amyloid (Wisniewski et al., 1991), polyclonal anti-κ and anti-λ light chains (Chemicon Int. Inc., Temecula), monoclonal anti-amylin (Pennisula Lab. Inc., Belmont, CA), and polyclonal anti-fibrinogen (Chemicon). Deparaffinized sections were either pretreated with 98% formic acid for 30 minutes or hydrated autoclaving for 20 minutes, followed by quenching of endogenous peroxidase activity with 0.3% H_2O_2 in methanol and blocking in 10% fetal calf serum in phosphate buffer, pH 7.4 for one hour at room temperature. The primary antibodies were diluted in the same buffer and incubated overnight at 4°C, followed by application of secondary biotinylated species specific antibodies (Amersham Corp. Airlington Heights, IL) and horseradish linked streptavidin (Sigma Chemical Co., St. Louis, MO) in the same buffer as above. Sections were developed in a staining mixture containing 0.01% 3,3'-diaminobenzidine in phosphate buffered saline with or without cobalt hexachloride ions (0.006%) (both reagents from Sigma Chemical Co., St. Louis, MO). Controls included preabsorption of the primary antibody to recombinant HB-GAM and N-terminus of the molecule with an excess of antigen and replacement of the primary antibody with preimmune serum. The purity of recombinant HB-GAM was greater than 99% by sodium dodecyl sulfate polyacrylamide gel electrophoresis.

Binding Studies

Recombinant HB-GAM (2 βg each or 0.36 × 10^{-4} M) was incubated at 37°C for 24 hours with Aβ1–40 (1–20 βg or 0.025–0.75 × 10^{-4} M) in 50 βl phosphate-buffered saline (PBS), pH = 7.4. Stock solutions of the peptides were prepared in 50% acetonitrile in deionized-distilled water with final concentrations of 5–10 mg/ml. Stock solutions were stored at −70°C prior to use. Aliquots of the stock solutions were mixed with the desired amount of proteins and incubated as described above. The protein-peptide solutions were analyzed by Tris-Tricine SDS-PAGE according to Schägger and Jagow. Incubations were stopped by the addition of a modified Laemmli sample buffer (containing 1%SDS) into each vial, under non-reducing conditions. Samples were not boiled but incubated at 37°C for 5–10 minutes. Protein-peptide complexes were electrophoresed on 16.5% Tris-Tricine gels as described in the figure legend.

Fluorometric Assay with Thioflavin T

Aliquots of peptides were incubated for different times at room temperature in 0.1M Tris/HCl, pH 7.4. Amyloid formation was quantified by using the Thioflavin T (ThT) fluorescence method (Naiki et al., 1991; Wisniewski et al., 1994). After incubation, Aβ1–40 peptides alone and in the presence of HB-GAM were added to 50 mM glycine, pH 9.2, containing 2 βM ThT in a final volume of 2 mL. As negative control BSA alone and in the presence of Aβ1–40 were used. Immediately thereafter, fluorescence was monitored at excitation 435 nM and emission 485 nM in a Hitachi F-2000 fluorescence spectrophotometer. A time scan of fluorescence was performed and three values (280, 290, 300s) were averaged after subtracting the background fluorescence of 2 μM ThT.

Determination of Binding Constant between HB-GAM and Aβ Peptides Using Fluorescence Quenching Method

HB-GAM (5 mM) was incubated with increasing concentrations of Aβ1–40, Aβ1–28 and Aβ1–42 peptides (1–500 nM) in 300 βl of 0.1 M Tris/HCl, pH 7.4. Fluorescence of HB-GAM solutions and HB-GAM in the presence of varying concentrations of Aβ peptides was measured after 20 min. of equilibration at emission 285 nM and excitation 290-415 nM on the spectrofluorimeter LS50S (Perkin-Elmer, San Francisco, CA, USA)(Soto et al., 1996b). The rate of quenching of endogenous fluorescence of HB-GAM in the presence of increasing concentrations of the Aβ peptides was further analysed by using the nonlinear regression algorithm (GraphPad Prism, v.2.0) .

RESULTS

Immunohistochemistry

Our GSS patient had PrP plaques in the cerebral and cerebellar cortex, as judged by positive Congo red and anti-PrP staining (not shown). Most of these plaques, with a central amyloid core were also positive for a presence of HB-GAM (Figure 1b). These patterns of immunoreactivity correlated well with anti-apoE staining (Figure 1a). The brains of 3 HCHWA-D cases did not contain neuritic plaques and NFTs as judged by negative Congo red and Thioflavin T staining. Positive Congo red staining was found in many of the cerebral, cerebellar and neuropil vessels. Amyloid laden vessels were also positive for Aβ protein. In addition many preamyloid (diffuse) deposits in the neuropil were also Aβ positive (Figure 2a). Antibodies anti-recombinant HB-GAM stained many of the leptomeningal, cortical and cerebellar vessels (Figure 1b), with faint staining of some diffuse deposits (arrow, Figure 2b).

The neuropathological features of the patients with ABri are the presence of amyloid in the form of congophilic angiopathy and non-neuritic plaques (Plant et al., 1990). Our cerebral sections were positively stained for the presence of amyloid using anti-apoE antibody (Figure 3a). The adjacent sections were stained with anti-HB-GAM rec. (Figure 3b) and faintly by an anti-HSPG antibody (Figure 3c). The staining of plaques by anti HB-GAM rec. antibody co-localized well with the presence of amyloid and staining with anti-apoE antibody.

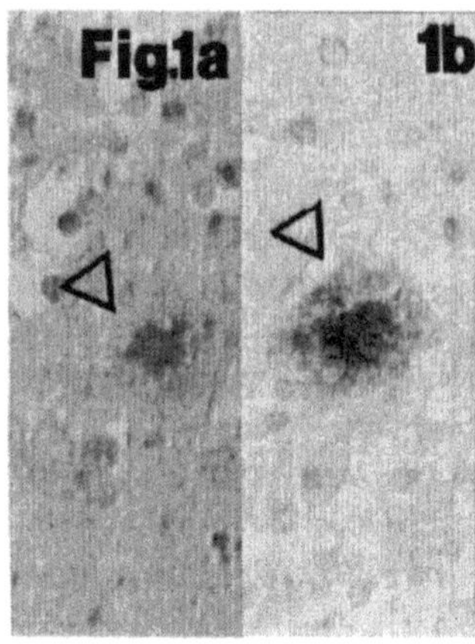

Figure 1. Gerstmann-Sträussman-Scheinker. Amyloid deposits in the cerebral cortex: a) PrP plaques (arrow) were immunoreactive with anti-HB-GAM: b) a sequential section to a) immunoreacted with monoclonal anti-apoE antibody. Magnification, × 400.

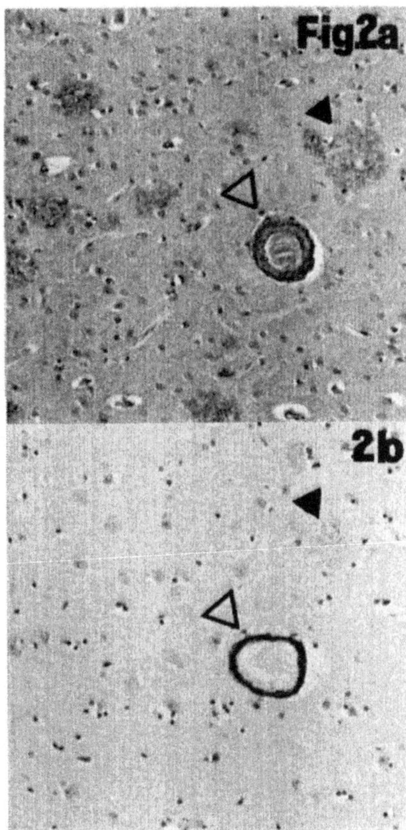

Figure 2. A section from frontal cortex of an HCHWA-D patient: a) immunoreacted with anti-Ab (MAb4G8), showing staining of diffuse plaques (black arrows) and amyloid laden vessel (see large open arrow); b) Sequential section to A) immunoreacted with anti-HB-GAM antibody recognizing amyloid laden vessel (large open arrow) and some diffuse Aβ lesions (black arrow). Magnification, × 200.

As expected, the AHun deposits in the meningeal vessels and subpial areas were strongly immunoreactive with antibodies to TTR (Figure 4b), and apo E (Figure 4c) (Vidal et al., 1996). The same deposits, were also strongly immunoractive with anti-HB-GAM antibodies (Figure 4a).

In all the sections stained with anti-HB-GAM rec. antibody was enhanced by pretreatment with 98% formic acid or hydrated autoclaving. The sections of systemic amyloidoses (light chain deposition and gelsolin-related amyloidosis) failed to show specific HB-GAM immunostaining, even when pretreated with 98% formic acid or hydrated autoclaving

Binding Studies

In order to determine if HB-GAM and Aβ can form a complex in vitro 2 μg of HPLC purified recombinant HB-GAM was incubated for 24 hours at 37°C, with increasing concentrations of Aβ1–40 peptide. Figure 5 shows the results of binding run on 16.5% Tris-Tricine gel. The HB-GAM/Aβ complex was formed in the presence of low percentage of SDS in sample buffer and absence of denaturating agents. Formation of the complex appeared to be concentration dependent (see Figure 5 and insert, lanes 2 and 3). This complex was also recognized by anti-Aβ and anti-HB-GAM antibodies (not shown). Fluorescence quenching studies revealed that HB-GAM can interact with several Aβ peptides

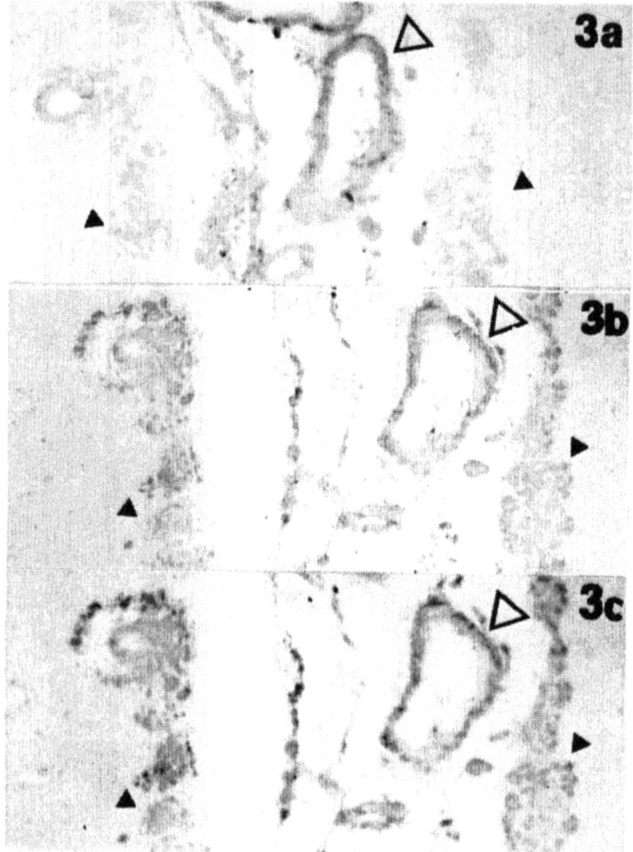

Figure 3. Meningiocerebrovascular amyloidosis of Hungarian type. a) Immunoreactivity of amyloid laden vessels (large open arrows) and subpial deposits (black arrows) with anti-HB-GAM; b) Sequential section immunoreacted with anti-TTR and anti-apoE; c). Magnification, × 100.

with high affinity. The dissociation constant (KD) for interaction of HB-GAM with Aβ1–40 was in low nanomolar range (KD = 12.1 nM) (Fig. 6B). A similar range for interaction of HB-GAM with Aβ1–28 (KD = 13.0 nM, B$_{max}$ = 192 ± 11.3 nM) and for Aβ1–42 (KD = 22.1 nM, B$_{max}$ = 141.5 ± 13.3 nM) was also noted, suggesting that HB-GAM can form high affinity complexes with different amyloid peptides.

DISCUSSION

Among the characteristic features of the amyloidoses is the invariant association with amyloid associated proteins. Many amyloid associated proteins are found in both systemic and cerebral amyloidoses, such as amyloid P component, proteoglycans, apoE, apoJ, apoA1 and complement components (Ghiso et al., 1994). Only a few amyloid associated proteins have been found to be more specific. Presenilin-1 and α1-antichymotrpsin have been reported to be specific for Aβ related deposits (Abraham et al., 1988). In the cases we studied immunohisto-chemically, HB-GAM was found only in cerebral amyloidoses, suggesting that it is a more specific amyloid associated protein. Since HB-GAM has been shown *in vitro* to binding proteoglycans (Li et al., 1990; Rauvala, 1989; Merenmies et al., 1991; Raulo et al., 1992; Hampton et al., 1992; Maeda et al., 1996), this is one possible reason for its presence in amyloid deposits. Proteoglycans are also

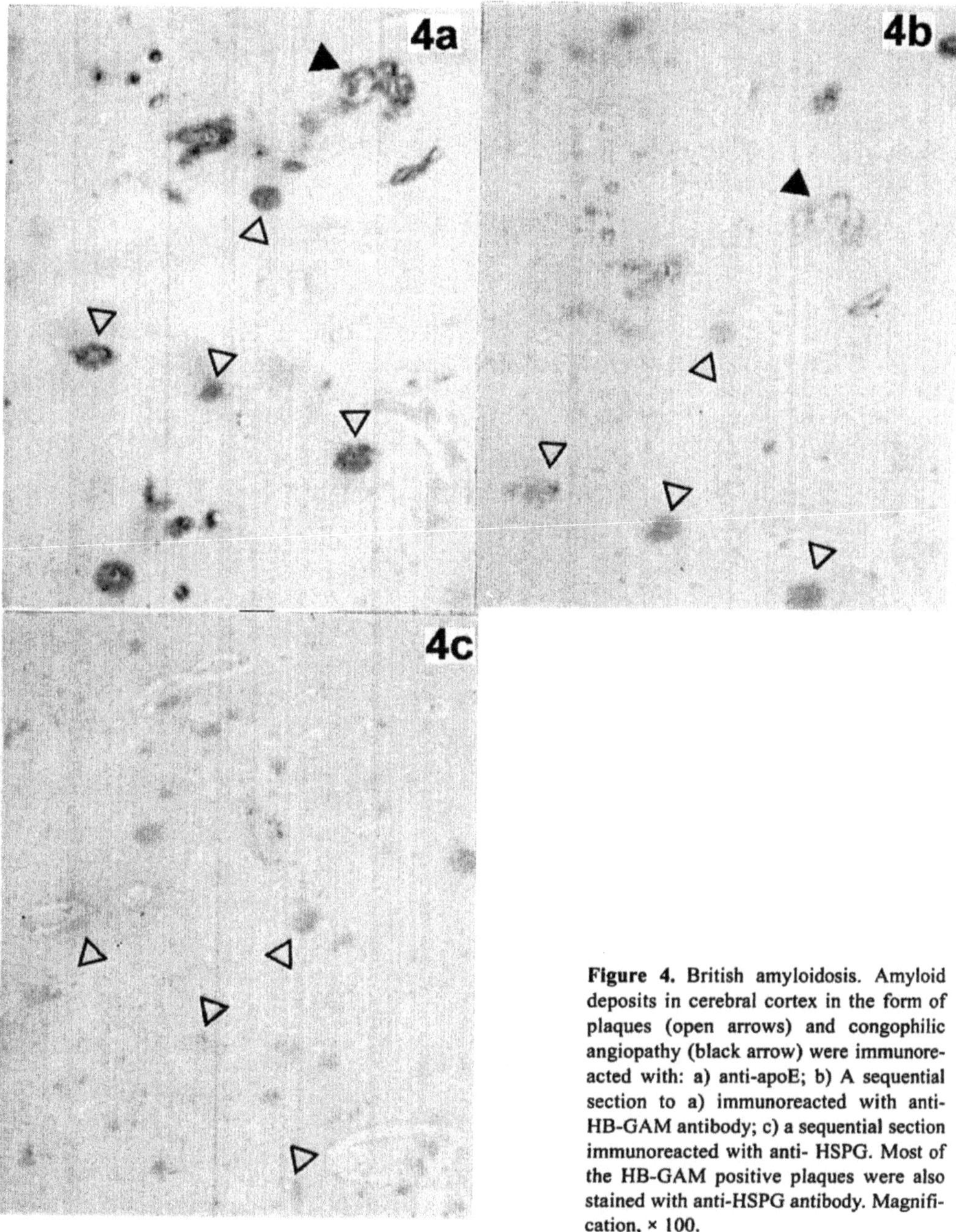

Figure 4. British amyloidosis. Amyloid deposits in cerebral cortex in the form of plaques (open arrows) and congophilic angiopathy (black arrow) were immunoreacted with: a) anti-apoE; b) A sequential section to a) immunoreacted with anti-HB-GAM antibody; c) a sequential section immunoreacted with anti- HSPG. Most of the HB-GAM positive plaques were also stained with anti-HSPG antibody. Magnification, × 100.

present in systemic amyloid deposits; however, HB-GAM is mainly expressed in the CNS, explaining its absence in systemic deposits. There are likely to be additional factors responsible for the presence of HB-GAM in cerebral amyloid deposits. We have demonstrated high affinity binding between Aβ peptides and HB-GAM; hence, in AD, HCHWA-D and DS related lesions HB-GAM may also be binding directly to the main component of the deposits.

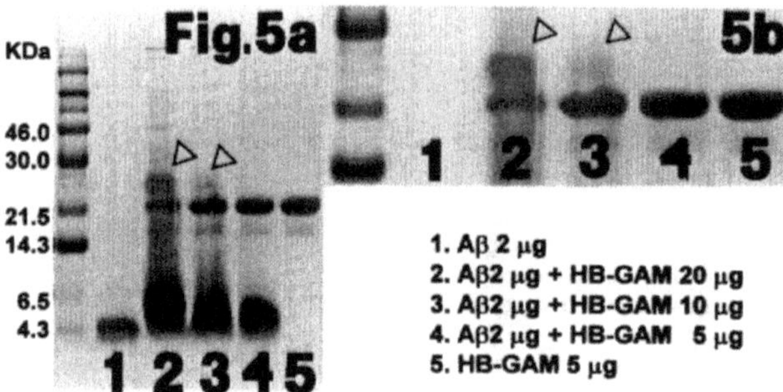

Figure 5. Binding studies. Results of binding between HB-GAM and Aβ1–40 run on 16.5% Tris-Tricine gel. The HB-GAM/Aβ complex was formed in the presence of low percentage of SDS in sample buffer and absence of denaturing agents. Formation of the complex appeared to be concentration dependent (see Figure 5 and insert, lanes 2 and 3).

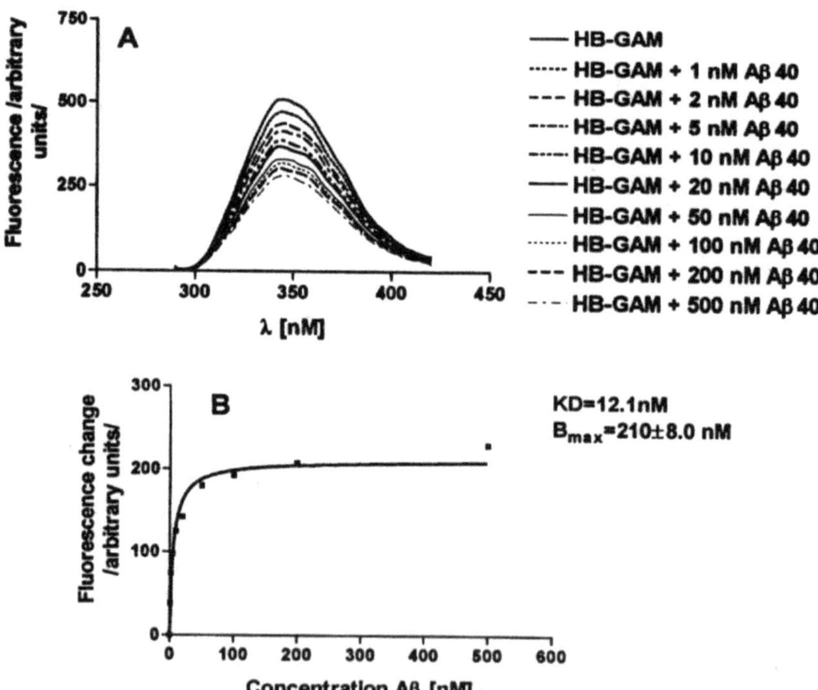

Figure 6. A) Endogenous fluorescence quenching of HB-GAM by increasing amounts of Aβ1–40 peptide. B) A binding constant between HB-GAM and Aβ1–40. The binding constant was found to be in low nanomolar range. The fluorescence quenching was performed as described in Material and Methods and analyzed further by fitting a nonlinear regression algorhitm (GraphPad Prism, v.2.0).

What the role of HB-GAM is within cerebral amyloid deposits is speculative. HB-GAM is known to be a cytokine that functions as a neurite outgrowth factor (Li et al., 1990; Rauvala, 1989; Merenmies et al., 1991; Raulo et al., 1992). Our previously published data showed that HB-GAM is upregulated in the AD brain and that the immuno-

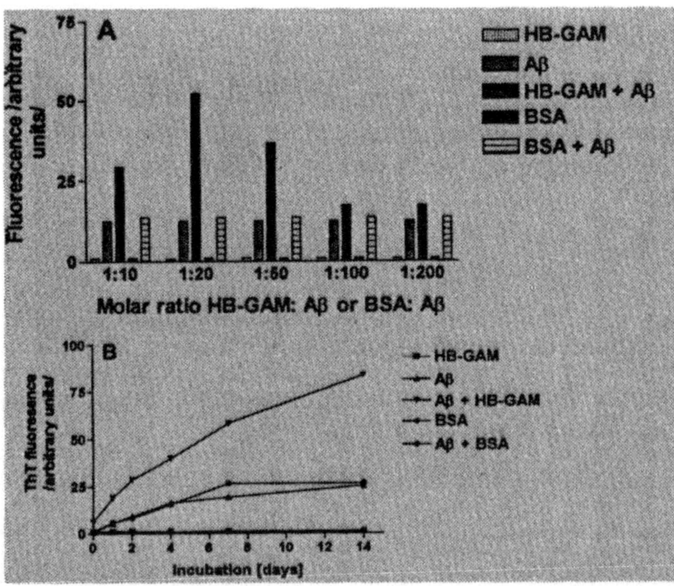

Figure 7. A) Molar ratio dependence of amyloid formation, by using Thioflavin T assay. For each experiment 30 μg of Aβ1–40 were used.The peptides alone and in the presence of HB-GAM or BSA (negative control) were incubated for 4 days at room temperature in 0.1M Tris-HCl, pH=7.4. Amyloid formation was quantitated by fluorometric assay. The values shown here correspond to average of three different samples. HB-GAM alone did not produce any fluorescence above ThT background. The highest increase was found at molar ratio HB-GAM: Aβ (1:50), B) Time dependent effect of HB-GAM on amyloid formation by Aβ1–40. The peptide alone and in the presence of HB-GAM was incubated as described above. Molar ratio used for these experiments was 1:50 (HB-GAM: Aβ). The values correspond to the average of three different experiments done in triplicates.

histochemical staining in Aβ related lesions co-localized with markers of neuronal injury (Wisniewski et al., 1996). Hence the presence of HB-GAM in AD and in other types of cerebral amyloid deposits may be regarded as part of a reactive process reflecting neuronal damage. In addition, we have shown that under certain *in vitro* conditions, where the Aβ peptide concentration is high, HB-GAM can be associated with greater amyloid-like fibril formation. Some amyloid associated proteins, such as apoE and α1-antichymotrypsin, have been proposed to function as a"pathological chaperone", acting to promote and/or stabilize a β-sheet conformation (Wisniewski et al., 1992; Ma et al., 1994; Wisniewski et al., 1994). In vitro it has been shown that apoE can induce a β-sheet conformation and amyloid-like fibril formation in Aβ peptides, when the experiments are done using a high concentration of Aβ peptides (Sanan et al., 1994; Wisniewski et al., 1994; Sanan et al., 1994; Soto et al., 1996a). In addition, it has been shown that apoE preferentially binds Aβ peptides that are in a β-sheet conformation (Golabek et al., 1996). Interestingly it has also been shown that when lower concentrations of Aβ peptide are used, apoE can inhibit amyloid-like fibril formation (Evans et al., 1995; Wood et al., 1996; Schwarzman et al., 1994; Naiki et al., 1997). We suggests that apoE, HB-GAM and some other amyloid associated proteins may be initially up-regulated in AD to serve a protective role; however, later in the pathological process under local conditions of high brain Aβ peptide concentrations, these proteins can have an opposite role and are associated with amyloid fibril formation by binding to a β-sheet conformation and rendering it resistant to degradation.

ACKNOWLEDGMENTS

This work was supported by NIH grants AG10953 and AG00542. M.L. is a recipient of Sandoz Foundation for Gerontological Research grant, grant from State Commitee for Scientific Research no. 4PO5A.0201.11 and a stipendist of the Foundation for Polish Science.

REFERENCES

Abraham, C.R., Selkoe, D.J., and Potter, H., 1988, Immunochemical identification of the serine protease inhibitor alpha 1-antichymotrypsin in the brain amyloid deposits of Alzheimer's disease, *Cell* 52:487–501.

Baumann, M., Wisniewski, T., Levy, E., Plant, G.T., and Ghiso, J., 1996, C-terminal fragments of α- and β- tubulin form amyloid fibrils *in vitro* and associate with amyloid deposits of familial cerebral amyloid angiopathy, British type. *Biochem.Biophys.Res.Commun.* 219:238–242.

Evans, K.C., Berger, E.P., Cho, C.G., Weisgraber, K.H., and Lansbury, P.T., Jr., 1995, Apolipoprotein E is a kinetic but not a thermodynamic inhibitor of amyloid formation: implications for the pathogenesis and treatment of Alzheimer disease, *Proc.Natl.Acad.Sci.USA* 92:763–767.

Ghiso, J., Wisniewski, T., and Frangione, B., 1994, Unifying features of systemic and cerebral amyloidosis, *Mol. Neurobiol.* 8:49–64.

Golabek, A.A., Soto, C., Vogel, T., and Wisniewski, T., 1996, The interaction between apolipoprotein E and Alzheimer's amyloid β-peptide is dependent on β-peptide conformation. *J.Biol.Chem.* 271:10602–10606.

Hampton, B.S., Marshak, D.R., and Burgess, W.H., 1992, Structural and functional characterization of full-length heparin-binding growth associated molecule, *Mol.Biol.Cell* 3:85–93.

Li, Y.S., Milner, P.G., Chauhan, A.K., Watson, M.A., Hoffman, R.M., Kodner, C.M., Milbrandt, J., and Deuel, T.F., 1990, Cloning and expression of a developmentally regulated protein that induces mitogenic and neurite outgrowth activity, *Science* 250:1690–1694.

Ma, J., Yee, A., Brewer, H.B., Jr., Das, S., and Potter, H., 1994, Amyloid-associated proteins alpha 1-antichymotrypsin and apolipoprotein E promote assembly of Alzheimer beta-protein into filaments, *Nature* 372:92–94.

Maeda, N., Nishiwaki, T., Shintani, T., Hamanaka, H., and Noda, M., 1996, 6B4 proteoglycan/ phosphacan, an extracellular variant of receptor-like protein-tyrosine phosphatase zeta/RPTPbeta, binds pleiotrophin/heparin-binding growth-associated molecule (HB-GAM), *J.Biol.Chem.* 271:21446–21452.

Merenmies, J., Pihlaskari, R., Laitinen, J., Wartiovaara, J., and Rauvala, H., 1991, 30-kDa heparin-binding protein of brain (amphoterin) involved in neurite outgrowth. Amino acid sequence and localization in the filopodia of the advancing plasma membrane, *J.Biol.Chem.* 266:16722–16729.

Naiki, H., Higuchi, K., Nakakuki, K., and Takeda, T., 1991, Kinetic analysis of amyloid fibril polymerization in vitro. *Lab.Inv.* 65:104–110.

Naiki, H., Gejyo, F., and Nakakuki, K., 1997, Concentration-dependent inhibitory effects of apolipoprotein E on Alzheimer's β-amyloid fibril formation *in vitro*. *Biochemistry* 36:6243–6250.

Plant, G.T., Révész, T., Barnard, R.O., Harding, A.E., and Gautier-Smith, P.C., 1990, Familial cerebral amyloid angiopathy with nonneuritic amyloid plaque formation, *Brain* 113:721–747.

Pras, M., Prelli, F., Franklin, E.C., and Frangione, B., 1983, Primary structure of an amyloid prealbumin variant in familial polyneuropathy of Jewish origin. *Proc. Natl. Acad. Sci. (USA)* 80:539–542.

Raulo, E., Julkunen, I., Merenmies, J., Pihlaskari, R., and Rauvala, H., 1992, Secretion and biological activities of heparin-binding growth-associated molecule. Neurite outgrowth-promoting and mitogenic actions of the recombinant and tissue-derived protein, *J.Biol.Chem.* 267:11408–11416.

Rauvala, H., 1989, An 18-kd heparin-binding protein of developing brain that is distinct from fibroblast growth factors, *EMBO J.* 8:2933–2941.

Rauvala, H., Vanhala, A., Castren, E., Nolo, R., Raulo, E., Merenmies, J., and Panula, P., 1994, Expression of HB-GAM (heparin-binding growth-associated molecules) in the pathways of developing axonal processes in vivo and neurite outgrowth in vitro induced by HB-GAM, *Brain Res.*. 157–176.

Sanan, D.A., Weisgraber, K.H., Russell, S.J., Mahley, R.W., Huang, D., Saunders, A., Schmechel, D., Wisniewski, T., Frangione, B., Roses, A.D., and Strittmatter, W.J., 1994, Apolipoprotein E associates with beta amyloid peptide of Alzheimer's disease to form novel monofibrils. Isoform apoE4 associates more efficiently than apoE3, *J.Clin.Invest.* 94:860–869.

Schwarzman, A.L., Gregori, L., Vitek, M.P., Lyubski, S., Strittmatter, W.J., Enghilde, J.J., Bhasin, R., Silverman, J., Weisgraber, K.H., Coyle, P.K., and Goldgaber, D., 1994, Transthyretin sequesters amyloid beta protein and prevents amyloid formation, *Proc.Natl.Acad.Sci.(USA)* 91:8368–8372.

Soto, C., Golabek, A.A., Wisniewski, T., and Castaño, E.M., 1996a, Alzheimer's soluble β-amyloid is conformationally modified by apolipoproteins in vitro. *Neuroreport* 7:721–725.

Soto, C., Kindy, M.S., Baumann, M., and Frangione, B., 1996b, Inhibition of Alzheimer's amyloidosis by peptides that prevent β-sheet conformation. *Biochem. Biophys. Res. Commun.* 226:672–680.

Vidal, R.G., Garzuly, F., Budka, H., Lalowski, M., Linke, R.P., Brittig, F., Frangione, B., and Wisniewski, T., 1996, Meningocerebrovascular amyloidosis associated with a novel transthyretin (TTR) missence mutation at codon 18 (TTRD18G), *Am.J.Pathol.* 148:361–366.

Wisniewski, T., Haltia, M., Ghiso, J., and Frangione, B., 1991, Lewy bodies are immunoreactive with antibodies raised to gelsolin related amyloid-Finnish type, *Am.J.Pathol.* 138:1077–1083.

Wisniewski, T., and Frangione, B., 1992, Apolipoprotein E: a pathological chaperone protein in patients with cerebral and systemic amyloid, *Neurosci.Lett.* 135:235–238.

Wisniewski, T., Castaño, E.M., Golabek, A.A., Vogel, T., and Frangione, B., 1994, Acceleration of Alzheimer's fibril formation by apolipoprotein E in vitro, *Am.J.Pathol.* 145:1030–1035.

Wisniewski, T., Lalowski, M., Baumann, M., Rauvala, H., Raulo, E., Nolo, R., and Frangione, B., 1996, HB-GAM is a cytokine present in Alzheimer's and Down's syndrome lesions, *Neuroreport* 7:667–671.

Wisniewski, T., Dowjat, W., Permanne, B., Palha, J.A., Kumar, A., Gallo, G., and Frangione, B., 1997, Presenilin is associated with Alzheimer's disease amyloid. *Am.J.Pathol.,* in press

Wood, S.J., Chan, W., and Wetzel, R., 1996, Seeding of Aβ fibril formation is inhibited by all three isotypes of apolipoprotein E. *Biochem.* 35:12623–12628.

19

REGULATION OF APP METABOLISM BY PROTEIN PHOSPHORYLATION

J. D. Buxbaum,[1,2] A. Ikin,[1] Y. Luo,[1] J. Naslund,[1] S. Sabo,[1] B. Vincent,[1] T. Watanabe,[1] and P. Greengard[1]

[1]Laboratory of Molecular and Cellular Neuroscience and
    Zachary and Elizabeth M. Fisher Center
The Rockefeller University
1230 York Avenue, New York, New York 10021
[2]Laboratory of Molecular Neuroscience
Mount Sinai School of Medicine
Department of Psychiatry
One Gustave Levy Place, New York, New York 10029

APP AND Aβ IN ALZHEIMER DISEASE

A hallmark of Alzheimer disease (AD) is the build-up of an amyloid protein (Aβ) (Glenner and Wong, 1984, Masters et al., 1985) in the brain parenchyma and in the cerebrovasculature (Tomlinson and Corsellis, 1984). Aβ is derived from a large transmembrane precursor, the amyloid protein precursor (APP) (Goldgaber et al., 1987, Kang et al., 1987, Kitaguchi et al., 1988, Ponte et al., 1988, Robakis et al., 1987, Tanzi et al., 1987, Tanzi et al., 1988). For a variety of reasons, many researchers believe that the build-up of Aβ in the brain causes the synaptic loss and associated dementia which occurs in AD. These reasons include the observation that one of the several mutations (hereafter referred to as the Swedish mutation, Mullan et al., 1992) in APP which cosegregate with AD is associated with abnormally high production of Aβ (Cai et al., 1993, Citron et al., 1992). It therefore seems plausible to argue that increased production of Aβ might underlie the symptoms of AD in individuals bearing this mutation. More recently it has been shown that an allele of apolipoprotein E (ApoE(4)) is associated with forms of AD (Corder et al., 1993, Strittmatter et al., 1993). This allele of ApoE is especially prone to inducing the aggregation and precipitation of Aβ in vitro. In the case of individuals with ApoE(4) it is possible that there is an associated increase in Aβ deposition (Schmechel et al., 1993) which again might underlie the symptoms of AD. Thus, there is evidence to suggest that both increased Aβ production and decreased Aβ clearance may contribute to AD. From these findings it is a small jump to argue that decreasing Aβ formation and/or increasing Aβ clearance might slow the progression of AD.

For some researchers this argument is sufficiently compelling to justify the study of the physiological regulation of APP processing and Aβ production. Regulation of APP processing might also give us insights into the function of APP and of its various products. For example, it might prove that the secreted form of APP (APPs) has an important role in the body's response to injury; the ability to regulate the secretion of APPs would then have important ramifications for its function.

REGULATION OF APP PROCESSING BY PROTEIN KINASE C

Protein Kinase C Regulates APP Processing

Soon after the discovery of APP it was noted that APP undergoes cleavage and secretion (Weidemann et al., 1989). This immediately raised the question as to whether this secretion was regulated by protein phosphorylation. To study this question, specific antibodies against the various parts of the APP molecule were used. The first experiments directed at studying the regulation of APP processing made use of a carboxyl-terminal antibody which precipitated full-length APP, as well as the carboxyl-terminal of APP which remains behind after the cleavage and secretion of APPs. It was observed that when cells were treated with phorbol dibutyrate (PBt2), an agent which activates protein kinase C, the levels of mature (fully glycosylated and sulfated) APP diminished significantly, while the levels of carboxyl-terminal derivatives of APP increased (Buxbaum et al., 1990). Because APPs production from full-length APP involves the loss of full-length APP and the generation of the carboxyl-terminal fragment, it was tempting to speculate that these results could be explained by arguing that APPs production was regulated by protein phosphorylation. When cells were incubated with H-7, an inhibitor of several protein kinases including protein kinase C, an increased recovery of cell-associated mature APP was observed, suggesting that protein phosphorylation played a role in basal APP processing in naive (untreated) cells. Maturation (glycosylation and sulfation) of APP, which is accompanied by a shift in apparent molecular weight in cultured cells, was not effected by phorbol esters.

Subsequent to the first study of the effects of protien phosphorylation on APP processing, the effects of protein phosphorylation on APPs production were studied by several groups. Using antibodies against the amino-terminal of APP and studying the APPs released into the extracellular space, it could be convincingly shown that phorbol esters and/or okadaic acid stimulate the production of APPs (Caporaso et al., 1992; Gillespie et al., 1992). More recently, H-7 was also demonstrated to inhibit APPs production (Gabuzda et al., 1993), again suggesting that basal APP processing in naive cells is under the control of protein phosphorylation.

After it was shown that Aβ was produced normally by cultured cells, the role of protein phosphorylation in the regulation of APP processing was extended to include a role in regulating the production of Aβ as well as p3. p3 is an Aβ fragment which is assumed to be derived after normal (alpha-) cleavage of APP (Haass et al., 1993). Several laboratories have shown that activation of protein kinase C leads to dramatically decreased production of Aβ with increased production of p3 (Buxbaum et al., 1993, Gabuzda et al., 1993, Hung et al., 1993). If p3 is in fact derived after alpha-cleavage of APP, then it is not surprising that increasing alpha-cleaved APPs production is associated with increased p3 production.

The decrease in Aβ production may be in part due to the amounts of full-length APP being limiting: increasing alpha-cleavage would decrease the amounts of APP available for β-cleavage (see ref. Buxbaum et al., 1993). Stimulation of APPs formation by protein kinase C decreases the levels of carboxyl-terminal APP fragments containing full-length Aβ (Fukushima et al., 1993), consistent with the hypothesis that Aβ is derived from such fragments. The effects of protein kinase C activation on Aβ production have been observed in a variety of cell types including primary human astrocytes (Gabuzda et al., 1993). H-7 could apparently cause decreased p3 production (accompanied by decreased APPs formation) and increased Aβ production in naive cells (Gabuzda et al., 1993). Cells expressing any of several mutations in APP which cosegregate with AD, including the Swedish mutation, still respond to protein kinase C activation with decreased Aβ production (Buxbaum et al., 1993, Hung et al., 1993), suggesting that regulating the production of Aβ as a therapeutic approach may be possible even in individuals with such mutations.

In summary, activators of protein kinase C stimulate APPs and p3 formation with a concomitant decrease in Aβ production and in the levels of cell-associated full-length APP. Phorbol esters can activate several different protein kinase C isozymes: there is currently evidence suggesting that protein kinase C-alpha may be an example of an isozyme of protein kinase C which can regulate APP processing (Slack et al., 1993).

The Cytoplasmic Domain of APP Does Not Mediate the Effects of Protein Kinase C

The mechanism(s) by which protein kinase C activation regulates APP processing were assumed to involve the phosphorylation of APP in the cytoplasmic domain by protein kinase C or other protein kinases. To test this assumption, APP molecules mutated in the cytoplasmic domain were studied for their response to protein phosphorylation. Point mutations of potential phosphorylation sites in the cytoplasmic domain had no effect on the phorbol ester regulation of APPs and Aβ formation (da Cruz e Silva et al., 1993, Hung and Selkoe, 1994). Even the deletion of the entire cytoplasmic domain of APP did not effect the phorbol ester-induced secretion of APPs. Thus, the well-characterized phosphorylation sites in the APP cytoplasmic domain apparently are not necessary in the regulation of APP processing by protein kinase C. A large portion of the extracellular domain (between residues 78 and 590 of APP695), which includes the major site of phosphorylation of APP in vivo, is also without an obvious role in the regulation of APP processing by protein kinase C (da Cruz e Silva et al., 1993, Hung and Selkoe, 1994). Furthermore, there is no major change in the phosphorylation of APP caused by protein kinase C activation (Gabuzda et al., 1993, Hung and Selkoe, 1994. These results indicate that protein kinase C regulates APP processing by the phosphorylation of some component of the processing pathway other than the amyloid precursor protein. This conclusion in turn raises two questions: 1) what is the role of the highly conserved putative phosphorylation sites in the cytoplasmic domain; and 2) what is the substrate for protein kinase C which is responsible for its effects on APP processing.

The mechanism by which protein kinase C regulates APP processing may be analogous to the way in which this enzyme regulates the processing of other transmembrane proteins, such as pro-TGF-alpha and the CSF-1 and TNF receptors, where phosphorylation of the transmembrane protein is apparently also not necessary. Studies with permeabilized and/or broken cells are being carried out to determine whether activation of a protease and/or modulation of a trafficking protein are the means by which protein kinase C regulates APP processing.

REGULATION OF APP PROCESSING BY PROTEIN PHOSPHATASE 1

In the first experiments directed at studying the regulation of APP processing, it was observed that when cells were treated with okadaic acid, an agent which inhibits protein phosphatases 1 and 2A, the levels of mature (fully glycosylated and sulfated) APP diminished significantly, while the levels of carboxyl-terminal derivatives of APP increased (Buxbaum et al., 1990). In addition, it was observed that maturation (glycosylation and sulfation) of APP, which was not effected by phorbol esters, was affected by okadaic acid. Furthermore, phorbol esters and okadaic acid, especially in combination, caused an increased recovery of an unusually large carboxyl-terminal fragment of APP in PC12 cells. It could also be convincingly shown that okadaic acid stimulated the production of APPs (Caporaso et al., 1992).

Okadaic acid inhibits both protein phosphatases 1 and 2A. It has recently been shown that protein phosphatase 1 is the enzyme which is primary involved in the effects of okadaic acid or calyculin A on APPs formation (da Cruz e Silva et al., 1994).

A role of protein phosphatases 1 and/or 2A in the regulation of APP processing was extended to include a role in regulating the production of Aβ as well as p3. Several laboratories have shown that inhibition of protein phosphatases 1 and 2A leads to dramatically decreased production of Aβ with increased production of p3 (Buxbaum et al., 1993, Gabuzda et al., 1993, Hung et al., 1993).

REGULATION OF APP PROCESSING BY CALCINEURIN (PROTEIN PHOSPHATASE 2B)

As indicated above, the inhibition of protein phosphatases 1 and 2A in a cell-free system did not affect Aβ formation (Desdouits et al., 1996). This contrasted with what was observed in intact cells, in which inhibition of these enzymes did inhibit Aβ formation. This could be explained as follows: the effects of inhibition of these phosphatases in intact cells on Aβ formation was due to depletion of substrate (full-length APP). In the cell free system, there was a direct effect of protein kinase C activation on Aβ formation: thus, as was observed in intact cells, activation of protein kinase C inhibited Aβ formation in the cell-free system. This raised the question as to the nature of the phosphatase which counteracts the direct effects of protein kinase C on Aβ formation. Studies with a specific peptide inhibitor of calcineurin (protein phosphatase 2B) indicated that calcineurin, like protein kinase C, had a direct effect on Aβ formation in a cell-free system (Desdouits et al., 1996). This observation was then extended to intact cells by the use of the cell-permeant calcineurin inhibitor cyclosporin A. Cyclosporin A inhibited Aβ formation in intact cells and the effect was magnified by the simultaneous addition of phorbol esters. A role for calcineurin, a calcium-calmodulin dependent enzyme, in Aβ formation was consistent with the effects of calmodulin antagonists (Desdouits et al., 1996) and compounds which regulate intracellular calcium levels (see below and Buxbaum et al, 1994; Querferth and Selkoe, 1995) on Aβ formation.

REGULATION OF APP PROCESSING BY PHOSPHOLIPASE C-LINKED FIRST MESSENGERS

With the demonstration of a role for protein kinase C in the regulation of APP processing, it was predicted that various first messengers which activate the phospholipase

C/protein kinase C cascade would also be capable of regulating APP processing. This prediction was confirmed in several subsequent studies. Cholinergic agonists were shown to regulate APPs formation by several groups: the effects could be mediated by muscarinic receptors, particularly muscarinic receptors known to be coupled to the phospholipase C/protein kinase C cascade (Buxbaum et al., 1992, Nitsch et al., 1992). Acetylcholine is altered in Alzheimer disease brain, making these studies particularly relevant. Interleukin 1 is also altered in Alzheimer disease brain and cerebrospinal fluid (Cacabelos et al., 1991, Griffin et al., 1989) and can activate the phospholipase C/protein kinase C cascade. In these early studies interleukin 1 too was shown to be able to regulate APPs formation (Buxbaum et al., 1992; also Buxbaum et al., 1994).

With the observation that Aβ is normally produced by cells, the effects of activation of the phospholipase C/protein kinase C cascade on Aβ formation were studied. Direct activation of this cascade by mastoparan and mastoparan X increased the formation of APPs while decreasing the formation of Aβ (Buxbaum et al., 1993). Similarly, muscarinic agonists could decrease Aβ production in cells overexpressing the M1 or M3 muscarinic receptors (Buxbaum et al., 1994, Hung et al., 1993). In human neuroglioma cells, cholinergic and muscarinic agonists, as well as interleukin 1, could regulate Aβ production to varying degrees (Buxbaum et al., 1994). The effect of cholinergic agonists was examined in cells in which the protein kinase C was down-regulated. No difference was observed in cells lacking phorbol ester stimulated protein kinase C when compared to control cells, when examined for muscarinic agonist regulation of APP processing (Buxbaum et al., 1994). This was interpreted as suggesting that the effects of the muscarinic agonists could be mediated by either the phospholipase C/protein kinase C cascade or by the phospholipase C/calcium cascade.

In summary various protein kinase C/phospholipase C linked first messengers have been shown to regulate APP processing. These include acetylcholine, other cholinergic agonists and interleukin 1, as well as bradykinin, thrombin and ATP. A recent report raises the possibility that the effects of phospholipase C-linked first messengers on APP processing may involve the activation of phospholipase A2 (Emmerling et al., 1993). While the activation of protein kinase C by various phospholipase C-linked first messengers may be sufficient to mediate the effects of these first messengers on APP processing it may not be necessary as increased cellular calcium in response to these first messengers may have effects similar to those resulting from activation of protein kinase C. Finally, comparing the relative efficiencies of different first messengers for their ability to regulate APPs and Aβ production indicates that, for a given cell, compounds which are better able to stimulate APPs production are generally better able to inhibit Aβ formation (see Table 2 in Buxbaum et al., 1994), consistent with APP being rate-limiting in the formation of Aβ (Buxbaum et al., 1993).

REGULATION OF APP PROCESSING BY CALCIUM

A Role for Calcium in the Regulation of APP Processing in Cultured Cells

A potential role for intracellular calcium in the regulation of APP processing was first demonstrated using the calcium ionophore A23187. Treating B-104 neuroblastoma cells or differentiated PC12 cells with A23187 led to increased production of APPs (Loffler and Huber, 1993). These data suggest that voltage or ligand-gated calcium channels could regulate APP processing. Calcium released from intracellular stores has also been implicated in the regulation of APP processing. Treating various cells with thapsigargin or cyclopiazonic acid, compounds which inhibit the endoplasmic reticulum calcium ATPase, leading to an increase in calcium into the cytoplasm, caused increased APPs formation (Buxbaum et al., 1994). Significantly, the effects of these compounds on APPs formation were still observed in cells which had been treated for 24 hr with phorbol esters to down-regulate protein kinase C, suggesting that the effects of these compounds are protein kinase C-independent. Under most conditions increased APPs formation induced with thapsigargin and cyclopiazonic acid was accompanied by decreased Aβ formation. However, in the presence of low concentrations of thapsigargin, increases in Aβ, or an Aβ-like peptide, were observed.

Evidence for a physiological role of calcium in the regulation of APPs and Aβ formation was mentioned above. In cells transfected with the M3 receptor and treated for 24 hr with phorbol esters to down-regulate protein kinase C, carbachol was able to stimulate APPs formation and inhibit Aβ production. This indicates that the phospholipase C/calcium cascade is able to regulate APP processing in a protein kinase C-independent manner (see Buxbaum et al., 1994).

Interestingly, elevations in cytoplasmic calcium levels can lead to either increases or decreases in Aβ formation (Buxbaum et al., 1994; Querferth and Selkoe, 1994). The evidence suggesting that inhibition of calcineurin can lead to decreased Aβ formation (Desdouits et al., 1996) is sufficient to explain the effects of calcium on increasing Aβ formation. A mechanism by which calcium can inhibit Aβ formation has not been identified yet (note that activation of phorbol sensitive protein kinase C by calcium has been ruled out by down-regulation of this enzyme; Buxbaum et al., 1994).

In summary, there is now compelling evidence that calcium, derived from either extracellular or intracellular sources, can regulate APP processing. The mechanisms by which calcium exerts its effects on APP processing are as yet unknown. The role of the cytoplasmic phosphorylation sites of APP in calcium-regulated APP processing is under investigation; preliminary studies indicate that they may not be necessary. It is interesting to consider the analogies between pro-TGFalpha and APP: both proteins can undergo secretory processing which is stimulated by protein kinase C or calcium (see Pandiella and Massague, 1991) and for neither protein is phosphorylation of the holoprotein required to mediate the effects of the stimulatory agent(s).

A Role for Calcium in the Regulation of APP Processing in Platelets

Calcium can apparently also regulate APP processing and secretion in platelets. Incubating platelets with either thrombin, calcium ionophore or collagen stimulates the release of APP or APP fragments from the cell (Bush et al., 1990, Gardella, et al., 1990, Schlossmacher et al., 1992, Smith et al., 1990, Van Nostrand et al., 1990). The release of APP from platelets involves cleavage of full-length APP, probably within the Aβ domain, although evidence for the release of full-length APP upon platelet activation has been reported by some (Bush et al., 1990, Gardella et al., 1990), but not other (Schlossmacher et al., 1992), researchers. The effects of thrombin and calcium ionophores on platelets probably involve a mechanism which is different from that which mediates their effects on neuronal and cultured cells because, for platelets, the APP is localized to alpha-granules where it is released upon degranulation. Interestingly, hyperacidification of platelets from patients with severe Alzheimer disease in response to thrombin has recently been reported (Davies et al., 1993); this abnormality may cause abnormal granule, and hence APP, secretion.

CONCLUSION

APP processing appears to be under complex regulation. This regulation is apparently important under both normal and pathological conditions. Of direct clinical interest is the observation that Aβ formation can be regulated by various means. This raises the possibility that altered APP processing may cause an increase in Aβ formation in AD, and suggests that it may be possible to regulate the production of Aβ as a therapeutic approach in AD. As an example of the utility of the latter approach, consider a patient carrying the Swedish APP mutation. If it is true that the cause of AD in such a patient is increased Aβ production, then decreasing Aβ production should delay the onset of the disease. As another example, in individuals where the cause of AD is the presence of ApoE(4) which causes Aβ accumulation and hence synaptic loss, decreasing Aβ formation may be beneficial.

ACKNOWLEDGMENTS

This work was supported by grants from the National Institute on Aging (PG), the American Health Assistance Foundation (JDB), and the Alzheimer Association (JDB).

REFERENCES

Bush A. I., Martins R. N., Rumble B., Moir R., Fuller S., Milward E., Currie J., Ames D., Weidemann A., Fischer P., Multhaup G., Beyreuther K. and Masters C. L., 1990, *J. Biol. Chem.* 265:15977–83.

Buxbaum J. D., Gandy S. E., Cicchetti P., Ehrlich M. E., Czernik A. J., Fracasso R. P., Ramabhadran T. V., Unterbeck A. J. and Greengard P. ,1990, *Proc. Natl. Acad Sci. U SA* 87:6003–6.

Buxbaum J. D., Koo E. H. and Greengard P. ,1993, *Proc. Natl. Acad. Sci. U SA* 90:9195–8.

Buxbaum J. D., Oishi M., Chen H. I., Pinkas-Kramarski R., Jaffe E. A., Gandy S. E. and Greengard P., 1992, *Proc. Natl. Acad. Sci. USA* 89:10075–8.

Buxbaum J. D., Ruefli A. A., Parker C. A., Cypess A. M. and Greengard P., 1994, *Proc. Natl. Acad. Sci.* USA, in press.

Cacabelos R., Barquero M., Garcia P., Alvarez X. A. and Varela de Seijas E., 1991, *Methods Find. Exp. Clin. Pharmacol.* 13:455–8.

Cai X. D., Golde T. E. and Younkin S. G., 1993, *Science* 259:514–6.

Caporaso G. L., Gandy S. E., Buxbaum J. D., Ramabhadran T. V. and Greengard P., 1992, *Proc. Natl. Acad. Sci.* USA 89:3055–9.

Citron M., Oltersdorf T., Haass C., McConlogue L., Hung A. Y., Seubert P., Vigo P. C., Lieberburg I. and Selkoe D. J, 1992, Nature 360:672–4.

Corder E. H., Saunders A. M., Strittmatter W. J., Schmechel D. E., Gaskell P. C., Small G. W., Roses A. D., Haines J. L. and Pericak-Vance M. A., 1993, *Science* 261:921–3.

da Cruz e Silva O. A. B., Iverfeldt K., Oltersdorf T., Sinha S., Lieberburg I., Ramabhadran T. V., Suzuki T., Sisodia S. S., Gandy S. and Greengard P., 1993, *Neuroscience* 57:873–7.

Davies T. A., Fine R. E., Johnson R. J., Levesque C. A., Rathbun W. H., Seetoo K. F., Smith S. J., Strohmeier G., Volicer L., Delva L. and al. e., 1993, *Biochem. Biophys. Res. Commun.* 194:537–43.

Emmerling M. R., Moore C. J., Doyle P. D., Carroll R. T. and Davis R. E. ,1993, *Biochem. Biophys. Res. Commun.*197:292–7.

Fukushima D., Konishi M., Maruyama K., Miyamoto T., Ishiura S. and Suzuki K., 1993, *Biochem. Biophys. Res. Commun.* 194:202–7.

Gabuzda D., Busciglio J. and Yankner B., 1993, *J. Neurochem.* 61:2326–9.

Gandy S., Czernik A. J. and Greengard P., 1988, *Proc. Natl. Acad. Sci. USA* 85:6218–21.

Gardella J. E., Ghiso J., Gorgone G. A., Marratta D., Kaplan A. P., Frangione B. and Gorevic P. D., 1990, *Biochem. Biophys. Res. Commun.* 173: 292–8.

Gillespie S. L., Golde T. E. and Younkin S. G., 1992, *Biochem. Biophys. Res. Commun.* 187:1285–90.

Glenner G. G. and Wong C. W., 1984, *Biochem. Biophys. Res. Commun.* 120:885–90.

Goldgaber D., Harris H. W., Hla T., Maciag T., Donnelly R. J., Jacobsen J. S., Vitek M. P. and Gajdusek D. C., 1989, *Proc. Natl. Acad. Sci. USA* 86:7606–10.

Griffin W. S., Stanley L. C., Ling C., White L., MacLeod V., Perrot L. J., White C. L. and Araoz C., 1989, *Proc. Natl. Acad. Sci. USA* 86:7611–5.

Haass C., Hung A. Y., Schlossmacher M. G., Teplow D. B. and Selkoe D. J., 1993, *J. Biol. Chem.* 268: 3021–4.

Hung A. Y., Haass C., Nitsch R. M., Qiu W. Q., Citron M., Wurtman R. J., Growdon J. H. and Selkoe D. J., 1993,. *J. Biol. Chem. 268*:22959–62.

Hung A. Y. and Selkoe D. J., 1994, *EMBO J.* 14.

Hunt H. H., Thinakaran G., Von Koch C., Lo A. C. Y., Tanzi R. E. and Sisodia S. S., 1994, *J. Biol. Chem.*269:2637–44.

Kang J., Lemaire H. G., Unterbeck A., Salbaum J. M., Masters C. L., Grzeschik K. H., Multhaup G., Beyreuther K. and Muller-Hill B., 1987, *Nature* 325:733–6.

Kitaguchi N., Takahashi Y., Tokushima Y., Shiojiri S. and Ito H., 1988, Nature 331:530–2.

Loffler J. and Huber G., 1993, *Biochem. Biophys. Res. Commun.* 195:97–103.

Masters C. L., Simms G., Weinman N. A., Multhaup G., McDonald B. L. and Beyreuther K., 1985, *Proc. Natl. Acad. Sci. USA* 82: 4245–9.

Mullan M., Crawford F., Axelman K., Houlden H., Lilius L., Winblad B. and Lannfelt L., 1992, *Nat. Genet.* 1:345–7.

Nitsch R. M., Slack B. E., Wurtman R. J. and Growdon J. H., 1992, *Science* 258:304–7.

Ponte P., Gonzalez-DeWhitt P., Schilling J., Miller J., Hsu D., Greenberg B., Davis K., Wallace W., Lieberburg I., Fuller F. and Cordell B., 1988, *Nature* 331:525–7.

Robakis N. K., Ramakrishna N., Wolfe G. and Wisniewski H. M., 1987, *Proc. Natl. Acad. Sci. USA* 84: 4190–4.

Schlossmacher M. G., Ostaszewski B. L., Hecker L. I., Celi A., Haass C., Chin D., Lieberburg I., Furie B. C., Furie B. and Selkoe D. J., 1992, *Neurobiol. Aging* 13:421–34.

Schmechel D. E., Saunders A. M., Strittmatter W. J., Crain B. J., Hulette C. M., Joo S. H., Pericak V. M. A., Goldgaber D. and Roses A. D., 1993, *Proc. Natl. Acad. Sci. USA* 90:9649–53.

Slack B. E., Nitsch R. M., Livneh E., Kunz G. M. J., Eldar H. and Wurtman R. J., 1993, *Ann. NY Acad. Sci.* 695:128–31.

Smith R. P., Higuchi D. A. and Broze G. J., 1990, *Science* 248:1126–8.

Strittmatter W. J., Saunders A. M., Schmechel D., Pericak V. M., Enghild J., Salvesen G. S. and Roses A. D., 1993, *Proc. Natl. Acad. Sci.* USA 90:1977–81.

Suzuki T., Nairn A. C., Gandy S. E. and Greengard P., 1992, *Neuroscience* 48, 755–61.

Suzuki T., Oishi M., Marshak D. R., Czernik A. J., Nairn A. C. and Greengard P., 1994, *EMBO J.* 13.

Tanzi R. E., Gusella J. F., Watkins P. C., Bruns G. A., St. George-Hyslop P., Van Keuren M. L., Patterson D., Pagan S., Kurnit D. M. and Neve R. L., 1987, *Science* 235:880–4.

Tanzi R. E., McClatchey A. I., Lamperti E. D., Villa-Komaroff L., Gusella J. F. and Neve R. L., 1988, *Nature* 331:528–30.

Tomlinson B. E. and Corsellis J. A. N. (1984). In: *Greenfield's Neuropathology,* J. H. Adams, J. A. N. Corsellis and L. W. Duchen, eds, Arnold, London, pp. 951–1025.

Van Nostrand W. E., Schmaier A. H., Farrow J. S. and Cunningham D. D., 1990, *Science* 248:745–8.

Weidemann A., Konig G., Bunke D., Fischer P., Salbaum J. M., Masters C. L. and Beyreuther K., 1989, *Cell* 57:115–26.

20

IDENTIFICATION OF PEPTIDES BINDING TO PRESENILIN 1 BY SCREENING OF RANDOM PEPTIDE DISPLAY LIBRARIES

Alexander Schwarzman,[1] Maria Tsiper,[1] Michael Vitek,[2]
Peter St. George-Hyslop,[3] and Dmitry Goldgaber[1]

[1]Department of Psychiatry
SUNY, Stony Brook, New York
[2]Department of Neurology
Duke University
Durham, North Carolina 27706
[3]Department of Medicine
University of Toronto
Toronto, Canada

INTRODUCTION

The genes encoding presenilin 1 (PS-1) on chromosome 14 and presenilin 2 (PS-2) on chromosome 1 have been identified as major causal genes for early onset familial Alzheimer's disease (FAD) (Sherington et al. 1995; Levy-Lahad et al., 1995). Genetic studies showed that early onset FAD linked to chromosomes 14 and 1 is caused by missence mutations in PS-1 and PS-2 (Sherington et al. 1995; Levy-Lahad et al., 1995). Patients with this form of FAD revealed increased levels of highly amyloidogenic species of amyloid beta protein ($A\beta_{1-42}$ and $A\beta_{1-43}$) in plasma and cerebral amyloid depositions (Scheuner et al. 1996; Mann et al. 1996). In addition, presenilins were shown to form stable complexes with amyloid precursor protein (APP) (Weidemann et al. 1997). Although mechanism of $A\beta_{1-42}$ and $A\beta_{1-43}$ accumulation in FAD is not clear the results above suggest that PS-1 and PS-2 are directly or indirectly involved in the APP metabolism and amyloid formation. Recently PS-2 gene was shown to contribute to apoptosis induced by trophic factor withdrawal, β-amyloid, and T cell receptor-induced apoptosis (Wolozin et al. 1996; Vito et al., 1996). Light and electron microscopy studies suggest predominant localization of PS-1 to the nuclear membrane, endoplasmic reticulum (ER)-Golgi compartments and coated transport vesicles (Cook et al., 1996; Kovacs et al., 1996; Lah et al., 1997).

Progress in Alzheimer's and Parkinson's Diseases
edited by Fisher *et al.*, Plenum Press, New York, 1998.

In spite of these new finding the biological functions of PS-1 and PS-2 remain unknown. Conceivably, identification of cellular proteins which interact with PS-1 and PS-2 will lead to understanding the biological role of presenilins and the mechanisms of AD pathogenesis. Furthermore, molecules which have different affinity for wild type and mutant FAD presenilins will delineate the metabolic pathways which are involved in FAD pathogenesis.

In order to identify PS-1 and PS-2 binding peptides and proteins, we screened random peptide display libraries using recombinant PS-1 as a binding target.

MATERIALS AND METHODS

Production of Recombinant PS-1

To obtain S-Tag-PS-1 fusion protein full length cDNA of wild type PS-1 and mutant PS-1 (Val 286)[1] was cloned into EcoR 1 site of the pET29a *E. coli* expression vector (Novagen). This vector contains sequence encoding S-Tag peptide and a thrombin cleavage site upstream of cloning insert. The S-Tag system is a protein tagging system based on the interaction of the S-Tag peptide (15 amino acids) with S protein (104 amino acids) derived from pancreatic ribonuclease A. Recombinant plasmids were expressed in *E. coli* strain BL21 (DE3). Cells were grown at 37°C in 50 ml of LB broth up to 0.7–0.8 OD_{600}. Induction of S-Tag-PS-1 synthesis was performed by addition of 1 mM IPTG with gentle shaking. After 3h induction bacterial cells were collected by centrifugation (5000 x g, 5min). Recombinant fusion protein was affinity purified from inclusion bodies using S-protein agarose (Novagen).

Screening of Random Peptide Display Libraries

Phage (fUSE2) displayed 15-mer random peptide library was kindly provided by Dr. G. P. Smith (University of Missouri-Columbia). Bacterial FliTrx™ 12-mer random peptide display library was obtained from Invitrogen. Recombinant fusion protein S-Tag-PS-1 (5μg) bound to the S-agarose was used as a binding target. In the first round of panning a mixture of 10^{13} phage particles or 10^{10} bacterial clones were mixed with 0.5 ml of S-protein agarose containing 5 μg of bound S-Tag-PS-1 and incubated overnight at 4°C on an orbital shaker. Agarose was washed five times with 100 ml of 0.05 N Tris-HCl, pH 7.8, 10 mM NaCl. Concentration of phages or cells in the final wash did not exceed 10^1 pfu/ml or 10^1 colonies/ml. Elution of phages bound to PS-1 was carried out by incubation of the agarose pellet with 5 units of biotinylated thrombin which cleavaged the amino acid sequence between S-Tag and PS-1. After incubation, thrombin was removed using a 0.5 ml column of Streptavidin-agarose. Eluted phages or cells were amplified up to the primary concentrations and the panning procedure was repeated. Three rounds of panning were performed for the fUSE2 displayed 15-mer random peptide library and five rounds of panning were performed for the FliTrx™ 12-mer random peptide display library. The detail characterization of the FliTrx™ 12-mer random peptide display library and the detailed method of biopanning is described in the Invitrogen manual. The detailed procedure of screening phage display peptide libraries was described by Smith and Scott (Smith and Scott, 1993). After final round of panning the sequences of binding peptides were identified by DNA sequencing of the insert in host DNA.

PS-1 Binding Assay

For analysis of PS-1 binding to peptides individual bacteriophages (10^{13} pfu) selected after final panning were immobilized overnight on polyvinyl 96-well microtiter plates (Costar). After aspirating of the media, wells were washed five times and blocked with PBS containing 2% bovine serum albumin, and 1% gelatin for 3 hours at room temperature. 0.5 µg of recombinant PS-1 in blocking solution was added to the wells and incubated for 2 hours at room temperature. Next, the wells were washed five times with PBS. Phage-bound PS-1 was eluted by Laemmli buffer at 90°C and analyzed by 10% SDS-PAGE in Tris-Glycine buffer. After electrophoresis, proteins were transferred onto 0.2 µ PVDF membrane (Bio-Rad). PS-1was visualized by ECL method (Amersham) using affinity purified rabbit polyclonal anti-PS-1 antibody which recognizes an epitope RSQNDNRERQEHNDRRSL, corresponding to residues 27–44 of PS-1.

RESULTS AND DISCUSSION

Electrophoretic analysis of purified recombinant PS-1 revealed a prominent band of about 18–19 kDa and a triplet of bands of about 45–52 kDa (Fig.1). Immunostaining of recombinant PS-1 demonstrated high molecular weight PS-1 aggregates and a band of about 35 kDa.

The electrophoretic PS-1 pattern is very similar to that found in transfected mammalian cells and transgenic animals (Thinakaran et al., 1996). 80–90% of recombinant PS-1 was extracted by 6M urea from inclusion bodies while the soluble cell fraction contained only insignificant amount of 18 kDa PS-1 fragment. (Not shown). Purified PS-1 easily aggregated in solutions without urea. At the same time fusion protein S-Tag-PS-1 bound on the S-protein agarose was stable for several days. Therefore, we used bound S-Tag-PS-1 for library screening as a protein target. The thrombin cleavage site located between S-Tag sequence and PS-1 sequence provided selective elution of phages and cells bound to PS-1.

The binding assay for individual clones was performed only for the fUSE2 displayed 15-mer random peptide library (Fig. 2). This procedure was not done for the FliTrx™ 12-mer random peptide display library because of a very high background of binding to immobilized cell clones.

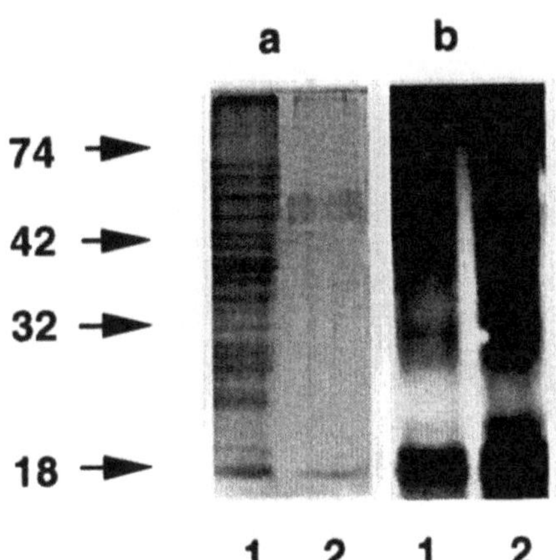

Figure 1. PS-1 Expression in *E. coli*. a. Coomassie staining of cell inclusion body proteins (1) and purified recombinant PS-1 (2). b. Western blot analysis of recombinant PS1: inclusion body proteins(1) and purified PS-1(2). Purification was performed using S-agarose as described in "Materials and Methods." Molecular weight markers (kDa) are marked by arrows.

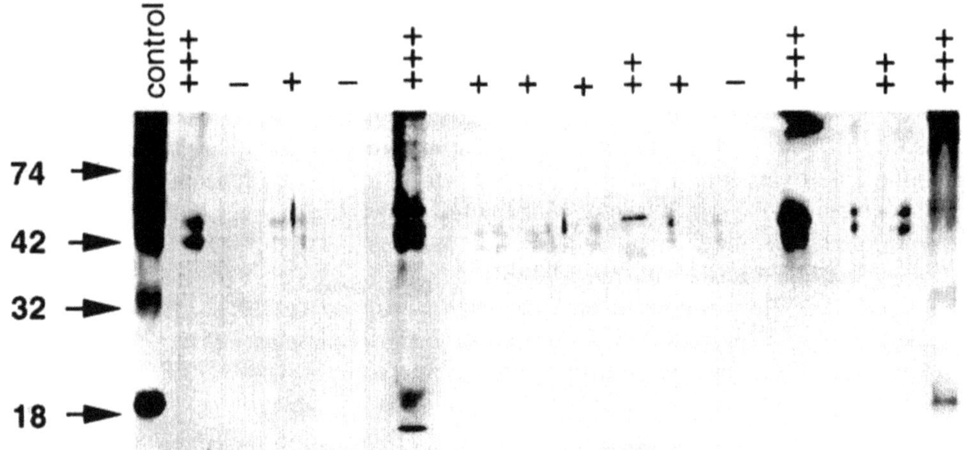

Figure 2. Screening of PS-1 binding phages, selected from 15-mer random peptide fUSE2 displayed library. Western blot analysis of recombinant PS-1 retrieved from complexes of PS-1 with immobilized selected phages (see "Binding assay" in "Materials and Methods"). Control: recombinant PS-1. "+++" = strong binding; "++" = moderate binding, "+" = weak binding. "–" = no binding. Molecular weight markers (kDa) are marked by arrows.

Peptides, selected from the phage displayed library were characterized by different binding capacity and binding specificity for purified PS-1 (Fig. 2).

Eight groups of peptides carrying common binding motifs were selected after final rounds of panning (Table 1).

Peptides of groups 1 and 2 (Table 1) revealed weak or moderate binding to full length PS-1 only (Fig. 2). On the contrary, peptide GPHFDYRTGLGWRFG (group 4) was characterized by very strong binding to both full length PS-1 and its 18 kDa N-terminal fragment. Moreover, this peptide has a stronger affinity to mutant PS-1(Val 286) than to wild type PS-1 (Fig. 3, lane 2).

Comparison of this peptide sequence with NCBI databases using BLASTp alignment models revealed amino acid similarity with the multiple hydrophobic domain (...294 EYRTGISWSFG 304...) of an integral membrane glycoprotein of human cytomegalovirus containing at least eight transmembraine domains (Chee et al., 1990). PS-1 is also predicted to be an integral membrane protein with seven hydrophobic transmembrane domains.[1] Mutation Leu286→Val is located in the transmembrane region of PS-1 and most likely alters its interaction with other hydrophobic components of cell membranes. Although human cell analog of viral integral membrane protein is not known our results clearly indicate that mutation Leu286→Val could lead to the alteration of interaction of PS-1 with hydrophobic membrane proteins. PS-1 is localized in the nuclear membrane, ER-Golgi compartments and coated transport vesicles (Kovacs et al., 1996; Lah et al., 1997). Several studies have identified overexpressed PS-1 in the plasma membrane of transfected cells (Takashima et al., 1996; Dewji et al., 1996). Conceivably, the altered structure of the transmembrane domain of PS-1 could destabilize the structural and/or functional integrity of cell membranes and/or impair intracellular protein trafficking. Recent finding that PS-2 forms complexes with the ER-localized immature APP shows that presenilins may be involved in APP trafficking and production of amyloidogenic species $A\beta_{1-42}$ and $A\beta_{1-43}$. However, no differences were observed between APP affinity for wild type and for mutant PS-2. On the other hand, mutant PS-2 was reported to enhance basal

Table 1. Amino acid sequences of peptides that interact with PS-1

Library[1]	Frequency[2]	Binding[3]	Sequence
			Group 1
1	1	+	F VSSMD LZZIIRDSS
1	3	++	TPVLIAF VSSGS WPV
2	1	ND	G VSSGG ARPVGR
2	1	ND	RPLRHLS GSSGE
1	2	++	VFHNLVL LSSGS DSS
2	1	ND	AGYI LSSKG PIE
1	1	+	FTS ASSGS RFRSHLF
2	1	ND	RIHSPVR PSCGG
1	1	+	SSGGT CDRDHRLRLP
1	1	+	GRQFVG VSLGS FGVL
			Group 2
2	2	ND	SEISA WSGGHPS
1	2	++	RPG VTGGSP SVDTSP
1	2	+	GNERSFAPW WFGGHA
2	1	ND	RWILPF WSGLR
1	1	+	LFRYG FSGPRL AEW
1	2	+	SGGRL DSIVGFFYAV
2	1	ND	GDGGHL AVADSP
1	1	+	HFR STGGRA SVPAS
2	1	ND	MAVGGRAI WLRD
2	1	ND	VGSKGL IASPIP
			Group 3
1	4	+++	TLIPRSFCPTHDRDC
			Group 4
1	4	+++	GPHFDYR TGLGWR FG
2	1	ND	LGLGWR VGNRKW
			Group 5
1	2	+	ALDGHCHL PRVTEEH
2	2	+	LPKVTDEH AN
			Group 6
1	3	++	RVALDGHCHLPRCSF
			Group 7
1	3	+++	MYLRVSPTLPGALLA
			Group 8
1	3	++	RNAPPL FNDVYWI AF
1	2	++	FASRI LFNDVYWVSF

[1]Library : 1: fUSE 2 - phage 15-mer peptide display library (G.Smith, University of Missouri-Columbia); 2: FliTrx™ - bacterial 12-mer peptide display library (Invitrogen).
[2]Frequency: Number of individual clones among 50 randomly sequenced clones after last panning.
[3]Binding: "+++" strong , "++" moderate, "+" weak, "ND"-not determined.
Consensus sequences are underlined

apoptotic activity in PC12 cells (Wolozin et al., 1996). Therefore, mutations may not interfere with the APP-preseniln complex formation, but effect interactions of presenilins with other proteins which are directly or indirectly involved in the APP metabolism and/or apoptosis.

We suggest that selection of PS-1 binding peptides from large and diversed peptide libraries provides opportunity to identify cellular proteins which interact with PS-1 and PS-2 and delineate metabolic pathways which are involved in FAD pathogenesis.

A. Schwarzman et al.

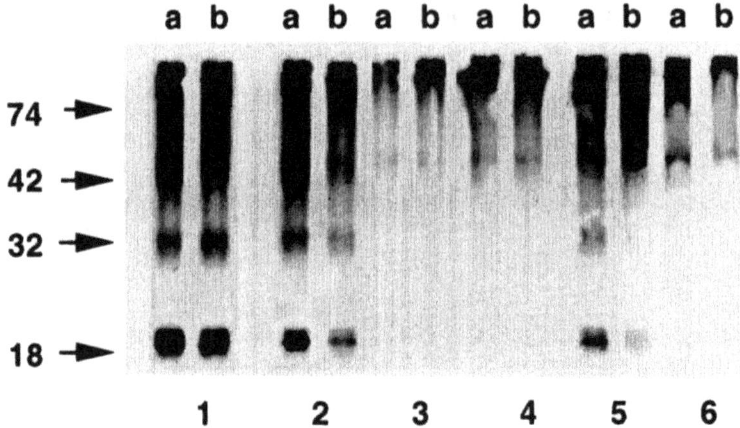

Figure 3. Effect of mutation Leu286→Val on interaction between PS-1 and peptides selected from 15-mer random peptide fUSE2 displayed library. Western blot analysis of recombinant PS-1 retrieved from complexes of Val 286 mutant PS-1(a) and wild type PS-1 (b) with immobilized selected phages (See "Binding assay" in "Materials and Methods"). 1. Recombinant PS-1(dilution 1:1000) used for the binding assay. 2–6. recombinant PS-1 retrieved from complexes of PS-1 with immobilized selected phages. Molecular weight markers (kDa) are marked by arrows.

ACKNOWLEDGMENTS

Supported in part by National Institute of Health, American Health Assistance Foundation, and Alzheimer's Association Grant.

REFERENCES

Chee, M.S., Bankier, A.T., Beck,S., Bohni, R., Brown, C.M., Cerny, R., Horsnell,T., Hutchison, C.A. III, Kouzarides,T., Martignetti, J.A., Preddie, E., Satchwell, S.C., Tomlinson, P., Weston, K.M. and Barrel, B.G.(1990). Analysis of the protein-coding content of the sequence of human cytomegalovirus strain AD169 *Microbiol. Immunol.* 154: 125–169.

Cook, D.G., Sung, J.C. Golde, T.E., Felsenstein, KM., Wojczyk, B.S., Tanzi, R.E., Trojanowski, J.Q., Lee, V.M.,Doms, R.W. (1996). Expression and analysis of presenilin 1 in a human neuronal system: localization in cell bodies and dendrites.*Proc.Natl.Acad.Sci.USA* 93: 9223–9228.

Dewji, N.N & Singer, S.J. (1996). Specific transcellular binding between membrane proteins crucial to Alzheimer's disease. *Proc.Natl.Acad.Sci.USA* 93:12575–12580.

Kovacs, D.M., Fausett, H.J., Page, K.J., Kim, T.W., Moir, R.D., Merriam, D.E., Hollister, R.D., Hallmark, O.G., Mancini, R., Felsenstein, K.M., Hyman, B.T., Tanzi, R.E., Wasco W. (1996). Alzheimer-associated presenilins 1 and 2: neuronal expression in brain and localization to intracellular membranes in mammalian cells. *Nature Med.* 2:224–229.

Lah, J.J., Heilman, C.J., Nash, N.R., Rees, H.D., Yi, H., Counts, S.E., & Levey, A. (1997). Light and Electron microscopic localization of presenilin-1 in primate brain. *J. Neurosci.,* 17:1971–1980.

Levy-Lahad, E., Wasco, W., Poorkaj, P., Romano, D.M., Oshima, J., Pettingel, W.H., Yu, C- E., Jondro, P.D., Schmidt, S.D., Wang, K., Crowley, A.C., Fu, Y-H., Guenette, S.Y., Galas, D., Nemens, E., Wijsman, E.M., Bird, T.D., Schellenberg, G.D., Tanzi R.E. (1995). Candidate gene for the chromosome 1 familial Alzheimer's disease locus. *Science* 269: 973–977.

Mann, D.M.A., Iwatsubo, T., Cairns, N.J., Lantos, P.L., Nochlin, D., Sumi, S.M., Bird,T.D., Poorkaj, J., Hardy, M., Hutton, M., Phihar,G., Crook, R., Rossor, M.N., & Haltia, M. (1996). Amyloid β protein (Aβ) depositions in cromosome 14-linked Alzheimer's Disease: Predominance of Aβ$_{42(43)}$ *Ann.Neurol.* 40: 149–156.

Scheuner, D., Eckman, C., Jensen, M., Song, X., Citron, M., Suzuki, N., Bird, T.D., Hardy, J., Hutton, M., Kukull, W., Larson, E., Levy-Lahad, E., Vitanen, M., Peskind, E., Poorkaj, P., Schellenberg, G., Tanzi, R., Wasco, W., Lannfelt, L., Selkoe, D., & Younkin, S. (1996). Secreted amyloid beta protein similar to that in the senile plaques of Alzheimer's disease is increased in vivo by presenilin 1 and 2 mutations linked to familial Alzheimer's disease. *Nature Med.* 2: 864–870.

Sherington, R., Rogaev, E.I., Liang, Y., Rogaeve, E.A., Levesque, G., Ikeda, M., Chi, H., Lin, C., Li, G., Holman, K., Tsuda, T., Mar, L., Foncln, J.-F., Bruni, A.C., Montesi, M.P., Sorbi, S., Rainero, I., Pinessi, L., Nee, L., Chumakov, I., Pollen, D., Brookes,A., Sanseau, P., Polinsky, R.J., Wasco, W., Da Silva, H.A.R., Hainess, J.L., Pericak-Vance, M.A., Tanzi, R.E., Roses, A.D., Fraser, P.E., Rommens, J.M. & St. George-Hyslop, P.H. (1995), *Nature* 375:754–759.

Smith, G.P. and Scott, J.K. (1993). Libraries of peptides and proteins displayed on filamentous phage. *Methods in Enzymol.* 217:228–257.

Takashima, A., Sato, M., Mercken, M., Tanaka, S., Kondo, S., Honda, T., Sato, K., Murayama, M., Noguchi, K., Nakazato, Y., Takahashi, H. (1996). Localization of Alzheimer- associated presenilin 1 in transfected COS-7 cells.(1996). *Biochem Biophys. Res. Commun.* 227:423–426.

Thinakaran, G. Borchelt, D.R., Lee, M.K., Slunt, H.H., Spitzer, L., Kim. G., Ratovitsky, T., Davenport, F., Nordstedt, C., Seeger, M., Hardy, J., Levey, A.I., Gandy, S.E., Jenkins, N.A., Copeland, N.G., Price, D.L., Sisodia, S.S.(1996). Endoproteolysis of presenilin 1 and accumulation of processed derivatives in vivo. *Neuron.* 17:181–190.

Vito, P. Lacana, E. D'Adamio, L. (1996). Interfering with apoptosis: Ca(2+)-binding protein ALG-2 and Alzheimer's disease gene ALG-3. *Science* 271, 521–525.

Weidemann , A., Paliga, K., Durrwang, U., Czech, C., Evin, G., Masters, C.L.& Beyreuther, K. (1997). Formation of stable complexes between two Alzheimer's disease gene products: Presenilin-2 and beta myloid precursor protein. *Nature Med.* 3:328–332.

Wolozin, B. Iwasaki, K. Vito, P. Ganjei, J.K. Lacana,E. Sunderland, T. Zhao, B. Kusiak, J.W. Wasco,W. D'Adamio, L. (1996). Participation of presenilin 2 in apoptosis: enhanced basal activity conferred by an Alzheimer mutation. *Science* 274: 1710–1713.

21

MATRIX-METALLOPROTEINASES (MMPS) IN ASTROGLIAL CELLS

Modulation by TNF-α and Interacting Cytokines

Nitza Lahat,[2] Sarah Shapiro,[1] Michael Inspector,[1] Reuben Reich,[3] Rosa Gershtein,[1] and Ariel Miller[2]

[1]Neuroimmunology and Immunology Research Units
Lady Davis Carmel Medical Center
Haifa, Israel
[2]Bruce Rappaport Faculty of Medicine
Technion, Israel
[3]Department of Pharmacology
Faculty of Medicine
Hebrew University
Jerusalem, Israel

INTRODUCTION

The matrix metalloproteinases (MMPs) have been implicated as contributing factors in the pathogenesis of injury and inflammation of the central nervous system including diseases such as Alzheimer (Gottschall & Yu, 1995), Multiple Sclerosis (MS) and its animal model, experimental autoimmune encephalitis (EAE) (Gijbels et al., 1992; Norga et al., 1995; Rosenberg et al., 1996). MMP activity has been associated with degradation of the extracellular matrix (ECM), activation of leukocytes, their extravasation and tissue infiltration, breakdown of the blood brain barrier (BBB) as well as nerve demyelination (Romanic & Madri, 1994). The process of regeneration and glial-scar formation also depends upon modulation of the ECM by MMPs, thus enabling glial cells to migrate to damaged areas of the brain (McKeon et al.,1995).

Based on their substrate specificities the MMPs are divided into three main families: the collagenases (MMP-1 and -8), the gelatinases (MMP-2 and -9) and the stromyelysins

(MMP-3, -7 and -10) (Romanic & Madri, 1994). Studies have demonstrated that the MMPs are regulated at different levels including transcriptional, by growth factors, oncogenes and cytokines (TNF-α, IL-1, IL-6 and others); post transcriptional by alteration of mRNA stability; post translational by alteration of latent zymogen to active form, as well as by specific endogenous tissue inhibitors, known as tissue inhibitors of metalloproteinases (TIMPs), comprising three types (Woessner, 1991).The imbalance of MMP activity and its inhibitors has been proposed to be responsible for various pathological conditions (Nuovo *et al.*, 1995; Rosenberg *et al.*, 1995).

The pro-inflammatory cytokines, TNFα and IL-1 have been found to be potent inducers of MMPs (Okalal *et al.*, 1990), while IL-6, an additional inflammatory cytokine, has been reported to induce the synthesis of TIMPs in different types of cells (Lotz & Guerne, 1991). Both enhancing and inhibitory capabilities have been observed for the anti-inflammatory cytokine TGFβ on MMPs and TIMPs activity, depending on the type of MMP and the tissue examined (Kerr *et al.*, 1990; Salo *et al.*, 1991; Overall *et al.*, 1989). An additional anti-inflammatory cytokine, interferon (IFN)-β, a drug shown to be efficacious in the treatment of MS patients, has been found to reduce the ability of activated T cells to synthesize MMP-9 (Stuve *et al.*, 1996). The effects of the Th1 type characteristic cytokine IFN-γ are however controversial, since it has been shown to have both inducive and suppressive influences on MMPs, perhaps dependent on the cell type and specific MMP examined, while not affecting or enhancing TIMPs' activity (Malik *et al.*, 1996; Tamai *et al.*, 1995; Gottschall *et al.*, 1995).

Astrocytes play a central role in autoimmune-inflammatory and regenerative process in the brain. Upon cytokine stimulation these cells express MHC Class II molecules, present antigens (Vidovic *et al.*, 1990), produce ECM components, a variety of MMPs (Gottschal & Yu, 1995) and TIMPs (Romanic & Madri, 1994), as well as inflammatory cytokines, which could participate in autocrine or in conjunction with immune cells, both in the pathology and remission of inflammatory processes. Understanding the relationship between cytokines and MMPs in activated astrocytes could deepen our knowledge on brain inflammation and recovery and may provide new approaches for drug design. In this study we investigated the response of astroglial cells to pro-inflammatory (TNF-α, IL-6, IFN-γ) and anti-inflammatory (TGFβ, IFN-β) cytokines, alone or in combinations, while focusing on the gelatinase activity of secreted MMP-2 and MMP-9.

METHODS AND RESULTS

Substrate specific zymography was performed for supernatants collected from astroglial cells (C6 cell line) exposed to pro- and anti-inflammatory cytokines. Constitutive activity of both MMP9 and MMP2 was observed in the supernatants as demonstrated in Figure 1 (lane 1). TNF-α did not affect MMP9 activity but induced a dose dependent elevation of MMP2 gelatinase activity (Figure 1). IFN-β alone (at different concentrations, from 0.1 to 100 U/ml) did not change the basal level of MMP2 proteolytic activity but enhanced the MMP9 activity. However increasing concentrations of IFN-β added to cells together with TNF-α, at a fixed concentration (250 U/ml), led to a moderate increase in both MMP9 and MMP2 activity (Figure 2). The induced MMP2 activity was significantly higher than the induced MMP9 activity. (These differences are apparent in the zymogram but not in the histogram which shows relative levels of activity for each MMP separately).

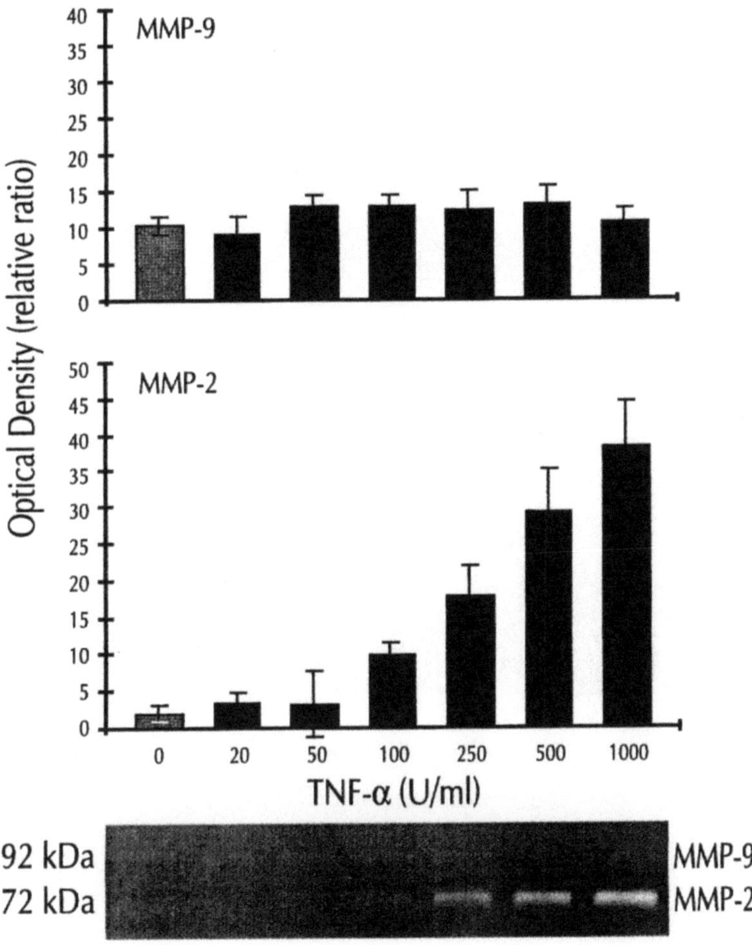

Figure 1. TNF-α induced differential modulation of MMPs in astroglial cells. Gelatin specific zymography was performed for supernatants collected from astroglial cells exposed to cytokines for 48 hours. The top histogram shows relative, computerized, optical density readings for each MMP observed separately. Numbers on the left are the molecular weights for observed MMPs.

In a similar manner IFN-γ alone at different concentrations, (0.1 to 100 U/ml) did not alter the level of basal MMP2 activity but significantly elevated MMP9 activity. When IFN-γ was added at different concentrations with a constant concentration of TNF-α, a moderate additive effect was observed in MMP9 activity, while a synergistic effect was observed on MMP2 activity (Figure 3).

IL-6 or TGFβ alone, also did not affect the activity of either MMP2 or MMP9, while the addition of both cytokines led to a dose dependent response in the activity of both the gelatinase specific MMPs examined (Figure 4). The combination of IL-6 (increasing concentrations) added to TNF-α (250 U/ml) led to a dose dependent enhancement in the activity of MMP2 and MMP9 (Figure 5). Similarly TGFβ together with TNF-α led to a dose dependent response in the activity of both MMPs. The highest

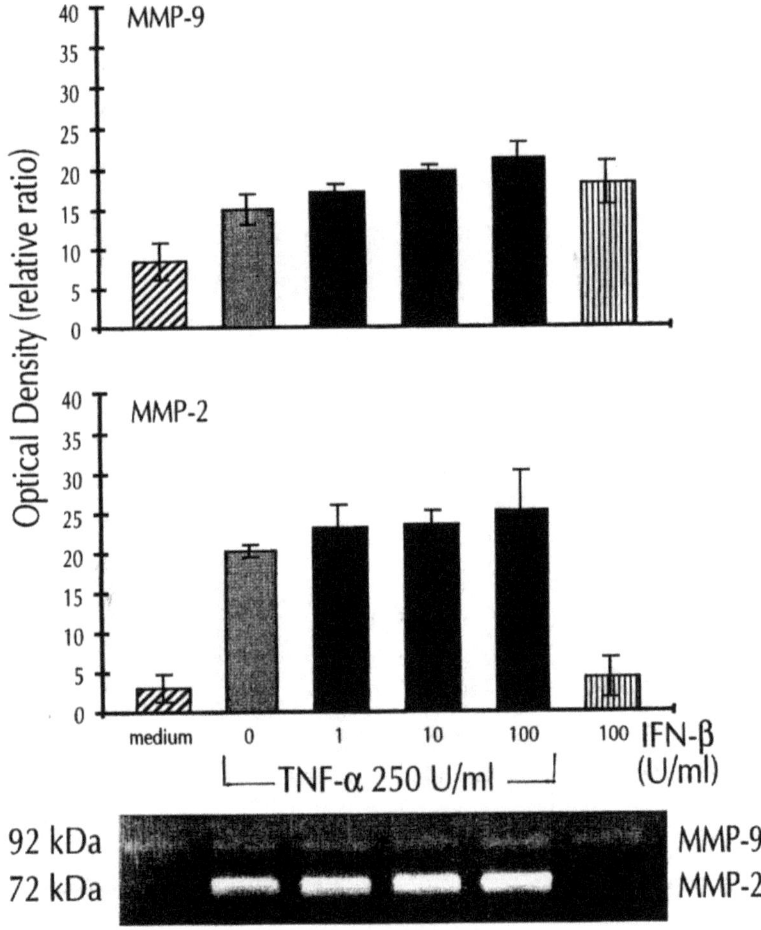

Figure 2. IFN-β induced differential modulation of MMPs in astroglial cells (see Figure 1).

TGFβ concentration examined (100 U/ml), slightly inhibited MMPs activity compared to the peak (1–5 U/ml) dosage (Figure 6).

DISCUSSION

The present study shows differential response to cytokines by the two gelatinases, MMP2 and MMP9, secreted from the astroglial cell line. Combinations of cytokines led to additive, synergistic or suppressive effects of the MMPs' activity. These findings stress the importance of the exact cytokine milieu in the micro-environment of the glial cells.

The cytokines investigated in this study have been associated with diseases of the CNS. TNF-α and IL-6 are pro-inflammatory cytokines known to be active in injury and inflammatory processes of the CNS. These cytokines are secreted by glial cells in addition to other cells, while TNF-α has been suggested as a marker of disease exacerbation

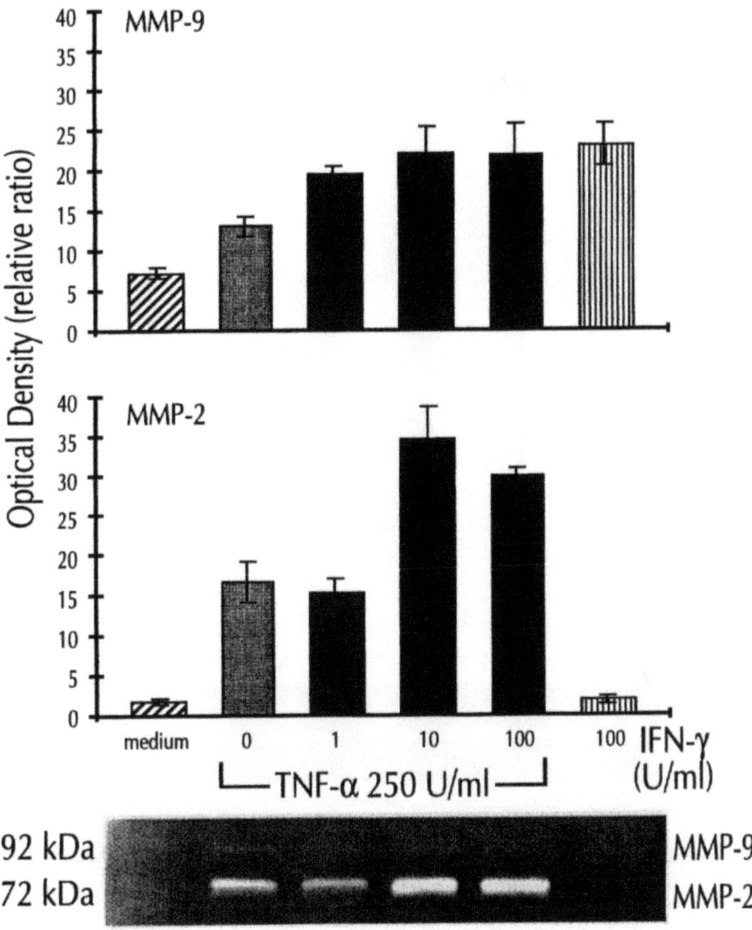

Figure 3. Combined effects of IFN-γ and TNF-α on MMPs' activity in astroglial cells (see Figure 1).

in MS patients. IFN-γ, a prominent Th1 cytokine, secreted from activated T cells in the vicinity of astrocytes, is believed to be responsible for the aberrant induction of antigen presentation by these cells and is also associated with MS. The efficacy of IFN-β in the treatment of MS patients has recently been reported (Rudick *et al.*, 1993; Paty, 1993). This cytokine is also known to possess anti-inflammatory properties such as reduction in the expression of class II molecules, resulting in the inhibition of antigen presentation (Miller *et al.*, 1996). TGFβ, an additional anti-inflammatory cytokine examined, secreted from Th3 cells and others cells, has been implicated in oral tolerance and copolymer-1 treatment of MS patients and EAE (Miller *et al.*, 1994; Whitacre *et al.*, 1996; Lahat *et al.*, 1997). The formation of glial scar, following CNS injury, is also dependent on the ability of TGFβ to stimulate astroglial cells, leading to extra-cellular matrix deposition (Logen *et al.*, 1992).

We observed constitutive expression of both MMP2 and MMP9 by astroglial cells in our study. Several investigators have defined MMP9 as an inflammatory metalloproteinase and correlate the ratio of MMP9/MMP2 with the severity of MS, while others do not make this distinction (Nog *et al.*, 1995). TNF-α enhanced the MMP2 activity in astroglial cells,

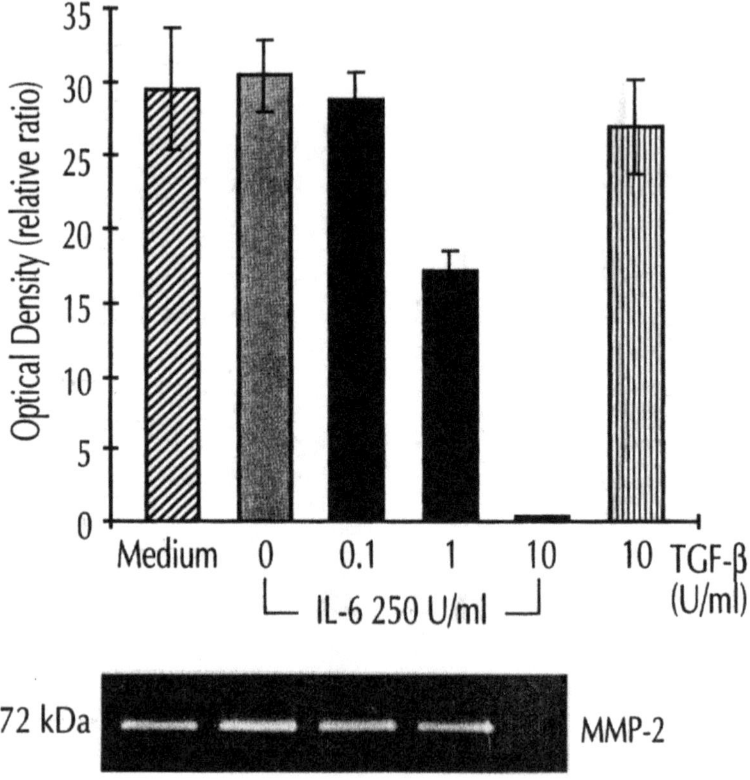

Figure 4. Synergistic inhibition of MMP2 by TGFβ and IL-6 (see Figure 1).

while IFN-γ and -β, when added alone, enhanced the activity of MMP9. TGFβ or IL-6 alone, on the other hand, did not affect any of the MMP activity. All these cytokines, when added together with TNF-α, enhanced the activity of both MMP2 and MMP9, either additively or synergistically (e.g., IFN-γ-MMP2). Thus TNF-α appears to define and dominate the inflammatory pattern of MMP secretion, even in the presence of cytokines that alone partly affect, do not affect, or reduce the activity of MMPs.

The gelatinase activity observed in the zymogram reflects the overall potential activity which includes in-vitro activation of pro-MMPs by the zymogram components and at the same time the activating or inhibitory effects of cytokines on TIMPs' activity. Most of the in-vivo counter-effects of MMPs on endogenous production and secretion of cytokines (Beckett *et al.*, 1996) as well as the effects of other factors on MMP activation and gene expression are neutralized in culture. The level of regulation of the observed MMP activity in the astroglial cells, whether transcriptional or post-transcriptional (i.e., RNA transcription, stability, TIMPs expression) are presently being studied. These physiological processes are important for understanding pathological processes in CNS inflammatory diseases and may have important implications for future approaches to cytokine mediated drug intervention in brain injury and glial scar formation. Our studies suggest that mixture of complementary cytokines rather than a single one should be taken into account.

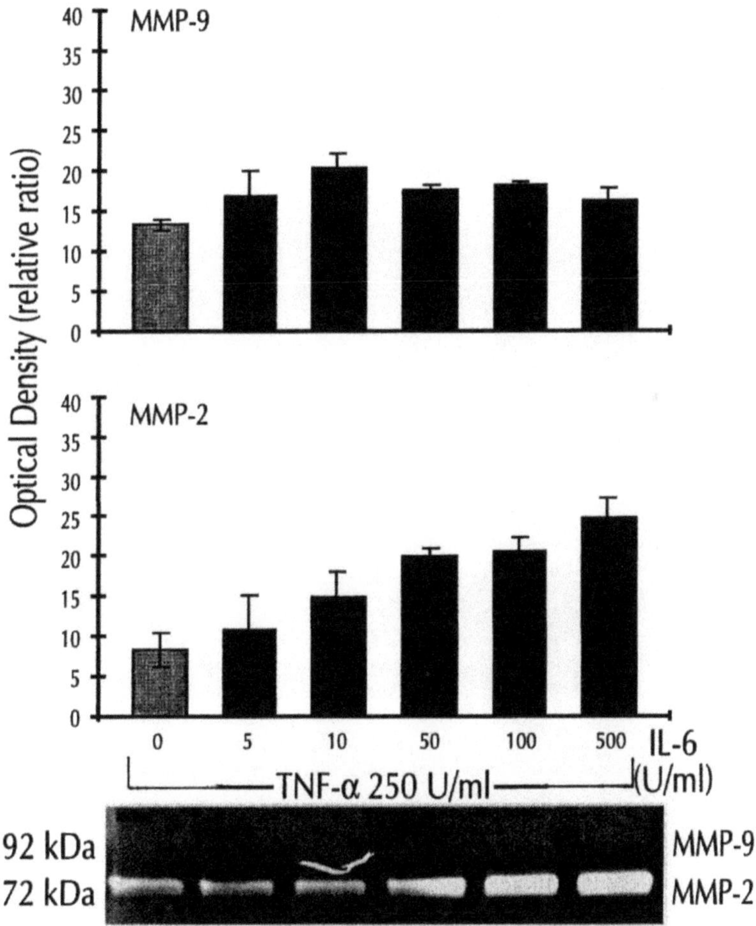

Figure 5. IL-6 enhances TNF-α induced MMPs' activity in astroglial cells (see Figure 1).

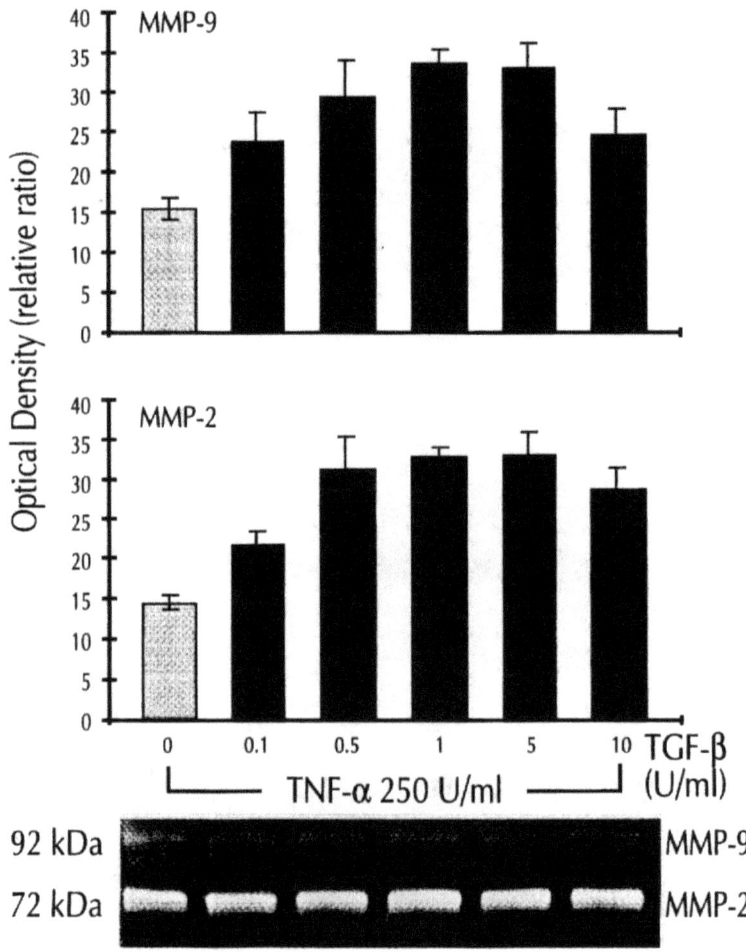

Figure 6. TGFβ enhances TNF-α induced MMPs' activity in astroglial cells (see Figure 1).

REFERENCES

Becket, R.P., Davidson, A.H., Drummond, A.H., Huxley, P., and Whittaker, M., 1996, Recent advances in matrix metalloproteinase inhibitor research, *DDT.* 1:16–26.

Gijbels, K., Masure, S., Carton, H., and Opdenakker, G., 1992, Gelatinase in the cerebrospinal fluid of patients with multiple sclerosis and other inflammatory neurological disorders, *J. Neuroimmunol.* 41:29–34.

Gottschall, P.E., and Yu, X., 1995, Cytokines regulate gelatinase A and B (Matrix Metalloproteinase 2 and 9) activity in cultured rat cells, *J. Neurochem.* 64:1513–1520.

Gottschall, P.E., Yu, X., and Bing, B., 1995, Increased production of MMP-9 and IL-6 by activated rat microglia in culture, *J. Neurosci. Res.* 42:335–342.

Kerr, L.D., Miller, D.B., and Matresian, L.M., 1990, TGFβ inhibition of transin/stromylysin gene expression is mediated through a FOS binding sequence, *Cell* 61:267–278.

Lahat, N., Shapiro, S.,Kinarty, A., Gershtein, R., Gurtovnick, A, Rawashdeh, H., Honigman, S., Miller, A., 1997, Copolymer-1 (Copaxone) driven anti-inflammatory cascade in multiple sclerosis patients, *J. Neurol.* 244 (suppl3):S32.

Logan, A., Frautschy, S.A., Gonzalez, A.M., Spoon, M.B., and Baird, A., 1992, Enhanced expression of TGFβ in the rat brain after a localized cerebral injury, *Brain Res.* 587:216–255.

Lotz, M., and Guerne, P.A., 1991, Interleukin 6 induces the synthesis of tissue inhibitor of metalloproteinases-1 (TIMP-1), *J. Biol. Chem.* 266:2017–2020.

Malik, N., Greenfeld, B.W., Wahl, A.F., and Kiener, P.A., 1990, Activation of human monocytes through CD40 induces matrix metalloproteinases, *J. Immunol.* 156:3952–3960.

McKeon, R.J., Hoke, A., and Silver, J., 1995, Injury induced proteoglycans inhibit the potential for laminin-mediated axon growth on astrocytic scars, *Exp. Neurol.* 136:32–43.9.

Miller, A., Lider, O., Roberts, A.B., Sporn, M.B., and Weiner, H.L., 1992, Suppressor T cells generated by oral tolerization to myelin basic protein suppress both in vitro and in vivo immune responses by the release of transforming growth factor beta after antigen-specific triggering, *Proc. Natl. Acad. Sci. USA.* 89:421–425.

Miller, A., Lanir, N., Shapiro, S., Revel, M., Honigman, S., Kinarty, A., and Lahat, N., 1996, Immunoregulatory effects of IFN-β and interacting cytokines on human vascular endothelial cells. Implications for MS and other autoimmune diseases, *J. Neuroimmunol.* 64:151–161.

Norga, K., Paemen, L., Masure, S., Dillen, C., Heremans, H., Billiae, A., Carton, H., Cuzner, L., Olsson, T., Van Damme, J., and Opdenaker, G., 1995, Prevention of acute autoimmune encephalomyelitis and abrogation of relapses in murine models of multiple sclerosis by the protease inhibitor D-penicillamine, *Inflamm. Res.* 44:529–534.

Nuovo, G. J., MacConnel, P.B., Sismir, A., Valea, F., and French, D.L., 1995, Correlation of the in-situ detection of PCR amplified metalloproteinase complementary DNAs and their inhibitors with prognosis in cervical cancer, *Cancer Res.* 55:267–275.

Okala, Y., Tsuchiga, H., and Shimizu, H., 1990, Induction and stimulation of 92 kDa gelatinase/type IV collagenase production in osteosarcoma and fibrosarcoma cell lines by tumor necrosis factor α, *Biochem. Biophys. Res. Commun.* 171:610–617.

Overall, C.M., Wrana, J.L., and Sodak, J., 1989, Independent regulation of collagenase, 72 kDa progelatinase and TIMP expression in human fibroblasts by TGFβ, *J. Biol. Chem.* 264:1860–1869.

Paty, D.W., MS/MRI Study Group, 1993, The IFNβ Multiple Sclerosis Study Group, Interferon beta-1b is effective in relapsing remitting multiple sclerosis II. MRI analysis of multicenter, randomized double-blind, placebo-controlled trial, *Neurology* 43:662–667.

Romanic, A.M., and Madri, J.A., 1994, Extracellular matrix degrading proteinases in the nervous system, *Brain Pathol.* 4:145–156.

Rosenberg, G.A., Kornfeld, M., Estrada, E., Kelley, R.O., Liotta, L.A., and Stetler-Stevenson, W.G., 1995, TIMP-2 reduces proteolytic opening of blood brain barrier by type IV Collagenase, *Brain Res.* 576:203–207.

Rosenberg, G.A., Dencoff, J.E., Correa, N., Reiners, M., and Ford, C.C. 1996, Effects of steroids on CSF matrix metalloproteinases in multiple sclerosis: relation to blood-brain barrier injury, *Neurology* 46:1626–1632.

Rudick, R.A., Carpenter, C.S., Cookfair, D.I., et al., 1993, In vitro and in vivo inhibition of mitogen-driven T cell activation by recombinant interferon beta. *Neurology* 43:2080–2087.

Salo, T., Lyons, J.G., Rahemtulla, F., Birkendal-Hansen, H., and Larjava, H., 1991, TGFβ1 upregulates type IV collagenase expression in cultured human keratinocytes, *J. Biol. Chem.* 266:11436–11441.

Stuve, O., Dooly, J.H., Uhm, J.H., Antel, J.P., Francis, G., Williams, G., and Yong V.W., 1996, Interferon beta 1b decreases the migration of T lymphocytes in-vitro: effects on matrix metalloproteinase-9, *Ann. Neurol.* 40:853–863.

Tamai, K., Ishikawa, H., Mauviel, A., and Vitto J., 1995, Interferon-gamma coordinately upregulates MMP-1 and MMP-3 but not TIMP expression in cultured keratinocytes, *J. Invest. Dermatol.* 140:384–390.

Vidovic, M., Spracio, S.M., Elovitz, M, and Benveniste E.E., 1990, Induction and regulation of class II MHC mRNA expression in astrocytes by IFN-γ and TNF-α, *J. Neuroimmunol.* 30:189–195.

Whitacre, C.C., Ginapp, I.Wý.E., Meyer, A., Cox, K.L., and Javed, N., 1996, Treatment of autoimmune disease by oral tolerance to autoantigens, *Clin. Immunol. Immunopathol.* 80:S31–39.

Woessner, I.F., 1991, Matrix metalloproteinase and their inhibitors in connective tissue remodeling, *FASEB J.* 5:2145–2154.

22

POLYAMINES AND RELATED COMPOUNDS IN NERVE CELL DEATH AND SURVIVAL

An Overview

Gad M. Gilad,[1] Varda H. Gilad,[1] Tatiana Prohorov,[2] and Jose M. Rabey[2]

[1]Laboratory of Neuroscience
[2]Department of Neurology
Assaf Harofeh Medical Center
Zrifin 70300, Israel

In addition to direct local tissue damage, brain and spinal cord injuries lead to numerous adverse reactions (e.g., energy depletion, disturbed calcium regulation, acidosis, increased excitatory neurotransmitter release, excess free radical accumulation, and increased lipid peroxidation) which, if not brought rapidly under control, lead to uncontrolled degradation of proteins, lipids, and nucleic acids and to the spread of neuronal damage (Hara et al., 1995; Mattson and Scheff, 1994).

As with the general adaptational (stress) syndrome, with its characteristic behavioral, physiological and neuroendocrine changes (Selye, 1936), so do cells respond rapidly to life-threatening stressful stimuli (e.g., mechanical injuries, cerebrovascular malfunctions, neurotoxins, or infections) by activating, via signal transduction pathways, a characteristic defensive molecular "stress program". The inductive expression of a universal set of stress proteins (Hightower, 1991; Dragunow and Robertson, 1988) and increased polyamine (PA) metabolism, termed the PA-stress-response (PSR) (Desiderio et al., 1988; Gilad and Gilad, 1992; Kanje et al., 1986; Paschen et al., 1988), are considered to be integral components of this survival molecular stress program (Gilad and Gilad, 1992). The intensity of the PSR appears to be proportional to the magnitude of the stressor.

THE BRAIN PA-STRESS-RESPONSE

Proper regulation of brain PA metabolism may be critical for an appropriate response to traumatic stress. A rapid, but short-lasting transient activation of the synthetic and degradative PA enzymes and a concomitant transient increase in all PAs is the hallmark of cells responding to various traumatic stressful stimuli (Tabor and Tabor, 1984). In

Progress in Alzheimer's and Parkinson's Diseases
edited by Fisher *et al.*, Plenum Press, New York, 1998.

the brain, however, traumatic stress leads to a transient elevation in the activity of ornithine decarboxylase (ODC), the enzyme that catalyzes putrescine formation in the first step of PA synthesis (Seiler and Bolkenius, 1985), and a concomitant reduction, or lack of change, in the activity of S-adenosylmethionine decarboxylase (SAM-DC), the enzyme that catalyzes the second stage of PA synthesis (Astancolle et al., 1991; Gilad and Gilad, 1992; Hietala et al., 1983; Zawia et al., 1991). This "incomplete" PSR may be the result of an altered pattern of gene expression, and/or restrictive cellular compartmentalization (Gilad and Gilad, 1992). It is interesting that putative binding sites (DNA sequences) for cyclic AMP-, phorbol ester (TPA)- and steroid hormone-responsive elements, were all found on the 5'-flanking region of the ODC gene (Abrahamsen and Morris, 1991). Apparently, therefore, the intensity of the PSR may depend on the balance between converging stress-activated signal transduction pathways. The activation of an incomplete PSR after brain trauma may be potentially harmful as it can result in the persistent accumulation of putrescine and reduction in PA concentrations.

THE CELLULAR FUNCTION OF PAs

Polyamines are small aliphatic compounds which are positively charged at physiological pH and avidly bind to negatively charged molecules (Tabor and Tabor, 1984). Several functions ascribed to PAs may assume importance in cellular defense. Thus, regulation of the ionic environment, modulation of signal pathways, control of cellular Ca^{2+} homeostasis, antioxidant effect (Lovaas, 1995), inhibition of lipid peroxidation, and interaction with nucleic acids are all putative sites for PA action (Gilad and Gilad, 1992). But the primary site(s) of PA action is still unclear. It should be emphasized that besides the injured neurons themselves, intact neurons and glial cells connected or associated with them may be potential targets where PAs exert their action; for example, by stimulating the production of neurotrophic factors (Gilad et al., 1989; Gilad and Gilad, 1992).

TREATMENT WITH PAs AFTER NEUROTRAUMA

It has been demonstrated in various systems that when increased demand for PA arises, not only does the biosynthetic capacity increase, but also the ability to take up extracellular PAs is greatly enhanced (Seiler and Dezeure, 1990). This, and the fact that extracellular PA concentrations are normally low (Seiler, 1991), are the rationale for using exogenous PAs in the attempts to enhance survival and rescue neurons from degeneration and cell death after traumatic stress. Several studies, using various experimental models of neurotrauma, demonstrate that administration of exogenous PAs after the insult can rescue neurons from cell death and enhance functional recovery (Gilad and Gilad, 1992).

AGMATINE

This guanidino compound, the product of arginine decarboxylation, is abundant in bacteria and plants where it serves as a precursor for PA synthesis. It was recently demonstrated that arginine can be decarboxylated in the brain by the enzyme ODC to form agmatine (Gilad et al., 1996a; Li et al., 1994), and that agmatine is present in the mammalian brain (Li et al., 1994). The decarboxylation of arginine is transiently increased during development and after ischemia, in parallel to ODC activity, indicating that agmatine formation may assume importance during development and after brain injury (Gilad et al., 1996a). Agmatine can be selectively metabolized in the rat brain into urea and putrescine, the precursor of polyamine synthesis (Gilad et al., 1996b).

AGMATINE TREATMENT AFTER NEUROTRAUMA

Several lines of evidence support our hypothesis that agmatine may be of therapeutic potential in neurotrauma (Gilad et al., 1995 and 1996a for references). First, agmatine has been implicated in a range of activities related to nervous system function; it can modulate several neurotransmitter receptors and interfere with second messenger pathways by inhibiting ADP-ribosylation of proteins. The latter process is implicated in processes underlying cell death. Second, agmatine can inhibit advanced glycosylation end-product formation, a process involved in damage to extracellular matrix proteins. Third, agmatine can inhibit brain nitric oxide (NO) synthase, but does not serve as a substrate for NO formation (Gilad et al., 1996b). Fourth, as mentioned above, agmatine in the brain may be a precursor for PA synthesis. And fifth, treatment with agmatine was reported to cause hypoglycemia and reduced serum lactate (i.e., insulin-like effects) in rodents. A recent series of studies demonstrate that systemic treatment with agmatine can exert potent neuroprotective effects in several experimental models of neurotrauma. Finally, and most importantly, agmatine treatment proved to be nontoxic (Gilad et al., 1995).

The extent of agmatine transport into the brain is unknown. But like PAs, agmatine may gain access into the brain via the blood brain barrier which becomes compromised quite early after traumatic injuries and remains so for long periods (Dietrich et al., 1991; Gilad et al., 1993), thus allowing exogenous compounds of limited transport easy access.

As clinically effective drug treatment is still unavailable, there is an intensive search for nontoxic agents to prevent neurological damage caused by CNS injury. Our studies now suggest that agmatine and novel "PA-based" compounds may prove to be such agents which should be tried for potential therapeutic use after neurotrauma and in neurodegenerative disorders.

ACKNOWLEDGMENTS

Supported by grants from the Israel Science Foundation, the German-Israeli Foundation for Scientific Research and Development, and the Theodore and Vada Stanley Foundation.

REFERENCES

Abrahamsen, M.S., and Morris, D.R., 1991, Regulation of expression of the ornithine decarboxylase gene by intracellular signal transduction pathways. In: *Perspectives on Cellular Regulation: From Bacteria to Cancer.* Wiley-Liss, Inc., New York, pp. 107–119.

Astancolle, S., Davalli, P., and Corti, A., 1991, Blockade of pp. 107–119, α-and β-adrenergic receptors can prevent stimulation of liver ornithine decarboxylase activity by glucocorticoid or laparotomy. *Biochem. Biophys. Res. Comm.* 174:915–921.

Desiderio, M.A., Zini, I., Davalli, P., Zoli, M., Corti, A., Fuxe, K., and Agnati, L.F., 1988, Polyamines, ornithine decarboxylase, and diamine oxidase in the substantia nigra and striatum of the male rat after hemitransection. *J. Neurochem. 51:*25–31.

Dietrich, W.D., Halley, M., Valdes, I., and Busto, R., 1991, Interrelationships between increased vascular permeability and acute neuronal damage following temperature-controlled brain ischemia in rats. *Acta Neuropathol. (Berl.)* 81:615–625.

Dragunow, M., and Robertson, H.A., 1988, Brain injury induces c-fos protein(s) in nerve and glia-like in adult mammalian brain. *Brain Res.* 455:295–299.

Gilad, G.M., Dornay, M., and Gilad, V.H., 1989, Polyamines induce precocious development in rats: Possible interaction with growth factors. *Int. J. Dev. Neurosci.* 7:641–653.

Gilad, G.M., and Gilad, V.H., 1992, Polyamines in neurotrauma; ubiquitous molecules in search of a function. *Biochem. Pharmacol.* 44:401–407.

Gilad, G.M., Gilad, V.H., and Rabey, J.M., 1996a, Arginine and ornithine decarboxylation in rodent brain; coincidental changes during development and after ischemia. *Neurosci. Lett.* 216:33–36.

Gilad, G.M., Gilad, V.H., and Wyatt, R.J., 1993, Accumulation of exogenous polyamines in gerbil brain after ischemia. *Mol. Chem. Neuropathol.* 18:197–210.

Gilad, G.M., Salame, K., Rabey, J.M., and Gilad, V.H., 1995, Agmatine treatment is neuroprotective in rodent brain injury models. *Life Sci.* 58:PL41-PL46.

Gilad, G.M., Wollman, Y., Iaina, A., Rabey, J.M., Chernihovsky, T., and Gilad, V.H., 1996b, Metabolism of agmatine into urea but not into nitric oxide in rat brain. *NeuroReport.* 7:1730–1732.

Hara, H., Sukamoto, T., and Kogure, K., 1993, Mechanism and pathogenesis of ischemia-induced neuronal damage. *Prog. Neurobiol.* 40:645–670.

Hietala, O.A., Laitinen, S.I., Laitnen, P.H., Lapinjoki, S.P., and Pajunen, A.E.I., 1983, The inverse changes of mouse brain ornithine and S-adenosylmethionine decarboxylase activities by chlorpromazine and imipramine. Dependence of ornithine decarboxylase induction on β-adrenoceptors. *Biochem. Pharmacol.* 32:1581–1585.

Hightower, L.E., 1991, Heat shock, stress proteins, chaperons, and proteotoxicity. *Cell* 66:191–197.

Kanje, M., Fransson, I., Edstrom, A., and Lowkvist, B., 1986, Ornithine decarboxylase activity in dorsal root ganglia of regenerating frog sciatic nerve. *Brain Res.* 381:24–28.

Li, G., Regunathan, S., Barrow, C.J., Eshraghi, J., Cooper, R., and Reis, D.J., 1994, Agmatine: An endogenous clonidine-displacing substance in the brain. *Science* 263:966–969.

Lovaas, E., 1995, Hypothesis: spermine may be an important epidermal antioxidant. *Med.Hypothesis* 45:59–67.

Mattson, M.P., and Scheff, S.W. 1994, Endogenous neuroprotection factors and traumatic brain injury: mechanisms of action and implications for therapy. *J. Neurotrauma* 11:3–33.

Paschen, W., Schmidt-Kastner, R., Hallmayer, J., and Djuricic, B., 1988, Polyamines in cerebral ischemia. *Neurochem. Pathol.* 9:1–20.

Seiler, N., 1991, Pharmacological properties of natural polyamines and their depletion by biosynthesis inhibitors as a therapeutic approach. *Prog.Drug Res.* 37:107–159.

Seiler, N., and Bolkenius, F.N., 1985, Polyamine reutilization and turnover in brain. *Neurochem. Res.* 10:529–544.

Seiler, N., and Dezeure, F., 1990, Polyamine transport in mammalian cells. *Int. J. Biochem.* 22:211–218.

Selye, H., 1936, A syndrome produced by diverse nocuous agents. *Nature* 138:32–37.

Tabor, C.W. and Tabor, H., 1984, Polyamines. *Ann. Rev. Biochem.* 53:749–790.

Zawia, N.H., Mattia, C.J., and Bondy, S.C., 1991, Differential effects of difluoromethylornithine on basal and induced activity of cerebral ornithine decarboxylase and MRNA. *Neuropharmacology* 30:337–343.

23

HALOPERIDOL INDUCES NEUROTOXICITY IN MOUSE EMBRYO BRAIN TISSUE

Evidence for Oxidative Damage Mechanism, and Implication for Tardive Dyskinesia

I. Gil-Ad,[1,4] D. Offen,[2,4] B. Shtaif,[1,4] R. Galili-Mosberg,[2,4] and A. Weizman[1,3,4]

[1]Laboratory of Biological Psychiatry
[2]Laboratory of Neurosciences
Felsenstein Medical Research Center
Beilinson Campus, Rabin Medical Center
Petah-Tiqva 49100, Israel
[3]Research Unit, Geha Psychiatric Hospital
Petah-Tiqva, Israel
[4]Sackler School of Medicine
Tel Aviv University
Tel-Aviv, Israel

BACKGROUND

Haloperidol (H) is a widely used drug in the treatment of schizophrenia and tics. It belongs to the butyrophenones class of neuroleptics which interferes with the DA transmission, often resulting in undesired adverse effects of which the most common are extrapyramidal symptoms and TD (Carlson, 1988; Carpenter et al., 1994).

Tardive movement disorder and parkinsonian symptoms are serious complications related to chronic neuroleptics therapy (Wolf & Moshaim, 1988). The mechanism underlying the development of the diseases is unknown. Imbalance in DA, D1 and D2 receptors, alteration in the gama amino butyric acid (GABA) system, and oxidative stress in the brain have been suggested (Davis, 1975; Kane & Marder,1993; Spivak et al., 1992). The typical neuroleptics e.g: H and chlorpromazine are potent inducers of extrapyramidal symptoms and TD, while clozapine and other atypical neuroleptics induce less extrapyramidal and TD symptoms.

Damage to the neuronal tissue mediated by an accumulation of reactive oxygen species (ROS) was suggested to be involved the undesired adverse effects of neuroleptics.

Some clinical studies proposed the use of alpha tocopherol (vitamin E) in patients with TD, showing a reduction of symptoms induced by chronic neuroleptic therapy (Spivak et al., 1992; Bischot et al., 1993).

Pharmacological studies suggest that chronic administration of the H is accompanied by the formation of neurotoxic pyridinium metabolites. (Rollema et al., 1994). Recent reports by Ben Shachar et al. (1993, 1994) have suggested that the neurotoxic effect of H and phenothiazines is mediated by mobilization of iron to the brain from its peripheral stores, leading to creation of an area highly susceptible to oxidative damage.

The important role of the glial cells in the protection of neurons from destructive processes has been demonstrated in some studies. Astrocytes were found to contain and secrete large amounts of antioxidative vitamins, such as ascorbate and vitamin E, as well as enzymes, such as glutathione peroxidase and superoxide dismutase (Makar et al., 1994). In addition, glial cells were found to synthesize and secrete neurotrophic factors such as glial cell-line derived neurotrophic factor (GDNF) and insulin- like growth factor 1 (IGF-1) which might also play a role in neuronal protection (Henderson et al., 1995).

AIMS OF THE STUDY

The study was designed to:

1. Determine the direct toxic effect of H on selected neuronal cells as compared to the effect on the whole brain tissue (glial and neuronal cells).
2. Evaluate the role of the DA receptor blocking activity in the mechanism of H induced neurotoxicity.
3. Screen and select antioxidative agents which can protect neurons from H-induced toxicity.

MATERIALS AND METHODS

Reagents

For tissue culture: minimum essential medium (MEM), horse serum 8%, fetal calf serum FCS 8%, glucose 0.6%, glutamine, gentamycin10 ug/ml, Leibowitch L-15 medium, DCCM medium (All obtained from Beith Haemek Israel). Poly d-lysine , uridine, 5 fluoro uridine, neutral red solution, DMSO, haloperidol, dopamine, alpha tocopherol, ascorbate, selenium, beta carotene, reduced glutathione (GSH), N-acetyl cysteine (NAC), and desferroxamine (All obtained from Sigma St. Louis, Mo USA).

Cell Culture

Pregnant ICR mice on day 14–15 of pregnancy (Harlan, Israel) were obtained and their brains dissected and homogenized in Leibowitch medium containing glucose, glutamine and gentamycine. Cells were distributed in wells previously dispensed with poly d-lysine (in 96 well microplate) 300,000–500,000 cell/well 0.48 hr later in half of the plates 5-fluoro deoxy uridine + uridine (FUDR) was added in order to obtain selected neuronal culture. The cells were treated with the different agents in triplicates for 24–72 hr. Controls served wells containing cells in medium only. Determination of cell viability in culture was performed using the neutral red method (Borenfreund & Puerner, 1984). Solution of neutral red 1% in DCCM medium was added for 24 hr at 37°C. Cells were visualized using phase microscope and quantitative determination was performed by washing excess reagent and eluting color from cells using specific alcoholic solution. The intensity of the stained lysosomes is positively correlated to the number of viable cells. Colorimetric determination was performed in an ELISA reader at 550 nm. Cell viability was expressed as percent of controls.

RESULTS

Figure 1 shows the effect of H at different concentrations 1–100 μM (Stock H preparation was 1 mM in 10% DMSO further diluted in PBS) on cell viability in neuronal culture as compared to neuron + glia cell culture. H induced neuronal cell death in selected neuronal culture leading to survival of 31–51% of cells, with maximal effect obtained at concentrations of 1–10 μM.

When the drug was added to culture containing mixed glial + neuronal cells, viability of cells was no different than control culture (cells embedded in medium only).

Figure 2 shows the effect DA 0.5 mM alone or combined with H 1μM on isolated neuronal cell viability and on viability of mixed glial and neuronal cells. DA alone caused a 40% decrease in neuronal viability. H alone caused a 60% decrease and the combination of both drugs resulted in only 18% survival of neuronal cells. In this experiment, glial cells in the culture inhibited toxicity induced by either DA alone or combined with H, which was similar to the effect of glial cells on H induced neurotoxicity.

Table 1 shows the effect of different antioxidants: vitamin E, beta carotene, selenium, vitamin C and desferrioxamine combined with H on neuronal cell viability. Our data demonstrate that among all these agents only vitamin E at concentrations of 0.1, 0.3 and 1 mM partially reversed H induced neurotoxicity.

Table 2 shows the effect of two antioxidative agents containing thiol groups, NAC and GSH, on neuronal cell viability after exposure to H (1 μM). Of the two agents, NAC was partially effective in suppressing H induced neurotoxicity at concentrations of 0.3 mM and 3.0 mM. GSH did not induce a statistically significant effect.

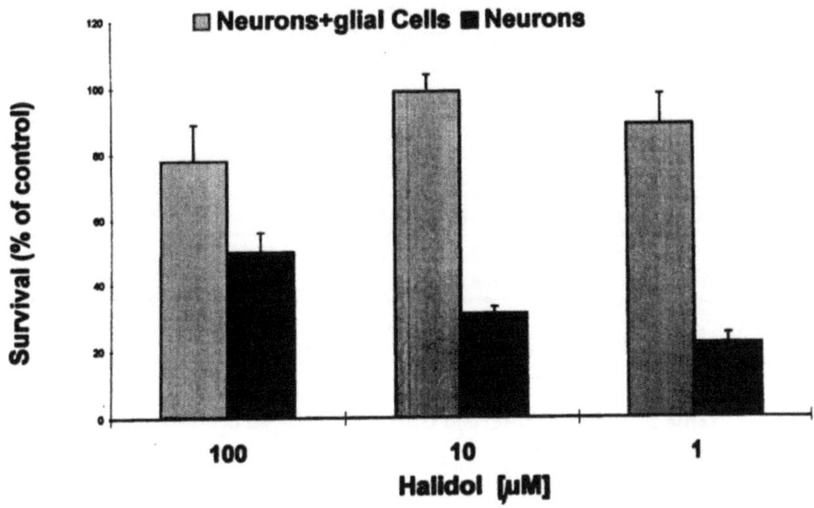

Figure 1. Dose effect of H on neurons and mixed neurons and glia cell viability.

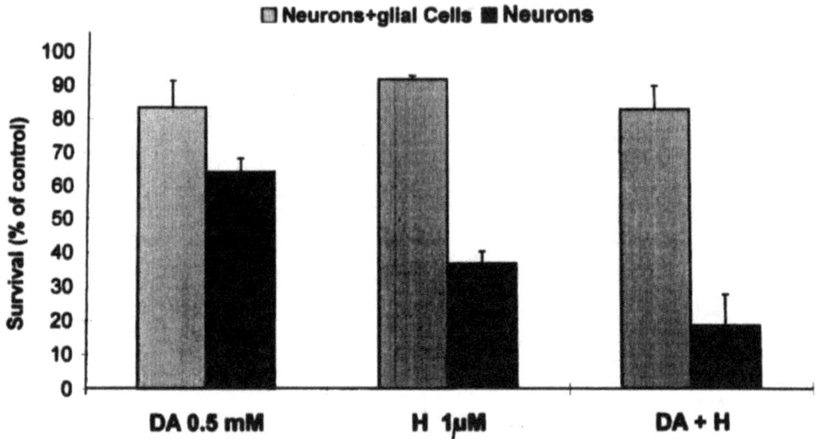

Figure 2. Effect of DA, H and combination of both on neurons and mixed neurons and glia cell viability.

All the antioxidants (at the concentrations mentioned above) were tested alone in culture and found ineffective in altering neuronal cell viability in basal conditions.

DISCUSSION

Our data provide further evidence for the direct in vitro neurotoxic effect of the widely used antipsychotic drug H on selected mouse embryonic neuronal cells in culture leading to cell death (30–70%), at concentrations of 1–100 µM. Previous reports showed cytotoxic activity of H on rat hippocampal neurons, as well as on mouse glioma and neuroblastoma cell lines (Behl et al., 1995; Vilner & Bowen, 1993). In our model, when H was added to mixed neurons and glial cells, its neurotoxic activity was markedly suppressed or eliminated. This finding suggests that glial cells possess a major role in the protection of neurons from damage induced by H and similarly structured drugs. Astrocytes

Table 1. Effect of antioxidants on H induced mouse embryo neuronal cell death[a]

H	H + Vit E			H + β carotene			H + Desferroxamine			H + Selenium	H + Vit C
1 µM	0.1 mM	0.3 mM	1 mM	1 mM	3 mM	10 mM	3 mM	10 mM	30 mM	0.1 mM	0.1 mM
52.0	86.0*	90.0**	90.0**	50.0	53.0	44.0	50.0	46.0	32.5	40	15.0**
±7.3	±12.6	±8.0	±2.8	±7.8	±8.8	±1.5	±6.7	±2.1	±0.5	±3.8	±6.3

[a]Cell viability (% of control).
Each value represents M ± SEM of 3 determinations except for H (n = 6).
*p < 0.05 vs H; **p < 0.01 vs H.

Table 2. Effect of NAC and GSH on H-induced neurotoxicity

H	H + NAC		GSH + H	
1 µM	0.3 mM	1 mM	0.3 mM	1 mM
52.0 ± 7.3	74.0 ± 5.2	72.0 ± 4.5	57.0 ± 8.8	65 ± 17.8

Each point represents M ± SEM of 3 determinations.

and oligodendrocytes were reported to contain high amounts of antioxidative vitamins and enzymes e.g. vitamin E, ascorbate, glutathione and enzymes of glutathione metabolism, as well as neurotrophic factors (Makar et al., 1994; Henderson et al., 1995; Scharr et al., 1993). These agents are important in combating oxygen insults in the brain, and therefore play a role in defending neurons from oxidative damage. ROS was suggested to be involved in the pathogenesis of several neurodegenrative diseases such as Parkinson's disease, Alzheimer's disease, and inherited forms of Amyotrophic Lateral Sclerosis (Chiueh et al., 1994; Joseph & Cutler, 1994; Adams & Odunze, 1991). Concerning neuroleptic induced TD, recent studies show that vitamin E treatment reduces the severity of involuntary movements in patients with TD but not in patients suffering from Parkinson's disease (Spivak et al., 1992; Bischot et al., 1993). Vitamin E was also found to attenuate the development of H-induced supersensitivity to dopaminergic agonists agents in the rat (Gattaz et al., 1993). All these studies support the concept of involvement of free radicals in the neuroleptics-induced involuntary movement disorders. Consistent with this idea are studies performed in rats and monkeys (Ben Shahar et al., 1993 and 1994), suggesting that increased iron concentration in basal ganglia could trigger in-vivo generation of hydroxyl radicals and oxidative stress, leading to the development of EPS and TD.

Supporting this notion too, is the finding that metabolism of H results in formation of neurotoxic agents such as the pyridinium metabolite HPP+, which induces parkinsonism in laboratory animals, by causing massive neuronal loss in the substantia nigra (Rollema et al., 1994). Other reports have demonstrated that some antioxidants: vitamin E analogs and DMSO and the monoamine B oxidase inhibitor, deprenyl, can protect nigral neurons from MPTP induced neurotoxicity (Wu et al., 1994). This finding supports the idea that neurotoxic symptoms induced by H and other typical neuroleptics are independent of their DA blockade activity, and result probably from oxidative damage in midbrain. Our results showed that simultaneous DA and H administration did not antagonize, but rather potentiated the neurotoxic activity of H on selected neuronal cells, which provide additional proof for the dissociation between the anti-DA (anti-psychotic) activity of the drug and its induced neurotoxicity.

Moreover DA alone was demonstrated to be a potent apoptotic agent in neuronal tissue, and in cell culture of mouse thymocytes (Ziv et al., 1994; Offen et al., 1996; Offen et al., 1995) and its neurotoxic activity was prevented in pheochromocytoma (PC12) cell culture by the thiol anti-oxidants: glutatione, N-acetyl cysteine and and dithiothreitol (Offen et al., 1995).

In our experiment DA alone, as expected, induced a marked neuronal cell death in isolated neuronal tissue, but in a similar manner to H it was not toxic in mixed glial and neuronal cell culture. DA toxicity was suggested to be involved in the pathogenic mechanism of Parkinson's disease (Adams & Odunze, 1991; Offen et al., 1995). The finding that in the presence of glial cells, toxicity of DA and H was prevented implies that defected mechanism of synthesis and/or secretion of anti-oxidants and/or growth factors from glial cells could be involved, at least in part, in the emergence of EPS and TD in patients.

With regard to the effect of different antioxidative agents, our data show that vitamin E and NAC were the most effective agents in protecting neurons from H toxicity. The other agents tested—beta-carotene, vitamin C, selenium and desferrioxamine were found ineffective. Beta- carotene was found to possess antiproliferative activity (Peram et al., 1996), vitamin C was reported to possess prooxidative effects in some conditions (Meyers et al., 1996; Leibler et al., 1986) and in our experiment combined administration of vitamin C and H resulted even in augmentation of the toxic effect of H. Desferrioxamine which is a potent chelator of iron, did not antagonize the effect of H. This finding implies that in isolated brain tissue, metabolism of H to unstable toxic molecules is independent of iron concentration in the tissue. NAC and GSH are antioxidants which contain a thiol group and were reported to prevent DA autooxidation, and DA induced DNA fragmentation in neuronal tissue (Vincent et al., 1994). Intracellular GSH activity constitutes an important defense system in living cells. NAC which is the precursor of GSH synthesis, prevents GSH depletion in response to drug induced oxidative stress (Aruma et al., 1990). GSH depletion was reported to occur following H therapy (Pai et al., 1994). Vitamin E prevents lipid peroxidation, which can be manifested by an increase in thiobarbituric acid reactive substances (TBARS), in TD patients. Positive correlation was found between severity of the syndrome and plasma levels of TBARS, and vitamin E was effective in ameliorating patients' symptoms (Peet et al., 1993). Ineffectiveness of vitamin C, beta carotene, selenium and desferrioxamine in rescuing neurons from H insult points to the specificity of interaction between the different antioxidants and unstable radicals formed following H treatment.

Of interest was the finding that H at high concentration of 100μM was less toxic than the more diluted solutions 10μM and 1μM. We assume that higher concentrations of DMSO in the medium of concentrated solution could account for the lesser toxicity of the drug, since DMSO is a potent scavenger of hydroxyl radicals and was found to protect nigral neurons from MPTP induced DA toxicity (Park et al., 1988; Willis et al., 1994). Supporting this observation is the finding that when H was dissolved in ethanol its toxicity was positively correlated to its concentration (Behl et al., 1995).

Finally our results indicate that oxidative damage to neuronal tissue is involved in the activity of H and possibly other neuroleptics. The finding that toxicity was evident only in the absence of glial cells, supports the hypothesis that manifestation of TD and neurotoxicity in patients on chronic neuroleptics therapy, involves defective glia cell protective activity due to decrease in antioxidative agents, and/or growth factors synthesis and release. Vitamin E , NAC and DMSO were found to be effective in partially antagonizing H-induced neurotoxicity and therefore these agents, or their analogs, may be valuable in preventing TD in patients undergoing chronic neuroleptic therapy.

ACKNOWLEDGMENTS

This research was in part supported by a Grant from the Adams Brain Super Center, Tel Aviv University, Tel Aviv, Israel and the Harry S. Stern Foundation for Psychiatric Research.

REFERENCES

Adams, J.D., Odunze, I.N., 1991, Oxygen free radicals and Parkinson's disease. *Free Rad. Biol. Med.* 10:161–169.

Aruma, O.I., Halliwell, B., Hoey, B.M., Butler, J., 1990, The antioxidant action of N-acetyl cystein: Its reaction with hydrogen peroxide, hydroxyl radicals, superoxide, and hypochlorus acid. *Free Radicals Biol. Med.* 6:593–597.

Behl, C., Rupprect, R., Skutella, T., Holsboer, F., 1995, Haloperidol induced cell death- mechanism and protection with vitamin E in vitro. *Neuroreport* 7:360–364.

Ben Shahar, D., Livne, E., Spanier, I., Leenders, K.L., Youdim, M.B., 1994, Typical and atypical neuroleptics induce alteration in blood brain barrier and brain 59Fe C13 uptake. *J. Neurochem.* 62: 1112–1118.

Ben Shahar, D., Livne, E., Spanier I., Zur, R., Youdim, M.B., 1993, Iron modulates neuroleptic induced effects related to the dopaminergic system. *Isr. J. Med. Sci.* 29:587–592.

Bischot, L., Van -den-Brink, G., Porsius, A.J., 1993, Vitamin E in extrapyramidal disorders. *Pharm. World Sci.* 15:146–150.

Borenfreund, E., Puerner, J.A., 1984, A simple quantitative procedure using monolayer cultures for cytotoxicity assays (HTD/NR -90). *J. Tissue Culture Methods* 9: 7–9.

Carlsson, A., 1988, The current status of dopamine hypothesis of schizophrenia. *Neuropsychother.* 1: 175–186.

Carpenter, W., Buchana, R.W., 1994, Schizophrenia. *New England J. Med.* 330:681–689.

Chiueh, C.C., Wu, R.M., Mohanakumar, K.P., Sternberger, L.M., Kirshna, G., Obata, T., Murphy, D.L., 1994, In vivo generation of hydroxyl radicals and MPTP induced dopaminergic toxicity in basal ganglia. *Ann. N.Y Acad Sci.* 17:738, 214–21.

Davis, J.M., 1975, Overview: Maintainance therapy in psychiatry: Schizophrenia. *Am. J. Psychiatry* 132:1237–45.

Gattaz, W.F., Emrich, A., Behrnes, S., 1993, Vitamin E attenuates the development of haloperidol - induced dopaminergic hypersensitivity in rats: Possible implication for tardive dyskinesia. *Neural. Transm. Gen. Sect.* 92:197–201.

Henderson, C.E., Philips, H.S., Pollock, R.A., Davies, A.M., Lemeulle, C., Armanini, M., Simpson, L.C., Moffet, B., Vandlen, R.A., Koliatsos, V E., Rosenthal, A., 1995, GDNF: a potent survival factor for motoneurons present in peripheral nerve and muscle. *Nature* 266:1062–64.

Joseph, J. A., Cutler, R., 1994, The role of oxidative stress in signal transduction changes and cell loss in senescence. *Ann. N.Y Acad Sci.* 17:738, 37–44.

Kane, J.M., Marder, S.D., 1993, Psychopharmacologic treatment of schizophrenia. *Schizo. Bull.* 19: 287–302.

Leibler, D.C., Kling, D.S., Reed, D.J., 1986, Antioxidant protection of phospholipid bilayers by alpha -tocopherol. Control of alpha -tocopherol status and lipid peroxidation by ascorbic acid and glutathione. *J. Biol. Chem.* 261:12114–12119.

Makar, T.K., Nedergraad, M., Preuss, A., Gelbard, A., Perumal, A.S., Cooper, A.J. L., 1994, Vitamin E., Ascorbate. Glutathione disulfide and enzymes of glutathione metabolism in cultures of chick astrocytes and neurons: Evidence that astrocytes play an important role in antioxidative processes in the brain. *J. Neurochemistry* 62: 45–53.

Meyers, D.G., Maloley, P.A., Weeks, D., 1996, Safety of antioxidants vitamins. *Arch Intern. Med.* 156: 925–935,

Offen, D., Ziv, I., Sternin, H., Melamed, E., Hochman, A., 1996, Prevention of dopamine induced cell death by thiol antioxidants: Possible implication for treatment of Parkinson's disease. Experiment. Neurology 141: 32–39.

Offen, D., Ziv, I., Gorodin, Z., Malik, Z., Barzilai, A., Melamed, E., 1995, Dopamine induced programmed cell death in mouse thymocytes. *Biochem. Biophys. Acta.* 1268: 171–177.

Pai, B.N., Janakiramaiah, N., Gangadhar, B.N., Ravindranath, V., 1994, Depletion of glutathione and lipid peroxidation in the CSF of acute psychotics following haloperidol administration. *Biol. Psychiat.* 36: 489–491.

Park, Y., Smith, R.D., Combs, AB., Kehrer, J.P., 1988, Prevention of acetaminophen induced hepatotoxicity by dimethyl sulfoxide. *Toxicology* 52 :156–175.

Peet, M., Laugarne, J., Rangranjan, N., Reynolds, G.P., 1993, Tardive Dyskinesia, lipid peroxidation and sustained amelioration with vitamin E treatment. *Int. Clin. Psychopharmacol.* 8, 151–153.

Peram, V., Iftikhar, S., Lietz, H., Mobarhan, S., Frommer,T.O., 1996, Cytotoxic effect of beta carotene in vitro is dependent on serum concentration and source. *Cancer Lett.* 106: (1)133–138.

Rollema, M., Shkolnik, M.D., 1994, Igarashi, K. MPP(+) like neurotoxicity of pyridinium metabolite derived from haloperidol. *J Pharmcol. Exp. Ther.* 268: 380–387.

Scharr, D.G., Seiber, B.A., Dreyfus, C.F., Black, I., 1993, Regional and cell specific expression of GDNF in rat brain. *Exp. Neurol.* 24: 368–371.

Spivak, B., Schwartz, B., Radwuan, M., Weizman, A., 1992, α-tocopherol treatment of tardive dyskinesia. *J. Nerve Ment Dis.* 180: 400–401.

Vilner, B.J., Bowen, W.D., 1993, Sigma receptors active neuroleptics are cytotoxic to c6 glioma cells in culture. *Eur. J. Pharmacol* 244: 188–201.

Vincent, M., Lafluer, M., Hoorweg, J., Joenje, H., Westmijze, E.J., Petel, J., 1994, The ambivalent role of glutathione in the protection of DNA against single oxygen. *Free Rad. Res.* 21, 9–17.

Willis, C.L., Meldrum, B.S., Nunn, P.B., Anderton, B.H., Leigh, P.N., 1994, Neuroprotective effect of free radical scavenger on beta N oxallylamine-L alanine (BOAA) induced neuronal damage in rat hyppocampus. *Neurosci. Lett.* 182:159–162.

Wolf, M. E., Moshaim A.D. (eds), 1988, Tardive Dyskinesia: Biological mechanism and clinical aspects. Washington DC, American Psychiatric Press Inc.

Wu, R.M., Mohanakumar, K.P., Murphy, D.L., Chieueh, C.C., 1994, Antioxidant mechanism and protection of nigral neurons against MPP+ toxicity by Deprenyl. *Ann. N.Y Acad Sci.* 17: 738, 214–221.

Ziv, I., Melamed, E., Nardi, N., Luria, D., Achiron, A., Offen, D., Barzilai, A., 1994, Dopamine induced apoptosis-like cell death in cultured chick sympathetic neurons- a possible novel pathogenetic mechanism in Parkinson's disease. *Neurosci. Lett.* 170: 136–140.

24

DIRECT EVIDENCE THAT LACTATE IS AN OBLIGATORY AEROBIC ENERGY SUBSTRATE FOR FUNCTIONAL RECOVERY POSTHYPOXIA IN VITRO

Avital Schurr,[1] Ralphiel S. Payne,[1] James J. Miller,[2] and Benjamin M. Rigor[1]

[1]Department of Anesthesiology
[2]Department of Pathology
Brain Attack Research Laboratory
University of Louisville School of Medicine
Louisville, Kentucky 40292

INTRODUCTION

Four decades ago, McIlwain showed that brain tissue *in vitro* is able to respire using lactate as energy substrate (McIlwain, 1953a and 1953b). More recent *in vitro* studies demonstrated that lactate is a preferred energy substrate over glucose in excised sympathetic chick ganglia (Larrabee, 1995 and 1996). Our own studies showed lactate's ability to support synaptic function in rat hippocampal slices as the sole energy substrate (Schurr and Rigor, 1995), results that were confirmed by several other investigators (Stittsworth and Lanthorn, 1993; Bueno et al., 1994; Izumi et al., 1994). Most recently, using the same preparation, we were able to show that when lactate is supplied exogenously it can support functional recovery after hypoxia (Schurr et al., 1997). Moreover, our experiments demonstrated that lactate is preferred over glucose for such recovery and, hence, we hypothesized that this glycolytic product is an obligatory aerobic energy substrate for functional recovery of brain tissue after prolonged hypoxia (Schurr et al., 1997). Our hypothesis is based on the assumption that due to ATP depletion during the hypoxic period the ability of brain tissue to phosphorylate glucose, a prerequisite for energy production, is lost. The lack of ATP thus makes lactate the only readily available precursor to pyruvate, the entry step to the tricarboxylic acid cycle. Many recent studies in humans and animals indicate that brain tissue produces lactate aerobically, especially under conditions of increased activity (Fox et al., 1988; Lear, 1990; Prichard et al., 1991; Raichle, 1991; Sappey-Marinier et al., 1992; Fellows et al., 1993). Studies with astrocytic and neuronal cultures led Magistretti and his colleagues to hypothesize that glutamate uptake by astrocytes stimulates the production of glycolytic lactate and its aerobic utilization by neurons (Magistretti et al., 1993, 1995; Pellerin and Magistretti, 1994 and 1996). Although our most recent results (Schurr et al., 1997) strongly support the postulated role of lactate as an obligatory energy substrate during recovery from hypoxia, verification of those results via a different experimental approach is needed to provide the necessary proof for our hypothesis.

Oldendorf (1973) demonstrated that the transport of short-chain monocarboxylic acids via the blood-brain barrier is carrier-mediated. This transport is stereo-specific (Nemoto and Severinghaus, 1974) and can be increased by kainate treatment in brain regions known to be activated by this excitotoxin (Lear and Kasliwal, 1991). A monocarboxylic acid carrier was shown to exist in chick sympathetic ganglia (Larrabee, 1983), and a carrier-mediated lactate transport at the cellular level in the striatum of freely moving rats was quantified (Kuhr et al., 1988). Measurements of lactate release from cultured neurons and astrocytes showed that only the latter cell type can produce substantial amounts of lactate from glucose under hypoxic or hypoglycemic conditions (Walz and Mukerji, 1988a, 1988b, and 1990). Several studies have suggested the existence of an astrocyte-neuron shuttle for lactate (Pellerin and Magistretti, 1994 and 1996; Tildon et al., 1993), an idea that has received much attention lately (Dringen et al., 1993a, 1993b, and 1995).

The present study assessed the role of astrocytic lactate and its neuronal inward transport in the recovery of synaptic function after hypoxia. Electrophysiological and biochemical measurements in the hippocampal slice preparation were employed along with the lactate transport inhibitor 4-CIN (Halestrap and Denton, 1975).

MATERIALS AND METHODS

Hippocampal Slice Preparation and Maintenance

Adult (200–350 g) male Sprague-Dawley rats were maintained and used according to the guidelines of the Institutional Animal Care and Use Committee. Hippocampal slices (400 µm thick) were prepared using a McIlwain tissue chopper. For each experiment one rat was used from which 20–30 slices were prepared and placed (10 to 15 per compartment) in a dual incubation (34 ± 0.3°C) chamber (Schurr et al., 1985 and 1988). Slices were supplied with a humidified gas mixture (95% O_2/5% CO_2) and perfused with artificial cerebrospinal fluid (aCSF, 60 ml/h) of the following composition (in mM): NaCl, 124; KCl, 5; NaH_2PO_4, 3; $CaCl_2$, 2.5; $MgSO_4$, 2; $NaHCO_3$, 23; D-glucose, 10. The pH of the aCSF was 7.3–7.4. In some experiments glucose was replaced with sodium lactate (20 mM). Where indicated 4-CIN (500 µM) was added. Chemicals were of analytical grade and obtained from Sigma Chemical Co. (St. Louis, MO). Hypoxia was produced by replacing O_2 in the gas mixture with N_2.

Electrophysiological Measurements

Extracellular recordings of electrically-evoked population spikes (synaptic function) in the stratum pyramidale of the CA1 region were made using borosilicate micropipettes (2–5 MΩ). Bipolar stimulating electrodes were placed in the Schaffer collaterals (orthodromic stimulation), and stimulus pulses of 0.1 ms in duration and of an amplitude 8 to 10 V (twice threshold) were applied once/min. A waveform analysis program was used to determine the amplitude of the evoked population spike. Any slice exhibiting an evoked response of an amplitude of 3 mV or larger was considered to be synaptically functional; a slice showing a response <3 mV was considered to be synaptically nonfunctional (Schurr et al., 1985 and 1997; Schurr and Rigor, 1995). Nonfunctional slices at 30-min post hypoxia were unresponsive even 6 h later, which signaled an irreversible neuronal damage (Schurr et al., 1985).

Measurements of Glucose and Lactate Concentration in Brain Slices

Lactate and glucose were measured as described elsewhere (Schurr et al., 1997) using the enzymatic kits of Sigma Chemical Co. (St. Louis, MO). Two slices per sample were taken out of the incubation chamber at the times indicated (Fig. 2), rinsed in ice cold aCSF containing no glucose and homogenized in 0.2 ml of 8% perchloric acid. The homogenate was then neutralized with 0.1 ml of 2 M $KHCO_3$ and centrifuged for 5 min at 8,000 x g. The supernatant (0.2 ml) was used for analysis of both lactate and glucose. Assays were automated on a Cobas Fara Centrifugal Analyzer (Roche Diagnostic Systems, Branchburg, NJ). In both assays, NADH was measured fluorometrically (excitation at 340 nm and emission at 450 nm).

Statistical Analysis

Each data point in the experiments described in this study was repeated at least 3 times. Values are means ± S.D. of the mean. Statistical analysis of electrophysiological data was performed using χ^2-test for significant differences. Biochemical data were tested for significant differences using a paired t-test.

RESULTS AND DISCUSSION

The effect of 4-CIN lactate-supported synaptic function is shown in Figure 1. Within 15 min 4-CIN (500 μM) completely inhibited, what presumably is, the utilization of lactate as the sole energy substrate when supplied at 20 mM, an equicaloric concentration of 10 mM glucose. This inhibition was evident from the decline in the population spike amplitude. When a lower concentration of 4-CIN (200 μM) was used, 30 min were required for complete inhibition of lactate-supported synaptic function (data not shown). Synaptic function supported by glucose was unaffected by 4-CIN (Fig. 1). These results suggest that 4-CIN is able to block synaptic function by blocking lactate utilization through the inhibition of its transport into neurons without any effect on glucose utilization. If lactate is

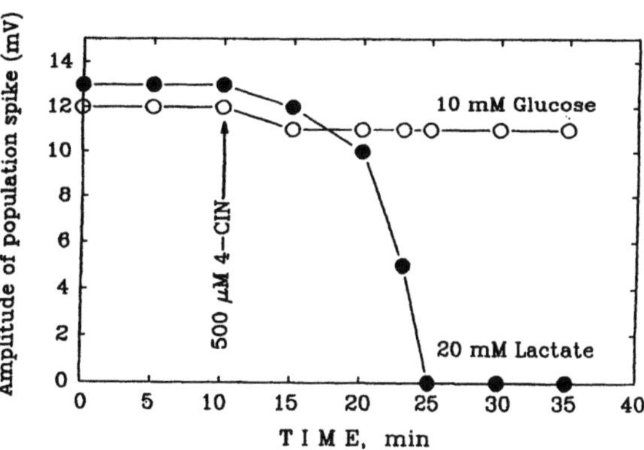

Figure 1. The effect of 4-CIN on lactate- and glucose-supported synaptic function (electrically-evoked CA1 population spike in rat hippocampal slices). Within 15 min of its addition to the perfusion medium, the lactate transporter inhibitor completely blocks lactate (20 mM) utilization without affecting the utilization of an equicaloric amount (10 mM) of glucose. This representitive experiment was repeated 3 times with identical results.

an obligatory neuronal aerobic energy substrate for recovery of synaptic function posthypoxia, as we have postulated (Schurr et al., 1997), then, inhibition of lactate transport by 4-CIN into neurons is expected to block this recovery.

Of control, untreated slices that were exposed to 10-min hypoxia, 77.8 ± 6.8% (56/72) exhibited recovery of synaptic function following 30-min reoxygenation. In contrast, a recovery rate of only 15 ± 10.9% (9/60) was measured in slices that were treated with 500 μM 4-CIN, starting at the beginning of the hypoxic period and through the end of the reoxygenation period (P < 0.0005). Prevention of functional recovery by 4-CIN upon reoxygenation occurred despite the continuous perfusion of slices with 10 mM glucose throughout the experimental period. This outcome strongly supports our hypothesis that lactate is an obligatory aerobic energy substrate for functional recovery after a period of oxygen deprivation (Schurr et al, 1997).

We have shown previously that inhibition of lactate production during hypoxia prevents functional recovery posthypoxia (Schurr et al., 1997). In the present study, 4-CIN should have no effect on the amount of lactate produced by slices during the hypoxic period. However, the lactate transporter inhibitor is expected to arrest lactate utilization during reoxygenation. Hence, slices treated with 4-CIN are expected to utilize only small amounts of lactate, if at all, and consequently retain higher levels of it during the reoxygenation period when compared with control, untreated slices.

The levels of lactate and glucose in slices were sampled at fixed time intervals during an identical experimental protocol to the one used for the electrophysiological meas-

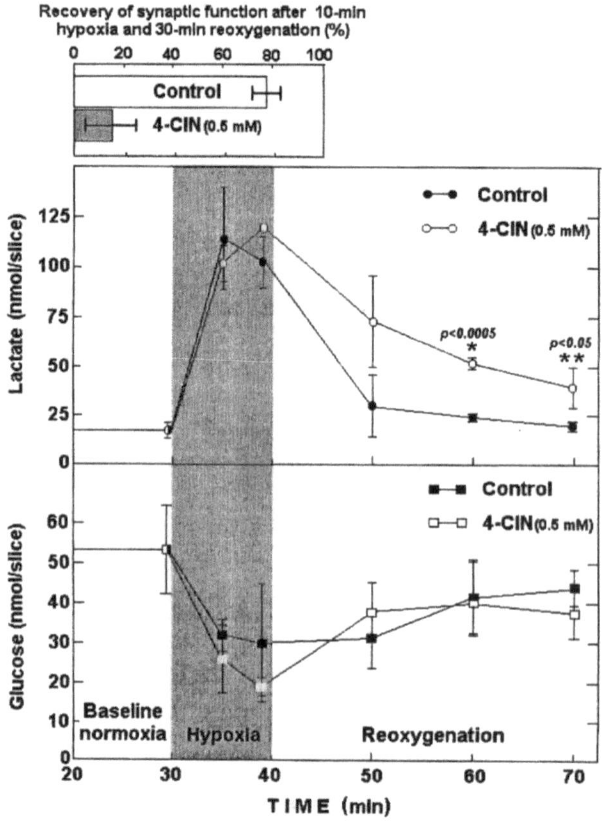

Figure 2. The effect of 10-min hypoxia on the levels of glucose and lactate in rat hippocampal slices. Of 60 slices supplemented with 500 μM 4-CIN, beginning at the onset of hypoxia and through the end of the reoxygenation period, only 9 slices recovered synaptic function (top histogram). Slices treated with 4-CIN retained higher concentrations of lactate during the reoxygenation period (minute 40 to minute 70 of the experiment). Of 72 control untreated slices, the majority (56) recovered synaptic function (top histogram) and utilized more of the lactate accumulated during hypoxia. Each data point represents at least three independent determinations of 2 slices/determination. *p < 0.001; **p < 0.05.

urements. The normoxic baseline levels of lactate (17 ± 2 nmol/slice) climbed to over 100 nmol/slice during the first 5 min of hypoxia whether or not 4-CIN (500 µM) was present. This indicates that the inhibitor did not affect the anaerobic glycolytic activity of hippocampal slices, a conclusion that also was confirmed by a corresponding drop in slice content of glucose, which occurred despite the abundance of extracellular glucose (10 mM). We deduce from these results that, during hypoxia, glucose uptake cannot keep up with glycolytic glucose consumption and hence the decline in tissue glucose levels. Upon reoxygenation of control, untreated slices, lactate tissue levels dropped to reach their prehypoxic levels. In 4-CIN-treated slices, lactate levels stayed significantly higher than those found in control slices (Fig. 2). There are three possible explanations for the difference in lactate levels between control, untreated and 4-CIN-treated slices: (a) lactate utilization in 4-CIN-treated slices decreased due to blockade of lactate transport into neurons; (b) lactate outward transport in astrocytes was inhibited by 4-CIN, making it unavailable to neurons; or (c) a combination of both (a) and (b). The results (Fig. 2) indicate that despite the presence of 4-CIN, tissue lactate levels declined upon reoxygenation. Assuming that most of the glycolytic lactate produced during hypoxia is astocytic, the decline of lactate level in the presence of 4-CIN suggests that outward astrocytic lactate transport was unaffected. Thus, we are tempted to favor explanation (a) as the most plausible. While the bulk of astrocytic lactate is due to the active role of astrocytes in ion pumping, neuronal lactate is possibly responsible for those 4-CIN-treated slices (15%) that did exhibit recovery of function posthypoxia. Glucose tissue levels, in contrast to lactate levels, return to normal during the first 20 min of reoxygenation, whether or not 4-CIN was present, underscoring the fact that aerobic lactate utilization is mandatory for functional recovery from hypoxia; glucose is unable to support such recovery (Schurr et al., 1997). Our findings also provide support for the proposed role that astrocytes play in shuttling lactate to neurons (Tildon et al, 1993; Dringen et al., 1993a, 1993b, and 1995; Magistretti et al., 1993 and 1995; Pellerin and Magistretti, 1994 and 1996; Volk et al., 1995; Korf, 1996).

REFERENCES

Bueno, D., Azzolin, I.R., and Perry, M.L.S., 1994, Ontogenic study of glucose and lactate utilisation by rat cerebellum slices, *Med. Sci. Res.* 22:631–632.

Dringen, R., Gebhardt, R., and Hamprecht, B., 1993a, Glycogen in astrocytes: possible function as lactate supply for neighboring cells, *Brain Res.* 623:208–214.

Dringen, R., Wiesinger, H., and Hamprecht, B., 1993b, Uptake of L-lactate by cultured rat brain neurons, *Neurosci. Lett.* 163:5–7.

Dringen, R., Peters, H., Wiesinger, H., and Hamprecht, B., 1995, Lactate transport in cultured glial cells, *Dev. Neurosci.* 17:63–69.

Fellows, L.K., Boutelle, M.G., and Fillenz, M., 1993, Physiological stimulation increases nonoxidative glucose metabolism in the brain of the freely moving rat, *J. Neurochem.* 60:1258–1263.

Fox, P.T., Raichle, M.E., Mintun, M.A., and Dence, C., 1988, Nonoxidative glucose consumption during focal physiologic neural activity, *Science* 241:462–464.

Halestrap, A.P., and Denton, R.M., 1975, The specificity and metabolic implications of the inhibition of pyruvate transport in isolated mitochondria and intact tissue preparations by α-cyano-4-hydroxycinnamate and related compounds, *Biochem. J.* 148:97–106.

Izumi, Y., Benz, A.M., Zorumski, C.F., and Olney, J.W., 1994, Effects of lactate and pyruvate on glucose deprivation in rat hippocampal slices, *Neuroreport* 5:617–620.

Korf, J., 1996, Intracerebral trafficking of lactate in vivo during stress, exercise, electro-convulsive shock and ischemia as studied with microdialysis, *Dev. Neurosci.* 18:405–414.

Kuhr, W.G., van der Berg, C.J., and Korf, J., 1988, In vivo identification and quantitative evaluation of carrier-mediated transport of lactate at the cellular level in the striatum of conscious, freely moving rats, *J. Cereb. Blood Flow Metab.* 8:848–856.

Larrabee, M.G., 1983, Lactate uptake and release in the presence of glucose by sympathetic ganglia of chicken embryos and by neuronal and nonneuronal cultures prepared from these ganglia, *J. Neurochem.* 40:1237–1250.

Larrabee, M.G., 1995, Lactate metabolism and its effects on glucose metabolism in an excised neural tissue, *J. Neurochem.* 64:1734–1741.

Larrabee, M.G., 1996, Partitioning of CO_2 production between glucose and lactate in excised sympathetic ganglia, with implications for brain, *J. Neurochem.* 67:1726–1734.

Lear, J.L., 1990, Glycolysis: Link between PET and proton MR spectroscopic studies of the brain, *Radiology* 174:328–330.

Lear, J.L., and Kasliwal, R.K., 1991, Autoradiographic measurement of cerebral lactate transport rate constants in normal and activated conditions, *J. Cereb. Blood Flow Metab.* 11:576–580.

Magistretti, P.J., Sorg, O., Yu, N., Martin, J.-L., and Pellerin, L., 1993, Neurotransmitters regulate energy metabolism in astrocytes: Implications for the metabolic trafficking between neural cells, *Dev. Neurosci.* 15:306–312.

Magistretti, P.J., Pellerin, L., and Martin, J.-L., 1995, Brain energy metabolism: An integrated cellular perspective, in *Psychopharmacology: The fourth generation of progress* (Bloom F.E. and Kupfer D.J., eds.), pp 657–670. Raven Press, New York.

McIlwain, H., 1953a, Glucose level, metabolism, and response to electrical impulses in cerebral tissues from man and laboratory animals, *Biochem. J.* 55:618–624.

McIlwain, H., 1953b, Substances which support respiration and metabolic response to electrical impulses in human cerebral tissues, *J. Neurol. Neurosurg. Psychiat.* 16:257–266.

Nemoto, E.M., and Severinghaus, J.W., 1974, Stereospecific permeability of rat blood-brain barrier to lactic acid, *Stroke* 5:81–84.

Oldendorf, W.H., 1973, Carrier-mediated blood-brain transport of short-chain mono-carboxylic organic acids, *Am. J. Physiol.* 224:1450–1454.

Pellerin, L., and Magistretti, P.J., 1994, Glutamate uptake into astrocytes stimulates aerobic glycolysis: A mechanism coupling neuronal activity to glucose utilization, *Proc. Natl. Acad. Sci. USA* 91:10625–10629.

Pellerin, L., and Magistretti, P.J., 1996, Excitatory amino acids stimulate aerobic glycolysis in astrocytes via activation of the Na^+/K^+ ATPase, *Dev. Neurosci.* 18:336–342.

Prichard, J., Rothman, D., Novotny, E., Petroff, O., Kuwabara, T., Avison, M., Howseman, A., Hanstock, C., and Shulman, R., 1991, Lactate rise detected by ^1H NMR in human visual cortex during physiologic stimulation, *Proc. Natl. Acad. Sci. USA* 88:5829–5831.

Raichle, M.E., 1991, The metabolic requirements of functional activity in the human brain: A positron emission tomography study, in *Fuel homeostasis and the nervous system.* Adv. Exp. Med. Biol. Vol. 291 (Vranic M., Efendic S., and Hollenberg C.H., eds.), pp 1–4. Plenum Press, New York.

Sappey-Marinier, D., Calabrese, G., Fein, G., Hugg, J.W., Biggins, C., and Weiner, M.W., 1992, Effect of photic stimulation on human visual cortex lactate and phosphates using ^1H and ^{31}P magnetic resonance spectroscopy, *J. Cereb. Blood Flow Metab.* 12:584–592.

Schurr, A., Reid, K.H., Tseng, M.T., Edmonds, H.L., Jr., and Rigor, B.M., (1985) A dual chamber for comparative studies using the brain slice preparation, *Biochem. Physiol.* 82A:701–704.

Schurr, A., West, C.A., and Rigor, B.M., 1988, Lactate-supported synaptic function in the rat hippocampal slice preparation, *Science* 240:1326–1328.

Schurr, A., and Rigor, B.M., 1995, The pharmacology of excitotoxins and energy deprivation in hippocampal slices, in *Brain Slices in Basic and Clinical Research* (Schurr A. and Rigor B.M., eds.), pp 221–241. CRC Press, Boca Raton.

Schurr, A., Payne, R.S., Miller, J.J., and Rigor, B.M., 1997, Brain lactate, not glucose, fuels the recovery of synaptic function from hypoxia upon reoxygenation: an in vitro study, *Brain Res.* 744:105–111.

Stittsworth, J.D., Jr., and Lanthorn, T.H., 1993, Lactate mimics only some effects of D-glucose on epileptic depolarization and long-term synaptic failure, *Brain Res.* 630:21–27.

Tildon, J.T., McKenna, M.C., Stevenson, J., and Couto, R., 1993, Transport of L-lactate by cultured rat brain astrocytes, *Neurochem. Res.* 18:177–184.

Volk, C., Kempski, B., and Kempski, O.S., 1995, Glial cells exhibit a specific transport system for lactate, *J. Cereb. Blood Flow Metab.* 15:S572.

Walz, W., and Mukerji, S., 1988, Lactate production and release in cultured astrocytes, *Neurosci. Lett.* 86:296–300.

Walz, W., and Mukerji, S., 1988, Lactate release from cultured astrocytes and neurons: A comparison, *Glia* 1:366–370.

Walz, W., and Mukerji, S., 1990, Simulation of ischemia in cell culture: Changes in lactate compartmentation, *Glia* 3:522–528

25

COMPARATIVE STUDY OF ANTIOXIDANTS' ACTION ON MEMBRANE-BOUND ACETYLCHOLINESTERASE (AChE) OF BLOOD ERYTHROCYTES AND BRAIN SYNAPTOSOMES

Faina I. Braginskaya, Elena M. Molochkina, Olga M. Zorina,
Irina B. Ozerova, and Elena B. Burlakova

Institute of Biochemical Physics
Russian Academy of Sciences
Moscow, Russia

INTRODUCTION

Membrane-bound AChE is widely used for the estimation of the inhibitory activity of various agents studied in AD therapy. The interpretation of both results is of great importance for clinical study and application of new drugs. Antioxidants (AO) inhibitors of free radical processes, present a promising group of compounds for AD treatment. We investigated the action of some AO on the kinetic properties of membrane-bound AChE of human erythrocytes and rat brain synaptosomes.

METHODS

Synaptosomes of rat brain were prepared in accordance with the sucrose density gradient centrifugation procedure (Gray and Whittaker, 1962).

The protein content in suspensions was determined by the method of Lowry et al. (1951). AChE activity was determined by Ellman's colorimetric technique with acetylthiocholine (ATCh) as a substrate (Ellman et al., 1961) and by means of potentiometric titration of CH_3COOH (both methods with continuous following by reaction kinetics).

To provide AO entering membrane lipids, "original" suspensions of synaptosomes or erythrocytes (containing 1.5–8 mg of subcellular or cellular protein per ml) were pre-incubated (at 4°C) with ethanolic solution of AO the concentration of which in the suspension was 2×10^{-4} M. The final concentration, calculated per ml of reaction medium was 1.3×10^{-6} M. Ethanol concentration in original suspensions did not exceed 0.5%. Reaction mixture contained 0.01–0.05 mg of protein per ml.

Progress in Alzheimer's and Parkinson's Diseases
edited by Fisher *et al.*, Plenum Press, New York, 1998.

RESULTS AND DISCUSSION

Classic phenolic AO 4-methyl-2,6-ditertiary butylphenol (ionol) did not influence membrane-bound AChE activity when added to the reaction medium directly before starting the reaction. After insertion of ionol into the erythrocyte lipid bilayer both maximal velocity Vmax and Michaelis constant K_M decreased; in this case membrane-bound AChE was inhibited at "high" and was activated at "low" substrate concentrations (Fig. 1, A). Being inserted into synaptosomal lipids ionol caused the increase both of K_M and of Vmax of the hydrolysis of ATCh by membrane-bound synaptosomal AChE in such a mode when low substrate concentrations corresponded to the inhibition and high concentrations—to the enzyme activation (Fig. 1, B).

Thus kinetic parameters of the erythrocyte AChE revealed reciprocal changes as compared with the enzyme of brain synaptosomes. The difference in the effects of the antioxidant on membrane AChE in erythrocytes and synaptosomes is well demonstrated

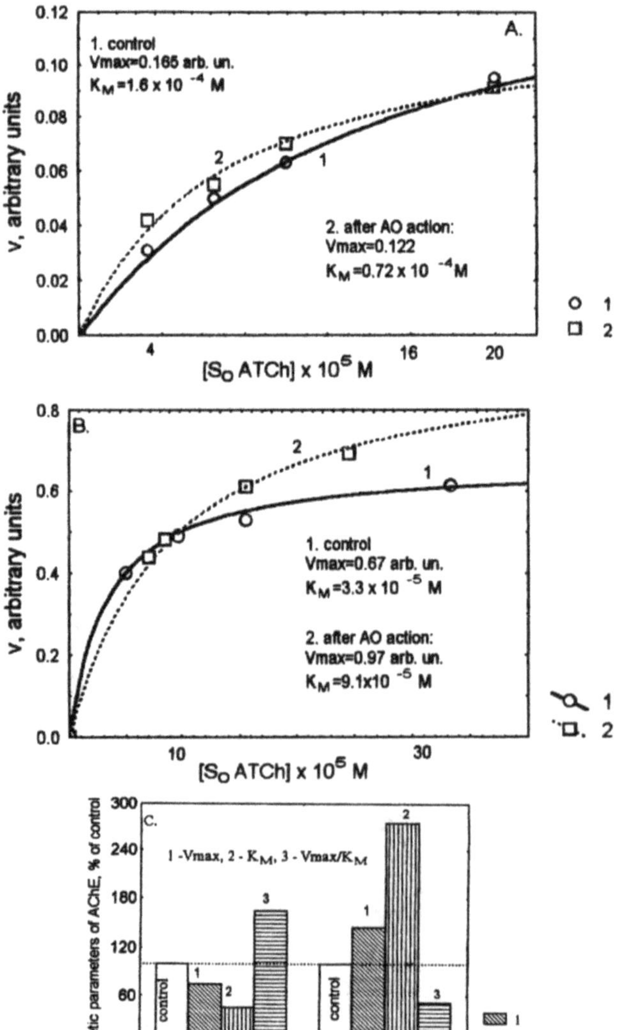

Figure 1. Substrate dependencies of AChE reaction rate (A, B) (at 37°C) and the changes of kinetic parameters of membrane-bound AChE (C) after insertion of ionol into erythrocyte (A) and synaptosomal (B) membranes. Original suspensions were preincubated (at 4°C) with ethanolic solution of ionol to provide AO entering membrane lipids. For A, B: 1 = control, 2 = after AO action. Initial reaction velocity and Vmax are given by arbitrary units i.d. by the changes in optical density of reaction mixture at 412 nm per min, calculated per 0.01 mg of protein; for C: 1 = Vmax, 2 = K_M, 3 = Vmax/K_M.

in Fig. 1, C. It is worth paying some attention to the alterations of AChE efficacy ($Vmax/K_M$). In accordance with Michaelis–Menten kinetics the rate of AChE reaction is proportional to $Vmax/K_M$ at small substrate concentrations. In accordance with literary data the content of ACh in the brain tissue is approximately 10^{-6}–10^{-8} M (Cuadra et al., 1994). So $Vmax/K_M$ can be considered as a parameter which probably determines the reaction rate at "real" concentrations of acetylcholine in brain.

Figure 1, C shows that $Vmax/K_M$ increased under the action of the AO in the case of erythrocyte AChE and significantly decreased in the case of synaptosomal enzyme. It is worth emphasizing that the enzyme efficacy changed in both cases mainly due to alterations in K_M value, however the latter decreased markedly in erythrocytes and increased in synaptosomes.

It is of interest to mention that intraperitoneal injection of ionol to rats resulted in alterations in the kinetic parameters of the synaptosomal AChE similar to those observed in vitro (Fig. 2).

We also studied the effects of so-called "hybrid" compounds which one can consider as "acetylcholine" where instead of acetic acid residue there is the radical of phenolic AO "phenozan" and neighbouring to N there is an alkyl radical of that or another "length" (C atoms number). Two substances were under investigation—containing 1 and 16 C atoms in the tail radical (we labelled them as 1 and 2 correspondingly). The "parent" AO phenozan with strong antioxidative effect also possesses a number of various biological activities. It is worth emphasizing its effects on learning and memory via the changes which the AO induces in the lipid phase of neuronal membranes (Burlakova, 1994). The applicability of those substances in AD therapy was considered earlier on the basis of their action on erythrocyte AChE (Braginskaya et al., 1996).

We studied the effect of those hybrid AO on the activity of soluble AChE of human erythrocyte origin (Braginskaya et al., 1996) and on the activity of AChE bound with erythrocyte and synaptosomal membranes. Fig. 3 demonstrates the influence of com-

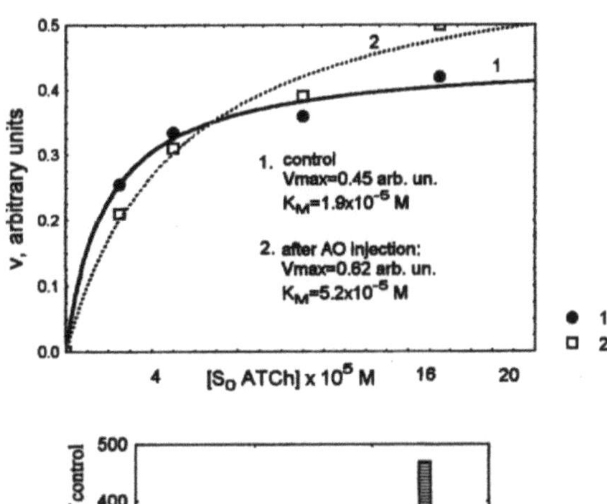

Figure 2. Substrate dependencies of AChE reaction rate (at 37°C) in the suspension of synaptosomes isolated 18 h after intraperitoneal injection of 20 mg/kg of ionol to Wistar rats. Reaction mixture contained 0.01–0.05 mg of synaptosomal protein per ml. Each point on the curves represents the mean of 5 assays.

Figure 3. Changes in kinetic parameters of AChE reaction (Vmax, K_M and efficacy $Vmax/K_M$) after in vitro action of "hybrid" AO without (1) and with hydrocarbon "tail" C-16 (2). The AO were added (4 × 10^{-5} M) into reaction medium without preincubation thus not providing entrance to membrane lipids.

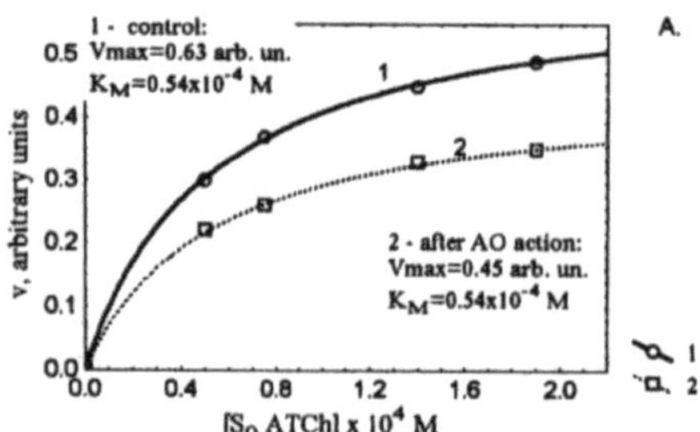

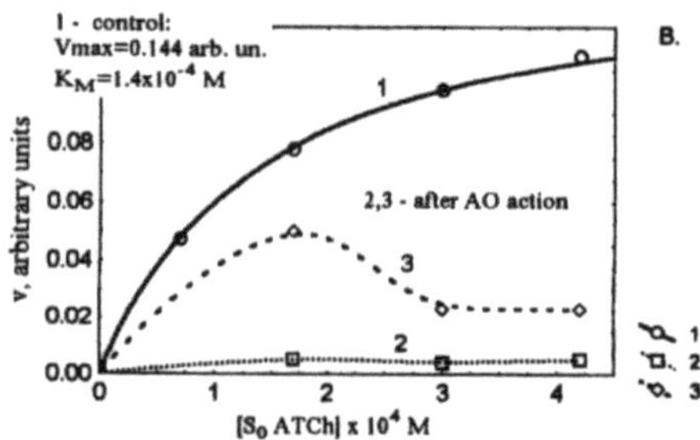

Figure 4. Influence of "hybrid" compound with C-16 "tail" on the rates of AChE reaction in synaptosomes (A) and erythrocytes (B) at AO insertion in membrane lipids with the help the preincubation of suspensions with ethanolic solution of AO (4°C). Reaction mixtures contained 0.01–0.05 mg of protein per ml. Each point on the curves represents mean of 5 assays. AO concentration in original suspension during preincubation was 1 mM, in reaction mixture 0.5×10^{-5} M (A, curve 2; B, curve 3) and 0.1 mM in original suspension, 0.5×10^{-6} M in reaction medium (B, curve 2).

pounds 1 and 2 on the kinetic parameters of soluble and membrane-bound AChE in the situation when the AO were added in reaction medium directly before starting the reaction and thus they did not insert into membrane lipid bilayers. The different mode and scale of the action of the tested AO on the AChE of different origin is evident. However AChE efficacy decreased in all three cases. Synaptosomal AChE underwent some more expressed diminution of Vmax/K_M than the erythrocyte enzyme. unlike the soluble enzyme the lowering of membrane-bound AChE efficacy did not intensify at introduction to the AO molecule of a long hydrocarbon tail. Apparently this might be connected to some extent with the invasive action of the tail on the membrane.

It is of the most interest to compare hybrid AO action on the enzyme of synaptosomes and erythrocytes at inclusion into membranes.

Figure 4 shows the changes in membrane AChE activity after inclusion of compound 2 (with a C-16 tail). As synaptosomal AChE is concerned one can see non-competitive-like inhibition of the membrane enzyme i.e., a decrease of Vmax and efficacy (~30%) (Fig. 4, A). A more complicated picture occurs in the case of the erythrocyte enzyme (Fig. 4, B). Under the same conditions (compare curves 2 and 3 on A and B) erythrocyte AChE was inhibited more effectively. Surprisingly a 10 times smaller concentration of AO inhibited AChE of erythrocytes entirely (curve 2 on Fig. 4, B). this fact is connected apparently with the effect of the long tail AO on the membrane structure.

The difference in the response to AO between synaptosomal and erythrocyte membranes must be taken into account using the erythrocyte model system for the evaluation of antiAChE properties of respective drugs. Thus for the choice of the compounds, experimental tests on synaptosomal AChE are of great importance.

REFERENCES

Braginskaya, F. I., Molochkina, E. M., Zorina, O. M., Ozerova, I. B., and Burlakova, E. B., 1996, New synthetic bioantioxidants - acetylcholinesterase (AChE) inhibitors. in: *Alzheimer Disease: From Molecular Biology to Therapy,* Becker,R..and Giacobini, E., eds., Birkhauser-Boston, p. 337–342.

Burlakova, E. B., 1994, Antioxidant drugs as neuroprotective agents. In: *Alzheimer Disease: Therapeutic Strategies*, Giacobini E., and Becker R., eds., Birkhauser: Boston, p. 313–317.

Cuadra, G., Summers, K., and Giacobini, E., 1994, Cholinesterase inhibitor effects on neurotransmitters in rat cortex in vivo. *J. Pharmacol. Exp. Ther.* 270:277–284.

Ellman, g. L., Courtney, K. D., Andres, V., Jr., and Featherstone, R. M., 1961, A new and rapid colorimetric determination of acetylcholinesterase activity. *Biochem. Pharmacol.* 7:88–96.

Gray, E. G., and Whittaker, V. P., 1962, Isolation of nerve endings from brain: an electron microscopic study of cell fragments derived by homogenization and centrifugation. *J.Anat.* 96:79–88.

Lowry, O. H., Rosebrough, N. J., Farr, A. K., and Randall, R.J., 1951, Protein measurement with the Folin phenol reagent. *J. Biol. Chem.* 193:265–275.

ULTRA-LOW DOSES OF ANTIOXIDANT AND ACETYLCHOLINE MODIFY THE LIPID PHASE AND KINETIC PROPERTIES OF ACETYLCHOLINESTERASE IN MURINE BRAIN MEMBRANES

E. M. Molochkina, I. B. Ozerova, and E. B. Burlakova

Institute of Biochemical Physics
Russian Academy of Sciences
Kosygin ul. 4, 117977, Moscow, Russia

INTRODUCTION

AntiAChE agents are well known to be the most effective drugs in AD therapy. Antioxidants (AO)—inhibitors of free radical processes—also present a promising group of compounds for AD treatment. There exists some information concerning the action of AO on learning and memory, the effect resulting from maintenance the proper composition and structure of brain membrane lipid bilayer through lipid peroxidation control (Burlakova, 1994). Some authors consider AO a new group of nootropic drugs (Voronina, 1994).

The capacity of ultra-low doses of many classes of physiologically active substances to influence various biological systems from biomacromolecules to organisms has now been widely investigated. It is of interest to explore the effects of ultra-low doses of AO and cholinergic agents in terms of their implication for AD treatment.

We investigated the effect of the phenolic AO phenosan and acetylcholine (ACh) on murine brain membrane acetylcholinesterase (AChE) in vitro and in vivo and the changes in brain membrane lipid phase, using a wide range of concentrations and doses of the substances (including ultra-low ones of 10^{-11}–10^{-15} M or mole/kg).

METHODS

Mice brain membranes were isolated from crude synaptosomal fractions (Prokchorova, 1982) by differential centrifugation after disruption with the help of osmotic shock.

The protein content was determined by the method of Lowry (Lowry et al., 1951).

Lipid extraction from subcellular fractions was carried out by Bligh and Dyer's technique (Bligh and Dyer, 1959). Determination of lipid phosphorus and evaluation of the total cholesterol content in the lipid extracts were carried out colorimetrically (Chen et al., 1956; Sperry and Webb, 1950). In order to estimate lipid peroxidation level we determined the content of primary oxidation products—conjugated lipid hydroperoxides (DK = diene conjugates) (Slater, 1984). Lipid peroxidation intensity was characterized also with malondialdehyde (Buege and Aust, 1978) accumulation velocity in the course of membrane oxidation in vitro: membrane suspensions in physiological solution (1–2 mg of protein per ml) were oxidized with air oxygen under shaking at 37°C. The potential capacity of lipids to oxidize was characterized by DB (double bonds) index. The latter was determined in lipid extracts by ozonation method with the help of special devices developed in the Institute of Biochemical Physics RAS (Razumovsky and Zaikov, 1975).

AChE activity was determined by Ellman's colorimetric method (Ellman et al., 1961) with permanent registration of the reaction kinetics.

RESULTS AND DISCUSSION

Figure 1 shows that the insertion of AO in the membrane lipid phase in vitro caused an increase of both Vmax and K_M with some decrease of AChE efficacy ($Vmax/K_M$). It is worth keeping in mind that the rate of AChE reaction is proportional to $Vmax/K_M$ at small concentrations of the substrate (including those corresponding to real content of ACh in brain). The maximal effect took place at the AO concentrations of 10^{-9} and 10^{-15} M.

Intraperitoneal injection of AO to mice resulted in similar and even more expressed alterations of the kinetic parameters of brain membrane AChE (1 h after injection), with the dose of 10^{-11} and 10^{-15} mole/kg being more effective than "usual" doses of 10^{-5} and 10^{-4} mole/kg.

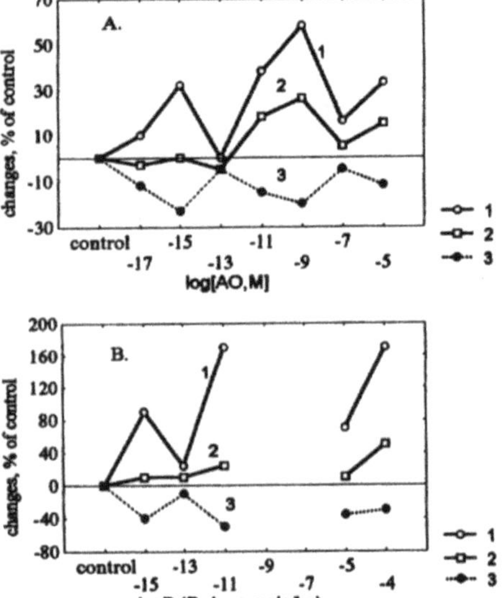

Figure 1. The effect of phenosan on mice brain membrane AChE. A. After insertion into membrane lipids in vitro through the incubation of membrane suspension with ethanolic solution of phenosan at 4°C during 20 h. Membrane protein concentration in suspension was 4 mg per ml. Ethanol concentration <0.5%. B. 1 h after in vivo administration of phenosan. The changes are shown as the differences between experimental and control values (% of control): 1 = K_M, 2 = Vmax, 3 = $Vmax/K_M$.

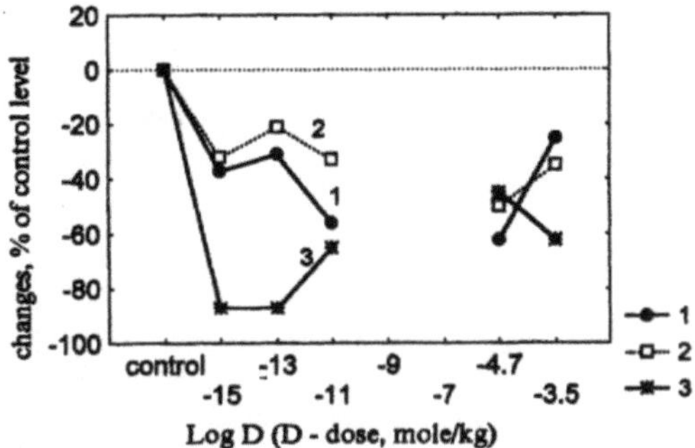

Figure 2. Changes in lipid peroxidation level and cholesterol content in murine brain membranes isolated 1 h after intraperitoneal injection of phenosan. 1 = DK/ total lipids, 2 = cholesterol/phospholipids, 3 = lipid peroxidation velocity in membrane suspension.

Injections of low doses of AO induced changes in brain membrane lipid phase which can be considered a typical effect of antioxidants: for example, an inhibition of lipid peroxidation and a decrease of cholesterol/phospholipids ratio were observed (Fig. 2).

It is of interest to mention that the decrease in this ratio suggests an increased fluidity of lipid bilayer in neuronal membranes. In accordance with some considerations (Shinitzky, 1987) this factor is favourable for the enhancement of memory and cognitive processes.

The mechanism of the observed effects of ultra-low doses of the phenolic AO is not yet clear. However one could state that AO usage at low doses might be fruitful in terms of implication for AD therapy. Low doses of AO may be promising on the basis of their action both on brain membrane lipid phase and on AChE activity.

Ellman's method of AChE activity assay (with acetyl*thio*choline as substrate) gave us the possibility to study the action of ACh as effector (not as substrate) on kinetic parameters of AChE reaction. As shown in Fig. 3 intraperitoneal injections of ACh iodide to mice resulted (1 h after injection) in the activation of brain membrane AChE, the effect being more expressed at the range of ultra-low doses. Injected ACh seemed not to be a competitive inhibitor of AChE as it might be expected. Administered in vivo ACh is likely to act indirectly. It is unknown now what does mediate the effect which is probably destined to maintain homeostasis of ACh level in brain.

As far as AD therapy is concerned, it is of some interest to consider the results on ACh effect on lipid phase of brain membranes. In vivo administration of ACh in mice caused alterations in membrane lipids (Fig. 4). ACh "simulated" the typical action of antioxidants and resulted in greater changes of lipid parameters than phenosan. As an example it is worth mentioning a 60% decrease of cholesterol/phospholipids ratio and strong inhibition of lipid peroxidation (evaluated by the content of primary oxidation products and DB index). Such type of influence of low doses of ACh on brain membrane lipids might

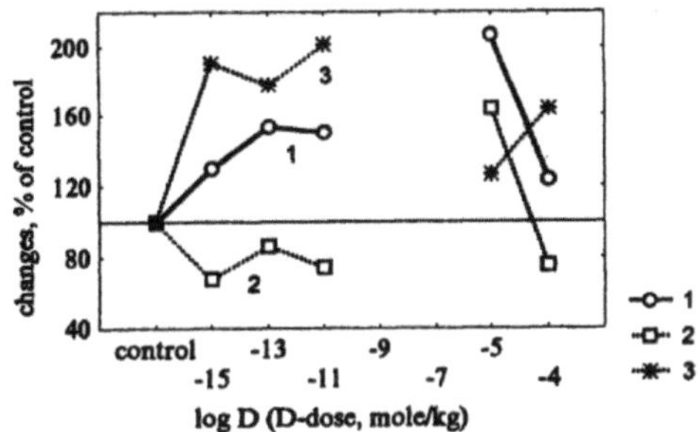

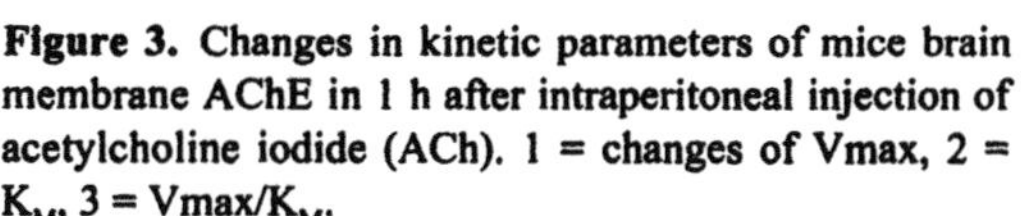

Figure 3. Changes in kinetic parameters of mice brain membrane AChE in 1 h after intraperitoneal injection of acetylcholine iodide (ACh). 1 = changes of Vmax, 2 = K_M, 3 = Vmax/K_M.

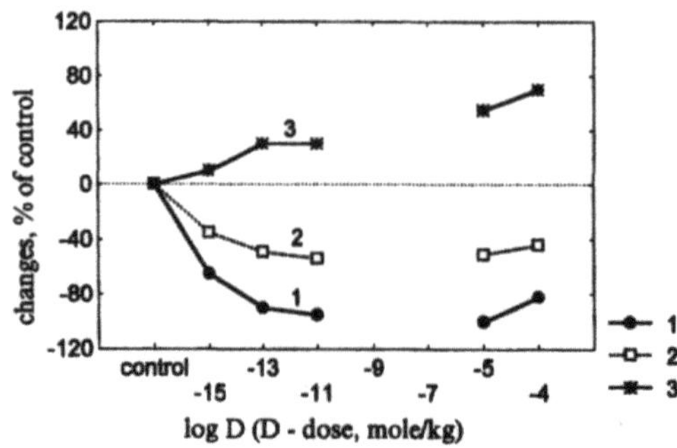

Figure 4. Changes in lipid peroxidation level and cholesterol content in murine brain membranes isolated 1 h after intraperitoneal injection of ACh. DK (primary oxidation products in lipids), 2 = cholesterol/phospholipids, 3 = DB index of lipids.

be useful in the treatment of memory and cognitive disorders in elderly persons and AD patients.

ACKNOWLEDGMENTS

The authors appreciate the kind assistance of V. D. Gaintseva in the determination of DB index.

REFERENCES

Bligh, E., and Dyer, N. A., 1959, A rapid method of total lipid extraction, *Can. J. Biochem.* 37:911.

Buege, J. A., and Aust St. D.,1978, Microsomal lipid peroxidation, *Meth. Enzymol.* 52:302.

Burlakova, e.b., 1994, Antioxidant drugs as neuroprotective agents, In: *Alzheimer Disease: Therapeutic Strategies*, Giacobini, E. and Becker, R., eds., Birkhauser : Boston, p. 313.

Chen , P. S., Toribara, T. J., and Warmer, H., 1956, Microdetermination of phosphorus, *Anal. Chem.* 28: 756.

Ellman, g. L., Courtney, K. D., Andres, V., Jr., and Featherstone, R. M., 1961, A new and rapid colorimetric determination of acetylcholinesterase activity, *Biochem. Pharmacol.* 7:88.

Lowry, O. H., Rosebrough, N. J., Farr, A. K., and Randall, R.J., 1951, Protein measurement with the Folin phenol reagent, *J. Biol. Chem.* 193:265.

Prokchorova, M. I., ed., 1982, Methods in biochemical research (rus), Leningrad State University publ., p.272.

Rasumovsky, S. D., and Zaikov, G. E., 1975, Ozone and its reactions with organic compounds (rus.), M. *Nauka*, p.365

Shinitzky, M., 1987, Patterns of lipid changes in membranes of the aged brain. *Gerontology* 33:149.

Slater, T. F., 1984, Overview of methods used for detecting lipid peroxidation. *Meth. Enzymol.* 105:283

Sperry, W. H., and Webb, M., 1950, A revision of Shoenheimer-Sperry method for cholesterol determination. *J. Biol. Chem.* 187:97.

Voronina, T. A., 1994, Nootropic drugs in Alzheimer disease treatment. New pharmacological strategies. In: *Alzheimer Disease: Therapeutic Strategies*, Giacobini, E. and Becker, R., eds, Birkhauser : Boston, p. 265.

27

AMYLOID-β HYPOTHESIS OF ALZHEIMER'S DISEASE

Mark S. Shearman

Merck Sharp & Dohme Research Laboratories
Neuroscience Research Centre
Harlow CM20 2QR, England

AD GENETICS

Recent progress in understanding the molecular basis of Alzheimer's disease (AD) can be attributed mainly to linkage analysis and positional cloning of gene mutations associated with familial AD (FAD) pedigrees. The majority of early-onset AD cases are familial, and co-segregate with mutations in three known genes: these are the amyloid precursor protein (APP) gene on chromosome 21; the presenilin-1 (PS-1) gene located on chromosome 14; and the presenilin homologue, PS-2, on chromosome 1. Mutations in APP, PS-1 and PS-2, are inherited as autosomal dominant traits with complete or a very high degree of penetrance. A significant proportion of early onset AD cannot be attributed to mutations in any one of these genes, however, and so it is clear that other loci remain to be identified.

The situation with late-onset AD is rather more complicated and less well understood at present. The apolipoprotein E (apoE) ε4 allele polymorphism represents a susceptibility marker with incomplete penetrance, that is known to be associated with up to 40–50% of late onset cases, mostly before the age of 65 (Corder et al., 1993). A susceptability marker has also been identified on chromosome 12, which may account for an additional 20% of late-onset cases (see Roses, A.D., this volume). Intronic mutations in PS-1 (Kehoe et al., 1996), and mutations in the maternally-inherited mitochondrial cytochrome oxidase CO1 and CO2 genes (Davis et al., 1997) indicate some familial association. Risk factors such as head trauma and environmental insults contribute to the remaining apparently sporadic late-onset AD.

Despite the obvious multifactorial contribution to AD, however, at the clinical and neuropathological level there are no gross features that demarcate disease groups.

AD PATHOPHYSIOLOGY

The "amyloid cascade hypothesis" attempts to explain the apparent convergence of the disease process in terms of the central role played by the APP molecule and the amy-

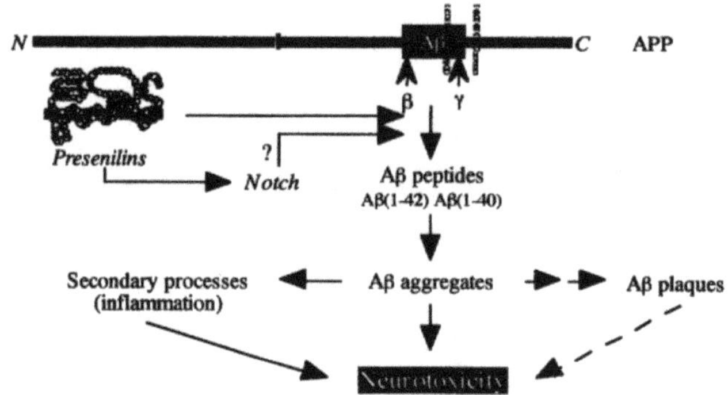

Figure 1. AD pathophysiology depicted in terms of a central role for APP and Aβ.

loid-β (Aβ) peptide (Figure 1). The sequential action of two proteases, as yet unidentified, termed β- and γ-secretase, release the Aβ peptide which exists mainly in two forms, of 40 and 42 amino-acids in length. The Aβ(1–42) molecule is particularly amyloidogenic, and is thought to initiate the aggregation and deposition of the peptides in brain, which ultimately leads to the formation of characteristic dense-core senile plaques. Aggregates of Aβ peptide can be directly neurotoxic, causing synaptic and neuronal cell loss. In addition, they are recognised by the immune system as foreign, resulting in microglial activation and astrocytosis. This inflammatory response in turn exacerbates the neurotoxicity.

The relative rate at which the Aβ(1–42) and Aβ(1–40) peptides are formed is critical to the onset and progression of the disease process. A number of factors can impinge directly or indirectly on this pathway and alter the normal processing in neurones. For example, mutations in the APP molecule that affect trafficking or processing, or mutations that alter the functioning of the presenilin proteins. More subtle influences on neuronal phenotype, such as those resulting from the interaction of presenilin proteins with the *Notch* receptor signalling pathway may also be found to be significant.

GENE MUTATIONS AND Aβ PHENOTYPE

The ability to specifically detect Aβ(1–42) and Aβ(1–40) peptides in biological samples has led to an important advance in the amyloid cascade hypothesis, linking FAD gene mutations to specific changes in Aβ peptide formation. Analysis of plasma and cell culture supernatants from patients with various forms of FAD (with a range of ages of onset) revealed increases in Aβ(1–42) or in the ratio of Aβ(1–42) to Aβ(1–40) (Scheuner et al., 1996). This finding has subsequently been confirmed by transfection experiments (Borchelt et al., 1996; Citron et al., 1997) and in transgenic animals (Duff et al., 1996; Borchelt et al., 1996; Citron et al., 1997). These observations fit well with the increased density of Aβ(1–42)-containing plaques that are a phenotype associated with the presence of apoE ε4 alleles (Schmechel et al., 1993) and support the proposal that increased generation of Aβ(1–42) represents the common denominator in AD pathogenesis (Selkoe, 1996; Hardy, 1997; and reference therein).

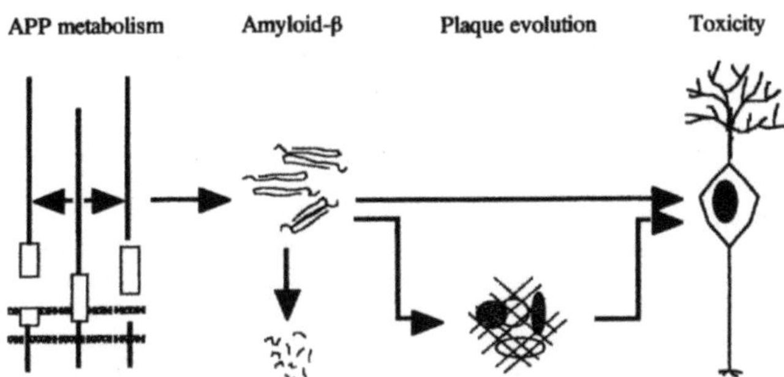

APP metabolism : APP expression , trafficking and processing
Amyloid-β : Aβ clearance, aggregation and sequestration; inflammation
Plaque evolution : Chaperone association and plaque mobilization
Toxicity : Aβ association and toxicity

Figure 2. Potential therapeutic strategies for Alzheimer's disease relating to APP and Aβ.

THERAPEUTIC STRATEGIES—Aβ AGGREGATION AND DEPOSITION

One of the attractions of the amyloid cascade hypothesis is that it suggests a number of defined targets at which therapeutic intervention can be considered and the outcome tested. Figure 2 depicts a schematic representation of the sequential and temporal events leading up to AD neuropathology.

At each hypothetical stage—APP metabolism, Aβ formation, plaque evolution and toxicity—a number of events could be disrupted by appropriate pharmacological agents with potential beneficial effects. The focus of the papers presented at this symposium is the identification and analysis of inhibitors that target the process of amyloid aggregation: the conversion of soluble, monomeric peptide into oligomeric and β-fibrillar structures. The rationale for pursuing such an approach being that to prevent or attenuate this process would enhance peptide clearance and so reduce the deleterious downstream effects that result from the formation of neurotoxic peptide species.

ACKNOWLEDGMENTS

This symposium was supported by grants from Merck Sharp & Dohme, Pharmacia-Upjohn, Cephalon Inc., Hoechst Marion Roussel, California Peptide Research Inc., Pfizer Inc., Glaxo-Wellcome, Eli Lilly & Co. and Boehringer Ingelheim KG.

REFERENCES

Borchelt, D.R., Thinakaran, G., Eckman, C.B., Lee, M.K., Davenport, F., Ratovitsky, T., Prada, C-M., Kim, G., Seekins, S., Yager, D., Slunt, H.H., Wang, R., Seeger, M., Levey, A.I., Gandy, S.E., Copeland, N.G., Jenkins, N.A., Price, D.L., Younkin, S.G., and Sisodia, S.S., 1996, Familial Alzheimer's disease-linked presenilin 1 variants elevate Aβ1–42/1–40 ratio in vitro and in vivo, *Neuron* 17: 1005–1013.

Citron, M., Westaway, D., Xia, W., Carlson, G., Diehl, T., Levesque, G., Johnson-Wood, K., Lee, M., Seubert, P., Davis, A., Kholodenko, D., Motter, R., Sherrington, R., Perry, B., Yao, H., Strome, R., Lieberburg, I., Rommens, J., Kim, S., Schenk, D., Fraser, P., St. George-Hyslop, P., and Selkoe, D., 1997, Mutant presenilins of Alzheimer's disease increase production of 42-residue amyloid β-protein in both transfected cells and transgenic mice, *Nature Med.* 3: 67–72.

Corder, E.H., Saunders, A.M., Strittmatter, W.J., Schmechel, D.E., Gaskell, P.C., Small, G.W., Roses, A.D., Haines, J.L., and Pericak-Vance, M.A., 1993, Gene dose of apolipoprotein E type 4 allele and the risk of Alzheimer's disease in late onset families, *Science* 261: 921–923.

Davis, R.E., Miller, S., Herrnstadt, C., Ghosh, S.S., Fahy, E., Shinobu, L.A., Galasko, D., Thal, L.J., Beal, M.F., Howell, N., and Parker Jr., W.D., 1997, Mutations in mitochondrial cytochrome c oxidase genes segregate with late-onset Alzheimer's disease, *Proc. Natl. Acad. Sci. USA* 94: 4526–4531.

Duff, K., Eckman, C., Zehr, C., Yu, X., Prada, C-M., Perez-Tur, J., Hutton, M., Buee, L., Harigaya, Y., Yager, D., Morgan, D., Gordon, M.N., Holcomb, L., Refolo, L., Zenk, B., Hardy, J., and Younkin, S., 1996, Increased amyloid-β42(43) in brains of mice expressing mutant presenilin 1, *Nature* 383: 710–713.

Hardy, J., 1997, The Alzheimer's family of diseases: many etiologies, one pathogenesis ?, *Proc. Natl. Acad. Sci. USA* 94: 2095–2097.

Kehoe, P., Williams, J., Holmans, P., Liddell, M., Lovestone, S., Holmes, C., Powell, J., Neal, J., Wilcock, G., and Owen, M., 1996, Association between a PS-1 intronic polymorphism and late onset Alzheimer's disease, *NeuroReport* 7: 2155–2158.

Selkoe, D.J., 1996, Amyloid β-protein and the genetics of Alzheimer's disease, *J. Biol. Chem.* 271: 18295–18298.

Scheuner, D., Eckman, C., Jensen, M., Song, X., Citron, M., Suzuki, N., Bird, T.D., Hardy, J., Hutton, M., Kukull, W., Larson, E., Levy-Lahad, E., Viitanen, M., Peskind, E., Poorkaj, P., Schellenberg, G., Tanzi, R., Wasco, W., Lannfelt, L., Selkoe, D., and Younkin, S., 1996, Secreted amyloid β-protein similar to that in the senile plaques of Alzheimer's disease is increased *in vivo* by the presenilin 1 and 2 and APP mutations linked to familial Alzheimer's disease, *Nature Med.* 2: 864–870.

Schmechel, D.E., Saunders, A.M., Strittmatter, W.J., Crain, B.J., Hulette, C.M., Joo, S.H., Pericak-Vance, M.A., Goldgaber, D., and Roses, A.D., 1993, Increased amyloid β-peptide deposition in cerebral cortex as a consequence of apolipoprotein E genotype in late-onset Alzheimer's disease, *Proc. Natl. Acad. Sci. USA* 90: 9649–9653.

28

DISCOVERY AND CHARACTERIZATION OF PEPTIDOORGANIC INHIBITORS OF AMYLOID β-PEPTIDE POLYMERIZATION

Mark A. Findeis and Susan M. Molineaux

Praecis Pharmaceuticals Incorporated
1 Hampshire Street
Cambridge, Massachusetts 02139-1572

INTRODUCTION

Polymerization of amyloid β-peptide (Aβ) results in neuronal toxicity *in vitro*, and the formation *in vivo* of Aβ-peptide plaque is associated with the onset and progression of Alzheimer's disease (AD) (Lorenzo and Yankner, 1994 and references therein). The precise mechanism by which AD-associated cellular toxicity and neurodegeneration occurs in humans is incompletely understood. Recent identification of the specific genetic defects that result in four classes of familial AD have the common feature of enhancing the production or deposition of Aβ (Selkoe, 1997). These data, in combination with additional observations regarding the progression of AD in Down syndrome patients or sporadic AD in older patients, the neurological and behavioral pathology of transgenic animal models of AD, and various biochemical properties of Aβ point to the production and subsequent polymerization of Aβ as an essential component of AD pathogenesis. This "Amyloid Hyposthesis" is reviewed in greater detail in the chapter by M. S. Shearman (see above). Thus, identification of compounds that slow, prevent, and possibly reverse the polymerization of Aβ has emerged as a goal in the development of therapeutic agents for AD.

A DESIGN STRATEGY FOR Aβ POLYMERIZATION INHIBITORS

Aβ assembles into oligomeric extended arrays of antiparallel β-sheet and eventually into cross β-fibril-like structure. The non-crystalline nature of these amyloid fibrils has precluded atomic-level resolution of their structures. Fibril diffraction (Inouye et al., 1993), solid-state nuclear magnetic resonance (NMR) (Lansbury et al., 1995) and atomic force microscopy (Harper et al., 1997) on polymerized native, non-native and truncated

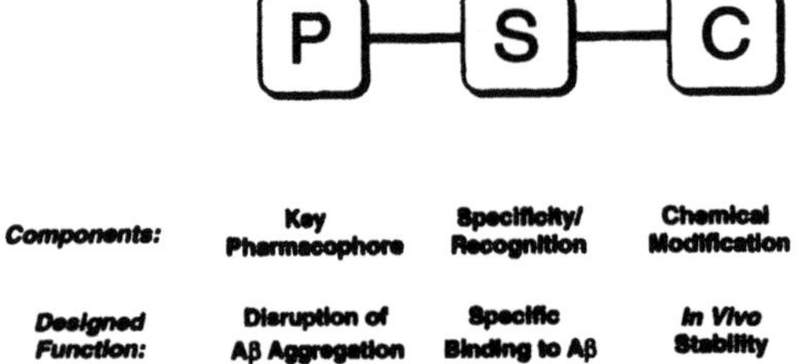

Figure 1. Strategy for design of inhibitors of Aβ polymerization in which binding specificity is derived from a peptidic component S based on the structure of Aβ, inhibition potency is added or enhanced by an organic modifying group P, and biological stability is enhanced by additional chemical modification C.

model sequence amyloidogenic peptides has revealed some details of amyloid structure. Solution-phase NMR has been used to obtain a structure of an Aβ fragment but these data do not directly inform us about fibril structure (Lee et al., 1995). In the absence of high-resolution structural data on fibrillar Aβ, the ability to pursue "structure-based" or "rational" drug design is limited. Aβ itself, however, provides a practical starting point in the pursuit of polymerization inhibitors.

Our strategy for developing an inhibitor of Aβ polymerization is summarized in Figure 1. The self-assembling properties of Aβ suggested that it would be possible to achieve binding to Aβ using a portion or analog of a portion of the Aβ sequence. Such an Aβ subsequence was expected to provide specific or selective binding affinity for Aβ (a specificity/recognition element, or "S" group). Organic modification of the S group was designed to enhance binding of the S group without adding amino acyl residues and to provide a non-peptidic key pharmacophore element (a "P" group) that would increase inhibition of polymerization through steric or conformational effects or both. Additional chemical modification of the resulting P–S combination with one or more "C" groups was anticipated to increase biochemical stability. Our initial assay for evaluating compounds is based on the Aβ polymerization assay previously reported by Lansbury (Jarrett et al., 1993). This assay uses an initially monomeric solution of Aβ(1–40) which is then stirred or shaken. After a period of mixing, during which Aβ monomers are forming oligomers, sufficient formation of a critical amount of an as yet uncharacterized higher molecular weight "seed" occurs resulting in rapid formation of amyloid fibril (Figure 2). Detection of polymer is achieved by measuring turbidity (Jarrett et al., 1993) or dye binding to fibrils (LeVine, 1993, 1995). Inhibitors of polymerization can be detected by the effect of delaying the onset of rapid polymerization (an increase in the "lag" period in the assay) or by reducing the amount of fibril formed (expressed as "% inhibition").

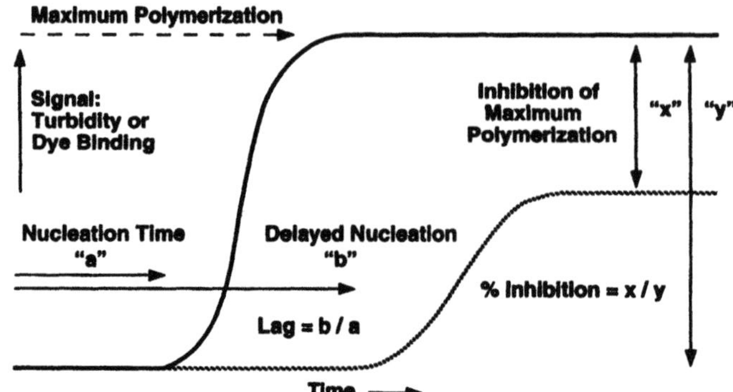

Figure 2. Assay for polymerization of Aβ. An inhibitor can delay the formation of oligomeric nuclei of Aβ that seed the formation of amyloid fibrils (an increase in "Lag") and the extent of polymerization at later time during the assay can be reduced (an increase in "% Inhibition").

Aβ POLYMERIZATION INHIBITORS

Our progression in the synthesis of inhibitors of Aβ polymerization from large analogs of Aβ (1–40) to small peptidoorganic compounds is summarized in Figure 3. The first series of compounds examined for inhibitor activity consisted of 34 to 40 residue derivatives of the Aβ (1–40) sequence, including some of the variations previously reported in the literature as having modified amyloidogenic potential or derivatives thereof (Hilbich et al., 1991 and 1992; Pike et al., 1995). These compounds and subsequent derivatives were prepared using standard chemistries for solid-phase and solution-phase synthesis. Generally, these compounds were modest to excellent inhibitors. In an effort to find a smaller portion of the Aβ sequence with anti-amyloidogenic properties we prepared peptides that corresponded to scanning Aβ (1–40) with a 15-residue window starting at five-residue intervals. Several of these peptides had comparable lag-delaying effects to the longer peptides, but also reduced the extent of polymerization observed at later times in the assay.

In an effort to enhance the inhibitory activity of peptides without extending the sequence, organic modification of Aβ (1–15), and to a lesser extent Aβ (1–40), at the amino terminus was performed using a selected group of reagents. These reagents were chosen to introduce a variety of structural elements varying in size, shape, polarity and charge. Most of the resulting modifications afforded compounds with reduced activity. Several of the activity-enhancing modifiers were then applied to the other members of the pentadecapeptide scan of Aβ (1–40) previously studied. Two trends were observed in this study. The best modifying group identified was cholyl. The best peptide core group was Aβ (6–20) with other sequences providing good inhibitors depending on the modification.

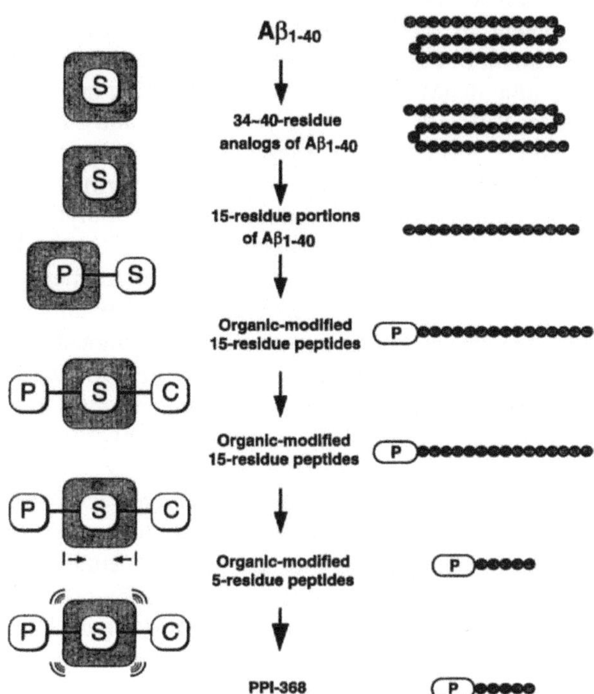

Figure 3. Summary of the progression of inhibitors from analogs of Aβ(1–40) to low molecular-weight peptidoorganic compounds (see text).

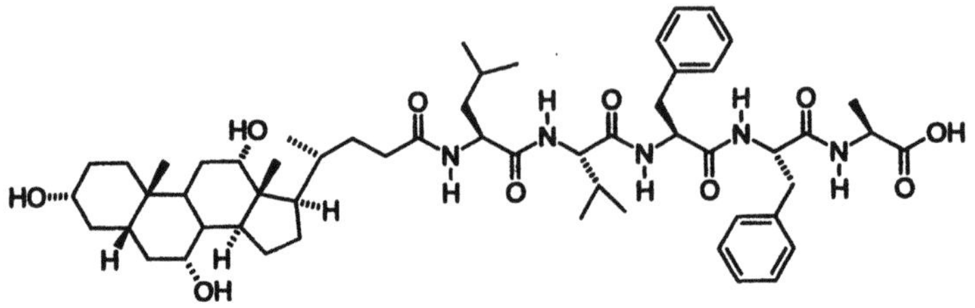

Figure 4. Structure of PPI-368, cholyl-L-leucyl-L-valyl-L-phenylalanyl-L-phenylalanyl-L-alanine.

Modified pentadecapeptides were considered as still rather large for practical drug leads. In an effort to obtain inhibitors still smaller in size, cholyl-modified-Aβ (6–20) was systematically reduced in size by deleting amino acyl residues from either the amino or carboxyl terminus. In this way, we were able to identify potent inhibitors containing as few as five amino acyl residues. Additional structure-activity studies allowed the refinement of the S group to a five-residue sequence with only non-polar sidechains. The resulting lead compound, PPI-368, is cholyl-LVFFA (Figure 4). The combination of the organic modifying P-group with the peptide element derived from Aβ is required for high activity. P group alone, cholic acid, was inactive in the screening assay, and the peptidic S group, LVFFA, had low activity, demonstrating the requirement of both groups acting synergistically. The analog of PPI-368 in which all amino acyl residues are replaced by alanine also lacked activity. Minor rearrangements or substitutions in the peptide S-group tended to have a negative effect on activity suggesting a significant level of specific intermolecular "molecular recognition" in the interaction of the inhibitors with Aβ.

PPI-368 is a potent inhibitor of Aβ polymerization and a promising lead for the development of therapeutic agents for the treatment of Alzheimer's disease through the mechanism of inhibition of Aβ polymerization. In a nucleation-dependent polymerization assay of a 50 μM Aβ (1–40) peptide solution monitored by turbidity, equimolar concentrations of PPI-368 blocked polymerization and submolar doses significantly delayed fibril formation. Electron microscopy confirmed that fibril formation did not occur in the presence of PPI-368. In nucleation assays performed at lower peptide concentrations (0.2–25 μM Aβ peptide) where formation of β-sheet polymers was monitored by thioflavin-T binding, high potency and dose-dependent inhibition by PPI-368 were observed. The ability of PPI-368 to inhibit the polymerization of monomeric peptide suggests that it binds directly to monomers or soluble oligomers. Trace amounts of radiolabeled PPI-368 were incorporated into fibrils during polymerization, demonstrating that the inhibitor can also bind to Aβ peptide within a fibrillar structure. PPI-368 was selective in that it did not inhibit the polymerization of the other amyloidogenic proteins transthyretin (TTR) (McCutchen et al., 1993) or islet amyloid polypeptide-(20–29) (IAPP(20–29)) (Ashburn and Lansbury, 1993).

In a polymerization extension assay seeded with pre-formed Aβ polymer, similar inhibition and dose-dependency phenomena were observed with PPI-368 in comparison with the nucleation assay. In gel-filtration studies using submolar concentrations of PPI-368, monomeric Aβ was still present and oligomers did not form, suggesting that PPI-368 would be effective at blocking the deposition of Aβ peptide onto pre-formed Aβ fibrils or plaque. PPI-368 is a potent, selective inhibitor of Aβ polymerization that coordinately delays the onset of polymerization and blocks the formation of all neurotoxic Aβ species for both Aβ (1–40) and Aβ (1–42) peptides.

REFERENCES

Ashburn, T. T., and Lansbury, P. T., Jr., 1993, Interspecies Sequence Variations Affect the Kinetics and Thermodynamics of Amyloid Formation: Peptide Models of Pancreatic Amyloid. *J. Am. Chem. Soc.* 115:11012–11013.

Harper, J. D., Wong, S. S., Lieber, C. M., and Lansbury, P. T., Jr., 1997, Observation of metastable Aβ amyloid protofibrils by atomic force microscopy. *Chem. Biol.* 4:119–125.

Hilbich, C., Kisters-Woike, B., Reed, J., Masters, C. L., and Beyreuther, K., 1991, Aggregation and Secondary Structure of Synthetic Amyloid βA4 Peptides of Alzheimer's Disease. *J. Mol. Biol.* 218:149–163.

Hilbich, C., Kisters-Woike, B., Reed, J., Masters, C. L., and Beyreuther, K., 1992, Substitutions of Hydrophobic Amino Acids Reduce the Amyloidogenicity of Alzheimer's Disease βA4 Peptides. *J. Mol. Biol.* 228:460–473.

Inouye, H., Fraser, P. E., and Kirschner, D. A., 1993, Structure of β-crystallite assemblies formed by Alzheimer β-amyloid protein anologues: analysis by x-ray diffraction. *Biophys. J.* 64:502–519.

Jarrett, J. T., Berger, E. P., and Lansbury, P. T., Jr., 1993, The Carboxy Terminus of the β Amyloid Protein Is Critical for the Seeding of Amyloid Formation: Implications for the Pathogenesis of Alzheimer's Disease. *J. Am. Chem. Soc.* 32:4693–4697.

Lansbury, P. T., Jr., Costa, P. R., Griffiths, J. M., Simon, E. J., Auger, M., Halverson, K. J., Kocisko, D. A., Hendsch, Z. S., Ashburn, T. T., Spencer, R. G. S., Tidor, B., and Griffin, R. G., 1995, Structural model for the β-amyloid fibril based on interstrand alignment of an antiparallel-sheet comprising a C-terminal peptide. *Nature Struct. Biol.* 2:990–998.

Lee, J. P., Stimson, E. R., Ghilardi, J. R., Mantyh, P. W., Lu, Y.-A., Felix, A. M., Llanos, W., Behbin, A., Cummings, M., Criekinge, M. V., Timms, W., and Maggio, J. E., 1995, ¹H NMR of Aβ Amyloid Peptide Congeners in Water Solution. Conformational Changes Correlate with Plaque Competence.*Biochemistry* 34:5191–5200.

LeVine, H., III, 1993, Thioflavine T interaction with synthetic Alzheimer's disease β-amyloid peptides: Detection of amyloid aggregation in solution. *Protein Sci.* 2:404–410.

LeVine, H., III, 1995, Thioflavine T interaction with amyloid β-sheet structures: Amyloid. *Int. J. Exp. Clin. Invest.* 2:1–6.

Lorenzo, A., and Yankner, B. A., 1994, β-Amyloid neurotoxicity requires fibril formation and is inhibited by Congo red. *Proc. Natl. Acad. Sci. USA* 91:12243–12247.

McCutchen, S. L., Colon, W., and Kelly, J. W., 1993, Transthyretin Mutation Leu-55-Pro Significantly Alters Tetramer Stability and Increases Amyloidogenicity. *Biochemistry* 32:12119–12127.

Pike, C. J., Walencewicz-Wasserman, A. J., Kosmoski, J., Cribbs, D. H., Glabe, C. G., and Cotman, C. W., 1995, Structure–Activity Analyses of β–Amyloid Peptides: Contributions of the β25–35 Region to Aggregation and Neurotoxicity. *J. Neurochem.* 64:253–265.

Selkoe, D. J., 1997, Alzheimer's Disease: Genotypes, Phenotype, and Treatment. *Science* 275:630–631.

29

ANTHRACYCLINES AND AMYLOIDOSIS

C. Post,[1] F. Tagliavini,[2] R. A. McArthur,[1] F. Della Vedova,[1] M. Gerna,[1] T. Bandiera,[1] M. Varasi,[1] A. Molinari,[1] and J. Lansen[1]

[1]Pharmacia & Upjohn S.p.A.
CNS Research
Nerviano (MI), Italy
[2]Istituto Nazionale Neurologico Carlo Besta
Milan, Italy

INTRODUCTION

Amyloidosis is defined as the cascade of structural changes of proteins leading to the formation of insoluble fibril aggregates that accumulate in tissue as amyloid plaques. All types of amyloidosis are structurally characterized by the cross β-pleated sheet conformation of the fibrils irrespective of their biochemical composition (reviewed by Glenner, 1980). This common structural feature of fibril aggregates is the basis of their insolubility and relative resistance to proteolytic digestion (Jarrett and Lansbury, 1993; Nordstedt et al., 1994). Amyloid plaque formation and deposition is believed to be the key event in nerve cell death in chronic and incurable neurodegenerative diseases such as Alzheimer's Disease (AD) (reviewed by Selkoe, 1996) and Creutzfeldt-Jakob Disease (CJD) (reviewed by Prusiner, 1996). One of the major therapeutic approaches to arrest, or at least slow down the progression of these devastating diseases, is to stop proteins from aggregating into amyloid fibrils.

Region specific amyloidosis is a key pathological feature in AD which is accompanied by astrogliosis, microgliosis, cytoskeletal changes and synaptic loss (Selkoe, 1991; Wisnieski and Terry, 1973; Wisnieski et al., 1981). These pathological alterations are thought to be linked to the cognitive decline that clinically defines the disease (Cummings et al., 1996). The major component of the amyloid plaque is amyloid-β (Aβ), a 39 to 43 residue peptide, which is a proteolytic fragment of a much larger integral membrane protein called amyloid precursor protein (APP) (Glenner and Wong, 1984; Masters et al., 1985). There is accumulating evidence that altered APP proteolytic processing can lead to an overproduction of Aβ peptide, in particular, the production of the highly hydrophobic and thus amyloidogenic Aβ 1–42 form. Altered APP proteolytic processing also leads to an overwhelming deposition of Aβ fibrils in the brain (reviewed by Price et al., 1995).

Progress in Alzheimer's and Parkinson's Diseases
edited by Fisher *et al.*, Plenum Press, New York, 1998.

The link between Aβ deposition and neurotoxicity comes from the observations that dystrophic neurites are found around senile plaques (Selkoe, 1991). Down's syndrome patients have 3 copies of the APP gene. These patients present Aβ deposits in late childhood or young adulthood and subsequently develop the classical neuropathological features of AD (Giaccone et al. 1989; Rumble et al., 1989). Missense mutations in the APP gene, clustered in the Aβ region of the precursor, are linked to familial AD (Chartier-Harlin et al., 1991; Goate et al., 1991; Mullan et al., 1992). These missense mutations have been shown to alter APP processing resulting in an increased production of Aβ peptide in transfected human cell lines (Cai et al., 1993; Citron et al., 1992; Haass et al., 1994; Suzuki et al., 1994), and in primary skin fibroblasts and plasma from patients harboring these mutations (Scheuner et al., 1996). Moreover, the recently described mutations in the presenilin 1 (PS_1) and presenilin 2 (PS_2) genes have also been shown to result in an overproduction of the longer forms of Aβ peptide. These too are linked with very early onset of neuropathological changes in familial AD (reviewed by Tanzi et al., 1996). On the other hand, transgenic mice expressing mutant forms of human APP exhibit numerous amyloid plaques as well as astrogliosis, microgliosis and synaptic loss in the brain (Games et al., 1995; Hsiao et al., 1996). In one transgenic model, correlation between memory deficits and Aβ plaque formation was also reported (Hsiao et al., 1996).

Prion diseases, such as scrapie of sheep, spongiform encephalopathy of cattle and CJD of humans, are transmissible neurodegenerative conditions characterized by the accumulation of protease-resistant forms of the prion protein (PrP), termed PrP^{res}, in the brain (Ghetti et al., 1996; reviewed by Prusiner, 1996). Unlike normal PrP, PrP^{res} has a large amount of β-sheet secondary structure and a strong tendency to aggregate into amyloid fibrils (Caughey et al., 1991; Jarrett and Lansbury, 1993; Prusiner, 1983). Deposition of PrP^{res} and PrP amyloid is accompanied by nerve cell degeneration and glial cell proliferation leading to the clinical signs of the disease (Forloni et al., 1993; Forloni et al., 1994). PrP like Aβ assembles into fibrils *in vitro*, and this aggregation process is a critical factor in the neurotoxicity observed in different cell culture systems (Forloni et al., 1993; Pike et al., 1993).

Recently, a number of small molecules have been reported to interfere with the *in vitro* aggregation of Aβ and PrP peptides. Due to the relationship between peptide aggregation and their neurotoxicity, these compounds were also found to inhibit or to reduce the neurotoxic effects of these peptides on different cell lines (reviewed by Bandiera et al., 1997). The anthracycline, 4'-iodo-4'-deoxydoxorubicin (IDX) (Figure 1) is a derivative of doxorubicin, a drug of proven efficacy in a large number of tumor malignancies (Barbiera et al., 1987).

The administration of IDX to patients with plasma cell dyscrasias complicated by immunoglobulin light chain amyloidosis resulted in the partial resorption of amyloid deposits. In addition, patients exhibited discernible clinical improvement, reduced symptoms

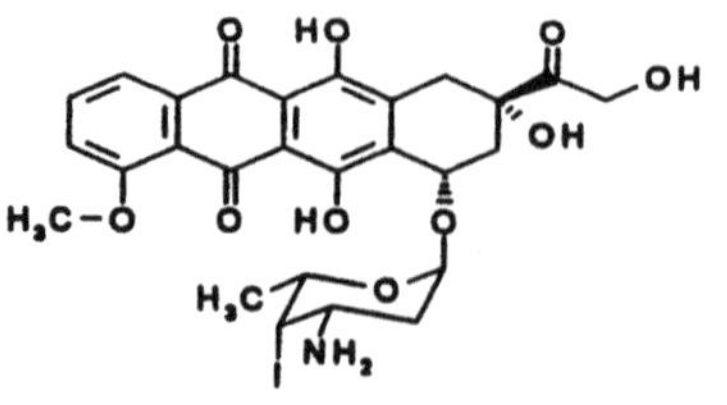

Figure 1. Chemical structure of 4'-iodo-4'-deoxydoxorubicin (IDX).

of the disease and two patients out of eight became clinically stabilized (Gianni et al., 1987). This unexpected effect of the compound on amyloidosis was confirmed by further studies showing that IDX binds strongly to natural amyloid fibrils of different chemical composition: immunoglobulin light chain, amyloid A, thransthyretin (methionine-30 variant) and β-microglobulin. IDX inhibits the assembly of insulin into amyloid fibrils *in vitro* and reduces amyloid deposits in a murine model of reactive amyloidosis (Merlini et al., 1995). On the basis of these results it was hypothesized that IDX could interfere with Aβ and PrP amyloidosis as well as with proteins causing peripheral amyloidosis.

RESULTS AND DISCUSSION

The ability of IDX to bind to Aβ and PrP amyloid was first investigated. Serial section of the cerebral cortex and cerebellum from patients with sporadic AD and CJD were incubated *in vitro* with 10^{-7} M aqeous solution of IDX or with the amyloid binding fluorochrome thioflavine-S. The sections were analyzed by fluorescence microscopy. The comparison of adjacent sections showed that all amyloid deposits revealed by thioflavine-S also exhibit the characteristic fluorescence of IDX (Figure 2).

The effect of IDX on the fibrilogenesis of the synthetic peptide (Aβ 25–35) homologous to residues 25–35 of human Aβ was then tested *in vitro*. Solutions of Aβ 25–35 (236 µM) were prepared in 1 mM phosphate buffer pH 7.4 containing increasing concentrations of IDX. The samples were incubated for different time intervals at room temperature, centrifuged at 10,000 × g for 15 min. at 4°C and the residual soluble Aβ monomer was measured in the supernatant by HPLC. In these conditions, IDX inhibited spontaneous aggregation of Aβ 25–35 in a dose-related manner (Figure 3).

Almost complete prevention of Aβ 25–25 aggregation was achieved at a molar concentration ratio Aβ peptide *versus* IDX of 5:1. In another set of experiments, a seed made from preformed Aβ 25–35 fibrils was incubated with increasing concentrations of IDX for 1 hour at room temperature. After this incubation period, the ability of the seed to trigger

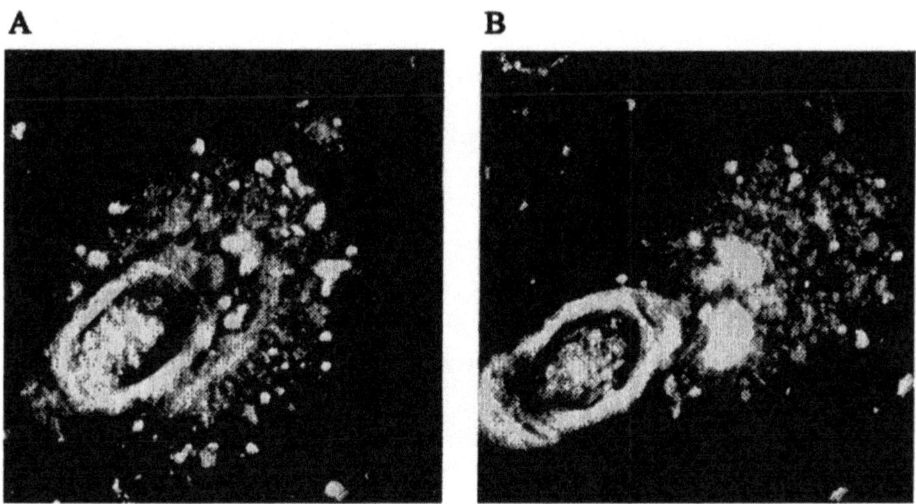

Figure 2. Binding of thioflavine S (A) and IDX (B) to parenchymal and vascular Aβ amyloid in brain section from a patient with AD.

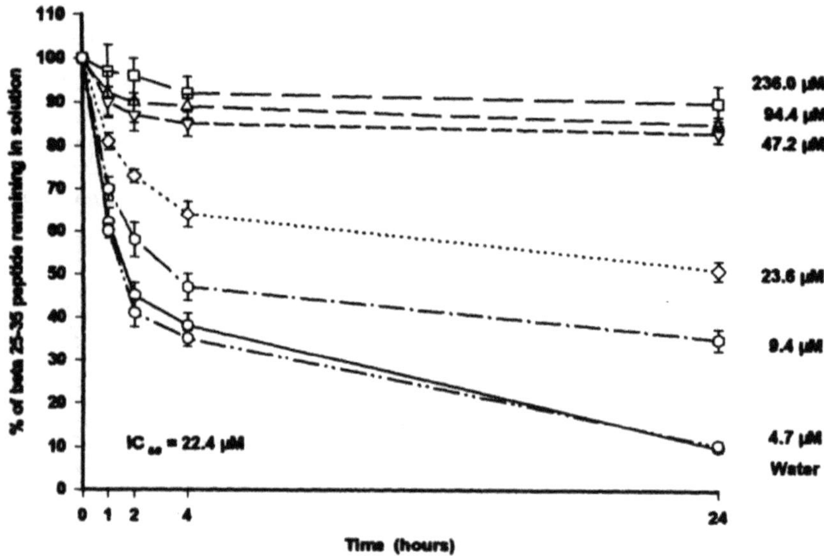

Figure 3. Effect of IDX on the spontaneous aggregation of Aβ 25–35 *in vitro*. Results are the mean ± SEM of three experiments performed each in triplicate.

the aggregation of a 40 µM solution of Aβ 25–35 monomer in 1 mM phosphate buffer pH 7.4 was investigated. Aggregation was allowed to take place for two hours at room temperature. Thereafter, the samples were centrifuged and the remaining soluble Aβ 25–35 monomer was measured in the supernatant by HPLC. In these conditions, pre-treatment of the seed with IDX inhibited its ability to trigger the aggregation of soluble Aβ 25–35 in a dose-dependent manner (Figure 4).

The effect of IDX on experimental scrapie, which is regarded as a model of prion diseases was then investigated (Tagliavini et al., 1997). In two separate experiments Syr-

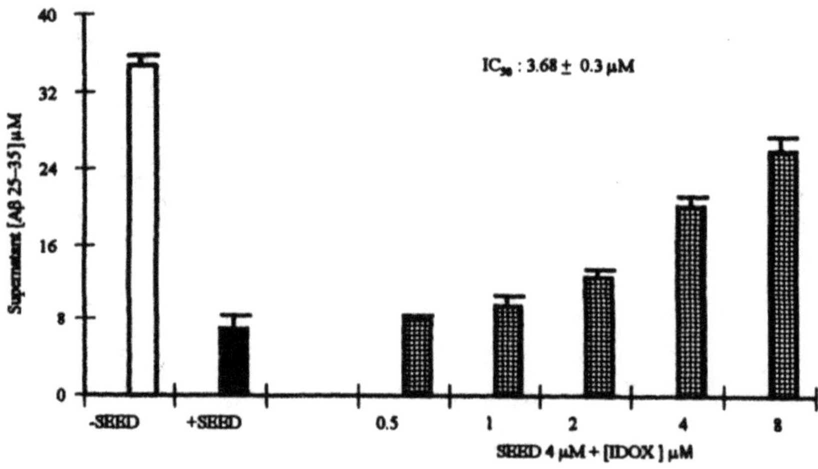

Figure 4. Effect of IDX on seed-triggered aggregation of Aβ 25–35. Results are the mean ± SEM of three experiments performed each in triplicate.

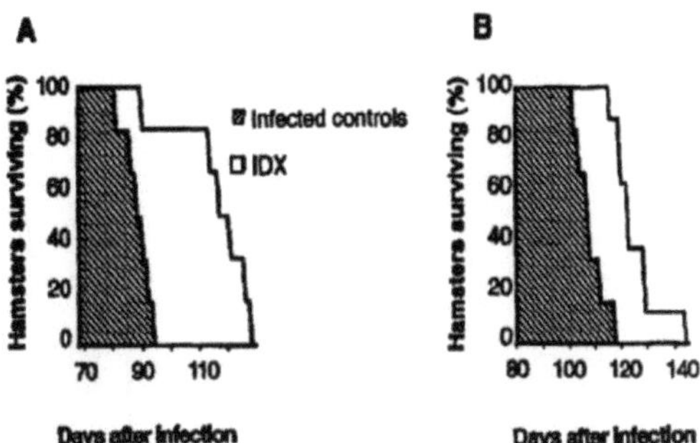

Figure 5. Effect on IDX on the survival of scrapie-infected hamsters. A and B survival time of infected controls (shared area) and of IDX-treated hamsters (white area) in the first (A) and second (B) experiment. Longevity was analyzed by Kaplan-Meier survival analysis. (Reproduced with permission from *Science*.)

ian hamsters were experimentally infected with the 263K scrapie strain, a pathological form of hamster prion protein. Other hamsters were inoculated with the scrapie strain co-incubated with 2.9 IDX for 1 h. In the first study the survival time as well as PrP^{res} accumulation in the brain were examined. In the second study, the same parameters were measured together with the accompanying neurological symptoms (tremors, balance, reactivity to sound and touch, and ability to escape from a closed environment). Hamsters infected with scrapie agent co-incubated with IDX lived significantly longer than those injected with scrapie strain alone in both experiments (Figure 5A and B). In the first study, all scrapie infected hamsters died by 94 days after infection (Mean ± SEM: 88.5 ± 1.9 days) while IDX treated animals lived up to 128 days (Mean ± SEM: 116 ± 5.6 days).

The key behavior alterations of scrapie infection in the second group of animals were at the initial phase of the disease. These were hyperreactivity to external stimuli and subsequent postural abnormalities affecting the ability of these animals to escape when placed in an enclosed area. IDX significantly increased the time before postural abnormalities and tremors appeared (Figure 6), and as a consequence retarded the progressive deterioration in their ability to escape from the cages (Figure 7).

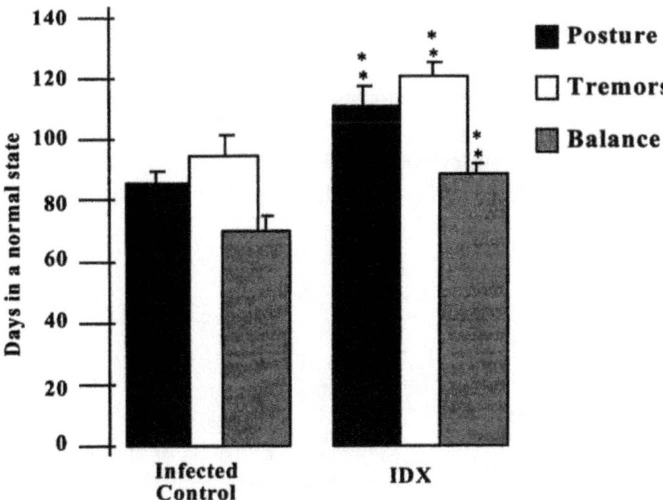

Figure 6. Effect of IDX on posture, balance and tremors of Syrian hamsters infected with scrapie. Mean number of days (± SEM) the infected controls and IDX treated hamsters of the second study remained in a state of normal posture and balance and had no tremors (**p < 0.01 versus infected controls, Tukey's q method for multiple comparison). (Reproduced with permission from *Science*.)

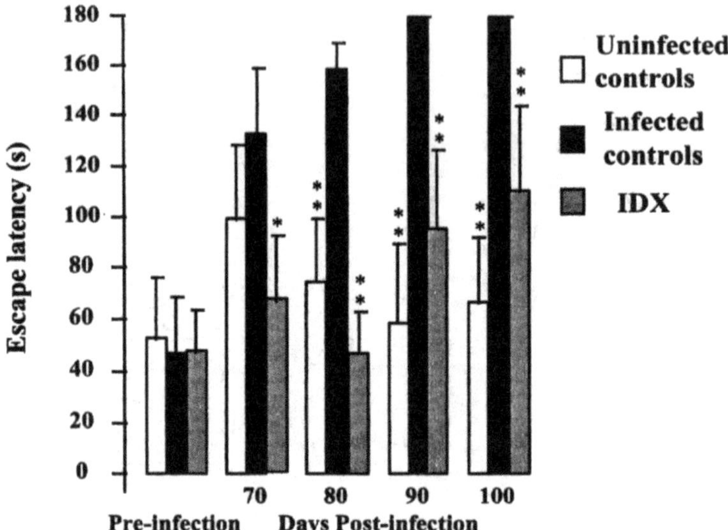

Figure 7. Effect of IDX on the ability of scrapie-infected Syrian hamsters to escape from an enclosed area. Mean latency (± SEM) with which uninfected controls, infected controls, and IDX-treated hamsters escaped from an enclosed area (*$p < 0.05$ and **$p < 0.01$ versus infected controls, Tukey's q method for multiple comparison). (Reproduced with permission from *Science*.)

This delay in the onset of the clinical symptoms was associated with a prolonged survival time confirming the results obtained in the first study (Figure 5B). Histological and immunohistochemical analysis of the brains of a subset of animals from each group culled when behavior changes were first apparent in the infected controls showed differences in PrP accumulation, spongiosis changes and astrogliosis. Quantitative analysis of PrP^{res} by immunoblotting, normalized for the levels of tubulin, indicated a decrease of approximately 80% in the brain of IDX treated hamsters (Figure 8). Notwithstanding the delay in appearance of neurological symptoms and death by IDX, however, all hamsters died from 263K scrapie infection.

The mechanism for proteins to aggregate as amyloid is only partially known, and the mechanism(s) by which IDX stops this process is not yet well understood. It may be speculated that the binding properties of IDX to the pathological form of the prion protein, or to the seed made from Aβ fibrils, may block further transformation of normal PrP and Aβ into amyloid fibrils.

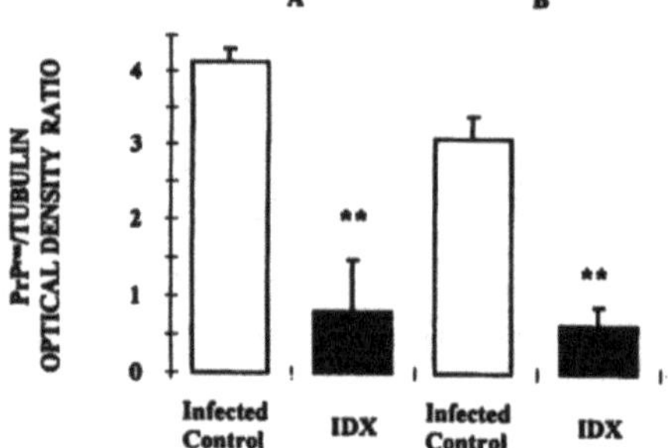

Figure 8. Effects of IDX on PrP^{res} accumulation in the brain of scrapie-infected hamsters. Quantitative densitometric analysis of PrP^{res} normalized for the levels of tubulin as revealed by protein immunoblotting. Immunoblot analysis was performed at day 68 (A) and day 80 (B) in infected controls and IDX-treated hamsters in the first and second experiment respectively. (**$p < 0.01$ by paired "t" test).

IDX is cytotoxic, and has poor blood–brain barrier penetration that make this a non-suitable compound for clinical use in cerebral amyloidosis. These results nevertheless indicate that anthracyclines can be effective in the treatment of amyloid diseases.

REFERENCES

Chartier-Harlin, M.C., Crawford, F., Houlden, H., Warren, A., Hughes, D., Fidani, L., Goate, A., Rossor, M., Roques, P., Hardy, J., and Mullan, M., 1991, Early-onset Alzheimer's Disease caused by mutations at codon 717 of the β-Amyloid Precursor Protein gene. *Nature* 353:844–846.

Citron, M., Oltersdorf, T., Haass, C., McConlogue, L., Hung, A.Y., Seubert, P., Vigo-Pelfrey, C., Lieberburg, I., and Selkoe D.J., 1992, Mutation of the β-Amyloid Precursor Protein in familial Alzheimer's Disease increases β-protein production. *Nature* 360:672–674.

Cummings, B.J., Pike, C.J., Shankle, R., and Cotman, C.W., 1996, β-Amyloid deposition and other measures of neuropathology predict cognitive status in Alzheimer's Disease. *Neurobiol. Aging* 17(6), 921–933.

Forloni, G., Angeretti, N., Chiesa, R., Monzani, E., Salmona, M., Bugiani, O., and Tagliavini, F., 1993, Neurotoxicity of a prion protein fragment. *Nature* 362:543–546.

Forloni, G., Del Bo, R., Angeretti, N., Chiesa, R., Smiroldo, S., Doni, R., Ghibaudi, A., Salmona, M., Porro, M., Verga, L., Giaccone, G., Bugiani, O., and Tagliavini, F., 1994, A neurotoxic prion protein fragment induces rat astroglial proliferation and hypertrophy. *Eur.J.Neurosci.* 6:1415–1422.

Games, D., Adams, D., Alessandrini, R., Barbour, R., Berthelette, P., Blackwell, C., Carr, T., Clemens, J., Donaldson, T., Gillespie, F., Guido, T., Hagoplan, S., Johnson-Wood, K., Khan, K., Lee, M., Leibowitz, P., Lieberburg, I., Little, S., Masliah, E., McConlogue, L., Montoya-Zavala, M., Mucke, L., Paganini, L., Penniman, E., Power, M., Schenk, D., Seubert, P., Snyder, B., Soriano, F., Tan, H., Vitale, J., Wadsworth, S., Wolozin, B., and Zhao, J., 1995, Alzheimer-type neuropathology in transgenic mice overexpressing V717F β-Amyloid Precursor Protein. *Nature* 373:523–527.

Ghetti, B., Piccardo, P., Frangione, B., Bugiani, O., Giaccone, G.,Young, K., Prelli, F., Farlow, M.R., Dlouhy, R., and Tagliavini, F., 1996, Prion protein amyloidosis. *Brain Pathol.* 6:127–145.

Giaccone, G., Tagliavini, F., Lindoli, G., Bouras, C., Frigerio, L., Frangione, B., and Bugiani, O., 1989, Down Patients: extracellular preamyloid deposits precede neuritic degeneration and senile plaques. *Neurosci.Lett.* 97:232–238.

Gianni, L., Bellotti, V., Gianni, A.M., and Merlini, G.P., 1995, New drug therapy of amyloidosis: Resorption of AL-type deposits with 4'-iodo-4'-deoxydoxorubicin. *Blood* 3:855–861.

Glenner, G.G.,1980, Amyloid deposits and amyloidosis (First part). *New Engl. J. Med.* 302(23):1283–1292.

Glenner, G.G.,1980, Amyloid deposits and amyloidosis (Second part). *New Engl. J. Med.* 302(24):1333–1343.

Glenner, G.G., and Wong, C.W., 1984, Alzheimer's Disease: initial report of the purification and characterization of a novel cerebrovascular amyloid protein. *Biochem.Biophys. Res.Comm.* 120(3):885–890.

Goate, A., Chartier-Harlin, M.C., Mullan, M., Brown, J., Crawford, F., Fidani, L., Giuffra, L., Haynes, A., Irving, N., James, L., Mant, R., Newton, P., Rooke, K., Roques, P., Talbot, C., Pericak-Vance, M., Roses, A., Williamson, R., Rossor, M., Owen, M., and Hardy, J., 1991, Segregation of a missence mutation in the Amyloid Precursor Protein gene with Familial Alzheimer's Disease. *Nature* 349:704–707.

Haass, C., Hung, A.Y., Selkoe, D.J., and Teplow D.B., 1994, Mutations associated with a locus for Familial Alzheimer's Disease result in alternative processing of Amyloid-β Protein Precursor. *J.Biol.Chem.* 269: 17741–17748.

Jarrett, J.L., and Lansbury, P.T.Jr, 1993, Seeding "one-dimensional crystallization" of amyloid: a pathogenic mechanism in Alzheimer's Disease and scrapie? *Cell* 73:1055–1058.

Hsiao, K., Chapman, P., Nilsen, S., Eckman, C., Harigaya, Y., Younkin, S., Yang, F., and Cole, G., 1996, Correlative memory deficits, Aβ elevation, and amyloid plaques in transgenic mice. *Science* 274:99–102.

Masters, C.L., Simms, G., Weinman, N.A., Multhaup, G., McDonald, B.L., and Beyreuther, K., 1985, Amyloid plaque core protein in Alzheimer Disease and Down Syndrome. *Proc. Natl. Acad. Sci. USA*, 82:4245–4249.

Merlini, G.P., Ascari, E., Amboldi, N., Bellotti, V., Arbastini, E., Perfetti, V., Ferrari, M., Zorzoli, I., Marinone, M.G., Garini, P., Diegoli, M., Trizio D., and Ballinari, D., 1995, Interaction of the anthracycline 4'-Iodo-4'-deoxydoxorubicin with amyloid fibrils: inhibition of amyloidogenesis. *Proc. Natl. Acad. Sci. USA*, 92:2959–2963.

Mullan, M., Crawford, F., Axelman, K., Houlden, H., Lillius, L., Winblad, B., and Lannfelt, L., 1992, A pathogenic mutation for probable Alzheimer's Disease in the APP gene at the N-terminus of β-amyloid. *Nat. Genet* 1:345–347.

Nordstedt, C., Näslund, J., Tjernberg, L.O., Karlström, A.R., Thyberg, J., and Terenius, L., 1994, The Alzheimer Aβ peptide develops protease resistance in association with its polymerization into fibrils, *J. Biol. Chem.* 269(49), 30773–30776.

Pike, C.J., Burdick, D., Walencewicz, A.J., Glabe, C.G., and Cotman, C.W., 1993, Neurodegeneration induced by β-amyloid peptides *in vitro*: the role of peptide assembly state. *J. Neurosci.* 13:1676–1687.

Price, D.L., Sisodia, S.S., and Gandy, S.E., 1995, Amyloid beta amyloidosis in Alzheimer's Disease. *Curr. Opin. Neurol.* 8:268–274.

Prusiner, S.B., McKinley, M.P., Bowman, K.A., Bolton, D.C., Bendeheim, B.E., Groth, D.F., and Glenner G.G., 1983, Scrapie prion aggregate to form amyloid-like birefringent rods. *Cell* 35:349–358.

Prusiner, S.B., 1991, Molecular biology of prion diseases. *Science* 251:1515–1522.

Prusiner, S.B., 1996, Prion biology and Diseases - Laughing cannibals, mad cows, and scientific heresy. *Med. Res. Rev.* 16(5):487–505.

Rumble, B., Retallack, R., Hilbich, C., Simms, G., Multhaup, G., Martins, R., Hockey, A., Montgomery, P., Beyreuther, K., and Masters, C.L., 1989, Amyloid A$_4$ protein and its precursor in Down's Syndrome and Alzheimer's Disease. *N. Engl. J. Med.* 320:1446–1452.

Scheuner, D., Eckman, C., Jensen, M., Song, X., Citron, M., Suzuki, N., Bird, T.D., Hardy, J., Hutton, M., Kukull, W., Larson, E., Levy-Lahad, E., Viitanen, M., Peskind, E., Poorkaj, P., Schellenberg, G., Tanzi, R., Wasco, W., Lannfelt, L., Selkoe, D., and Younkin, S., 1996, Secreted amyloid β-protein similar to that in the senile plaques of Alzheimer's Disease is increased *in vivo* by the presenilin 1 and 2 and APP mutations linked to Familial Alzheimer's Disease. *Nat. Med.* 2(8):864–869.

Selkoe, D.J., 1991, The molecular pathology of Alzheimer's Disease. *Neuron* 6:487–488.

Selkoe, D.J., 1996, Amyloid β-protein and the genetics of Alzheimer's Disease. *J. Biol. Chem.* 271(31), 18295–18298.

Suzuki, N., Cheung, T.T., Cai, X.D., Odaka, A., Otvos, L.Jr, Eckman C., Golde, T.E., and Younkin, S.G., 1994, An increased percentage of long amyloid-β protein secreted by Familial Amyloid-β Precursor Protein (βAPP$_{717}$) mutants. *Science* 264:1336–1340.

Tagliavini, F., McArthur, R.A., Canciani, B., Giaccone, G., Porro, M., Bugiani, M., Lievens, P.M., Bugiani, O., Peri, E., Dall'Ara, P., Rocchi, M., Poli, G., Forloni, G., Bandiera, T., Varasi, M., Suarato, A., Cassutti, P., Cervini, M.A., Lansen, J., Salmona, M., and Post, C., 1997, Effectiveness of anthracycline against experimental Prion Disease in Syrian Hamsters. *Science* 276:1119–1122.

Tanzi, R.E., Kovacs, D.M., Kim, T.W., Moir, R.D., Guenette, S.Y., and Wasco, W., 1996, The Presenelin Genes and their Roler in Early-Onset Familial Alzheimer's Disease. *Alz. Dis. Rev.* 1:91–98.

Wisniesky, H.M., and Terry, R.D., 1973, Reexamination of the pathogenesis of the senile plaques. *Prog. Neuropathol.* 11:1–26.

Wisniesky, H.M., Morets, R.C., Lossinsky, A.S., 1981, Evidence for induction of localized amyloid deposits and neuritic plaques by an infectious agent. *Ann. Neurol.* 10:517–522.

30

THE AMINO TERMINUS OF THE β-AMYLOID PEPTIDE CONTAINS AN ESSENTIAL EPITOPE FOR MAINTAINING ITS SOLUBILITY

Beka Solomon,[1] Eilat Hanan,[1] Rela Koppel,[1] Dan Frankel,[1] Ilana Ophir,[2] and Dale Schenck[3]

[1]Department of Molecular Microbiology and Biotechnology
[2]Department of Cell Research and Immunology
Faculty of Life Sciences
Tel-Aviv University
Ramat Aviv 69978, Tel-Aviv, Israel
[3]Athena Neuroscience Inc.
800 Gateway Blvd., South San Francisco, California 94080

INTRODUCTION

Amyloid β-peptide (Aβ) is a normal metabolite of ~4-kDa that is produced by processing a large, transmembrane glycoprotein called amyloid β-protein precursor (AβPP). Once released by proteolytic cleavage of AβPP, the β-peptide may exist in solution (Haas et al. 1992; Seubert et al., 1992). The pathological conditions and mechanisms that transform soluble β-amyloid peptide into the fibrillary, toxic, β-sheet form that is found in plaques and vessels of patients with Alzheimer's disease is not yet completely understood, but clearly the same amino acid sequence of Aβ can have both a fibrillar and a soluble structure.

Many investigators have studied the propensity of Aβ or its fragments to assemble into insoluble aggregates (see Maggio and Mantyh, 1996, for review). The Aβ can exist in two alternative conformations, depending on the secondary structure adopted by the N-terminal domain (Hollossi et al., 1989; Soto et al., 1995) under various environmental conditions (Barrow and Zagorsky, 1991). The N-terminal domain contains sequences that permit the existence of a dynamic equilibrium between the α-helix and the β-strand conformations (Soto et al., 1995). The perturbations of the equilibrium of various conformational states of the β-amyloid peptide can be caused by local pH changes, alterations of environmental hydrophobicity, or binding of other proteins (Soto et al., 1995; Kirschenbaum and Daggett, 1995).

Progress in Alzheimer's and Parkinson's Diseases
edited by Fisher *et al.*, Plenum Press, New York, 1998.

The existence of sequences that are kinetically involved in the folding process has previously been suggested in other systems and has been demonstrated by *in-vitro* denaturation-renaturation experiments (Silen & Agard, 1989). Such sequences, which may play a role in the folding pathway, suggests the possibility that they serve not only for the folding process but also may contribute to the conformational stabilization. Monoclonal antibodies (mAbs) which are able to stabilize the conformation of an antigen against incorrect folding may also recognize an incompletely folded epitope- and induce native conformation in a partially unfolded protein (Blond & Goldberg, 1987; Solomon & Schwartz, 1995). Appropriate mAbs may interact at such strategic sites where protein unfolding is initiated, thereby stabilizing the protein and preventing further precipitation (Solomon & Balas, 1991; Katzav-Gozansky et al., 1996).

We recently reported that the binding of mAbs, which were raised against the synthetic β-amyloid peptide (1–28) prevented the fibrillar aggregation and partially maintained solubility of the β-peptide (Solomon et al., 1996; Hanan & Solomon, 1996). In the present study, we confirmed the presence of the epitopes that exhibit conformational sensitivity and are essential for maintaining peptide solubility. The binding of high-affinity mAbs to such regions may disturb the equilibrium between the end conformations of the peptide and thereby modulate its aggregation.

MATERIALS AND METHODS

The *in-vitro* formation of β-amyloid was induced by incubating β-peptide (1–40) for 3 h at 37°C. To study β-amyloid formation and its inhibition, we prepared immune complexes with a panel of monoclonal antibodies raised against β-amyloid fragments, spanning intact or partial fragments of the N-terminal region of the β-amyloid peptide.

Antibodies

The aggregation of β-amyloid was monitored using a panel of the following five mAbs prepared by Athena Neuroscience, San Francisco, CA. USA: 6C6 and 10D5 were raised against β–peptide (1–28); 2H3, 1C2 and 266 were raised against the respective peptides (1–12) and (13–28). These mAbs have been extensively characterized (Hyman et al., 1992; Seubert et al. 1992: Games et al., 1995) for their specificity for Aβ fragments. The mAb CP4 represents a panel of mAbs raised against carboxypeptidase A selected as unrelated antibody in the following studies (Solomon et al., 1989).

Binding Profile of the Various Monoclonal Antibodies to β-Amyloid Peptide

The β-amyloid peptide used as coating antigen (50 ng/well) was covalently bound to epoxy-coated ELISA plates of 96 wells by incubation for 24 h at 4°C in coating buffer (1M potassium phosphate, pH 7.5) (Solomon et al., 1993). The residual epoxy groups were blocked by incubation with 1% fat milk. Increasing concentrations of the studied mAbs in 100µl final volume were added to wells containing β-peptide bound on the ELISA plates and then incubated for 1 h at 37°C. The apparent binding constants of the antibodies were derived from the reciprocal of the free mAb concentration, at which 50% of maximal binding to β-amyloid peptide was measured (Pinkard and Weir, 1978).

β-Amyloid Peptide Aggregation and Immunocomplexation

The synthetic β-amyloid peptide (Aβ 1–40) was obtained from Sigma Chemical Co., St. Louis, Missouri, USA. Amyloid formation was performed in test-tubes containing 200 μl of a phosphate buffered solution (pH 7.7) of β-amyloid peptide (0.5×10^{-3} M) by incubating for 3 hr at 37°C. Insoluble β-amyloid fractions were removed by centrifugation at 10,000 × g for 5 min, using an Eppendorf centrifuge. To measure the residual soluble β-amyloid peptide, increasing amounts of the appropriate mAbs were added until saturation was reached. In another set of experiments, mAbs at equimolar antibody/antigen ratio were added to the reaction mixtures before the first incubation period of 3 hr at 37°C. The amount of soluble β-amyloid peptide remaining after exposure to 37°C for 3 h in the presence and absence of the various mAbs was determined by an ELISA assay using rabbit polyclonal anti-β-amyloid as the coating antibody (Solomon et al., 1996).

β-Amyloid Fibril Formation Was Assessed by

Electron Microscopy. Negatively stained amyloid fibrils were prepared by floating carbon-coated grids on aqueous peptide solutions (1 mg/ml) and air drying. β-amyloid samples, either alone or immunocomplexed to mAb 6C6 (molar ratio 4:1) exposed for 3 h at 37°C, were negatively stained with aqueous uranyl acetate (2 wt/vol) and then visualized using a JEOL-1200 EX electron microscope operated at 80/KV, at a magnification of 80,000.

Fluorimetry. Fluorimetric analysis of soluble β-amyloid peptide and the immunocomplexes of all the studied antibodies (molar ratio Aβ/Ab 4:1) stained with Thioflavin T (Sigma Chemical Co., Lt. Louis, MO., USA) were performed by standard methods (LeVine, 1993). Fluorescence was measured using a Perkin-Elmer LS-50 fluorimeter at λ_{ex} = 435 nm and λ_{em} = 485 nm. Aliquots of aqueous solutions of β-amyloid peptide, 15 μg/50 μl alone or complexed with the respective monoclonal antibodies were exposed for the 7 days at 37°C. The fluorescence of each reaction mixture was measured after addition of 1 ml ThT (3 μM in 50 mM sodium phosphate buffer pH 6.0).

RESULTS

Characterization of Monoclonal Antibodies against β-Amyloid Peptide

The specificity of the studied monoclonal antibodies towards various peptides located in the N-terminal region of Aβ is summarized in Table 1. The apparent binding constant of the antibodies that bind to regions (1–12) and (1–16) are at least of two orders of magnitude higher than those that bind to regions (13–28) of the β-peptide (Table 1).

Effect of Immunocomplexation on the *in-Vitro* Aggregation of β-Amyloid Peptide

The panel of monoclonal antibodies used in this study maintain at different extents the solubility of the β-amyloid peptide under the experimental conditions employed. The mAbs 6C6 and 10D5, which recognize an epitope spanning the amino acid residues 1–16 (Seubert et al., 1992) of the β-amyloid peptide, inhibited the formation of β-amyloid by

Table 1. Relation between the binding characteristics
of site-directed monoclonal antibodies and prevention
of β-amyloid-peptide aggregation

Monoclonal antibody	Epitope location	Approximate binding constant (M^{-1})	Soluble β-amyloid peptide detected in the presence of antibodies (%)[b]
6C6	1–16[a]	≈4.0 × 10⁹	70 ± 10
10D5	1–16	≈1.5 × 10⁹	75 ± 5
2H3	1–12	≈2.5 × 10⁹	30 ± 10
266	13–28	≈8.0 × 10⁷	20 ± 5
1C2	13–28	≈1.50 × 10⁸	10 ± 10

[a]Sequence of amino acids related to respective fragments of Aβ.
[b]The percentage of soluble β-amyloid peptide found in the supernatant is related to the same amount of soluble peptide bound directly to the antibody-coated ELISA plate.

maintaining 70% to 80% of the β-peptide in solution relative to the aggregation occurring in the absence of the respective antibodies (Table 1). The antibodies 1C2 and 266, directed to the region comprising peptides 13–28, had a considerably low solubilization effect. The mAb 2H3, despite a high binding constant, is less effective, in spite of epitope proximity to the mAbs 6C6 and 10D5.

Monoclonal Antibodies Inhibit the Formation of Fibrillar β-Amyloid

Electron microscopy of negatively stained β-amyloid and its immunocomplex with mAb 6C6 revealed that the fibrillar β-amyloid conformation, which formed in the absence of antibodies, was converted to an amorphous state in the presence of the mAbs (Fig. 1). Thioflavin T, a suitable probe for the quantitative evaluation of the fibrillar aggregation of β-amyloid peptide, confirmed the electron microscopy results (Fig. 2). Binding to the fibrillar β-amyloid enhanced the fluorescence emission of Thioflavin T at 485 nm as a function of incubation time at 37°C and concentration of β-amyloid (see insert of Fig. 2). Thioflavin T based fluorometric assay of β-amyloid aggregation was measured in the presence of mAbs raised against β-amyloid peptide and CP4 selected as representative of a panel of unrelated antibodies. Adding each of the studied antibodies at relatively low concentrations to the solution of Aβ before exposure to 37°C inhibited the fluorescence at 485 nm to a different extent and interfered with fibril formation, despite the failure to maintain peptide solubility. The addition of unrelated antibody did not interfere with the ThT fluorescence intensity (Fig. 2).

DISCUSSION

The involvement of the N-terminal region in the conformational transformations of Aβ was confirmed by studies using synthetic peptides bearing the Aβ sequence in various solvents and in studies with synthetic Aβ peptides containing single amino acid substitutions (Kirschner et al., 1987; Wood et al., 1995). The polar domain of Aβ (1–28) is capable of stable self-association to form fibrils at acid pH, even in the absence of the stabilizing influence of the hydrophobic carboxyl terminus (Kirshenbaum & Daggett, 1995). The importance of the N-terminal region in maintaining the solubility of the β-pep-

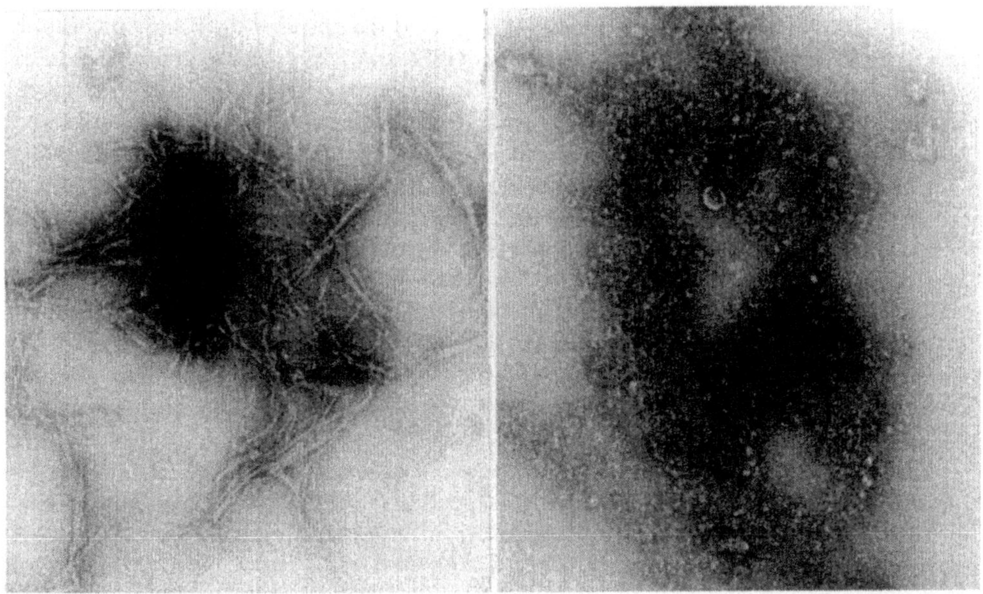

Figure 1. Electron micrographs of β-amyloid aggregates in the absence (left) and in the presence of mAb 6C6 (right) at magnification × 80,000.

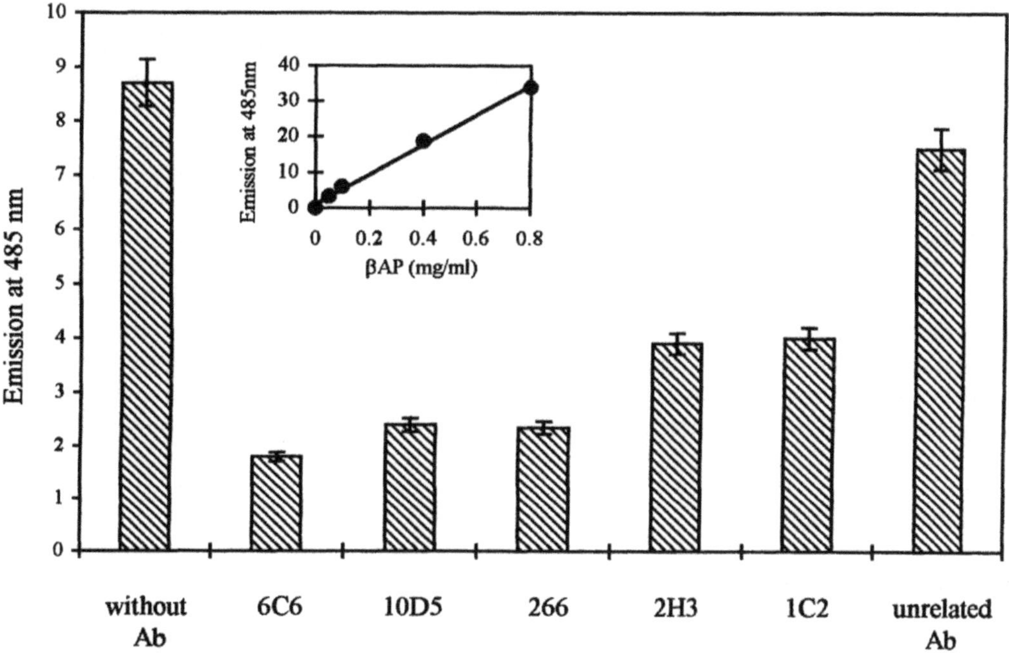

Figure 2. Thioflavin T based fluorometric assay of β-amyloid aggregation measured in the presence of mAbs. The insert represents the dependence of ThT fluorescence intensity on the β-amyloid concentration.

tide has recently been confirmed by studies demonstrating that amino-terminal deletions within the (1–12) and (1–17) peptides enhance the aggregation of the β-amyloid peptide *in vitro* in parallel with the neurotoxicity effect (Pike et al., 1995). The conformation of the β-peptide in solution is mostly random coil, seeded with a low percentage of β-sheet and α-helical conformations and the N-terminal domain permits the existence of a dynamic equilibrium between the α-helix and β strand. A single mutation of Val-18 to Ala induces a significant increment of the α-helical content of Aβ and reduces its ability to form amyloid fibrils (Soto et al, 1995). By contrast, the exchange of glutamine for glutamic acid at residue 22 (Dutch variant) leads to an increase in amyloid formation. These local substitutions did not significantly modify the ionic and hydrophobic properties of Aβ but increased the α-helical or β-sheet content of Aβ. It is possible that small changes in the secondary structure of the N-terminus are directly related to amyloid formation. It should be mentioned that the difference between rodent and human Aβ, which differ at positions 5, 10, and 13, suggest the importance of this region of Aβ in amyloidosis because rodents did not develop brain amyloid (Dyrks et al., 1993).

In view of the importance of the N-terminal fragment in amyloid formation we investigated the interaction of synthetic β-amyloid-peptide (1–40) with a panel of monoclonal antibodies raised against the region comprising amino acids (1–28) as well as other small related peptides. Binding studies performed suggested that at least one epitope is essential for maintaining the solubility of the whole peptide. This epitope was revealed only when large fragments of the β-amyloid peptide were used for immunization. The mAbs 6C6 and 10D5, which bound to an epitope located in the (1–16) region, prevented *in-vitro* β-amyloid (1–40) formation and maintained the peptide's solubility. Monoclonal antibody 2H3, which binds to an epitope located in region (1–12), which is different from the epitopes recognized by mAbs 6C6 and 10D5, interfered with fibrillar formation but did not maintain peptide solubility. The other mAbs studied, 266 and 1C2 (raised against β-peptide amino acids 13–28) exhibited only a low protective effect on β–amyloid peptide solubility.

That a peptide obtains a definite conformation when interacting with a molecule inducing conformational change is well established (Chaiken et al., 1987). Such a molecule can be a protein that interacts with the peptide, a surface, or changes in solvent polarity. When interacting with an antibody, the peptide changes its conformation from random coil to an "end conformation" that is recognized by the antibody. The antibody, which maintains the solubility of the peptide may shift the equilibrium toward a soluble conformation and increase the α-helix content, which it recognizes and stabilizes.

If amyloid formation is indeed sensitive to the secondary structure that is adopted by the N-terminal domain of Aβ as recently proposed (Soto et al., 1995), then the compounds that promote the α-helical or other soluble and stable conformations could prevent the fibrillar deposition of β-amyloid peptide. Pathological chaperones increase the content of β-sheet conformation (Soto et al., 1996) parallel to amyloid formation, while site-directed mAbs may promote the soluble conformation and thus have therapeutic importance.

REFERENCES

Barrow, C.J., and Zagorski, M.G., 1991, Solution structures of β-peptide and its constituent fragments: Relation to amyloid deposition. *Science* 253:179.

Blond, S., and Goldberg, M., 1987, Partly native epitopes are already present on early intermediates in the folding of tryptophan synthase. *Proc. Natl. Acad. Sci. USA* 84:1147.

Chaiken, I, Chiancone, E., Fontana, A., and Neri, P. ,eds., 1987, *Macromolecular Biorecognition, Principles and Methods.* The Humana Press Inc., Clifton, NJ.

Dyrks, T., Dyrks, E., Masters, C.L., and Beyreuther, C., 1993, Amyloidogenicity of rodent and human β-amyloid sequences. *FEBS Lett* 324:231.

Games, D., Adams, D., Alessandrini, R., Barbour, R., Berthelette, P., Blackwell, C., et al., 1995, Alzheimer-type neuropathology in transgenic mice overexpressing V717F β-amyloid precursor protein. *Nature* 373:523.

Haass, C., Schlossmacher, M.G., Hung, A.Y., Vigo-Pelfrey, C., Mellon, A., Ostaszewski, B. L., Lieberburg, I., Koo, E.H., Schenk, D., Teplow., D.B., and Selkoe D.J., 1992, Amyloid β-peptide is produced by cultured cells during normal metabolism. *Nature* 359:322.

Hanan, E., and Solomon, B., 1996, Protective effect of monoclonal antibodies against Alzheimer's β-amyloid aggregation. *Amyloid. Int. J. Exp. Clin. Invest.* 3:130.

Hollosi, M., Otvos, L., Kajtar, J., Percell, A., and Lee, V.M.Y., 1989, Is amyloid deposition in Alzheimer's disease preceded by an environment induced double conformational transition? *Pept. Res.* 2:109.

Hyman, B.T., Tanzi, R.B., Marxloff, K., Barbour, R., and Schenk, D.B., 1992, Kunitz protease inhibitor-containing amyloid β-protein precursor immunoreactivity in Alzheimer's disease. *J. Neuropath. Exp. Neurol.* 51:76.

Katzav-Gozansky, T., Hanan, E., and Solomon, B., 1996, Effect of monoclonal antibodies in preventing carboxypeptidase A aggregation. *Biotechnol. Appl. Biochem.* 23:227.

Kirschner, D.A., Inouye, H., Duffy, L.K., Sinclair, A., Lind, M., and Selkoe, D.J., 1987, Synthetic peptide homologous to β-protein from Alzheimer disease forms amyloid-like fibers *in vitro. Proc. Natl. Acad. Sci. USA*, 84:6953.

Kirshenbaum, K., and Daggett, V., 1995, pH-Dependent conformations of the amyloid β(1–28) peptide fragment explored using molecular dynamics. *Biochemistry* 34:7629.

LeVine II, H., 1993, Thioflavine T interaction with synthetic Alzheimer's disease β-amyloid peptides: Detection of amyloid aggregation in solution. *Protein Science* 2:404.

Maggio, J.E., and Mantyh, P.W., 1996, Brain amyloid—A physicochemical perspective. *Brain Pathol.* 6: 147.

Pike, C.J., Overman, M.J., and Cotman, C.W., 1995, Amino-terminal deletions enhance aggregation of β-amyloid peptides *in vitro. J. Biol. Chem.* 270:23895–23898.

Pinkard, R.N., and Weir, D.M., 1978, In: *Handbook of Experimental Immunology*, Weir, D.M., ed., *Blackwell Scientific*, Oxford, 16:1–16.20.

Seubert, P., Vigo-Pelfrey, C., Esch, F., Lee, M., Dovey, H., Davis, D., Sinha, S., Schlossmacher, M., Whaley, J., Swindlehurst, C., McCormack, R., Wolfert, R., Selkoe, D., Lieberburg, I., and Schenk, D., 1992, Isolation and quantification of soluble Alzheimer's β-peptide from biological fluids, *Nature* 359: 325.

Silen, J.L., and Agard, D.A., 1989, The x-lytic protease pro-region does not require a physical linkage to activate the protease domain *in vivo*. Nature 341:462.

Solomon, B., Koppel, R., Kenett, D., and Fleminger, G., 1989, Localization of a highly immunogenic region of carboxypeptidase A recognized by three different monoclonal antibodies and their use in the detection of subtle conformational alterations in this enzyme region. *Biochemistry,* 28:1235.

Solomon, B., and Balas, N., 1991, Thermostabilization of carboxypeptidase A by interaction with its monoclonal antibodies. *Biotechnol. Appl. Biochem.* 14:202.

Solomon, B., Schmitt, S., Schwartz, F., Levi, A., and Fleminger, G., 1993, Eupergit C- coated membranes as solid support for a sensitive immunoassay of human albumin. *J. Immunol. Meth.* 157:209.

Solomon, B., and Schwartz, F., 1995, Chaperone-like effect of monoclonal antibodies on refolding of heat-denatured carboxypeptidase A. *J. Mol. Recogn.* 8:72.

Solomon, B., Koppel, R., Hanan, E., and Katzav, T., 1996, Monoclonal antibodies inhibit *in-vitro* fibrillar aggregation of the Alzheimer's β-amyloid peptide. *Proc. Natl. Acad. Sci. USA.,* 93:452.

Soto, C., Castano, E.M., Frangione, B., and Inestrosa, N.C, 1995, The α-helical to β-strand transition in the amino-terminal fragment of the amyloid β-peptide modulates amyloid formation. *J. Biol. Chem.* 270: 3063.

Soto, C., Golabek, A., Wisniewski ,T., and Castano, E.M., 1996. Alzheimer's β-amyloid peptide is conformationally modified by apolipoprotein E *in vitro. Mol. Neurosci.* 7:721.

Wood, S.J., Wetzel, R., Martin, J.D., and Hurle, M.R., 1995 Prolines and amyloidogenicity in fragments of the Alzheimer's peptide β/A4. *Biochemistry* 34:724.

31

ANIMAL MODELS OF AMYLOID AGGREGATION AND DEPOSITION

Robert Kisilevsky

Department of Pathology
Queen's University
and
The Syl and Molly Apps Research Center
Kingston General Hospital
Kingston, Ontario, Canada, K7L 3N6

INTRODUCTION

Amyloid was for more than a century considered to be an interesting, unique, but inconsequential tissue deposit which rarely caused significant clinical problems. We now recognize that there are many forms of amyloid. Amyloid represents a uniform organization of a disease-, or pathological process-, specific protein which is combined with a set of common structural components. Furthermore, amyloid is not the rare entity it was originally thought to be. It has become implicated in the pathogenesis of diseases which affect millions of patients. These range from common disorders such as Alzheimer's diseases, adult-onset diabetes, and consequences of prolonged dialysis, to the historically recognized rare systemic forms associated with inflammation and plasma cell disturbances. Strong evidence is emerging that even when amyloid is deposited in local organ sites significant physiologic effects may ensue. By all criteria, such as scientific curiosity, incidence, medical importance, and commercial markets, amyloid has come of age.

Definition of Amyloid

Amyloid is defined by its tinctotrial, ultrastructural, and protein conformational features. These include; a) an amorphous appearance by light microscopy when using routine protein stains; b) positive staining with Congo red which when viewed in polarized light imparts to the amyloid a red/green birefringence (i.e. changing the orientation of the polarized light by 90° reverses the two colors); c) a fibrillar appearance ultrastructurally with the fibrils being on average 10 nm in diameter and of varying length; and d) the fibrils ex-

Progress in Alzheimer's and Parkinson's Diseases
edited by Fisher *et al.*, Plenum Press, New York, 1998.

amined by infra-red or X-ray diffraction techniques exhibit spectra characteristic of proteins with a predominance of crossed-β-pleated sheets. It is precisely these common characteristics that originally led to the faulty conclusion that amyloid was a single entity.

Classification

Amyloid, as we now recognize it, is a generic term for usually extracellular tissue deposits with the defining characteristics outlined above. At least 17–18 different proteins have been identified as being responsible for these deposits (Husby, 1994). Each protein is associated with a different disease. Where there is a common protein in seemingly different diseases a common pathologic process is operating in these different disorders. For example, the AA form of amyloid occurs in leprosy, osteomyelitis, tuberculosis, and cystic fibrosis. The common pathologic process in each of these diseases is persistent acute inflammation, the antecedent of AA amyloidosis.

The classification of the amyloids is no longer based on their clinical features. Rather, the nature of the protein responsible for the amyloid has become the determining criterion. A modification of the World Health Organization's Classification is illustrated in Table 1 (Kazatchkine et al., 1993), which illustrates the diversity of the proteins capable of amyloid formation, that many are normal proteins, and that proteolytic processing of precursors is not a universal feature of all forms of amyloidogenesis.

ANIMAL MODELS

Though 18 forms of amyloid have been identified to date, only 7 are described as occuring naturally in animals. Among these are two that are found only in animals and

Table 1. Classification of amyloids

Amyloid protein	Protein precursor	Protein variant	Clinical setting
AA	SAA	SAA1/SAA2	Persistent acute inflammation
AL	κ or λ light chain		Multiple myeloma, plasma cell dyscrasias, and primary amyloid
AH	γ chain		Waldenstom's macroglobulinemia
ATTR	Transthyretin (TTR)	60 mutants	Familial amyloid polyneuropathy (FAP)
		normal TTR	Senile systemic amyloid
AApoAI	apoAI	Arg 26	FAP Iowa
AGel	Gelsolin	Asn 187	Familial amyloid, Finnish
ACys	Cystatin C	Gln 68	Hereditary cerebral hemorrhage with amyloid (HCHWA), Icelandic
ALys	Lysozyme	Thr 56	Hereditary systemic amyloid, Ostertag-type
AFib	Fibrinogen	Leu 554	Hereditary renal amyloid
Aβ	β-protein precursor	several mutants	Alzheimer's disease
			Down's syndrome, HCHWA Dutch
APrP	Prion protein	several mutants	CJD*, scrapie, BSE*, GSS*, Kuru
APro	Prolactin		Pituitary amyloid in the aged
ACal	(Pro)calcitonin		Medullary carcinoma of the thyroid
AANF	Atrial naturetic factor		Isolated atrial amyloid
AIAPP	Islet amyloid polypeptide		Type II Diabetes, insulinomas
AIns	Insulin		Islet amyloid in the degu (a rodent)
AApoAII	ApoAII (murine)	Gln 5	Amyloid in senescence accelerated mice

*CJD: Creutzfelt Jacob Disease; BSE: Bovine Spongiform Encephalopathy; GSS: Gerstmann Straussler Sheinker Syndrome.

Table 2. Animal models of amyloidosis

Form of amyloid	Animal model
AIns	Degu
AApoA-II	Murine Accelerated Senescence
AL	Natural/human L-chain infusion
APrP	Natural/intra- and inter species transfer
ATTR	Transthyretin transgenics
AIAPP	Natural/amylin transgenics
Aβ	Natural/βPP transgenics
AA	Natural/rapid induction regimen

which from a human perspective may therefore be strictly of scientific interest. Five forms mimic their human counterpart, three of which can be induced with appropriate protocols in susceptible species. Among these five, two successful transgenics have been generated, and an additional transgenic has been successfully raised in one form of amyloid which is normally found only in humans. The strength and weaknesses of each of these 8 animal models (Table 2) is considered briefly below.

Insulin (AIns)

This form of amyloid has been described only in the Degu (a rodent) (Hellman et al., 1990). It may be associated with diabetes in these animals, and it illustrates that insulin may be amyloidogeneic. At present it is a curiosity and as a model of amyloidogenesis does not offer any advantages over other animal models.

Apolipoprotein A-II (AApoA-II)

AApoA-II amyloidosis is associated with murine accelerated senescence (Higuchi et al., 1986a; Higuchi et al., 1991). In this murine disorder a mutation in ApoA-II at Gln5/Pro is responsible for the amyloidogenic properties of ApoA-II (Higuchi et al., 1986b). The amyloid is deposited in a systemic fashion, but not in the CNS. These animals do not develop amyloid until 8–12 months of age. The mutation is also responsible for a more rapid turnover of plasma ApoA-II (Naiki et al., 1988), and it is this feature rather than amyloid deposition that may be responsible for the accelerated senescence. At present it is not possible to manipulate this murine disease, which restricts the investigation of accelerated senescence to one of observation. This disorder does not have a human counterpart.

Light Chain (AL)

AL amyloidosis is the form found in humans associated with plasma cell dyscrasias and primary amyloidosis, which is probably a variant in which the amyloid appears before the plasma cell disturbance. This form of amyloid is deposited in a systemic, or local, distribution, but not the CNS. It has also been described naturally in dogs, cats, and horses (Linke et al., 1991; Breuer et al., 1993; Liepnieks et al., 1996), all of which are unwieldy as animals models. The precursor protein is the immunoglobulin L-chain (both kappa and lambda) only some of which are amyloidogenic. The amyloidogenicity resides in the variable end of the L-chain. This structural difference means that the protein varies from patient to patient as well as species to species. It introduces a confounding factor, namely a different amyloid protein for each patient or individual animal, that is clearly difficult to control. Nevertheless, there are bone marrow and macrophage culture systems of AL amyloid which can be manipulated experimentally so as to investigate the factors responsible AL amyloidogenesis (Durie et al., 1982; Tagouri et al., 1996). Attempts have also been made to produce a murine model of AL amyloid by the intravenous infusion of human amyloidogenic L-chains (Solomon et al., 1992). Unfortunately the quantity of protein required is large (100 mg/day for 12 weeks). Such treatment does lead to murine AL amyloid deposited in a systemic fashion. Administration of non-amyloidogenic L-chains fails to elicit this response. The reproducibilty of this protocol has been questioned by investigators.

Prion (APrP)

Prions, their relationship to various forms of human and animal spongioform encephalopathy (SE), and their potential for causing epidemic degenerative neurological disease, have been the subject of several recent reviews (Ghetti et al., 1996; Prusiner et al., 1996; Prusiner, 1996). Whether the degenerative brain disease is due to the prion protein's amyloidogenic potential is still contentious. Nevertheless, this protein does have the potential to form brain amyloid deposits, and the process (as well as the SE) may be induced by the injection of exogenous prion particles. The injected exogenous prion protein in its amyloid(?) conformation appears to serve as a template for endogenously synthesized prion protein to reconfigure itself into particles with neuropathological properties. APrP and AA amyloid (to be described below) are the only two animal models of amyloidogenesis in which the induction may be manipulated. This is a significant advantage in that one is not dependent on the natural occurence of this disorder for its study. However, in contrast to AA, which may be induced in 18–48h, APrP takes weeks to months to appear in tissues. APrP animal models may be supplemented with *in-vitro* and culture systems, which allows one to study this form of amyloidogenesis at varying levels of complexity, from "simplified" pure protein systems to intact living organisms. Because this form of amyloid occurs in the CNS it may prove useful as a model to examine anti-amyloid agents not only for their efficacy, but also their ability to cross the blood brain barrier. These feature are significant advantages. The "infectious" nature, and cross-species infectivity of this form of amyloid may, however, pose a problem for investigators.

Transthyretin (ATTR)

In humans ATTR falls into two braod categories, those in which transthyretin posseses a mutation and those in which ATTR is composed of the "wild type" protein (Saraiva, 1995; Benson and Uemichi, 1996). The former are usually associated with familial amyloid polyneuropathy (FAP) or familial cardiac amyloid, whereas the latter are seen in senile cardiac and senile systemic amyloid. This disorder has not been described as a natural one in animals. Transgenic animal models have been developed. In particular the met30/val mutation, the most common cause of FAP has been established in mice (Yamamura et al., 1993; Nagata et al., 1995). Animals manifest amyloid only 8–10 month following birth. Rather than developing amyloid primarily in the peripheral nervous system, as in humans, these animals show a systemic distribution. The factors responsible for the specific anatomic distribution of ATTR have not been established. Transgenics mice involving the "wild type" transthyretin have been developed recently (J. Buxbaum, personal communication). Little additional information is available at this in time. At present neither of these models can be manipulated experimentally and one is restricted to the use of observational techniques over time.

Significant work has been accomplished with *in-vitro* models of ATTR. Transthyretin circulates as a tetramer, and there is a body of information demonstrating that the stability of the tetramer is inversely related to the amyloidogenic potential of transthyretin (Mccutchen et al., 1993; Colon et al., 1996). The more stable the complex the less likely ATTR will occur. *In-vivo* and *in-vitro* comparisons will therefore be possible.

Amylin/IAPP (AIAPP)

In Humans the AIAPP form of pancreatic amyloid is associated with adult onset diabetes mellitus. This form of amyloid has also been described in cats, and monkeys (Johnson et al., 1996). The amyloidogenic potential resides in the sequence -GAILS- found in residues 25–29 of amylin which is found only in those species which develop AIAPP (Westermark et al., 1990). Rodents amylin does not normally carry this sequence, but human IAPP (hIAPP) base sequences coupled to a rodents insulin promoter have been established in mice. Such transgenics produce large quantites of the potentially amyloidogenic hIAPP in the islets of Langerhans. They do not, however develop pancreatic AIAPP and diabetes unless they are on a fat diet greater than 4.5% (Verchere et al., 1996). This provides a model to study AIAPP and its possible relationship to diabetes. Dependency on the diet allows the initiation of AIAPP and diabetes to be induced at the will of the investigator. It is not yet clear what will happen to existing amyloid deposits, and the diabetes, if the fat content of the diet is reduced. In vitro islet culture techniques and IAPP fibrillogenic procedures are available to study amyloidogenesis in simpler systems, and provide an important supplement to the animal model (Clark et al., 1993).

β-Protein (Aβ)

The study of Aβ amyloidogenesis has become a, if not the, prime focus of Alzheimer's (AD) research. Genetic evidence (Roses, 1996; Levy-Lahad and Bird, 1996), as well as toxicity of Aβ vis-a-vis neuronal cells in culture (Lorenzo and Yankner, 1994), indicate that Aβ, just as other forms of amyloid, are noxious to cells in their immediate microenvironment. Aβ is probably the most common form of amyloid, and is associated not only with AD but with familial forms of congophilic angiopathy. The amyloid associated with AD has been described in naturally aged dogs and primates (Martin et al., 1991; Bons et al., 1992; Cummings et al., 1993; Gearing et al., 1994). However, these species do not develop these features for many years after birth, and are unwieldy as experimental subjects. Notwithstanding the information being generated from in-vitro studies, the lack of an experimentally manipulatable animal model for the *in-vivo* study of AD has slowed pathogenetic understanding as well as efforts to intervene with this disease process. It is for this reason that attempts have been made to construct murine transgenics with sequences coding for Aβ, or significantly larger portions of the human β-protein precursor (βPP) gene. The subject has been reviewed in great depth recently (Greenberg et al., 1996). With the exception of two recent reports many past attempts have been deficient in one or more respects. These have ranged from a failure to express the relevant mRNA, the relevant protein, the relevant pathology or the behavioral alterations.

The reports by Games et al (Ikeda et al., 1994), and Hsiao et al (Hsiao et al., 1996), appear to have met many of the criteria necessary for a valid transgenic rodent model of AD. In the first report full length βPP-695 containing the human mutant Val717/Phe (i.e near the gamma-secretase site) was expressed as a chimeric cDNA transgene. A PDGF-β promoter was used to drive neuron specific expression. These mice over-expressed the transgene and the 1–40 and 1–42 Aβ peptides. After 6–9 months Aβ amyloid deposits appeared which with time increased in quantity, and were associated with an astrocytic reaction and a reduction of synaptic density. Deficits in learning have yet to be reposted. In the second report a murine transgenic of a βPP-695 human isoform containing two mutations, Lys670/Asn and Met671/Leu, (i.e. near the β-secretase site) deveolped impaired learning by 9–10 months, accompanied by a 5 fold increase in Aβ(1–40) and a 14 fold increase in Aβ(1–42). These mice also exhibited Aβ amyloid deposits in the limbic and cortical structures.

These transgenic murine models, in conjuction with *in-vitro* studies with purified peptides, and associated components common to all amyloids, may provide the basis for pathogenetic understanding and pharmacological interference of AD. Nevertheless, the relatively long period of time necessary for these animals to develop Aβ amyloid and the features of AD, and the present inability to experimentally manipulate the induction of Aβ amyloid, tempers the use of these animal models for pathogenetic studies and as screens for anti-amyloid agents.

Inflammation-Associated (AA)

Animal models of AA amyloidosis have been available for over 100 years. They mimic the human situation closely and are probably the best studied form of amyloidosis. Sufficient information has been gathered to understand AA amyloidogenesis *in-vivo* in fair detail (Kisilevsky and Young, 1994), which in turn has provided pathogenetic understanding of other forms of amyloid. This information has allowed investigators to induce histologically demonstrable murine AA amyloid in 36–48h (Axelrad et al., 1982). With more sophisticated techniques amyloid is detectable in 18h (Graether et al., 1996). Furthermore, one can turn the induction process on and off at will so that amyloid deposition and removal may both be studied. The speed of induction has allowed the separation of important from epigenetic factors. These studies have shown that AA induction requires an adequate precursor pool, but a pool even 1000 fold higher than normal is, on its own, insufficient to cause amyloidosis (Kisilevsky and Young, 1994). Micrenvironmental facctors are critical. A nucleating step for fibrillogenesis is required (Kisilevsky and Boudreau, 1983). This *in-vivo* feature matches *in-vitro* data obtained from the study of many other amyloids. These AA models have also identified a set of components which are found in all amyloid. These include the structural components of basement membranes; namely heparan sulphate proteoglycan (HSPG), laminin, collagen IV and serum amyloid P (SAP), and apo E (Baltz et al., 1986; Lyon et al., 1991; Gallo et al., 1994). With these models it was possible to show that the interaction of heparan sulphate with the AA precursor, serum amyloid A, prompted the precursor to change conformation taking on the increased β-sheet characteristics common to amyloid (McCubbin et al., 1988). Similar studies have now been done with Aβ and βPP [(Narindrasorasak et al., 1995), and Fraser and Kisilevsky unpublished results]. The HSPG perlecan has now been identified in most amyloids. The heparan sulphate binding motif is common to more than half the known forms of amyloid precursors, which has suggested that agents that mimic aspects of heparan sulphate structure may prove to have anti-amyloid properties. This has been substantiated with many forms of amyloid (Kisilevsky, 1996).

Several short-comings of this model include the lack of a good *in-vitro* counterpart for AA amyloidogenesis. And, from the perspective of AD, this form of amyloid does not affect the CNS. Nevertheless, the speed with which anti-amyloid compounds may be assessed *in-vivo* (1 week), the involvement of components apparently common to all amyloids, and a satisfying correlation between effects seen *in-vivo* with AA and *in-vitro* with Aβ (Kisilevsky, Fraser, Chakrabarthy, and Szarek, unpublished results) attest to its usefulness.

SUMMARY

In the last 5 years much progress has been made in developing murine models of several forms of amyloid. In most cases these models reflect their human counterparts, and show not only amyloid's diversity, but the common structural and pathogenetic aspects of amyloidogenesis. It is these shared featured, and common pathogenetic mechanisms, that should encourage investigators to borrow concepts and observations from among the various models and apply them to their own particular interests.

REFERENCES

Axelrad, M.A., Kisilevsky, R., Willmer, J., Chen, S.J., and Skinner, M., 1982, Further characterization of amyloid enhancing factor, *Lab. Invest.* 47:139–146.

Baltz, M.L., Caspi, D., Evans, D.J., Rowe, I.F., Hind, C.R.K., and Pepys, M.B., 1986, Ciculating amyloid P component is the precursor of amyloid P component in tissue amyloid deposits, *Clin. Exp. Immunol.* 66:691–700.

Benson, M.D., and Uemichi, T., 1996, Transthyretin amyloidosis, *Amyloid* 3:44–56.

Bons, N., Mestre, N., and Petter, A., 1992, Senile Plaques and Neurofibrillary Changes in the Brain of an Aged Lemurian Primate, Microcebus-Murinus, *Neurobiol. Aging* 13:99–105.

Breuer, W., Colbatzky, F., Platz, S., and Hermanns, W., 1993, Immunoglobulin-Producing Tumours in Dogs and Cats, *J. Comp. Pathol.* 109:203–216.

Clark, A., Dekoning, E.JP., and Morris, J.F., 1993, Formation of Islet Amyloid from Islet Amyloid Polypeptide, *Biochem. Soc. Trans.* 21:169–176.

Colon, W., Lai, Z.H., Mccutchen, S.L., Miroy, G.J., Strang, C., and Kelly, J.W., 1996, FAP mutations destabilize transthyretin facilitating conformational changes required for amyloid formation, *Ciba Foundation Symposium* 199:228–242.

Cummings, B.J., Su, J.H., Cotman, C.W., White, R., and Russell, M.J., 1993, beta-Amyloid Accumulation in Aged Canine Brain - A Model of Early Plaque Formation in Alzheimer's Disease, *Neurobiol. Aging* 14:547–560.

Durie, B.G.M., Persky, B., Soehnlen, B.J., Grogan, T.M., and Salmon, S.E., 1982, Amyloid production in human myeloma stem-cell culture, with morphologic evidence of amyloid secretion by associated macrophages, *N. Engl. J. Med.* 307:1689–1692.

Gallo, G., Wisniewski, T., Choi-Miura, N.H., Ghiso, J., and Frangione, B., 1994, Potential role of apolipoprotein-E in fibrillogenesis, *Am. J. Pathol.* 145:526–530.

Gearing, M., Rebeck, G.W., Hyman, B.T., Tigges, J., and Mirra, S.S., 1994, Neuropathology and apolipoprotein E profile of aged chimpanzees: Implications for Alzheimer disease, *Proc. Natl. Acad. Sci. USA* 91:9382–9386.

Ghetti, B., Piccardo, P., Frangione, B., Bugiani, O., Giaccone, G., Young, K., Prelli, F., Farlow, M.R., Dlouhy, S.R., and Tagliavini, F., 1996, Prion protein amyloidosis, *Brain Pathol.* 6:127–145.

Graether, S.P., Young, I.D., and Kisilevsky, R., 1996, Early detection of inflammation-associated amyloid in murine spleen using thioflavin T fluorescence of spleen homogenates: Implications for amyloidogenesis, *Amyloid* 3:20–27.

Greenberg, B.D., Savage, M.J., Howland, D.S., Ali, S.M., Siedlak, S.L., Perry, G., Siman, R., and Scott, R.W., 1996, APP transgenesis: Approaches toward the development of animal models for Alzheimer disease neuropathology, *Neurobiol. Aging* 17:153–171.

Hellman, U., Wernstedt, C., Westermark, P., Obrien, T.D., Rathbun, W.B., and Johnson, K.H., 1990, Amino Acid Sequence from Degu Islet Amyloid-Derived Insulin Shows Unique Sequence Characteristics, *Biochem. Biophys. Res. Commun.* 169:571–577.

Higuchi, K., Yonezu, T., Kogishi, K., Matsumura, A., Takeshita, S., Higuchi, Ka., Kohno, A., Matsushita, M., Hosakawa, M., and Takeda, T., 1986a, Purification and characterization of a senile amyloid related antigenic substance (apoSASsam) from mouse serum. ApoSASsam is an apoA-II apolipoprotein of mouse high density lipoproteins, *J. Biol. Chem.* 261:12834–12840.

Higuchi, K., Yonezu, T., Tsunasawa, S., Sakiyama, F., and Takeda, T., 1986b, The single proline-glutamine substitution at position 5 enhances the potency of amyloid fibril formation of murine apoA-II, *FEBS Lett.* 207:23–27.

Higuchi, K., Naiki, H., Kitagawa, K., Hosokawa, M., and Takeda, T., 1991, Mouse Senile Amyloidosis - ASSAM Amyloidosis in Mice Presents Universally As a Systemic Age-Associated Amyloidosis, *Virchows Arch. B Cell Pathol.* 60:231–238.

Hsiao, K., Chapman, P., Nilsen, S., Eckman, C., Harigaya, Y., Younkin, S., Yang, F.S., and Cole, G., 1996, Correlative memory deficits, Aβ elevation, and amyloid plaques in transgenic mice, *Science* 274:99–102.

Husby, G., 1994. Classification of Amyloidosis. In: *Clinical Rheumatology: Vol.8 No.3, Reactive Amyloidosis and the Acute Phase Response*, Husby, G., Ed., Bailliere Tindall, London, pp. 503–511.

Ikeda, S., Tokuda, T., Yanagisawa, N., Kametani, F., Ohshima, T., and Allsop, D., 1994, Variability of beta-amyloid protein deposited lesions in Down's syndrome brains, *Tohoku J. Exp. Med.* 174:189–198. Johnson, K.H., Westermark, P., Sletten, K., and Obrien, T.D., 1996, Amyloid proteins and amyloidosis in domestic animals, *Amyloid* 3:270–289.

Kazatchkine, M.D., Husby, G., Araki, S., Benditt, E.P., Benson, M.D., Cohen, A.S., Frangione, B., Glenner, G.G., Natvig, J.B., and Westermark, P., 1993, Nomenclature of Amyloid and Amyloidosis - WHO-IUIS Nomenclature Sub-Committee, *Bull. WHO* 71:105–108.

Kisilevsky, R., 1996, Anti-amyloid drugs: Potential in the treatment of diseases associated with aging, *Drug Aging* 8:75–83.

Kisilevsky, R., and Boudreau, L., 1983, The kinetics of amyloid deposition: I. The effect of amyloid enhancing factor and splenectomy, *Lab. Invest.* 48:53–59.

Kisilevsky, R., and Young, I.D., 1994. Pathogenesis of amyloidosis. In: *Clinical Rheumatology: Vol.8 No.3, Reactive Amyloidosis and the Acute Phase Response*. pp. 613–626. Husby, G., Ed., Bailliere Tindall, London.

Levy-Lahad, E., and Bird, T.D., 1996, Genetic factors in Alzheimer's disease: A review of recent advances, *Ann. Neurol.* 40:829–840.

Liepnieks, J.J., DiBartola, S.P., and Benson, M.D., 1996, Systemic immunoglobulin (AL) amyloidosis in a cat: Complete primary structure of a feline lambda light chain, *Amyloid* 3:177–182.

Linke, R.P., Geisel, O., and Mann, K., 1991, Equine Cutaneous Amyloidosis Derived from an Immunoglobulin lambda-Light Chain – Immunohistochemical, Immunochemical and Chemical Results, *Biol. Chem. Hoppe-Seyler* 372:835–843.

Lorenzo, A., and Yankner, B.A., 1994, beta-amyloid neurotoxicity requires fibril formation and is inhibited by Congo red, *Proc. Natl. Acad. Sci. USA* 91:12243–12247.

Lyon, A.W., Narindrasorasak, S., Young, I.D., Anastassiades, T., Couchman, J.R., McCarthy, K., and Kisilevsky, R., 1991, Co-deposition of basement membrane components during the induction of murine splenic AA amyloid, *Lab. Invest.* 64:785–790.

Martin, L.J., Sisodia, S.S., Koo, E.H., Cork, L.C., Dellovade, T.L., Weidemann, A., Beyreuther, K., Masters, C., and Price, D.L., 1991, Amyloid Precursor Protein in Aged Nonhuman Primates, *Proc. Natl. Acad. Sci. USA* 88:1461–1465.

McCubbin, W.D., Kay, C.M., Narindrasorasak, S., and Kisilevsky, R., 1988, Circular dichroism and fluorescence studies on two murine serum amyloid A proteins, *Biochem. J.* 256:775–783.

McCutchen, S.L., Colon, W., and Kelly, J.W., 1993, Transthyretin Mutation Leu-55-Pro Significantly Alters Tetramer Stability and Increases Amyloidogenicity, *Biochemistry* 32:12119–12127.

Nagata, Y., Tashiro, F., Yi, S., Murakami, T., Maeda, S., Takahashi, K., Shimada, K., Okamura, H., and Yamamura, K., 1995, A 6-kb upstream region of the human transthyretin gene can direct developmental, tissue-specific, and quantitatively normal expression in transgenic mouse, *J. Biochem. Tokyo* 117:169–175.

Naiki, H., Higuchi, K., Yonezu, T., Hosokawa, M., and Takeda, T., 1988, Metabolism of Senile Amyloid Precursor and Amyloidogenesis: Age-related Acceleration of Apolipoprotein A-II Clearance in the Senescence Accelerated Mouse, *Am. J. Pathol.* 130:579–587.

Narindrasorasak, S., Altman, R.A., Gonzalez-DeWhitt, P., Greenberg, B.D., and Kisilevsky, R., 1995, An interaction between basement membrane and Alzheimer amyloid precursor proteins suggests a role in the pathogenesis of Alzheimer's disease, *Lab. Invest.* 72:272–282.

Prusiner, S.B., 1996, Prion biology and diseases—Laughing cannibals, mad cows, and scientific heresy, *Med. Res. Rev.* 16:487–505.

Prusiner, S.B., Telling, G., Cohen, F.E., and DeArmond, S.J., 1996, Prion diseases of humans and animals, *Semin. Virol.* 7:159–173.

Roses, A.D., 1996, The Alzheimer diseases, *Curr. Opin. Neurobiol.* 6:644–650.

Saraiva, M.J.M., 1995, Transthyretin mutations in health and disease, *Hum. Mutat.* 5:191–196. Solomon, A., Weiss, D.T., and Pepys, M.B., 1992, Induction mice of human light-chain-associated amyloidosis, *Am. J. Pathol.* 140:629–637.

Tagouri, Y.M., Sanders, P.W., Picken, M.M., Siegal, G.P., Kerby, J.D., and Herrera, G.A., 1996, *In vitro* AL-Amyloid formation by rat and human mesangial cells, *Lab. Invest.* 74:290–302.

Verchere, C.B., D'Alessio, D.A., Palmiter, R.D., Weir, G.C., Bonner-Weir, S., Baskin, D.G., and Kahn, S.E., 1996, Islet amyloid formation associated with hyperglycemia in transgenic mice with pancreatic beta cell expression of human islet amyloid polypeptide, *Proc. Natl. Acad. Sci. USA* 93:3492–3496.

Westermark, P., Engstrom, U., Johnson, K.H., Westermark, G.T., and Betsholtz, C., 1990, Islet Amyloid Polypeptide—Pinpointing Amino Acid Residues Linked to Amyloid Fibril Formation, *Proc. Natl. Acad. Sci. USA* 87:5036–5040.

Yamamura, K., Tashiro, F., Yi, S., Wakasugi, S., Araki, S., Maeda, S., and Shimada, K., 1993, Transgenic Mouse Model for Human Genetic Diseases, *Mol. Reprod. Dev.* 36:248–250.

32

THE CONFORMATIONS OF TAU PROTEIN AND ITS AGGREGATION INTO ALZHEIMER PAIRED HELICAL FILAMENTS

Eckhard Mandelkow, Peter Friedhoff, Jacek Biernat, and Eva-Maria Mandelkow

Max-Planck
Unit for Structural Molecular Biology
c/o DESY, Notkestrasse 85
D-22603 Hamburg, Germany

INTRODUCTION

Alzheimer's disease is accompanied by a number of structural and metabolic alterations in the brain. Two characteristic hallmarks are the protein aggregates in amyloid plaques (made up mostly of the Aβ peptide, a derivative of the membrane protein APP) and in the neurofibrillary tangles (consisting largely of the microtubule-associated protein tau). Certain forms of AD are related to mutations in the APP gene so that much of current Alzheimer research is aimed at clarifying the chain of events that lead from the altered gene to the aggregated gene product. On the other hand, no Alzheimer-related mutations are known for tau in the coding region (Froelich et al., 1997) so that the protein cannot be implicated directly in inherited forms of the disease. Nevertheless, in contrast to amyloid plaques the distribution of neurofibrillary deposits correlates well with the clinical progression of the disease (Braak and Braak, 1991; Arriagada et al., 1992; Dickson et al., 1995) and thus can used to subdivide the disease into 6 stages. In this regard, tau deposits have a comparable diagnostic value to the loss of synapses (Terry, 1996 and this volume). In addition the levels of tau in the cerebrospinal fluid become elevated in Alzheimer's disease which opens up a potential route to early diagnosis (Jensen et al., 1995; Vigo-Pelfrey et al., 1995).

The Aβ peptide contains a hydrophobic domain normally inserted into the membrane, and this makes it intuitively understandable why an overproduction of the peptide would lead to insoluble aggregates. By contrast, tau is one of the most soluble proteins known; it survives heat, denaturating agents or acid treatment without losing its biological function, the binding to microtubules and the stimulation of their assembly (Weingarten et

Progress in Alzheimer's and Parkinson's Diseases
edited by Fisher *et al.*, Plenum Press, New York, 1998.

al., 1975; Lindwall and Cole, 1984). The fact that this protein can aggregate into insoluble fibers is therefore counterintuitive. Over the past few years we have studied the structure and assembly of tau, its phosphorylation by various kinases, and its interaction with microtubules (review, Mandelkow et al., 1995). Phosphorylation tends to dissociate tau from its natural partner, the microtubule (e.g. Biernat et al., 1993; Illenberger et al., 1996; Drewes et al., 1997), and since this increases the soluble pool of tau it is an important first step in generating protein for the assembly of PHFs. However, the assembly itself appears to depend mainly on other factors (conformation, oxidation, nucleation by other components, see below). Here we will restrict ourselves to the question of tau and PHF structure, and the possible roles of different tau conformations.

Structure and Conformations of the Tau Monomer

In the human central nervous system there are up to 6 isoforms of tau protein, arising from a single gene by alternative splicing (Goedert et al., 1988; Lee et al., 1988; Himmler, 1989, Fig. 1). They have between 352 and 441 residues. There are either 0, 1, or 2 inserts of 29 residues each near the N-terminus, and 3 or 4 homologous stretches of 31 residues each, the "repeats" in the C-terminal half (repeat R2 may be missing). Thus the longest isoform has four repeats and two inserts, the shortest (fetal) isoform has 3 repeats and no inserts. The 4 repeats are followed by a poorly conserved "fifth" repeat (R'). A "big tau" isoform containing ~300 additional residues (exon 4a) is expressed in peripheral nerves (Couchie et al., 1992). Tau contains either one or two cysteines, residue 322 in repeat 3 (always present), and residue 291 in repeat 2 (present only in 4-repeat isoforms). This difference has an influence on PHF assembly (see below). The amino acid composition of tau is dominated by hydrophilic and charged residues, an acidic stretch near the N-terminus followed by mostly basic domains. The repeats are flanked by regions rich in prolines. The C-terminal half of tau (repeats plus flanking regions) constitutes the microtubule-binding domain.

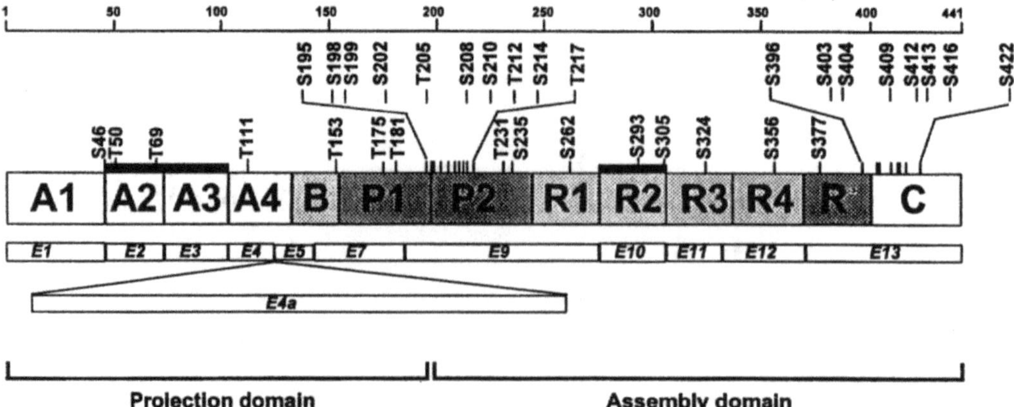

Figure 1. Bar diagram of tau protein, showing the domains, isoforms generated by alternative splicing, exons, and phosphorylation sites. The microtubule binding domain consists of repeats R1-R4 and the flanking regions P (P1, P2, proline-rich) and R' ("fifth" repeat, see Gustke *et al.*, 1994). Exons are listed below; exon 4a is present in the "big tau" isoform of peripheral nerves. Exons E2, E3, and E10 (highlighted with black bars) can be absent due to alternative splicing, generating the 6 isoforms in human CNS. A number of potential phosphorylation sites reported in the literature are listed above (see Friedhoff & Mandelkow, 1997).

Tau has resisted all efforts of crystallization so far (precluding an X-ray crystallographic analysis), and it is too large for a structural analysis by magnetic resonance methods. Therefore, details of the folding of the polypeptide chain are unknown. Most of the available structural data comes from electron microscopy, spectroscopy, or small angle X-ray scattering of tau in solution. Additional information comes from antibodies which sense the three-dimensional folding of the polypeptide chain.

Electron microscopy of tau particles imaged by the glycerol-spray rotary shadowing technique (Wille et al., 1992) shows them to be rod-like, with lengths around 35 nm. These images prove that tau can be highly elongated. However, this picture may be over-simplified since the technique tends to straighten out particles that are flexible. Solution X-ray scattering shows that tau may assume many different conformations, reminiscent of a random ("Gaussian") coil (Schweers et al., 1994). In this regard tau differs from most proteins which typically have a well-folded structure which ensures uniform particle dimensions. In fact, the persistence length of tau is 2 nm, similar to that of a denatured protein. In other words, tau may be likened to a "natively unfolded" protein. This loose, open structure may explain why tau is resistant to heat, denaturants, or acids, because these treatments destroy the compact folding of other proteins but cannot harm tau. The Stokes radius (2.5 nm for the repeat domain, Wille et al., 1992) also indicates an elongated structure with an axial ratio around 10.

The same theme is reiterated by spectroscopic data. Circular dichroism suggests that tau has a "random coil" structure, with at most 4% ordered secondary structure (α helix or β sheet). This low value is close to the error of the method and therefore not significant. In agreement with this, computer-based predictions of individual tau sequences show the near-absence of secondary structure as well. However, short stretches of beta strands emerge from computer modeling if one uses as a data base the collection of known repeat sequences of tau or related MAPs from different species (following the algorithm of Rost and Sander, 1993). In this case, a short β-strand emerges just behind the PGGG motif at the end of each repeat (Fig. 2). In general, β sheets can be formed from β- strands running either parallel or antiparallel. In the case of tau we favor a parallel arrangement since this would allow the second repeat to be spliced out without interrupting the structure (Fig. 3a).

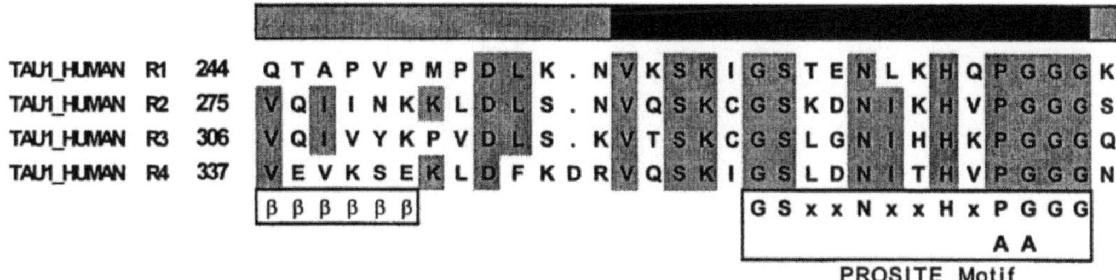

Figure 2. Sequence of tau in the repeat region, and predicted secondary structure derived from the ensemble of all known repeats of tau and MAP2. The more homologous 18-mer region is highlighted with the black bar, the less conserved "linker" region (13 residues) with a gray bar. The first column indicates the protein (SWISS-Prot name), the second column the number of the repeat and the third column the number of the first amino acid residue based on the longest isoforms for each protein. Residues with >60% identity are shaded gray. The bottom line indicates the secondary structure prediction for the aligned sequences using the program PHD (Rost and Sander, 1993) and the location of the PROSITE motif for tau and related MAPs. Most of the prediction is for random coil, except the six residues in β conformation at the beginning of the repeats (see arrows in Fig. 3a).

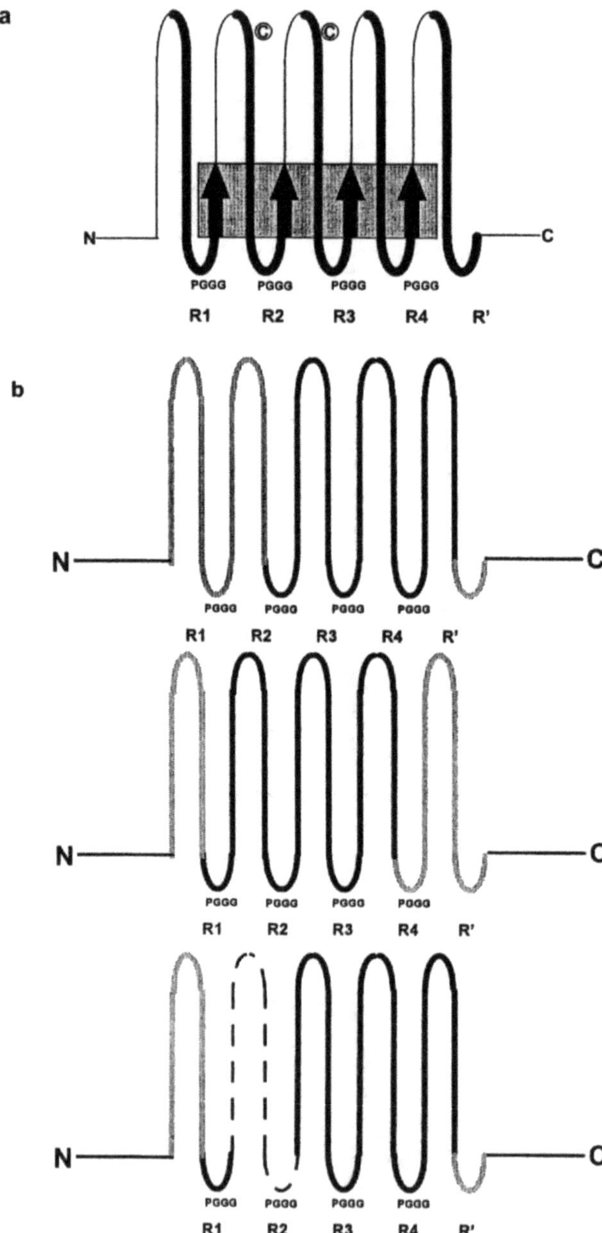

Figure 3. Models depicting the folding of the repeat domain of tau. (a) Model derived from structure predictions. The repeated sequences are shown as S-shapes, terminating at a PGGGX motif (bottom loops). The following residues are predicted to form short β strands (arrows). Assuming that the strands are parallel they could possibly join into a β sheet. The parallel arrangement would allow repeat 2 to be excised while keeping the same basic structure. The model also would allow cysteines 291 and 322 to approach each other closely, consistent with the fluorescence energy transfer results. (b) Model illustrating the peptides found in the pronase-resistant core of Alzheimer PHFs (Jakes *et al.*, 1991). The observed peptides (black) begin shortly before the PGGG motif at the end of either repeats R1 or R2. They contain the equivalent of 3 repeats, derived from either 3-repeat or 4-repeat isoforms. Thus, the top model contains the end of R2+R3+R4+most of R', the middle contains end of R1+R2+R3+most of R4, the bottom contains end of R1+R3+R4+most of R' (R2 is missing because this peptide is from a 3-repeat isoform).

The methods described above are sensitive to the overall conformation of the protein, but there are also other methods which probe the local environment. One of them is fluorescence energy transfer. When the two cysteines in tau are labeled with pyrene these groups form an excimer in solution, indicating that they are less than 1 nm apart. Thus, the polypeptide chain must be folded up in solution so that cysteines 291 and 322 become close neighbors (Schweers et al., 1995). This would be compatible with the folding shown in Fig. 3a and would correspond to the shape of the "compact monomer" described below.

Antibodies provide another tool to assess the protein folding, provided that their epitopes are formed from non-contiguous parts of the chain which must come together in space. One example is SMI34, originally raised against phosphorylated neurofilaments (Sternberger et al., 1985) which crossreacts with Alzheimer tau and requires the repeats plus either of the flanking regions in phosphorylated form (Lichtenberg-Kraag et al., 1992). Another case is that of antibody Alz50 which recognizes a conformation of tau typical of Alzheimer's disease (Wolozin et al., 1986). It is independent of phosphorylation but requires a region near the N-terminus (residues 7–9) and one of the repeats (any repeat according to Carmel et al., 1996; or preferably repeat 3, Jicha et al., 1997, see contribution by P. Davies, this volume). Antibody MC-1 raised against Alzheimer PHFs also requires a similar discontinuous epitope as Alz50 (Jicha et al., 1997). It is remarkable that the three antibodies against "pathological" tau recognize a special folded conformation which brings regions outside the repeats into close vicinity of the repeats, and it is likely that this folding is important for the assembly of tau into PHFs. By contrast, the internal folding of the repeats leading to the vicinity of cysteines 291 and 322 occurs in non-pathological (recombinant) tau (Fig. 4).

Conformation of the Tau Dimer, an Intermediate of PHF Formation

Dimeric tau derives its importance from the fact that it is an important intermediate in the assembly of PHFs. Dimers are formed by disulfide crosslinking, they are therefore not observed in reducing conditions and not expected in healthy nerve cells as long as they maintain their reducing potential. In vitro, dimers can be induced by cysteine crosslinkers (such as MBS, Wille et al., 1992) or by allowing the cysteines to oxidize spontaneously (e.g. in the absence of reducing agents such as DTT, Schweers et al., 1995).

In the electron microscope, tau dimers are seen as rod-like particles, similar to the monomers. Dimers with antibody labels at both ends appear dumbbell-shaped, with anti-

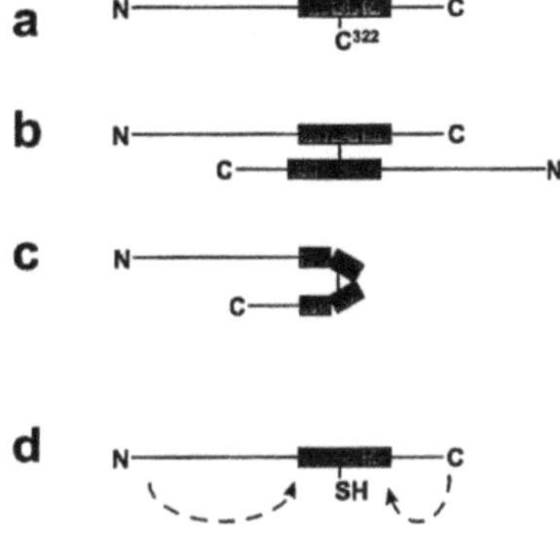

Figure 4. Models illustrating tau and tau dimerization. (a) Monomer of tau with 3 repeats (shaded). There is only one cysteine (residue 322 in the third repeat) since the second repeat is absent. (b) Dimer of tau crosslinked via cysteine 322 in oxidizing conditions. Note the antiparallel arrangement. (c) Model of compact tau monomer with 4 repeats. Note the intrachain disulfide bridge (cysteines 291 and 322) formed in oxidizing conditions. In this configuration the monomer cannot contribute to PHF assembly. (d) Model of tau monomer as in (a), indicating how regions in the N- or C-terminal tails might interact with the repeats to generate a folded conformation recognized by antibodies against Alzheimer tau.

bodies attached to both ends. This suggests that the two monomers of the dimer are arranged in an antiparallel fashion and roughly in register (Fig. 4a, b). However, this shape may be oversimplified by the technique used, as in the case of the monomers, since in solution the dimers also adopt a mostly random structure, as judged by CD spectroscopy. The Stokes radius of the dimeric repeat domain is 3.0 nm and supports a similar axial ratio of ~10 as the monomer.

Native gels reveal remarkable differences between monomers and dimers, depending on disulfide oxidation. In a reducing environment, different constructs of tau have electrophoretic mobilities roughly as expected from their molecular weights. In an oxidizing environment, 3-repeat constructs or isoforms (containing only the single cysteine 322) appear with twice their normal mass, indicating their covalent crosslinking into dimers via intra-molecular disulfide bridges. In striking contrast, 4- repeat constructs (containing the two cysteines 291 and 322) have a strongly reduced apparent mass. This is explained by the formation of intra-molecular disulfide bridges between the two cysteines of a monomer. It precludes the formation of dimers (since the free SH groups have been used up) and forces the molecule into a more compact shape, as evidenced by the lower apparent mass (Fig. 3a, 4c). This result, together with the data from pyrene labeling mentioned above, show that the two cysteines in repeats 2 and 3 tend to be close together in solution and are therefore easily crosslinked in an oxidizing environment.

Structure of Paired Helical Filaments

The name of PHFs is derived from their electron microscopic appearance as two strands (Fig. 5). They are twisted around one another, such that the cross-over repeats are around 75–80 nm and their apparent width varies between 10 and 22 nm, as if each strand had a diameter of about 10 nm (Crowther and Wischik, 1985). A fraction of PHFs isolated

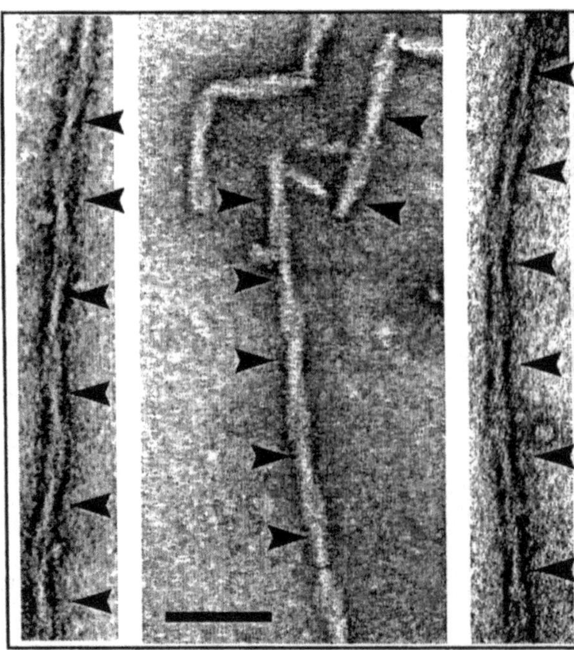

Figure 5. Electron micrograph of paired helical filaments assembled in vitro from a 3-repeat construct of tau. Note twisted appearance with cross-over repeats around 80 nm. Bar = 100 nm.

from Alzheimer brains are not twisted but straight, as if the two protofibrils ran parallel to each other. Image reconstructions suggest that both appearances can be explained by a similar domain structure of the protofibrils (Crowther, 1991). The PHFs usually terminate in an abrupt fashion without fraying out, suggesting that the two strands are not separate entities on a molecular level. This would be explained if the constituent subunits of tau protein were distributed over both subfibers. Images from atomic force scanning microscopy emphasize a ribbon- like structure, twisting with the same cross-over distance of ~80 nm, but without the subdivision into two strands (Pollanen et al., 1994). The main problem in all models of PHFs thus far is that their protein subunits cannot be clearly delineated so that the packing of molecules is still unknown. There is a debate on the subunit composition, but it is widely accepted that all tau isoforms occur in PHFs (Kosik et al., 1988; Jakes et al., 1991) while other tangle proteins are only peripherally associated (e.g. ubiquitin, Morishima-Kawashima et al., 1993).

Important constraints for structural models come from proteolytic cleavage and antibody labeling. The cleavage experiments show that PHFs contain a pronase resistant core which roughly coincides with the repeat domain (Kondo et al., 1988; Wischik et al., 1988). The N- and C-terminal regions outside the repeats contribute to the "fuzzy coat" and can be cleaved off. Antibody labeling of PHFs before or after pronase digestion reinforces this conclusion (Ksiezak-Reding and Yen, 1991). An intriguing result was obtained by analyzing the peptides remaining in the core after pronase digestion (Novak et al., 1993). The peptides contained the equivalent of about 3 repeats, but were derived from both 3-repeat or 4-repeat isoforms (Fig. 3b). Thus, pronase was able to nick the chain at certain points (N-terminally near the ends of repeats R1 or R2) but left 3-repeat blocks of tau physically intact within the core of the filaments.

A common motif of many "amyloid" fibers is their assembly via interacting β strands, often in a "cross-beta" configuration where the β strands run perpendicular to the fiber axis. Examples are the fibers made from the Aβ peptide in Alzheimer's disease (Kirschner et al., 1986), or fibers from transthyretin in systemic amyloidosis (Blake & Serpell, 1996). Such fibers can be stained with certain dyes such as Congo red or Thioflavin S which are thought to interact with the repeating β strands (Glenner et al., 1972). Since PHFs react with these dyes to some extent it had been assumed that PHFs had a cross-β structure of subunits. However, the results from X-ray diffraction and Fourier transform infrared spectroscopy (FTIR) speaks against this model. Repeated β strands should reveal a periodicity of about 0.47 nm which is not detectable by X-rays, and similarly they should generate a maximum around 1620–1630 cm^{-1} in FTIR, in contrast to the observed maximum at 1658 cm^{-1} which is typical of random coil (Schweers et al., 1995). These results are consistent with the near-absence of secondary structure observed with tau in solution noted above. But unfortunately they also leave open the question of tau's packing within a PHF; in particular, it remains unknown how a "random" molecule packs into a fiber which has a "random" substructure and yet shows a well-defined overall shape and periodicity.

Assembly of Tau into PHFs

To understand the principles by which PHFs or other biological fibers are formed it is necessary to assemble the subunits into the fibers in vitro and study the structure both in the subunit and in the polymeric states. For PHFs the progress has been slow, primarily because tau is soluble in most circumstances. Many peptides have the tendency to aggregate in some conditions, but the significance remains unclear if the aggregates do not resemble the native fiber (for examples see Geisler et al., 1993). Thus, tau isolated from brain tissue can form fibers of homogeneous diameter (Montejo de Garcini et al., 1988; Lichtenberg-Kraag and Mandelkow, 1990), but the relationship to PHFs remained unclear. Bona fide PHFs, showing the appropriate diameter and periodicity, were first assembled from recombinant tau constructs containing essentially the repeats (Wille et al., 1992). This PHF assembly was obtained mainly from cross-linked tau dimers. However, the efficiency was low, and it was nearly impossible to obtain PHFs from full-length tau.

The next step was elucidation of the role of disulfide bridges (Schweers et al., 1995). Three-repeat tau constructs, having one cysteine, can be dimerized by oxidation and form PHFs readily, while 4-repeat constructs form intra-molecular cross-bridges which inhibits dimerization and assembly. Nevertheless, even with dimerized 3-repeat constructs the assembly was slow and inefficient. Moreover, the difficulty remained that full length tau would not assemble, and that native PHFs contained both 3-repeat and 4-repeat isoforms.

A further important step was the recent discovery of polyanionic cofactors that greatly facilitate the nucleation of PHFs. They stimulate the assembly of full-length tau, both with 3 or 4 repeats. Perez et al. (Perez et al., 1996) and Goedert et al. (Goedert et al., 1996) used heparin or other sulfated glycosaminoglycans which are components of the extracellular matrix. By contrast, we used intracellular factors such as RNA (Kampers et al., 1996), arguing that the assembly of a cytosolic protein would require an interaction with other cytosolic components (Fig. 6). A systematic variation of the domain composition showed that all tau proteins would assemble into PHFs provided that they contain at least two repeats. This emphasizes the role of the repeat domain of tau in PHF assembly, consistent with their presences in the cores of Alzheimer PHFs. Secondly, the assembly still required disulfide cross-linking and could be prevented by reducing agents such as DTT.

The role of RNA or other polyanionic cofactors can probably be explained by their effect on the conformation of tau, particularly on the domains outside the repeats. Without RNA, these domains appear to inhibit the dimerization and PHF assembly, so that only smaller constructs could be assembled successfully by Wille et al. (Wille et al., 1992). With RNA the conformation is changed such that it is no longer inhibitory. The result is that full-length tau can be assembled, and that tau dimers can be formed even from 4-re-

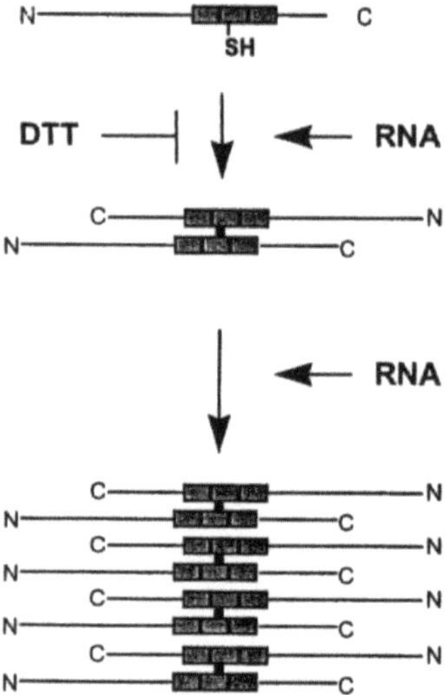

Figure 6. Model of assembly of tau into PHFs. Monomers (top) first pair up into dimers (middle) via the formation of disulfide bridges, dimers then assemble into PHFs (bottom). In this diagram the repeat domain is shaded, the axis of the PHF is vertical in order to enhance the visibility of the PHF core (repeats, shaded) and the "fuzzy" coat (N- and C-terminal regions outside the repeats, shown as lines). Reducing agents (DTT) prevent dimerization and thus PHF assembly. RNA strongly promotes both dimerization and PHF assembly. 3-repeat tau isoforms assemble more efficiently because they have a single cysteine 322 which forms inter-dimer disulfide bridges. 4-repeat tau isoforms (with cysteines 291 and 322) tend to form intra-chain disulfide bridges which block dimerization and PHF assembly. However, in the presence of RNA even 4-repeat tau and full length isoforms are incorporated into PHFs.

peat tau, presumably because the disulfide cross-links between two tau molecules are now preferred over the intra-chain cross-links. In short, assembly of tau protein in oxidizing conditions and in the presence of cytosolic nucleating agents fulfill all the requirements for bona fide PHF formation (full length molecules, all isoforms). This opens the way for new and detailed studies of the kinetic properties of PHF assembly, for analyzing PHF assembly in cell models, and for studying the structure of PHFs.

A crucial question remains—how does the assembly pathway outlined above pertain to neurons in Alzheimer' brain tissue? Cells normally have a reducing environment maintained by an excess of glutathione. This ensures the successful scavenging of reactive oxygen species and free radicals, and it depends on a well-functioning energy metabolism. Alzheimer's disease appears early in large pyramidal neurons of the hippocampus which have a high metabolic rate and thus might be expected to be most vulnerable to toxic effects (e.g. glutamate excitotoxicity, toxic $A\beta$, radicals generated by activated microglia, etc). In addition, mitochondrial DNA lacks the repair system of nuclear DNA so that oxidative phosphorylation becomes less efficient with age, as seen from experiments involving the mitochondria from Alzheimer tissue (Davis et al., 1997). The relative longevity of man may explain why other animals, including aged sheep or monkeys (Nelson et al., 1996) or transgenic mice overexpressing the amyloid precursor protein (Games et al., 1995) or human tau (Götz et al., 1995) do not show neurofibrillar pathology comparable to that of Alzheimer's disease. Finally, a recent report (Ginsberg et al., 1997) showed that RNA is present in virtually all neurofibrillary tangles, supporting the potential role of RNA as a nucleating factor in PHF assembly.

REFERENCES

Arriagada, P.V., Growdon, J.H., Hedley-Whyte, E. and Hyman, B.T., 1992, Neurofibrillary tangles but not senile plaques parallel duration and severity of Alzheimers disease. *Neurology* 42:631–639.

Biernat, J., Gustke, N., Drewes, G., Mandelkow, E.M. and Mandelkow, E., 1993, Phosphorylation of serine 262 strongly reduces the binding of tau protein to microtubules: Distinction between PHF-like immunoreactivity and microtubule binding. *Neuron* 11:153–163.Braak, H. and Braak, E., 1991, Neuropathological staging of Alzheimer-related changes. *Acta Neuropath.* 82:239–259.

Carmel, G., Mager, E.M., Binder, L.I. and Kuret, J., 1996, The structural basis of monoclonal-antibody Alz50s selectivity for Alzheimers-disease pathology. *J. Biol. Chem.* 271:32789–32795.

Couchie, D., Mavilia, C., Georgieff, I., Liem, R., and Shelanski, M., 1992, Primary structure of high molecular weight tau present in the peripheral nervous system. *Proc. Natl. Acad. Sci. USA* 89:4378–4381.

Crowther, R.A., 1991, Straight and paired helical filaments in Alzheimer disease have a common structural unit. *Proc. Natl. Acad. Sci. USA* 88:2288–2292.

Crowther, R.A. and Wischik, C.M., 1985, Image reconstruction of the Alzheimer paired helical filament. *EMBO J.* 4:3661–3665.

Davis, D.R., Anderton, B.H., Brion, J.P., Reynolds, C.H. and Hanger, D.P., 1997, Oxidative stress induces dephosphorylation of tau in rat-brain primary neuronal cultures. *J. Neurochem.* 68:1590–1597.

Dickson, D., Crystal, H., Bevona, C., Honer, W., Vincent, I. and Davies, P., 1995, Correlations of synaptic and pathological markers with cognitive of the elderly. *Neurobiol. Aging* 16:285–304.

Drewes, G., Ebneth, A., Preuss, U., Mandelkow, E.-M. and Mandelkow, E., 1997, MARK - a novel family of protein kinases that phosphorylates microtubule-associated proteins and disrupts the microtubule cytoskeleton. *Cell* 89.

Froelich, S., Basun, H., Forsell, C., Lilius, L., Axelman, K., Andreadis, A. and Lannfelt, L., 1997, Linkage to chromosome 17q12–21 and sequencing of the tau gene in familial rapidly progressive frontotemporal dementia. *Am. J. Med. Genet.*, in press.

Games, D., Adams, D., Alessandrini, R., Barbour, R., Berthelette, P., Blackwell, C., Carr, T., Clemens, J., Donaldson, T., Gillespie, F., Guido, T. and Hagopian, S., 1995, Alzheimer-type neuropathology in transgenic mice overexpressing V717F beta-amyloid precursor protein. *Nature* 373:523–527.

Geisler, N., Heimburg, T., Schünemann, J. and Weber, K., 1993, Peptides from the conserved ends of the rod domain of desmin disassemble intermediate filaments and reveal unexpected structural features: A circular-dichroism, fourier-transform infrared, and electron-microscopic study. *J. Struct. Biol.* 110:205–214.

Ginsberg, S.D., Crino, P.B., Lee, V.M.Y., Eberwine, J.H. and Trojanowski, J.Q., 1997, Sequestration of RNA in Alzheimers-disease neurofibrillary tangles and senile plaques. *Annals Neurol.* 41:200–209.

Glenner, G.G., Eanes, E.D. and Page, D.L. (1972) The relation of the properties of Congo red-stained amyloid fibrils to the b-conformation. *J. Histochem. Cytochem.* 20:821–826.

Goedert, M., Jakes, R., Spillantini, M.G., Hasegawa, M., Smith, M.J. and Crowther, R.A., 1996, Assembly of microtubule-associated protein tau into Alzheimer-like filaments induced by sulfated glycosaminoglycans. *Nature* 383:550–553.

Goedert, M., Wischik, C., Crowther, R., Walker, J. and Klug, A., 1988, Cloning and sequencing of the cDNA encoding a core protein of the paired helical filament of Alzheimer disease: Identification as the microtubule-associated protein tau. *Proc. Natl. Acad. Sci. USA* 85:4051–4055.

Götz, J., Probst, A., Spillantini, M.G., Schafer, T., Jakes, R., Burki, K. and Goedert, M. (1995) Somatodendritic localization and hyperphosphorylation of tau-protein in transgenic mice expressing the longest human brain tau-isoform. *EMBO J.* 14:1304–1313.

Gustke, N., Trinczek, B., Biernat, J., Mandelkow, E.M. and Mandelkow, E., 1994, Domains of Tau protein and interactions with microtubules. *Biochemistry* 33:9511–9522.

Himmler, A., 1989, Structure of the bovine tau gene: Alternatively spliced transcripts generate a protein family. *Mol. Cell. Biol.* 9:1389–1396.

Illenberger, S., Drewes, G., Trinczek, B., Biernat, J., Meyer, H.E., Olmsted, J.B., Mandelkow, E.M. and Mandelkow, E., 1996, Phosphorylation of Microtubule Associated Proteins MAP2 and MAP4 by the Protein Kinase p110 ^{mark}: Phosphorylation Sites and Regulation of Microtubule Dynamics. *J. Biol. Chem.* 271:10834–10843.

Jakes, R., Novak, M., Davison, M. and Wischik, C.M., 1991, Identification of 3- and 4-repeat tau isoforms within the PHF in Alzheimer's disease. *EMBO J.* 10:2725–2729.

Jensen, M., Basun, H. and Lannfelt, L., 1995, Increased cerebrospinal-fluid tau in patients with Alzheimers-disease. *Neurosci. Lett.* 186:189–191.

Jicha, G.A., Bowser, R., Kazam, I.G. and Davies, P., 1997, Alz-50 and MC-1, a new monoclonal-antibody raised to paired helical filaments, recognize conformational epitopes on recombinant-tau. *J. Neurosci. Res.* 48: 128–132.

Kampers, T., Friedhoff, P., Biernat, J. and Mandelkow, E.M., 1996, RNA stimulates aggregation of microtubule-associated protein-tau into alzheimer-like paired helical filaments. *FEBS Lett.* 399:344–349.

Kirschner, D.A., Abraham, C. and Selkoe, D.J. , 1986, X-ray diffraction from intraneural paired helical filaments and extraneural amyloid fibers in Alzheimer disease indicates cross-~b conformation. *Proc. Natl. Acad. Sci. USA* 83:503–507.

Kondo, J., Honda, T., Mori, H., Hamada, Y., Miura, R., Ogawara, M. and Ihara, Y., 1988, The carboxyl third of tau is tightly bound to paired helical filaments. *Neuron* 1:827–834.

Kosik, K., Orecchio, L., Binder, L., Trojanowski, J., Lee, V. and Lee, G., 1988, Epitopes that span the tau molecule are shared with paired helical filaments. *Neuron* 1:817–825.

Ksiezak-Reding, H. and Yen, S.H., 1991, Structural stability of paired helical filaments requires microtubule-binding domains of tau: A model for self-association. *Neuron* 6:717–728.

Lee, G., Cowan, N. and Kirschner, M., 1988, The primary structure and heterogeneity of tau protein from mouse brain. *Science* 239:285–288.

Lichtenberg-Kraag, B. and Mandelkow, E.M., 1990, Isoforms of tau protein from mammalian brain and avian erythrocytes: Structure, self-assembly, and elasticity. *J. Struct. Biol.* 105:46–53.

Lichtenberg-Kraag, B., Mandelkow, E.M., Biernat, J., Steiner, B., Schröter, C., Gustke, N., Meyer, H.E. and Mandelkow, E., 1992, Phosphorylation dependent interaction of neurofilament antibodies with tau protein: Epitopes, phosphorylation sites, and relationship with Alzheimer tau. *Proc. Natl. Acad. Sci. USA* 89:5384–5388.

Lindwall, G. and Cole, R.D., 1984, Phosphorylation affects the ability of Tau protein to promote microtubule assembly. *J. Biol. Chem.* 259:5301–5305.

Mandelkow, E.M., Biernat, J., Drewes, G., Gustke, N., Trinczek, B. and Mandelkow, E., 1995, Tau domains, phosphorylation, and interactions with microtubules. *Neurobiol. Aging* 16:355–362.

Montejo de Garcini, E., Carrascosa, J., Correas, I., Nieto, A. and Avila, J., 1988, Tau factor polymers are similar to paired helical filaments of Alzheimer's disease. *FEBS Lett.* 236:150–154.

Morishima-Kawashima, M., Hasegawa, M., Takio, K., Suzuki, M., Titani, K. and Ihara, Y., 1993, Ubiquitin is conjugated with amino-terminally processed tau in paired helical filaments. *Neuron* 10:1151–1160.

Nelson, P.T., Stefansson, K., Gulcher, J. and Saper, C.B., 1996, Molecular evolution of tau-protein - implications for Alzheimers-disease. *J. Neurochem.* 67:1622–1632.

Novak, M., Kabat, J. and Wischik, C.M., 1993, Molecular characterization of the minimal protease resistant tau-unit of the Alzheimer's-disease paired helical filament. *EMBO J.* 12:365–370.

Perez, M., Valpuesta, J.M., Medina, M., Degarcini, E.M. and Avila, J., 1996, Polymerization of tau into filaments in the presence of heparin: The minimal sequence required for tau-tau-interaction. *J. Neurochem.* 67:1183–1190.

Pollanen, M.S., Markiewicz, P., Bergeron, C. and Goh, M.C., 1994, Twisted ribbon structure of paired helical filaments revealed by atomic-force microscopy. *Am. J. Pathol.* **144**, 869–873.

Rost, B. and Sander, C. (1993) Prediction of protein secondary structure at better than 70% accuracy. *J. Mol. Biol.*, **232**, 584–599.

Schweers, O., Mandelkow, E.M., Biernat, J. and Mandelkow, E., 1995, Oxidation of cysteine 322 in the repeat domain of microtubule-associated protein tau controls the assembly of Alzheimer paired helical filaments. *Proc. Natl. Acad. Sci. USA* 92:8463–8467.

Schweers, O., Schönbrunn-Hanebeck, E., Marx, A. and Mandelkow, E., 1994, Structural studies of tau protein and Alzheimer paired helical filaments show no evidence for ß- structure. *J. Biol. Chem.* 269:24290–24297.

Sternberger, N.H., Sternberger, L.A. and Ulrich, J., 1985, Aberrant neurofilament phosphorylation in Alzheimer's disease. *Proc. Natl. Acad. Sci. USA* 82:4274–4276.

Terry, R.D.,1996, The Pathogenesis of Alzheimer Disease - an Alternative to the Amyloid Hypothesis. *J. Neuropathol Exp Neurol* 55:1023–1025.

Vigo-Pelfrey, C., Seubert, P., Barbour, R., Blomquist, C., Lee, M., Lee, D., Coria, F., Chang, L., Miller, B., Lieberburg, I. and Schenk, D., 1995, Elevation of microtubule-associated protein tau in the cerebrospinal-fluid of patients with Alzheimers-disease. *Neurology* 45:788–793.

Weingarten, M.D., Lockwood, A.H., Hwo, S.Y. and Kirschner, M.W., 1975, A protein factor essential for microtubule assembly. *Proc. Natl. Acad. Sci. USA* 72:1858–1862.

Wille, H., Drewes, G., Biernat, J., Mandelkow, E.M. and Mandelkow, E., 1992, Alzheimer-like paired helical filaments and antiparallel dimers formed from microtubule-associated protein tau in vitro. *J. Cell. Biol.* 118:573–584.

Wischik, C., Novak, M., Thogersen, H., Edwards, P., Runswick, M., Jakes, R., Walker, J., Milstein, C., M., R. and Klug, A., 1988, Isolation of a fragment of tau derived from the core of the paired helical filament of Alzheimer disease. *Proc. Natl. Acad. Sci. USA* 85:4506–4510.

Wolozin, B.L., Pruchnicki, A., Dickson, D.W. and Davies, P., 1986, A novel antigen in the Alzheimer brain. *Science (Wash.)* 232:648–650.

33

ROLE OF NEUROFIBRILLARY DEGENERATION IN ALZHEIMER'S DISEASE

Inge Grundke-Iqbal and Khalid Iqbal

New York State Institute for Basic Research in Developmental Disabilities
1050 Forest Hill Road
Staten Island, New York 10314

INTRODUCTION

Independent of the etiology, i.e., whether genetic or non-genetic, Alzheimer's disease (AD) is characterized by a specific type of neuronal degeneration, called neurofibrillary degeneration. The neuronal cytoskeleton in AD is progressively disrupted and displaced by the appearance of bundles of paired helical filaments (PHF), the neurofibrillary tangles. In addition to the neuronal perikaryon the PHF also accumulate in the neuropil as neuropil threads and as dystrophic neurites surrounding wisps or a core of β-amyloid in the neuritic plaques. To date, the exact relationship between the neurofibrillary degeneration and the β-amyloidosis, the two hallmark lesions of AD, is not understood. The bulk of the data suggests that these two lesions can be formed independent of each other and that neither might be the cause of the formation of the other in AD. The number of neurons undergoing neurofibrillary degeneration increases with the progression of the disease and correlates with the degree of dementia (Tomlinson et al., 1970; Alafuzzoff et al., 1987; Arigada et al., 1992; Dickson et al., 1991). β-amyloidosis alone, in the absence of neurofibrillary degeneration does not produce the disease clinically. Thus understanding the molecular mechanism of the neurofibrillary degeneration is critical to devising a rational therapeutic treatment of all forms of AD.

BREAKDOWN OF THE MICROTUBULE NETWORK AND THE FORMATION OF NEUROFIBRILLARY TANGLES IN AFFECTED NEURONS

Neurons with neurofibrillary tangles lack microtubules, and microtubule assembly from AD brain cytosol is not observed (Iqbal et al., 1986). PHF are comprised mainly of the microtubule associated protein (MAP) tau in an abnormally hyperphosphorylated state (Grundke-Iqbal et al., 1986a, 1986b). In addition to PHF there is a pool of cytosolic abnormally phosphorylated tau in the affected neurons (Iqbal, et al., 1986; Köpke et al., 1993). This pool of the abnormal tau seen immunocytochemically as the "stage 0" tangles (Bancher et al., 1989) is most likely the precursor to PHF since the neurofibrillary tangles have very little turnover, if any, and survive even after the death of the affected neurons as the "ghost tangles."

Tau promotes the assembly of tubulin into microtubules and maintains the structure of microtubules. Microtubules in turn are required for the axonal transport. These functions of tau are regulated by its degree of phosphorylation. The normal brain tau, which is optimally active, has 2–3 moles of phosphates per mole of the protein. Tau in PHF and in AD brain, which is abnormally hyperphosphorylated, contains 5–9 moles of phosphate per mole of the protein (Köpke et al., 1993). Unlike normal tau, the AD abnormally hyperphosphorylated tau (AD P-tau) does not promote the in vitro assembly of microtubules, bind to microtubules or stabilize their structure (Iqbal et al., 1994; Alonso et al., 1994; 1996). The AD P-tau competes with tubulin in binding to normal tau and inhibits the assembly of microtubules. The association of AD P-tau with normal tau results in tangles of ~3.3 nm straight filaments. Unlike normal tau, the abnormally phosphorylated tau in AD brain is glycosylated and deglycosylation of AD neurofibrillary tangles by endoglycosidase F/N glycosidase F converts them into tangles of thin straight filaments (Wang et al., 1996a) similar to those formed by the association of the AD P-tau and the normal tau (Alonso et al., 1996).

In addition to tau, the neuron contains high molecular weight-microtubule associated proteins (HMW-MAPs) MAP1 and MAP2 which also promote microtubule assembly and maintain the structure of microtubules. Like tau, MAP1 and MAP2 associate to AD P-tau and the sequestration of the HMW-MAPs from microtubules by AD P-tau results in the disassembly of microtubules (Alonso et al., 1997) . Both the disassembly of microtubules and the sequestration of tau, MAP1 and MAP2 by AD P-tau are inhibited by its dephosphorylation. However, the affinity of the binding between the AD P-tau and normal tau is higher than that between AD P-tau and the HMW-MAPs. Furthermore, unlike the association between the AD P-tau and the normal tau, the binding of AD P-tau to MAP1 or MAP2 does not result in the formation of tangles or individual long filaments. This explains the degeneration of many neurites without any accumulation of PHF in AD brain. HMW-MAPs have not been observed in isolated PHF.

ROLE OF PROTEIN PHOSPHATASES IN THE HYPERPHOSPHORYLATION OF TAU

Employing phosphorylation dependent antibodies and mass spectrometry, twenty-one phosphorylation sites in the AD abnormally phosphorylated tau have been identified (Morishima-Kawashima et al., 1995; Iqbal et al., 1995). Ten of the 21 sites are canonical sites for proline directed protein kinases (PDPKs) and the rest are the non-PDPK sites. Tau can be phosphorylated by several PDPKs and non-PDPKs (e.g. Baudier et al., 1987; Roder et al., 1991; Drewes et al., 1992; Ledesma et al., 1992; Ishiguro et al., 1992; Litersky et al., 1992; Singh et al., 1994). However, in AD the exact role of any of these kinases in the abnormal hyperphosphorylation of tau is not yet known and to date, the activity of none of these kinases has been found to be upregulated.

The state of phosphorylation of protein is the function of the activities of protein kinases and as well as the protein phosphatases that regulate its phosphorylation. The hyperphosphorylation of tau in AD might be the result of either higher activities of protein kinases or lower activities of protein phosphatases, or both. A large number of phosphoprotein phosphatases have been described in mammalian tissues (for review, see Cohen, 1989). These enzymes can be divided into two broad types, i.e. phosphoseryl/phosphothreonyl-protein phosphatases (PSPs) and phosphotyrosyl protein phosphatases (PTPs). The PSPs have been further subclassified into four subtypes, i.e. protein phosphatase (PP)-1, PP-2A, PP-2B, and PP-2C. These phosphatase activities differ in substrate specificity, dependence on divalent cations, and sensitivities to specific inhibitors (Ingebritsen and Cohen, 1983; Cohen, P., 1989) To date, only phosphorylation of serines and threonines has been observed in normal tau and AD abnormally hyperphosphorylated tau. Thus only PSPs are expected to dephosphorylate tau.

Employing phosphorylation dependent antibodies to tau, site specific dephosphorylation of the AD P-tau has been investigated (Ingebritsen and Cohen, 1983; Gong et al., 1994a, 1994b; Wang et al., 1995, 1996b). The AD P-tau can be rapidly dephosphorylated by PP-2B at the abnormal sites Ser 46, Ser 198/Ser 199/Ser 202, Thr 231, Ser 235 and Ser 396/Ser 404, by PP-2A at all the above sites except Ser 235, and by PP-1 at only Ser 198/Ser 199/Ser 202, Thr 231 and Ser 396/Ser 404. The activities of all the three phosphatases, i.e. PP-2B, PP-2A and PP-1 towards the abnormally phosphorylated tau are markedly increased by the presence of Mn^{2+}. Unlike tau *in vitro* phosphorylated by MAP kinase (Goedert et al., 1992) which is the more preferred substrate to $PP\text{-}2A_1$ than $PP\text{-}2A_2$, the AD abnormal tau is an equally good substrate to both isoforms of PP-2A. Dephosphorylation by PP-2C of the abnormal tau at none of the above sites has been detected.

The rapid dephosphorylation of the AD abnormally phosphorylated tau by alkaline phosphatase (Iqbal et al., 1986; Grundke-Iqbal et al., 1986b; Iqbal et al., 1989) and by PP-2A, PP-2B and PP-1 (Gong et al., 1994a, 1994b, 1994c) *in vitro* had suggested that the abnormal hyperphosphorylation of tau might in part be the result of a deficiency of the phosphoprotein phosphatase system in brains of AD patients. To have a direct effect on the regulation of phosphorylation of tau, PP-2A, PP-2B and PP-1 should be present in the affected neurons. Immunocytochemical studies have revealed that these protein phosphatases are present both in granular and pyramidal neurons, including the tangle-bearing neurons (Pei et al., 1994). Employing ^{32}P-labeled (with protein kinase A) phosphorylase kinase as substrate and specific inhibitors, it has been shown, 1) that the activities of PP-1, PP-2A, PP-2B and PP-2C can be determined in autopsied (2–7 hours) and frozen human brains; and 2) that the activities of PP-1 and PP-2A are decreased in AD neocortex (Gong et al., 1993). Furthermore, the studies on dephosphorylation of the AD abnormally phosphorylated tau have revealed: 1) that PP-2A and PP-2B and, to a lesser extent PP-1, are involved in the dephosphorylation of tau; and 2) that the phosphatase activity towards dephosphorylation of Ser 198/Ser 199/Ser 202, major abnormal phosphorylation sites in the abnormal tau is decreased by ~30% in the brain of patients with AD (Gong et al., 1995). These findings have suggested that a decrease of tau phosphatase activity might be the cause of the abnormal hyperphosphorylation of tau in AD.

TAU-PHOSPHATASE ACTIVITY AS A THERAPEUTIC TARGET

Dephosphorylation by PP-2A, PP-2B and to a lesser extent by PP-1 restores the microtubule assembly promoting activity of AD P-tau (Wang et al., 1996b). Furthermore, the

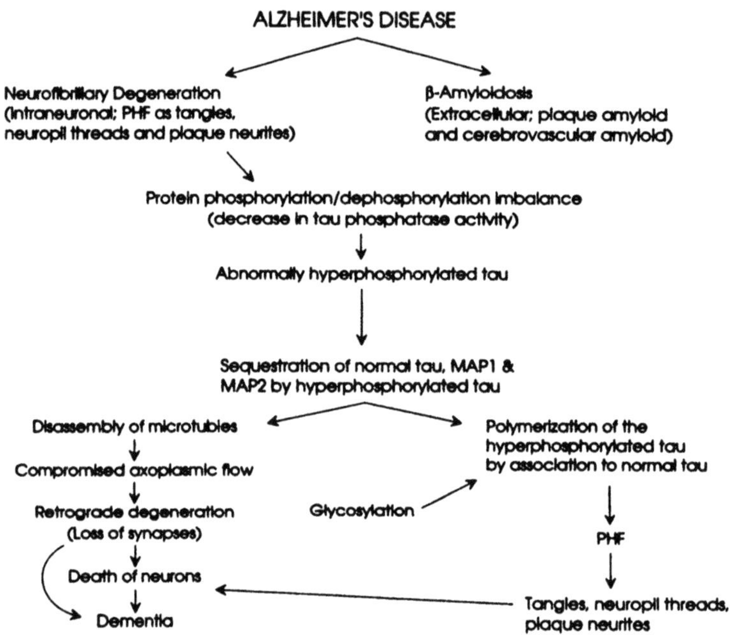

Figure 1. Alzheimer's disease, independent of the etiology, is histopathologically characterized by neurofibrillary degeneration and β-amyloidosis. A protein phosphorylation/dephosphorylation imbalance in the affected neurons, at least partly by reduction of protein phosphatase activity(s) leads to an abnormal hyperphosphorylation of tau. The abnormal tau sequesters normal microtubule associated proteins (MAPs) and causes disassembly of microtubules. The breakdown of the microtubule network in the affected neurons compromises axonal transport, leading to retrograde degeneration, which in turn results in dementia.

dephosphorylation of neurofibrillary tangles of PHF by the two major tau phosphatases, PP-2A and PP-2B, produces marked biochemical, biological and structural alterations (Wang et al., 1995). Both PP-2A and PP-2B dephosphorylate PHF-tau at the sites of Ser 198/Ser 199/Ser 202 and only partially dephosphorylate it at Ser 396/Ser 404; in addition, PHF-tau is dephosphorylated at Ser 46 by PP-2A, and Ser 235 by PP-2B. The relative electrophoretic mobility of PHF-tau increases after dephosphorylation by either enzyme. Divalent cations, manganese, and magnesium increase the activities of PP-2A, and PP-2B toward PHF-tau. Dephosphorylation both by PP-2B and PP-2A, decreases the resistance of PHF-tau to proteolysis by the brain calcium-activated neutral proteases, the calpains. The ability of PHF-tau to promote the *in vitro* microtubule assembly is restored after dephosphorylation by PP-2A$_1$ and PP-2B. Microtubules assembled by the dephosphorylated PHF -tau are structurally identical to those assembled by normal tau. The dephosphorylation both by PP-2A$_1$ and PP-2B causes dissociation of the tangles and the PHF; some of the PHF dissociate into straight protofilaments/subfilaments. Approximately 25% of the total tau is released from PHF on dephosphorylation by PP-2A$_1$. These observations have demonstrated that tau in PHF is accessible to dephosphorylation by PP-2A$_1$ and PP-2B, and dephosphorylation makes PHF dissociate, accessible to proteolysis by calpain, and biologically active in promoting the assembly of tubulin into microtubules. Thus by increasing the activities of one or more of these tau phosphatases it might be possible to prevent and inhibit the neuronal degeneration and consequently both the sporadic as well as the familial AD.

ACKNOWLEDGMENTS

We thank Ms. Janet Biegelson for secretarial assistance and the Biomedical Photography Unit for the preparation of the figure.

Supported in part by the New York State Office of Mental Retardation and Developmental Disabilities; National Institutes of Health grants NS 18105, AG 05892, AG 08076, and Zenith Award (to K.I.) From the Alzheimer's Association, Chicago, Illinois.

REFERENCES

Alafuzoff, I., Iqbal, K., Friden, H., Adolfsson, R., Winblad, B., 1987, Histopathological criteria for progressive dementiadisorders: clinical-pathological correlation and classification by multivariate data analysis, *Acta Neuropathol.* (Berl.). 74:209–225.

Alonso, A. del C., Zaidi, T., Grundke-Iqbal, I., Iqbal, K., 1994, Role of abnormally phosphorylated tau in the breakdown of microtubules in Alzheimer disease, *Proc. Natl. Acad. Sci. USA.* 91:5562–5566.

Alonso, A. del C., Grundke-Iqbal, I., Iqbal, K., 1996, Alzheimer's disease hyperphosphorylated tau sequesters normal tau into tangles of filaments and disassembles microtubules, *Nature Med.* 2:783–787.

Alonso, A. del C., Grundke-Iqbal, I., Barra, H.S., Iqbal, K., 1997, Abnormal phosphorylation of tau and the mechanism of Alzheimer neurofibrillary degeneration: Sequestration of MAP1 and MAP2 and the disassembly of microtubules by the abnormal tau, *Proc. Natl. Acad. Sci. USA.* 94:298–303.

Arigada, P.A., Growdon, J.H., Hedley-White, E.T., Hyman, B.T., 1992, Neurofibrillary tangles but not senile plaques parallel duration and severity of Alzheimer's disease, *Neurology* 42:631–639.

Bancher, C., Brunner, C., Lassmann, H., Budka, H., Jellinger, K., Wiche, G., Seitelberger, F., Grundke-Iqbal, I., Iqbal, K., Wisniewski, H.M., 1989, Accumulation of abnormally phosphorylated tau precedes the formation of neurofibrillary tangles in Alzheimer's disease, *Brain Res.* 477:90–99.

Baudier, J., Cole, D., 1987, Phosphorylation of tau proteins to a state like that in Alzheimer's brain is catalyzed by a calcium/calmodulin-dependent kinase and modulated by phospholipds, *J. Biol. Chem.* 262:17577–17583.

Cohen, P., 1989, The structure and regulation of protein phosphatases, *Ann. Rev. Biochem.* 58:453–508.

Dickson, D.W., Crystal, H.A., Mattiace, L.A., Masur, D.M., Blau, A.D., Davies, P., Yen, S.H., Aronson, M., 1991, Identification of normal and pathological aging in prospectively studied nondemented elderly humans, *Neurobiol. Aging* 13:179–189.

Drewes, G., Lichtenberg-Kraag, B., Döring, F., Mandelkow, E.-M., Biernat, J., Goris, J., Doree, M., Mandelkow, E., 1992, Mitogen activated protein (MAP) kinase transforms tau protein into an Alzheimer-like state, *EMBO J.* 11:2131–2138.

Goedert, M., Cohen, E.S., Jakes, R., Cohen, P., 1992, P^{42} map kinase phosphorylation sites in microtubule- associated protein tau are dephosphorylated by protein phosphatase $2A_1$: Implications for Alzheimer's disease, *FEBS Lett.* 312:95–99.

Gong, C.-X., Singh, T.J., Grundke-Iqbal, I., Iqbal, K., 1993, Phosphoprotein phosphatase activities in Alzheimer disease, *J. Neurochem.* 61:921–927.

Gong, C.-X., Singh, T.J., Grundke-Iqbal, I., Iqbal, K., 1994a, Alzheimer disease abnormally phosphorylated tau is dephosphorylated by protein phosphatase 2B (calcineurin), *J. Neurochem.* 62: 803–806.

Gong, C.-X., Grundke-Iqbal, I., Iqbal, K., 1994b, Dephosphorylation of Alzheimer disease abnormally phosphorylated tau by protein phosphatase-2A, *Neuroscience* 61:765–772.

Gong, C.-X., Grundke-Iqbal, I., Damuni, Z., Iqbal, K., 1994c, Dephosphorylation of microtubule-associated protein tau by protein phosphatase-1 and -2C and its implication in Alzheimer disease, *FEBS Lett.* 341:94–98.

Gong, C.-X., Shaikh, S., Wang, J.-Z., Zaidi, T., Grundke-Iqbal, I., Iqbal, K., 1995, Phosphatase activity toward abnormally phosphorylated τ: decrease in Alzheimer disease brain, *J Neurochem.* 65:732–738.

Grundke-Iqbal, I., Iqbal, K., Quinlan, M., Tung, Y.C., Zaidi, M.S., Wisniewski, H.M., 1986, Microtubule- associated protein tau: A component of Alzheimer paired helical filaments, *J. Biol. Chem.* 261:6084–6089.

Grundke-Iqbal, I., Iqbal, K., Tung, Y.C., Quinlan, M., Wisniewski, H.M., Binder, L.I., 1986, Abnormal phosphorylation of the microtubule associated protein τ(tau) in Alzheimer cytoskeletal pathology, *Proc. Natl. Acad. Sci. USA.* 83:4913–4917.

Ingebritsen, T.S., Cohen, P., 1983, The protein phosphatases involved in cellular regulation: Classification and substrate specificities, *Eur. J. Biochem.* 132:255–261.

Iqbal, K., Grundke-Iqbal, I., Zaidi, T., Merz, P.A., Wen, G.Y., Shaik, S.S., Wisniewski, H.M., Alafuzoff, I., Winblad, B., 1986b, Defective brain microtubule assembly in Alzheimer's disease, *Lancet* 2:421–426.

Iqbal, K., Grundke-Iqbal, I., Smith, A.J., George, L., Tung, Y.C., Zaidi, T., 1989, Identification and localization of a tau peptide to paired helical filaments of Alzheimer disease, *Proc. Natl. Acad. Sci. USA*. 86:5646–5650.

Iqbal, K., Zaidi, T., Bancher, C., Grundke-Iqbal, I., 1994, Alzheimer paired helical filaments: Restoration of the biological activity by dephosphorylation, *FEBS Lett.* 349:104–108.

Iqbal, K., Grundke-Iqbal, I., 1995, Alzheimer abnormally phosphorylated tau is more hyperphosphorylated than the fetal tau and causes the disruption of microtubules, *Neurobiol. Aging* 16(3):375–379.

Ishiguro, K., Takamatsu, M., Tomizawa, K., Omori, A., Takahashi, M., Arioka, M., Uchida, T., Imahori, K., 1992, Tau protein kinase I converts normal tau protein into A68-like component of paired helical filaments, *J. Biol. Chem.* 267:10897–10901.

Köpke, E., Tung, Y.C., Shaik, S., Alonso, A. del C., Iqbal, K., Grundke-Iqbal, I., 1993, Microtubule associated protein tau: abnormal phosphorylation of a non-paired helical filament pool in Alzheimer disease, *J. Biol. Chem.* 268:24374–24383.

Ledesma, M.D., Correas, I., Avila, J., Diaz-Nido, J., 1992, Implication of brain cdc2 and MAP2 kinases in the phosphorylation of tau protein in Alzheimer's disease, *FEBS Lett.* 308:218–224.

Litersky, J.M., Johnson, G.V.W., 1992, Phosphorylation by cAMP-dependent protein kinase inhibits the degradation of tau by calpain, *J. Biol. Chem.* 267:1563–1568.

Morishima-Kawashima, M., Hasegawa, M., Takio, K., Suzuki, M., Yoshida, H., Watanabe, A., Titani, K., Ihara, Y., 1995, Hyperphosphorylation of tau in PHF, *Neurobiol. Aging* 16:365–380

Pei, J.-J., Sersen, E., Iqbal, K., Grundke-Iqbal, I., 1994, Expression of protein phosphatases PP-1, PP-2A, PP-2B and PTP-1B and protein kinases MAP kinase and P34^{cdc2} in the hippocampus of patients with Alzheimer disease and normal aged individuals, *Brain Res.* 655:70–76.

Roder, H.M., Ingram, V.M., 1991, Two novel kinases phosphorylate tau and KSP site of heavy neurofilament subunits in high stoichiometric ratios, *J. Neurosci.* 11:3325–3343.

Singh, T.J., Grundke-Iqbal, I., McDonald, B., Iqbal, K., 1994, Comparison of the phosphorylation of microtubule associated protein tau by non-proline dependent protein kinases, *Mol. Cell Biochem.* 131:181–189.

Tomlinson, B.E., Blessed, G., Roth, M., 1970, Observations on the brains of demented old people, *J. Neurol. Sci.* 11:205–242.

Wang, J.-Z., Gong, C.-X., Zaidi, T., Grundke-Iqbal, I., Iqbal, K., 1995, Dephosphorylation of Alzheimer paired helical filaments by protein phosphatase-2A and -2B, *J. Biol. Chem.* 270:4854–4860.

Wang, J.-Z., Grundke-Iqbal, I., Iqbal, K., 1996a, Glycosylation of microtubule-associated protein tau: An abnormal post-translational modification in Alzheimer's disease, *Nature Med.* 2:871–875.

Wang, J.-Z., Grundke-Iqbal, I., Iqbal, K., 1996b, Restoration of biological activity of Alzheimer abnormally phosphorylated τ by dephosphorylation with protein phosphatase-2A, -2B and -1, *Mol. Brain Res.* 38:200–208.

34

CYTOSKELETAL PROTEIN GENE EXPRESSION AFTER NEURONAL INJURY RECAPITULATES DEVELOPMENTAL PATTERNS

Implications for Tau Protein in Alzheimer's Disease

Nancy A. Muma and Christopher B. Chambers

Department of Pharmacology
Loyola University Chicago Stritch School of Medicine
2160 S. First Avenue
Maywood, Illinois 60153

INTRODUCTION

Cytoskeletal proteins play a crucial role in providing the structural support for all eukaryotic cells. Neurons, in particular, require an intact and well-organized cytoskeleton to perform their normal function of transmitting information throughout the nervous system. Neurons are specialized for this function by virtue of their unique structure: a central cell body, numerous dendritic extensions which receive information from other neurons, and an elongated axon which can transmit information to other neurons. Cytoskeletal proteins are vital to maintaining the integrity of these specialized processes. Disruptions of the cytoskeleton perturb neuronal structure and cause dysfunction of the nervous system.

Cytoskeletal proteins are perturbed in Alzheimer's disease (AD). Tau protein is a cytoskeletal protein and more specifically it is a microtubule associated protein. In AD, tau protein is redistributed to the somatodendritic compartment from its normal location in axons. Furthermore, tau proteins are an integral component of the straight and paired helical filaments which compose neurofibrillary tangles, neuropil threads, and the neuritic aspect of the senile plaques in AD (Lee *et al.*, 1991; Trojanowski and Lee, 1994; Kosik, 1992).

Previous studies on the regulation of the major cytoskeletal proteins during development and in simple models of neuronal injury have provided insights into the complex changes that occur in these proteins during neurodegenerative diseases. Similar strategies could be used to study tau protein expression in neurons during development and in models of neuronal injury to lay a foundation for understanding the dysregulation and perturbations of tau in AD.

Progress in Alzheimer's and Parkinson's Diseases
edited by Fisher *et al.*, Plenum Press, New York, 1998.

RESULTS AND DISCUSSION

Cytoskeletal proteins are developmentally regulated in the nervous system. We and others have demonstrated that gene expression of the major neuronal cytoskeletal proteins actin, tubulin, and neurofilament proteins are developmentally regulated (Muma *et al.*, 1991). For example, in the dorsal root ganglia of rats, the levels of mRNA encoding the low and high molecular weight neurofilament protein subunits are low at birth and increase during the first post-natal month of life (Figure 1). In contrast, the levels of β-tubulin mRNA are higher at birth than after 28 days of age (Figure 1). Furthermore, the levels of these proteins in the corresponding axons of the dorsal roots follow the alterations in the levels of their mRNA.

Following injury to an axon in the peripheral nervous system, protein gene expression is dramatically altered while the axon regenerates. The levels of mRNA encoding the major neuronal cytoskeletal proteins actin, tubulin, and the neurofilament protein subunits as well as the levels of the corresponding proteins are altered to support regeneration of the axon (Muma *et al.*, 1990). For example, a crush injury to the rat sciatic nerve (a regeneration-permissive injury) produces an increase in the levels of β-tubulin mRNA which returns to normal when the axons have reached their targets at approximately 56 days after injury (Figure 2). In contrast, as early as four days after this type of injury, the levels of mRNA encoding the low and high molecular weight neurofilament protein subunits decrease and then slowly return back toward normal levels while axonal outgrowth occurs (Figure 2).

From these and other similar studies (Hoffman and Cleveland, 1988; Tetzlaff *et al.*, 1991), it is clear that during axonal regeneration the expression of the major cytoskeletal proteins recapitulates the patterns of expression used during early development. Far from being static, the injured neuron is capable of modifying its cytoskeleton to mirror a developmental period when contacts among neurons are being established. This lead to the hypothesis that tau protein expression following axonal injury would also recapitulate the changes which occur during early development.

Microtubule associate proteins such as tau proteins are also developmentally regulated (Matus, 1988; Binder *et al.*, 1984). Tau is a group of proteins which arise from alternative splicing of a single gene (Himmler, 1989; Goedert *et al.*, 1992) and various post-translational modifications. Both the alternative splicing and the post-translational modifications of tau are developmentally regulated. For example, the phosphorylation of tau has been intensely studied. In fetal animals tau has been found to be highly phosphorylated while in adults it is phosphorylated to a lesser extent (Goedert *et al.*, 1993; Brion *et al.*, 1993).

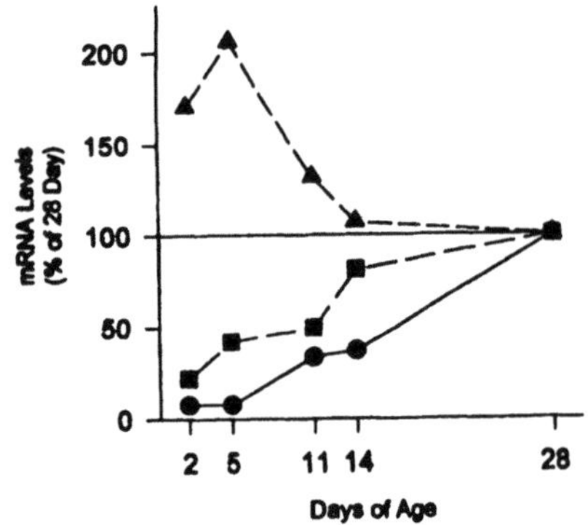

Figure 1. Northern blotting was used to examine cytoskeletal protein mRNA expression during early post-natal development of rat dorsal root ganglia. During early post-natal development, the levels of mRNA coding for β-tubulin (triangles) decrease whereas the levels of mRNA coding for the low (circles) and the high molecular weight neurofilament (squares) protein subunits gradually increase in the rat dorsal root ganglia.

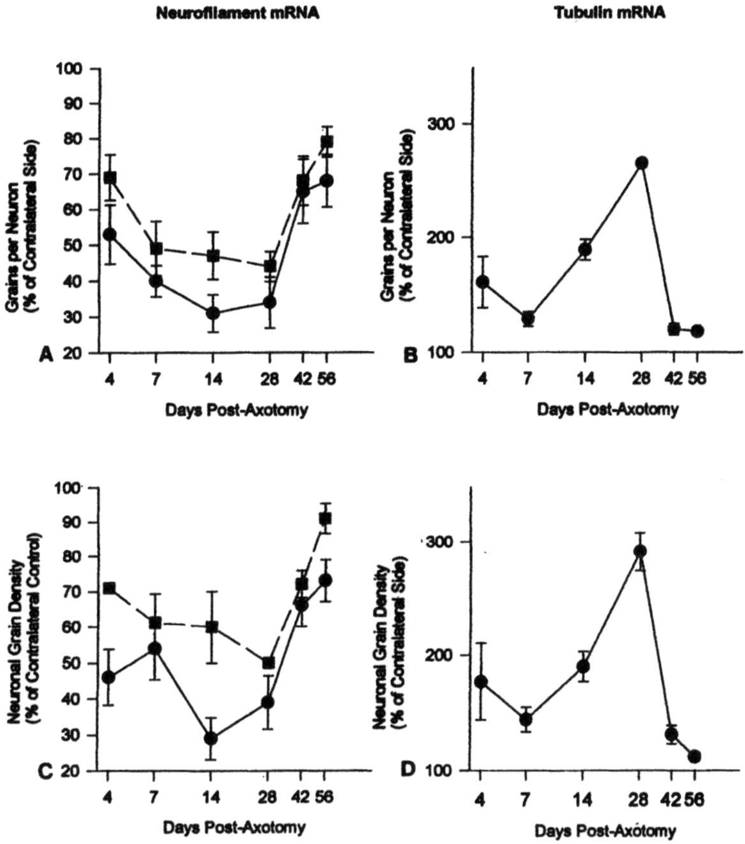

Figure 2. In situ hybridization was used to examine the levels of mRNA coding for cytoskeletal proteins during regeneration of rat sciatic nerve. During regeneration, the levels of mRNA coding for the low molecular weight neurofilament (circles) and high molecular weight neurofilament (squares) protein subunits decrease and gradually return toward normal levels at 56 days after injury (A,B). In contrast, the levels of β-tubulin mRNA increase during regeneration and return to normal when the axons have reached their targets (C,D). mRNA levels can be measured as either grains per neurons (A,C) or as neuronal grain density (B,D).

Six tau mRNA isoforms result from alternative splicing of tau pre-mRNA (Himmler, 1989; Goedert *et al.*, 1992). In the carboxyl-terminal end of tau, either three or four repeated 31 amino acid sequences (which compose the microtubule binding domains) can be expressed by the addition or deletion of a fourth repeat domain coded for by exon 10. Alternative splicing also occurs in the amino-terminal end of tau in which either a single 29 amino acid sequence (coded for by exon 2) or two 29 amino acid sequences (coded for by exons 2 and 3) are inserted. The second 29 amino acid insert (exon 3) is never expressed in the absence of the first 29 amino acid insert (Andreadis *et al.*, 1995). Other than this restricted combination, all other combinations of exons can result and thus give rise to the six tau mRNA isoforms.

The developmental expression of tau mRNA isoforms has been examined in human and rats. Tau mRNA isoforms with three carboxyl-terminal repeats are abundant in human fetal brain whereas tau mRNA isoforms with four repeats was not detected (Goedert *et al.*, 1989). Both the three- and four-repeat tau isoforms exist in neurons in adult human brain

(Goedert *et al.*, 1989). In rat brain, expression of tau mRNA with three carboxyl-terminal repeats is detectable at embryonic day 14 and increases during embryonic development (Kosik *et al.*, 1989). During post-natal development, the levels of tau mRNA containing three carboxyl-terminal repeats decrease to low levels by 20 days of age (Figure 3; Kosik *et al.*, 1989; Chambers and Muma, 1997). Furthermore, the expression of tau mRNA containing four carboxyl-terminal repeats is inversely related to the pattern of expression of the three-repeat isoform. Only trace levels of tau mRNA with four repeats are detectable until 8–10 days of age (Figure 3; Kosik *et al.*, 1989; Chambers and Muma, 1997). The levels of the three-repeat tau mRNA isoform are also high in rat spinal cord during early post-natal development but decrease sharply by 10 days of age (Figure 4) (Chambers and Muma, 1997). The expression of the four repeat tau mRNA is very low in rat spinal cord through 20 days of age (Figure 4).

Our studies demonstrate that tau protein mRNA expression is also altered during regeneration of axons in the peripheral nervous system (Chambers and Muma, 1997). The levels of tau mRNA containing either three or four carboxyl-terminal repeats are significantly decreased 2 and 3 days after a crush injury to the sciatic nerve of rats (Figure 5). Therefore, the expression pattern of tau mRNA for the four carboxyl-terminal repeat isoform during regeneration briefly recapitulates the pattern which occurs during development but the expression of the three carboxyl-terminal repeat isoform does not.

If an axon is injured and is not allowed to regenerate, the pattern of cytoskeletal protein gene expression differs from that which occurs during regeneration. During this abortive regenerative process, the pattern of expression of several cytoskeletal proteins is altered such that the changes which occur after a regeneration-permissive injury are greater and are prolonged (Tetzlaff *et al.*, 1988; Jiang *et al.*, 1994). For example, during abortive regeneration, the decreases in neurofilament mRNA levels are maintained rather than gradually returning back toward normal levels (Tetzlaff *et al.*, 1988; Jiang *et al.*, 1994). Surprisingly, during abortive regeneration of the rat sciatic nerve (i.e. after transection of the nerve without permitting regeneration) the pattern of expression of the three carboxyl-terminal repeat tau mRNA isoform recapitulates the pattern of expression seen during early development (Figure 6; Chambers and Muma, 1997). The levels of the three repeat isoform increase and the ratio of the four repeat to three repeat isoform decrease during abortive regeneration. The mechanisms regulating the differences in gene expression following successful regeneration and during abortive regeneration for these cytoskeletal proteins are unclear.

These and other studies on cytoskeletal protein gene expression during development and following axonal injuries suggest that cytoskeletal proteins participate in different aspects of maintaining axons; tubulin plays an important role in axonal outgrowth whereas neurofilaments participate in maintaining axonal caliber. For example, during sciatic nerve regeneration, while the levels of neurofilament proteins (and their mRNAs) are low, the caliber of the sciatic nerve is diminished (Hoffman *et al.*, 1988). Tau acts to polymerize and stabilize microtubules. If the levels of tau protein decrease as the levels of tau mRNA decrease, then microtubules and the axons they support should be less stable and more dynamic (Hall *et al.*, 1991). A dynamic neuronal cytoskeleton is likely to be a desirable condition for axonal regeneration. Furthermore, the different isoforms of tau vary in their capability to stabilize and polymerize microtubules (Scott *et al.*, 1991; Litersky *et al.*, 1993). The four-repeat isoform of tau binds to tubulin better than the three-repeat isoform and is better at inducing polymerization. A decrease in the ratio of four repeat to three repeat tau proteins would further confer flexibility to the growing axons.

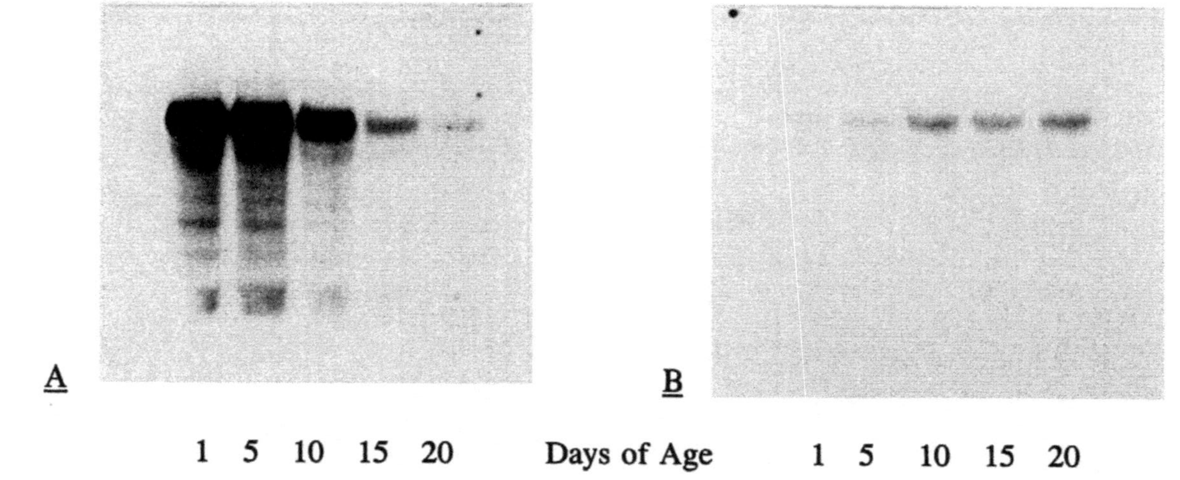

Figure 3. The three and four repeat tau isoforms are developmentally regulated during post-natal development of rat brain. Polyadenylated mRNA was extracted from brains of rats at early post-natal ages and 20 µg samples were separated on denaturing agarose gels. Blots were hybridized with oligonucleotide probes for the three repeat (A) and four repeat (B) tau mRNA isoforms.

N. A. Muma and C. B. Chambers

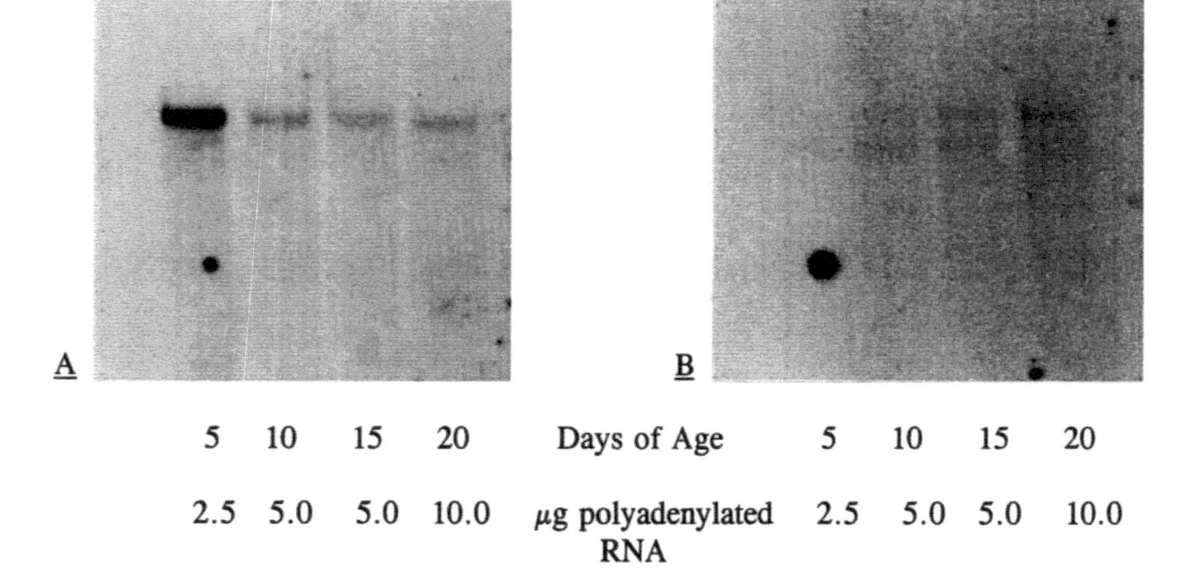

Figure 4. The three and four repeat tau isoforms are also developmentally regulated during post-natal development of rat spinal cord. Varying amounts of polyadenylated RNA extracted from spinal cords of rats at early post-natal ages were used to prepare Northern blots. Blots were hybridized with oligonucleotide probes for the three repeat (A) and four repeat (B) tau mRNA isoforms.

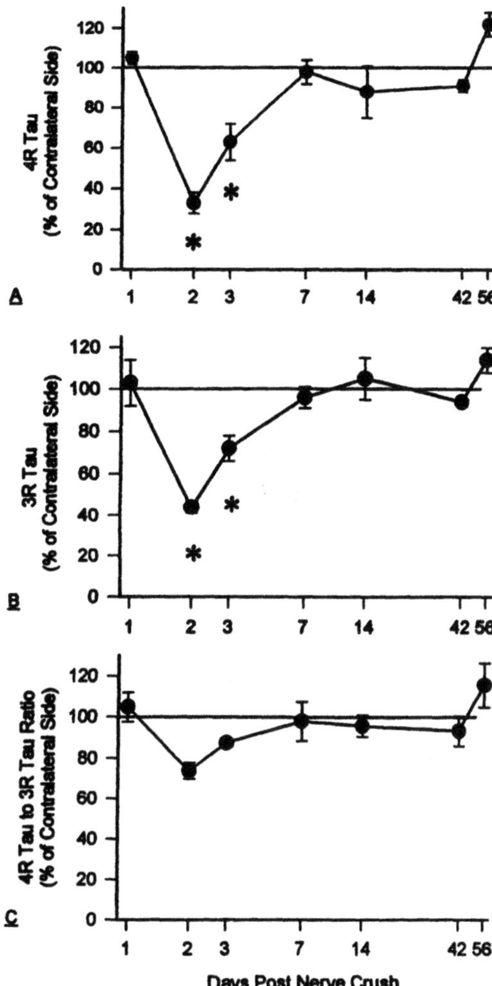

Figure 5. Reverse-transcription polymerase chain reaction method was used to measure the levels of the four repeat (A) and three repeat (B) tau mRNA isoforms during regeneration of rat sciatic nerve. The levels of both isoforms were significantly (* indicates $p < 0.05$) lower at two and three days after a crush injury; however, there were no significant differences in the ratios of the three and four repeat tau mRNA isoforms (C).

An understanding of the regulation of tau protein expression in neurons during development and following neuronal injury lays the foundation for understanding the regulation of tau in AD. In AD, neuronal sprouting and abortive regeneration of axons may be occurring (Geddes *et al.*, 1990; Cotman *et al.*, 1990; Masliah *et al.*, 1991; Kowall and McKee, 1993). Axonal injury via a disruption in calcium homeostasis, beta amyloid toxicity, or oxidative or physical injury could initiate changes in cytoskeletal protein gene expression which occur during abortive regeneration (since regeneration does not occur in the brain). Indeed, the re-expression of a fetal isoform of α-tubulin occurs in the brain in Alzheimer's disease (Geddes *et al.*, 1990). Therefore, the three repeat isoform of tau protein may be expressed at higher levels in neurons in Alzheimer's disease. In paired helical filaments purified from AD brain, the levels of tau with three-repeats is higher than that which occurs in normal brain tissue (Greenberg *et al.*, 1992). Since the three repeat isoform of tau interacts with tubulin less well than the four repeat isoform, higher levels of expression of the three repeat isoform of tau may lead to a pool of tau that can more readily self-associate and form paired helical filaments. Experiments are underway to determine if the levels of the three repeat isoforms of tau mRNA are over-expressed in neurons in Alzheimer's disease.

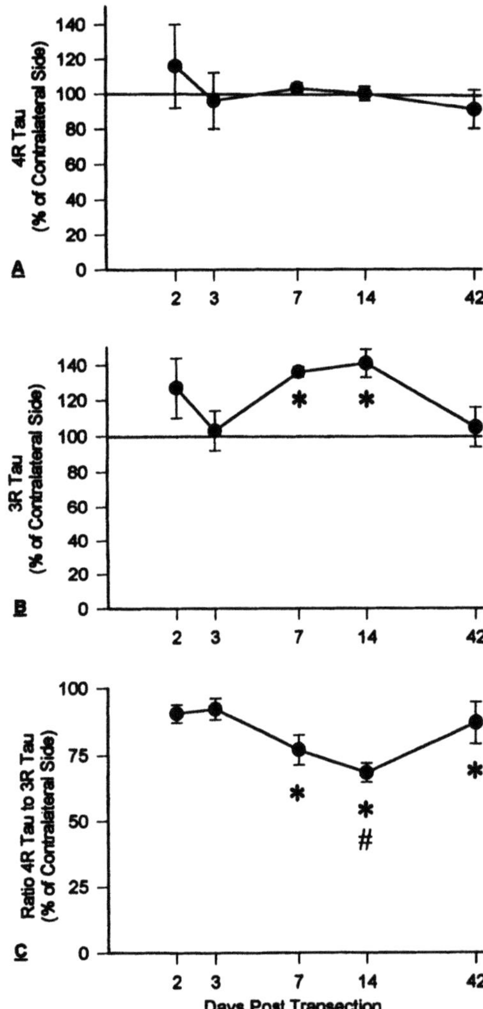

Figure 6. Reverse-transcription polymerase chain reaction methods were used to measure the levels of the four repeat (A) and three repeat (B) tau mRNA isoforms during abortive regeneration of rat sciatic nerve. The levels of the three repeat tau mRNA are increased at 7 and 14 days following nerve transection (* p < 0.05); the ratio of four repeat to three repeat tau mRNA is significantly decreased at 7, 14, and 42 days (* p < 0.05) and the ratio at 14 days is significantly decreased compared to 2 and 3 days following nerve transection (# p < 0.05).

ACKNOWLEDGMENTS

Supported by the Retirement Research Foundation and the National Institutes of Health (grant NS30460).

REFERENCES

Andreadis, A., Broderick, J. A., and Kosik, K. S., 1995, Relative exon affinities and suboptimal splice cite signals lead to non-equivalence of two cassette exons. *Nucleic Acids Res.* 23:3585–3593.

Binder, L. I., Frankfurter, A., Kim, H., Caceres, A., Payne, M. R., and Rebhun, L. I., 1984, Heterogeneity of microtubule associated protein 2 during rat brain development. *Proc. Natl. Acad. Sci.* USA 81:5613–5617.

Brion, J., Smith, C., Couck, A., Gallo, J., and Anderton, B., 1993, Developmental changes in tau phosphorylation: fetal tau is transiently phosphorylated in a manner similar to paired helical filament-tau characteristic of Alzheimer's disease. *J. Neurochem.* 61:2071–2080.

Chambers, C. B. and Muma, N. A., 1997, Tau mRNA isoforms following sciatic nerve axotomy with and without regeneration. *Mol. Brain Res.* 48:115–124, 1997.

Cotman, C. W., Geddes, J. W., and Kahle, J. S., 1990, Axon sprouting in the rodent and Alzheimer's disease brain a reactivation of developmental mechanisms. In: *Progress in Brain Research*, Storm-Mathisen, J., Zimmer, J., and Ottersen, O. P., eds., Elsevier, vol. 83, (30), pp. 427–434.

Geddes, J. W., Wong, J., Choi, B. H., Ki, Cotman, C. W., and Miller, F. D., 1990, Increased expression of the embryonic form of a developmentally regulated mRNA in Alzheimer's disease. *Neurosci. Lett.* 109:54–61.

Goedert, M., Spillantini, M. G., Potier, M. C., Ulrich, J., and Crowther, R. A., 1989, Cloning and sequencing of the cDNA encoding an isoform of microtubule-associated protein tau containing four tandem repeats: differential expression of tau protein mRNAs in human brain. *EMBO J* 8: 393–399.

Goedert, M., Spillantini, M. G., Cairns, N. J., and Crowther, R. A., 1992, Tau proteins of Alzheimer paired helical filaments: abnormal phosphorylation of all six brain isoforms. *Neuron* 8:159–168.

Goedert, M., Jakes, R., Crowther, R. A., Six, J., Lubke, U., Vandermeeren, A., Cras, P.,Trojanowski, J. Q., and Lee, V. M.-Y. 1993, The abnormal phosphorylation of tau protein at Ser-202 in Alzheimer disease recapitulates phosphorylation during development. *Proc. Natl. Acad. Sci.* U S A 90:5066–5070.

Greenberg, S. G., Davies, P., Schein, J. D., and Binder, L. I., 1992, Hydrofluoric acid-treated tau PHF proteins display the same biochemical properties as normal tau. *J. Biol. Chem.*267:564–569.

Hall, G. F., Lee, V. M.-Y., and Kosik, K. S., 1991, Microtubule destabilization and neurofilament phosphorylation precede dendritic sprouting after close axotomy of lamprey central neurons. *Proc. Natl. Acad. Sci.* U S A 88:5016–5020.

Himmler, A., 1989, Structure of the bovine tau gene: alternately spliced transcripts generate a protein family. *Mol. Cell. Biol.* 9:1389–1396.

Hoffman, P. N., Koo, E. H., Muma, N. A., Griffin, J. W., and Price, D. L., 1988, Role of neurofilaments in the control of axonal caliber myelinated nerve fibers. In: *Intrinsic determinants of neuronal form and function.* Lasek, R.J., Black, M.M., eds., Alan R. Liss Inc., New York, p p. 389–402.

Hoffman, P. N. and Cleveland, D. W., 1988, Neurofilament and tubulin expression recapitulates the developmental program during axonal regeneration: induction of a specific beta tubulin isotype. *Proc. Natl. Acad. Sci.* U S A 85:4530–4533.

Jiang, Y. Q., Pickett, J., and Oblinger, M. M.,1994, Comparison of changes in β-tubulin and NF gene expression in rat DRG neurons under regeneration-permissive and regeneration-prohibitive conditions. *Brain Res.* 637:233–241.

Kosik, K. S., Orecchio, L. D., Bakalis, S., and Neve, R. L.,1989, Developmentally regulated expression of specific tau sequences. *Neuron* 2:1389–1397.

Kosik, K. S. 1992, Alzheimer's disease: a cell biological perspective. *Science* 256:780–783.

Kowall, N. W. and McKee, A. C., 1993, The histopathology of neuronal degeneration and plasticity in Alzheimer's disease. *Adv. Neurol.* 59:5–33.

Lee, V. M.-Y., Balin, B. J., Otvos, L. ,Jr., and Trojanowski, J. Q., 1991, A68: a major subunit of paired helical filaments and derivatized forms of normal tau. *Science* 251:675–678.

Litersky, J. M., Scott, C. W., and Johnson, G. V. W., 1993, Phosphorylation, calpain proteolysis and tubulin binding of recombinant human tau isoforms. *Brain Res.* 604:32–40.

Masliah, E., Mallory, M., Hansen, L., Alford, M., Albright, T., DeTeresa, R., Terry, R., Baudier, J., and Saitoh, T., 1991, Patterns of aberrant sprouting in Alzheimer's disease. *Neuron* 6:729–739.

Matus, A., 1988, Microtubule associated proteins their potential role in determining neuronal morphology: *Ann. Rev. Neurosci.* 11:29–44.

Muma, N. A., Hoffman, P. N., Slunt, H. H., Applegate, M. D., Lieberburg, I., and Price, D. L., 1990, Alterations in levels of mRNAs coding for neurofilament protein subunits during regeneration. *Exp. Neurol.* 107:230–235.

Muma, N. A.,Slunt, H.H., and Hoffman, P. N., 1991, Postnatal increases in neurofilament gene expression correlate with the radial growth of axons. *J. Neurocytol.* 20:844–854.

Scott, C. W., Blowers, D. P., Barth, P. T., Lo, M. M. S., Salama, A. I., and Caputo, C. B., 1991, Differences in the abilities of human tau isoforms to promote microtubule assembly. *J. Neurosci. Res.* 30:154–162.

Tetzlaff, W., Alexander, S. W., Miller, F. D., and Bisby, M. A., 1991, Response of facial and rubrospinal neurons to axotomy changes in mRNA expression for cytoskeletal proteins and GAP-43. *J. Neurosci.* 11:2528–2544.

Tetzlaff, W., Bisby, M. A., and Kreutzberg, G. W., 1988, Changes in cytoskeletal proteins in the rat facial nucleus following axotomy. *J. Neurosci.* 8:3181–3189.

Trojanowski, J. Q. and Lee, V. M.-Y., 1994, Phosphorylation of neuronal cytoskeletal proteins in Alzheimer's disease and Lewy body dementias. *Ann. N. Y. Acad. Sci.* 747:92–109.

35

HYPERPHOSPHORYLATION OF TAU IN APOLIPOPROTEIN E-DEFICIENT MICE

Idit Genis and Daniel M. Michaelson

Department of Neurobiochemistry
The George S. Wise Faculty of Life Sciences
Tel Aviv University, Israel

INTRODUCTION

Genetic studies of familial and sporadic Alzheimer's disease (AD) suggest that this disease is associated with several genetic factors which include the amyloid precursor protein gene, the allele E4 of apolipoprotein E (apoE) as well as the presinilin 1 and presinilin 2 genes (Clarke et al., 1993; Levy-Lahad., 1995; Roses, 1994; Sherrington et al., 1995). Of these genes only the apoE4 allele has been linked thus far to sporadic AD (Corder et al., 1993; Roses, 1994). Further studies revealed a gene dosage dependent reduction in the age of onset of AD which in subjects homozygote to the E4 allele can start up to fifteen years earlier than in those who lack apoE4 (reviewed by Roses, 1996).

Animal model studies suggest that apoE plays an important role in repair mechanisms both in the peripheral and in the central nervous systems (Ignatius et al., 1986; Poirier et al., 1995). This assertion is supported by cell culture studies (Bellosta et al., 1995; Pitas, 1996; Nathan, 1994) and by the recent observation that apoE-deficient mice are deranged in their ability to withstand and to recover from head injury (Chen et al., 1997). These findings and the fact that the deleterious effects of apoE4 are manifested mainly by lowering of the age of onset of the disease, suggest that apoE plays an important role in neuronal maintenance and repair and that the effectiveness of these mechanisms is reduced in subjects which carry the E4 allele.

Three hypotheses have been proposed to explain the isoform specific effects of apoE on neuronal function. The first theory asserts that the allele specific effects of apoE in AD are due to derangements in the ability of apoE4 to support membrane repair and biosynthesis mechanisms, which are required for synaptic maintenance and remodeling. This theory is based on the known role of apoE as a lipid transporter (Poirier, 1995; Mahley, 1988); on the differential effects of the apoE3 and apoE4 on neurite outgrowth in culture (Pitas, 1996; Nathan, 1994) and on the finding that brain cholinergic nerve terminals of

Progress in Alzheimer's and Parkinson's Diseases
edited by Fisher *et al.*, Plenum Press, New York, 1998.

AD patients carrying the apoE4 are markedly more affected than those of patients who lack this allele.

The second theory hypothesizes that the deleterious effects of apoE4 are due to its diminished capacity to counteract oxidative phenomena which occur during aging and injury. This theory is based on *in vitro* studies which revealed that apoE has anti-oxidative capacity and that apoE4 has a markedly lower reducing capacity than the other apoE alleles (Miyata and Smith, 1996; Lomnitski et al., 1997).

The third hypothesis regarding the allele specific effects of apoE in AD is that *in vivo* apoE3 interacts with tau more effectively than apoE4 and that tau is thereby protected from being hyperphosphorylated and from destabilizing the neuronal cytoskeleton. This theory stems from the findings that: tau hyperphosphorylation is a neuropathological hallmark of AD and is presumed to destabilize the neuronal cytoskeleton; AD neurofibrilary tangles contain apoE immunoreactive material (Namba et al., 1991); that *in vitro* apoE3 binds to purified tau more effectively than does apoE4; and that under suitable experimental conditions apoE3 but not apoE4 is able to block tau phosphorylation (Strittmatter et al., 1994). This apoE-tau theory implies that some, though not necessarily all, the deleterious effects of apoE4 are mediated by a lack of function of the good apoE3 allele.

ApoE deficient mice provide a useful model for studying the role of apoE in neuronal function (Gordon et al., 1995; Chen et al., 1997; Lomnitski et al., 1997). In particular this model can be used for inquiring whether the loss of function associated with apoE deficiency affects tau phosphorylation. Indeed we have recently shown, utilizing specific anti phosphorylated tau abs, that tau of apoE deficient mice is hyperphosphorylated (Genis et al., 1995). This finding is consistent with the assertion that apoE and tau can interact *in vivo*. However, further studies are required for determining the mechanism underlying this effect and whether it is isoform specific. The experiments described below are a first step in this direction and investigate the brain area specificity and age dependency of tau hyperphosphorylation in apoE-deficient mice.

RESULTS

The levels of tau phosphorylation in different brain areas of newly born and adult apoE-deficient and control mice were probed utilizing the following mAb: AT8 which recognizes a specific tau serine residue in its phosphorylated state (202 in human tau & 193 in rodent tau; Mawal-Dewan et al., 1994; Goedert et al.,1994); anti tau mAb T46 which binds to a phosphorylation insensitive epitope on the C terminal of tau (Goedert et al., 1994); and ALZ50 which binds to tau epitopes highly enriched in AD paired helical filaments [Ksiezac-Reding et al., 1990].

Figure 1 depicts the mAbs AT8, T46 and ALZ50 immunoblots thus obtained of tau from the cortex and cerebellum of 3 adult apoE-deficient and 3 adult control mice. As can be seen AT8 reacted with a prominent tau bond (~55 kDa) whose intensity was higher in both the cortex and the cerebellum of the apoE-deficient mice. In contrast anti tau Ab134 yielded immunoblot bands whose intensities in the two mouse groups were similar. These results are similar to those previously obtained with whole brain homogenates (Genis et al., 1995). They suggest that the total tau contents of the cortex and cerebellum of the two mice groups are similar and that in both brain areas the level of phosphorylated epitopes recognized by AT8 is higher in the apoE-deficient than in control mice. Furthermore, the ALZ50 immunoblots of the two brain areas were also similar and yielded, as was observed with whole brain homogenates (Genis et al., 1995), more intense staining in the upper

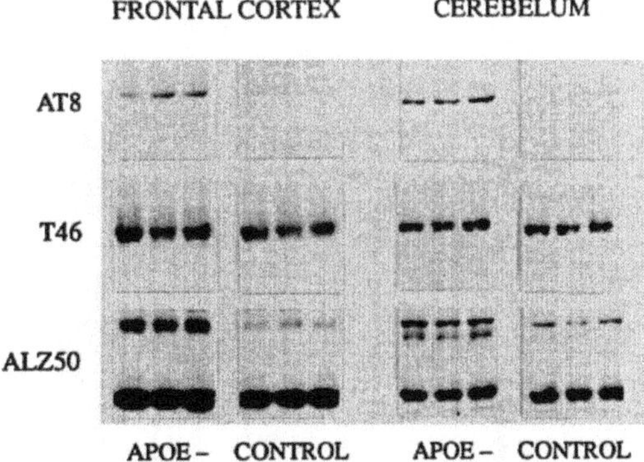

Figure 1. Immunoblot analysis of cortical and cerebellar tau of apoE-deficient and control mice utilizing the anti-tau mAbs T46, AT8 and ALZ50. The cortical and cerebellar immunoblots shown are from two experiments each of which contained three adults (four months old) mice per group. The experiment was performed as previously described (Genis et al., 1995).

band of the apoE-deficient mice than in that of the controls. Examination of hippocampal homogenates revealed differences between the apoE-deficient and control mice similar to those obtained with the cortex and cerebellum (not shown). These findings suggest that the effects of apoE deficiency on tau phosphorylation are not brain area specific.

The effects of age on tau phosphorylation in apoE-deficient and control mice are depicted in Figure 2. As can be seen the levels of AT8 phosphorylation of newly born apoE-deficient and control mice were similar, whereas by 3 months tau of the apoE-deficient mice was more extensively phosphorylated than that of the corresponding controls. A similar time dependency was observed with aAb ALZ50 (Fig. 2).

These findings imply that the apoE deficiency mediated changes in tau phosphorylation evolve postnatally during life. This suggests that effects of apoE deficincy are not due to developmental changes but rather, and as is believed to be the case in AD, to functional derangements of the mature system.

The difference in tau phosphorylation between the two adult mice groups may be due either to an increase in tau phosphorylation of the apoE-deficient mice during maturation,or alternatively to enhanced dephosphorylation of control tau. This issue can not be addressed by the immunoblots depicted in Figure 2 as they were obtained by two separate immunoblots experiments each corresponding to one of the age groups and the resulting AT8 immunoreactivity was monitored. The samples of both age groups were therefore reblotted together such that similar tau levels (i.e mAbT46 immunoreactions) were run simultaneously for all four groups. Comparison of the resulting age dependent tau im-

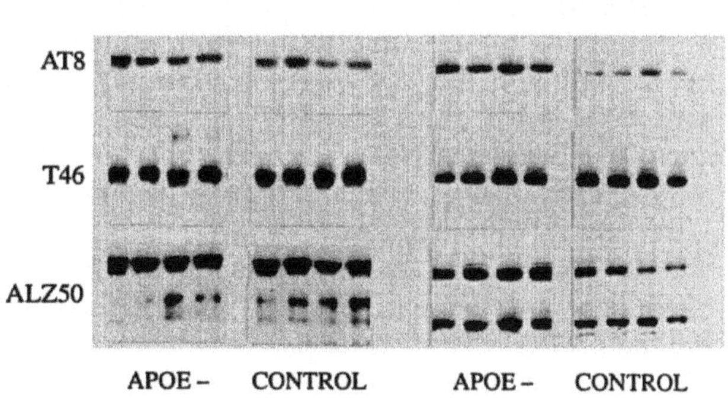

Figure 2. Age dependency of tau phosphorylation of neonate and adult apoE-deficient and control mice. Immunoblot analysis of tau of 2 weeks and 4 months old apoE-deficient and control mice was performed utilizing anti tau mAbs T46, AT8 and ALZ50, as previously described (Genis et al., 1995). Immunoblots presented correspond to two separate experiments each of which contained 4 mice per group, at ages 2 weeks and 3 months.

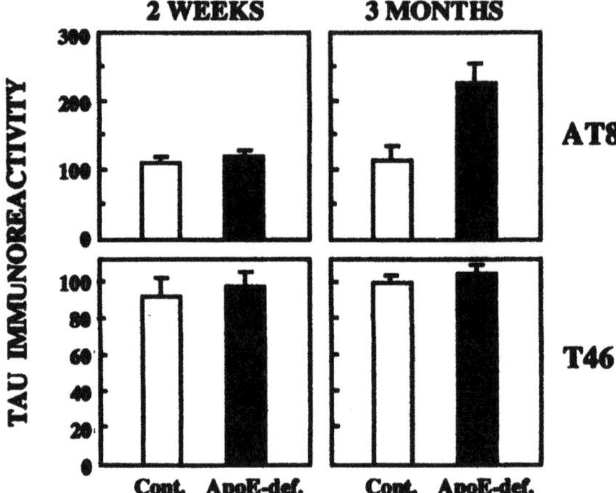

Figure 3. Quantitative comparison of the levels of tau phosphorylation of neonate and adult apoE-deficient and control mice. Immunoblot analyses of adult (4 months) and newly born (2 weeks) apoE-deficient and control mice (n = 3 in each group) were performed utilizing mAb146 and mAb AT8 as presented in Fig 2, except that the samples of both mice and age groups were blotted simultaneously and that the amounts of tau (i.e. T46 immunoreactivities) loaded on the blots were the same for the newly born and adult apoE-deficient and control mice. Sister immunoblots that were loaded with the same amount of tau were reacted with AT8, after which intensities of all the resulting immunoblots bands were quantitated utilizing the TINA PCgel computer software.

munoreactivities thus obtained is depicted in Figure 3. As can be seen the two neonate mice groups had similar levels of AT8 phosphorylation and the differences between them at adulthood was due to an age-dependent increase in AT8 tau phosphorylation in the apoE-deficient mice and not to dephosphorylation of control tau.

DISCUSSION

The observation that tau of apoE deficient mice is hyperophosphorylated raises two key issues, namely what is the cellular and biochemical mechanisms underlying this effect and whether tau hyperphosphorylation affects the phenotype of the apoE-deficient mice. This study represents an initial attempt to address these issues.

The level of tau phosphorylation in a given cell is determined by the intracellular interplay between its kinase and phosphatase activities as well as by putative interactions of tau with other cytoplasmic constituents. Thus the observed age dependent tau hyperphosphorylation in apoE-deficient mice may be due to the lack of direct apoE-tau interactions in these mice, which based on *in vitro* studies are presumed to be protective against tau hyperphosphorylation *in vivo*. Alternatively, it is possible that apoE represses a kinase (or activates a phosphatase) in control mice and that derepression of this activity in apoE-deficient mice is responsible for tau hyperphosphorylation in these animals. The former possibility is consistent with the finding that tau hyperphosphorylation in apoE-deficient mice is not brain area specific.Additional tau phosphorylation mapping studies will further our understanding of this issue by revealing whether the tau epitopes whose extents of phosphorylation are altered in apoE-deficient mice cluster at a given tau locus, and by unraveling the kinases and phosphatases which specifically affect tau phosphorylation. It is of interest to note that tau is not hyperphosphorylated in all strains of apoE-deficient mice

(Mercken and Brion, 1996) suggesting that additional, genetic, factors may be required for the phenotypic expression of the effects of apoE on tau phosphorylation in the mouse. Such a possibility is in accordance with the clinical data that not all AD patients homozygote for apoE4 get the disease.

It is not yet known whether tau phosphorylation in apoE deficient mice has neuropathological consequences. Our recent description of distinct neurochemical and cognitive deficits in apoE-deficient mice (Gordon et al., 1995; Chapman et al., 1997). some of which can be alleviated by suitable pharmacological treatment (Fisher et al., 1997) and of derangements in their brain repair mechanisms, now provide experimental tools necessary for investigating the functional consequences of tau hyperphosphorylation in apoE-deficient mice.

ACKNOWLEDGMENTS

This work was supported in part by grants to DMM from the United States-Israel Binational Science Foundation (grant no. 95116), from the Fund for Basic Research of the Israel Academy of Sciences and Humanities (grant no 670/96), from the Revah-Kabelli Fund and from the Jo and Inez Eichenbaum Foundation.

DMM is the incumbent of the Myriam lebach Chair in Molecular Neurodegeneration.

REFERENCES

Bellosta, S., Nathan, B.P., Orth, M., Dong, L.M., Mahley, R.W., and Pitas, R.E., 1995, Stable expression and secretion of Apolipoproteins E3 and E4 in mouse neuroblastoma cells produces differential effects on neurite outgrowth. *J. Biol. Chem.* 270:63–71.

Chapman, S., and Michaelson, D.M., 1997, Specific neurochemical derangements of brain projecting neurons in apolipoprotein E-deficient mice. Submitted.

Chen, Y., Lomnitzki, L., Michaelson, D.M., and Shohami, E., 1997, Moto and cognitive deficits in apolipoprotein E-deficient mice after closed head injury. *Neurosci.*, in press.

Clarke, G.A., White, C.A., and Moss, D.J., 1993, Substrate-bound GP130/F11 will promote neurite outgrowth: evidence for a cell surface receptor. *Eur. J. Cell Biol.* 61:108–115.

Corder, E.H., Saunders, A.M., Strittmatter, W.J., Schmechel, D.E., Gaskell, P.C., Small, G.W., Roses, A.D., Haines, J.L., and Pericak-Vance, M.A., 1993, Gene dose of apolipoprotein E type 4 allele and the risk of Alzheimer's disease in late onset families. *Science* 261: 921–923.

Fisher, A., Brandeis, R., Chapman, S., Pittel, Z., and Michaelson, D.M., 1997, M1 muscarinic agonist treatment reverses cognitive and cholinergic impairments of apolipoprotein E-deficient mice, in press.

Genis, I., Gordon, I., Sehayek, E., and Michaelson, D.M., 1995, Phosphorylation of tau in Apolipoprotein E-deficient mice. *Neurosci. Lett.* 199:5–8.

Goedert, M., Jakes, R., Crowther, R.A., Cohen, P., Vanmechelen, E., Vandermeeren, M., and Cras, P., 1994, Epitop mapping of monoclonal antibodies to the paired helical filaments of Alzheimer's disease: identification of phosphorylation sites in tau protein. *Biochem. J.* 301:871–877.

Gordon, I., Grauer, E., Genis, I., Sehayek, E., and Michaelson, D.M., 1995, Memory deficits and cholinergic impairment in apolipoprotein E-deficient mice. *Neurosci. Lett.* 199:1–4.

Ignatius, M.J., Gebicke-Harter, P.J., Skene, J.H., Schilling, J.W., Weisgraber, K.H., Mahley, R.W., and Shooter, E.M., 1986, Expression of apolipoprotein E during nerve degeneration and regeneration. *Proc. Natl. Acad. Sci.* 83:1125–1129.

Ksiezac-Reding, H., Chien, C.H., Lee, V.M-Y., and Yen, S.H., 1990, Mapping of the Alz-50 epitope in microtubule-associated protein tau. *J. Neurosci. Res.* 25:412–419.

Levy-Lahad, E., Wisman, E.M., Nemens, E., Anderson, L., Godart, K.A., Weber, J.L., Bird, T.D., and Schellenberg, G.D., 1995, A familial Alzheimer's disease locus on chromosome 1. *Science* 269:970–972

Lomnitski, L., Kohen, R., Chen, Y., Shohami, E., Trembovler, V., Vogel, T., and Michaelson, D.M., 1997, Reduced levels of antioxidants in brains of Apolipoprotein E-deficient mice following closed head injury. *Phar. Biochem Behav.* 56:669–673.

Mahley, R.W., 1988, Apolipoprotein E: cholesterol transport protein with expanding role in cell biology. *Science* 240:622–630.

Mawal-Dewan, M., Henley, J., Van de Voorde, A., Trojanovski, J.Q., and Lee, V.M.-Y., 1994, The phosphorylation state of tau in the developing rat brain is regulated by phosphoprotein phosphatase. *J. Biol. Chem.* 269:30981–30987.

Mercken,L., and Brion, J.P., 1995, Phosphorylation of tau protein is not affected in mice lacking apolipoprotein E. *NeuroReport* 6:2381–2384.

Miyata, M., and Smith, J., 1996, Apolipoprotein E allele-spesific antioxidant activity and effects on cytotoxicity by oxidative insults and β-amyloid peptides. *Nature* 14:55–61.

Namba, Y., Tomanaga, M., Kawasaki, H., Otomi, E., and Ikada, K., 1991, Apolipoprotein E immunoreactivity in cerebral amyloid deposites and neurofibrillary tangles in Alzheimer's disease and Kuru plaque amyloid in Creutzfeld-Jacob disease. *Brain Res.* 542:163–166.

Nathan, B.P., Bellosta, S., Sanan, D.A., Weisgraber, K.H., Mahley, R.W., and Pitas, R.E., 1994, Differential effects of apolipoproteins E3 and E4 on neuronal growth *in vitro*. *Science* 264:850–852.

Pitas, R.E., 1996, Microtubule formation and neurite extension are blocked by apolipoprotein E4. *Cell Devel. Biol.* 7:725–731.

Poirier, J., 1995, Apolipoprotein E in animal models of CNS injury and in Alzheimer's disease. Trends. *Neurosci.* 17:525–530.

Roses, A.D., 1994, Apolipoprotein E affects the rate of Alzheimer disease expression: beta-amyloid burden is a secondary consequence dependent on APOE genotype and duration of disease. *J. Neuropathol. Exp. Neurol.* 53:429–437.

Roses, A.D., 1996, Apolipoprotein E alleles as risk factors in Alzheimer's disease. *Ann. Rev. Med.* 47:378–400.

Sherrington, R., Rogaev, E.I., Liang, Y., Rogaeva, E.A., Levesque, G., Ikeda, M., Chi, H., Lin, C., Li, G., Holman, K., Tsuda, T., Mar, L., Foncin, J.f., Bruni, A.C., Montesi, M.P., Srobi, S., Rainero, I., Pinessi, L., Nee, L., Chumakov, I., Pollen, D., Brooks, A., Sanseau, P., Polinsky, R.J., Wasco, W., Dasilva, H.A.R., Hains, J.L., Pericak-Vance, M.A., Tanzi, R.E., Roses, A.D., Fraser, P.E., Rommence, J.M., and St. George-Hyslop, P.H., 1995, Cloning of a gene bearing missence mutations in early-onset familial Alzheimer's disease. *Nature* 375:754–760.

Strittmatter, W.J., Saunders, A.M., Godert, M., Weisgraber, K.H., Dong, L. M., Jacks, R., Huang, D.Y., Schmechel, D., Pericak-Vance, M., and Rose, A.D., 1994, Isoform spesific interaction of Apolipoprotein E with tau and phosphorylated tau: implications for Alzheimer's disease. *Proc. Natl. Acad. Sci.* 91:243–249.

36

Aβ INDUCES CELL DEATH IN PC12 CELLS AND TAU-TRANSFECTED CHO CELLS, BUT ONLY TAU PHOSPHORYLATION IN PC12 CELLS

Lone Fjord-Larsen, Jens D. Mikkelsen, and Ole F. Olesen

Department of Neurobiology
H. Lundbeck A/S
Ottiliavej 9, DK-2500 Copenhagen-Valby

INTRODUCTION

Brains from patients with Alzheimer's disease are characterized by extracellular depositions of β-amyloid peptide (Aβ) and an intracellular accumulation of paired helical filaments (PHF) consisting of hyperphosphorylated tau proteins. The normal phosphorylation of tau protein controls microtubule polymerisation and stabilization, whereas its abnormal phosphorylation probably favours its dissociation from microtubules, its self-aggregation into PHF and its location in the somato-dendritic compartment. Aβ peptides have been shown to induce cell death in vitro and in vivo (Loo et al., 1993; Li et al., 1996.; Chen et al., 1996), but the connection between Aβ and tau phosphorylation is not clear. To shed light on this issue, tau phosphorylation was studied in rat PC12 pheochromocytoma cells and Chinese hamster ovary (CHO) cells transfected with human tau-cDNA. Here we report a different phosphorylation pattern of tau in PC12 and transfected CHO cells. Moreover, we examined the expression pattern in the two cell lines of glycogen synthase kinase-3β (GSK-3β) and the mitogen activated protein kinase (MAPK), both of which have been implicated in tau phosphorylation (Ishiguro et al., 1993; Mandelkow et al., 1992; Drewes et al., 1992).

MATERIALS AND METHODS

Cell Cultures

CHO cells were maintained in Dulbecco's modified Eagle's Medium (DMEM)/ Hams F12 supplemented with 10% fetal calf serum, 1% Mem Eagle and 1% penicillin/

streptavidin. PC12 cells were maintained in DMEM supplemented with 10% horse serum, 5% fetal calf serum and 1% penicillin/streptavidin. Cultures were maintained at 37°C in 5% CO_2.

Transfection

A 1100 bp cDNA fragment containing the open reading frame of human tau (shortest isoform) was inserted into the pSG5 mammalian expression vector (Stratagene). This plasmid was co-transfected with the mammalian expression vector pZeo (Invitrogen) which contains the Zeomycin resistance gene. Stable clones were selected in 125 μg/ml Zeocin (Invitrogen). Clones were screened for high level tau expression by immunocytochemistry.

Preparation of Interphase and Mitotic Cells

Cells were arrested in the mitotic phase by incubation with 50 ng/ml Nocodazole (Sigma) for 14 hours. Mitotic cells were then collected by mechanical shake-off and gentle pipetting. The adherent cells were used as interphase cells. A sample of the cells was stained with Hoechst 33258 to confirm that the separation of mitotic and interphase cells was efficient.

Antibodies

Primary antibodies used in this study include polyclonal phosphorylation independent tau antibody (Sigma), AT8 (Innogenetics) directed towards tau that is hyperphosphorylated on Ser-202, Tau-1 (Boehringer Mannheim) directed towards tau that is unphosphorylated on Ser-199 and Ser-202, and antibodies directed towards GSK-3β (Transduction Laboratories), ERK1 and ERK2 (Santa Cruz Biotechnology, Inc.).

Immunocytochemistry

Cells were fixed using 4% paraformaldehyde/0.15 M Soerensen buffer, washed three times in phosphate buffered saline (PBS), and permeabilized in 0.1% Triton X-100/PBS. The cells were blocked with 10% horse serum/1% BSA/PBS, washed in PBS and incubated with primary antibody. After washing, the cells were reacted with a secondary anti-mouse Ig antibody conjugated to biotin, followed by an avidin-biotin complex conjugated to horseradish peroxidase. The complex was visualized with 0.32 mg/ml diaminobenzidine/0.01% hydrogen peroxide.

Western Blot Analysis

Extracts of PC12 or CHO-tau cells were prepared by lysing cells on ice in buffer containing 10 mM Tris-HCl, pH 7.4, 2 mM EDTA, 0.5 mM EGTA, 20 μg/ml Leupeptin, 10 mM Benzamidine, 0.1 mM PMSF and 500 mM NaCl. Cell extracts were centrifuged at 16.000 x g for 20 min and protein content in supernatants were determined according to Lowry. Samples were electrophoresed on 12.5% SDS-polyacrylamide gels and transferred to PVDF-membranes. Residual protein-binding sites were blocked with 1% non-fat drymilk in PBS. Membranes were incubated overnight with primary antibody, followed by incubation with a secondary anti-mouse Ig antibody conjugated to biotin, followed by an avidin-biotin complex conjugated to horseradish peroxidase. Immunostaining was visualized using enhanced chemoluminiscence (ECL) according to the manufacturer's instructions (Amersham).

RESULTS

Aβ Inhibits MTT Reduction in Both Cell Lines

$A\beta_{25-35}$ induced a dose-dependent decrease in the ability of both PC12 and CHO cells to reduce MTT. After 24 h incubation with 10 μM Aβ, the MTT reduction of PC12 cells decreased to 40% of control cells. CHO cells treated similarly responded with a 50% decrease in MTT reduction (Figure 1).

Different Phosphorylation Pattern of Tau in Untreated Cells

Immunocytochemistry showed that a minor fraction of the cells was positive with AT8, thus demonstrating that tau was phosphorylated at Ser-202 (Figure 2A). However, most transfected CHO cells were Tau-1 positive and thus contained tau unphosphorylated at Ser-199/202 (Figure 2B). The cells containing phosphorylated tau were all rounded, indicating that they were in the mitotic phase. This observation was confirmed by Western blotting of cells separated into mitotic and interphase cells, showing a strong phosphorylation of the AT8 epitope in the mitotic CHO cells and no tau phosphorylation in interphase cells (Figure 3A). In contrast, immunocytochemistry of PC12 cells showed that differentiated as well as undifferentiated cells contained both tau phosphorylated at Ser-202 as well as tau unphosphorylated at Ser-199/202 (Figure 2C, 2D). Mitotic PC12 cells showed some increase in tau AT8 immunoreactivity compared to interphase cells (Figure 3B).

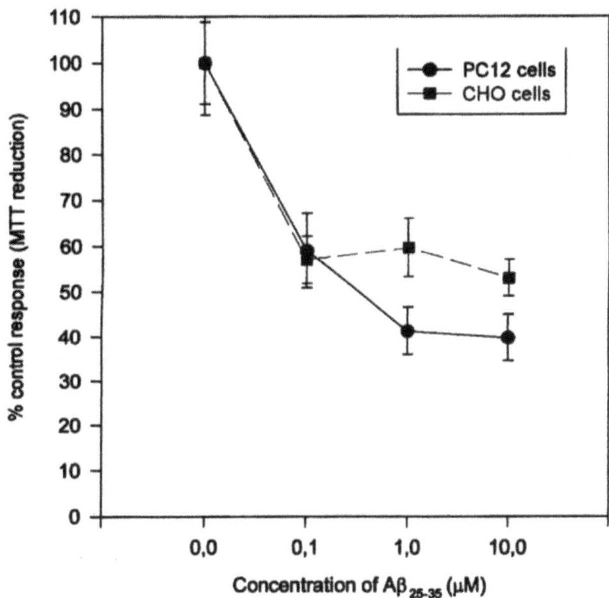

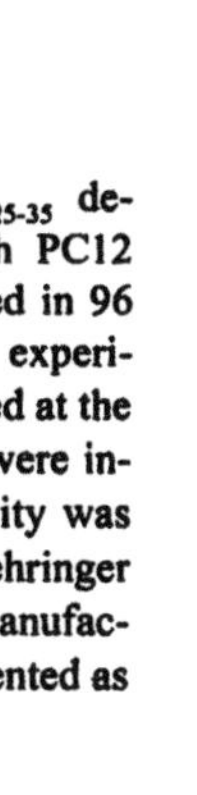

Figure 1. Incubation with $A\beta_{25-35}$ decreases MTT reduction in both PC12 and CHO cells. Cells were plated in 96 well plates the day before the experiment. $A\beta_{25-35}$ (Bachem) was added at the indicated concentrations. Cells were incubated for 24 hours and viability was assessed using MTT assay (Boehringer Mannheim) according to the manufacturers instructions. Data are presented as mean ± SD.

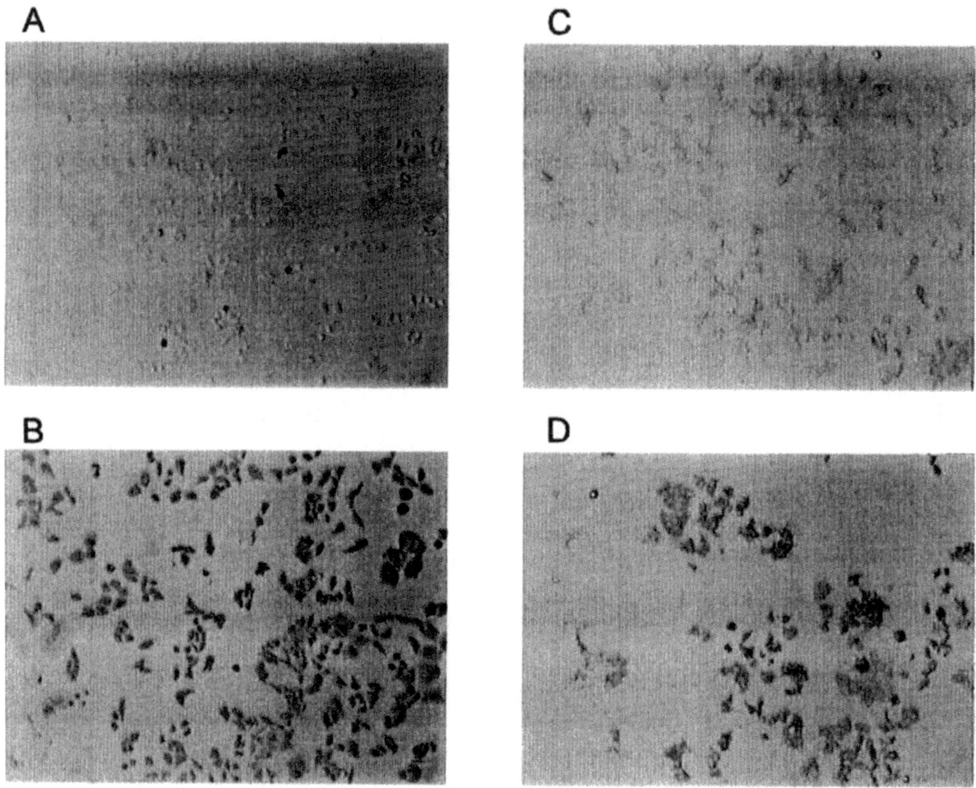

Figure 2. Immunostaining with Tau-1 and AT8 in transfected CHO cells and PC12 cells. A) Staining with AT8 in CHO cells. Some of the cells contain tau phosphorylated at Ser202. B) Staining with Tau-1 in CHO cells. The majority of cells contains tau unphosphorylated at Ser199/202. C) Staining with AT8 in PC12 cells. D) Staining with Tau-1 in PC12 cells. All cells contain both phosphorylated and unphosphorylated tau.

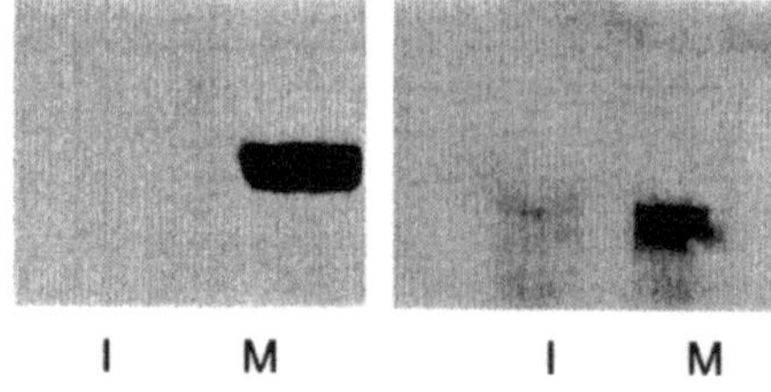

Figure 3. Tau phosphorylation in mitotic versus interphase cells. Cells were separated into mitotic and interphase cells and extracts were immunoblotted using the AT8 antibody. A) Western blot of cell extracts from transfected CHO cells showing that tau is phosphorylated during the mitotic phase. B) Western blot of cell extracts from PC12 cells showing that tau phosphorylation to some extent is affected of cell cycle status.

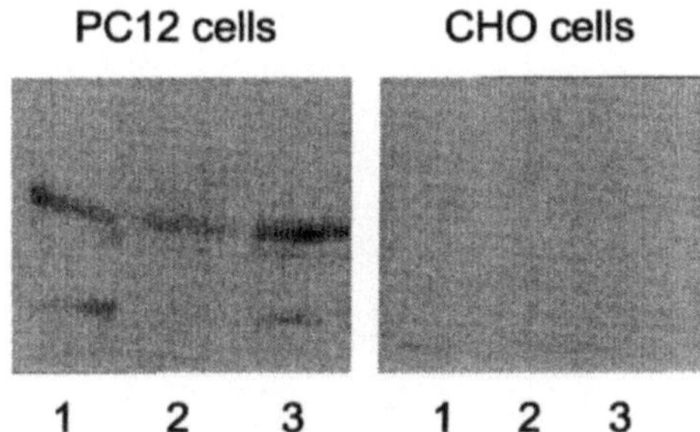

Figure 4. Aβ induces tau phosphorylation in PC12 cells (left), but not in CHO cells (right). Cells were plated in 100 mm dishes the day before experiments. Cells were incubated with 0, 1 or 10 μM Aβ for 48 h (lanes 1, 2 and 3, respectively). Extracts of the treated cells were immunoblotted using the AT8 antibody.

Aβ Induces Tau Phosphorylation in PC12 Cells, but Not in CHO Cells

Western blotting using the AT8 antibody showed that incubation with $A\beta_{25\text{-}35}$ induced a dose-dependent increase in tau phosphorylation in PC12 cells, whereas it had no effect on tau phosphorylation in CHO cells (Figure 4). Cell extracts were also immunoblotted with a phosphorylation independent tau antibody to ensure that the same amount of tau protein was loaded in each lane (data not shown).

Phosphatase (PP) Inhibitors Induce Tau Phosphorylation in Both Cell Lines

Treatment of PC12 and CHO cells with either of the phosphatase inhibitors Okadaic acid (OA) or Calyculin A (CA) increased AT8 immunoreactivity significantly. The most dramatic effect was seen with CA, even at concentrations ten times less than OA (Figure 5). As CA has a higher affinity for PP1 and the same affinity for PP2A as OA, these results indicate that PP1 as well as PP2A are important for maintaining tau in a dephosphorylated state. There was no difference in the effect of phosphatase inhibitors between PC12 and CHO cells.

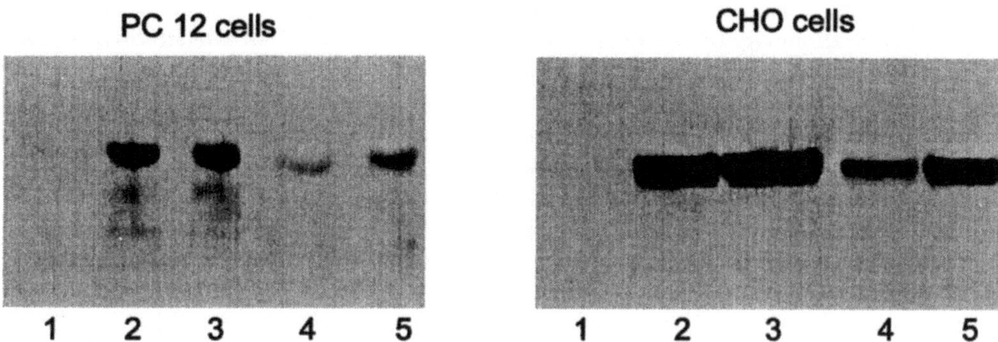

Figure 5. OA and CA induces tau phosphorylation in both cell lines. Cells were plated in 100 mm dishes the day before experiments. Cells were exposed to CA in concentrations of 0, 0.05 and 0.1 μM (lanes 1, 2 and 3), and OA in concentrations of 0.5 and 1 μM (lanes 4 and 5) for 2 h. Extracts of the treated cells were immunoblotted using the AT8 antibody.

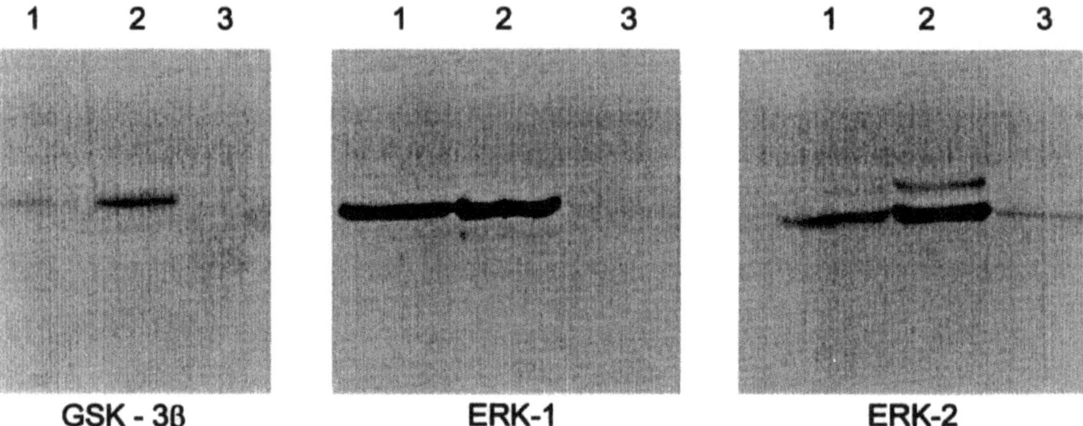

Figure 6. Expression of kinases in PC12 cells, undifferentiated (1) or differentiated (2) and CHO cells (3). PC12 cells expressed a higher level of ERK-1 and GSK-3β than CHO cells, whereas there was no significant difference in expression of ERK-2.

The Two Cell Lines Express Different Levels of Kinases

The expression of kinases in the cell lines was examined by immunocytochemistry and Western Blot using antibodies against GSK-3β, ERK-1 and ERK-2. The CHO cells expressed a lower level of ERK1 and GSK-3β than PC12 cells, whereas no significant difference in expression of ERK2 was found. Moreover, 5 days differentiation of PC12 cells in 50 ng/ml NGF led to increased levels of ERK-2 and GSK-3β (Figure 6).

DISCUSSION

A different phosphorylation pattern of tau was revealed in PC12 and transfected CHO cells. Tau phosphorylation in CHO cells was completely dependent on cell cycle status, whereas PC12 cells contained phosphorylated tau as well as unphosphorylated tau, independently of cell cycle. The data thus suggest that PC12 cells, in contrast to CHO cells, express tau phosphorylating kinase(s), which are activated during interphase. Incubation with $A\beta_{25-35}$ decreased MTT reduction in both cell lines, but induced an increase in tau phosphorylation only in PC12 cells. Analysis of the expression of kinases revealed that PC12 cells have a higher expression level of GSK-3β and ERK-1. Apart from kinases, the other important factor for regulation of phosphorylation is phosphatases. In the presence of inhibitors of PP1 and PP2A, the majority of tau accumulates in a phosphorylated state in both PC12 cells and CHO-tau cells, showing that both cell lines possess pathways leading to tau phosphorylation, and that PP1 and PP2A are necessary for maintaining tau in a dephosphorylated state. However, the Aβ-induced tau phosphorylation cascade appears to be specific for neuronal cells, as seen only in PC12 cells, possibly due to the higher levels of ERK-1 and GSK-3β.

REFERENCES

Chen, S.Y., Harding, J.W. and Barnes C.D. 1996. Neuropathology of synthetic β-amyloid peptide analogs in vivo. *Brain Res.* 715:44.

Drewes G., Lichtenberg-Kraag, B., Döring, F., Mandelkow and E.M., Mandelkow, E. 1992. Mitogen activated protein (MAP) kinase transforms tau protein into an Alzheimer-like state. *EMBO J.* 11: 2131.

Ishiguro, K., Shiratsuchi, A., Sato, S. Omori, A., Arioka, M., Kobayashi, S., Uchida, T. And Imahori, K. 1993. Glycogen synthase kinase 3β is identical to tau protein kinase I generating several epitopes of paired helical filaments. *FEBS Lett.* 148:202.

Li, Y.P., Bushnell, A.F., Lee, C.M., Perlmutter, L.S. and Wong, S.K.F. 1996. β-Amyloid induces apoptosis in human-derived neurotypic SH-SY5Y cells. *Brain Res.* 738:196.

Loo, D.T., Copani, A., Pike, C.J., Whittemore, E.R., Walencewitz, A.J. and Cotman, C.W. 1993. Apoptosis is induced by β-amyloid in cultured central nervous system neurons, *Proc. Natl. Acad. Sci. USA* 90:7951.

Mandelkow, E.M., Drewes, G., Biernat, J., Gustke, N., Van Lint, J., Vandenheede, J.R. and Mandelkow, E. 1992. Glucogen synthase kinase 3 and the Alzheimer disease-like state of microtubule-associated protein tau. *FEBS Lett.* 314:315.

37

DIFFERENT COGNITIVE PROFILES ON MEMORY TESTS IN PARKINSON'S DISEASE AND ALZHEIMER'S DISEASE

Ricardo F. Allegri,[1] Paula Harris,[1] and Raúl L. Arizaga[2]

[1]Department of Neuropsychology (SIREN)
CEMIC — University of Buenos Aires Associated Hospital
Galvan 4102
(1431) Buenos Aires, Argentina
[2]Department of Neuroepidemiology
INSSPJP — PAMI
Ecuador 650
(1428) Buenos Aires, Argentina

INTRODUCTION

It is well know that dementia, a clinical syndrome characterized by an acquired and persistent loss of intellect, is not a single entity or the outcome of one specific etiology. It should be noted, however, that within the dementia syndrome, some distinctive profiles of cognitive impairment are associated with different etiologies (Ross et al., 1992).

Two major patterns of neuropsychological decline, identified as cortical and subcortical subtypes of dementia, have been described (Cummings and Benson, 1984). Although controversial (Cummings, 1986; Withehouse, 1986), this distinction is useful for neuropsychological diagnosis. In both subtypes, memory function in affected in different ways (Beatty, 1992; Helkala et al., 1988; Moss et al., 1986). While memory disturbances associated with Parkinson's disease (PD) are similar to those characteristic of subcortical disorders (such as Huntington's disease and Multiple Sclerosis), memory impairments most commonly found in Alzheimer's disease (AD) are prototypical of a cortical dementia (Beatty, 1992).

In order to further investigate the memory disturbances associated with AD and PD, we performed this clinical study examining whether changes in episodic memory are present at an early stage of these diseases. A second goal of this research protocol was to characterize the episodic memory profiles in AD and PD.

Progress in Alzheimer's and Parkinson's Diseases
edited by Fisher *et al.*, Plenum Press, New York, 1998.

PATIENTS

A hundred and ten patients, 60 with diagnosis of probable AD (NINCDS-ADRDA; McKhann, et al., 1984), and 50 with PD (United Kingdom PD Society Brain Bank Clinical Criteria for PD; Hughes, 1992), matched for age, sex and education, were included in this study. Patients with PD displayed typical clinical features of this condition and all of them responded to levodopa. Average scores in the Hoen Yahr scale (Hoen and Yahr, 1967) was 3.2 ± 0.4. All patients underwent a complete neurological and clinical examination. Neuroimaging (CT scan or MRI) disclosed no focal lesions; ischaemia scores were < 4. Patients with major depression (according to the DSM IV criteria) or treated with anticholinergics were excluded. 30 normal controls, most of them spouses of patients, were also evaluated; none of them had history of alcoholism nor of neurological or psychiatric disorders. Demographic and clinical data of the studied subjects are presented in Table 1.

METHODS

Global Measures

Global assessment of cognitive functioning and deterioration was evaluated with the Mini Mental State Examination (MMSE; Folstein et al., 1975), and Global Deterioration Scale (GDS; Reisberg, et al., 1982). Cutoff levels were > 14 (MMSE) and ≤ 4 (GDS).

Memory Tests

Episodic memory was assessed by: (a) logical memory tasks (immediate and delayed recall of a story) (Signoret et al., 1979); (b) auditory verbal learning of a list of twelve non related words (three trials); (c) free recall of the list; (d) cued recall: a semantic cue is given to facilitate recall of lacking items; (e) recognition: items still not restored are prompted by a four item multiple-choice task; (f) digit span, forward and backward (Wechsler, 1988). Primacy (number of items recalled among the first four in the verbal learning list of words (first trial)), and recency effects (numbers of items recalled among the last four in the verbal learning list of words (first trial)) were calculated. Confabulations produced during the recall of the story and the word list, were also taken into account. Digit span and recency effect was used for measuring short-term memory; while long-term memory was estimated through primacy effect.

Table 1. Clinical and demographic data

	Controls	AD	PD	F	p
No. of patients	30	60	50		
Age (years)	72.0 (8.3)	71.7 (7.9)	71.6 (9.0)	0.014	NS
Education (years)	10.9 (3.2)	11.0 (4.2)	10.2 (4.3)	0.435	NS
Time from onset of the disease (months)	—	23.04	30.27		
MMSE	28.5 (0.9)	24.0 (2.8)	24.8 (0.9)	2.126	NS[1]
GDS	—	3.6 (0.6)	—		

[1]AD vs PD; NS = not significant.

STATISTICAL ANALYSIS

Results are expressed as means ± SD. The calculated means were then tested for statistically significant differences using a one way analysis of variance (ANOVA), (BMDP Statistically software; Dixon, 1990). A $p < .05$ was considered significant.

RESULTS

As shown in Table 1, global cognitive performance was significantly better ($p < 0.001$) in control subjects than in AD and PD patients who exhibited similar scores in the MMSE ($F = 2.12$; p = not significant).

As regards episodic memory (Table 2), extremely significant differences ($p < 0.001$) between AD and control subjects were detected in most of the tasks. Interestingly, patients with PD showed a different and particular mnesic profile: they performed poorly, like AD patients, in the immediate and delayed free recall of newly verbal information, but almost as accurately as controls in the recognition tasks (multiple choice) ($F = 2.27$; p = not significant).

As compared to control subjects, AD and PD patients (Table 3) revealed severe impairments in long term memory (primacy effect: $p < 0.001$). Short term memory (recency effect and forward digit span) was also affected ($p < 0.001$ vs controls) in AD but PD performed like controls (p = not significant, PD vs controls).

DISCUSSION

According to our results, episodic memory profiles differ in subjects suffering from AD and PD. Comparison of neuropsychological test scores obtained in these patients and

Table 2. Episodic memory performance

	Controls	AD	PD	F	p
Story recall (n = 12)					
Immediate	8.8 (1.7)	3.0 (2.1)	7.1 (1.7)	55.05[1]	<0.001
				8.28[2]	=0.005
				74.87[3]	<0.001
Delayed	8.7 (1.5)	2.2(2.3)	6.3 (3.0)	12.17[1]	<0.001
				157.40[2]	<0.001
				55.05[3]	<0.001
Word list (n = 12)					
Immediate (3rd. trial)	8.8 (1.4)	4.3 (2.2)	5.7 (2.1)	44.00[1]	<0.001
				85.21[2]	<0.001
				8.93[3]	<0.050
Delayed (free recall)	7.3 (2.0)	1.4 (1.9)	3.8 (2.0)	45.36[1]	<0.001
				153.0[2]	<0.001
				33.02[3]	<0.001
Delayed (cued recall)	10.5 (1.5)	3.7 (2.9)	8.5 (2.5)	11.84[1]	<0.001
				117.50[2]	<0.001
				72.64[3]	<0.001
Delayed recognition	11.0 (1.3)	6.1 (3.2)	10.5 (1.3)	2.27[1]	NS
				50.12[2]	<0.001
				63. 97[3]	<0.001

[1]Controls vs PD; [2]controls vs AD; [3]AD vs PD; NS = not significant.

Table 3. Differences in short term memory (recency effect and digit span) and long term memory (primacy effect)

	Controls	AD	PD	p
Primacy effect	8.3 (1.9)	2.5 (2.3)	5.4 (2.4)	<0.001[1]
				<0.001[2]
				<0.001[3]
Recency effect	7.4 (2.4)	5.2 (2.4)	5.6 (2.1)	<0.01[1]
				<0.001[2]
				NS[3]
Digit span (forward)	6.5 (0.8)	5.8(1.1)	6.2 (1.2)	NS[1]
				<0.01[2]
				NS[3]

[1]Controls vs PD; [2]controls vs AD; [3]AD vs PD; NS = not significant.

in normal controls reveals that both patients groups performed significantly below controls in story recall and in the verbal learning tasks. Patients with PD restore the story more succesfully than AD patients. These performed worse in the story recall (immediate and delayed) probably due to the impairment of semantic link that characterizes AD (Chetkow and Bub, 1992). This fact indicates that the presence or absence of a semantic bond connecting the items to be retained, clearly modifies memory achievements in PD patients. The story to be recalled includes this semantic link, an element that is lacking in verbal learning tasks.

Patients with PD performed poorly, like AD patients, in the free recall of newly verbal information, but almost as accurately as controls in the recognition tasks. Memory can be conceived as a process entailing the flow of information between interrelated stores. Consequently, entering data would pass through different stages: acquisition, consolidation and retrieval (Signoret, 1985). According to this view, a sort of retrieval difficulty (e.g. an inability of the memory system to locate a memory trace) could be responsible of the memory deficits observed in PD patients; hence, the acquisition and consolidation stages would be preserved in this condition. Other investigators (Butters et al., 1984; Brown and Marsden, 1988; Helkala et al., 1988; Allegri et al., 1992) have discussed this possibility in previous reports. Failure in the retrieval process with unharmed storage capabilities would be then the causative mechanism underlying this "forgetting pattern" that characterize the memory disturbances observed in PD patients.

On other hand, patients with AD would suffer from an encoding impairment. As a consequence, new information is not being transferred from the short term store into the long term store ("amnesia pattern"). Data would remain temporarily in this short term store and would then be "sweeped off" by new entering information (interference). This could be supported by the differences in the "primacy and recency" effects detected in AD patients, and by the significant loss of information observed when a non related task is to be performed between the verbal learning and the delayed recall.

Not only quantitative but also important qualitative differences were noted during neuropsychological testing: when asked to restore the story, 24 out of 60 AD patients produced confabulations. This manifestation was not observed in PD patients (nor in controls).

From the presented results we may conclude that: 1) episodic memory profiles differ in patients with AD and PD, showing the latter merely a retrieval difficulty and preserved acquisition and storage processes, benefit from the semantic facilitation, and display a normal recognition pattern; and 2) A near normal performance in the cued recall and recognition tasks constitues a relavant tool for the neuropsychological diagnosis of dementia syndrome and related disorders, being the hallmark of the subcortical type of cognitive decline.

SUMMARY

Memory impairment is observed both in cortical and subcortical types of dementing conditions such as AD, and PD. We evaluated episodic memory performance in 60 patients with AD, in 50 patients with PD, as well as in 30 age and education matched control subjects (CON).

Both groups of patients scored poorly in the story recall (p < 0.001 vs CON). However, the presence of a semantic link in the given task (story recall, cued recall), significantly improved the outcome of the tests in PD patients. Moreover, recognition was almost normal in these subjects (PD vs CON; not significant). The loss of information (probably due to interference effect) was very important in AD patients.

Our results suggest that patients with PD are still able to translocate information into the long term storage. This is not the case with AD patients. Possibly, then, a retrieval failure is responsible for the memory impairments observed in patients with PD; on the other hand, an encoding difficulty would underly the characteristic "amnesia" of AD patients.

ACKNOWLEDGMENTS

Supported in part by Fundación de Estudios Epidemiológicos e Investigaciones Clínicas en Neurología y Psiquiatría, Buenos Aires, Argentina.

REFERENCES

Allegri, R.F., Ranalli, C.G., DeDaras, A., Fascetto, V., Gallegos, M., Scarlatti, A., and Tamaroff, L., 1992, Evaluación Neuropsicológica en la Enfermedad de Parkinson. *Medicina (Buenos Aires)* 52:141–144.

American Psychiatric Association, 1994, *Diagnostic and Statistical Manual of Mental Disorders.* 4th ed., Washington, D.C.

Beatty, W.W., 1992, Memory disturbances in Parkinson's disease. In: *Parkinson's disease: Neurobehavioral aspects.* Huber, S.J. and Cummings, J.L., eds, Oxford University Press, pp. 49–58.

Brown, R.G. and Marsden, C.D., 1988, Subcortical dementia: the neuropsychological evidence. *Neuroscience* 25:363–387.

Butters, N., Miliotis, P., Albert, M., and Sax, D., 1984, Memory assessment: evidences of the heterogeneity of amnesic symptoms. In: *Clinical Neuropsychology,* Goldstein, G., ed., Plenum, New York, 127–159.

Chetkow, H. and Bub, D., 1992, Semantic memory loss in dementia of Alzheimer's type. *Brain* 113:397–417.

Cummings, J.L, and Benson, F.D., 1984, Subcortical dementia. review of an emerging concept. *Arch. Neurol.* 41:874–879.

Cummings, J.L., 1986, Subcortical dementia: neuropsychology, neuropsychiatry and pathophysiology. *Br. J. Psychiatry* 149:682–687.

Dixon, W.J., 1990, BMDP Statistical software. University of California (UCLA), PC 90.

Folstein, M.S., Folstein, S.E., McHugh, P.R., 1975, "Mini Mental State". A practical method for grading the cognitive state of patients for the clinician. *J. Psychiat. Res.* 12:189–198.

Hachinski, V.C., Illif, L.D., and Zilhka, E., et al., 1975, Cerebral blood flow in dementia. *Arch.Neurol,* 32:632–637.

Helkala, E.L., Laulumaa, V., Soininen, H., and Riekkinen, P.J., 1988, Recall and recognition memory in patient with Alzheimer's and Parkinson's disease. *Ann. Neurol.* 24:214–217.

Hoen, M., and Yahr, M.D., 1967. Parkinsonism: onset, progression and mortality. *Neurology* 17:427–442.

Hughes, A.J., Daniel, S.E., Kilford, L., Lees, A.J., 1992, Accuracy of clinical diagnosis of idiopathic Parkinson's disease: a clinicopathological study of 100 cases *J. Neurol. Neurosurg Psychiatry* 55:181–184.

McKhann, G., Drachman, D., Folstein, M. et al., 1984, Clinical diagnosis of Alzheimer's disease: report of NINCDS -ADRDA Work Group under the auspices of Department of Health and Human Service Task Force on Alzheimer's disease. *Neurology* 34:939–944.

Moss, M.B., Albert, M.S., Butters, N., and Payne, M., 1986. Differential patterns of memory loss among patients with Alzheimer's disease, Huntington's disease and alcoholic Korsakoff's syndrome. *Arch. Neurol.* 43:239–246.

Reisberg, B., Ferris, S.H., DeLeon, M.J. et al., 1982. The global deterioration scale of assessment of primary degenerative dementia. *Am. J. Psychiatry* 139:1136–1139.

Signoret, J.L., 1985. Memory and Amnesias. In: *Principles of Behavioral Neurology*. M-M Mesulam, FA Davis Company Philadelphia, pp 169–192.

Signoret, J.L., and Whiteley, A., 1979. Memory battery scale. *Inter. Neuropsych. Soc. Bull.* 2–26.

Wechsler, D., 1988. *Test de inteligencia para adultos* (WAIS). Paidos, Buenos Aires.

Whitehouse, P.J., 1986. The concept of subcortical dementia: another look. *Ann. Neurol.* 19:1.

38

NEUROPSYCHOLOGICAL SUBTYPES AND RATE OF PROGRESSION IN ALZHEIMER'S DISEASE

C. Piccini, D. Campani, M. Piccininni, G. Manfredi, L. Amaducci, and L. Bracco

Department of Neurological and Psychiatric Sciences
University of Florence
Policlinico di Careggi
85 Viale Morgagni, 50134 Florence, Italy

INTRODUCTION

In the latest years, a debated question is whether the different clinical patterns of Alzheimer's Disease (AD) are due to the presence of subtypes or, rather, to stages of the disease (Mayeux, 1985; Chui et al., 1985; Jorm, 1985; Mohr et al., 1990; Richte & Touchon, 1992; Yesavage et al., 1991, 1993; Joanette et al., 1994). Thus, an ever greater emphasis has been paid to the necessity of longitudinal studies (Berg et al., 1984; Jorm, 1985; Yesavage et al., 1991; Haxby et al., 1992; Richte & Touchon, 1992; Morris et al., 1993) and to detailed description of cognitive deficits in AD patients (Haxby et al., 1992).

In our opinion, published data and clinical experience, make plausible the hypothesis that AD includes some neuropsychological subtypes, expressed by generalized or focal mental impairment, where focal refers to prevalent impairment of language or visuo-spatial functions.

In this paper we describe the approach we developed to verify the presence and, if any, the rate of these neuropsychological subtypes, taking into account the severity of mental deterioration. Furthermore, we evaluated them in terms of their clinico-demographic features as well as of rate of progression of mental decline.

METHODS

As part of a longitudinal survey on primary degenerative dementia, we studied 119 consecutive patients with a diagnosis of probable Alzheimer's Disease who were referred to our Neurological Department between April 1982 and April 1994. We based the clinical diagnosis on a standardized protocol (Bracco, 1981; Bracco et al., 1992) that does not differ substantially from the NINCDS-ADRDA guidelines (McKhan et al., 1984) and used data from a patient's clinical history, neurological examination, laboratory tests and CT/MRI scans to exclude forms of dementia other than AD.

Cognitive functions were evaluated using an extensive neuropsychological battery including scales examining daily-living activities as well as tasks exploring verbal and spatial memory, orientation, calculation, language, writing, reading capacities, and visuo-motor functions. The battery consisted of: Information-Memory-Concentration Test (IMCT), Blessed Dementia Scale for Daily Living Activity, Digit Span, Corsi Tapping Test, Randt Memory Test, Babcock Story, Set Test (category fluency), Token Test, reading, writing, Gibson Maze, Copying Drawings. This battery, standardized on a group of 146 normal elderly subjects (Bracco et al., 1990), allows us to classify the level of mental impairment as absent, minimal, mild, moderate, severe or very severe according to five tests selected through discriminant analysis (Bracco et al., 1986). All tests scores were adjusted for each subject's age and educational level.

In this study we administered the neuropsychological battery to each of the 119 patients on the initial and each follow-up observation (every six months). Therefore we collected a total of 679 neuropsychological evaluations: 40 corresponded to a minimal level of mental impairment, 87 to mild, 175 to moderate, 168 to severe and 209 to very severe impairment. Since the last category (n = 209) was equivalent to a state of untestability (floor effect), the data from patients so classified were not included in the analysis. Hence, our findings are based on 470 neuropsychological observations.

In order to make comparable tests differing for score ranges, we transformed raw scores into coefficients by the formula: coeff. = $(x - X)/X$, where x is the patient's raw score and X the mean score of the normal elderly subjects. The resulting value, which ranges from plus to minus 1, was multiplied by minus 1 so that a score of zero corresponds to normal performance, a positive value represents impaired performance and a negative value performance better than the mean of normal controls.

To verify the presence of the hypothesized cognitive subtypes ("generalized impairment," "prevalent language impairment," "prevalent visuo-spatial impairment") we computed so-called Indices of Prevalent Impairment of Performance (IPIP). To measure how much linguistic as opposed to visuo-spatial skills were compromised we subtracted the coefficients for constructional praxis (Copying Drawings) and visuomotor ability (Gibson Maze) from coefficients for tests exploring the language domain (Set Test and Token Test). Tests were chosen among those for which there was evidence from studies carried out in patients with unilateral focal damages that the performance differed significantly according to the side of lesion. Furthermore they have been chosen as the more feasable in terms of properties of the scale: all the tests have a closed scale (including verbal fluency–Set Test). These index values ranged from +1 to −1. The more positive the index, the greater the impairment in linguistic as compared to visuo-spatial performance whereas more negative indices describe the reverse situation; a value of zero corresponds to equal impairment in these two cognitive domains, that is a generalized impairment.

To establish how atypical the IPIPs profile are in respect to global mental impairment, we converted these indices in z-scores: such a conversion has been computed by means of the mean and standard deviation of IPIP stratified for the degree of the cognitive impairment; thus, the atypicity has been evaluated for a specific level of dementia severity. We obtained 5 groups of z-scores depending on the level of mental impairment.

Rate of change of mental decline was calculated for each patient as the difference between his/her final and initial score at the IMCT divided by the number of intervening years.

RESULTS

Our study population had a mean age at onset of 58.8 (7.0) years, with a mean length of illness at the entry into the study of 3.5 (2.4) years and a mean score at the Blessed Dementia Scale of 8.3 (4.9). No differences were found in these variables between males (n = 39) and females (n = 80). The conversion of the IPIPs into z-scores for each level of cognitive impairment made it possible to identify patients whose behavior was atypical and to classify their pattern of cognitive impairment as "generalized" or "with prevalent L/V impairment." The percentages of patients with language or visuo-spatial prevalent impairment were 0% and 7%, 9% and 21%, 7% and 10%, 14% and 4% for the four considered levels of dementia severity.

Table 1 lists the clinico-demographic features of the three groups. Gender turned out to be the only significantly different variable (p = 0.02) in that there was a higher percentage of males (61%) among language impaired patients. In particular, the three groups didn't display any difference in terms of rate of progression on the IMCT.

DISCUSSION

Given the known instability of statistical clustering procedures and the often somewhat arbitrary decision-making process involved in determining the number of groups, we decided to use an alternative method in order to assess the presence of neuropsychological subtypes and to validate previous published data.

Our data confirm the presence of cognitive subtypes in AD. The total percentage of patients with prevalent Language or Visuospatial impairment falls between 20 and 30%, and they can be detected at all stages of dementia. Our values are lower than the 40% reported in previous studies (Martin et al., 1987; Spinnler & Della Sala, 1988) and this discrepancy might be due to our procedure which defines as "atypical" a patient whose performance differs significantly from his group mean, taking into account that he/she himself/herself forms part of that group.

In agreement with some (Lorin & Largen, 1985; Becker et al., 1988; Yesavage et al., 1992), though by no means all (Seltzer & Sherwin, 1983; Filley et al., 1986; Faber-Lagen-

Table 1. Clinical-demographic features of patients with "generalized," "prevalent language," or "prevalent visuo-spatial" impairment

	Generalized (n = 84)	Language (n = 18)	Visuo-spatial (n = 17)	p
M:F	0.4	1.6	0.4	0.02
Age at onset (yrs)	59.4 (7.1)	58.0 (5.1)	58.5 (6.6)	n.s.
Length of illness at entry (yrs)	3.4 (2.0)	3.7 (3.3)	3.4 (1.8)	n.s.
Schooling (yrs)	6.7 (3.5)	8.4 (5.1)	5.9 (3.0)	n.s.
Rate of change on the IMCT *	4.8 (4.15)	5.5 (2.52)	5.0 (3.55)	n.s.

Values in parentheses are standard deviations.
*Mean annual rate of change on the Information-Memory-Concentration test (points/years).

                                      C. Piccini *et al.*

doen et al., 1988, Binetti et al., 1993) published findings, we found no difference in age at onset for our groups of globally and focally impaired patients. Likewise we found no difference in terms of annual rate of change on the IMCT.

A group difference, instead, was found in sexual composition: among our language impaired patients there was a significantly higher percentage of males, suggesting that it could reflect differences in patterns of cerebral lateralization in the two sexes (Witelson 1976; Rugg, 1995; Shaywitz et al., 1995). Visuo-spatially impaired patients appeared more frequently in the early stages of AD while linguistically impaired ones appear more often in the advanced stages, as reported also by Rassmusson (Rassmusson & Brandt, 1995). This difference may reflect the way in how the degree of mental impairment is classified since it depends in large part on verbal measures.

In conclusion, our results, on one hand, confirm the possibility to identify neuropsychological suptypes not depending from differences in disease severity; on the other hand, they lack to point to a different clinical course of such neuropsychological subtypes.

REFERENCES

Becker, J.T., Huff, F.J., Nebes, R.D., Holland, A., and Boller, F., 1988, Neuropsychological function in Alzheimer's disease: Pattern of impairment and rates of progression. *Arch. Neurol.* 45:263–268.

Berg, L., Danziger, W.L., Storandt, M., Coben, L.A., Gado, M., Hughes, C.P., Knesevich, J.W., and Botwinick, J., 1984, Predictive features in mild senile dementia of the Alzheimer type. *Neurology* 34:563–569.

Binetti, G., Magni, E., Padovani, A., Cappa, S.F., Bianchetti, A., and Trabucchi, M., 1993, Neuropsychological heterogeneity in mild Alzheimer's Disease. *Dementia* 321–326.

Bracco, L., 1981, Un protocollo italiano per le demenze, Atti del XXI della SIN.

Bracco, L., Tiezzi, A., Lippi, A., and Amaducci, L., 1986, Staging of mental impairment by means of discriminant analysis. *Int. J. Ger. Psychiat.* 1:99–106.

Bracco, L., Amaducci, L., Pedone, D., Bino, G., Lazzaro, M.P., Carella F., D'Antona, R., Gallato R., and Denes G., 1990, Italian Multicentre Study on Dementia (SMID): a neuropsychological test battery for assessing Alzheimer's Disease. *J. Psychiat. Res.* 24:213–226.

Bracco, L., Amaducci, L., and SMID group, 1992, Italian Multicenter Study on Dementia: a protocol for data collection and clinical diagnosis of Alzheimer's disease. *Neuroepidemiology* 11:39–45.

Chui, H.C., Lee teng, E., Henderson, V., and Moy, A.C., 1985, Clinical subtypes of dementia of the Alzheimer type. *Neurology* 35:1544–1550.

Faber-Langendoen, K., Morris, J.C., Knesevich, J.W., LaBarge, E., Miller, P., and Berg, L., 1988, Aphasia in senile dementia of the Alzheimer Type. *Ann. Neurol.* 23:365–370.

Filley, C.M:, Kelly, J., and Heaton, R.K., 1986, Neuropsychologic features of early and late onset Alzheimer's disease. Arch. Neurol. 43:575–576.

Haxby, J.V., Raffaele, K., Gillette, J., Schapiro, M.B., and Rapoport, S.I., 1992, Individual trajectories of cognitive decline in patients with dementia of Alzheimer type. J. Clin. Exp. Neuropsych. 14:575–592.

Joanette, Y., Ska, B., Poissant, A., and Giroux, F., 1994, Vers une multiplicité des profils des atteintes cognitives dans la demence de type Alzheimer. In: *Actualités sur la maladie d'Alzheimer et les syndromes apparentés*, Poncet, M., Michel, B. and Nieoullon, A., ed., Solal éditeurs, Marseille, France, pp. 229–233.

Jorm, A.F., 1985, Subtypes of Alzheimer's Dementia: a conceptual analysis and critical review. Psychological Medicine, 15:543–553.

Lorin, D.W., and Largen, J.W., 1985, Neuropsychological patterns of presenile and senile dementia of the Alzheimer type. Neuropsychologia 23:351–357.

Martin, A., Browers, P., Lalonde, F., Cox, C., Teleska, P., Fedio, P., Foster, N.L. and Chase, T.N., 1987, Towards a behavioral typology of Alzheimr's patients. J. Clin. Exper. Neuropsychology 8:594–610.

Mayeux, R., Stern, Y., and Spanton, S., 1985, Heterogeneity in dementia of the Alzheimer type: Evidence of subgroups. *Neurology* 35:453–461.

McKhann, G., Drachman, D., Folstein, M., Katzman, R., Price, D., and Stadlan, E.M., 1984, Clinical diagnosis of Alzheimer's disease: report of the NINCDS-ADRDA Work Group under the auspices of the Department of Health and Human Services Task Force on Alzheimer's Disease. *Neurology* 34:939–944.

Mohr, E., Mann, U.M., and Chase,T.N., 1990, Subgroups in Alzheimer's disease: fact or fiction? Univ Ottawa, *Psychiatr. J.* 15:203–206.

Morris, J.C., Edland, S., Clark, C., Deland, S., Clark, C., Galasko, D., Koss, E., Mohs, R., van Belle ,G., Fillenbaum, G., and Heyman, A., 1993, The Consortium to Establish a Registry for Alzheimer's Disease (CERAD): Part IV. Rates of cognitive change in the longitudinal assessment of probable Alzheimer's Disease. *Neurology* 43: 2457–2465.

Rasmusson, X.D., and Brandt, J., 1995, Instability of cognitive asymmetry in Alzheimer's Disease. *J. Clin. Exp. Neuropsychology* 17: 449–458.

Ritche, K., and Touchon, J., 1992, Heterogeneity in senile dementia of the Alzheimer type:individual differences, progressive deterioration or clinical subtypes? *J. Clin. Epidemiol.* 45: 1391–1398.

Rugg, M., 1995, La difference vive. *Nature* 373: 561–562.

Seltzer, B., and Sherwin, I., 1983, A comparison of clinical features in early and late onset primary degenerative dementia. One entity or two? *Arch. Neurol.* 40:143–146.

Shaywitz, B.A., Sharwitz, S.E., Pugh, K.R., Constable, R.T., Skudlarsky, P., Fulbright, R.K., Bronen, R.A., Fletcher, J.M., Shankweller, D.P., Katz, L., and Gore, J.C., 1995, Sex differences in the functional organization of the brain for language. *Nature* 373:607–609.

Spinnler, H., and Della Sala, S., 1988, The role of clinical neuropsychology in the Alzheimer's disease, *J. Neurol.* 235:258–271.

Witelson, S.F., 1976, Sex and the single hemisphere: specialization of the right hemisphere for spatial processing. *Science* 193: 425–27.

Yesavage, J.A., and Brooks, J.O., 1991, On the importance of longitudinal research in Alzheimer's Disease. *J. Am. Geriatr. Soc.* 39:942–944.

Yesavage, J.A., Brooks, J.O., Taylor, J., and Tinklenberg, J., 1993, Development of aphasia, apraxia and agnosia and decline in Alzheimer's Disease. *Am. J. Psychiatry* 150:742–747.

39

BRAIN BANKING IN AGING AND DEMENTIA RESEARCH—THE AMSTERDAM EXPERIENCE

R. Ravid,[1] D. F. Swaab,[2] W. Kamphorst,[3] and A. Salehi[2]

[1]The Netherlands Brain Bank
Meibergdreef 33
1105 AZ Amsterdam, The Netherlands
[2]The Netherlands Institute for Brain Research
Meibergdreef 33
1105 AZ Amsterdam, The Netherlands
[3]Pathological Institute, Free University
de Boelelaan 1117
1081 HV Amsterdam, The Netherlands

INTRODUCTION

Collecting human brain for research on Alzheimer's disease (AD) and related disorders should put emphasis on the development of a rapid autopsy system, *e.g.*, as practised by the Netherlands Brain Bank (NBB) and guarantee the quality of the tissue by proper matching and measuring the pH of the brain or cerebrospinal fluid (CSF) (Ravid and Swaab, 1993; Ravid et al., 1992). Specimens from diseased and control brains are properly matched for the various ante and post-mortem factors in addition to Apo-E typing and the quality of the tissue is guaranteed by measuring the pH of the CSF. This is performed on CSF drawn during the rapid autopsy from the lateral ventricles and subsequently stored for the development and evaluation of diagnostic tests for AD and Parkinson's disease (PD).

Due to the large variability of the collected material, there are various pitfalls; many patient-related factors may introduce a huge variation or systematic errors. Therefore, collecting and providing post-mortem human brain samples for research should include accurate matching for ante and post-mortem factors. Each area dissected from the brain of a diseased patient, needs to be matched with an identical area from a control patient. Depending on the brain area and parameters studied, tissues must, *e.g.*, be matched for age, sex, agonal state, month of death, clock time of death, use of medicines, etc. The post-mortem factors which should be taken into account are: post-mortem delay (PMD), right or left part of the brain, fixation and storage time. The need and importance of controls

Progress in Alzheimer's and Parkinson's Diseases
edited by Fisher *et al.*, Plenum Press, New York, 1998.

cannot be overemphasized. In many instances, various neuroscientists who work on AD, require in addition to the non-demented controls also specimens from patients who suffered from other neurological or psychiatric disorders to be able to control for disease specific and non-specific phenomena (Figs. 1 and 2). Accordingly, a comprehensive brain bank should include a variety of neurological and psychiatric disorders.

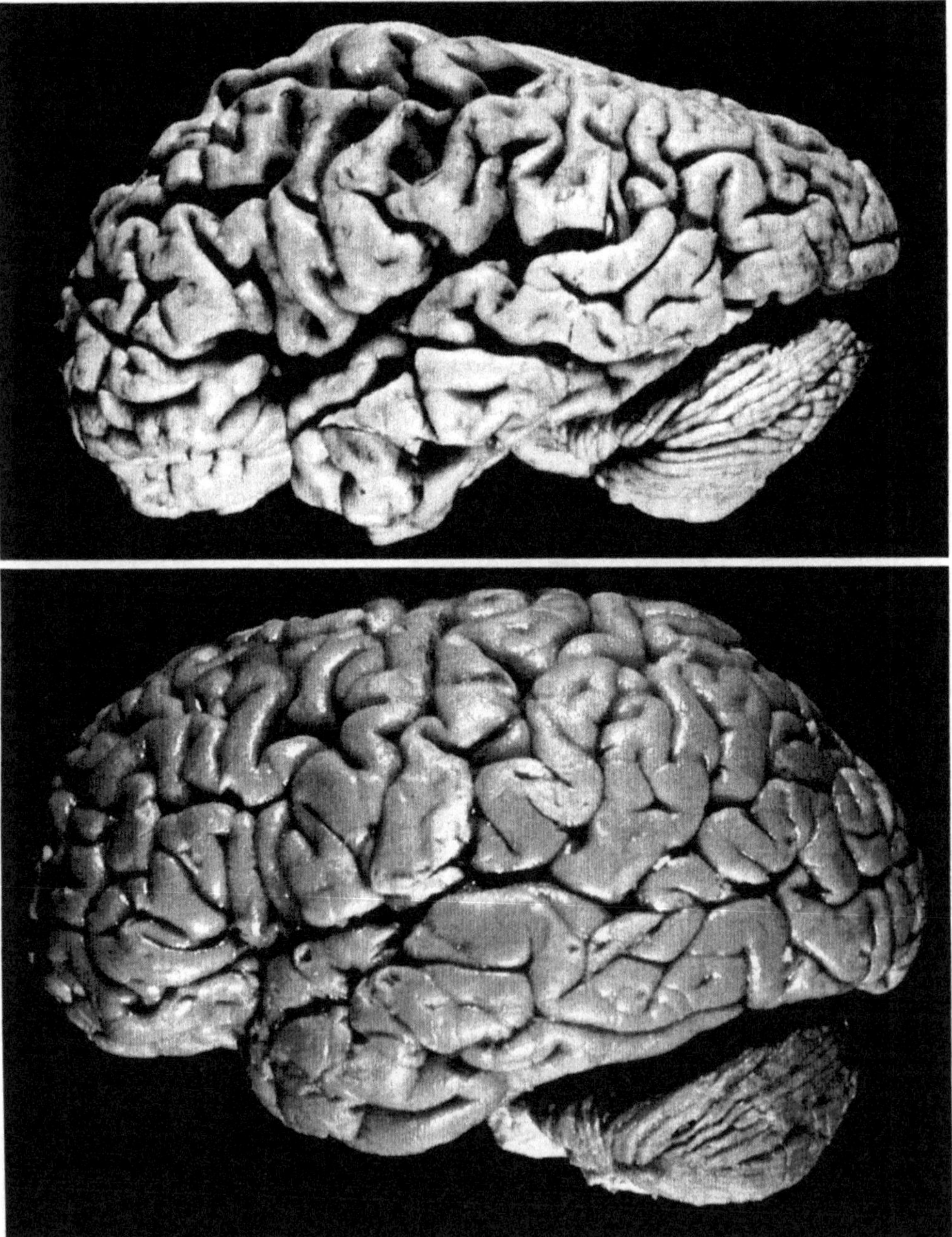

Figure 1. A comparison of the gross features of a brain obtained at autopsy from an Alzheimer's disease patient (top) and an age-matched non-demented control. Note the difference in size and the extreme degree and pattern of atrophy in the AD brain.

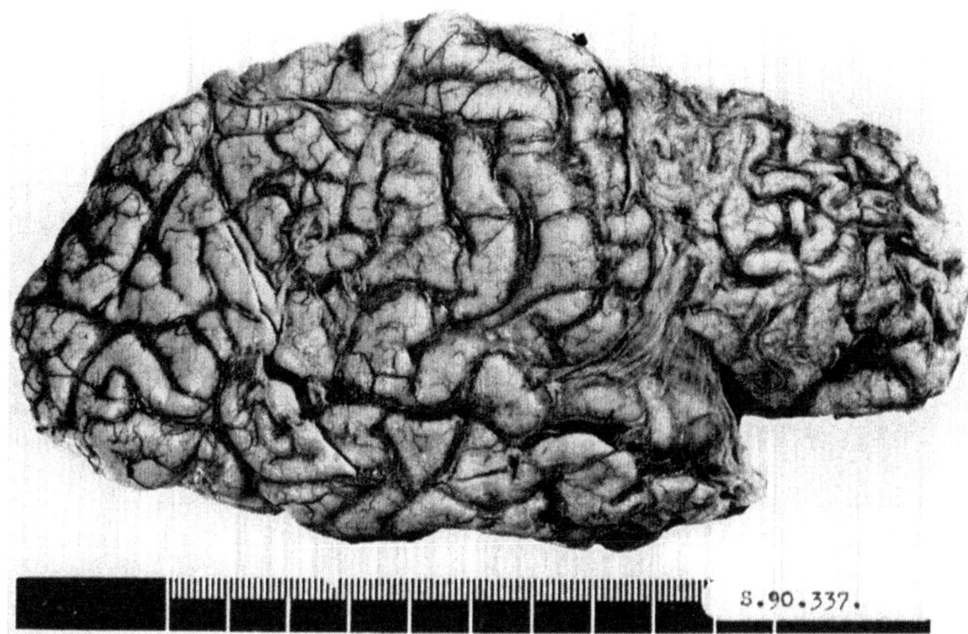

Figure 2. A brain obtained at autopsy from a patient with Pick's disease. Note the extreme frontal atrophy.

In collaboration with other European brain banks, the Netherlands Brain Bank (NBB) is attempting to set up standardized protocols for the clinical and neuropathological diagnosis as well as standard procedures for the collection and dissection of tissue for research purposes. These procedures include protocols for sampling, dissection, tissue preparation and factors for matching.

Age, Disease

The nucleus basalis of Meynert (NBM) which is severely affected in various neurological disorders, such as AD, PD, Creutzfeldt-Jakob disease (CJD), Pick's disease, Korsakoff's disease and progressive supranuclear palsy (PSP) can serve as an excellent example for illustrating the importance of matching. Significant differences have been shown in this nucleus between AD patients when compared to controls, using *e.g.,* Alz-50 monoclonal antibody as a marker for cytoskeletal abnormalities (Swaab et al., 1992; Van de Nes et al., 1993). In PD this nucleus has been found to contain Lewy bodies (Purba et al., 1994). Recently, the general concept of major cell loss in the NBM in AD made place to a new concept namely that neuronal atrophy is the major hallmark of AD in the NBM (Swaab et al., 1994; Salehi et al., 1994).

Decreased neuronal activity in the NBM has been reported in AD. This nucleus is one of the major sources of cholinergic innervation of the cortex and is severely affected in AD as well as in other neurodegenerative diseases. Measuring the size of the Golgi apparatus (GA) has been earlier reported to be a good parameter for the neuronal activity (Lucassen et al., 1993). In order to establish whether neuronal activity is related to the degenerative changes in the NBM in AD, the activity of NBM neurons was estimated by quantification of the size of the GA in immunocytochemically stained formalin-fixed sections using an image analyzer (Salehi et al., 1994). Qualitative microscopic analysis had shown that the area occupied by the GA in the cytoplasm of NBM neurons is generally smaller in AD patients (Fig. 3c,d) than in controls (Fig. 3a,b). A highly significant reduction of 49% was observed in the mean area of the GA in AD patients as compared to controls (Fig. 4). The frequency distribution of the cross-sectional area of the GA in AD patients was significantly (p < 0.001) shifted to the lower digits compared with controls (Fig. 5).

The agonal state may influence the pH and a number of chemical substances in the brain. Subjects who died after a long terminal illness have a lower pH in the brain, CSF and blood, and this acidosis corresponds to increased lactic acid concentrations (Perry et al., 1982; Hardy et al., 1985). Lower levels of pH were found throughout the brain in cases of death following protracted illness, as compared to sudden death (Spokes, 1979). Various enzymatic activities were found to be related to pH and lactate in post-mortem brain in Alzheimer's disease and Down's syndrome as well as other dementias (Yates et al., 1990). These authors found that lactate levels were higher and phosphate-activated glutaminase and glutamic acid decarboxylase levels were lower in brain tissue of agonal controls than in the sudden death controls.

The pH values measured in CSF obtained by rapid autopsies performed by the NBB on non-demented controls (a) and Alzheimer's disease patients (b) did not change significantly with post-mortem delay (Fig. 6), and we concluded that the pH of brain tissue CSF obtained at autopsy is influenced by agonal state and not by post-mortem delay and thus is very useful for brain banking routine procedures (Ravid et al., 1992). Tissue pH has recently been reported to be a fair indicator of mRNA preservation in human post-mortem brain as well (Kingsbury et al., 1995).

In human studies, prolonged diseases such as respiratory distress may influence a number of biochemical parameters. Whenever possible, subjects should thus be matched for premorbid state. This is a particularly difficult criterium to satisfy in studies of aging, since most young donors die from accidents, suicides or drug overdose whereas older donors die from various chronic disease states. A similar problem exists in studies of Alzheimer's disease patients, who frequently suffer from pneumonia and cachexia in the terminal stage.

Lateralization

Fixing one hemisphere and freezing the other is current practice in many brain banks. It prevents, however, the recognition of possible left-right differences in the brain. Several functions and transmitters are asymmetrically represented in the left or right hemisphere; lateralization of norepinephrine has been demonstrated in the human brain (Oke et al., 1978) and there is evidence for a left prominence in the distribution of thyroid releasing hormone (TRH) in several hypothalamic nuclei with higher concentrations in the left side (Borson-Chazot et al., 1986). The hemispherical lateralization has also a functional and pathological significance, *e.g.*, the absence of left TRH predominance for hypothalamic structures may be of pathological significance (Jordan et al., 1992).

Left-right asymmetries have also been reported for glutamic acid decarboxylase (GAD) and gamma-aminobutyric acid (GABA). Positive correlations were found between left-right asymmetries of various neurotransmitters within the same brain structure whereas correlations between different structures were negative. These findings indicate that a greater or lesser degree of asymmetry characterizes each particular brain (Glick et al., 1982). Consequently it is preferential to sample bilaterally and if not possible, mention on which hemisphere the measurements have been performed.

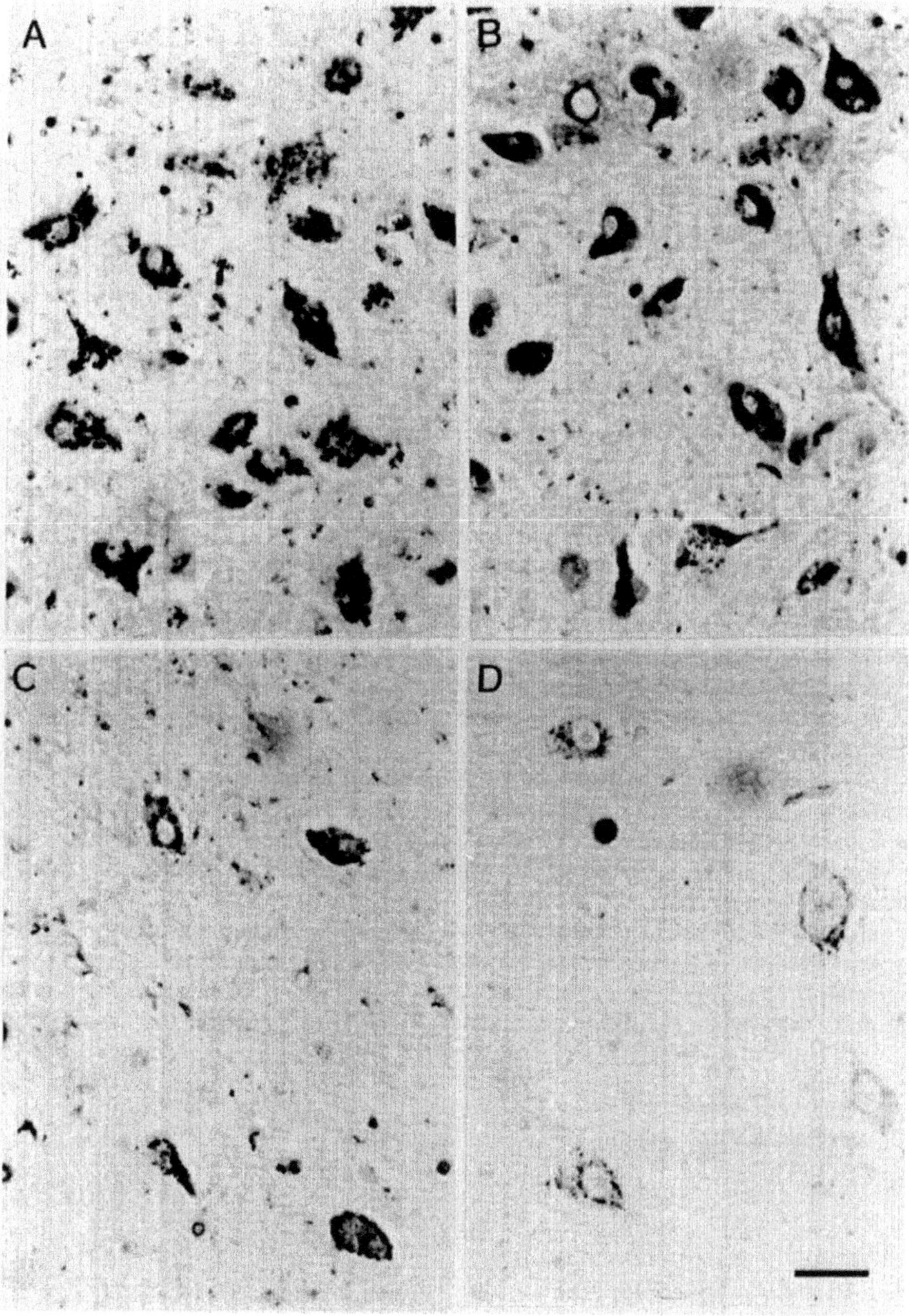

Figure 3. Immunocytochemical staining of the GA in young (A) and old (B) controls and AD (C,D) patients. Note the clear reduction in size of the GA in AD patients when compared to the old controls. Scale bar = 30 μm.

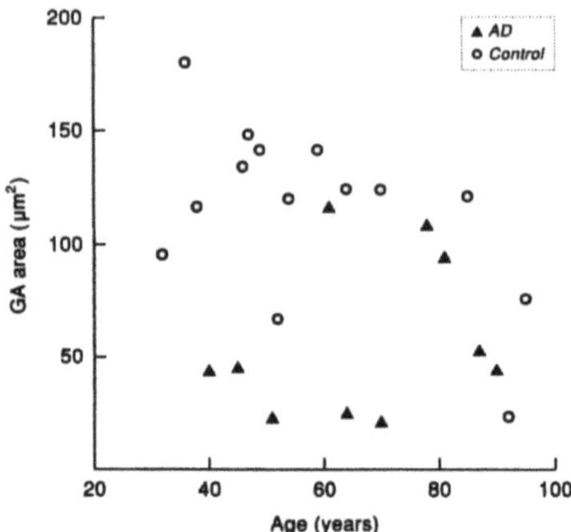

Figure 4. The mean GA area per neuron in various age groups of controls and AD patients. Note the clear difference in size of the old GA between controls and AD patients.

Fixation and freezing procedures, storage and fixation time may affect many of the parameters used to assess changes in the brain and the potentialities of staining procedures considerably. On the other hand, some tissue components are not very sensitive to these factors. Human brain tissue used for biochemical studies is usually rapidly frozen and slowly thawed. However, to isolate synaptosomes which are morphologically well preserved and have retained their metabolic performance one should use the opposite procedure as snap-freezing generally yields metabolically and functionally inactive preparations (Hardy et al., 1982).

It is noteworthy that a large number of metabolic and functional processes as well as binding capacity of various receptors are retained surprisingly well in frozen tissue. That way it becomes possible to study regional variations, distribution and comparative activities of various transmitters or drugs in normal and diseased brain and correlate them to the anatomical changes.

Fixation in formalin causes an increase in brain weight and the subsequent washing in water introduces a systematic error in brain weight, *e.g.*, larger brains gain more weight than small brains. However, brains from younger individuals do not gain more in weight than older ones when the difference in fresh brain weight between the two groups was

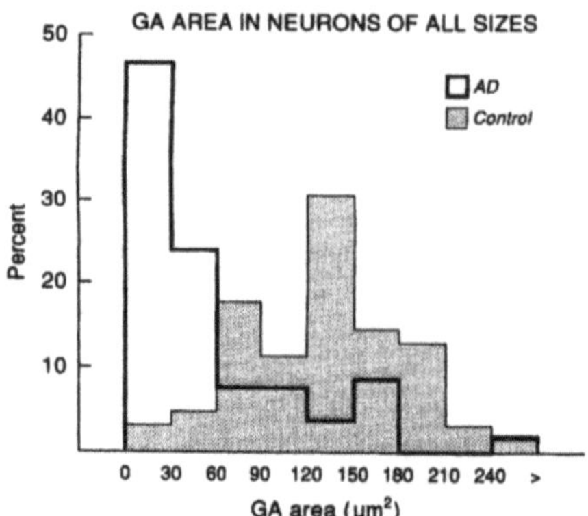

Figure 5. A histogram of the frequency distribution of the size of the GA in all NBM neurons in controls and AD subjects. There is a significant shift to low digits in AD (p < 0.001) indicating a strong decrease in the size of the GA.

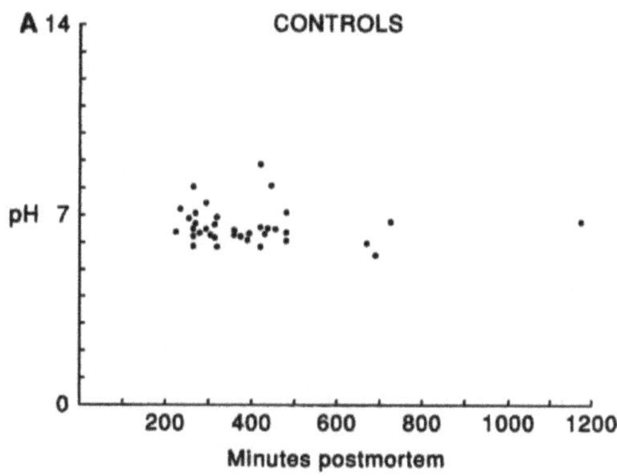

Figure 6. The pH of brain tissue collected by The Netherlands Brain Bank during three years as a function of post-mortem delay. Statistical analysis of the data was performed by applying the two-tailed Pearson correlation analysis. There was no significant correlation between pH and post-mortem delay neither in the control group (A) (ρ = 0.1069; P = 0.529) nor in the Alzheimer's disease group (B) (ρ = 0.1678; P = 0.09).

taken into account. Similarly, the increase in brain weight during fixation is not sexually dimorphic when the fresh brain weight is taken into account (Skullerud, 1985). Duration of fixation and the type of fixative used have implications for the quality of immunocytochemical staining of various peptides.

Storage time of tissue may be important for in situ hybridization and in situ end labelling.

All the data on the effects of ante and post-mortem factors mentioned in the above section have clear consequences for the daily practice and methodologies of brain banking. It makes it evident that brain banks need to guarantee high quality material for research by apriori keeping all this variables in mind when setting up the standard procedures for documenting, collecting, sampling, storing and providing the diagnosis of the tissue samples used for research.

CONCLUSIONS

As newer and more sophisticated research methods are introduced, the demand for human brain will continue to increase. This trend mirrors a growing realization that an increasing number of processes occurring in the human brain can be studied on autopsy material. The availability of this material, whether fresh, frozen or fixed, makes it possible to develop methodologies for studying the neuroanatomical and neurochemical aspects of the human brain. It has also become possible in recent years to correlate functional changes with neurochemical and neuroanatomical abnormalities in disease states.

Some compounds in the brain are damaged irreversibly within minutes after death and others are known to disintegrate within seconds. This led to the widespread idea that autopsy material would not be suitable for basic research purposes and would not supply the necessary answers on the various fundamental questions regarding processes occurring in normal or diseased brain. However, from data published in recent years in which autopsy material has been routinely used, it is evident that this is a misconception. It also became evident that when using the proper fixation procedures, sufficient structural integrity is retained in the tissue to allow morphological and morphometrical studies (Swaab and Uylings, 1988). Electron microscopic examination of synaptosomal preparations from post-mortem human brain showed them to be only slightly less pure than preparations from fresh tissue although there was some degree of damage (Hardy et al., 1982).

Agonal state affects the stability of brain compounds and causes brain hypoxia. This again forms a tremendous difficulty for the study of human neurological and psychiatric diseases as one of the frequent causes of death is bronchopneumonia which leads to brain hypoxia and results in pronounced lactic acidosis. Collecting human brain for research purposes should put emphasis on the development of a rapid autopsy system, as practised *e.g.,* by The Netherlands Brain Bank since 1985 (Ravid and Swaab, 1993) and guarantee the quality of the tissue by proper matching for the various ante and post-mortem factors and measuring the pH (Ravid et al., 1992). This provides a simple means to screen the dissected tissue and match the right case control cases for neurodegenerative disorders.

The analysis of post-mortem human brain data remains extremely difficult; the interpretation of the various results must be done with great care to exclude confounding factors due to the heterogeneity of the material with respect to the various factors mentioned in detail in the previous sections.

It is evident that numerous possible pitfalls remain to be encountered especially when human brain tissue is studied with the conventional neuroanatomical techniques. A concerted effort is needed to ensure that the samples would not differ systematically. Matching for the various ante and post-mortem factors is an essential step towards obtaining meaningful results. Without it, differences observed between groups of samples may be wrongly attributed to the disease process.

The NBB has developed in the past 11 years an efficient rapid autopsy programme and uses a fresh dissection procedure which is advantageous in increasing the range of conventional as well as modern neurobiological techniques to be applied on human post-mortem specimens in aging and dementia research.

ACKNOWLEDGMENTS

We thank the Netherlands Brain Bank for supplying the human brain tissue, and Anke de Boer for her work regarding the lay-out of this manuscript.

REFERENCES

Borson-Chazot, F., Jordan, D., Fevre-Montagne, M., Kopp, N., Tourniaire, J., Rouziux, J.M., Veisseire, M., and Mornex, R., 1986, TRH and LH-RH distribution in discrete nuclei of the human hypothalamus: evidence for a left prominence of TRH, *Brain Res.* 382:433–436.

Glick, S.D., Ross, D.A., and Hough, L.B., 1982, Lateral asymmetry of neurotransmitters in human brain, *Brain Res.* 234:53–63.

Hardy, J.A., Dodd, P.R., Oakley, A.E., Kidd, A.M., Perry, R.J., and Edwardson, J.A., 1982, Use of post-mortem human synaptosomes for studies of metabolism and transmitter amino acid release, *Neurosci. Lett.* 33:317–322.

Hardy, J.A., Wester, P., Winblad, B., Gezelius, C., Bring, G., and Eriksson, A., 1985, The patients dying after long terminal phase have acidotic brains: implications for biochemical measurements on autopsy tissue, *J. Neural Transm.* 61:253–264.

Jordan, D., Borson-Chazot, F., Veisseire, M., Deluermoz, S., Malicler, D., Dalery, J., and Kopp, N., 1992, Disappearance of hypothalamic TRH asymmetry in suicide patients, *J. Neural Transm.* 89:103–110.

Kingsbury, A.E., Foster, O.J.F., Nisbet, A.P., Cairns, N., Bray, L., Eve, D.J., Lees, A.J., and Marsden, C.D., 1995, Tissue pH as an indicator of mRNA preservation in human post-mortem brain, *Molecular Brain Res.* 28:311–318.

Lucassen, P.J., Ravid, R., Gonatas, N.K., Swaab, D.F., 1993, Activation of the human supraoptic and paraventricular neurons with aging and in Alzheimer's disease as judged from increasing size of the Golgi apparatus, *Brain Res.* 632:10–23.

Oke, A., Keller, R., Mefford, Y., and Adams, R.N., 1978, Lateralization of norepinephrine in human hypothalamus, *Science* 200:1411–1413.

Perry, E.K., Perry, R.H., and Tomlinson, B.E., 1982, The influence of agonal states on some neurochemical activities of post-mortem human brain tissue, *Neurosci. Lett.* 29:303–309.

Purba, J.S., Hofman, M.A., and Swaab, D.F., 1994, Decrease in number of oxytocin neurons in the paraventricular nucleus of human hypothalamus in Parkinson's disease, *Neurology* 44:84–89.

Ravid, R., Van Zwieten, E.J., and Swaab, D.F., 1992, Brain banking and the human hypothalamus - factors to match for, pitfalls and potentials. In D.F. Swaab, M.A. Hofman, M. Mirmiran, R. Ravid and F.W. Van Leeuwen (Eds), *Progress in Brain Res.* 93:83–95.

Ravid, R., and Winblad, B., 1993, Brain Banking in Alzheimer's disease: factors to match for, pitfalls and potentials. Alzheimer's disease: Advances in clinical and basic research.

Corain, B., Iqbal, K., Nicolini, M., Winblad, B., Wisniewsky, H., and Zatta, P. (Eds), John Wiley and Sons Ltd., pp. 213–218.

Ravid, R., and Swaab, D.F., 1993, The Netherlands Brain Bank - a clinico-pathological link in aging and dementia research, *J. Neural Transm.* Suppl. 39:143–153.

Salehi, A., Lucassen, P.J., Pool, Ch.W., Gonatas, N.K., Ravid, R., and Swaab, D.F., 1994, Decreased neuronal activity in the Nucleus Basalis of Meynert in Alzheimer's disease as suggested by the size of the Golgi apparatus, *Neuroscience* 59:871–880.

Skullerud, K., 1985, Variations in the size of the human brain, *Acta Neurol. Scand.*, 71 (No. 102):14–15.

Spokes, E.G.S., 1979, An analysis of factors influencing measurements of dopamine, noradrenaline, glutamate decarboxylase and choline acetylase in human post-mortem brain tissue, *Brain* 102:333–346.

Swaab, D.F., Fliers, E., and Partiman, T.S., 1985, The suprachiasmatic nucleus of the human brain in relation to sex age and senile dementia, *Brain Res.* 342:37–44.

Swaab, D.F., and Uylings, H.B.M., 1988, Potentialities and pitfalls in the use of human brain material in molecular neuroanatomy. In: Van Leeuwen, Buys and Pach (Eds), Molecular Neuroanatomy, Elsevier Science Publishers, pp. 403–416.

Swaab, D.F., Grundke-Iqbal, I., Iqbal, K., Kremer, H.P.H., Ravid, R., and Van de Nes, J.A.P., 1992, Tau and ubiquitin in the human hypothalamus in aging and Alzheimer's disease, *Brain Res.* 590:239–249.

Swaab, D.F., Hofman, M.A., Lucassen, P.J., Salehi, A., and Uylings, H.B.M., 1994, Neuronal shrinkage is the major hallmark in Alzheimer's disease, *Neurobiol. Aging* 15:369–371.

Van de Nes, J.A.P., Kamphorst, W., Ravid, R., and Swaab, D.F., 1993, The distribution of Alz-50 immunoreactivity in the hypothalamus and adjoining areas of Alzheimer's disease patients, *Brain* 116:103–115.

Yates, C.M., Butterworth, J., Tennant, M.C., and Gordon, A., 1990, Enzyme activities in relation to pH and lactate in post-mortem brain in Alzheimer-type and other dementias, *J. Neurochem.* 55(5):1624–30.

40

INSULIN, INSULIN RECEPTORS, AND IGF-I RECEPTORS IN POST-MORTEM HUMAN BRAIN IN ALZHEIMER'S DISEASE

F. Frölich,[1] D. Blum-Degen,[2] S. Hoyer,[3] H. Beckmann,[2] and P. Riederer[2]

[1]Department of Psychiatry I
University of Frankfurt/Main, Germany
[2]Department of Psychiatry
University of Würzburg, Germany
[3]Department of Pathochemistry and
General Neurochemistry
University of Heidelberg, Germany

INTRODUCTION

In dementia of Alzheimer type (SDAT), reductions in glucose metabolism in vivo (Kumar et al., 1991). reduced activities of enzymes involved in glycolytic and oxidative glucose breakdown were reported in post-mortem brain tissue (Perry et al., 1980, Gibson et al., 1988). These reductions appeared to be more severe than the "nonspecific" reductions in a number of biochemical constituents that had been related to brain atrophy (Bowen et al., 1979). Thus, the hypothesis has been forwarded that defects in the regulation of glucose metabolism, i.e. due to changes in CNS insulin receptor function, might be an early contributing event to the onset of SDAT (Hoyer, 1996). Brain insulin regulates enzymes of cerebral glucose metabolism via specific high-affinity insulin receptors, which differ from peripheral insulin receptors in the amount of glycosylation (Baskin et al., 1988, Wozniak et al., 1993, dePablo & de la Rosa, 1995). Furthermore, insulin also binds to insulin-like growth factor I receptors and via these receptors possibly exerts trophic effects on neuronal cells and interacts with cholinergic neurotransmission (Calissano et al., 1993, Quirion et al., 1991, Rotwein, 1991, Kyriakis et al., 1987).

It may be hypothesized that: 1) Insulin acts as a neurotrophic/regulatory peptide in human brain tissue; 2) In normal brain aging, the insulin/insulin receptor system undergoes changes which correspond to the known changes of brain glucose metabolism; 3) The changes of insulin and insulin receptors in normal aging differ from those in SDAT;

and 4) The changes of the cerebral insulin receptor system in SDAT are compatible with the known deficits of cellular glucose metabolism in SDAT.

We have investigated whether immunoreactivities of insulin and c-peptide in the brain change with normal aging and, whether the respective levels in SDAT differ from those in an age-matched control group. Furthermore we investigated whether density and affinity of both insulin and insulin-like growth factor I receptor-binding change with normal aging, and whether the respective levels in SDAT differ from those in an age-matched control group.

MATERIALS AND METHODS

Clinical diagnosis of dementia was made according to DSM-IIIR and had a severe dementia. The patients fulfilled the diagnostic criteria of the NINCDS/ADRDA for probable SDAT (McKhann et al., 1984). Control patients without a history of neurological or psychiatric disease were hospitalized and died from somatic disorders. The sample consisted of 17 patients with SDAT (mean age: 79.8 ± 2.0 years) and 21 controls (mean age: 64.5 ± 5.1 years). An age-matched group of 13 samples was selected form controls (mean age 80.1 ± 2.5). Post mortem delay was 24.7 ± 4.1 hours for SDAT, and 25.4 ± 4.0 hours for the age-matched controls. Brain lactate content was 20.7 ± 1.5 mg/dl in SDAT and 21.7 ± 1.4 mg/dl in age-matched controls.

Brains were removed at autopsy and divided by mid-sagittal section for neurochemical analysis and for histological examination. The final diagnosis of SDAT was established histologically. In control brains, the histological examination of the cerebral cortex and the hippocampus did not show more senile plaques and tangles than could be explained by age. Brain tissue was obtained using an anatomical atlas and followed a standard procedure. For radioimmuno-assays, this tissue was homogenized at 4°C in a medium containing 10 mM MOPS (pH 7.6), 120 mM NaCl, 1mM EDTA, 0.1mM benzethonium chloride, 1 mM benzamidine and 0.1% trasylol. For radioligand binding assays, this tissue was homogenized in MOPS/sucrose buffer and washed twice.

Insulin and c-peptide were determined with commercially available RIA's (Bierman Diagnostics, Bad Nauheim, Germany). Radioligand binding assays were performed as "cold" saturation assays with ^{125}J-insulin or ^{125}J-IGF-I, respectively. Tracer (10^{-10}M) was displaced by increasing amounts (9 steps) of cold ligand, and unspecific binding was determined by 10^{-7} M cold ligand. Separation of bound and free ligand was achieved by centrifugation. Preliminary estimations of binding parameters (B_{max} and K_D values) for both receptors were calculated with the PC softwares "EBDA" and "LIGAND". For the analysis of binding experiments a two-site model without cooperativity was used, which is known to reflect best the insulin and IGF-I binding situation (Desoye et al., 1992).

RESULTS

Both insulin and c-peptide could be demonstrated reliably in human post-mortem brain tissue. There were significant regional differences in the insulin concentration (1-factorial ANOVA, $F = 2.66$, df = 8, $p < 0.01$), and insulin and c-peptide levels were correlated significantly with each other ($r = 0.294$, $p < 0.001$).

In normal aging, both insulin and c-peptide decreased significantly with advancing age $r = 0.508$ for insulin, $r = 0.531$ for c-peptide). Accordingly, insulin receptor densities

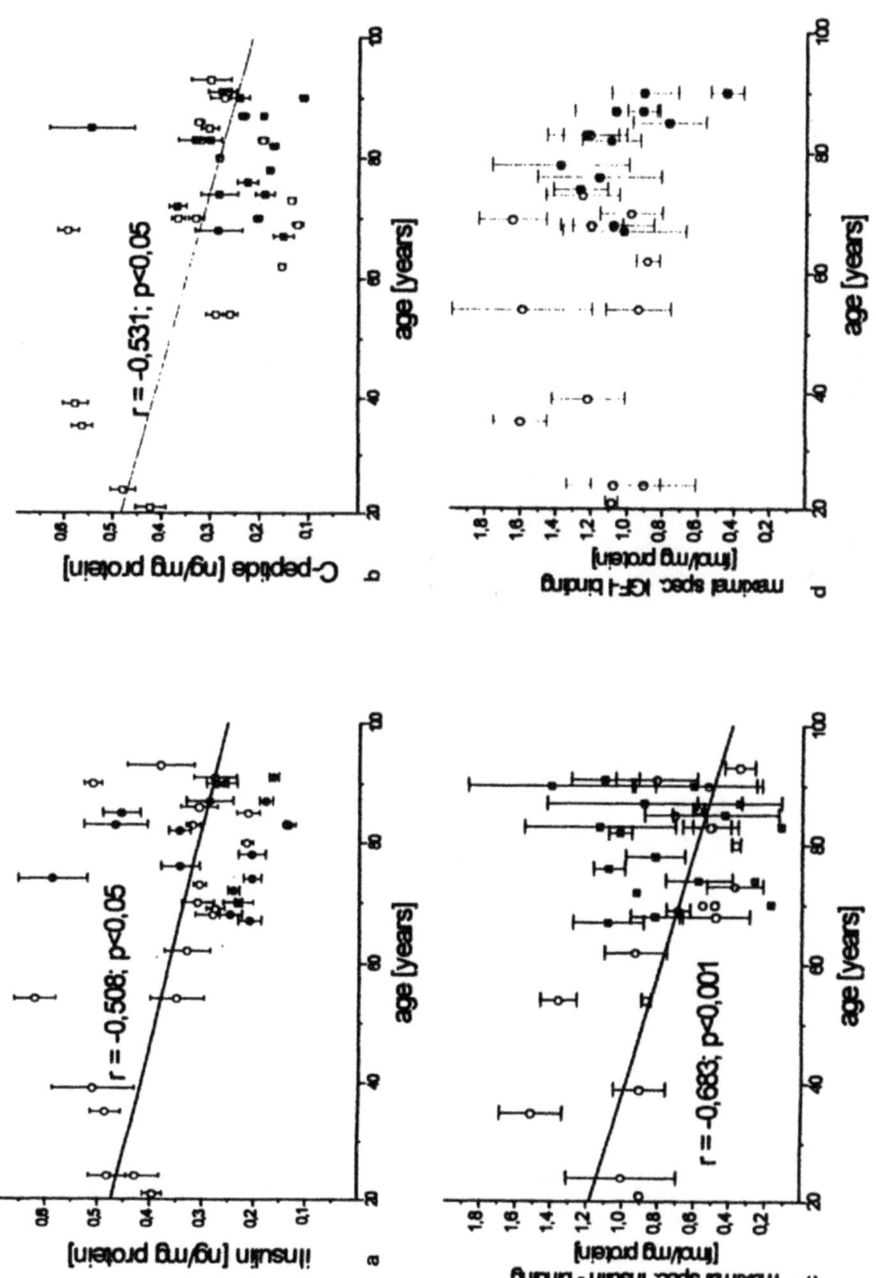

Figure 1a–d. Insulin [a], c-peptide [b], density of insulin receptor-binding [c], density of IGF-I receptor binding [d] in post-mortem human brain in relation to normal aging. Values are means of the individual brain over 9 brain areas (for receptor only 4 brain areas) ± SEM, given as ng/mg protein for insulin and c-peptide, and fmol/mg protein for receptor densities; sample size is n = 21 for controls, n = 17 for SDAT. Significant correlations were calculated by Pearson's product moment correlation coefficient (r value and p level are stated on the graph) and are marked by a regression line.

also decreased with advancing age (r = 0.683) without changing their ligand affinity. In contrast, another structurally related peptide receptor, the IGF-I receptor, did not show decreased receptor densities with aging, which demonstrates some specifity of the changes in the insulin/insulin receptor system.

In dementia of Alzheimer type, insulin and c-peptide levels did not differ significantly from an age-matched control group. Neither did IGF-I receptor densities or affinities differ

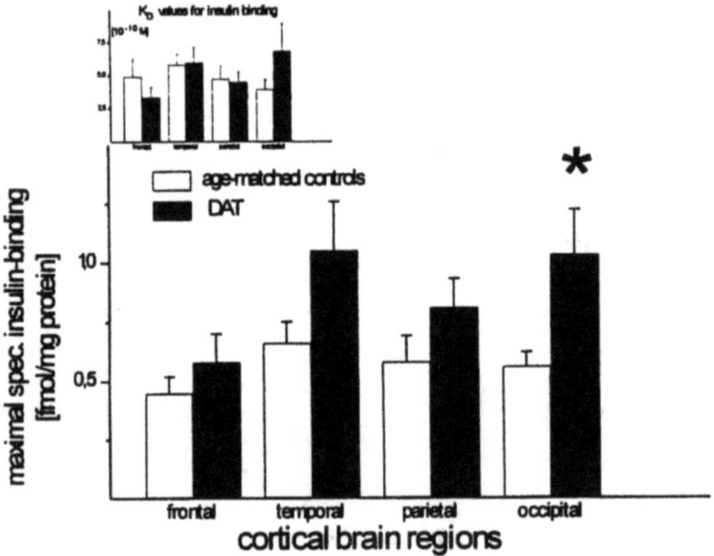

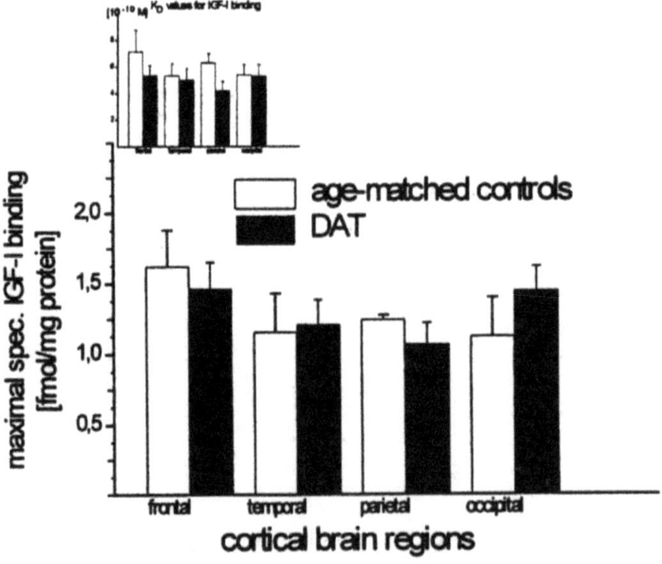

Figure 2. Density (Bmax) and affinity (KD) of insulin [a] and IGF-I [b] receptor-binding in post-mortem human brain cortex in SDAT and age-matched controls. Main graph indicates receptor densities, insert indicates ligand affinities. Values are means ± SEM, given as fmol/mg protein for receptor density and 10^{-10} M for ligand affinity; sample size is n = 13 for age-matched controls, n = 17 for SDAT. Significant differences from control values (p < 0.05 by Mann-Whitney U-test) are marked by an asterisk.

from their respective control values. However, insulin receptor densities increased, most notably in the occipital cortex. Insulin receptor affinities did not differ significantly from their control values. These changes may indicate a compensatory up-regulation of receptor number, possibly as a response to impaired signal transduction.

DISCUSSION

Insulin and c-peptide are both derived from a common precursor, proinsulin, from which these peptides are released in equimolar amounts by proteolytic cleavage (Polonsky et al., 1984). Only insulin has biological activity and only insulin is degraded by proteases. It has been shown by cell culture and animal experiments that insulin in the brain has potent effects on neuronal glucose metabolism and cell differentiation (Knusel et al., 1990, Puro & Agardh, 1984, Hoyer et al., 1994) via the mitochondrial citric acid cycle (Bessmann et al., 1986). Our experiments with post-mortem human brain provide further indirect evidence for a biological role of insulin in the brain, because of the demonstration of c-peptide in brain. This suggests an expression of proinsulin, from which c-peptide (and insulin) is released. Second, insulin levels correlate significantly with c-peptide, which also suggests active release of both peptides.

We have demonstrated that both peptides and the number of insulin receptors decrease with advancing age. During human ontogenesis, insulin receptors have been shown to decrease (Potau et al., 1991). However, data on aging changes have been lacking. In contrast, a structurally related receptor system, the IGF-I receptor, does not decrease during aging indicating that the changes of the insulin receptor system reflect not merely an unspecific cellular loss, but may have biological significance.

In dementia of Alzheimer type, we compared samples with histopathologically confirmed dementia of Alzheimer type with an age-matched control group without neuropsychiatric disorders. Because of a close matching of both groups with respect to several important factors in addition to age, i.e. sex, post-mortem delay, storage time of the brain tissue, and lactate content of the brain as a measure of the agonal period, any major artifacts may be excluded (data not shown). Neither insulin nor c-peptide levels differed from their control values. However, we showed for the first time that the number of insulin receptors were increased, indicative of an up-regulation of this receptor system most likely due to impaired signal transduction, because the availability of the ligand was not reduced. Our data thus demonstrate that the changes of the insulin / insulin receptor system in normal aging and in dementia of Alzheimer type differ from each other. Interestingly, insulin receptors in the substantia nigra in Parkinson's disease have recently been shown to be reduced (Moroo et al., 1993), which suggested an involvement in neurodegenerative disorders. We could confirm that IGF-I receptor densities in dementia of Alzheimer type remain constant, as had been shown earlier (DeKayser et al., 1994, Crews et al., 1992).

REFERENCES

Baskin, D.G., Wilcox, B.J., Figlewicz, D.P., and Dorsa, D.M., 1988, Insulin and insulin-like growth factors in the CNS. *TINS* 11:107–111.

Bessmann, S.P., Mohan, C., and Zaidise, I., 1986, Intracellular site of insulin action: Mitochondrial Krebs cycle. *Biochemistry* 83:5067–5070.

Bowen, D.M., White, P., Spillane, J.A, Goodhart, M.J., Curzon, G., Iwangoff, P., Mayer-Ruge, W. and Davison, A.N., 1979, Accelerated aging or selective neuronal loss as an important cause of dementia? *Lancet* 1:11–14.

Calissano, P., Ciotti, M.T., Battistini, L., Zona, C., Angelini, A., Merlo, D., and Mercanti, D., 1993, Recombinant insulin-like growth factor I exerts a trophic action and confers glutamate sensitivity on glutamate-resistant cerebellar cells. *Proc. Natl. Acad. Sci USA* 90:8752–8756.

Crews, F.T., McElhaney, R., Freund, G., Ballinger, W.E.J., and Raizada, M.K., 1992, Insulin-like growth factor I receptor binding in brains of Alzheimer's and alcoholic patients. *J. Neurochem.* 58:1205–1210.

de Pablo, F., de la Rosa, E., 1995, The developing CNS: a scenario for the action of proinsulin, insulin and insulin-like growth factors: *Trends Neurosci.* 18:143–150.

DeKayser, J., Wilczak, N., and Goosens, A., 1994, Insulin-like growth factor-1 receptor densities in human frontal cortex and white matter during aging, in Alzheimer's disease, and in Huntington's disease. *Neurosci. Lett.* 172:93–96.

Desoye, G., Schmon, B., Gmoser, G., Friedl, H., Urdl, W., and Weiss, P.A.M., 1992, Insulin binding to erythrocytes of nonpregnant women: a reevaluation, underlining the importance of body weight even in nonobese subjects. *Clin. Chim. Acta* 207:57–71.

Gibson, G.E., Sheu, K.F., Blass, J.P., Baker, A., Carlson, K.C., Harding, B. and Perrino, P., 1988, Reduced activities of thiamine-dependent enzymes in the brains and peripheral tissues of patients with Alzheimer's disease. *Arch. Neurol.* 45:836–840.

Henneberg, N., and Hoyer, S., 1994, Short-term or long-term intracerebroventricular (i.c.v.) infusion of insulin exhibits a discrete anabolic effect on cerebral energy metabolism in the rat. *Neurosci. Lett.* 175:153–156.

Hoyer, S., Prem, L., Sorbi, S., and Amaducci, L., 1993, Stimulation of glycolytic key enzymes in cerebral cortex by insulin. *Neuroreport* 4:991–993.

Hoyer, S., 1996, Oxidative metabolism deficiencies in brains of patients with Alzheimer's disease. *Acta Neurol. Scand.* [Suppl 165]:18–24.

Knusel, B., Michel, P.P., Schwaber, J.S., and Hefti, F., 1990, Selective and nonselective stimulation of central cholinergic and dopaminergic development in vitro by nerve growth factor, basic fibroblast growth factor, epidermal growth factor, insulin and the insulin-like growth factors I and II. *J. Neurosci.* 10:558–570.

Kumar, A., Schapiro, M.B., Grady, C., Haxby, J.V., Wagner, E., Salerno, J.A., Friedland, R.P. and Rapoport, S.I., 1991, High-resolution PET studies in Alzheimer's disease. *Neuropsychopharmacology.* 4:35–46.

Kyriakis, J.M., Hausman, R.E., and Peterson, S.W., 1987, Insulin stimulates choline acetyltransferase activity in cultured embryonic chicken retina neurons. *Proc. Natl. Acad. Sci. USA* 84:7463–7467.

McKhann, G., Drachman, D., Folstein, M., Katzman, R., Price, D. and Stadlan, E., 1984, Clinical diagnosis of Alzheimer's disease: report of the NINCDS-ADRDA work group under the auspices of department of health and human services task force on Alzheimer's disease. *Neurology* 34:939–944.

Moroo, I., Yamada, T., Makino, H., Tooyama, I., McGeer, P.L., McGeer E.G., and Hirayama, K., 1993, Loss of insulin receptor immunoreactivity from the substantia nigra pars compacta neurons in Parkinsons's disease. *Acta Neuropathol.* 87:343–348.

Perry, E.K., Perry, R.H., Tomlinson, B.E., Blessed, G. and Gibson, P.H., 1980, Coenzyme A-acetylating enzymes in Alzheimer's disease: possible cholinergic "compartment" of pyruvate dehydrogenase. *Neurosci. Lett.* 18:105–110.

Polonsky, K.S., and Rubenstein, A.H., 1984, C-peptide as a measure of the secretion and hepatic extraction of insulin; pitfalls and limitations. *Diabetes* 33:486–493.

Potau N., Escofet, M.A., and Martinez, M.C., 1991, Ontogenesis of insulin receptors in human cerebral cortex. *J. Endocrinol. Invest.* 14:53–58.

Puro, D., and Agardh, E., 1984, Insulin-mediated regulation of neuronal maturation. *Science* 225:1170–1172.

Quirion R, Araujo DM, Lapehak PA, Seto D, Chabot JG, 1991. Growth Factors and Lymphokines: Modulators of Cholinergic Neuronal Activity. *Can. J. Neurol. Sci.* 18:390–393.

Rotwein P, 1991. Structure, evolution, expression and regulation of insulin-like growth factors I and II. *Growth Factors* 5:3–18.

Wozniak, M., Rydzewski, B., Baker, S.P., and Raizada, M.K., 1993, The cellular and physiological actions of insulin in the central nervous system. *Neurochem. Int.* 22:1–10.

41

DEMONSTRATION OF ALUMINUM IN THE BRAIN OF PATIENTS WITH ALZHEIMER'S DISEASE

Sakae Yumoto,[1] Shigeo Kakimi,[2] Hideki Matsushima,[3] Akira Ishikawa,[3] and Yoshikazu Homma[4]

[1]Yumoto Institute of Neurology
Kawadacho 6-11, Shinjuku-ku, Tokyo 162, Japan
[2]Department of Anatomy, School of Medicine
Nihon University
Qyaguchi, Itabashi-ku, Tokyo 173, Japan
[3]Department of Physics
College of Humanities and Sciences
Nihon University
Sakurajousui 156, Setagaya-ku, Tokyo, Japan
[4]NTT Interdisciplinary Research Laboratories
Musashino-shi, Tokyo 180, Japan

INTRODUCTION

Epidemiological studies have revealed that increased aluminum (A1) concentration in drinking water increases the incidence of Alzheimer's disease (senile dementia of Alzheimer's disease type) (Martyn et al., 1989; Flaten, 1990; Neri and Hewitt, 1991). A1 is a highly neurotoxic substance, and induces degeneration and death of nerve cells in the brains of humans and experimental animals (Mahurkar et al., 1973; Alfrey et al., 1976; Yumoto et al., 1992). We have reported that after subcutaneous injection of Al into rats, the numbers of dendrites and spines (postsynaptic structures of axodendritic synapses) of cortical nerve cells decreased markedly (Yumoto et al., 1992, 1993). These morphological changes were similar to those reported in the brains of patients with Alzheimer's disease (Purpura, 1975).

High Al concentrations have been reported in the brains of patients with Alzheimer's disease (Crapper et al., 1976, 1980; Perl and Brody, 1980; Good et al., 1992; Yumoto et

Progress in Alzheimer's and Parkinson's Diseases
edited by Fisher *et al.*, Plenum Press, New York, 1998.

al., 1992). However, Landsberg et al. (1991, 1992) did not detect any Al in the brains of these patients using proton (2 MeV) microprobe particle-induced X-ray emission (PIXE) analysis, and concluded that Al has no pathogenic role in this disease. Recently, we demonstrated Al in the isolated brain cell nuclei from Alzheimer's disease patients using heavy ion (5 MeV Si^{3+}) microprobe PIXE analysis (Yumoto et al., 1996a). Heavy ion (3 MeV Si^{3+}) microprobe PIXE analysis has a several fold higher sensitivity for Al detection than the 2 Mev proton microprobe PIXE analysis (Horino et al., 1993a, 1993b).

In this study, we further examined the presence of Al in the brains (hippocampus) of patients with Alzheimer's disease using secondary ion mass spectrometry (SIMS) and energy dispersive X-ray spectroscopy (EDX) to investigate the cause of Alzheimer's disease.

MATERIALS AND METHODS

Isolation of Brain Cell Nuclei

Brain tissue (hippocampus) was removed at autopsy from patients with Alzheimer's disease (5 cases), and from age matched controls without neurological disorders (3 cases). Brain cell nuclei were isolated from samples by sucrose density gradient centrifugation according to the method reported previously (Yamamoto and Takahashi, 1978; Yumoto et al., 1992), and suspended in 0.2 M sucrose. Isolated nuclei were not fixed or stained with dyes or heavy metals.

Preparation of Frozen Sections

The hippocampi from Alzheimer's disease patients and controls were cut into small blocks, fixed with 2.5%, glutaraldehyde in 0.1 M veronal-acetate buffer (pH 7.4) for 2 hours, transferred to a series of 0.3, 0.7, 1.2, 1.8, and 2.3 M sucrose solutions, successively, and frozen with liquid nitrogen. The concentrations of Al in 2.5% glutaraldehyde solution and sucrose solutions were less than 5 ppb as assayed by inductively coupled plasma (ICP) mass spectrometry. Frozen sections (approximately 0.1 μm thick) were cut on a cryo-ultramicrotome using glass knives at −140°C.

SIMS Analysis

The isolated nuclei were mounted on carbon wafers instead of silicon wafers as in the previous report (Yumoto et al., 1997a). Use of carbon wafers allowed Si in the samples to be detected by SIMS analysis. Secondary ion images of isolated nuclei were observed using a Cameca IMS 4f ion microscope under 10.5 keV 0_2^+ bombardment with positive ion detection as reported previously (Yumoto et al., 1997a).

EDX Analysis

Frozen sections were picked up on Nylon grids covered with Formvar film, and dried in a clean desiccator. The EDX spectra of the samples were measured using a Noran Instruments TN 2000 X-ray microanalyser and JEM 200EX transmission electron microscope at an acceleration voltage of 100 KeV. Point analyses were made in regions identified as the nuclei, nucleoli and cytoplasm of nerve cells in frozen sections.

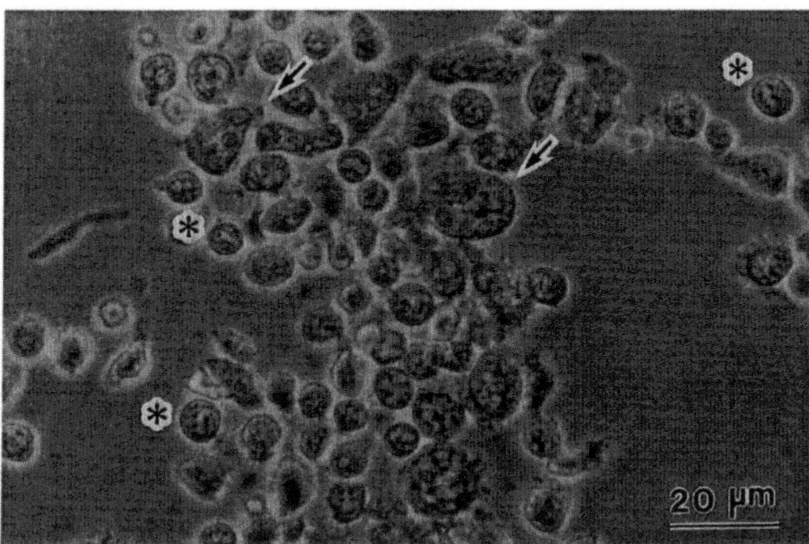

Figure 1. Isolated nuclei from the brain (hippocampus) of a patient with Alzheimer's disease. Nuclei derived from nerve cells (arrows) and nuclei from non-neural cells (arrowheads) are observed.

RESULTS

Isolated Nuclei

Figure 1 shows a phase contrast microscopy picture of isolated nuclei from the hippocampus of a patient with Alzheimer's disease. Nuclei derived from nerve cells (arrows) and nculei from non-neural cells (astericks) were observed.

SIMS Analysis

Secondary ion images of isolated cell nuclei from the hippocampus of a patient with Alzheimer's disease are shown in Figure 2. Al was detected in the spherical regions 5–15 μm in diameter (upper left, arrows). P (upper right, arrows) was co-localized with Al in the spherical regions.

Nuclei contain high concentrations of DNA and RNA which both have phosphate groups. Therefore, the regions where P was detected were identified as isolated nuclei. The size and shape of these regions were the same as those of the brain cell nuclei.

Ca (lower left) was co-localized with Al and P in the isolated nuclei, while Si could not be detected in the nuclei.

On the other hand, regions which had high Al and Si concentrations in the absence of P were occasionally observed (asterisks in upper left and in lower right). These regions were probably contaminated by aluminosilicate, the main component of dust in the environment (Landsberg et al., 1992).

These findings in the isolated brain cell nuclei of Alzheimer's disease patients were in complete agreement with those obtained by PIXE analysis (Yumoto et al., 1992), by microprobe PIX analysis (Yumoto et al., 1996), and by SIMS analysis (Yumoto al., 1997a).

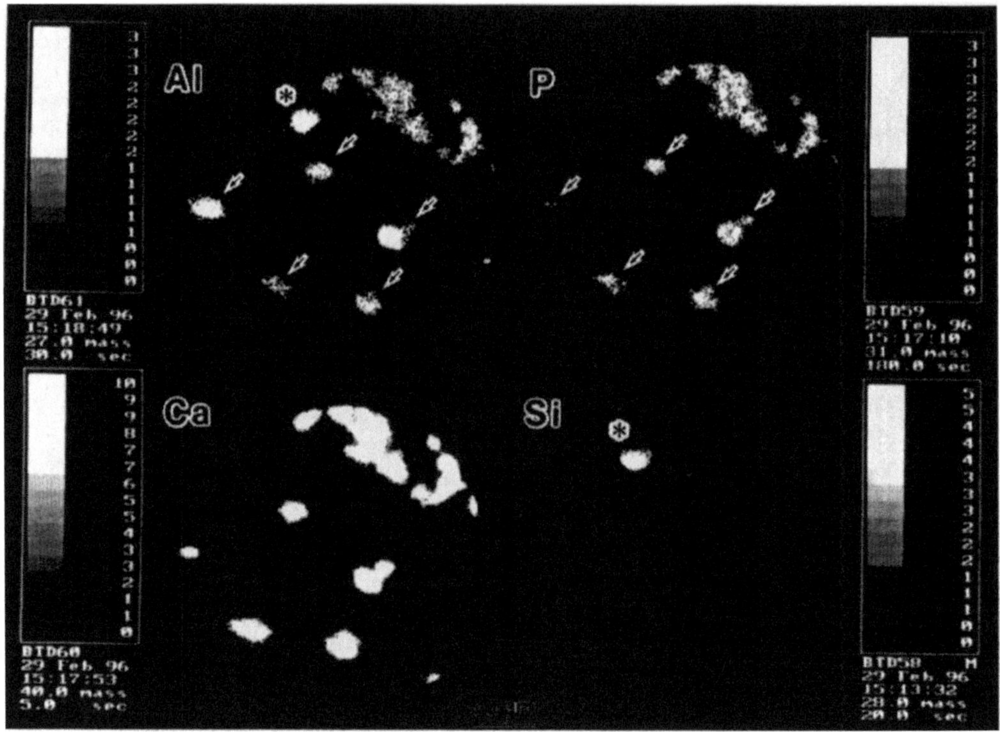

Figure 2. Secondary ion images of isolated cell nuclei from the brain (hippocampus) of an Alzheimer's disease patient. Al (upper left, arrows) was co-localized with P (upper right, arrows) and Ca (lower left) in the isolated nuclei.

P and Ca also were co-localized in isolated cell nuclei from the hippocampus of an age-matched control (Figure 3, arrows). On the other hand, neither Al nor Si could be detected in the isolated nuclei form the control brain.

EDX Analysis

A frozen section of a nerve cell from the hippocampus of a patient with Alzheimer's disease is shown in Figure 4. An elevated level of Al was demonstrated on the nucleolus of the nerve cell (Figure 4, arrow) by EDX point analysis (Figure 5). An Al peak was also detected in other components of the nuclei in nerve cells such as heterochromatin, euchromatin and the nuclear envelope. However, the highest Al peak within the nucleus in a nerve cell was always demonstrated in the nucleolus.

Al was demonstrated in the cytoplasm of the nerve cell (Figure 4, arrowhead) by point analysis (Figure 6). Al could not be detected in the extracellular space (Figure 4, asterisk, and Figure 7), or on the surface of the Formvar membrane.

On the other hand, high Si peaks were observed in the extracellular space (Figure 7) and on the Formvar membrane where no samples were mounted. Since Si could not be detected by SIMS analysis in the isolated brain cell nuclei from Alzheimer's disease patients (Figure 2) or in those from age-matched controls (Figure 3), it seems likely that the Si peaks detected by EDX analysis were mainly derived from the Formvar membrane itself.

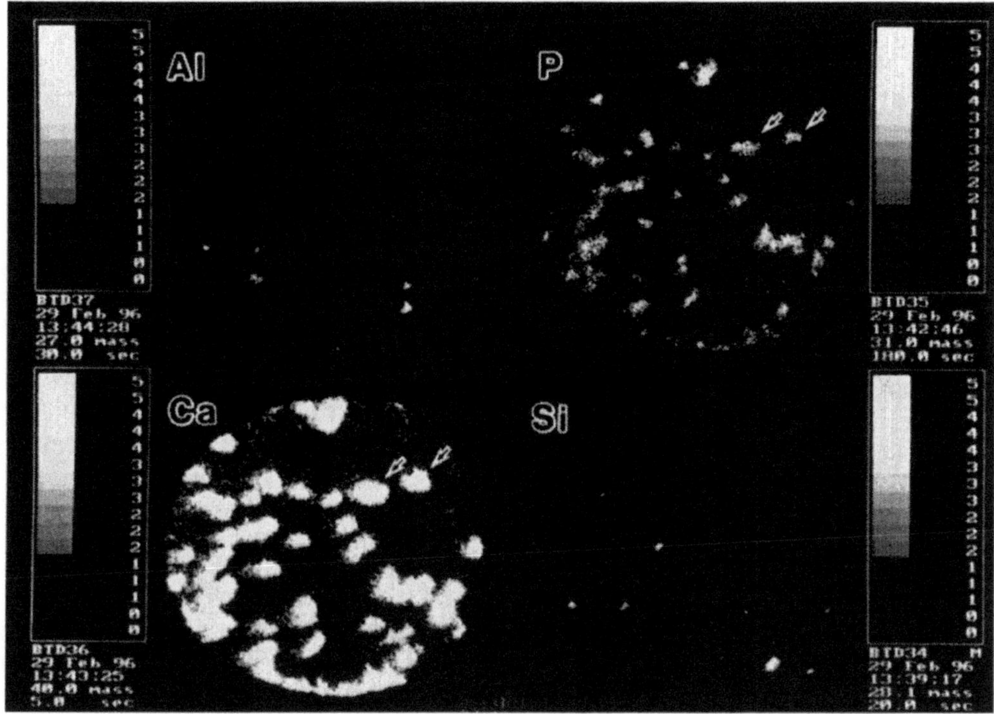

Figure 3. Secondary ion images of isolated cell nuclei from the brain of an age-matched control. P (upper right, arrows) was colocated with Ca (lower left, arrows) in the isolated nuclei. Neither Al nor Si could be detected in the isolated nuclei.

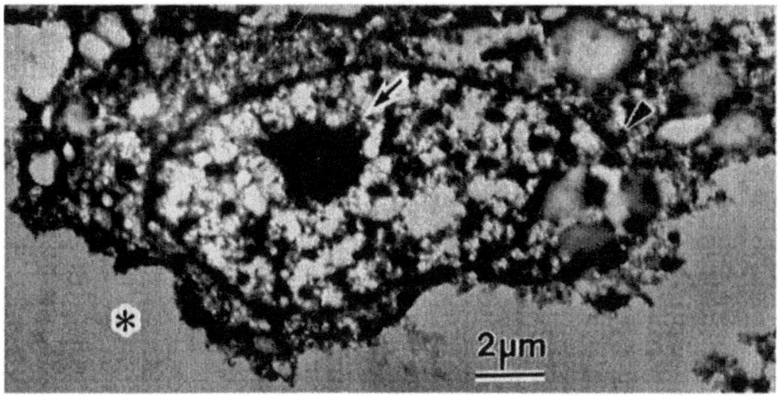

Figure 4. An electron micrograph of a nerve cell in a frozen section from the brain (hippocampus) of a patient with Alzheimer's disease. A well-developed, large nucleolus (arrow) was observed in the nucleus of the nerve cell. The section was mounted on a Nylon grid covered with the Formvar membrane. EDX spectra in the nucleolus (arrow), in the cytoplasm (arrowhead), and in the extracellular space (asterisk) are shown in Figures 5, 6, and 7, respectively.

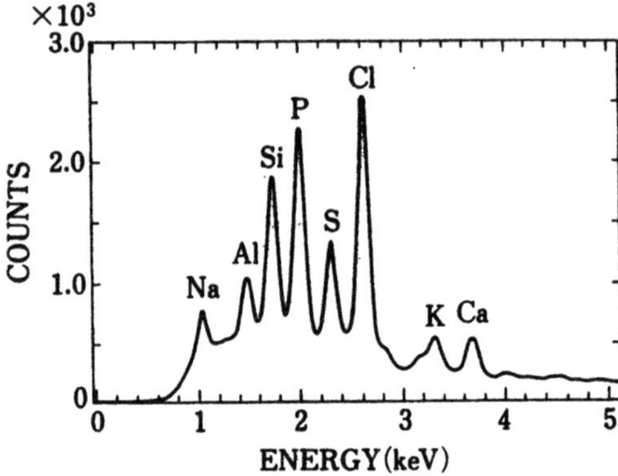

Figure 5. EDX spectrum obtained in the nucleolus of a nerve cell (shown in Figure 4, arrow) in a frozen section prepared from the brain of an Alzheimer's disease patient. A high Al peak was observed.

In frozen sections prepared from the control brains, Al could not be detected by EDX analysis.

DISCUSSION

The present study, using SIMS and EDX analyses, demonstrated A1 accumulation in the cell nuclei of brains (hippocampus) from patients with Alzheimer's disease. However, Edwardson et al. (1992) have reported that nuclear accumulation of Al in postmortem tissue results from redistribution following cell death and acidification of intracellular pH.

We previously reported that after an intraperitoneal injection of ^{26}Al (10 dpm) to healthy rats, 0.002% of the injected ^{26}Al was incorporated into the cerebrum through the blood-brain barrier (Kobayashi et al., 1990), and that 17% of the ^{26}Al ingested in the cerebrum was measured in the nuclei by accelerator mass spectrometry (Yumoto et al., 1995). We also demonstrated that most (approximately 89%) of the ^{26}Al taken in by the nuclei was bound to chromatin (Yumoto et al., 1997b). Therefore, we conclude that Al accumulation in the brain cell nuclei is not the result of exogenous contamination or redistribution related to postmortem processing of the tissues. Crapper et al. (1980) also demonstrated high Al concentrations in isolated brain cell nuclei from Alzheimer's disease patients, using atomic absorption spectrophotometry. They reported that 81% of Al within the nucleus

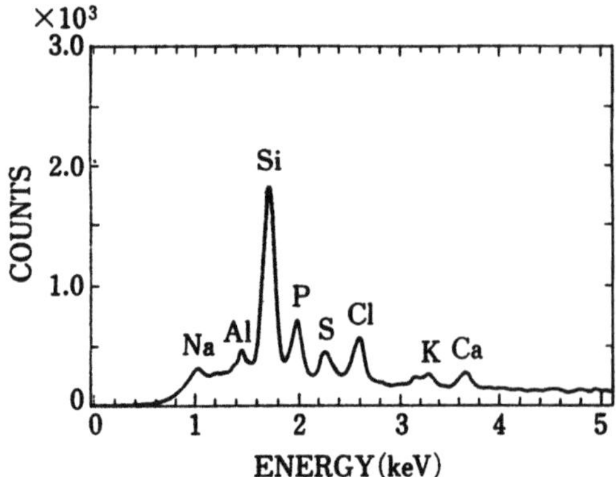

Figure 6. EDX spectrum obtained in the cytoplasm of a nerve cell (shown in Figure 4, arrowhead) in a frozen section from the brain of an Alzheimer's disease patient.

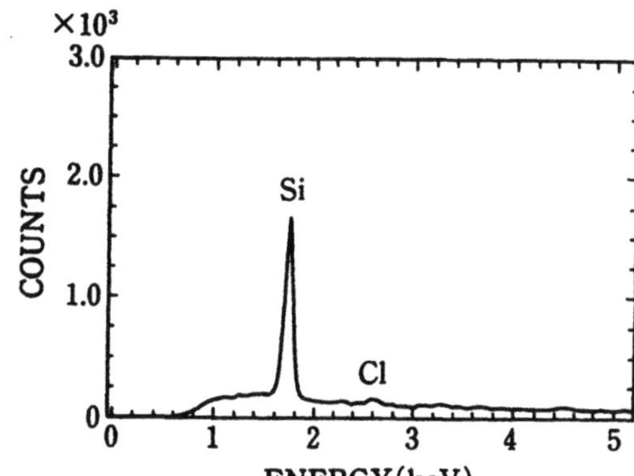

Figure 7. EDX spectrum obtained in the extracellular space (shown in Figure 4, asterisk) in a frozen section from the brain of a patient with Alzheimer's disease. The section was mounted on a Nylon grid covered with the Formvar membrane.

was associated with the highly condensed heterochromatin, which is generally considered to be transcriptionally inactive.

Al is a trivalent cation, and has high affinity for negatively charged groups in the proteins and DNA which comprise chromatin (Martin, 1986). It has been postulated that Al incorporated into the nuclei cross-links proteins and DNA, and represses gene expression irreversibly in brain cells, especially in nerve cells (McLachlan et al., 1988; Muma et al., 1988; Yumoto et al., 1997b). In this study, using EDX analysis, we demonstrated significant binding of Al to the nucleoli of nerve cells in the brains of Alzheimer's disease patients. The nucleolus is mainly composed of nucleolar chromatin and synthesizes ribosomal RNA, hence playing an essential role in the production of new ribosomes. Nerve cells have a characteristically large well-developed nucleolus in the nucleus, and possess a large number of ribosomes (Nissl bodies) in their cytoplasm. The nucleoli have been reported to synthesize more than 80% of all cellular RNA (Busch and Schildkraut, 1988). Sarkander et al. (1983) reported that Al markedly inhibited RNA synthesis in cultured nerve cells.

It seems likely that Al binding to the nucleoli of nerve cells represents one of the major target sites of Al neurotoxicity, and plays an important role in the pathogenesis of Alzheimer's disease. Our results strongly support the theory that Alzheimer's disease is caused by irreversible accumulation of Al in the nuclei of brain cells, especially nucleoli of nerve cells (Crapper et al., 1980; McLachlan et al., 1988; Yumoto et al., 1992, 1996b, 1997b).

REFERENCES

Alfrey, A. C., LeGrendre, G. R. and Kaehny, W. D., 1976, The dialysis encephalopathy syndrome. *N. Engl. J. Med.* 294:184–188.

Busch, H. and Schildkraut, C., 1988, Nucleus, DNA, and chromatin. In: *The Liver: Biology and Pathobiology*, Arias, I.M., Jakoby, W. B., Popper, H., Schachter, D. and Shafritz, D. A., eds., Raven Press, second edition, New York, pp. 47–82.

Crapper, D. R., Krishnan, S. S. and Quittkat, S., 1976, Aluminum, neurofibrillary degeneration and Alzheimer's disease. *Brain* 99:67–80.

Crapper, D. R.,Quittkat, S., Krishnan, S. S. Dalton, A. J. and DeBoni U., 1980, Intranuclear aluminum content in Alzheimer's disease, dialysis encephalopathy and experimental aluminum encephalopathy. *Acta Neuropathol.* (Berlin) 50:19–24.

Edwardson, J. A., Candy, J. M., Ince, P. G., McArthur, F. K. M., Morris, C. M., Oakley, A. E., Taylor, G.A. and Bjertness, E., 1992, Aluminium accumulation, β-amyloid deposition and neurofibrillary changes in the central nervous system. In: *Aluminium in Biology and Medicine*, John Wiley and Sons, Chichester, pp. 165–185.

Flaten, T. P., 1990, Geographical associations between aluminium in drinking water and death rates with dementia (including Alzheimer's disease), Parkinson's disease and amyotrophic lateral sclerosis in Norway. *Environ. Geochem. Health* 12:152–167.

Good, P. F., Perl, D. P., Bierer, L. M. and Schmeidler, J., 1992, Selective accumulation of aluminum and iron in the neurofibrillary tangles of Alzheimer's disease: A laser microprobe (LAMMA) study. *Ann. Neurol.* 31:286–292.

Horino, Y., Mokuno, Y. and Fujii, K., 1993a, Microanalysis of materials by PIXE using focused MeV heavy ion beams. *Nucl. Instr. Meth.* B75:535–538.

Horino, Y., Mokuno, Y., Kinomura, A., Fujii, K. and Yumoto, S., 1993b, Micro-PIXE (particle induced X-ray emission) analysis of aluminium in rat-liver using MeV heavy ion microprobes. *Scanning Microsc.* 7:1215–1220.

Kobayashi, K., Yumoto, S., Nagai, H., Hosoyama, Y., Imamura, M., Masuzawa, Sh., Koizumi, Y. and Yamashita, H., 1990, ^{26}Al tracer experiment by accelerator mass spectrometry and its application to the studies for amyotrophic lateral sclerosis and Alzheimer's disease. I, *Proc. Japan Acad.* 66 B: 189–192.

Landsberg, J. P., McDonald, B., Roberts, J. M., Grime, G.W. and Watt, F., 1991, Identification and analysis of senile plaques using nuclear microscopy. *Nucl. Instr. Meth.* B 54: 180–185.

Landsberg, J. P., McDonald, B. and Watt, F., 1992, Absence of aluminium in neuritic plaque cores in Alzheimer's disease. *Nature* 360: 65–68.

Mahurkar, S.D., Salta, R., Smith, E.C., Dhar, S.K., Meyers, L. and Dunea, G., 1973, Dialysis dementia. *Lancet* 1:1412–1415.

Martin, R.B., 1986, The chemistry of aluminum as related to biology and medicine, *Clin. Chem.* 32: 1797–1806.

Martyn, C. N., Barker, D. J. P., Osmond, C., Harris, E. C., Edwardson, J. A. and Lacey, R.F., 1989, Geographical relation between Alzheimer's disease and aluminium in drinking water. *Lancet* 1:59–62.

McLachlan, D.R.C., Lukiw, W.J., Wong, A.L., Bergeron, C. and Bech-Hansen, N.T., 1988, Selective messenger RNA reduction in Alzheimer's disease. *Mol. Brain Res.* 3:255–262.

Muma, N. A., Troncoso, J. C., Hoffman, P., Koo, E.H. and Price, D., 1988, Aluminum neurotoxicity - altered expression of cytoskeletal genes. *Mol. Brain Res.* 3:115–122.

Neri, L.C. and Hewitt, D., 1991, Aluminium, Alzheimer's disease, and drinking water. *Lancet* 338: 390.

Perl, D.P. and Brody, A.R., 1980, Alzheimer's disease: X-ray spectrometric evidence of aluminium accumulation in neurofibrillary tangle bearing neurons. *Science* 208:297–299.

Purpura, D.P., 1975, Dendritic differentiation in human cerebral cortex: Normal and aberrant developmental patterns. *Adv. Neurol.* 12: 91–116.

Sarkander, H.-I., Balss, G., Schloesser, R., Stoltenburg, G. and Lux, R.M., 1983, Blockade of neuronal brain RNA initiation sites by aluminum: A primary molecular mechanism of aluminum-induced neurofibrillary changes? *Aging* 21:259–274.

Yamamoto, H. and Takahashi, Y., 1978, Isolation and characterization of DNA-dependent RNA polymerase A, B, and C from rat brain nuclei. *J. Neurochem.* 31:449–456.

Yumoto, S., Ohashi, H., Nagai, H., Kakimi, S., Ogawa, Y., Iwata, Y. and Ishii, K., 1992, Aluminum neurotoxicity in the rat brain. *Int. J. PIXE* 2:493–504.

Yumoto, S., Ohashi, H., Nagai, H., Kakimi, S., Ishikawa, A., Kobayashi, K., Ogawa, Y. and Ishii, K., 1993, Aluminium toxicity in the rat liver and brain. *Nucl.Instr. and Meth.* B 75:188–190.

Yumoto, S., Kakimi, Y., Ogawa, Y., Nagai, H., Imamura, M. and Kobayashi, K., 1995, Aluminium neurotoxicity and Alzheimer's, disease. In: *Alzheimer's and Parkinson's Diseases: Recent Developments,* Hanin, I., Yoshida, M. and Fisher, A., eds., Plenum Publishing Corporation, New York, pp. 223–229.

Yumoto, S., Horino, Y., Mokuno, Y., Kakimi, S. and Fujii, K., 1996a, Microprobe PIXE analysis of aluminium in the brains of patients with Alzheimer's disease. *Nucl. Instr. and Meth.* B 109/110: 362-367.

Yumoto, S., 1996b, Acid rain, aluminium and Alzheimer's disease. In: *Global Environment and Human Activity,* Watanuki, K. and Yoshioka, K. eds., Maruzen Planet, Tokyo, pp. 41–57.

Yumoto, S., Maekawa, C. and Homma, Y., 1997a, SIMS analysis of aluminium in the brains of patients with Alzheimer's disease. In: *Secondary Ion Mass Spectrometry SIMS X,* Benninghoven, A., Hagenhoff B. and Werner H.W., eds., John Wiley and Sons, Chichester, pp. 819–822.

Yumoto, S., Nagai, H., Imamura, M., Matsuzaki, H., Hayashi, K., Masuda, A., Kumazawa H., Ohashi H. and Kobayashi K., 1997b, ^{26}Al uptake and accumulation in the rat brain. *Nucl. Instr. Meth.* B 123: 279–282.

42

LIPID COMPOSITION OF DIFFERENT BRAIN REGIONS IN PATIENTS WITH ALZHEIMER'S DISEASE AND MULTI-INFARCT DEMENTIA

D. Řípová,[1] V. Němcová,[1] C. Höschl,[1] E. Fales,[2] E. Majer,[2] and A. Strunecká[3]

[1]Psychiatric Center Prague
Ústavní 91
[2]Psychiatric Hospital of Bohnice
Ústavní 91, 181 03 Prague 8, Czech Republic
[3]Faculty of Sciences, Charles University
Viničná 7, Prague 2, Czech Republic

INTRODUCTION

In membranes phospholipids are in a highly dynamic state, altering membrane functions and participating actively in the regulation of cell metabolism. Changes of the phospholipid head group as well as heterogenous acyl chain composition influence and regulate the structure, stability and fluidity of the membranes. Phospholipids serve as important mediators in the transduction of extracellular signals.

Recent progress in the neurochemistry of Alzheimer's disease (AD) has led to the suggestion that changes in lipid composition and metabolism of brain lipids could contribute to the deterioration of central nervous system functioning. The cholinergic system is the predominantly affected neurotransmitter system in AD and senile dementia (Bartus et al., 1982). It has been proposed that cholinergic neurons are selectively vulnerable to the degenerative process (Wurtman, 1992). Membrane phosphatidylcholine (PC) has been considered as the potential pool of choline for acetylcholine synthesis, which could be maintained by excessive PC depletion. This hypothesis has been supported by Bárány et al. (1985), who reported increased glycerol-3-phosphorylcholine in postmortem AD brains. The study of Nitsch et al. (1991) reported a 15% decrease in PC level in the frontal cortex of AD patients and the increased level of glycerophosphocholine. The total phospholipid content was slightly decreased in AD brains. These authors recently found a 12–15% decrease in the level of PC in frontal and parietal cortex, and no change in the primary auditory cortex (Nitsch et al., 1992).

To determine whether the pathogenesis of AD is associated with alterations in phospholipid composition, levels of the major phospholipid classes were measured in different areas in the postmortem brains of AD patients. Although changes in the lipid content have been reported by many authors, the available data are sometimes controversial. In this study the total phospholipid content as well as the level of PC, phosphatidylethanolamine (PE), sphingomyelin (SPM), phosphatidylserine (PS), phosphatidylinositol (PI), and the composition of saturated and unsaturated fatty acids in total phospholipids were examinated in AD and an age- and postmortem interval-matched nondemented group (C). To determine the specificity of alterations for AD type dementia, the brains of age- and postmortem interval-matched patients with multi-infarct dementia (MID) were examined for all the parameters mentioned above.

MATERIALS AND METHODS

Human Brain Tissue

Histological and neurochemical studies were carried out on postmortem brains of 30 demented and nondemented subjects. At autopsy, the hemispheres were separated and both hemispheres were used for microscopical and biochemical examinations. Four brain areas (gyrus frontalis medius, gyrus temporalis superior et medius, lobus parietalis inferior, cornu Ammoni et gyrus parahippocampalis) were obtained from the left hemisphere and one of cerebellum (lobulus semiluminaris inferior) was obtained from the right hemisphere. All brain areas were dissected on a cold plate and divided according to the atlas of Borovansky et al. (1973). Using a silver stain technique (Cross, 1983), the clinical diagnosis of AD was confirmed histologically, based on the distribution of numerous senile plaques and neurofibrillary tangles. Criteria were consistent with those used in the classification of Mirra et al. (1991). Plaque density was counted in five microscopic fields and was expressed as plaques per square milimeter (in cortical and hippocampus sections). Only brain samples with plaque density >20 (frequent) were chosen for biochemical examinations.

All samples were divided into three groups: 1) AD group (clinically diagnosed dementia, number of senile plaques and tangles in given areas of the cortex and in the hippocampus higher than would be expected for age), 12 subjects: mean age 79.17 ± 1.47 years, postmortem interval 5.43 ± 0.58 hours; 2) MID group (clinically diagnosed dementia, number of senile plaques and tangles corresponds to normal aging, vascular changes, neuropathological lesions, gliosis), 12 subjects: mean age 79.75 ± 2.42 years, postmortem interval 5.25 ± 0.54 hours; and 3) control group (no clinical manifestation of dementia, number of senile plaques and tangles corresponds to normal aging), 6 subjects: mean age 76.68 ± 2.83 years, postmortem interval 5.17 ± 1.34 hours.

Biochemical Methods

Lipid Extraction. Brain regions chosen for lipid analysis were immediately homogenized in 0.25 M sucrose with an Ultra-Turrax blender and the resulting 10% homogenate was stored at −70°C until assayed. To extract lipids, chloroform-methanol 1:1 (v/v) was added to the homogenate to obtain a final chloroform-methanol-water ratio of 1:1:0.1 (v/v/v). After 5 min extraction, tubes were centrifuged 10 min at 1200 g. The lower phase was then reextracted twice with chloroform-methanol 2:1 (v/v). Combined extracts were evaporated. The lipid residue was dissolved in 5 ml chloroform and placed onto a Silica-SepPack cartridge (Millipore) which was then washed with 25 ml chloroform to remove neutral lipids. Phospholipids were eluted from the Silica-SepPack with 25 ml methanol. The solvent was evaporated and phospholipids were dissolved in 500 µl chloroform/ methanol 2:1 (v/v). Twenty µl of the extract were used for the separation.

Separation of Phospholipids and Fatty Acids. High performance liquid chromatography (HPLC) for the separation of phospholipids was accomplished on a microparticulate silica column using isocratic elution and UV detection by absorbance at 203 nm, with acetonitrile: 85% phosphoric acid (98:2) as solvent mixture (flow rate 1.5 ml/min). Using HPLC, saturated: 12:0, 14:0, 16:0, 17:0 (internal standard), 18:0 and mono- and polyunsaturated: 18:1, 18:2, 20:4, 20:5, 22:4, 22:6 fatty acids were determined as their hydrazides (Miwa and Yamamoto, 1991). Separation of hydrazides was carried out on a C_8 Ultrasphere column (the column temperature was kept constant at 30°C), using isocratic elution and UV detection by absorbance at 400 nm, with acetonitrile:methanol:water (73:12:15) at a flow rate of 1.2 ml/min. The quantification of phospholipids and their fatty acids was calculated from calibration curves for authentic phospholipid and fatty acid standards.

Concentration of Proteins

Proteins were estimated according to Lowry et al. (1951) with bovine serum albumin as a standard.

Data and Statistical Evaluation

Results are expressed as mean value ± S.E.M. Experimental data were analyzed using the BMDP software (Dixon et al., 1992). The analysis of variance (ANOVA) was utilized for the global multiple groups comparison (program 7D). Pairwise group comparisons were performed using the separate variance version of the t-test.

RESULTS

In the cortex, hippocampus and the cerebellum the content of phospholipid phosphorus (P) did not significantly differ in control, AD and MID subjects (in µgP/mg prot.- frontal cortex: C- 7.94 ± 0.92, AD- 8.48 ± 0.24, MID- 8.74 ± 0.70; parietal cortex: C- 9.78 ± 0.64, AD- 9.03 ± 0.64, MID- 9.40 ± 0.68; temporal cortex: C- 8.66 ± 0.76, AD- 8.05 ± 0.47, MID- 8.38 ± 0.41; hippocampus: C- 8.18 ± 1.14, AD- 8.55 ± 0.45, MID- 9.52 ± 0.36; cerebellum: C- 7.60 ± 0.77, AD- 6.91 ± 0.48, MID- 7.03 ± 0.62).

No significant changes were found in protein content of different brain regions in control, AD and MID subjects (in mg prot./g of wet tissue—frontal cortex: C- 110.83 ± 0.83, AD- 112.17 ± 0.69, MID- 106.67 ± 0.32; parietal cortex: C- 111.83 ± 0.30, AD- 106.08 ± 0.41, MID- 105.50 ± 0.39; temporal cortex: C- 113.33 ± 0.84, AD- 116.00 ± 0.69, MID- 107.36 ± 0.33; hippocampus: C- 120.00 ± 0.97, AD- 107.58 ± 0.62, MID- 101.67 ± 0.31; cerebellum: C- 114.17 ± 0.52, AD- 110.42 ± 0.79, MID- 109.82 ± 0.45).

Table 1 documents the composition of phospholipids and their fatty acids in five brain regions in control nondemented, AD and MID subjects. In the temporal cortex a slight decrease in the 20:5 fatty acid composition was measured (statistically significant pairwise comparisons by t-test: p = 0.0123; insignificant global comparison by ANOVA: p = 0.0568) in the MID group as compared to AD group. The PC composition was slightly

Table 1. Phospholipid and fatty acid composition of different regions in postmortem brain of control (CONT.), Alzheimer's disease (AD) and multi-infarct dementia (MID) subjects

%		Frontal Cortex			Parietal Cortex			Temporal Cortex			Hippocampus			Cerebellum		
		CONT.	AD	MID	CONT.	AD	MID	CONT.	AD	MID	CONT.	AD	MID	CONT.	AD	MID
TOTAL PL	PI	3.8 ±0.2	3.9 ±0.2	4.3 ±0.2	3.5 ±0.2	3.6 ±0.1	4.0 ±0.2	4.2 ±0.6	3.5 ±0.2	3.8 ±0.2	3.6 ±0.2	4.0 ±0.4	4.0 ±0.2	3.4 ±0.3	4.0 ±0.3	4.0 ±0.2
	PS	10.3 ±0.8	10.5 ±0.3	10.3 ±0.3	11.0 ±0.4	10.6 ±0.3	10.9 ±0.3	10.2 ±0.6	10.8 ±0.2	10.6 ±0.2	11.2 ±0.3	10.4 ±0.4	11.0 ±0.2	8.5 ±0.3	7.9 ±0.2	8.6 ±0.4
	PE	35.1 ±2.1	37.1 ±0.4	36.9 ±0.7	36.9 ±1.1	36.6 ±0.5	36.7 ±0.6	36.9 ±1.1	36.3 ±0.5	37.5 ±0.5	32.9 ±0.8	34.4 ±0.6	34.8 ±0.6	31.4 ±0.6	29.4 ±1.0	31.9 ±0.6
	PC	40.1 ±1.2	40.2 ±0.5	40.2 ±0.6	39.1 ±1.5	40.7 ±0.5	38.8 ±1.2	40.6 ±1.4	40.7 ±0.5	40.1 ±0.5	41.9 ±0.8	40.2 ±0.6	39.3 ±0.7	46.7 ±0.5	47.5 ±0.6	45.2 ±0.9
	SPM	9.0 ±0.7	8.3 ±0.4	8.4 ±0.3	9.6 ±0.5	8.4 ±0.4	8.7 ±0.4	8.2 ±0.7	8.7 ±0.5	8.1 ±0.4	10.5 ±1.1	11.0 ±0.5	11.0 ±0.4	10.0 ±0.6	11.2 ±0.5	10.3 ±0.3
TOTAL FA	12:0	0.2 ±0.04	0.2 ±0.05	0.2 ±0.04	0.2 ±0.06	0.2 ±0.04	0.1 ±0.03	0.2 ±0.07	0.2 ±0.04	0.1 ±0.04	0.2 ±0.07	0.2 ±0.04	0.1 ±0.04	0.2 ±0.07	0.3 ±0.04	0.2 ±0.04
	14:0	1.0 ±0.12	0.8 ±0.07	0.9 ±0.06	0.9 ±0.06	1.0 ±0.08	1.1 ±0.07	0.8 ±0.09	1.0 ±0.06	0.9 ±0.05	0.9 ±0.09	0.8 ±0.05	1.0 ±0.08	0.9 ±0.07	1.1 ±0.06	1.0 ±0.05
	16:0	23.1 ±0.4	22.5 ±0.2	22.8 ±0.3	22.0 ±0.4	22.3 ±0.4	21.5 ±0.3	22.3 ±0.4	22.1 ±0.5	22.7 ±0.6	21.2 ±0.4	21.9 ±0.3	21.5 ±0.3	24.3 ±0.3	25.0 ±0.5	24.2 ±0.4
	18:0	21.4 ±0.8	21.4 ±0.6	21.6 ±0.3	21.5 ±0.5	21.8 ±0.3	21.6 ±0.4	22.4 ±0.4	21.0 ±0.5	23.3 ±0.9	21.0 ±0.4	20.8 ±0.4	21.8 ±0.3	20.5 ±0.3	19.8 ±0.3	20.4 ±0.3
	18:1	21.8 ±0.5	21.7 ±0.5	21.3 ±0.4	22.7 ±0.6	22.8 ±0.6	23.2 ±0.8	21.5 ±0.6	21.7 ±0.8	20.8 ±0.7	24.9 ±1.0	24.3 ±0.5	24.3 ±0.6	23.2 ±0.6	23.3 ±0.3	22.4 ±0.3
	18:2	1.7 ±0.2	2.2 ±0.1	1.9 ±0.1	2.0 ±0.2	2.0 ±0.2	1.9 ±0.1	1.7 ±0.3	2.0 ±0.1	1.8 ±0.1	1.9 ±0.2	1.8 ±0.2	1.7 ±0.1	1.9 ±0.2	1.8 ±0.2	1.9 ±0.1
	20:4	9.8 ±0.1	9.9 ±0.2	9.7 ±0.2	9.2 ±0.2	9.0 ±0.2	8.9 ±0.2	9.8 ±0.5	9.7 ±0.4	9.2 ±0.3	10.2 ±0.3	10.2 ±0.2	10.0 ±0.2	9.4 ±0.3	9.5 ±0.3	9.8 ±0.2
	20:5	0.3 ±0.12	0.5 ±0.09	0.3 ±0.09	0.3 ±0.17	0.5 ±0.10	0.2 ±0.07	0.4 ±0.15	0.5 ±0.09	0.2 ±0.07	0.3 ±0.15	0.4 ±0.07	0.2 ±0.07	0.3 ±0.13	0.5 ±0.11	0.3 ±0.12
	22:4	4.9 ±0.3	5.0 ±0.2	4.8 ±0.2	4.7 ±0.3	4.5 ±0.2	5.0 ±0.1	4.9 ±0.2	5.2 ±0.2	4.9 ±0.2	6.5 ±0.2	5.9 ±0.2	5.6 ±0.2*	3.4 ±0.2	3.4 ±0.1	3.5 ±0.3
	22:6	16.0 ±0.5	16.0 ±0.5	16.7 ±0.3	16.5 ±0.3	15.9 ±0.5	16.4 ±0.6	16.0 ±0.3	15.8 ±0.3	16.1 ±0.6	13.0 ±0.7	13.6 ±0.4	13.8 ±0.4	16.3 ±0.4	15.5 ±0.4	16.3 ±0.3

means ± S.E.M.; * p = 0.0089 by t-test; ANOVA: p = 0.0211; PL = phospholipids; FA = fatty acids

reduced in the hippocampus of MID subjects compared to the control group (statistically significant pairwise comparisons by t-test: p = 0.0302; insignificant ANOVA). A significantly decreased composition of 22:4 fatty acid was estimated in this brain area in MID subjects compared to the controls (significant pairwise p = 0.0089 and global comparison by ANOVA: p = 0.0211).

DISCUSSION

The proposal that altered phospholipid metabolism might result in neuropathology of AD has been investigated by many authors. Postmortem phospholipid analysis of human brains performed so far, has resulted in heterogenous data. The increased level of glycerophosphocholine (Bárány et al., 1985; Nitsch et al., 1992) and the decreased content of PC seems to be consistent with the hypothesis that membrane PC could serve as the storage pool of choline for acetylcholine synthesis. The study of Kanfer et al. (1993) demonstrated elevated glycerol-3-phosphorylcholine phosphodiesterase and decreased choline kinase activities in AD brains as compared to non-AD demented controls. Also in vitro ^{31}P NMR spectroscopy on brain samples detected increased levels of glycerophosphorylcholine and glycerophosphorylethanolamine, while levels of the phosphomonoesters phosphocholine and phosphoethanolamine were decreased in frontal and parietal regions of AD patients compared to control subjects (Bárány et al., 1985).

On the other hand, in vivo ^{31}P NMR study of 24 patients with mild AD showed a significant increase in the phosphomonoester-total phosphorus ratio in the prefrontal regions of their brains (Cuenod et al., 1995). Wells et al. (1995) found a lower level of ethanolamine glycerophospholipids in the plasma membrane fraction from synaptosomes from postmortem AD brains, but no differences were observed in PC.

Some other studies, however, revealed only a mild decrease in total phospholipids or individual phospholipid classes in various regions of AD brain (Brooksbank and Martinez, 1989). Söderberg et al. (1992) analyzed the lipid composition of 10 different brain regions in AD and found that the total phospholipid amount slightly decreased only in white matter and in nucleus caudatus, while in most brain regions the total amount of phospholipids remain unchanged. The elevated content of PI was found in the areas that are morphologically affected by AD, such as the frontal and temporal cortex and the hippocampus.

The analysis of postmortem brains of AD patients enables the investigation of the target organ and the diagnosis of the terminal stage of AD based on clinical observation and on the histological examination of morphological changes in neuronal tissue. On the other hand, the process of dying and the postmortem interval can affect the metabolism of phospholipids in neuronal membranes. Řípová et al. (1996) reported that the composition of the major phospholipid classes in rat brain, namely PC and PE, remains unchanged in the postmortem interval of 0–12 hours. In our study, samples from human brain regions, namely frontal, parietal and temporal cortex, hippocampus and cerebellum, were analyzed in the same average time interval in AD, MID and control groups. Only tissue samples of AD brains with plaque density higher than 20 in one square millimeter were chosen for biochemical examination. No differences in the total phospholipid content, absolute concentrations and the proportions of the major phospholipid classes were found in five selected brain areas in AD, MID and control subjects. The concentrations of the major phospholipids are in general accord with values reported by previous studies (Brooksbank and Martinez, 1989; Söderberg et al., 1992). Also the analysis of the total phospholipid fatty acid composition did not reveal any substantial differences between the AD brains and controls. The decreased content of polyunsaturated component 22:4 was observed in the hippocampus of MID brains in comparison with controls. Our finding is in general agreement with the investigation of Brooksbank and Martinez (1989), while other authors reported that the fatty acid composition of brain phospholipids varied (Jellinger et al., 1993). A decreased content of polyunsaturated fatty acids and a substantial increase in the relative amount of the saturated components of different brain regions was found in AD (Söderberg et al., 1991).

In the search for the etiology of AD several hypotheses have been postulated. However, none of them has been fully confirmed by experimental results. The heterogenous and often controversial data provided by laboratory research cannot be accounted for by experimental errors. It reveals the multiple character of AD etiology and probably the subtlety of the regulatory mechanisms. There is an open question if the availability of substrate for acetylcholine and PC synthesis-choline has a regulatory role. Moreover, the alterations in the metabolism of PC may occur in some small pool and may be masked by the bulk of this major membrane phospholipid. It seems, however, that the estimation of the levels of major phospholipids in postmortem brains does not serve as an indicator of AD or MID type dementia.

The reductionistic approach trying to find alteration in one enzyme or one reaction cannot explain the pathophysiological changes occurring in the brain, operating as neural events massively coupled in parallel. Potentially, every chemical event could be influenced by every other event. Explanatory models for such parallel-coupled systems are likely to involve a type of non-linear dynamics. An abundance of laboratory reports reveals potentiating interactions of this kind. Currently we have no conceptual framework to integrate them.

ACKNOWLEDGMENTS

This work and presentation has been supported by the Internal Grant Agency of the Ministry of Health of the Czech Republic (Grant No. 2877-3) and by the Ministry of Education of the Czech Republic (Presentation Programme).

REFERENCES

Bartus, R.T., Dean, R.L., Beer, B., and Lippa, A.S., 1982, The cholinergic hypothesis of geriatric memory dysfunction, *Science* 217:408–417.

Borovansky, L., Hromada, J., Kos, J., Zrzavy, J., and Zlabek, K., 1973, Soustavna anatomie cloveka II, Prague, Avicenum.

Brooksbank, B.W.L., and Martinez, M., 1989, Lipid abnormalities in the brain in adult Down's syndrome and Alzheimer's disease, In: *Molecular and Chemical Neuropathology*, Horrocks, L.A. ed., Humana Press Inc. 157–185.

Cross, R.B., 1983, Demonstration of neurofibrillary tangles in paraffin sections: a quick and simple method using a modification of Palmgren's method, *Med.Lab.Sci.* 39:67–69.

Cuenod, C.A., Kaplan, D.B., Michot, J.L., Jehenson, P., Leroy-Willig, A., Forette, F., Syrota, A., and Boller, F., 1995, Phospholipid abnormalities in early Alzheimer's disease. In vivo phosphorus 31 magnetic resonance spectroscopy, *Arch.Neurol.* 52:89–94.

Dixon, W.J., Brown, M.B., Engelman, L., and Jennrich, R.I., 1992, Multiple comparison tests, In: *BMDP Statistical Software Manual*, Dixon, W.J., ed, University of Carolina Press, Berkley, Los Angeles, Oxford:196–200.

Jellinger, K., Kienzl, E., Puchinger, L., and Stachelberger, H., 1993, Changes of phospholipids in Alzheimer's disease brain, In: *Alzheimer's Disease:Advances in Clinical and Basic Research*, Corain,B. et al., eds., Wiley, .& Sons Ltd,:315–323.

Kanfer, J.N., Pettergrew, J.W., Moossy, J., and McCartney, D.G., 1993, Alterations of selected enzymes of phospholipid metabolism in Alzheimer's disease brain tissue as compared to non-Alzheimer's demented controls, *Neurochem.Res.* 18:331–334.

Lowry, O.H., Rosenbrough, N.J., Farr, A.L., and Randal, .J., 1951, Protein measurement with the Folin phenol reagent, *J.Biol.Chem.* 192:265–275.

Mirra, S.S., Heyman, A., McKeel, D., Sumi, S.M., Crain, .J., Brownlee, .M., Vogel, F.S., Hughes, J.P., Van Belle, G., and Berg, L., 1991, The consortium to establish a registery for Alzheimer's disease (CERAD), *Neurology* 41:479–486.

Miwa, H., and Yamamoto, M., 1991, High-performance liquid chromatographic analysis of fatty acid compositions of platelet phospholipids as their 2-nitophenylhydrazides, *J.Chromatogr.* 568:25–34.

Nitsch, R., Blusztajn, J.K., Wurtman, R.J., and Growdon, J.H.,1991, Membrane phospholipid metabolites are abnormal in Alzheimer's disease, *Neurology* 41:269.

Nitsch, R., Bluzstajn, J .K., Pittas, A.G., Stack, B.E., Growdon, J.H., and Wurtman, R.J., 1992, Evidence for a membrane defect in Alzheimer's disease brain, *Proc.Natl.Acad.Sci.* USA 89:1671–1675.

Řípová, D., Němcová, V., and Höschl, C., 1996, Effect of postmortem interval on phospholipid and fatty acid composition in the rat brain, *Eur.Neuropsychopharmacol.* 6:192.

Söderberg, M., Edlund, C., Alafuzoff, I., Kristensson, K., and Dallner, G., 1992, Lipid composition in different regions of the brain in Alzheimer's disease/senile dementia of Alzheimer's type, *J.Neurochem.* 59:1646–1653.

Söderberg, M., Edlund, C., Kristensson, K., and Dallner, G., 1991, Fatty acid composition of brain phospholipids in aging and in Alzheimer's disease, *Lipids* 26:421–425.

Wells, K., Farooqui, A.A., Liss, L., and Horrocks, L.A., 1995, Neural membrane phospholipids in Alzheimer's disease, *Neurochem.Res.* 20:1329–1333.

Wurtman, R.J., 1992, Choline metabolism as a basis for the selective vulnerability of cholinergic neurons, *TINS* 15:117–122.

43

VERBAL AND MOTOR MEMORY IN ALZHEIMER'S DISEASE: RELEASE FROM PROACTIVE INHIBITION

Joseph Harris,[1] Malcolm Dick,[2] Veronica Sandoval,[3] Daniel Gallegos,[3] Sean Lozano,[3] Sergio Rangel,[3] and Mary-Louise Kean[1]

[1]Psychology Program, Institute of Technology, Arts and Sciences
Holon, Israel
Neuropsychology Unit for Treatment and Rehabilitation
Tel-Aviv, Israel
Herczeg Institute on Aging, Tel-Aviv University
Ramat Aviv, Israel
[2]Department of Psychobiology
University of California
Irvine, California
[3]Neuropsychology Program
University of California
Berkeley, California

INTRODUCTION

The first and most prominent clinical manifestation of Alzheimer's disease (AD) is memory loss. Previously it was believed that memory loss occurred "across the board", that is, all types of memory (i.e., verbal, visual, spatial memory, etc.) were severely impaired. The primary purpose for this study is to provide an answer to a relatively simple question, namely, can the recall of AD patients be facilitated on a motor memory task by changing the distance and/or direction of the last of a series of movements, thereby producing the "release from proactive inhibition effect (RPI)". It would be expected that proactive inhibition would build up as the subject's memory of a recent movement is interfered with by his memory of previous movements. However, if there is a noticeable change in the character of a final movement, the reproduction accuracy would be improved. The superior reproduction accuracy of an altered movement (termed manipulated) over a non-altered movement (termed control) after a repeated movement series (termed constrained) has been called the "release from proactive inhibition effect" and appears to be a highly reliable finding occurring not only in the motor memory of young adults (Shif-frin & Schneider, 1977), but also in that of children as young as age five and the mentally retarded (Kelso et al., 1979). Given the beneficial effect that RPI has on retention in these different populations, might this same process provide a useful method for enhancement of memory with AD patients? As a review of the literature can find no comparable study performed with this patient group, the goal of the study was simply to demonstrate either the presence or absence of the RPI effect in AD patients. While the outcome of this experiment would provide further evidence as to the generality of the RPI effect, it would also address the more important question of whether or not manipulations designed to improve encoding in AD patients can have a facilitory effect on memory.

Despite the robust nature of the RPI effect, work by Martin and colleagues (1985) suggests that this phenomenon might not be present in motor memory of AD patients. According to these authors, the observed episodic memory impairment results from a combination of two factors: 1) an abnormally rapid loss of information due to damage to the medial-temporal regions of the brain, and 2) a generalized failure to encode critical stimulus attributes due to the fact that the cognitive system responsible for such an analysis has been compromised by the disease. Consequently, manipulations designed to aid encoding such as inducing patients to encode a greater number of stimulus attributes, or to encode the more salient or distinguishing features of the stimulus will be unsuccessful. The findings from other studies (e.g., Miller, 1977; Graf and Mandler, 1995) showing that verbal memory performance of AD patients cannot be improved by providing them with instructions to the use of mediators, imagery, rehearsal, nor can it benefit from the use of other elaborate strategies lend support to Martin and colleagues' encoding limitation hypothesis.

If motor and verbal memory are isomorphic, that is affected by similar processes and follow the same general laws, then we would expect that efforts to enhance encoding through the RPI process should not benefit the AD patient. However, others disagree with the idea of a single parsimonious system, and contend that the verbal and motor domains are governed by different sets of rules and involve separate memory stores (Albert & Moss, 1994; Cohen & Bean, 1983; Dick et al., 1988 & 1991; Harris, 1993 & 1996). In the present study, the RPI process may facilitate encoding in AD subjects and thereby improve recall accuracy. Should this occur, the encoding limitation hypothesis would be applicable to situations involving the processing of verbal and visual/spatial materials and not necessarily to information in the motor domain.

METHODS

Subjects

Twenty-four community-dwelling older adults, 14 females and 10 males, with a diagnosis of probable AD, participated in this study. Diagnosis was based on DSM IV criteria (American Psychiatric Association, 1994). Physician's reports were used to exclude patients who had a history of chronic alcoholism, major psychiatric illness, or neurological or cardiovascular disease. To exclude patients with possible multi-infarct dementia, no subjects were accepted who attained an ischemic score of 4 or above (Rosen et al., 1980).

Severity of the patient's dementing illness was defined in terms of scores on a variety of psychological tests including the Mini-Mental State Exam (MMSE; Folstein et al., 1975); the Brief Cognitive Rating Scale (BCRS: Reisberg, 1983); and the Verbal Scale of the Wechsler Adult Intelligence Scale-Revised (WAIS-R: Wechsler, 1981).

The MMSE scores of the patients ranged between 14 and 22 (M = 18.3, SD = 4.0). On the BCRS the average performance of the patients in each of five areas assessed was (M = 4.54, SD = 0.8) indicative of a moderately severe decline. Five of the subtests from the WAIS-R (i.e., Information, Digit Span, Vocabulary, Comprehension, and Similarities) were used to determine the patient's level of intellectual functioning. The VIQ scores ranged from 70 to 108 (M = 86.1, SD = 10.1). This represents a significant decline from their estimated premorbid IQ (cf. Wilson, Rosenbaum, & Brown, 1979) of 111.2. The mean age and number of years of education of the patients were 82.0 (SD = 7.4) and 13.2 (SD = 2.1), respectively.

Forty-eight young adults and 48 healthy elderly adults served as subjects in the two control groups. The young adults were college students who participated for course credit. Their average age was 19.7 (SD = 2.1), and they had completed an average of 13.9 (SD = 1.1) years of education. The elderly adults were community dwelling volunteers. They were selected so as to overlap with the AD patients in both age (M = 77.2, SD = 6.8) and education (M = 13.0, SD = 6.4). All of the older controls had a MMSE score of 21 or above (M = 28.3, SD = 1.7) and stated that they were in good health.

For the Verbal portion of the study, subjects were presented a set of eight words, one at a time, on 8.5 in. by 11 in. flashcards. They were instructed to read each word out loud and to attempt to remember the list of words. A final ninth card in the set contained a series of question marks ("?????") instead of a word. The question marks served to prompt the subject to recall the set of eight words. This process was repeated over four trials. For the fifth trial, the set of words presented was from one of four conditions: a) control—the word category color of the cards remained the same; b) semantic—the word category changed; c) perceptual—the colors of the cards and print were changed; d) multiple—both a word category change and colors of the cards and print were changed.

Using a linear positioning apparatus, blindfolded subjects performed a series of movements. The apparatus consists of a movable slide, which runs on top of two parallel bars (two meters in length). In the center of the slide is a handle that the subjects hold while performing movements. On the side of the slide is a pointer that moves along a scale allowing the experimenter to measure the length of a movement in millimeters. The slide pivots from 0 to 180 degrees. The handle can be moved in distances ranging from 10 to 400 mm.

For each trial, subjects performed five movements: four criterion movements that were all of the same distance and direction (e.g. 300 mm at 105°). and a fifth movement that was performed in one of four conditions: (a) control—same distance and direction as in the previous four movements; (b) distance—shift in distance (e.g. 200 mm at 105°); (c) direction—shift in direction (e.g. 300 mm at 45°); (d) multiple—shift in direction and distance (e.g. 200 mm at 45°). After performing each of the five movements, they were asked to recall and reproduce each movement. All movements were performed with the dominant hand. For all 4 conditions, subjects performed 4 trials consisting of 5 movements and reproductions, for a total of 80 movements with reproductions.

Data Analysis

Three error measures: absolute error (AE), constant error (CE), and variable error (VE) were examined. Two analyses of variance were performed. The first analysis was a 3 (Group: young vs. old vs. AD) × 4 (Verbal: control vs. semantic vs. perceptual vs. multiple) ANOVA. The second was a 3 (Group: young vs. old vs. AD) × 4 (Movement: control vs. distance vs. direction vs. multiple) ANOVA.

RESULTS

For all analyses, results were considered statistically significant with a $p < .01$. Subsequent analyses using the Scheffe procedure confirmed significance. Differences were found in verbal memory among the three groups. The mean no. of words recalled for young adults was 5.4 (SD = 1.7), healthy older adults 4.8 (SD 1.7), and AD patients 2.0 (SD = 1.2). The results of the ANOVA for the verbal tasks were as follows: Group main effect F = (2, 76) 430.31, $p < 0.0001$; Verbal main effect F = (4, 76) 8.10, $p < 0.01$; Interaction between group X Verbal F = (6, 76) 3.35, $p < 0.01$.

Significant results were also found in motor memory tasks. The average absolute error for young adults were 37.8 (SD = 44.35), for healthy older adults 52.2 (SD = 50.30), and AD patients is 55.5 (SD = 34.37). There were no significant main interaction effects for CE. In general, the analysis produced three notable effects. First there was a significant main effect for group- VE, $F(2, 76) = 70.2$; AE, $F(2, 76) = 63.2$. This difference occurred even during criterion movements where memory plays a less important role than in the manipulated movements. The differences between the young and older controls was not significant.

The second and more important finding concerns whether or not AD patients were able to reproduce the fifth movement more accurately in the distance, direction and multiple conditions than for the control condition. The presence of a significant main effect for movement condition for VE, $F(2, 76) = 74.1$, in conjunction with the nonsignificant interaction of group by movement condition $(F < 1.00)$ indicates that the superiority of experimental movements over control movements was consistent across all three subject groups. Similarly, the AE data revealed a strong effect for movement condition, $F(2, 76) = 109.3$. However, the findings based on VE, the interaction of group X movement condition was significant $F(2, 76) = 18.4$. Nevertheless, the presence of this interaction does not mean that AD patients were unaffected by the RPI process. To the contrary, the difference between the manipulated and control movements was significantly larger in the AD than in the control groups. Collapsing across retention conditions, the mean difference between the manipulated and control movements was 8.6 cm for the young adults, 12.4 for the elderly, and 26.4 for the AD patients. It is evident that the facilitory effect stemming from the RPI process does indeed occur both in cognitively intact and demented adults.

Finally, while there was a significant main effect for the movement condition using both VE, $F(2, 76) = 58.6$ and AE, $F(2, 76) = 64.8$, the interaction between this effect and subject group was only significant for AE, $F(2, 76) = 14.9$. Inspection of the data reveals that for all three groups, the size of the reproduction error increased in a linear fashion across the four conditions: the size of the error being smallest during the multiple condition, larger during the distance condition, even larger during the direction condition and largest when the fifth movement was a control condition movement. The group by movement condition interaction found for AE simply indicates that error size increased at a faster rate in AD than in controls.

DISCUSSION

The major findings of this study are that if individuals with AD perform a series of similar movements, proactive inhibition occurs. When the condition for a final movement is manipulated, their recall accuracy for that movement is greatly facilitated. The fact that RPI effect occurs in the motor memory of the AD subjects is further proof to the generality and robust nature of this phenomenon. More importantly, the findings suggest that, at least in the motor domain, efforts to enhance encoding in AD patients can have a positive effect on recall. Given that the AD patient can utilize the RPI process to facilitate recall, how should this finding be interpreted? More specifically, can an examination of the memory codes underlying the RPI effect shed additional light on the nature of the encoding deficit present in AD?

In general, two different hypotheses have been proposed to account for the superior reproduction accuracy of the manipulated movement conditions (see Kelso et al., 1979, for a review). One view emphasizes "cognitive" aspects of RPI. That is, there is a failure of a plan or encoding strategy as a result of the heavy influence on recall of new items by the number of items previously tested. The result being that the greater the number of previous items tested, the poorer the recall (e.g., Naire et al., 1995; Kelso et al., 1979; Herlitz & Bäckman, 1993; Herlitz et al., 1994). The effect of this cognitive component is to generate confusing signals that impair the subject's ability to accurately recall a recent similar movement from a prior one. In contrast to the cognitive view with its emphasis on higher order encoding, the focus of the "motor" view (e.g., Bell, 1950; Eslinger & Damasio, 1986; Graf, et al., 1986; Corkin, et al 1986) is on lower level, efferent based mechanisms. According to this latter view, when a movement is made, the resulting efferent discharge is stored in the form of an efferent copy. At recall, the subject monitors the efferent commands and matches them to the stored copy. The reason for why the manipulated movements are reproduced more accurately than the initial four movements is that their efferent commands are more efficiently monitored and stored.

Perhaps the best way to conceptualize the differences between the two hypotheses is in terms of level of processing theory (c.f., Underwood, 1983). In essence, the level of processing theory suggests that input can be coded at different levels, and the deeper the encoding, the less the forgetting. Deeper encoding implies a greater degree of cognitive or meaningful analysis, and can be contrasted to encoding at a shallow, sensory level which can give rise to only a transient memory trace. From this perspective, a cognitive view could maintain that information derived from the manipulated conditions is more "meaningful" to the subjects (since they are cognizant of a change in the movements) and is subjected to a deeper level of analysis than are control condition movements, where subjects have no unique knowledge about that specific movement. In return, the motor view could maintain that subjects process information contained in both manipulated and control condition movements to the same shallow depth of analysis (i.e., sensory or perceptual level), but manipulated movements undergo more elaborate processing within that level. Therefore, while both hypotheses attribute the superior recall accuracy of manipulated movement to events occurring at encoding, they differ in that the motor view stresses the more efficient coding of kinesthetic features, while the cognitive view allocates the advantage to the role played by more meaningful, conceptual codes.

Given the two alternative explanations for the RPI effect, the question now asked is whether or not AD patients encoded the manipulated movements in the same fashion as did the normal subjects. In previous studies of verbal memory (c.f., Corkin, 1982; Wilson, et al., 1983), AD patients are impaired in their ability to code the deeper, more meaningful attributes of words (i.e., semantic or conceptual properties). If this processing limitation extends to the motor domain, then it is possible that the patients in this study were relying primarily on kinesthetic or perceptual sorts of information in order to reproduce the movements. A reliance on lower-level physical or perceptual codes may explain why these individuals were less accurate than their nondemented peers at recall of all movements. On the other hand, it is also possible that the demented patients were encoding manipulated movements in terms of higher-order conceptual features (i.e., image, plans) and those codes were better formed and decayed less rapidly than during the control movement condition.

ACKNOWLEDGMENTS

Supported in part by the Ford Foundation, American Psychological Association, NIA Grant #1RO3AG12780-01, and the Howard Hughes Center for Academic Excellence, University of California, Irvine.

REFERENCES

Albert, M. and Moss, M., 1994, The assessment of memory disorders in patients with Alzheimer's disease. In: *The Neuropsychology of Memory,* Butters, N. and Squire, L. R., eds., New York, Guilford Press 236–246.

American Psychiatric Association, 1994. *Diagnostic and Statistical Manual of Mental Disorders,* 4th ed., Washington, D.C., *Am. Psychiatric Assoc.*

Bayles, E., 1992, Language function in senile dementia. *Brain and Lang.* 16:265–280.

Beatty, W. W., 1988, Preserved cognitive functions in dementia. In: *Cognitive Approaches to Neuropsychology,* Williams, J. M. and Long, C. J., eds., Plenum Press: New York.

Bell, H., 1950, Retention of pursuit rotor skill after one year. *J. Exp. Psychol.* 40:648–649.

Cohen, R. L., 1981, On the generality of some memory laws. *Scand. J. Psychol.*22:267–281.

Cohen, R. L. and Bean, G., 1983, Memory in educable mentally retarded adults: Deficit in subject or experimenter. *Intelligence* 7:287–298.

Corkin, S., 1982, Some relationships between global amnesia and the memory impairments in Alzheimer's disease. In: *Alzheimer's Disease: A Report of Progress in Research,.* Corkin, S., Davis, K. L., Gordon, J. H., and Wurtman,R. J., eds., New York: Raven Press. pp. 149–164.

Corkin, S., Gabrieli, J. D., Stanger, B. Z., Mickel, T., Rosen, J., Sullivan, E. V. and Growdon, J. H., 1986, Skill learning and priming in Alzheimer's disease. *Neurology* 36:296.

Dick, M. B., Harris J. and Kean, M.L., 1990, Recall and memory of motor movements in dementia-Alzheimer's type. *Proc. 4th Neurobiol. Learning and Memory Conf.* Costa Mesa, CA.

Dick, M. B., Kean, M.L. and Sands, D., 1988, The preselection effect on recall facilitation of motor movements in Alzheimer-Type dementia. *J. Geront.,* 43:127–135.

Eslinger, P. J. and Damasio, A.R., 1986, Preserved motor learning in Alzheimer's disease: Implications for anatomy and behavior. *J. Neurosci.*6:3006–3009.

Folstein, M. F., 1983. The mini-mental state examination. In: *Assessment in Geriatric Pharmacology,* New Canaan: Crook,T. and Bartus,R., eds., Mark Powley Association. pp. 47–51.

Graf, P., Squire, L. and Mandler, G.,1986, The information that amnesiac patients do not forget. *J. Exp. Psychol: Learn. Mem. Cog,* 9:164–178.

Graf, P. and Mandler, G.,1995, Activation makes words more accessible, but not necessarily more retrievable *J. Verb. Learn. Verb. Behav,* 23:553–568.

Harris, J., 1993, *Assessing Dementia in Alzheimer's Disease.* Berkeley, CA.: University of California Press.

Harris, J., 1996, *Verbal and Motor Memory in Alzheimer's Disease.* Berkeley, CA.: University of California Press.

Herlitz, A., Adofsson, R., Bäckman, L., and Nilsson, L.G., 1994, Cue utilization following different forms of encoding in mildly, moderately, and severely demented patients with Alzheimer's disease. *Brain and Cogn.,* 15:119–130.

Herlitz, A. and Bäckman, L.,1993, Recall of names and colors of objects in normal aging and Alzheimer's disease. *Arch. Geront. Geriat.,* 11:147–154.

Kelso, J. A. S., Goodman, D., Stamm, C. L., and Hayes, C., 1979, Movement coding and memory in retarded children. *Am. J. Ment. Def.* 63:601–611.

Martin, A., Brouwers, P., Cox,. C. and Fedio, P., 1985, On the nature of the verbal memory deficit in Alzheimer's disease. *Brain Lang.* 25:323–341.

Naire, J. S., Puser. C. and Widner, R. L., Jr., 1995, Representations in the mental lexicon: Implications for theories of the generation effect. *Mem.and Cogn.* 13:183–191.

Reisberg, B., 1983, Clinical presentation, diagnosis, and symptomatology of age-associated cognitive decline in Alzheimer's disease. In: *Alzheimer's disease,* Reisberg, B., ed., New York: Free Press. pp. 173–187.

Rosen, W. C., Terry. R. D., Fuld, P. A., Katzman, R. and Peck, A., 1980, Pathological verification of ischemic score in differentiation of dementias. *Ann. Neurol.* 7:486–488.

Shiffrin, R. M. and Schneider, W., 1977, Controlled and automatic human information processing: II. Perceptual learning, automatic attending, and a general theory. *Psychol. Rev.* 84:127–162.

Underwood, B. J., 1983, *The Attributes of Memory.* New York; Wiley.

Wechsler, D., 1981, *Wechsler Adult Intelligence Scale-Revised.* New York: Psychological Corporation.

Wilson, R. S., Bacon, L. D., Fox, J. H., and Kaszniak, A. W., 1983, Primary and secondary memory in dementia of the Alzheimer type. *J. Clin. Neuropsychol.* 5:97–104.

Wilson, R. S., Rosenbaum. G. and Brown, G., 1979, The problem of premorbid intelligence in neuropsychological assessment. *J. Clin. Neuropsychol.* 1:49–53.

Wilson, R. S., Kaszniak, A. W., Bacon, L. D., Fox, J H. and Kelly, M. P.,1982, Facial recognition memory in dementia. *Cortex* 18:329–336.

44

COGNITIVE AND NON-COGNITIVE SYMPTOMS IN SENILE DEMENTIA

A. Sellers, L. Pérez, C. Carrera, J. C. Bustos, J. M. Caamaño, B. Rodríguez,
R. Mouzo, P. Pérez, J. I. Lao, K. Beyer, X. A. Álvarez, and R. Cacabelos

Biomedical Research Center
Santa Marta de Babío
15166 Bergondo, La Coruña, Spain

INTRODUCTION

Behavioral changes, mood-related disturbances and sleep disorders are the major cause of institutionalization and caregiver concern in families with Alzheimer's disease (AD) (Rabins et al., 1982; Steele et al., 1990; Morris et al., 1996). The estimated prevalence of psychiatric symptoms in AD accounts for 40–60% of the cases (Ballard et al., 1995). Psychiatric symptoms are associated with lower total MMSE scores (Cooper et al., 1990) and overall cognitive deterioration (Drevets et al., 1989; Forstl et al., 1993). In general, psychotic symptoms run in parallel with an accelerated cognitive deterioration, in some cases partially induced by psychotropic drugs. In many other cases, behavioral changes do not seem to be associated with exogenous factors. Psychotic symptoms, especially delusions, hallucinations and misidentifications, are positively correlated with agressive behavior and institutionalization (Deutsch et al., 1991). Agitation and wandering are also associated with rapid cognitive decline in dementia (Tinklenberg et al., 1990).

Mood-related symptoms, including depression, anxiety, slowed thinking, irritability, apathy, social withdrawal and suicidal talk are also very frequent in AD (Gilley, 1993). The major depressive syndrome occurs in approximately 15–30% of patients with dementia and in older medical inpatients (Folstein et al., 1994; Fenton et al., 1994). Although 40–60% of the patients respond to antidepressant and/or anxiolytic medication, both depression and anxiety-like symptoms contribute to a deterioration in living conditions of the patients and their relatives. Sleep disorders are another important factor for patient and family discomfort, and occasionally also for institutionalization.

Since AD is a heterogeneus entity, we postulate that behavioral changes, mood disorders and sleep disorders can be associated with both endogenous and exogenus factors such as: 1) dementia type; 2) disease stage; 3) environmental factors; 4) medical conditions; and 5) drug-induced behavioral, mood and sleep disorders.

Progress in Alzheimer's and Parkinson's Diseases
edited by Fisher *et al.*, Plenum Press, New York, 1998.

In the present report we discuss the frequency of cognitive and non cognitive symptoms in dementia according to disease staging and type of dementia, in order to elucidate the potential influence on major clinical features present in dementia.

PATIENTS AND METHODS

We have studied the predominant clinical symptoms in the evolution of 231 patients with senile dementia [72 males (31%) and 159 females (69%); age: 73 ± 12.45 years], including Alzheimer's Disease (AD, N= 55), vascular dementia (VD, N = 73), mixed dementia (MXD, N = 93) and other dementias (N = 10).

According to the Global Deterioration Scale (GDS), the patients were divided into three subgroups: 1) mild dementia (GDS = 3; N = 76); 2) moderate dementia (GDS = 4–5; N = 111); and 3) severe dementia (GDS = 6–7; N = 44).

All the patients met criteria for dementia according to the DSM-IV (American Psychiatric Association, 1994) and NINCDS-ADRDA (Mc Khann et al., 1984) scales. They were submitted to the same research protocol: clinical and neuropsychological assessment, EEG and brain mapping, EKG, laboratory examination, neuroimaging (CT-Scan), TCD evaluation and genetic testing (Cacabelos, 1991).

Neuropsychological evaluation and psychometric assessment were performed with the EuroEspes Neuropsychological Battery including MMSE, BCRS, FAST, GDS, BE-HAVE-AD, ADAS, Hamilton-A/D, Hachinski scale, and the Senile Dementia-Associated Sleep Disorders Scale (SDASDS).

Data were analyzed using the Chi-squared analysis.

RESULTS

The total frequency of clinical symptoms found in dementia is shown in Table 1. Globally, cognitive symptoms (memory loss, apraxia, aphasia, agnosia, disorientation) and motor dysfunction are the most frequent symptoms in dementia (more than 90% of the cases). Anxiety (76%), depression (70%), behavioral changes (68%) and agitation (66%) were very frequent clinical findings, while sleep disorders were present in 40–45% of the cases at the time of diagnosis.

DISCUSSION

This study investigated the frequency of major clinical symptoms in senile dementia according to dementia type, as well as their association with the progression of the disease. The results indicate that most symptoms (cognitive and non-cognitive) progress in frequency in parallel with the natural course of the disease.

Interestingly, cerebrovascular symptoms as assessed by clinical evaluation, neuroimaging and transcranial Doppler ultrasonography were significant more frequent in VD (86%) than in MXD (77%) and AD (64%), remaining stable in frequency from mild (76%) to severe (73%) dementia.

It is also evident that the most important non-cognitive symptoms in dementia include anxiety, depression, behavioral changes, agitation and psychotic symptoms, with motor disorders being the most frequent finding in any type of dementia, with a frequency of 80% in mild dementia, 95% in moderate dementia and 100% in severe dementia. Sev-

Table 1. Cognitive and non-cognitive
symptoms in senile dementia[a]

	Frequency
Cognitive symptoms	
Memory decline	231 (100%)
Aphasia	219 (95%)
Apraxia	228 (99%)
Agnosia	216 (94%)
Disorientation	209 (90%)
Non-cognitive symptoms	
Anxiety	175 (76%)
Depression	161 (70%)
Behavioral changes	156 (68%)
Psychotic symptoms	97 (42%)
Agitation	153 (66%)
Insomnia	103 (45%)
Circadian rhythm disorders	92 (40%)
Motor dysfunction	210 (91%)
Incontinence	51 (22%)
Myoclonus	18 (8%)
Convulsions	5 (2%)
Other neurological symptoms	38 (16%)
Cerebrovascular symptoms	177 (77%)
Other medical conditions	133 (58%)
Age	73 ± 12.45
N	231
Female	159 (69%)
Male	72 (31%)

[a]Concerning clinical symptoms associated with dementia type, neurological manifestations, cerebrovascular symptoms, (migraine, sickness) and other medical conditions were more frequent in vascular and mixed dementias than in Alzheimer's Disease.

eral studies support the idea that extrapyramidal signs are a frequent finding currently associated with late-life dementia. Parkinsonism and extrapyramidal signs may be an early preclinical manifestation of dementia, and in many patients with AD, the presence of extra pyramidal signs accelerate cognitive decline and shorten survival times. In agreement with our results, most studies indicate that motor dysfunction and extrapyramidal signs progress in parallel with cognitive decline and dementia severity.

Psychotic symptoms are very disruptive for the patient and caregiver and require psychotropic treatment because they contribute to an increase in reactions and behavioral pathology. Disruptive behavioral and psychotic symptoms are the most important factors contributing to nursing home admissions (Ellis et al., 1996) and also contribute to an increase in direct and indirect costs in dementia. However, they have received much less attention than cognitive symptoms since they are considered secondary events in dementia. In addition, most drugs for treating behavioral changes and psychotic symptoms increase memory decline, motor dysfunction and general disability. Several authors have reported a more rapid deterioration in demented patients with psychotic symptoms (Forstl et al., 1993; Drevets et al., 1989). Psychotic symptoms are associated with an increase in agression, agitation, emotional incontinence, irritability, wandering and family problems (Ballard et al., 1995).

Table 2. Clinical symptoms according to dementia type[a]

	VD	MXD	AD
Cognitive symptoms			
Memory decline	73 (100%)	93 (100%)	55 (100%)
Aphasia	69 (95%)	89 (96%)	54 (98%)
Apraxia	73 (100%)	91 (98%)	54 (98%)
Agnosia	69 (95%)	85 (91%)	53 (96%)
Disorientation	65 (89%)	82 (88%)	53 (96%)
Non-cognitive symptoms			
Anxiety	56 (77%)	67 (72%)	43 (78%)
Depression	46 (63%)	70 (75%)	37 (67%)
Behavioral changes	50 (68%)	66 (71%)	32 (58%)
Psychotic symptoms	31 (42%)	40 (43%)	22 (40%)
Agitation	44 (60%)	68 (73%)	35 (64%)
Insomnia	38 (52%)	41 (44%)	19 (35%)
Circadian rhythm disorders	34 (47%)	37 (40%)	17 (31%)
Motor dysfunction	67 (92%)	87 (94%)	48 (87%)
Incontinence	16 (22%)	25 (27%)	8 (15%)
Myoclonus	4 (5%)	10 (11%)	4 (7%)
Convulsions	3 (4%)	1 (1%)	1 (2%)
Other neurological symptoms	15 (21%)	11 (12%)	12 (22%)
Cerebrovascular symptoms	63 (86%)[#,*]	72 (77%)	35 (64%)[#]
Other medical conditions	50 (68%)[*]	57 (61%)	19 (35%)[#]
Age	74 ± 14.50	73 ± 10.36	69 ± 13.04
N	73	93	55
Female	55 (75%)	62 (67%)	34 (62%)
Male	18 (25%)	31 (33%)	21 (38%)

[a]The frequency and intensity of cognitive and non-cognitive symptoms, such as anxiety, behavioral changes, psychotic symptoms, agitation, and insomnia, increases with the progression of the disease from mild to severe dementia. As expected, convulsions, motor disfunction, incontinence, and various neurological symptoms also increased in frequency with disease progression. Medical conditions other than those typically present in demented patients were also more frequent in severe dementia.
[*]$p < 0.05$ vs AD.
[#]$p < 0.05$ vs MXD.

According to some authors, primary and secondary mood states are the most frequent symptoms in dementia (Folstein et al., 1994). In the present study, anxiety and depression were present in 76% and 70% of the cases, respectively, progressing with cognitive deterioration during the natural course of the disease. In 10–15% of the cases, a depressive state emerges as a primary symptom. In approximately 60% of the cases depression responds to antidepressant therapy, but in the remaining 40% the disease conditions evolve into a dementia state during the following 3–5 years.

In summary, cognitive symptoms are more prevalent than non-cognitive symptoms in early stages of dementia. Behavioral changes and mood-related disturbances in demented patients are very frequent and constitute a major concern for relatives and caregivers. They are also a negative predictor of survival and quality of life for the patients and contribute to an increase in direct and indirect costs for relatives and institutions.

Since treatments for controlling behavioral changes accelerate the dementia process, new drugs for effectively treating behavioral disorders in SD are needed. These drugs should be devoid of negative effects on neuronal survival in order to preserve memory function, cognition and psychomotor activity.

Table 3. Clinical symptoms according to dementia severity

	Mild	Moderate	Severe
Cognitive symptoms			
Memory decline	76 (100%)	111 (100%)	44 (100%)
Aphasia	65 (86%)[#,*]	110 (99%)	44 (100%)[#]
Apraxia	73 (96%)[#,*]	111 (100%)	44 (100%)[#]
Agnosia	63 (83%)[#,*]	109 (98%)	44 (100%)[#]
Disorientation	55 (72%)[#,*]	110 (99%)	44 (100%)[#]
Non-cognitive symptoms			
Anxiety	49 (64%)[*]	89 (80%)	37 (84%)[#]
Depression	52 (68%)	74 (67%)	35 (80%)
Behavioral changes	39 (51%)[#,*]	79 (71%)	38 (86%)
Psychotic symptoms	19 (25%)[*]	50 (45%)	28 (64%)
Agitation	41 (54%)[*]	76 (68%)	36 (82%)[#]
Insomnia	29 (38%)	55 (50%)	19 (43%)[#]
Circadian rhythm disorders	24 (32%)	43 (39%)	25 (57%)
Motor dysfunction	61 (80%)[*]	105 (95%)	44 (100%)[#]
Incontinence	7 (9%)[*]	24 (22%)	20 (45%)
Myoclonus	3 (4%)	11 (10%)	4 (9%)
Convulsions	0 (0%)	2 (2%)	3 (7%)
Other neurological symptoms	8 (11%)	19 (17%)	11 (25%)
Cerebrovascular symptoms	59 (76%)	87 (78%)	32 (73%)
Other medical conditions	44 (58%)	62 (56%)	27 (61%)
Age	74 ± 7.32	71 ± 16.08	74 ± 7.52
N	76	111	44
Female	49 (64%)	80 (72%)	30 (68%)
Male	27 (36%)	31 (28%)	14 (32%)

[*]p < 0.05 vs Severe.
[#]p < 0.05 vs Moderate.

REFERENCES

American Psychiatric Association, *Diagnostic and Statistical Manual of Mental Disorders. DSM-IV,* Fourth Edition, *Am. Psychiat. Assoc.,* Washington, D.C. 1994.

Ballard,C., Oyebode, F., 1995, Psychotic symptoms in patients with dementia. *Int. J. Geriat. Psychiat.* 10: 743–752.

Cacabelos, R., 1991, Marcadores diagnósticos, In: *Enfermedad de Alzheimer,* Prous Science Publishers, Barcelona., pp. 249–279.

Cooper, J., Mungas, D., Weiler, P., 1990, Relation of cognitive status and abnormal behaviors in Alzheimer's disease. *J. Am. Geriat. Soc.* 38:867–870.

Deutsch, L., Bylsma, F., Rovner, B., Steele, C., Folstein, M., 1991, Psychosis and physical aggression in probable Alzheimer's disease. *Am. J. Psychiat.* 148:1159–1163.

Drevets, W.C., Rubin, E.H. , 1989, Psychotic symptoms and the longitudinal course of senile dementia of the Alzheimer type. *Biol.Psychiat.* 25:39–48.

Ellis, R.J., Caligiuri, M., Galasko, D., Thal, L.J., 1996, Extrapyramidal motor signs in clinically diagnosed Alzheimer disease. *Alzheimer Dis. Assoc. Disord.* 10:103–114.

Fenton, F.R., Cole, M.G., Engelsmann, F., Mansouri, I. , 1994, Depression in older medical inpatients. *Int. J. Geriat. Psychiat* 9:279–284.

Folstein, M.F., Bylsma, F.W., 1994, Noncognitive symptoms of Alzheimer's disease. In: *Alzheimer's Disease,* Terry, R.D., Katzman, R., Bick, K.L. (Eds.), Raven Press, New York:27–40.

Forstl, H., Bisthorn, C., Gligen-kelisch, C., Sattel, H., Schreiber-Gasser, U., 1993, Psychotic symptoms and the course of Alzheimer's disease: Relationship to cognitive, electroencephalographic and computerised CT findings. *Acta Psychiat. Scand.* 87:395–399.

Gilley, D.W., 1993, Behavioral and affective disturbances in Alzheimer's disease: In: *Neuropsychology of Alzheimer's Disease and other Dementia,* Parks, R.W., Zec, R.F., Wilson, R.S., eds., Oxford Univesity Press, Oxford, 112:137.

Mc Khann, G., Drachman, D., Folstein, M. et al. , 1984, Clinical diagnosis of Alzheimer's disease: Report of the NINCDS-ADRDA Work Group under the auspices of Department of Health and Human Services Task Force on Alzheimer's Disease. *Neurology* 34:939–944.

Morris, R.K., Rovner, B.W., German, P.S., 1996, Factors contributing to nursing home admission because of disruptive behavior, *Int. J. Geriat. Psychiat.* 11:243–249.

Rabins, P., Mace, N.L., Lucas, M.J., 1982, The impact of dementia on the family. *J. Am. Med. Assoc.* 248: 333–335.

Steele, C., Rovner, B., Chase, G.A., Folstein, M., 1990, Psychiatric symptoms and nursing home placement of patients with Alzheimer's disease. *Am. J. Psychiat.* 147:1049–1051.

Tinklenberg, J., Brooks, J.O., Tanke, E.D., 1990, Factor analysis and preliminary validation of the Mini-Mental State Examination from a longitudinal perspective. *Int. Psychogeriatr.* 2:123–134.

45

DEMENTIA ASSOCIATED SLEEP DISORDERS

A. Sellers, L. Pérez, B. Rodríguez, V. M. Pichel, J. M. Caamaño, M. Laredo,
M. Alcaraz, X. A. Álvarez, and R. Cacabelos

Biomedical Research Center
Santa Marta de Babío
15166 Bergondo, La Coruña, Spain

INTRODUCTION

Sleep disorders, together with behavioral disturbances and lost functions of the activities of daily living, are the most important predictor in the decision to institutionalize demented patients, as well as an important factor for patient and family discomfort (Rabins et al., 1982; Steele et al., 1990; Morriss et al., 1996). In most countries, the institutionalization of demented patients ranges from 10–70% (Preston,1986, Ballard et al., 1995). The frequency of sleep disorders in senile dementia has not been well studied. In fact, while behavioral impairment and mood disorders were traditionally studied in Alzheimer's disease (AD) with validated psychometric tools, no reliable scale can be used for the assessment of sleep disorders in senile dementia (Cacabelos et al., 1996). This fact has led us to elaborate a psychometric test for their evaluation: The Senile Dementia-Associated Sleep Disorders Scale (SDASDS), based upon the International Classification of Sleep Disorders (American Sleep Disorders Association).

In cross-sectional studies it has been reported that several psychiatric symptoms were associated with lower total MMSE scores (Cooper et al., 1990) and overall cognitive deterioration (Drevets and Rubin, 1989; Forstl et al., 1993). Sleep disorders in dementia are related to the severity of the disease. The sleep of AD patients is often disturbed by medications, depression, and circadian rhythm changes (Anconi-Israel et al., 1994). Since AD is a heterogeneus entity, we postulated that clinical features such as sleep disorders can be associated with both endogenous and exogenous factors depending upon the following: 1) dementia type; 2) disease stage; 3) environmental factors (home conditions, ablities of the caregiver, admission to nursing homes); 4) medical conditions (surgery, cardiovascular and cerebrovascular disorders, metabolic and endocrine diseases, malnutrition); and 5) drug-induced sleep disorders. In this report we show the frequency of sleep disorders in dementia according to disease staging and type of dementia.

Progress in Alzheimer's and Parkinson's Diseases
edited by Fisher *et al.*, Plenum Press, New York, 1998.

PATIENTS AND METHODS

We have evaluated the predominant sleep disorders in the evolution of 231 patients with senile dementia [72 males (31%) and 159 females (69%); age: 73 ± 12.45 years], including Alzheimer's Disease (AD, N = 55); vascular dementia (VD, N = 73); mixed dementia (MXD, N = 93) and other dementias (N = 10).

According to the Global Deterioration Scale (GDS), the patients were divided into three subgroups: 1) mild dementia (GDS = 3; N = 76); 2) moderate dementia (GDS: 4–5; N = 111); and 3) severe dementia (GDS: 6–7; N = 44).

All the patients met criteria for dementia according to the DSM-IV (American Psychiatric Association) and NINCDS-ADRDA (McKhann et al., 1984) scales. They were submitted to the same research protocol: clinical and neuropsychological assessment, EEG and brain mapping, EKG, laboratory examination, neuroimaging (CT-Scan), and TCD evaluation and genetic testing (Cacabelos, 1991; Cacabelos et al., 1996).

Neuropsychological evaluation and psychometric assessment were performed with the EuroEspes Neuropsychological Battery including MMSE, BCRS, FAST, GDS, BEHAVE-AD, ADAS, Hamilton A/D, Hachinski Scale, and the Dementia-Associated Sleep Disorders Scale (SDASDS).

The SDASDS consists of two subscales, with a score from 0 to 3 in increasing intensity: (a) Subscale-1: 15 items associated with sleep disorders. (b) Subscale-2: 15 items associated with dementia.

Data were analyzed by using the Chi-squared test.

RESULTS

The gobal frequency of sleep disorders found in dementia is as follows: The major sleep disorders were insomnia (45%), fragmented 24-hr sleep disorders (37%) and nocturnal sleep disruption (32%). Drug administration and other medical conditions appeared to be the most important factors in causing sleep disorders in dementia. The association of sleep disorders with other medical conditions is higher in MXD than VD and AD, respectively. No significant differences were found in sleep disorders when analyzed as a function of drug-induced sleep disorders.

According to the dementia type sleep disorders showed a higher frequency in patients with VD than MXD and AD (Fig. 1). No significant differences were found between vascular dementia-associated sleep disorders and mixed dementia associated-sleep disorders. Circadian rhythm sleep disorders such as fragmented 24-hr sleep pattern and irregular sleep-wake pattern were most frequent in VD than MXD and AD. Alterations in sleep quality are less frequent in EA than VD and MXD, respectively.

The frequency of sleep disorders, alteration in sleep quality and sleep disorders due to other medical conditions corresponded to the severity of dementia, increasing their frequency from mild to severe dementia (Fig. 2). Circadian rhythm alterations are the predominant sleep disorders in severe dementia, and insomnia is the highest symptom in moderate dementia.

DISCUSSION

Sleep disorders in dementia have been neglected as a matter of specific research despite their frequency and risk of institutionalization (Pollak and Perlick, 1991). However,

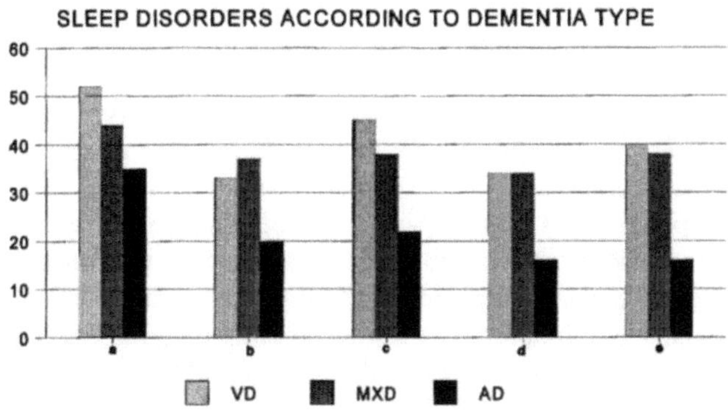

Figure 1. Sleep disorders according to dementia type.

clear changes in endogenous circadian rhythms have been reported in AD and aging (Myers and Badia, 1995; Satlin et al., 1995). Sleep disorders are closely associated with depressive symptoms, but AD patients may show changes in the sleep pattern with no symptoms of apparent depression, which suggests that sleep disorders are an independent feature in AD psychopathology. Insomnia was the most frequent sleep disorder in our cases (45%). It was more frequent in moderate dementia (50%) than in mild (38%) and severe dementia (43%). Our results indicate that most symptoms progress in frequency in parallel with the disease staging. Circadian rhythm alterations are the predominant sleep disorders in severe dementia, and insomnia is the highest symptom in moderate dementia. In most cases, agitation, nocturnal disorientation and the administration of several types of drugs have been attributed to alterations in sleep conditions. Interestingly, external conditions other than drug administration and circumstantial habits do not seem to influence sleep disturbances in our study.

It is also evident that the frequency of sleep disorders is higher in VD than MXD and AD, respectively. Among sleep disorders more frequent in VD we found fragmented 24-hours sleep pattern and irregular sleep-wake pattern.

The circadian rhythm dysfunction may be partially responsible for the fragmented nocturnal sleep in AD patients (Myers and Badia, 1995). In fact, alterations in the number and function of neurons have been found in the suprachiasmatic nucleus (Swaab et al., 1985). Changes in melatonin production from the pineal gland as well as a deficient activ-

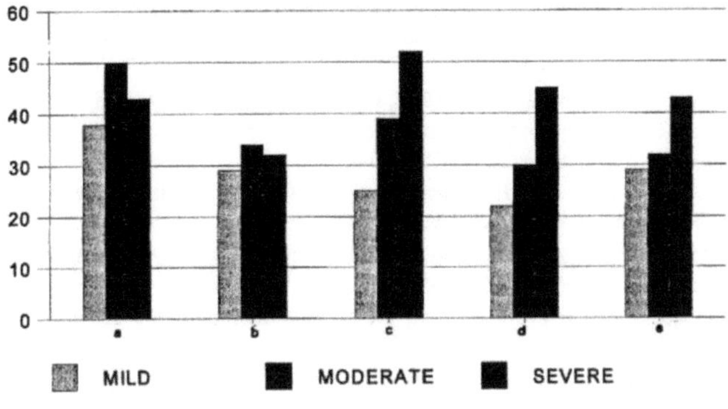

Figure 2. Sleep disorders according to dementia severity.

ity of melatonin on the endogenous circadian clock might also account for disarrangements in the sleep-wake cycle (Bonn, 1996). Changes in circadian rhythms are currently associated with a reduction in nightime sleep quality, daytime alertness and mental performance. Some of these deleterious effects might be potentially reversed by increasing melatonin levels (Myers and Badia, 1995). Is very likely that neurochemical dysregulations in the pathways converging in the suprachiasmatic nucleus to regulate circadian rhythms might be responsible, at least in part, for idiophatic sleep disorders in dementia.

Sleep disorders in demented patients are very frequent and constitute a major concern for relatives and caregivers. They are also a negative predictor of survival and quality of life for SD patients. Their frequency is higher in patients with VD than MXD and AD. Sleep disorders are positively correlated with the progression of the disease. Circadian rhythm alterations are the predominant sleep disorders in severe dementia and insomnia is the highest symptom in moderate dementia. Since treatments for controlling sleep disorders accelerate the dementia process, new drugs for effectively treating sleep disorders in SD are needed. These drugs should be devoid of negative effects on neuronal survival in order to preserve memory function, cognition and psychomotor activity. In this sense, melatonin analogous substances could be an alternative.

REFERENCES

Anconi-Israel, S., Klauber, M.R., Gillin, J.C., Campbell, S.S., Hofstetter C.R., 1994, Sleep in non-institutionalized Alzheimer's disease patients. *Aging* 6: 451–458.

American Psychiatric Association, 1994. Diagnostic and Statistical Manual of Mental Disorders. Fourth Edition. DSM-IV. Am. Psychiatric Assoc. Washington, D.C.

American Sleep Disorders Association.,1990, The International Classification of Sleep Disorders. Ame.Sleep Disorders Assoc. Rochester, Minesota, USA.

Ballard,C., Oyebode, F., 1995, Psychotic symptoms in patients with dementia. *Int. J. Geriat. Psychiat.* 10:743–752.

Bonn, D., 1996; Melatonin's multifarious marvels: Miracle or myth? *Lancet* 347:184.

Cacabelos, R., 1991, Alzheimer's disease. Prous Science Publishers; Barcelona.

Cacabelos, R., Rodríguez, B., Carrera, C., Beyer,K., Lao, J.I., Sellers, M.A., 1996, ApoE-related dementia symptoms: Frequency and progression. In: *Annals of Psychiatry*, Cacabelos, R., ed., 6:189–205.

Cacabelos, R., Lao, J.I., Beyer, K., Álvarez, X.X., Franco-Maside, A., 1996, Genetic testing in Alzheimer's disease: ApoE genotyping and etiopathogenic factors. *Methods Find. Exp. Clin. Pharmacol.* 18 (A):161–179.

Cooper, J., Mungas, D., Weiler,P., 1990, Relation of cognitive status and abnormal behaviors in Alzheimer's disease. *J. Am. Geriatr. Soc.* 38: 867–870.

Drevets, W. C., Rubin, E.H., 1989, Psychotic symptoms and the longitudinal course of senile dementia of the Alzheimer type. *Biol. Psychiatry* 25:39–48.

Forstl, H., Bisthorn, C., Gligen-Kelisch, C., Satte l, H., Schreiber-Gasser, U., 1993, Psychotic symptoms and the course of Alzheimer's disease: Relationship to cognitive, electroencephalographic and computerised CT findings. *Acta Psychiatr. Scand.*87:395–399.

Mc Khann, G., Drachman, D., Folstein, M. et al., 1984, Clinical diagnosis of Alzheimer's disease: Report of the NINCDS-ADRDA Work Group under the auspices of Department of Health and Human Services Task Force on Alzheimer's Disease. *Neurology* 34:939–944.

Morriss, R.K., Rovner, B.W., German, P.S., 1996, Factors contributing to nursing home admission because of disruptive behavior. *Int. J. Geriat. Psychiatry* 11:243–249.

Myers, B.L., Badia, P., 1995, Changes in circadian rhythms and sleep quality with aging: Mechanisms and intervetions. *Neurosci. Biobehav. Rev.* 19: 553–571.

Pollak, C.P., Perlick, D., 1991, Sleep problems and institutionalization in the elderly. *J. Geriatr. Psychiatry Neurol.* 4: 204–210.

Preston, G.A.N., 1986, Dementia in elderly acdults: Prevalence and institutionalization. *J. Gerontol.* 41:261–267.

Rabins, P., Mace, N.L., Lucas, M.J., 1982, The impact of dementia on the family. *J. Am. Med. Assoc.* 248: 333–335

Satlin, A., Volicer, L., Stopa, E.G., Harper, D., 1995, Circadian locomotor activity and core-body temperature rhythms in Alzheimer's disease. *Neurobiol. Aging* 16:765–771.
Steele, C., Rovner, B., Chase, G.A., Folstein, M., 1990, Psychiatric symptoms and nursing home placement of patients with Alzheimer's disease. *Am. J. Psychiatry* 147:1049–1051.
Swaab, D.F., Fliers, E., Partiman, T.S., 1985, The suprachiasmatic nucleus of the human brain in relation to sex, age and senile dementia. *Brain. Res.* 342:37–44.

46

FREEZING PHENOMENON, THE FIFTH CARDINAL SIGN OF PARKINSONISM

Nir Giladi[1] and Stanley Fahn[2]

[1]Movement Disorders Unit
Department of Neurology
Tel-Aviv Medical Center
Tel-Aviv, Israel
[2]Neurological Institute
Columbia Presbyterian Medical Center
New York, New York

INTRODUCTION

Freezing is a common motor disturbance in patients with parkinsonism (Giladi et al., 1992; Fahn, 1995; Giladi et al., 1997). It most frequently affects gait (Giladi et al., 1992) and speech (Ackermann et al., 1993); writing and brushing teeth (Barbeau, 1976) are less commonly affected. Freezing phenomenon refers to transient episodes, usually lasting seconds, in which the motor activity being attempted by an individual is halted. This motor blockade is best described in relation to gait as if the feet seem "glued" to the floor or in other motor acts as a "block" in the execution of a task. It is typical that during the freezing episode the patient exerts increased effort to overcome the block with voluntary increased muscle tone (Andrews, 1973), but the movements are ineffective. Freezing episodes are unrelated to any weakness, flaccidity or decreased muscle tone, and once freezing has cleared, the patient moves or performs the task at the usual pace (Fahn, 1995).

The clinical evaluation and quantification of freezing has been difficult because of the highly variable nature of this motor disturbance from minute to minute, day to day and in different tasks. This feature is partly related to the important influence of sensory input or mental state on the expression or severity of freezing (Stern et al., 1980; Fahn, 1995).

The freezing phenomenon is a common symptom in Parkinson's disease (PD) (Giladi et al., 1992; 1996) and has been reported in most other hypokinetic movement disorders (parkinsonian syndromes) as well (Giladi et al., 1997). In contrast, freezing has not been reported in disorders which are unrelated to the extrapyramidal system. Considering the wide range of parkinsonian syndromes which are associated with freezing episodes and the classical association with the extrapyramidal system, Fahn has recently added freezing as the fifth cardinal symptom of parkinsonism (Fahn, 1994).

Progress in Alzheimer's and Parkinson's Diseases
edited by Fisher *et al.*, Plenum Press, New York, 1998.

FREEZING PHENOMENON AND PARKINSONISM

Charcot (1877) appears to have been the first to describe the freezing phenomenon—both start hesitation and freezing when arising—in patients with PD. Wechsler 50 years later (1927) gave the first detailed description of start hesitation in a parkinsonian patient, and during the next 40 years, in the pre-levodopa period, freezing was mentioned by several authors as part of parkinsonian akinesia (Luria 1932; Schwab 1954; Martin 1967). Recently, Giladi et al., (1992; 1996) have reported that about 7% of untreated parkinsonian patients experience freezing of gait as part of their early, pre-levodopa, extrapyramidal syndrome. This percentage grows up to 30% just prior to the introduction of levodopa and strengthens the association between freezing of gait and the progression of Parkinson's disease (Giladi et al., 1996). Two studies which have recently been presented as abstracts, reported about similar percentages (Nakamura et al., 1997; Kizkin et al., 1997). Freezing episodes were reported to be common in other neurodegenerative disorders like Progressive Supranuclear Palsy (PSP), and vascular parkinsonism (Giladi et al., 1997) to further support its association with hypokinetic movement disorders.

Barbeau (1972) and Ambani & Van Woert (1973) were the first to notice a significant increase in freezing frequency starting about a year after the introduction of high dosage levodopa treatment and to relate it to the "long term levodopa syndrome". Over the last 25 years, when levodopa has became the main symptomatic treatment for PD, freezing became a common symptom of advanced parkinsonism due to disease progression and long duration of levodopa treatment (Giladi et al., 1992; Nakamura et al., 1997; Kizkin et al., 1997).

NOMENCLATURE

Start hesitation as well as episodes of block in motion have been given many different names over the years. In the earlier days, researchers simply described in detail the clinical symptom. Schwab et al (1959) were the first to include start hesitation as part of parkinsonian "akinesia" and to use the term "freezing" for the "difficulties patients experience shifting from one motor task to another". When Barbeau (1972; 1976) first reported the increased frequency of start hesitation and block on turns or in the middle of motion, secondary to levodopa treatment, he also chose to use the term freezing, even though the dopa related freezing episodes seemed to be shorter and more sudden in their appearance. Narabayashi (1980) and Lakke (1981) further used "freezing" when they defined akinesia as a "disorder characterized by poverty and slowness of initiation and execution of willed and associated movements and difficulty in changing one motor pattern to another, in the absence of paralysis".

Following that line, several authors have chosen to use the term "pure akinesia" or "pure freezing syndrome" when they describe a unique form of parkinsonism dominated by freezing episodes (Narabayashi et al., 1980; Quinn et al., 1989; Riely et al., 1994). A very similar clinical picture dominated by freezing of gait was called by others "gait ignition failure" (Atchison et al., 1993) or "primary progressive freezing of gait" (Achiron et al., 1994). Giladi et al., (1992) have suggested the general term "motor blocks" trying to create a term which is more correct and uniform for all the different types of freezing episodes. However, the term "freezing" is so strongly engrained in the medical and the movement disorders specialist community that we came back to the term "freezing" and strongly suggest that this unambiguous term be used by all researchers in the field.

PATHOPHYSIOLOGY

Freezing of gait is a symptom which is frequently associated with other parkinsonian symptoms and signs but the underlying mechanism of its appearance is poorly understood. It seems to be part of the general slowness of movement (bradykinesia) seen in PD, or more precisely related to abnormal execution of complex motor tasks such as repetitive, simultaneous, or sequential motor acts (Schwab et at, 1954; Marsden, 1989). It is suggested that the primary underlying abnormality is related to the inability to deliver (execute) or hold a pre-programmed, continuous, complex motor performance in response to an established and correct internal plan of action (Marsden, 1989).

There are three general types of freezing episodes. The first is in direct association with parkinsonism and is seen in PD and a variety of other parkinsonian syndromes (Giladi et al., 1997). This type of freezing not always improves by levodopa treatment, for example in patients with PSP or vascular parkinsonism. The others are related to levodopa induced motor fluctuations in patients with Parkinson's disease. "Off" freezing, which is frequently confused with akinetic state, is classically improved by dopaminergic therapy to relate it to a hypodopaminergic state (Linazasoro, 1996). In contrast, "on" freezing which is briefer and appears when the patient walks almost normally, does not improve by apomorphine injections, suggesting another mechanism unrelated to dopaminergic stimulation (Linazasoro, 1996).

It has been reported that freezing of gait was associated with decreased concentrations of monoamines in the spinal fluid of patients with "pure freezing syndrome" (Narabayashi, 1983; Tohgi et al., 1993). As a result, L-threo-DOPS (an artificial precursor of norepinephrine) was administered to patients with reported improvement of the freezing phenomenon (Narabayashi et al., 1981).

The only study which tried to characterize the neurophysiology of freezing at the peripheral nervous system was published by Andrews (1973) who recorded electromyographic activity by surface electrodes in five PD patients who suffered from frequent freezing episodes in gait. All five patients had typical electromyographic activity during freezing of gait episode which was an initial activity of the gastrocnemius-soleus muscles followed approximately 7 msec. later by activity of the tibialis posterior muscle. This activity of flexors and shortly later co-activation of flexors and extensors were observed during freezing episodes in the muscles of the knee as well.

CLINICAL FEATURES

Freezing episodes classically appear in complex, highly synchronized, automatic motor tasks like gait and speech. They can usually be overcome by switching from automatic to non-automatic movements like stepping over lines when gait is affected. Emotional stress may also affect the motor disturbance. One of the classical features of freezing episodes is the way patients can overcome the freezing by different motor or behavioral tricks (Stern et. al., 1980).

The most common form of gait freezing is start hesitation (Giladi et al., 1992). It is seen when the patient initiates walking. The patient attempts to lift a foot and to step forward, but the foot is "glued" to the ground. A similar block in an attempt to move can be experienced when the patient is making a turn in place ("turn hesitation"). Interestingly, such freezing on turning is direction related, worse when the patient turns either right or left, an observation which demonstrates the laterality aspects of freezing. Such differences in the degree of freezing between the two legs is also seen in gait. Another type of gait freezing is typically seen in narrow spaces like walking through door ways. Such episodes are experienced most commonly at home or in most familiar places. The higher frequency of freezing episodes at home may be explained by an association with automatic motor acts. One tends to move at home with less attention and with low stress due to familiarity of the place. Such conditions seems to contribute to the occurrence of freezing. In contrast, at the doctor's office most patients have the best performance and least freezing, a phenomena which leaves the care giver frequently amazed.

As mentioned before, freezing can be a very disabling symptom in parkinsonism or in the "off" state. It is especially difficult when it appears on every attempt to move with very short breaks in between the episodes. At such situations it can be distinguished from akinesia of the "off" state by the "normal" motor function in other non-automatic tasks or in between the freezing episodes as well as by its response to tricks. In contrast, freezing that is experienced at the "on" state, when the patient is enjoying the benefit of dopaminergic treatment, tends to be much shorter, and with better motor performance in between the episodes. Freezing is frequently associated with foot dystonia or levodopa induced dyskinesias (Giladi et al., 1992).

There is an increased risk for gait freezing in PD if one's initial motor symptoms were on the left side of the body, with gait difficulties, speech or balance problems. Interestingly, the risk to develop freezing is significantly decreased if the initial motor symptom was tremor (Giladi et al., 1996).

TREATMENT OF FREEZING OF GAIT

Freezing phenomenon is considered as one of the more resistant symptoms in Parkinson's disease. The "off" freezing might respond to dopaminergic treatment, while the "on" freezing sometimes improves by lowering the dosage of dopaminergic medications. Behavioral treatment is often an effective and safe approach, using tricks to overcome the freezing.

Selegiline is the only drug that has been specifically reported to decrease the risk of gait freezing in the early stages of PD (Giladi et al., 1996). The mechanism of selegiline action on freezing is poorly understood and theoretically can be explained by its known dopaminergic like activity, amphetaminergic activity of its metabolite or through an undefined, non-aminergic/non-monoamine oxidase - B inhibitory effect. Whether other antiparkinsonian drugs have a similar effect (compared to placebo) has not yet been evaluated.

There is very little published data regarding the effect of levodopa on "off" freezing, but apomorphine injections had a good symptomatic response (Linazasoro, 1996). In contrast, others (Weiner et at, 1993; Ahlskog et al., 1992) have reported increased frequency of freezing in patients who were treated with dopamine agonists. Similarly, patients who were treated with selegiline in the DATATOP study had slightly higher frequency of freezing after several years of levodopa treatment (Parkinson Study Group, 1996).

L-threo DOPS (a chemical precursor of norepinephrine) has been reported to be of moderate symptomatic effect for freezing, mainly in those patients who had "pure freezing syndrome" in Japan (Narabayashi et al., 1981; Ogawa et al., 1984). A similar study with PD patients in USA (Oribe et al., 1993) reported a complete disappearance of freezing in 2 patients, an improvement that lasted 3 weeks and disappeared without any additional response even to higher dosages of L-threo-Dops. Two additional patients had transient subjective improvement for 4 weeks. Another two studies at Columbia Presbyterian Medical

Center in New York and Queen Square in London, did not find any benefit from L-threo-DOPS treatment for freezing in advanced PD (Fahn, personal communication; Quinn et al., 1984). Interestingly, one patient who improved, continued to improve for several months when placebo was substituted (Fahn personal communication). The role of L-threo DOPS in freezing of gait in parkinsonian patients is still controversial, but it seems to help only patients with pure freezing syndrome, an entity that today is believed to be a subtype of PSP (Imai et al., 1993).

One of the most characteristic features of freezing is its response to tricks (Martin, 1967; Stern et al., 1980; Dietz et al., 1990; Mizuno et al., 1994). Stern et al., (1980) were the first to report in details about those tricks, dividing them into: 1) Gait modification by the patient alone or with the assistance of another person; and 2) an assistance by auditory (non-verbal), verbal or visual stimuli. The use of motor tricks is highly recommended because of their effectiveness, safety and availability while needed.

Stereotactic neurosurgery has become an increasingly common approach to treat patients with advanced PD. The most frequently used stereotactic neurosurgery for PD today is posterior medial pallidotomy, but its effect on gait, postural reflexes and freezing episodes is controversial. Dogali et al (1996), following 33 patients for 1 year after medial pallidotomy; Lozano et al (1995), following 14 PD patients for 3 months; and Sutton et al (1995), who operated on 15 PD patients and followed them for only 8 weeks, came to the same conclusion that internal globus pallidus lesioning did not improve freezing of gait. In addition, Latinen reported about 259 patients who underwent medial pallidotomy, but there is only limited data on the actual effect of pallidotomy on freezing (1995).

In contrast, Iacono, who reported about his experience with 126 patients (1994), 58 with unilateral lesioning and 68 patients with bilateral lesions, stated that by a subjective follow-up assessment through the telephone 1 year after surgery, there was significant improvement in freezing of gait. Baron et al (1996) have recently reported their pilot study result of 15 PD patients. A very thorough 1 year follow-up has also observed improvement in freezing in 9 of 13 patients who had "off" freezing and in 3 of 7 patients with "on" freezing. These differences might be attributed to differences in location of the lesion in the GPi and partially to the quality of follow-up assessment. One can conclude from the available literature that GPi pallidotomy in most centers did not improve either "off" or "on" gait freezing.

Preliminary results from high frequency, deep brain stimulation (DBS) of the subthalamic nucleus (STN) have shown good response of freezing of gait (FOG) to stimulation (Pollack, personal communication). Benabid and Pollack have claimed that STN high frequency stimulation causes the same effect as levodopa (Pollack personal communication), to suggest that "off" freezing is the type which should respond to STN-DBS.

REFERENCES

Achiron A., Ziv I., Goren M., Goldberg H., Zoldan Y., Sroka H., Melamed E., 1993 Primary progressive freezing gait, *Mov. Disord.* 8:293–297.

Ackermann H., Grone B.F., Hoch G., Schonle PW., 1993, Speech freezing in Parkinson's disease: a kinematic analysis of orofacial movements by means of electromagnetic articulography, *Folia Phoniatr. Basel* 45(2):84–89.

Ahlskog J.E., Muenter M.D., Bailey P.A., Stevens P.M., 1992, Dopamine agonist treatment of fluctuating parkinsonism. D-2 (controlled-release MK-458) vs combined D-1 and D-2 (pergolide), *Arch. Neurol.* 49:560–568.

Ambani L.M., Van Woert M.H., 1973, Start hesitation - a side effect of long-term levodopa therapy, *N. Eng. J. Med.* 288:1113–1115.

Andrews C.J., 1973, Influence of dystonia on the response to long-term L-dopa therapy in Parkinson's disease, *J. Neurol. Neurosurg. Psychiatry* 36:630–636.

Atchison P.R., Thompson P.D., Frackowiak R.S.J., Marsden C.D., 1993, The syndrome of gait ignition failure: A report of six cases, *Mov. Disord.* 8:285–292.

Barbeau A., 1972, Long-term appraisal of levodopa therapy, In: *Neurology*, McDowell F, ed., 22(suppl):22–24.

Barbeau A., 1976, Six years of high level levodopa therapy in severely akinetic parkinsonian patients, *Arch. Neurol.* 33:333–338.

Baron M.S., Vitek J.L., Bakay R.A.E., Green J., Kaneoke Y., Hashimoto T., Turner R.S., Woodard J.L., Cole S.A., Mcdonald W.M., DeLong M.R., 1996, Treatment of advanced Parkinson's disease by posterior Gpi pallidotomy: 1-year results of a pilot study, *Ann. Neurol.* 40:355–366.

Charcot J.M., 1877, Clinical lectures on disease of the nervous system. Sigerson G: translator. Vol. I. *L. Sydenham Soc.* 145–146.

Dietz M.A., Goetz C.G., Stebbins G.T., 1990, Evaluation of a modified inverted walking stick as a treatment for parkinsonian freezing episodes, *Mov. Dis.* 5:243–247.

Dogali M., Fazzini E., Kolodny E., Eidelberg D., Sterio D., Devinsky O., Beric A., 1995, Stereotactic ventral pallidotomy for Parkinson's disease, *B. M. Neurology* 45:753–761.

Fahn S., 1994, Parkinsonism. In: *Merritt's Textbook of Neurology*, Rowland, L.P., ed:, 9th Ed. Philadelphia, Lea & Febiger.

Fahn S., 1995, The freezing phenomenon in parkinsonism. In:.*Advances in Neurology*, Fahn, S, Hallett, M., Lüder, H.O., and. Marsden, C.D, eds., Lippincott - Raven Publishers, Philadelphia, Vol. 65, p. 53–63.

Giladi N., McMahon D., Przedborski S., Flaster E., Guillory S., Kostic V., Fahn S., 1992, Motor blocks in Parkinson's disease, *Neurology* 42:333–339.

Giladi N., McDermott M., Fahn S., Przedborski S., and the Parkinson Study Group, USA, 1996, Freezing of gait in Parkinson's disease, *Neurology* 46(suppl 2):A377 (P05.130).

Giladi N., Kao R., Fahn S., 1997, Freezing phenomenon in patients with parkinsonism, *Mov. Disord.*, in press.

Iacono R.P., Lonser R.R., Mandybur G., Morenski J.D., Yamada S., Shima F., 1994, Stereotactic pallidotomy results for Parkinson's exceed those of fetal graft, *Am. Surg.* 60:777–783.

Imai H., Nakamura T., Kondo T., Narabayashi H., 1993, Dopa-unresponsive pure akinesia or freezing. A condition within a wide spectrum of PSP? In: *Advances in Neurology*, Narabayashi H., Nagatsu T., Yanagisawa N., Mizuno Y. eds., , Vol. 60, Raven Press, Ltd., New York, 622–625.

Kizkin S., Özer F., Ufacik M., Hanoglu L., Karsidag S., Arpaci B., 1997, Motor blocks in Parkinson's disease, *Mov. Disord.* 12(suppl 1):101(P378).

Laitinen L.V., 1995, Pallidotomy for Parkinson's disease, *Neurosurg. Clin. North Am.* 6:105–112.

Lakke P.W.F., 1981, Classification of extrapyramidal disorders, *J. Neurol. Sci.* 51:311–327.

Linazasoro G., 1996, The apomorphine test in gait disorders associated with parkinsonism. *Clin. Neuropharmacol.* 19:171–176.

Lozano A.M., Lang A.E., Galvez-Jimenez N., Miyasaki J., Duff J., Hutchinson W.D., 1995, Effect of Gpi pallidotomy on motor function in Parkinson's disease, *Lancet* 346:1383–1387.

Luria A.R., 1932, The nature of human conflicts, *Liverghite*, p.153.

Marsden C.D., 1989, Slowness of movement in Parkinson's disease, *Mov. Disord.* 4(suppl 1):S26-S37.

Martin J.P., 1967, Disorder of locomotion associated with disease of the basal ganglia. In: *The Basal Ganglia and Posture*, Philadelphia: J.B. Lippincott, 24–35.

Mizuno Y., Kondo T., Mori H., 1994, Various aspects of motor fluctuations and their management in Parkinson's disease, *Neurology* 44(suppl 6):S29-S34.

Nakamura Y., Yoshinaga J., Sasaki T., Endo S., Mantani T., Hikiji A., 1997, Multiple analysis of the problems of long-term levodopa therapy in Parkinson's disease, *Mov. Disord.* 12(suppl 1):110(P417).

Narabayashi H., Kondo T., Hayashi A., Suzuki T., Nagatzu T., 1981, L-threo- 3,4,dihydroxyphenylserine treatment for akinesia and freezing of parkinsonism, *Proc. Jap. Acad.* 57(B):351–354.

Narabayashi H., 1980, Clinical analysis of akinesia, *J. Neural. Transm.* 16(suppl):129–136.

Narabayashi H., 1983, Pharmacological basis of akinesia in Parkinson's disease, *J. Neural. Transm.* Suppl. 19:143–151.

Ogawa N., Kuroda H., Yamamoto M., Nukina I., Ota Z., 1984, Improvement in freezing phenomenon of Parkinson's disease after DL-*threo*-3,4- dihydroxyphenylserine, *Acta Med. Okayama* 38:301–304.

Oribe E., Kaufmann H., Yahr M.D., 1993, Freezing phenomena in Parkinson's disease: clinical features and effect of treatment with L-*threo*-DOPS. In: *Norepinephrine deficiency and its treatment with L-threo-DOPS in Parkinson's disease and the related disorders*, Narabayashi H and Mizuno, Y., eds., *Parthenon Publishing Group*, New York, p.89–96.

Parkinson Study Group., 1996, Impact of deprenyl and tocopherol treatment on Parkinson's disease in DATATOP patients requiring levodopa, *Ann. Neurol.* 39:37–45.

Quinn N.P., Perlmutter J.S., Marsden C.D., 1984, Acute administration of DL- *threo* DOPS does not affect the freezing phenomenon in parkinsonian patients, *Neurology* 34(suppl 1):149.

Quinn N.P., Luther P., Honavar M., PýMarsden C.D., 1989, Pure akinesia due to Lewy body Parkinson's diasease: A case with pathology, *Mov. Disord.* 4:85–89.

Riley D.E., Fogt N., Leigh R.J., 1994, The syndrome of "pure akinesia" and its relationship to progressive supranuclear palsy, *Neurology* 44:1025–1029.

Schwab R.S., Chafetz M.E., 1954, Control of two simultaneous voluntary motor acts in normals and in parkinsonism, *Arch. Neurol. Psychiatry* 72:591–598.

Schwab R.S., England A.C., Peterson E., 1959, Akinesia in Parkinson's disease, *Neurology* 9:65–72.

Stern G.M., Lander C.M., Lees A.J., 1980, Akinetic freezing and trick movements in Parkinson's Disease, *J. Neural. Transm.* 16 (Suppl):137–141.

Sutton J.P., Couldwell W., Lew M.F., Mallory L., Grafton S., Degiorgio C., Welsh M., Apuzzo M.L.J., Ahmadi J., Waters C.H., 1995, Ventroposterior medial pallidotomy in patients with advanced Parkinson's disease, *Neurosurgery* 36:1112–1117.

Tohgi H., Abe T., Takahashi S., Takahashi J., Nozaki Y., Ueno M., Kikuchi T., 1993, Monoamine metabolism in the cerebrospinal fluid in Parkinson's disease: relationship to clinical symptoms and subsequent therapeutic outcomes, *J. Neural. Transm. Park Dis Dement. Sect.* 5(1):17–26.

Wechsler I.S., 1927, Text Book of Clinical Neurology. Philadelphia: W.B. Saunders p.516–520.

Weiner W.J., Factor S.A., Sanches-Ramos J.R., Singer C., Sheldon C., Cornelius L., Ingenito A., 1993, Early combination therapy (bromocriptine and levodopa) does not prevent motor fluctuations in Parkinson's disease, *Neurology* 43:21–27.

47

COGNITIVE IMPAIRMENT IN PATIENTS WITH PARKINSONISM

C. N. Homann, K. Suppan, K. Polmin, R. Schmidt, E. Floh, S. Horner, and
E. Ott

Department of Neurology
University of Graz
Austria

INTRODUCTION

180 years ago James Parkinson in his original description of paralysis agitans, stated "the senses and intellect are uninjured" by the disease (Parkinson, 1817). Since then many have disputed this part of the description. In recent years it has become accepted that cognitive impairment is a prominent feature of parkinsonism with a prevalence of 10–15% and an incidence of 48–69/1000 person years of observation (Mayeux et al., 1990; Biggins et al., 1992). Typical patterns of cognitive impairment, named subcortical dementia have been thoroughly discussed by several authors. These changes have been described in parkinsonism and IPD. and in scanty reports in postencephalytic, vascular or Parkinson Plus Syndromes (Cummings et Benson, 1984). So far very little has been said on Atypical Parkinson Syndromes (APS) not fitting in the previous categories. APS in a previous study (Aarsland et al., 1996) was found to by 0.8 as frequent as IPD.

Cognitive impairment is said to increase the likelihood for PD patients to be institutionalized (Aarsland et al., 1996). Therefore it would be important to know more about this disabling symptom in all of the parkinsonian subgroups.

SUBJECTS AND METHODS

We applied vigorously the existing criteria for IPD (Hughes et al., 1992), MSA (Watts et al., 1994), PSP (Quinn, 1994) and CBGD (Lees, 1987) on 50 parkinsonian patients consecutively admitted to our wards who gave consent to neurophysiological testing. This way we diagnosed 32 patients as having primary PD and 3 patients (1 MSA, 1 vascular PD and 1 toxic PD) as having secondary PS. The remaining 15 patients were con-

Table 1. Age, gender ,and distribution according to mental
performance of patients with Parkinson's Syndrome (PS),
Alzheimer's Disease (AD), and normal healthy controls (Norm)

Variable	PS (n = 50)	AD (n = 18)	Norm (n = 26)
Age, y	71.2	67.2	63.6
Gender, m/f	31/19	5/13	19/7
m-f ratio	1:0.6	1:3.9	1:2.7
Mental impairment			
none	37 (74%)	0 (0%)	26 (100%)
mild	10 (20%)	6 (33%)	0 (0%)
moderate	3 (6%)	9 (50%)	0 (0%)
severe	0 (0%)	3 (14%)	0 (0%)

sidered having APS. 26 Normal controls were recruited from 2000 healthy subjects taken from the Austrian Stroke Prevention Study, 18 Alzheimer patients from our Dementia Clinic (Table 1).

Extensive laboratory investigations, CT and/or MRI scan were performed in all, Apomorphine testing in 16 patients. Clinical examination was performed by 2 neurologists experienced in the field of movement disorders. Neuro-psychological testing, Minimental State Examination and Mattis Dementia Rating Scale, was carried out by the same neuropsychologist in all patients. In order to be able to compare subgroups of equal level of cognitive impairment we divided—based on MMSE performance—the 13 mentally impaired parkinsonian and the 18 Alzheimer's patients into mild (MMSE: 21–25) moderate (MMSE: 11–20) and severely (MMSE: 0–10) affected. The 37 mentally intact parkinsonian patients were matched on a one by one basis, according to their exact MMSE total score, their gender and age (± 2 years).This way we found 26 matching normal subjects. We then applied comparative analyses using the Mann Whitney U test on the different subgroups.

RESULTS

Contrary to the study by Aarsland and co-investigator (1996) our analysis revealed no difference of significance between the parkinsonian subgroups. We did find a lower age in our atypical patients (60.8 vs. 67.6) but this did not reach the level of significance (p = 0.07). Instead of finding a higher number of demented atypical parkinson patients we found nearly two times as many typical parkinsonians (25% vs. 13%) in the mildly mentally impaired group. Taking the mean values of the entire group there was no real difference in the performance of the MMSE (p = 0.84) nor of the Mattis (p = 0.65) tests between the two groups however (Table 2).

Mentally intact PS patients scored worse regarding "initiation and preservervation" (35.4 vs. 36.5; p = 0.045) assigning them a lower MDRS score (137.7 vs. 141.3; p = 0.045) than normal controls (Figure 1). Although matched by MMSE total score there was an unexpected highly significant deficit in "orientation in time" (4.7 vs. 5; p = 0.004) of the PS group (Figure 2).

Mildly impaired PS patients differed from Alzheimer's patients in specific tasks like "inhibition and perseveration" (31.7 vs. 23.7; p = 0.038) and "combination" (37.8 vs. 25.0; p = 0.041) giving them a higher MDRS total score (126.3 vs. 97.2; p = 0.025) A

Table 2. Age, gender, and Mini Mental State Examination/
Mattis Dementia Rating Scale total scores of patients with
Idiopathic Parkinson's Disease and with Atypical Parkinson's
Syndrome[a]

Variable	IPD (n = 32)	APS (n = 15)	p
Age, y	67.6 (13.1)	60.8 (13.7)	0.07
Sex m/f ratio	1:0.5	1:0.9	n.a.
MMSE total	26.2 (3.0)	26.7 (2.7)	0.84
MDRS total	133.4 (13.3)	137.4 (5.5)	0.65

[a]The number in parentheses indicates the Standard Deviation, those without the mean values.

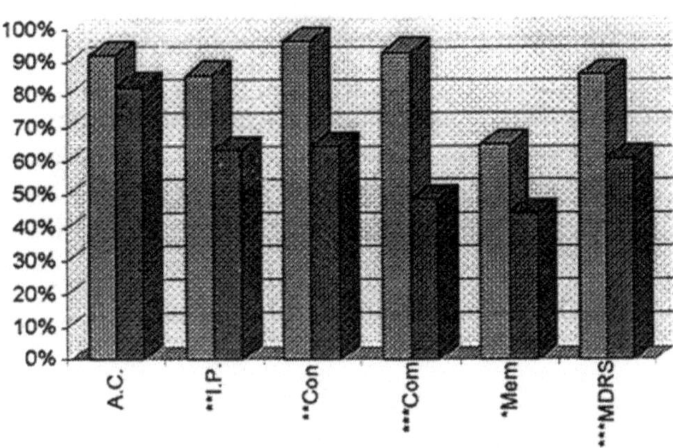

Figure 1. MDRS scores of patients with PS and normal controls. p < 0.05; A.C: attention/concentration, maximal score 37; I.P.: initiation and perseveration, maximal score 37, Con: construction, maximal score 6; Com: combination, maximal score 39; Mem: memory, maximal score 25; Total, maximal score 144.

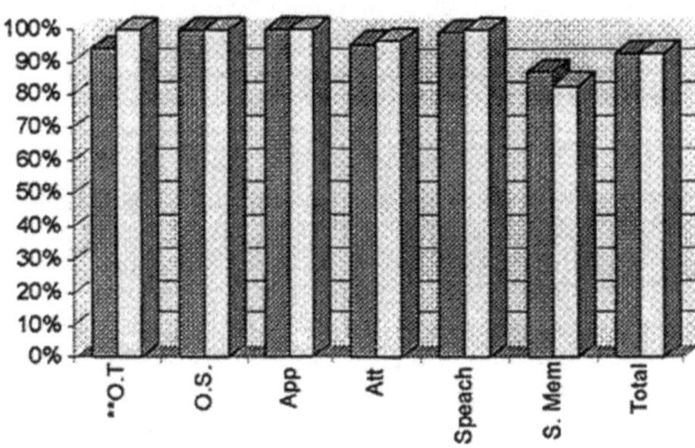

Figure 2. MMSE scores of patients with PS and normal controls. p < 0.005; O.T: orientation in time; maximal score 5; O.S.: orientation in space, maximal score 5; App.: apprehension, maximal score 3; Att: attention/calculation, maximal score 5; speech, maximal score 8, S. Mem.: spatial memory, maximal score 1, Total, maximal score 30.

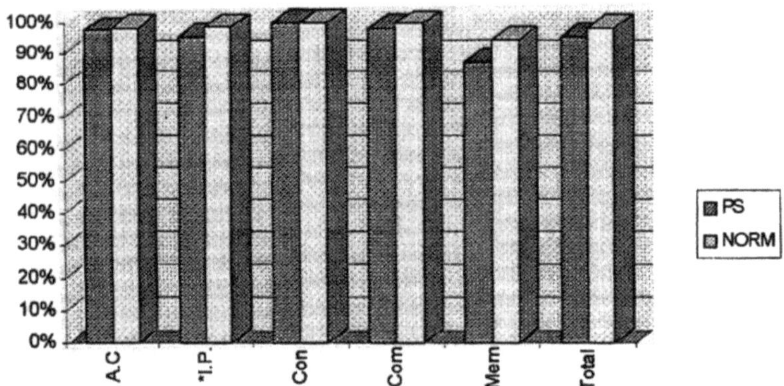

Figure 3. MDRS scores of PS and AD patients (p < 0.05; p < 0.005; p < 0.000).

group comparison between mild and moderately impaired PS vs. AD resulted in yet greater differences in the above mentioned tasks as well as in "construction" and the MRDS total score (124.3 vs. 87.7; p = 0.000) (Figure 3). The poorer mental performance in the AD group could not be explained by a lack of attention or concentration (34.2 vs. 30.5; p = 0.125), nor an ageing effect as they were younger (75.7 vs. 68.5; p = 0.024).

CONCLUSION

Our study did not confirm the finding by Aarsland and co-investigators (1996) that additional atypical symptoms are associated with a greater frequency in cognitive decline. Hence we can not support the hypothesis that this would be an expression of a more widespread disease in these patients either.

On the contrary our findings would lead us to the conclusion that there are quantitative and qualitative distinctive features of cognitive impairment common to all non-secondary Parkinsonian syndromes, suggesting the involvement of identical receptor systems. Previous researchers have pointed out a defect of the norepinephrinic system in the nucleus coeruleus being the possible cause of dementia in IPD (Cast et al., 1987). This will probably be true for APS as well. Future large scale neuropathological studies will hopefully provide answers to these issues.

REFERENCES

Aarsland, D., Tandberg, E., Larsen, J.P., and Cummings J.L., 1996, Frequency of Dementia in Parkinson Disease, Arch. Neurol. 538–542.

Biggins, C.A., Boyd, J.L., Harrop, F.M., Madeley Potentialen, Mindham, R.H.S., Randall, J.I., Spokes, E.G.S., 1992, A controlled, longitudinal study of dementia in Parkinson's disease 55:566–571

Cast, R, Dennis, T. L'Heureux, Raismann, Javoy-Agid, K., Scatton, B, 1987, Parkinson's disease and dementia: norepinephrine and dopamine in locus coeruleus.

Cummings, J.L., Benson, D.F., 1984, Subcortical Dementia, Review of an Emerging Concept Arch. Neurol. 41.

Hughes, A.J., Daniel, S.E., Kilford, L., Lees, A.J., 1992, Accuracy of clinical diagnosis of idiopathic Parkinson's disease: a clinico-pathological study of 100 cases. J. Neurol. Neurosurg. Psychiatry 55:181–184.

Lees, A.J., 1987, The Steel-Richardson Olszewski-Syndrom (progressive supranuclear palsy). In: *Movement Disorders 2*, Marsden C.D., S. Fahn., eds, chapter 13. London, Butterworths 272–287.

Mayeux, B., Chen, J., Mirabello, E., Marder, K., Bell, K., Dooneief, G., Cote, L., Stern, Y., 1990, An estimate of the incidence of dementia in idiopathic Parkinson's disease 40:1513–1517.

Parkinson, J, 1817, An essay on the shaking palsy. London, Sherwood, Neely and Jones.

Quinn N, 1994, Multiple system atrophy. In: Movement Disorders 3, Marsden, C.D,. Fahn, S., eds., chapter 13. London: Butterworths-Heinemann, 262–281.

Watts, R.L., Mirra, S.S., and Richardson, E.P., 1994, Corticobasal ganglionic degeneration. In: Movement Disorders 3., Marsden, C.D., Fahn, S., eds, Butterwort-Heinemann, Oxford, 282–299.

48

COGNITIVE IMPAIRMENT WITHOUT DEMENTIA IN PARKINSON'S DISEASE

Abraham Lieberman

Muhammad Ali Parkinson's Center at the Barrow Neurological Institute
Phoenix, Arizona
National Parkinson Foundation (NPF)
Miami, Florida

INTRODUCTION

Cognitive changes are an integral part of Parkinson's disease (PD). Dementia, defined as a global impairment in cognition, occurs in 27% of PD patients, range 14–32% (Lieberman et al., 1979; Lieberman, 1997, in press). A selective impairment in cognition called cognitive impairment without dementia, frontal lobe dysfunction, fronto-striatal dysfunction, or bradyphrenia also occurs (Cooper et al., 1991; Rogers., 1986). Although cognitive impairment without dementia has been extensively studied, it's prevalence is unknown, and it's relationship to dementia unclear. Is cognitive impairment without dementia an independent entity, or is it a fore-runner of dementia?

Dementia may not be recognized by the patient, but it will be recognized by the patient's family, friends, or care-givers, because its behavioral consequences are painfully evident. Futhermore, most demented patients can be distinguished from non-demented patients on standardized neuropsychological tests (Lieberman, 1997; Prigatano., 1986). Cognitive impairment without dementia, however, may not be recognized by the patient's family, friends, or business associates (many of these patients continue working). Patients with cognitive impairment without dementia can, as a group, be distinguished from age-matched, education matched controls on standardized neuropsychological tests. However, an individual patient who has cognitive impairment without dementia may not be readily distinguished from an individual age-matched, education matched control.

Recently, in a review, the prevalence of dementia in PD was analyzed (Lieberman, 1997 in press). Among 1907 PD patients, 27% were demented (range 14–32%). The incidence of dementia increased with age and varied from 2.7% per year for ages 55 to 65, to 13.7% per year for ages 70 to 79 years. The pathology of PD dementia was also analyzed (Lieberman, in press). Among pathologically verified PD patients who were demented,

10% of the demented patients had only subcortical changes. However, 90% of the demented patients had both subcortical and cortical changes. The present review was undertaken to estimate the prevalence of cognitive impairment without dementia, and to study it's relationship to dementia.

RESULTS AND DISCUSSION

A computerized MEDLINE search was conducted to identify articles in English in peer-reviewed journals pertaining to dementia, cognitive impairment, frontal lobe dysfunction, and bradyphrenia. The period included 1972 to the present. The year 1972 was chosen for two reasons:

1. In 1972 levodopa was readily available. Prior to levodopa, the severity of the motor signs of PD usually precluded cognitive testing except in patients with less advanced disease.
2. By 1972 most patients with post-encephalitic parkinsonism had died. Post-encephalitic Parkinson patients, with rare exceptions, had more wide-spread cognitive and behavioral changes than idiopathic PD patients (Brown et al., 1990).

Nine reports encompassing 407 patients with untreated PD are reviewed in Table 1 (Cooper et al., 1991; Jordan et al., 1992; Lees et al., 1989; Owen., 1992; Reid et al., 1989; Bayles et al., 1996; Matthews et al., 1979; Rogers et al., 1987; Garron et al., 1972). To determine if a patient had dementia, defined as a global decline in cognition, most reports used Wechsler's Adult Intelligence Scale (WAIS), and/or the Mini-Mental Status Examination (MMSE). To determine if a patient had cognitive impairment without dementia, most reports used the Wisconsin Card Sorting Test (WCST) or subtests of the WAIS such as block design or picture completion. The tests used and the details of the testing are summarized in the footnotes to Tables 1 and 2.

In most reports the authors compared a group of untreated PD patients with a group of age-matched, education-matched controls and determined whether the PD patients, as a group, had cognitive impairment without dementia. Most reports did not distinguish the number of individual patient with cognitive impairment without dementia, nor did they estimate the prevalence of cognitive impairment without dementia (Cooper et al., 1991; Jordan et al., 1992; Reid et al., 1989; Bayles et al., 1996; Matthews et al., 1979; Rogers et al., 1987; Garron et al., 1972). This is because there is disagreement as to what constitutes cognitive impairment without dementia, which tests are sensitive to it, and what criteria should be used to diagnose it (Taylor et al., 1989).

Nine reports in recently diagnosed, untreated, PD patients encompassed 407 patients. Mean age of the patients was 60.8 years, mean duration of their PD was 2.9 years. In seven of the nine reports, encompassing 314 patients, the authors determined, or I could estimate the number and percent of patients who had dementia. The mean age of these patients was 61.7 years, while the mean duration of their PD was 3.0 years. Among these patients, 24% were demented (range 17–35%). In only two of the nine reports, did the authors determine, or could I estimate, the number and percent of patients who had cognitive impairment without dementia. These patients were usually defined by a score of at least two standard deviations from controls on the Wisconsin Card Sorting Test (WCST). The mean age of these patients was 57.3 years, while the mean duration of their PD was 2.1 years. Nine of the 45 patients, 20%, had cognitive impairment without dementia.

Table 1. Cognitive changes in recently diagnosed, untreated, Parkinson's disease patients

Study	Number of patients	Age (years)	PD duration (years)	Global cognitive decline (number) (a)	CIND (number) (b)
Bayles 1996 (1)	77	65	5.6	16 (21%)	
Cooper 1991 (2)	60	60	1.3	21 (35%)	
Garron 1972 (3)	47	63.5	5.5	9 (19%)	
Jordan 1992 (4)	32	58	1.6		
Lees 1983 (5)	30	58	2.4		6 (20%)
Matthews 1979 (6)	16	57	2.0		
Owen 1992 (7)	15	56	1.5		3 (20%)
Reid 1989 (8)	72	58	2.1	6 (8%)	
Reid 1989	28	73	1.2	11 (39%)	
Rogers 1987 (9)	30	59	1.0	10 (33%)	
Total 407		60.8	2.9	74/314 (24%)	9/45 (20%)

PD duration, 5.6 years, longer than others in Table 1, reflecting longer PD duration in treated patients. Bayles excluded depressed patients. Nine of 77 patients had a MMSE score between 24–26 (Bayles, Table 2). This was considered by Bayles as questionable dementia. Seven of 77 patients had a MMSE less than 23. This was considered by everyone as dementia. I considered all 16 patients as having minimal dementia. Bayles didn't test for cognitive impairment without dementia.

a. Decline on at least one test of Global Cognitive Function: Mini-Mental Status Examination (MMSE) or Wechsler Adult Intelligence Scale (WAIS). The MMSE and WAIS were often supplemented by the Normalized Adult Reading Test (NART), an Aphasia Screening Test, Benton's Visual Retention Test, de Renzi's Token Test, Raven's Matrices, or Wechsler's Memory Scale (WMS).

b. Decline on at least one test of cognitive impairment without dementia usually the Wisconsin Card Sorting Test (WCST). The WCST was usually supplemented by the WAIS picture completion, block design, and object assembly. The WCST was occasionally supplemented by Austin Maze Task, Luria's Frontal Lobe Tests, the Tower of London Task, a Trail Making Task.

Several authors supplemented the tests of global function and cognitive impairment without dementia with tests of psychomotor skills including tests of Simple Reaction Time, Choice (Complex) Reaction Time, the Purdue Peg-Board. Several authors screened for depression with the Beck, Hamilton, or Zung Scale.

1. Bayles reported 77 patients, 43 controls, in a prospective clinic based study, 18% of patients received anti-PD drugs. Because 82% of patients were untreated.

2. Cooper reported 60 patients, 37 controls, in a prospective clinic based study. Tests included MMSE, Blessed's Dementia Rating Scale, WMS, and WCST. Fifty two patients were depressed but this was considered by author not to have affected outcome. As a group PD patients had cognitive impairment without dementia. 21 of the 60 patients, 35%, had minimal dementia (Cooper Table 1). I could not determine the number of patients, %, who had CIND. Four months later, Cooper assessed the effects of levodopa and anti-cholinergics. Levodopa and anti-cholinergics modified several test sub-groups, but did not change over-all results.

3. Garron reported 47 patients, 47 controls, in a prospective clinic based study. Tests included an automated battery that assessed dementia and CIND. As a group PD patients had CIND. Nine of the 47 patients had minimal dementia (Garron, Table 2). I could not determine the number of patients, %, who had cognitive impairment without dementia. In 1972 levodopa had only recently become available. This explains the long disease duration before treatment.

4. Jordan reported 32 patients, 24 controls, in a prospective clinic based study. This study was followed by a second study of the same 32 patients after levodopa treatment (Table 2). Tests included Blessed's Dementia Rating Scale, NART, WMS, WCST, Simple, and Complex Reaction Time. Jordan didn't test for depression. Jordan reported that the PD patients as a group were impaired on tests of global cognitive function. I could not determine, from the data, the number, %, of patients who were demented.

5. Lees reported 30 patients, 37 controls, in a prospective clinic based study. Tests included NART, WAIS, and WCST. Lees did not test for depression. Six of 30 patients, 20%, completed two or less WCST sets (Lee's histograms). I considered that these six patients had cognitive impairment without dementia.

6. Matthews reported 16 patients, 16 controls, in a prospective clinic based study. This study was conducted simultaneously with Matthew's study of patients with advanced PD (Table 2). I included this study of less than 20 patients because Matthew's combined studies had 42 patients. Tests included WAIS and Trail Making Tasks. Matthews did not test for depression. Matthews reported that PD patients as a group had global impairment or cognitive impairment without dementia. I could not determine, from the data, the number, %, of patients who had dementia or cognitive impairment without dementia.

7. Owen reported 15 patients, 15 controls, in a prospective clinic based study. This study was conducted simultaneously with Owen's study of patients with advanced PD (Table 2). Tests included MMSE and Cambridge Neuropsychological Automated Battery: tests of executive function including planning, sequencing, and set-shifting. Owen tested patients for depression and considered that this did not influence cognition. PD patients as a group had Cognitive impairment without dementia. Three patients, 20%, had cognitive impairment without dementia.

8. Reid studied 100 PD patients and 50 controls in a prospective clinic based study. Reid divided the patients into two groups: 72 patients with a mean age 58 years, and 28 patients with a mean age 73 years. Tests included WAIS, WMS, Benton's Visual Retention Test, Raven's Matrices, Austin Maze Task. Reid did not do WCST, excluded depressed patients, and considered patients who deviated 2 standard deviations from the mean of a particular test as being demented or having cognitive impairment without dementia.

9. Rogers reported 30 patients, 30 controls, and 30 non-PD depressed patients, in a prospective clinic based study. Tests included WAIS, NART, digit arrangement, and simple and complex reaction times. Rogers reported that 10 PD patients had a significant decline in expected IQ. I considered this as minimal dementia. The PD group as a whole had cognitive impairment without dementia. I could not determine the number, %, who had cognitive impairment without dementia. Rogers did not consider depression as having influenced the tests.

Table 2. Cognitive changes in treated PD patients

Study	Number of patients	Age (years)	PD duration (years)	Global cognitive decline (number)	CIND (number)
Boyd 1991 (1)	47	64	not available	15 (32%)	
Canavan 1989 (2)	19	58	2.8		10 (53%)
Jordan 1992 (3)	32	60	4.1		
Loranger 1972 (4)	63	63	7.2	23 (37%)	
Levin 1989 (5)	41	63	not available		
Matthews 1979 (6)	26	59	5.0		
Mindham 1982 (7)	40	70	9.0	8 (20%)	
Owen 1992 (8)	29	62	8.5		6 (20%)
Piccirilli 1989 (9)	30	61.5	7.4		8 (27%)
Piccirilli 1989	30	64.9	10.8	7 (23)	1 (3%)
Pillon 1991 (10)	164	62		29 (18%)	28 (17%)
Pirozzolo 1991 (11)	60	62.6	9.4		
Total 581		62.7	6.9	81/422 (19%)	53/272 (19%)

1. Boyd reported 47 patients, 47 controls, in a prospective clinic based study. Tests included WAIS, NART, WMS. Boyd tested for depression but did not exclude depression. 15 PD patients had dementia. Six controls had dementia.
2. Canavan reported 19 patients, 20 controls, in a prospective clinic based study. Tests included WAIS and WCST. Although Canavan reported only 19 patients, I included his report. Canavan did not test for depression. 11 PD patients, 53%, had cognitive impairment without dementia.
3. Jordan reported 32 levodopa treated patients, 24 controls, in a prospective clinic based study. This report followed Jordan's report on same 32 patients before treatment (Table 1). All of Jordan's patients were similarly tested.
4. Loranger reported 63 patients, and an unspecified number of controls, in a prospective clinic based study. Levodopa only became widely available in 1972 and, at the time of the study, most patients hadn't been treated. This explains the long disease duration before treatment. Twenty three of 63 patients, 37%, were minimally demented.
5. Levin reported 41 patients, 41 controls, in a prospective clinic based study. Thirty seven of 41 patients, 90% were treated with levodopa. Tests included WAIS, WMS, WCST. Levin reported PD patients as a group that had cognitive impairment without dementia. I could not determine, from the data, the number of patients, (%), who were demented or had cognitive impairment without dementia.
6. Matthews reported 26 patients, 16 controls, in a prospective clinic based study. This study was conducted simultaneously with Matthew's study on 16 untreated patients (Table 1). Matthews reported that the PD patients as a group had cognitive impairment without dementia. I could not determine, from the data, the number of patients, (%), who had a dementia or cognitive impairment without dementia.
7. Mindham reported 40 patients, 40 controls, in a prospective clinic based study. Three of Mindham's patients had postencephalitic parkinsonism but were included with his patients with idiopathic PD. Thirty of 37 patients, 81%, were treated with levodopa. Mindham did not test for depression. I could not determine, from the data the, number of patients, (%), who had cognitive impairment without dementia.
8. Owen reported 29 levodopa treated patients, 29 controls, in a prospective clinic based study. This study conducted simultaneously with Owen's study on 15 untreated patients (Table 1). Fourteen of 29 patients, 28%, had cognitive impairment without dementia.
9. Piccirilli conducted two studies. The first study evaluated 30 newly diagnosed PD patients who were treated with levodopa. The second study evaluated same 30 patients 3.4 years later. Tests included WAIS, WMS, Scale, Raven's Matrices, di Renzi Token Test, Luria's Frontal Lobe Test, but not WCST. Eight of 22 patients, 63%, with cognitive impairment without dementia had bilateral PD. After 3.4 years 6/8 patients, 75%, with cognitive impairment without dementia became demented. Only one patient without cognitive impairment without dementia eventually became demented.
10. Pillon reported 164 patients in a prospective clinic based study. Tests included WAIS, WMS, Raven's Matrices, WCST. Pillon tested for depression. Twenty nine of 164 patients, 18%, were demented and 28 patients, 10%, had cognitive impairment without dementia.
11. Pirozzolo reported 60 patients in a prospective clinic based study. Tests included WAIS, WMS, Bender Gestalt, Trail-making A and B. Pirozzolo found a correlation between radykinesia and visual spatial skills.

Eleven reports in more advanced, levodopa treated PD patients encompassed 581 patients. The mean age of these patients was 62.7 years, while the mean duration of their PD was 6.9 years. In eight of 11 reports, encompassing 422 patients, the prevalence of dementia was calculated. The mean age of these patients was 63.1 years, and the mean duration of their PD was 4.4 years. Among these patients, 19% (range 18% to 37%) had dementia. In four of 11 reports, encompassing 272 patients, the authors determined or I could estimate the prevalence of cognitive impairment without dementia. The mean age of these patients was 61.0 years. The mean duration of their PD was 4.0 years. Among these 422 patients, 82 patients, 19% (range 10% - 53%), had cognitive impairment without dementia.

Extrapolating to both groups as a whole, and assuming patients who are demented could not be tested for cognitive impairment without dementia, the combined prevalence of dementia or cognitive impairment without dementia in all PD patients, untreated or treated is 40%.

Several reports studied the relationship of dementia or cognitive impairment without dementia to disease severity (Lieberman, 1979; Lieberman, 1997, in press; Bayless et al., 1996; Boyd et al., 1991; Canavan et al., 1989; Loranger et al., 1972; Levin et al., 1972; Mindham et al., 1982; Piccirilli et al., 1989; Pillon et al., 1991; Pirozzolo et al., 1982; Mortimer et al., 1982), depression (Cummings, 1992; Starkstein et al., 1989), side of onset of PD, right side of brain versus left side of brain versus bilateral (Levin et al., 1989; Piccirilli et al., 1989; Tomer et al., 1993) and medication (Jordon et al., 1992; Owen et al., 1992; Levin et al., 1989; Mindham et al., 1982; Piccirilli et al., 1989; Pillon et al., 1991; Pirozzolo et al., 1982; Cooper, 1992). No consistent relationships were found.

Within the limits of estimating cognitive impairment without dementia, there were no differences in age between untreated and treated patients: 60.8 years versus 62.7 years. However, the treated patients had, as expected, a longer duration of disease: 6.9 years versus 2.9 years. This was significant at $p < .001$. The increased number of patients with cognitive impairment without dementia as a reflection of disease duration, rather than patient age, suggests cognitive impairment without dementia begins, as does PD, as a subcortical process. Then as PD progresses, cognitive impairment without dementia evolves into dementia. An alternative possibility is that cognitive impairment without dementia does not evolve into dementia, but that the cortical changes of dementia "overwhelm" it, and make it impossible to assess. I favor the first explanation because in the one report where the evolution of cognitive impairment without dementia was studied, eight of 30 patients, 27%, initially had cognitive impairment without dementia (Piccirilli et al., 1989). Three years later, six of the eight patients who had cognitive impairment without dementia, 75%, had dementia. Only one of the 30 patients became demented without having had cognitive impairment without dementia.

PD is considered, pre-eminently, as a movement disorder, one associated with a loss of dopamine neurons in the substantia nigra, and noradrenaline neurons in the locus ceruleus. These dead and dying subcortical neurons contain Lewy bodies, considered essential in diagnosing PD (Hughes et al., 1992). As the cause, or causes, of PD is unknown, PD is diagnosed clinically by:

1. finding two of four cardinal signs of a movement disorder including rigidity, resting tremor, bradykinesia, and postural instability; and
2. demonstrating an unequivocal response to levodopa (Hughes et al., 1992).

If PD patients then develop cognitive impairment without dementia, or dementia, these mental changes are considered as part of PD. However, if mental changes appear first then PD may be diagnosed as diffuse Lewy body disease (DLBD), or AD with extra-pyramidal features, or fronto-temporal dementia with parkinsonism (Lieberman, 1997 in press; Foster et al., 1997).

While the personality changes and behavioral manifestations of dementia are obvious, the personality changes and behavioral manifestations of cognitive impairment without dementia are not. Thus, cognitive impairment without dementia is rarely detected in the absence of signs of PD movement disorder. Rather, cognitive impairment without dementia is usually appreciated, in retrospect as a loss of initiative, a declining job performance, or as difficulty in performing previously learned tasks such as balancing a checkbook, completing a crossword puzzle, or programming a VCR.

It is postulated that cognitive impairment without dementia results from the loss of dopamine neurons in the medial nigra (Rinne et al., 1989), noradrenaline neurons in the locus ceruleus (Zweig et al., 1993), or cholinergic neurons in the nucleus basalis of Meynert (Whitehouse et al., 1983). It is further postulated that this neuronal loss disrupts one of several fronto-striatal loops (Taylor et al., 1986; Cummings, 1993) . The relevant loops include:

1. A loop from the dorsolateral prefrontal cortex to the dorsolateral caudate nucleus, then to the globus pallidus, then to the ventral anterior and dorsal median thalamus, then back to the prefrontal cortex. This loop is thought to subserve the executive functions of innovating, planning, sequencing and organizing;
2. A loop from the lateral orbito-frontal cortex to the ventral median caudate nucleus, then to the globus pallidus, then to the ventral anterior and dorsal median thalamus, then back to the orbito-frontal cortex. This loop may also subserve executive functions; and
3. A loop from the anterior cingulate gyrus to the nucleus accumbens, then to the globus pallidus, then back to the cingulate gyrus. Dysfunction in this loop may be manifested as abulia, anergia, and apathy, symptoms often confused with depression. However, these patients are not depressed, do not feel sorry for themselves, have no guilt-feeling, and usually do not respond to anti-depressants.

It is of historical interest to note that bradyphrenia, a term that is often used as a synonym for cognitive impairment without dementia, was originally described in patients with encephalitis lethargica with parkinsonism but without dementia (Rogers, 1986; Rogers et al., 1987). Bradyphrenia, like cognitive impairment without dementia, was described as consisting of cognitive changes such as slowed thinking and difficulty innovating. However, bradyphrenia, unlike cognitive impairment without dementia was also described as consisting of abulia, anergia, and apathy. Bradyphrenia, as originally described, probably involved all three fronto-striatal loops. Cognitive impairment without dementia, may involve only one or two loops.

Its is postulated that cognitive impairment without dementia arises from damage to subcortical neurons that, in turn, disrupt one or more fronto-striatal loops. It is further postulated that cognitive impairment without dementia is not independent of dementia but is a fore-runner of dementia.

The finding of a Parkinson gene on chromosome 4 in an Italian family (the Contursi kindred) and in three unrelated Greek kindreds and the gene's association with the protein alpha-synuclein raises hope that the relationship between cognitive impairment without dementia, dementia, and PD will be unraveled (Polymeropoulos et al., 1997). The Italian and Greek patients had the cardinal signs of PD, responded to levodopa, and, at post-mortem, had subcortical Lewy bodies. Except for an early age of onset, as expected in an autosomal dominant disease, the Contursi and Greek kindreds resemble idiopathic PD. Two Parkinson patients from the Contursi kindred became demented and died (Golbe et al., 1990). At post-mortem, both had subcortical Lewy bodies. One patient had no cortical pathology, and one had an AD-like cortical pathology. If a gene can code for an abnormal protein, and if the protein can, like alpha-synuclein "clump" in the presynaptic nerve terminals of motor "loop" neurons and damage these cells, then it can also clump in cognitive "loop" neurons and damage these cells. If this is shown to be true, then the implied relationship between cognitive impairment without dementia and dementia will be substantiated.

REFERENCES

Bayles, K.A., Tomoeda, C.K., and Wood, J.A., 1996, Change in Cognitive Function in Idiopathic Parkinson Disease. *Arch. Neurol.* 53:1140–1146.

Boyd, J. L., Cruickshank, C., and Kenn, C.W., 1991, Cognitive impairment and dementia in Parkinson's disease: A controlled study. *Psych. Med.* 21:911–921.

Brown, R.G., and Marsden, C.D., 1990, Cognitive Function in Parkinson's Disease: From Description to Theory. *Trends Neurosci.* 13:21–29.

Canavan, A.G.M., Passingham, R.E., and Marsden, C.D., 1989, The Performance on Learning Tasks of Patients in the Early Stages of Parkinson's Disease. *Neuropsychologia* 27:141–156.

Cooper, J.A., Sagar, H. J., Jordan, N., and Harvey, N. S., 1991, Cognitive Impairment In Early, Untreated Parkinson's Disease And Its Relationship To Motor Disability. *Brain* 114:2095–2122.

Cooper, J.A., Sagar, H.J., and Doherty, S.M., 1992, Different Effects of Dopaminergic and Anticholinergic Therapies on Cognitive and Motor Function in Parkinson's Disease: A Follow-up Study of Untreated Patients. *Brain* 115:1701–1725.

Cummings, J.L., 1993, Frontal-Subcortical Circuits and Human Behavior. *Arch. Neurol.* 50:873–880.

Cummings, J.L., 1992, Depression and Parkinson's Disease: A Review. *Am. J. Psychiatr.* 149:443–454.

Foster, N.L, Wilhelmsen, K, and Anders, A.F., 1997, Frontotemporal Dementia and Parkinsonism Linked to Chromosome 17: A Consensus Conference. *Ann. Neurol.* 41:706–715.

Garron, D.C., Klawans, H.L., and Narin, F., 1972, Intellectual Functioning of Persons with Idiopathic Parkinsonism. *J. Nerv. Ment. Dis.* 154:445–452.

Golbe, L.I., Di Iorio, G., and Bonavita, V., 1990, A Large Kindred with Autosomal Dominant Parkinson's Disease. *Ann. Neurol.* 27:276–282.

Hughes, A. J., Daniel, S. E., Kilford, L., and Lees, A. J., 1992, Accuracy of clinical diagnosis of idiopathic Parkinson's disease: a clinico-pathological study of 100 cases. *J. Neurol. Neurosurg. Psychiatry* 55:181–184.

Jordan, N., Sagar, H., and Cooper, J.A., 1992, Cognitive Components of Reaction Time in Parkinson's Disease. *J. Neurol. Neurosurg. Psychiatry* 55: 658–664.

Lieberman, A., Dziatolowski, M., and Kupersmith, M., 1979, Dementia in Parkinson Disease. *Ann. Neurol.* 6:355–359.

Lieberman, A., 1997, Point of View: Dementia in Parkinson's Disease. In: *Parkinsonism & Related Disorders,* in press.

Lees, A. J., and Smith, E., 1983, Cognitive Deficits in the Early Stages of Parkinson's Disease. *Brain* 106:257–270.

Levin, B. E., Llabre, M.M., and Weiner, W.J., 1989, Cognitive impairments associated with early Parkinson's disease. *Neurology* 39:557–561.

Loranger, A.W., Goodell, H., and McDowell, F.H., 1972, Intellectual Impairment in Parkinson's Syndrome. *Brain* 95:405–412.

Matthews, C. G., and Haaland, K Y., 1979, The effect of symptom duration on cognitive and motor performance in Parkinsonism. *Neurology* 29:951–956.

Mindham, R.H.S., Ahmed, S.W.A., and Clough, C.G., 1982, A Controlled Study of Dementia in Parkinson's Disease. *J. Neurol. Neurosurg, Psychiatry* 45: 969–974.

Mortimer, J.A., Pirozzolo, F.J., and Hansch, E.C., 1982, Relationship of Motor Symptoms to Intellectual Deficits in Parkinson Disease. *Neurology* 32:133–137.

Owen, A.M., James, M., and Leigh, P.N., 1992, Fronto-striatal Cognitive Deficits at Different Stages of Parkinson's Disease. *Brain* 115:1727–1751.

Piccirilli, M., D' Alexandro, P., and Finali, G., 1989, Frontal Lobe Dysfunction in Parkinson's Disease: Prognostic Value for Dementia. *Eur. Neurol.* 29:1–76.

Polymeropoulos, M.H., Lavedan, C., and Leroy, E., 1997, Mutation in the Alpha-Synuclein Gene Identified in Families with Parkinson's Disease. *Science* 276:2045–2047.

Prigatano, G. P., 1986, Higher Cerebral Deficits: The History of Methods of Assessment and Approaches to Rehabilitation: Part I. *Barrow Neurological Institute (BNI) Quarterly* 3:15–26.

Pillon, P., Dubois, B., Ploska., 1991, Severity and Specificity of Cognitive Impairment in Alzheimer's, Huntington's, and Parkinson's Disease and Progressive Supranuclear Palsy. *Neurology* 41:634–643.

Pirozzolo, F.J., and Hansch, E.C., Mortimer, J.A., 1982, Dementia in Parkinson's Disease: A Neuropsychological Analysis. *Brain Cogn.* 1:71–83.

Reid, W.G.J., Broe, A., and Hely, A., 1989, The Neuropsychology of De Novo Patients with Idiopathic Parkinson's Disease: The Effects of Age of Onset. *Int. J. Neurosci.* 48:205–217.

Rinne, J.O., Rummukainen, J., and Paljarvi, L., 1989, Dementia in Parkinson's Disease is Related to Neuronal Loss in the Medial Substantia Nigra. *Ann. Neurol.* 26:47–50.

Rogers, D., 1986, Bradyphrenia in Parkinsonism: A Historical Review. *Psychol Med.* 16:257–265.

Rogers, D., Lees, A. J., and Smith, E., 1987, Bradyphrenia In Parkinson's Disease and Psychomotor Retardation In Depressive Illness. *Brain* 110:761–776.

Starkstein, S.E., Berthier, M.L., and Bolduc, P.L., 1989, Depression in Patients with Early Versus Late Onset of Parkinson's Disease. *Neurology* 39:1441–1445.

Taylor, A. E., Saint-Cyr, J. A., and Lang, A. E., 1986, Frontal Lobe Dysfunction in Parkinson's Disease; *Brain* 109:845–883.

Tomer, R., Levin, B. E., and Weiner W J., 1993, Side of Onset of Motor Symptoms Influences Cognition in Parkinson's Disease. *Ann. Neurol.* 34:579–584.

Whitehouse, P.J., Hedreen, J.C., and White, C.L., 1983, Basal Forebrain Neurons in the Dementia of Parkinson's Disease. *Ann. Neurol.* 13:242–248.

Zweig, R.M., Cardillo, J., Cohen, M., 1993, The Locus Ceruleus and Dementia in Parkinson's Disease. *Neurology* 43:986–991.

NEUROLEPTIC MALIGNANT SYNDROME AND DEMENTIA WITH LEWY BODIES

A Case Study

Howard Feldman,[1] Kevin Solomons,[2] Tom Cooney,[3] and Thomas G. Beach[4]

[1]Division of Neurology, University of British Columbia and
The Clinic for Alzheimer's Disease and Related Disorders
Vancouver Hospital and HSC
Vancouver, Canada
[2]Division of Geriatric Psychiatry
Riverview Hospital and University of British Columbia
Vancouver, Canada
[3]Department of Anatomical Pathology
Royal Columbian Hospital
New Westminster, Canada
[4]Division of Neuropathology
University of British Columbia
Vancouver Hospital and HSC
Vancouver, Canada

INTRODUCTION

The clinical criteria for Dementia with Lewy bodies (DLB) as proposed by the International Working Group include neuroleptic hypersensitivity as a "supportive feature" (McKeith et al.,1996). The spectrum of this neuroleptic hypersensitivity continues to be elucidated, as cases are reported where the use of neuroleptics has been associated with a dramatically accelerated rate of decline and death (McKeith et al., 1992a). This observation emerges on the more general background of elderly patients having a greater risk to develop fatal Neuroleptic Malignant Syndrome (NMS) particularly in the context of underlying neurologic disease (Shalev and Munitz, 1986; Pearlman, 1986). In the descriptions of severe neuroleptic hypersensitivity in DLB, NMS has been reported as part of the DLB hypersensitivity spectrum. The incidence of NMS in the setting of dementia with Lewy bodies is not presently known. Similarly, the effects of neuroleptic use in younger patients with DLB and the risks of NMS are not fully characterized.

Progress in Alzheimer's and Parkinson's Diseases
edited by Fisher *et al.*, Plenum Press, New York, 1998.

In this chapter, we present a pathologically proven case study of dementia with Lewy bodies where NMS occurred with a more benign course and where ultimately survival could not be demonstrated to have been shortened by this event. Inadvertent rechallenge with neuroleptics occurred subsequent to the NMS without undue effect and ECT was a successful modality of behavioral management for a time during this illness suggesting the possibility that this treatment modality may be worth further investigation.

CASE REPORT

A 59 year old university educated professional presented with a five year history of gradual and progressive cognitive impairment. His initial cognitive symptoms included anomia and lexical retrieval difficulties. He developed impairment in his problem solving and comprehension and he appeared confused to friends. Behaviorally he was noted to be uncharacteristically irritable. Early on there were no hallucinations or delusions. He developed a sleep disorder several years into his illness which was investigated and diagnosed as a REM sleep behavior disorder with EMG augmentation. This led to a trial of Clonazepam that improved his sleep but resulted in a further decline in his cognitive function. He was described to have poor balance but there were no falls.

His medical history included maternally inherited Stargardt's disease which had left him with some reduced peripheral vision and with central vision to light only. He had known hypercholesterolemia. There was no family history of neurodegenerative disease and no dementia risk factors were otherwise noted. He used a mild to moderate amount of alcohol.

His initial general examination was unremarkable. On mental status examination he was temporally, but not spatially disoriented. He had impairment of retrieval greater than acquisition and retention of newly learned information. There was difficulty noted with his calculations and abstractions. In testing language he had lexical retrieval difficulties with normal spelling and writing. His neurological examination apart from his visual findings demonstrated only mild tandem instability. On neuropsychological assessment, his Verbal-IQ was prorated at 96 (lower than predicted). His word fluency was low normal. He scored impaired on the Rey Auditory Verbal Learning Test and paired associate verbal learning. He was distractible, irritable and performed poorly on sequence tests. His verbal processing was impaired and he had difficulty in maintaining concentration on two parallel tasks.

His investigations included a CT head scan that showed mild cerebral and cerebellar cortical atrophy. EEG showed generalized fast activity over both hemispheres as well as generalized slowing of the background activity.

The diagnostic impression was that he had "clinically probable Alzheimer's disease "(NINCDS ADRDA criteria). There was no clinical or lab evidence of Refsum's disease or Bassen Kornzweig syndrome that might be associated with his ocular disease.

Roughly six months following the above assessment he was admitted to hospital with confusion, agitation, and uncontrolled aggression. He was treated with loxapine (up to 175 mg/day) and lorazepam (up to 6 mg/day). He did not develop extrapyramidal side effects. There was a concurrent fairly precipitous decline of cognitive function. When his behavioral symptoms stabalized over the next 4–6 weeks his psychoactive medications were tapered. Maintenance dosages of loxapine (15 mg) and lorazepam (2 mg) were reached. His behavior then escalated again and he was treated with a combination of loxapine (100 mg/day) and methotrimeprazine (50 mg daily). Within two weeks of this flare-up he developed classical features of NMS with leukocytosis (11.2×10^9), CPK (1954 U/L), hyperpyrexia, rigidity, and increased agitation. His neuroleptics were discontinued and with conservative support this state resolved over a further two weeks. He was placed on trazodone (350 mg daily) and alprazolam (4.25 mg daily) but he went on to have recurrent relapses of disturbed behavior thereafter. Following his NMS, he was treated with ECT as well to address a comorbid agitated depression. This was well tolerated and effective until maintenance ECT was discontinued. Neuroleptics were generally avoided thereafter though he was inadvertently rechallenged with thioridazine (25 mg tid) during a flare up of difficult to manage agitated and aggressive behavior. He did not develop any adverse effects from this rechallenge of neuroleptics.

Cognitively, he went on to develop a striking loss of language with impaired reception and paraphasias. Executive function continued to decline and he developed cognitive slowing and marked preservation. He had reflex grasping that was very prominent. Over the next six months his posture became stooped, and he developed cogwheeling of his arms. A clinical diagnosis of dementia with Lewy Bodies was made in longitudinal follow-up. He died of aspiration pneumonia and chest abscess twelve months following his initial NMS.

POST MORTEM FINDINGS

His brain weighed 1475 grams. There was some noted cortical cerebral atrophy particularly over the posterior frontal gyri and temporal lobes. On microscopy, there were both diffuse and neuritic plaques with a moderate density of neuritic plaques in the frontal sections (Figure 1). By CERAD criteria the density of plaques was sufficient for an Alzheimer's disease diagnosis. There were additionally frequent ubiquitin positive Lewy bodies in the deeper cortical layers with the greatest numbers in the temporal cortex and cingulate gyrus (Figures 3 and 4).

Tangles were rare or absent in the neocortex and hippocampus. There were moderate plaques, frequent tangles and spongiform change in the parahippocampal gyrus (Figure 5). There was no neuronal loss evident or astrocytic gliosis. In the substantia nigra there was a marked decrease in pigmented neurons, with increased Lewy bodies and with scattered pigmented macrophages (Figure 2). Lewy body score according to the Consensus Working Group criteria was 9/10.

DISCUSSION

McKeith et al. (1992a, 1992b) reported a series of twenty subjects ages 69–87 diagnosed with dementia with Lewy bodies. Neuroleptic exposure and adverse responses were noted in 13/16 neuroleptic exposed subjects, including seven with severe reactions who died between 2–19 weeks later. Severe reactions were characterized as sudden onset of sedation, increased confusion, rigidity, and immobility with features including those of NMS. The mean time from neuroleptic induced symptoms to death was 6–8 weeks in those with severe reactions. The neuroleptics implicated in that series included thioridazine, haloperidol, trifluoperazine, and flupenthixol.

We present a case study of a younger subject with dementia with Lewy bodies whose illness lasted an estimated 7 years from its onset at age 55. This course parallels the known natural history of DLB (McKeith et al., 1992a). He had the onset of agitated and

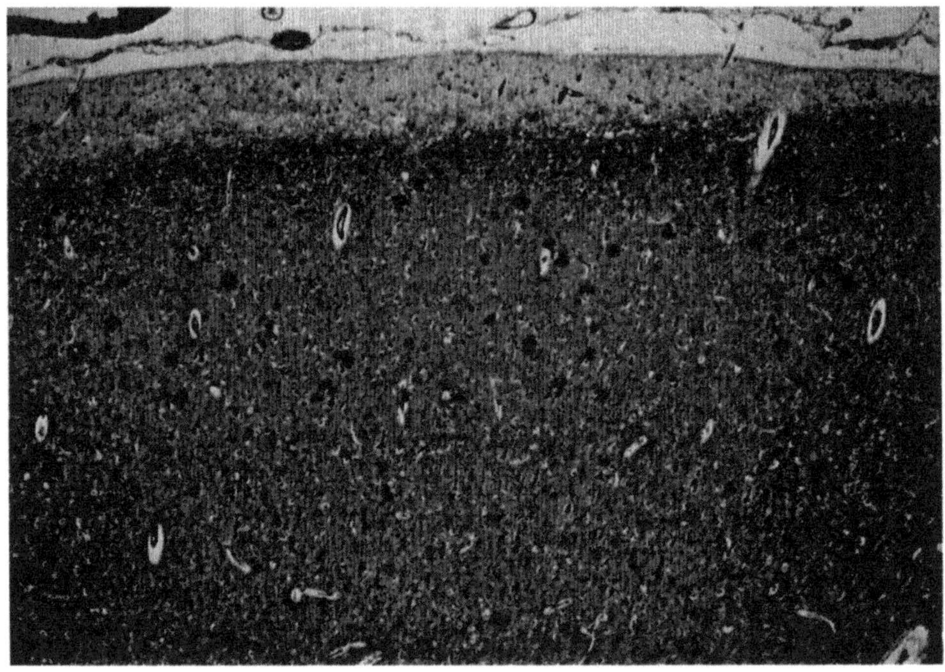

Figure 1. Neuritic plaques, frontal cortex (Bielschowsky).

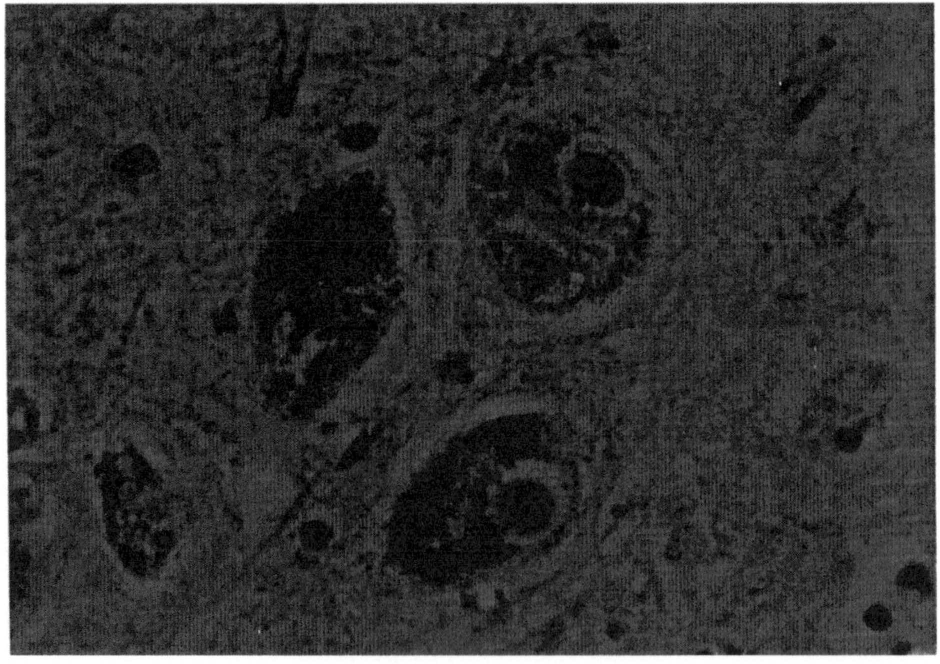

Figure 2. Substantia nigra Lewy Bodies (H & E).

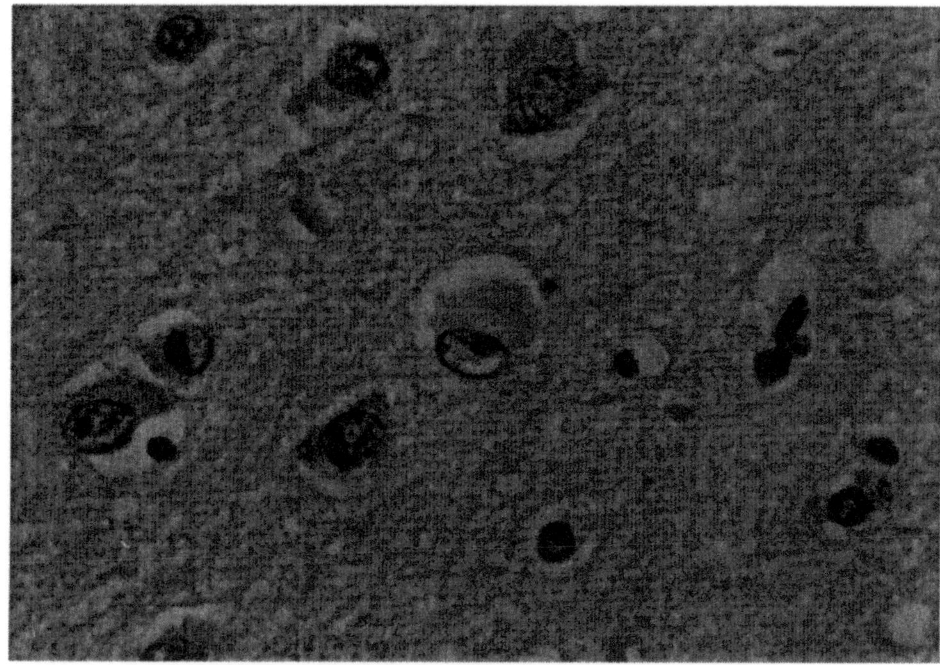

Figure 3. Cortical Lewy Body, Cingulate Gyrus (H & E).

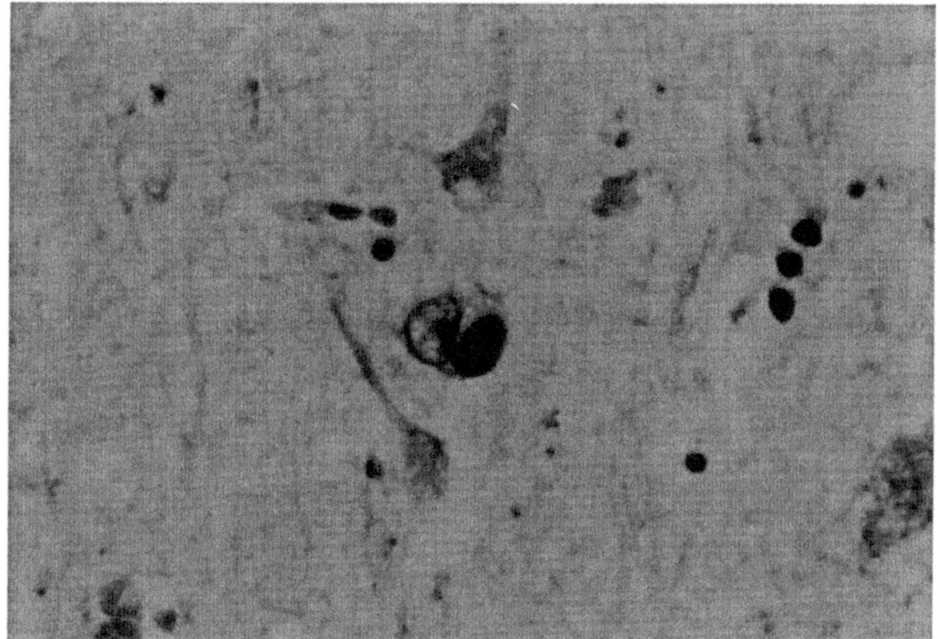

Figure 4. Cortical Lewy Body, Cingulate Gyrus (Ubiquitin).

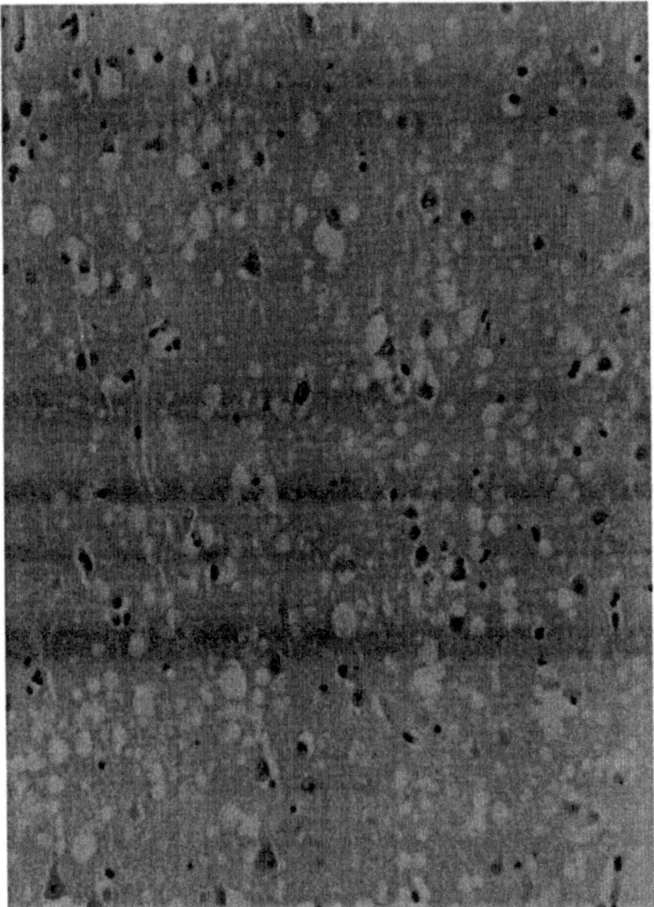

Figure 5. Cortical Spongiosus, Transentorhinal cortex (H & E).

aggressive behavior with visual hallucinations at roughly 5 years into his illness, late for the typical descriptions of DLB. He was treated with high dose neuroleptics loxapine (up to 175 mg/day) and lorazepam (up to 6 mg/day) without any movement disorder or other clearly related neuroleptic adverse events for a treatment period of 4 weeks. His psychoactive medications were tapered to maintenance levels and he was not noted to have extrapyramidal signs at this point. A flare up of difficult behaviors followed which lead to a rapid dose increase of loxapine (100 mg/day) and methotrimeprazine (50 mg daily). He developed NMS within the next 2 weeks which led to his discontinuation of neuroleptics. His NMS resolved with conservative management over a further 2 weeks. At a later point in his illness, he was inadvertently rechallenged with thioridazine without redeveloping NMS and without inducing significant side effects. From the time that his behavior deteriorated his management remained difficult. He responded favorably to ECT which was used to treat associated agitated depression. He survived for twelve months after his bout of NMS. Neuropathologically, he fulfilled diagnostic criteria for DLB and had a high Lewy body score with features of brainstem, limbic and neocortical disease.

His neuroleptic sensitivity reaction would be classified as being severe in relation to prior reports. However, there is no convincing evidence that his death was hastened by either this sensitivity or by his NMS which ran a benign course. This more benign outcome with severe neuroleptic sensitivity has not been reported previously. Whether this is an observation that will prove to be more generalizable to younger patients is not presently known and further study is required. With the management challenges that arise, this clarification of the course of younger patients treated with neuroleptics in DLB will be important.

CONCLUSIONS

This younger patient with clinically and pathologically typical DLB had a course of severe neuroleptic sensitivity that included NMS. His survival following NMS and severe neuroleptic sensitivity was longer than that characterized in older patients and there did not appear to be a significant effect of this sensitivity on his ultimate survival. A rechallenge with thioridazine was not associated with NMS. This suggests that there may be a differential age response to neuroleptics in DLB that will be worth additional observation.

Therapeutically his clinical response to ECT was additionally favorable and this may represent a treatment modality option for consideration in this setting where treatment options are limited. It is possible that cholinergic enhancing therapy may be useful in this setting. This is currently being investigated.

ACKNOWLEDGMENTS

The authors are grateful to Agnes Sauter for her helpful assistance in this work and to Novartis Canada for their support in its presentation.

REFERENCES

McKeith, I.G., Fairbairn, A., Perry, R.H., Thompson, P., & Perry, E., 1992a, Neuroleptic sensitivity in patients with senile dementia of Lewy body type. *Br. Med. J.* 305:673–678.

McKeith, I.G., Perry, R.H., Fairburn, A.F., Jabeen, S., Perry, E.K., 1992b, Operational criteria for senile dementia of Lewy body type. *Psychol. Med.* 22:911–922.

McKeith, I.G., Galasko, D., Kosaka, K., Perry, E.K., Dickson, D.W., Hansen, L.A., Salmon, D.P., Lowe, J., Mirra, S.S., Byrne, E.J., Lennox, G., Quinn, N.P., Edwardson, J.A., Ince, P.G., Bergeron, C., Burns, A., Miller, B.L., Lovestone, S., Collerton, D., Jansen, E.N.H., Ballard, C., deVos, R.A.I., Wilcock, G.K., Jellinger, K.A., Perry, R.H., 1996, For the Consortium on Dementia with Lewy Bodies. Consensus guidelines for the clinical and pathological diagnosis of dementia with Lewy Bodies (DLB): report of the consortium on DLB international workshop. *Neurology* 47:1113–1124.

Pearlman, C.A., 1986, Neuroleptic malignant syndrome:a review of the literature. *J. Clin. Psychopharmacol.* 6:257–273.

Shalev, A., and Munitz, H., 1986, The neuroleptic malignant syndrome: agent and host interaction. *Acta Psychiatr. Scand.* 73:337–347.

50

CASE REPORT ON A GENERALIZED EPILEPSY IN A PATIENT SUFFERING FROM PARKINSON'S DISEASE

Emanuel Kogan, Irma Schöll, and Alexandra E. Henneberg

Hospital for Parkinson's Disease
Franz-Groedel-Str. 6
D - 61231 Bad Nauheim, Germany

INTRODUCTION

A "loss of postural reflexes" is well-known in patients suffering from Parkinson's disease. So far, this symptom has been regarded as an entity that is connected with the pathology of Parkinson's disease itself and never questioned as being a distinct syndrome. However, two case reports describe single patients suffering from myoclonic attacks and Parkinson's disease (Scarpino et al., 1990; Yoshida et al., 1993). We below describe a further patient, suffering from myoclonic attacks, EEG alterations and Parkinson's disease.

PATIENT'S CASE HISTORY

A 60-year-old patient, who had a four-year history of Parkinson's disease was submitted to our hospital. He complained of severe akinesia at day and night, retropulsion, gait difficulties as well as speech and swallowing disturbances. On examination in an, "on state" he showed severe rigidity, bradydysdiadochokinesia, walking difficulties and antero- and retropulsion. He had been treated by 6 × 100 mgs of L-DOPA (with decarboxylaseinhibitor), 5 mgs of selegiline, 6 × 0.125 mgs of pergolide and 50 mgs of amantadine sulfate.

THERAPY AND SPECIAL OBSERVATIONS

The patient was treated by an increase of the selegiline (7.5 mgs) and the amantadine sulfate medication (300 mgs) and an additional 100 CR-L-DOPA at night. Intensive physiotherapy and speech therapy was performed. After a week's time we observed a

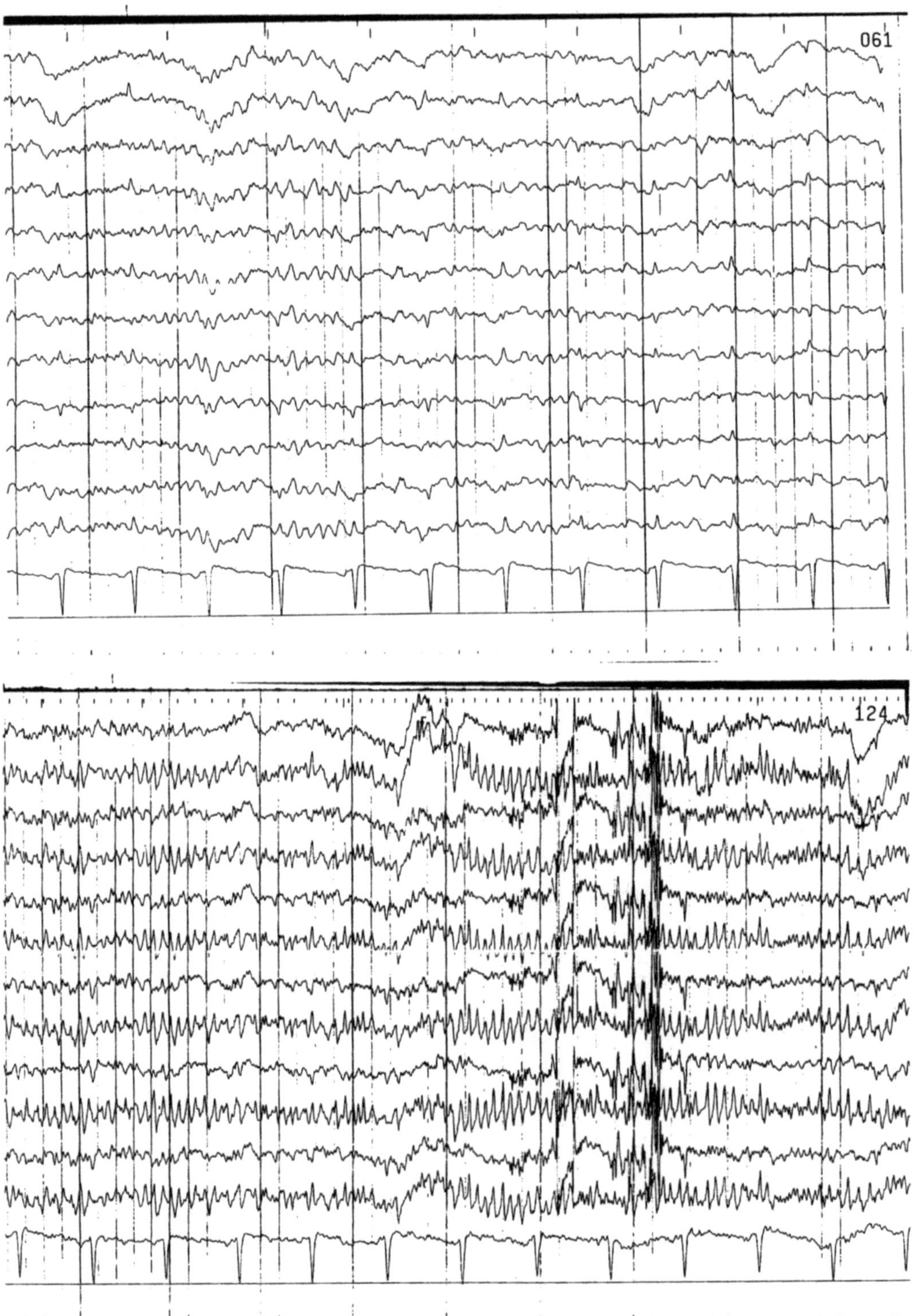

Figure 1. EEG from the patient described above. A) Normal without photic stimulation; B) after five minutes of hyperventilation and during photic stimulation with generalized polyspike wave complexes.

myoclonic astatic attack. An EEG with hyperventilation and photic stimulation was performed and showed generalized polyspikes and polyspike waves under more than 10/sec photic stimuli.

Therefore an additional therapy on sodium valproate was begun, that was increased stepwise up to 2 × 300 mgs without further complications. The attacks disappeared and the EEG returned to normal.

DISCUSSION

The patient described above seemed to have developed myoclonic astatic attacks during an increase of the anti-Parkinsonian medication in our hospital. However, only D 1 agonists and clozapine have been claimed so far to induce seizures (Neufeld et al., 1996; Starr, 1996), whereas the same has not been described for selegiline and amantadines. Moreover, in the meantime, we have observed another 17 patients suffering from Parkinson's disease, myoclonic attacks and EEG alterations, who were on different drugs and will be described elsewhere. Therefore we conclude, that we might have found a subgroup of patients suffering from Parkinson's disease and generalized epilepsy, who are easily treated by an additional anticonvulsive drug treatment and by that get rid of their drop attacks.

REFERENCES

Neufeld, M.Y., Rabey, J.M., Orlov, E., and Korczyn, A.D., 1996, Electroencephalographic findings with low-dose clozapine treatment in psychotic parkinsonian patients. *Clin. Neuropharmacol.* 19:81.

Scorpino, O., Pelliccioni, G., Guidi, M., Mauro, A.M., and Mercante, O., 1990, Maladie de Parkinson et epilepsie photosensible. *Rev. Neurol.* 146:36.

Starr, M.S., 1996, The role of dopamine in epilepsy. *Synapse* 22:159.

Yoshida, K., Moriwaka, F., Matsuura, T., Hamada, T., and Tashiro, K., 1993, Myoclonus and seizures in a patient with parkinsonism: induction by levodopa and its confirmation on SEPs, *Japan. J. Psychiatry Neurol.* 47:621.

51

PATHOPHYSIOLOGY OF HEREDITARY PROGRESSIVE DYSTONIA WITH MARKED DIURNAL FLUCTUATION—ITS CHARACTERISTICS IN CONTRAST TO OTHER DOPA-RESPONSIVE DISORDERS

Masaya Segawa and Yoshiko Nomura

Segawa Neurological Clinic for Children
2-8 Surugadai Kanda
Chiyoda-ku, Tokyo 101, Japan

INTRODUCTION

Hereditary progressive dystonia with marked diurnal fluctuation (Segawa et al., 1976; 1986) or strictly defined dopa responsive dystonia (Nygaard et al., 1993a) (HPD/DRD) is a female predominant, autosomally dominantly inherited, dopa-responsive postural dystonia caused by heterozygotic abnormalities of GTP cyclohydrolase I gene located on 14q22.1–q22.2 (Ichinose et al., 1994). Clinically, it is characterized by marked diurnal fluctuation of symptoms and marked and sustained response to levodopa without any side effects. Although postural tremor appears later in adulthood, no parkinsonian resting tremor or plastic rigidity develops throughout the course of the illness. Moreover, there is no mental or psychological abnormality or dysfunction of the autonomic nervous system.

In this presentation, we would like to discuss the pathophysiology of HPD/DRD based on clinical characteristics, clinical-neuro-physiological, biochemical, and neuropathologial and histochemical findings, and finally discuss why this disorder does not develop the pathophysiology of Parkinson's disease or show psychomental abnormalities.

PATHOGNOMONIC CLINICAL AND LABORATORY FINDINGS

The main symptom is postural dystonia throughout the course of illness and plastic rigidity do not appear even in advanced stages (Segawa et al., 1986). Postural tremor develops later but parkinsonian resting tremor is not observed (Segawa et al., 1986).

Progress in Alzheimer's and Parkinson's Diseases
edited by Fisher *et al.*, Plenum Press, New York, 1998.

Although movement becomes bradykinetic in the advanced stage, it is due to the increase of muscle tone of both agonist and antagonist and not due to the poverty of movement or failure in the initiation of movement (Segawa et al., 1986). Interlimb coordination is preserved and freezing phenomenon is not observed even in the advanced stage (Segawa et al., 1986; Segawa and Nomura, 1991a). Psychomental functions are preserved normally. DTRs are exaggerated with ankle clonus and striatal toe, but without Babinski sign (Segawa et al., 1986).

The clinical course is characterized by its age-dependency (Segawa et al., 1986; 1993b). In cases with clinical onset in the 1st decade, marked progression is observed until the middle of the 2nd decade, but it attenuates with age and it almost ceases from the 4th decade. Along with this course, diurnal fluctuation reduces its grade and becomes almost inapparent in the 4th decade, while postural tremor develops later from adolescent, mostly from the 4th decade. On the contrary, in cases with onset in adulthood, symptoms start with gait disturbance and postural tremor. They are mild and their progression is very slow. Moreover, in these cases, the diurnal fluctuation is slight or inapparent.

These symptoms respond to levodopa completely without any relation to the longevity of the clinical course or age of onset and the effects sustain without any side effects (Segawa et al., 1986; 1990).

Besides these, in cases with onset in the 1st decade the body length fails to gain with the onset of dystonia (Segawa et al., 1976; 1986). But this is also recovered by levodopa if it is administrated before adolescence (Segawa et al., 1976; 1986).

Polysomnographies (PSGs) revealed abnormalities only in parameters modulated by NS•DA neurons and normal preservation of those modulated by the serotonergic (5HT) and noradrenergic (NA) neurons (Segawa et al., 1976; 1987; Segawa and Nomura, 1991b; 1993b). Moreover, these PSGs showed no feature suggesting DA receptor supersensitivity (Segawa et al., 1987).

Twitch movements (TMs); short muscle activity localized to one muscle and lasting less than 0.5 seconds with an amplitude of more than 20 μV on the surface EMG, in REM stage (sREM) reduced their numbers to around 20% of normal values and with these values followed the decremental age variation and the incremental nocturnal variation during sleep observed in normal children (Segawa and Nomura, 1993b).

As the numbers of TMs in sREM reflect the activities of the NS•DA neurons (Segawa et al., 1987; Segawa and Nomura, 1993b), these results of PSGs revealed that in HPD activities of the NS•DA neuron decreased to around 20% of normal values and followed the age and nocturnal variations of normal subjects (children) with these reduced levels but without any further decrement (Segawa and Nomura, 1993b; 1995).

Neuroimaging studies showed no abnormalities in CT and MRI. ^{18}F-Dopa PET revealed no (Snow et al., 1993) or slight (Sawle et al., 1991) reduction in cooperation rates. [^{11}C] raclopride PET for detecting D_2 receptors showed no upward or downward regulation in patients of the 3rd decade (Leenders et al., 1995).

The CSF examination revealed the decrease in neopterin and biopterin levels to around 20% of normal values (Fujita et al.,1990; Furukawa et al., 1993). This naturally suggests the deficiency of GTP cyclohydroxylase I (GCH-I) as a cause of HPD/DRD (Fujita et al.,1990, Furukawa et al., 1993).

Neuropathologies of an autopsied sporadic case with dopa responsive dystonia (Rajput et al., 1994) proved to be HPD/DRD after DNA analysis of the brain (Furukawa et al., 1996) and revealed no degenerative morphological changes in the substantia nigra (SN) (Rajput et al., 1994). But neurohistochemical examination showed a reduction of DA content in the SN and the striatum with regional caudate/putamen distribution and subregional rostrocaudal distribution similar to iPD; however, the subregional dorso ventral distribution was different from iPD with its predominant reduction in the ventral part (Rajput et al., 1994, Hornykiewicz, 1995). This suggests predominant involvement of the striatal direct pathway which is located in the ventral area (Gibb, 1996). Furthermore, TH was decreased in its activities and protein levels only in the striatum and they were normal in the SN (Rajput et al., 1994; Hornykiewicz, 1995). In the putamen, both biopterin and neopterin reduced tó 17% and 35% of normal levels, respectively (Furukawa, in press).

Studies of molecular biology of HPD showed no linkage to the gene of TH (Flecher et al., 1989; Tsuji et al., 1993). But linkage to the long arm of the 14th chromosome was detected by Nygaard et al (Nygaard et al., 1993b). Ichinose et al found that the gene of HPD/DRD is located on GCH-I gene in 14q22.1–q22.2 (Ichinose et al., 1994).

Up to now 25 mutations and frame shift have been detected (Segawa in press). They differ among cases, but identical in one family as shown in the first report (Ichinose et al., 1994). However, no abnormalities have been detected in other families with HPD/DRD, including the one in which linkage to 14q was detected.

Levels of GCH-I activities in stimulated peripheral mononuclear cells revealed reduction of less than 20% of normal range in affected cases, while they were 37 and 38% in two asymptomatic carriers (Ichinose et al., 1994). The levels of neopterin in CSF were less than 20% in affected subjects and 35% in an asymptomatic carrier (Takahashi et al., 1994). The ratio of mutant RNA of GCH-I gene against normal RNA was 28% in the affected cases and 8% in the asymptomatic carrier (Hirano et al., 1995; 1996). These show that HPD is dominant GCH-I gene abnormalities with low penetance and that partial GCH-I reduction of less than 20% develops symptoms while subjects with more than 30% are asymptomatic.

PATHOPHYSIOLOGY OF HPD

Partial deficiency of BH_4 activities due to heterozygotic abnormalities of GCH-I gene might affect the TH synthesis rather selectively, as the affinity for TH of BH_4 is lowest among aromatic acid hydroxylases (Nomura, in press).

This causes a decrease of TH at the terminal of the NS•DA neuron because BH_4 predominantly exists at the terminal (Levine et al., 1981; Sawada et al., 1987) and as GCH-I in the brain modulates synthesis of TH only in the catecholamine neuron (Nagatsu et al., 1997).

Studies on MPTP monkeys (Crossman 1990; Mitchell et al., 1990; Sambrook et al., 1994) revealed non-involvement of the indirect pathways, the nucleus ventralis lateralis (VL) of the thalamus and the pedunculopontine nucleus (PPN) for development of peak dose dystonia.

The pathophysiologies considered for HPD/DRD are shown on Figure 1.

Decrease in TH at the terminal of NS•DA neuron disfacilitates D_1 receptors and the striatal direct pathways located in the ventral area of the striatum and consequently disinhibits the inhibitory descending efferents of the basal ganglia and develops postural dystonia. For this modulation, particular descending efferents of the basal ganglia to the reticulospinal tract is suspected (Nomura, in press), which may also be involved in the exaggeration of DTR. As the PPN is left uninhibited, locomotion is preserved normally, and with preservation of the D_2 receptors, the indirect pathways and the VL nucleus of the thalamus, plastic rigidity and dopa induced dyskinesia do not develop (Segawa et al., 1993a, Segawa and Nomura, 1995). Although postural tremor may develop later through an ascending pathway of the thalamus, the VL thalamus might not be involved in this pathophysiology.

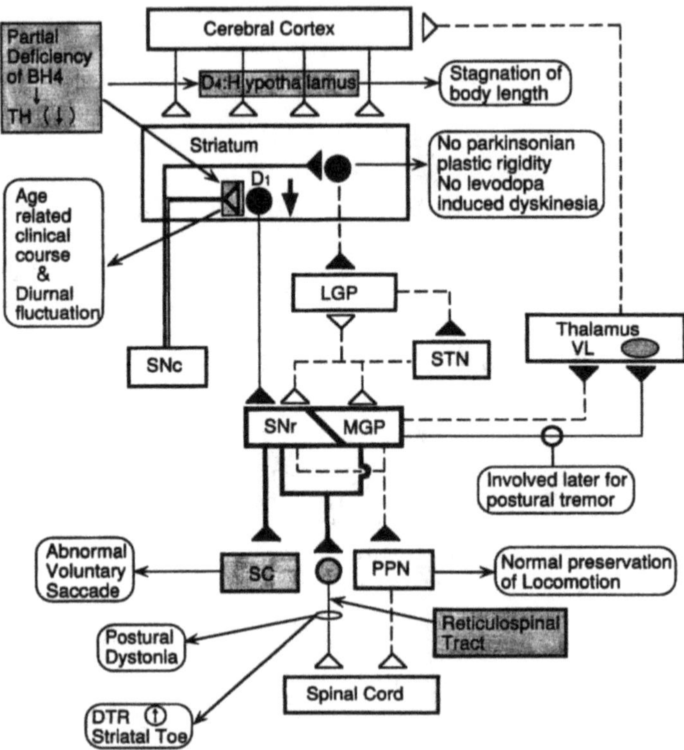

Figure 1. Pathophysioloy of HPD/DRD (hypothesis) Gray areas indicate causative process and primary locus and the target structures that develop symptoms particular for each. The short and wide downward arrow indicates hypoactivity of the neuron. The upward small arrow in circle indicates the exaggeration of DTR. Open triangles and closed triangles are the terminals of excitatory and inhibitory neurons, respectively. Dotted lines show pathways or neurons not involved in the pathophysiology of HPD/DRD. SNc: pars compacta of the substantia nigra; SNr: pars reticulata of the substantia nigra; LPG: lateral globus pallidus; MGp: medial globus pallidus; STR: subthalamic nucleus; SC: superior colliculus; PPN: pedunculopontine nucleus; VL: ventral lateral nucleus of the thalamus.

TH levels in the striatum show exponential decremental variation in the first three decades (McGeer and McGeer, 1973). TH levels in the brain (McGeer and McGeer, 1973) or DA secretion at the terminal of the NS•DA neuron (Phillips, 1989) show circadian variation; decremental in the active phase and incremental in the resting phase. These variations are well reflected in the variations of the number of TMs during sREM. On the other hand, TH activities of the substantia nigra (NS) show no apparent age variation (McGeer and McGeer, 1973) and the neuronal activities of the NS are stable without phase related alteration (Steinfels et al., 1983).

In HPD/DRD, the terminals of the NS•DA neuron are considered to follow these age and circadian variations with levels of TH less than 20% of normal values (Segawa and Nomura, 1993a; 1993b; 1995).

High levels of monoaminergic transmitters in the early developmental course have roles for synaptogenesis or corticogenesis, besides roles for neural transmission (LeWitt et al., 1997). So the values of 20% do not cause failure of the neural transmission in early childhood, but at around 6 years they are reduced below the critical level of neural transmission in the late afternoon when the TH activities are lower with decremental diurnal fluctuation (Segawa, in press). At early ages indirect pathways are functionally immature and D_2 receptors exist in large numbers. These situations might mask or minimize the effects of disinhibition of the efferents of the basal ganglia, induced by the dysfacilitation of the D_1 receptors. For the marked progression in the first one and one half decade the functional maturation of the indirect pathway at these ages also might have an important role (Nomura, in press, Segawa, in press). For the delay in the onset of postural tremor in the 2nd decade, particularly in the 4th decade, marked reduction of the number of D_2 receptors in these decades (Antonini et al., 1993) might have roles.

As this tremor responds completely to levodopa, different pathophysiologies other than parkinsonian resting tremor or essential tremor might be involved for it.

WHY DOES HPD/DRD NOT APPEAR AS PARKINSON'S DISEASE OR DOES NOT INVOLVE THE INDIRECT PATHWAYS?

In the first three decades, there are particular levodopa responsive disorders which show dystonia and parkinsonism. They are, dystonic juvenile parkinsonism (dJP) (Yokochi 1979; 1995) and autosomal-recessive early onset parkinsonism with diurnal fluctuation (AR-EPDF) (Yamamura et al., 1973; 1993). dJP has age of onset in the early half of the 2nd decade and AR-EPDF in the 3rd decade.

Both have particular neuropathology and histochemistry for each and each is considered as a disease entity. AR-EPDF has recently been detected to be linked to 6-q 25.2–27 (Matsumine et al., 1997). They may develop as postural dystonia when symptoms start in childhood. But soon parkinsonian features overcome the dystonia. All of them respond to levodopa but in contrast to HPD/DRD levodopa induced dyskinesia develops soon.

Neuropathologically, dJP (Yokochi, 1984; Gibb et al., 1991) and AR-EPDF (Yokochi, 1995) differ from HPD/DRD with degenerative changes in SNc, similar to iPD, though Lewy bodies are not observed in AR-EPDF (Yokochi, 1995).

Histochemistry of one of the sibling cases of dJP showed decrease in TH and DA only at the terminal (Yokochi et al., 1984). Histochemistry of AR-EPDF revealed a decrease in the TH levels both in the SN and the striatum but it was more marked in the latter, in which it is predominant in the dorsal part (Kondo et al., 1997). Biopterin and neopterin levels in the striatum were within normal range in AR-EPDF (Kondo et al., 1997).

Pathognomonic importance of the distribution of TH levels in the striatum is shown in the following sporadic male case of JP with onset at 23 years, whose symptoms were parkinsonism but not dystonia (Kondo et al., 1997). Histochemistry showed decrease of TH only in the striatum, predominantly in the putamen, and the decrement was observed only in the dorsolateral part of the striatum. The biopterin levels were normal compared with an age matched control.

These evidences suggest that the pathological lesion in the SNc causes involvement of the NS•DA neuron affecting the D_2 receptors and the indirect pathways and develop parkinsonism and levodopa induced dyskinesia. Alternatively, TH deficiency due to abnormal pteridine metabolism or BH_4 deficiency may cause dystonia through the D_1 receptors and the direct pathway located in the ventral area of the striatum, while the primary TH deficiency may cause parkinsonism through the D_2 receptors and the indirect pathway located in the dorsal part of it (Segawa, in press).

This might be due to the difference of the period of the age of developmental variation of pteridine metabolism and that of TH itself. The former is highest in infancy and shows marked decremental age variation in early childhood (Shintaku, 1994) while the latter still remains in higher levels in the second decade (McGeer and McGeer, 1973). So

BH_4, the final product of the pteridine metabolism, may modulate DA receptors which appears early in the developmental course, that is, D_1 receptors of the striatum and D_4 receptors of the tuberoinfundibular system and TH may have roles in modulating D_2 receptors later in the early half of the second decade (Segawa, in press).

Disorders with abnormal pteridine metabolism other than HPD also show dystonia as the main feature (Nomura, in press). These clinical evidences support the above hypothesis.

WHY ARE PSYCHOMENTAL FUNCTIONS PRESERVED IN HPD/DRD?

HPD/DRD with primary BH_4 abnormalities and without the primary abnormalities of TH develop dystonia but not Parkinson's disease. But this could not explain the preservation of the psychological activities, because dJP and AR-EPDF show no mental or psychological abnormalities. While recessive deficiency of GCH-I and other enzymes of pteridine metabolism develop mental disabilities besides postural dystonia. This is due to the marked decrease in 5HT as well as in DA due to complete deficiency of BH_4 (Nomura, in press) as the 5HT neuron in the early developmental course modulates synaptogenesis or corticogenesis with its axons broadly projecting all over the brain with layer specificity (LeWitt et al., 1997).

Although a few cases of HPD/DRD show depressive state or autistic tendency (personal communication), suggesting hypofunction of 5HT neurons, in most cases of HPD/DRD with minimum or no involvement of 5HT neurons, the psychomental functions.

SUMMARY

HPD with partial deficiency of BH_4 due to heterozygotic abnormalities of GCH-I gene, reduces TH levels selectively at the terminals of NS•DA neuron. This abnormality develops postural dystonia through the D_1 receptors and the direct pathway but does not show features of Parkinson's disease as D_2 receptors and the indirect pathways are not involved. These are dependent on the particular developmental course of BH_4 metabolism and the location of it in the brain. Without marked reduction of 5HT activities, psychomental activities are preserved in HPD.

However, it is left unclarified why one mutant or abnormal gene causes symptomatic and asymptomatic cases, making differences in the levels of GCH-I activities and why female predominance develops.

REFERENCES

Antonini, A., Leenders, K.L., Reist, H., Thomann, R., Beer, H-F., and Locher, J., 1993, Effect of age on D_2 dopamine receptors in normal human brain measured by positron emission tomography and ^{11}C-raclopride. *Arch. Neurol.* 50:474–480.

Crossman, A.R. Animal models of movement disorders. Paper presented at the First International Congress on Movement Disorders, April, 1990, Washington, D.C.

Fletcher, N.A., et al. 1989, Tyrosine in hydroxylase and levodopa responsive dystonia. *J. Neuro. Neurosurg. Psychiatr.* 52:112–144.

Fujita, S., and Shintaku, H.,1990, Etiology and pteridin metabolism abnormality of hereditary progressive dystonia with marked diurnal fluctuation (HPD: Segawa disease). *Med. J. Kushiro City Hosp.* 2: 64–67.

Furukawa, Y., Nishi, K., Kondo, T., Mizuno, Y., and Narabayashi, H., 1993, CSF biopterin levels and clinical features of patients with juvenile parkinsonism, In: *Advances in Neurology,* Volume 60, H. Narabayashi, T. Nagatsu, N. Yanagisawa, and Y. Mizuno, eds., Raven Press, New York, pp.562–567.

Furukawa, Y., Shimadzu, M., Rajput, A.H. et al., 1996, GTP-cyclohydrolase I gene mutations in hereditary progressive and dopa responsive dystonia, *Ann. Neurol.* 39:609–617.

Furukawa, Y., Shimadzu, M., Hornykiewicz, O., and Kish, J. Molecular and biochemical aspects of hereditary progressive and dopa-responsive dystonia, In: *Advances in Neurology ,* in press.

Gibb, W.R.G., Narabayashi, H., Yokochi, M. Izuka, R., and Lees, A.J., 1991, New pathologic observations in juvenile onset parkinsonism with dystonia, *Neurology* 41:820–822.

Gibb, W.R.G., 1996, In: Selective pathology, disease pathogenesis and function in the basal ganglia, In: *Recent Advances in Clinical Neurophysiology,* J. Kimura and H. Shibasaki, eds., Elsevier, Amsterdam, pp.1009–1015.

Hirano, M., Tamura, Y., Nagai, Y., Ito, H., Imai, T. and Ueno, S., 1995, Exon skipping caused by a base substitution at a splice site in the GTP cyclohydrolase I gene in a Japanese family with hereditary progressive dystonia/dopa responsive dystonia, *Biochem. and Biophys. Res. Commun.* 213:645–651.

Hirano, M., Tamura, Y., Ito, H., Matsumoto, S., Imai, T. and Ueno, S., 1996, Mutant GTP cyclohydrolase I mRNA levels contribute to dopa-responsive dystonia onset, *Ann. Neurol.* 40:796–798.

Hornykiewicz, O.,1995, Striatal dopamine in dopa-responsive dystonia: Comparison with idiopathic Parkinson's disease and other dopamine-dependent disorders, In: *Age-Related Dopamine-Dependent Disorders, Monogr. Neural. Sci.,* Vol. 14., M. Segawa and Y. Nomura, eds., Karger, Basal, pp. 101–108.

Ichinose, H., Ohye, T., Takahashi, E., Seki, N., Hori, T., Segawa, M., Nomura, Y., Endo, K., Tanaka, H., Tsuji, S., Fujita, K., and Nagatsu, T., 1994, Hereditary progressive dystonia with marked diurnal fluctuation caused by mutations in the GTP cyclohydrolase I gene, *Nature Genetics* 8:236–242.

Kondo, T., Mori, H., Sugita, Y., Mizuno, Y., Mizutani, Y. and Yokochi, M., 1997, Juvenile Parkinsonian - A clinical, neuropathological and biochemical study. *Mov. Disord* 12 Suppl 1: 32.

Leenders, K.L., Antonini, A., Meinck, H-M., and Weindl. A., 1995, Striatal dopamine D2 receptors in dopa-responsive dystonia and Parkinson's disease, In: *Age-Related Dopamine-Dependent Disorders, Monogr. Neural. Sci.,* Volume 14, M. Segawa, and Y. Nomura, eds., Karger, Basel, pp .95–100.

Levine, R.A., Miller, L.P. and Lovenberg, W., 1981, Tetrahydrobiopterin in striatum; localization in dopamine nerve terminals and role in catecholamine synthesis, *Science,* 214:919–921.

LeWitt, P., Harvey, J.A., Friedman E., Simansky, K. and Murphy, H.E., 1997, New evidence for neurotransmitter influences on brain development, *Trends Neurosci.* 20:269–274.

McGeer, E.G, and McGeer, P.L., 1973, Some characteristics of brain tyrosine hydroxylase, In: *New Concepts in Neurotransmitter Regulation,* J. Mandel, ed., Plenum Press, New York, London, pp. 53–68.

Matsumine, M., Saito, M., Shimoda-Matsubayashi, S. et al., 1997, Localization of a gene for an autosomal recessive form of juvenile parkinsonism to chromosome 6q25.2–27, *Am. J. Hum. Genet.* 60:588–596.

Mitchell, I.J., Luquin, R, Boyce, S., Clarke, C.E., Robertson, R.G., Sambrook, M.A. and Crossman, A.R., 1990, Neural mechanisms of dystonia: Evidence from a 2-deoxyglucose uptake study in a primate model of dopamine agonist-induced dystonia, *Mov. Disord.* 5:49–54.

Nagatsu, I., Sakai, M., Takeuchi, T., Arai, R., Karasawa, N., Yamada, K. and Nagatsu, T., 1997, Tyrosine hydroxylase (TH)-only-immunoreactive non-catecholaminergic neurons in the brain of wild mice or the human TH transgenic mice do not contain GTP cyclohydrolase I, *Neurosci. Lett.* 228: 55–57.

Nomura, Y., Uetake, K., Yukishita, S., Hagiwara, H.,Tanaka, T., Tanaka, R., Hachimori, K., Nishiyama, N. and Segawa, M. Dystonias responding to levodopa and failure in biopterin metabolism, *Advances in Neurology,* in press.

Nygaard, T.G., Snow, B.J., Fahn, S. and Calne, D.B., 1993a, Dopa-responsive dystonia: clinical characteristics and definition, In: *Hereditary Progressive Dystonia with Marked Diurnal Fluctuation,* M. Segawa, ed., Parthenon, Carnforth, UK, pp. 21–35.

Nygaard, T.G., Wihelmsen, K.C., Risch, N.J., Brown, D.L., Trugman, J.M., Gilliam, T.C., Fahn S. and Weeks D.E., 1993b, Linkage mapping of dopa-responsive dystonia (DRD) to chromosome 14q, *Nature Genetics* 5: 386–391.

Phillips, A.G., Paper presented at the 3rd International Basal Ganglia Society Meeting, Gagliari, Italy, 1989.

Rajput, A.H., Gibb, W.R.G., Zhong, X.H, Shannak, K.S., Kish S. and Chang L.G., 1994, Dopa-responsive dystonia: pathological and biochemical observations in one case, *Ann. Neurol.* 35:396–402.

Sambrook, M.A., Crossman, A.R. and Mitchell, I.J., 1994, Experimental models of basal ganglia disease, In: Movement Disorders 3, C .D. Marsden, and S. Fahn, eds, Butterworth-Heinemann Ltd., Oxford, pp. 28–45.

Sawada, M., Hirata, Y., Arai,H., Iizuka, R. and Nagatsu, T., 1987, Tyrosine hydroxylase, tryptophan hydroxylase, biopterin, and neopterin in the brains of normal controls and patients with senile dementia of Alzheimer type, *J. Neurochem.* 48:760–764.

Sawle, G.V., Leenders. K. L., Brooks, D.J. et al., 1991, Dopa-responsive dystonia: [F-18] Dopa positron emission tomography, *Ann. Neurol.* 30:24–30.

Segawa, M., Hosaka, A., Miyagawa, F., Nomura, Y. and Imai, H, 1976, Hereditary progressive dystonia with marked diurnal fluctuation, in: *Advances in Neurology,* Volume. 14, R. Eldridge and S. Fahn, eds., Raven Press, New York, pp. 215–233.

Segawa, M., Nomura, Y. and Kase M., 1986, Diurnally fluctuating hereditary progressive dystonia, In: *Handbook of Clinical Neurology: Extrapyramidal Disorders* Volume 5 (49), P.J. Vinken, and G.W. Bruyn, eds., Elsevier, Amsterdam, pp. 529–539.

Segawa, M., Nomura Y, Hikosaka, O., Soda, M., Usui, S. and Kase M., 1987, Roles of the basal ganglia and related structures in symptoms of dystonia, In: *The Basal Ganglia II*, M.B.Carpenter and A. Jayaraman, eds., Plenum Publishing Corp., New York, pp.489–504.

Segawa, M., Nomura, Y., Yamashita, S., Kase, M., Nishiyama, N. Yukishita, S., Ohta, H., Nagata, K and Hosaka, A., 1990, Long term effects of L-Dopa on hereditary progressive dystonia with marked diurnal fluctuation, In: *Motor Disturbance II*, A. Berardelli, R. Benecke, M. Manfredi and C.D. Marsden, eds., Academic Press, London, pp. 305–318.

Segawa, M. and Nomura, Y., 1991a, in Pathophysiology of human locomotion: Studies on pathological cases, In: *Neurobiological Basis of Human Locomotion,* M. Shimamura, S. Grillner and V.R. Edgerton, eds., Japan Scientific Societies Press, Tokyo, pp 317–328.

Segawa, M. and Nomura, Y., 1991b, Rapid eye movements during stage REM are modulated by nigrostriatal dopamine (NS-DA) neuron? In: *The Basal Ganglia III* , G. Bernardi , M.B. Carpenter, G. Di Chiara, M. Morelli, and P. Stanzione, eds., Plenum Press, New York, pp 663–671.

Segawa, M. and Nomura, Y., 1993a, Hereditary progressive dystonia with marked diurnal fluctuation, In: *Hereditary Progressive Dystonia with Marked Diurnal Fluctuation,* (M. Segawa, ed., Parthenon, Carnforth, UK, pp. 3–19.

Segawa, M. and Nomura, Y., 1993b, Hereditary progressive dystonia with marked diurnal fluctuation: Pathophysiological importance of the age of onset, In *Advances in Neurology,* Volume 60, H. Narabayashi, T. Nagatsu, N. Yanagisawa, and Y. Mizuno, eds., Raven Press, New York, pp. 568–576.

Segawa, M. and Nomura, Y., 1995, Hereditary progressive dystonia with marked diurnal fluctuation and dopa-responsive dystonia: Pathognomonic clinical features, In: *Age-Related Dopamine-Dependent Disorders, Monogr. Neural. Sci.,* Vol. 14, M. Segawa and Y. Nomura, eds., Karger, Basel, pp. 10–24.

Segawa, S., Nishiyama, N. and Nomura, Y. Dopa responsive dystonia parkinsonism - Pathophysiological consideration in Parkinson's disease - *Advances in Neurology,* G. Stern, ed., in press.

Shintaku, H., 1994, Early diagnosis of 6-pyruvoyl-tetradropterin synthase deficiency, *Pteridines* 5:18–27.

Snow, B.J., Okada, A., Martin, W.R.W., Duvoisin, R.C. and Calne, D.B., 1993, Positron-emission tomography scanning in dopa-responsive dystonia, parkinsonism-dystonia, and young-onset parkinsonism, In: *Hereditary Progressive Dystonia with Marked Diurnal Fluctuation,* M. Segawa, ed., Parthenon, Carnforth, UK, pp. 181–186.

Steinfels, G.F., Heym, J., Strecker, R.E, and Jacobs B.L., 1983, Behavioural correlates of dopaminergic unit activity in freely moving cats, *Brain Res.* 258:217–228.

Takahashi, H., Levine, R.A., Galloway, M.,P., Snow, B.J., Calne, D.B. and Nygaard, T.G., 1994, Biochemical and fluorodopa positron emission tomographic findings in an asymptomatic carrier of the gene for dopa-responsive dystonia, *Ann. Neurol.* 35: 354–356.

Tsuji, S., Tanaka, H., Miyatake, T., Ginns, E.I., Nomura, Y.,and Segawa, M., 1993, Linkage analysis of hereditary progressive dystonia to the tyrosine hydroxylase gene locus, In: *Hereditary Progressive Dystonia with Marked Diurnal Fluctuation,* M. Segawa, ed. Parthenon, Carnforth, UK, pp. 107–114.

Yamamura, Y., Sobue, I., Ando, K., Iida, M., Yanagi, T.and Kono, C., 1973, Paralysis agitans of early onset with marked diurnal fluctuation of symptoms, *Neurology* 23:239–244.

Yamamura, Y., Hamaguchi, Y., Uchida, M., Fujioka, H., and Watanabe, S., 1993, Parkinsonism of early-onset with diurnal fluctuation, In: *Hereditary Progressive Dystonia with Marked Diurnal Fluctuation,* M. Segawa, ed., Parthenon, Carnforth, UK, pp. 51–59.

Yokochi, M., 1979, Juvenile Parkinson's disease - Part I, clinical aspects, *Adv.Neurol. Sci.* (Tokyo) 23:1060–1073.

Yokochi, M., Narabayashi, H., Izuka, R., and Nagatsu, T, 1984, Juvenile parkinsonism - some clinical, pharmacological and neuropathological aspects, In: *Advances in Neurology,* Vol. 40, R.G. Hassler and J.F. Christ, eds., Raven Press, New York, pp. 407–413.

Yokochi, M.,1995, Juvenile parkinsonism and other dopa-responsive syndromes, In: *Age-Related Dopamine-Dependent Disorders, Monogr. Neural .Sci.,* Vol. 14, M. Segawa and Y. Nomura, eds., Karger, Basel, pp. 25–35.

52

EFFECTS OF PROGRESSIVE NEUROLOGICAL DISEASE ON INTERPERSONAL RELATIONS BETWEEN PATIENTS AND FAMILY MEMBERS

L. L. Sprinzeles

Parkinson's Disease Foundation
New York, New York 10032

INTRODUCTION

This paper addresses the deleterious effects of neurological disorder on interpersonal relations between patients and family members. Although the theme focuses primarily on Parkinson's disease (PD), many of its implications are relevant to Alzheimer's disease (AD) and/or other chronic disorders (Beck et al., 1985; Langston et al., 1992).

Definition: PD (and AD) are uniquely human diseases, (although animal models do exist). They are progressive, neurological disorders of unknown etiology. While climatic or cultural factors do not appear to influence the development of the disorder, there are gender and ethnic differences. The prevalence of PD of men vs. women is an estimated 60:40 ratio. There is also a preponderance of Caucasians afflicted with PD compared to Afro-Americans. PD and AD may coexist, and prevalence increases with age. PD may be caused by: 1- genetic predisposition; 2- exo- or endotoxins; 3- a combination thereof. Research is ongoing, but to date, treatment is palliative. While chromosomes 1, 14, and 21 are thought to carry the mutated gene(s) responsible for the development of some neurological disorders; namely, AD, (and 21 for Down syndrome), mutation of genes on chromosome 4 may lead to the development of PD; and several other chromosomes may carry the mutated genes causing Parkinson plus syndromes (Polymeropoulos et al., 1996). Whereas the onset of PD occurs in approximately 65% or more to people in midlife or later, more than 30% are afflicted at an earlier age. An estimated half to one million people in the U.S. have idiopathic PD which is a form of parkinsonism. The neuronal damage of PD occurs in the substantia nigra in the basal ganglia of the brain. Symptoms are most often controlled for several years, pharmacomedically, and in selective cases surgically. Degeneration in other forms of parkinsonism may take place in the substantia nigra but affects also varied other segments of the brain, and usually, is not responsive to anti-PD medication (Fahn, 1992).

Progress in Alzheimer's and Parkinson's Diseases
·edited by Fisher *et al.*, Plenum Press, New York, 1998.

From a relational perspective, psychological problems and personality difficulties are as diverse among the neurologically afflicted as in the general population. Psychosocial ramifications and impact of PD on interpersonal relations are influenced by many factors (Ellring, 1992). The uncertainty of disease progression, chronicity, unknown etiology and no known cure engender emotional issues which can have a negative impact upon family dynamics (Rosenthal, 1985). This is most aptly expressed by the logo of the Well Spouse Foundation, "Where one is sick two (or more) need help."

Additionally, for the parkinsonian patient, disturbance in neurotransmission by the depletion of dopamine, compounded by deficiency of serotonin, a mood regulating amine in the Raphe nucleus in the brain, and disturbance in other enzymatic functions may cause endogenous depression. Reactive depression may ensue upon receiving a diagnosis of PD. Thus one finds depression as a frequent premorbid or concomitant phenomenon of PD (Mayeux, 1990). It is less "visible" than motor symptoms, is only too often overlooked and receives less attentions than motor symptoms. However, depression may be due to a combination of physiological and psychological factors. Moreover, psychosocial components are known to influence the development and/or resolution of depression.

METHOD

In order to assess the effects of neurological disease on interpersonal relations between patients and family members, the data of two separate investigations were collected and analyzed. The purpose was explained to the participants, and they were given assurance of non-disclosure of information without their consent. 1) Thirty patients with PD and their caregivers who were support group members were individually interviewed on four separate occasions over a forty-two months' timespan. Also, medical records were examined for determination of the patients' level of disability, age range, reported effects of these data on interpersonal relations, and patients' disposition status at the end of the forty-two months (Mace 1992). 2) A one-time interview of twenty-four spouses was conducted to determine the prevalence of depression among them. They were seen during the waiting period of patients' medical visits, given a questionnaire and a Minnesota Multiphasic Personality Inventory (MMPI) for completion, and were requested to rate partners' present functionality compared to the previous year. The findings are described in Discussion or Results, respectively, and MMPI data are listed in Table 1 (Gilberstadt, 1965).

DISCUSSION

The surveyed population of patients with PD and family members reported the following personality characteristics and other manifestations which they perceived to have caused disturbance in family relations: 1) Patients' diminished functional ability, be it physical, mental or both (Stern, 1993), and family members' limitation to pursue personal, social or occupational goals (Duvoisin, 1991); 2) Depression, loss of communication and partnership; 3) Fear of social unacceptability or embarrassment by either party because of inability to conform to perceived social norms with resultant social isolation (A. Strauss, 1984); 4) Financial problems due to the inverse ratio of increased health care cost and decreased income (P.J. Strauss, 1994); 5) Role reversal; 6) Sexual dysfunction (Lipe, 1992);

7) Increased workload of caregiver; 8) Incontinence; 9) Sleep disturbance (Pollak, 1991); and, 10) dementia (Stern, 1993).

Communication with and education of patients and families focused on PD and its ramifications. This was particularly important in dealing with newly diagnosed patients and their families who were often overwhelmed by the implications of the disease and reacted with feelings of loss and mourning. Confusing also is the patients' functional unpredictability, being able to perform a task one minute and not the next; or being unable to engage in two concurrent tasks. These variations are sometimes misinterpreted as unwillingness, lack of motivation, self-pity or dependency (Huber, 1990).

Age at onset of the disease may also influence interpersonal relations. Young patients may face loss of employment and income, worry about children's education, fear inadequate personal, social or sexual performance, increasing dependency of long duration, role reversal, guilt about the uncertainty of transmission of defective genes to their offspring, and so on. Family members may resent the imposition of additional tasks and limitations of pursuits or may also fear heredity. When the disease strikes at an older age, earlier stage of life issues hopefully have been resolved (Strong, 1990). Usually, older couples have had more time together to cement their relationship. Children have at least reached chronological independence. Retirement is not as threatening anymore. In the rarer situation of parents caring for an afflicted child, guilt about having caused the affliction may result in total absorption in caregiving to the exclusion of other activities, and in the case of younger families often to the detriment of patients' siblings (Waite, 1990).

It is invariably more difficult for family members than for patients to cope with patients' declining cognitive functions or dementia than with physical impairment, since meaningful communication is rarely possible (Stern, 1993). Dementia may be due to: 1) The progression of the disease; 2) An underlying different disease; or 3) The response to the anti-PD medication. In the first situation, palliative measures such as exposure to premorbidly enjoyed or other stimulating activities, socialization in a protected environment, etc. have often been found beneficial for patients (and may lighten the burden of family members). Depending on the cause of the second condition, treatment needs to be adjusted to the specific disease. In the third situation, decrease of anti-PD medication may improve mentation but worsen motor symptoms. Unfortunately, dementia is hardly, if ever, responsive to currently available treatment. Physiostigmine or Tacrine, the substances used to treat dementia in AD were found only minimally effective for AD or PD. Assessment of the long-term effectiveness of the newer substance Aricept, has not yet been tested for a sufficient length of time to evaluate the results. While pharmacological and/or surgical treatment reduce the morbidity of PD, adjunctive modalities tend to enhance therapeutic results. For example: 1) Physical therapy and exercise help maintain or improve mobility and circulation (Steefel, 1997); 2) Psychological counseling is designed to mitigate emotional pain (Brown, 1997); 3) Music therapy is often beneficial in lifting depression; 4) Occupational therapy, and in some cases assistive devices are useful in overcoming impairment of activities of daily living (ADL); 5) Respiratory and/or speech therapy may make the difference in patients' breathing technique, intelligibility of speech and voice projection; 6) support group participation reduces social isolation (Atwood, 1991); 7) Some patients need protein re-distribution to derive full benefit from their medication, etc. (Scheider et al., 1997).

Premorbid personality and the quality of family support system will to an extent determine coping effectiveness. It is likely that premorbidly self-assertive people will aim at retaining maximum independence and optimum level of functioning, while passive individuals are more apt to regress to childlike dependency. On the other hand, physically active or socially conscious people may feel embarrassed by visible symptoms, retreat into the confines of their homes with resultant social isolation. Depression and loss of initiative may ensue in patients and family members. Freedom of action of the non-afflicted family members may be seriously curtailed. These phenomena often cause anger, resentment, frustration and varied negative feelings which undermine family dynamics. It is important for the non-afflicted individuals, particularly the caregivers to eke out some time for themselves. Caregivers who are totally immersed in attending to the patients' nursing needs may themselves suffer physical or mental breakdown. Support group members are able to impact upon such individuals by pointing out to them their modus operandi. Constructive criticism from peers is often more readily accepted than from professionals because of shared experiences and empathy (Conti, 1996).

RESULTS

Of the thirty caregivers who were support group members, twenty-one were able to keep the patients at home; nine were institutionalized. The results of the initial investigations are as follows: Patients' age at diagnosis ranged from forty-seven to seventy years, and disease duration from two to twenty-three years.

Patients who were former group participants, now institutionalized, were compared to institutionalized patients who were non-support group members. The first group of institutionalized patients were no longer kept at home because of physical and mental decline (stages four to five). Their ages ranged from forty-seven to seventy years with a disease duration of ten to twenty-three years. The institutionalized non-support group patients were in the approximate age range at the time of onset of the disease as their counterparts in the first group, but were placed in homes at an earlier (average) stage of disease, (stages three to five), five to twelve years after diagnosis of PD. The second investigation dealt with the prevalence of depression among caregivers of non-institutionalized patients. The questionnaire was completed by twenty-four caregivers (twenty-three were the patients' spouses). It included their rating of patients' present functionality compared to the previous year. Only mild deterioration was reported by caregivers which was documented by medical records. Of particular note is the value of maintaining the patients' occupational pursuits. This may require work modification compatible with their abilities but within their limitations (Nagler, 1990). There may be additional advantages in facilitating caregivers' occupational pursuit, reducing financial pressure, alleviating anger, resentment, boredom, depression, etc. Although the twenty-four interviewees denied feelings of depression, of the ten MMPI scales, the spouses scored highest on depression. However, the scores of twelve individuals were above the seventieth percentile which is statistically significant. The itemized scores on the MMPI scales are listed in Table 1.

Table 1. Itemized scores on the MMPI scales

Hypochondriasis	Hs	8–26	Depression	D	27–64
Hysteria	Hy	20–35	Psychopathic deviate	Pd	10–26
Masculinity/femininity	Mf	21–38	Paranoia	Pa	5–15
Psychathenia	Pt	4–34	Schizophrenia	Sc	8–17
Hypomania	Ma	4–19	Social introversion	Si	24–48
Cannot say?		1–9	Lie	L	1–9
Validity	F	9–28	Correction	K	6–21

CONCLUSIONS

Although to date, there is no cure for PD, symptoms can usually be controlled for several years. education about the intricacies of the disease and timely intervention often helped families identify problems and acquire workable coping mechanisms. Adjunctive treatment modalities have been found to improve or maintain patients' functionality. Also, support groups helped people become or remain involved in personal, occupational or social activities, enabled them to communicate openly, reduced social isolation and mitigated deleterious effects on interpersonal relations between patients and family members. Furthermore, the data of the two aforementioned investigations showed a decrease in the rate of institutionalized patients compared to their non-support group counterparts.

REFERENCES

Atwood, G.W.A.T., 1991, Support Groups: Where You Learn What Your Doctor Hasn't Time To Tell You, In: Living Well With Parkinson's Disease, *Wiley& Sons*, NY, pp 149–156.

Beck, A.T. et al., "Depression,"In: Clinical Handbook of Psychological Disorders, D.H. Barlow, ed., *The Guilford Press*, NY, pp 205–225.

Brown, L.S., 1997, Exile and Redemption in Psychology, *Journal of the American Psychological Association.* 54:4–452.

Conti, V.L., 1996, The Heartache of Stress, National Center for Research Resources (NCRR) Report.20:5–7.

Duvoisin, R.C., 1991, Parkinson's Disease: A Guide for Patient and Family, Third Edition, *Raven Press,* NY, pp 1–169.

Ellring, H., 1992, Psychological Aspects in Parkinson's Disease, Movement Disorders, Supplement 1, *Raven Press,* NY, 7:181–191.

Fahn, S., 1992, "Adverse Effects of Levodopa," in: The Scientific Basis for Treatment of Parkinson's Disease, R. Olanow and A. Lieberman, eds., *The Parthenon Publishing Group,* Park Ridge, pp 89–112.

Gilberstadt, H., et al., 1965, A Handbook for Clinical and Actuarial MMPI Interpretation, *W.B. Saunders Company*, Philadelphia, pp 3–6.

Huber, S.J., 1990, "Management of Behavioral Symptoms in Parkinson's Disease," in: Handbook of Parkinson's Disease, W.C. Koller and G. Paulson, eds., *Marcel Dekker,* Inc., NY, pp 557–566.

Langston, W.C., et al., 1992, "Etiology of Parkinson's Disease," in: The Scientific Basis for the Treatment of Parkinson's Disease, op. cit., pp 33–58.

Lipe, H. et al., 1990, Sexual Function of Married Men with Parkinson's Disease Compared to Sexual Function of Married Men with Arthritis, *Neurology*, 40:1347–1349.

Mace, N.L., et al., 1992, A Family Guide to Caring for Persons with Alzheimer's Disease, *Warren Brooks Edition,* NY, pp 211–216.

Mayeux, R., et al., 1990, "Assessment of Depression in Parkinson's Disease," in: Parkinson's Disease, C. Rose, ed., *Demos Publishers,* NY, pp 43–49.

Nagler, M., 1990, What It Means To Be Different: Perspective of the Disabled, in: Perspective on Disability, *Health Market Research,* Palo Alta, pp 587–594.

Pollak, C.P., et al., 1991, Sleep Problems and Institutionalization of the Elderly, *Journal of Psychiatry and Neurology*, 4:204–218.

Polymeropoulos, M.H., et al., 1996, Mapping of a Gene for Parkinson's Disease to Chromosome 4q21-q23, in: *Science,* 274:1197–1199.

Rosenthal, T.L., et al., 1985, "Clinical Stress Management," in: *Clinical Handbook of Psychological Disorders,* op. cit., pp 145–205.

Scheider, I., et al., 1997, Dietary Oxidants and Other Dietary Factors in the Etiology of Parkinson's Disease. *Movement Disorders,* 12:2:190–196.

Steefel, L.,1997, Massage Therapy as an Adjunct Healing Modality in Parkinson's Disease, *Alternative Complementary Therapies,* 2:6–13.

Stern, Y., et al., 1993, "Mental Dysfunction in Parkinson's Disease" in: Mental Dysfunction in Parkinson's Disease, E.C.Wolters and P. Scheltems, eds., Vrije Universiteir, *The Netherlands,* pp 123–132.

Strauss, A., 1984, Chronic Illness and the Quality of Life, C.V. Mosby Company, Baltimore.

Strauss, P.J., 1994, Medical Coverage for the Middleclass Elderly, in: *New York Times*, Section B, pp 1–5.
Strong, M., 1990, Mainstay, *Little Brown & Co.*, Boston, pp 557–566 .
Waite, L., 1990, Coping Responses to the Stresses of Parkinson's Disease, Master's Thesis, University of California.

53

COGNITIVE DEFICITS IN ALZHEIMER'S DISEASE, PARKINSON'S DISEASE, AND HUNTINGTON'S CHOREA

Elka Stefanova,[1] Vladimir Kostic,[1] Gordana Ocic,[1], and Ljubomir Ziropadja[2]

[1]Institute of Neurology CCS
ul. Dr Subotica 6, 11000 Belgrade, Yugoslavia
[2]Faculty of Philology
University of Belgrade
Yugoslavia

INTRODUCTION

Since the description of the currently somewhat controversial distinction between "cortical" and "subcortical" dementia (Albert et al., 1974), it is an important issue whether dementias arising from different causative factors exhibit qualitatively different patterns of cognitive deficit. Despite many differences, dementia of Alzheimer's type (DAT), dementia in Parkinson's disease (PD), and Huntington's disease (HD) share many common neuropathological, neurochemical and neuropsychological features (Brown and Marsden, 1988).

The aim of this study was to compare patients in the early stage of DAT, HD and PD, matched for the level of dementia on different cognitive abilities, applying extensive neuropsychological tests which covered memory, intellectual abilities, language, visuospatial and executive functions.

METHODS

The study comprised 10 outpatients in each of the three groups: with DAT, HD and PD, and with the Mini Mental State Examination (MMSE) score between 17 and 24. The NWSE score did not differ between the DAT, HD and PD groups (being 20.8 ± 2.1, 21.1 ± 2.0, and 21.7 ± 2.0, respectively) and suggested the existence of mild to moderate dementia. The patients with HD were younger (38.4 ± 13.2 years) than the patients with DAT (63.3 ± 7.8 years), and with PD (63.7 ± 6.6 years). The groups of DAT, HD and PD patients had the same educational level with a mean of 12.5, 10.2, and 10.9 years, respectively.

Progress in Alzheimer's and Parkinson's Diseases
edited by Fisher *et al.*, Plenum Press, New York, 1998.

The diagnosis of probable DAT was determined according to the DSM-IV and NINDSADRDA criteria (McKhann et al., 1984), as well as the Hachinski ischemic score < 4. All patients with HD were in functional stage 2 (Shoulson and Fahn, 1979); i.e. they could manage in daily life without help. The mean stage of PD patients according to Hoehn and Yahr was 2.8. Anticholinergic therapy was an exclusion criterion. To gauge the absolute levels of impairment in the groups with DAT, HD and PD we used control data from our neuropsychological department, obtained from age-matched healthy controls with comparable educational level.

General intellectual abilities were assessed by the Wechsler Adult Intelligence Scale-Revised form (WAIS-R). IQ scores [full IQ (FIQ), verbal IQ (VIQ), and performance IQ (PIQ)], as well as scaled scores from 11 subtests of the WAIS-R were calculated. For general memory testing the Wechsler Memory Scale-Revised (WMS-R) was used. In addition, the following complementary tests were administered: Wisconsin Card Sorting Test (WCST), Rey-Osterieth Complex Figure Test (R-OCFT), Rey Auditory Verbal Learning Test (R-AVLT), adapted to the Serbian Language Phonemic Fluency Test with the letters S, K, and L chosen; Category Fluency Test; Trail Making Test (TMT) form A and B; and Boston Naming Test (BNT).

Statistical analyses were performed using Statistical Packages for Social Sciences (SPSS, 1994). Discriminant analysis was performed in order to determine whether the observed profile difference was sufficiently consistent to classify correctly patients with DAT, HD and PD.

RESULTS

The patients in all three groups were significantly worse than their matched healthy controls on the tests we used in this study (data not shown).

Considering different MMSE items score, 90% of DAT patients compared to 40% of PD and 20% of HD patients who gave insufficient data on the time orientation item ($\chi^2 = 18.2$; df = 4; p < 0.001). Analyses of the place orientation ($\chi^2 = 10.6$; df = 4; p < 0.05) and the short delay recall ($\chi^2 = 27.6$; df = 4; p < 0.001) items revealed a similar insufficiency in the DAT group: 80% of DAT patients did not recall one word on short delay recall item, while noone within the HD and PD groups showed such impairment. On the repetition item only 60% of subjects with HD gave a correct answer ($\chi^2 = 9.2$; df = 2; p < 0.01), in comparison to 100% in the DAT and PD groups. The DAT (90%) and PD (100%) patients correctly performed the three-demand praxis task, in comparison to only 30% in the HD group ($\chi^2 = 14.9$; df = 4; p < 0.01).

The results of the WAIS-R measures are shown in Table 1. On FSIQ the post hoc Scheffé procedure proved only the difference between PD and HD patients. On the VIQ score the PD group was superior to patients with DAT and HD. For the digit symbol performance the post hoc Scheffé procedure revealed a significant difference only between the PD and HD patients.

One way ANOVA showed significant intergroup differences on several measures of WMS-R (Table 2). The post hoc Scheffé procedure indicated clear superiority of the PD group on attention-concentration measure in comparison to patients with DAT and HD. The lowest performance on the verbal paired associates learning task, as well as on the delayed visual reproduction subtest and visual span task was found in the DAT group. For the visual paired associates task, DAT patients were insufficient only in comparison to the PD group.

Table 1. Overall achievements on WAIS-R in patients with Alzheimer's disease, Huntington's disease, and Parkinson's disease, ANOVA F values, and significance

Variable	DAT	HD	PD	$F_{(2,27)}$	Significance
FSIQ	86.9 ± 7.3	80.5 ± 5.9	95 ± 10.4	8.03	p = 0.0018***
VIQ	97.5 ± 10.3	83.2 ± 4.9	101 ± 8.9	13.07	p = 0.0001***
Information	8.4 ± 1.7	7.3 ± 2.3	9.2 ± 2.5	1.80	ns
Digit span	6.5 ± 1.2	6.7 ± 2.9	7.3 ± 2.0	0.36	ns
Vocabulary	8.2 ± 2.8	7.5 ± 1.7	8.0 ± 1.7	0.28	ns
Arithmetic	5.9 ± 2.3	5.6 ± 1.7	7.9 ± 2.1	3.57	p = 0.04*
Comprehension	7.6 ± 2.0	6.9 ± 2.2	8.0 ± 3.1	0.51	ns
Similarities	5.9 ± 1.9	7.2 ± 1.8	7.2 ± 2.9	1.05	ns
PIQ	79.5 ± 5.7	79.3 ± 8.5	86.4 ± 8.7	2.69	ns
Picture completion	5.1 ± 1.1	6.7 ± 1.3	6.4 ± 1.8	3.40	p = 0.048*
Picture arrangement	5.1 ± 1.4	6.0 ± 0.9	5.8 ± 1.3	1.41	ns
Block design	2.5 ± 2.3	4.8 ± 1.7	4.4 ± 2.4	3.17	ns
Object assembly	4.0 ± 1.2	6.0 ± 2.2	5.0 ± 1.7	3.21	ns
Digit symbol	3.0 ± 1.5	4.4 ± 1.7	2.4 ± 1.3	4.67	p = 0.018**

DAT = dementia of Alzheimer's type; HD = Huntington disease; PD = Parkinson's disease; FSIQ = full scale IQ; VIQ = verbal IQ; PIQ = performance IQ; ns = not significant.

On the R-AVLT, the groups differ significantly in learning only on the third [$F_{(2,27)}$ = 3.7; p < 0.05] and fourth trial [$F_{(2,27)}$ = 5.6; p < 0.01]: the PD group was superior to the DAT patients on the third and fourth trial, while HD patients were superior to the DAT group only on the fourth trial (Figure 1). The performance on the R-AVLT delay task was significantly different among the groups [$F_{(2,27)}$ = 7.0; p < 0.01], with significant insufficiency of DAT in comparison to PD and HD groups. At the recognition trial a strikingly different main group effect was obtained [$F_{(2,27)}$ = 21.1; p < 0.001]. The patients with DAT failed to recognize the

Table 2. Overall achievements on WMS-R in patients with Alzheimer's disease, Huntington's disease, and Parkinson's disease, F values, significance

Variable	DAT	HD	PD	$F_{(2,27)}$	Significance
Img	63.3 ± 16.3	50 ± 13.3	81.4 ± 18.6	3.98	p = 0.03*
Imv	75.5 ± 18.4	71.7 ± 11.03	85.4 ± 17.9	1.91	ns
Logical memory	13.2 ± 8.0	14.6 ± 5.8	18.3 ± 8.4	1.23	ns
Verbal paired associates	7.3 ± 3.3	13.3 ± 2.5	16.1 ± 5.2	13.5	p = 0.0001***
Imvis	63.0 ± 20.5	63.7 ± 16.6	72.2 ± 16.6	0.80	ns
Figural memory	4.2 ± 2.1	5.5 ± 1.5	5.1 ± 1.8	1.28	ns
Visual paired associates	3.6 ± 2.0	4.7 ± 2.1	6.8 ± 2.4	5.4	p = 0.01**
Visual reproduction	11.8 ± 12.3	18.7 ± 7.4	19.5 ± 9.1	1.86	ns
Ia/c	64.0 ± 11.2	63.1 ± 13.0	80.1 ± 13.2	5.80	p = 0.008**
Mental control	3.0 ± 1.9	3.1 ± 0.9	4.4 ± 1.1	2.98	ns
Digit span	9.6 ± 1.7	9.9 ± 3.6	11.4 ± 2.0	1.39	ns
Visual span	6.6 ± 2.7	10.3 ± 2.4	12.1 ± 2.5	11.7	p = 0.0002***
Imdg	63.0 ± 10.0	60.9 ± 7.5	73.8 ± 13.7	4.49	p = 0.02*
Logical memory	7.1 ± 5.0	10.8 ± 6.1	13.5 ± 7.6	2.55	ns
Visual paired associates	1.9 ± 1.1	1.6 ± 1.0	3.3 ± 2.1	3.52	p = 0.044*
Verbal paired associates	3.4 ± 1.7	4.3 ± 1.8	5.0 ± 1.8	1.88	ns
Visual reproduction	0.4 ± 0.6	10.8 ± 6.8	10.8 ± 8.5	8.96	p = 0.001***

DAT = dementia of Alzheimer's type; HD = Huntington's disease; PD = Parkinson's disease; Img = general memory index; IMv = verbal memory index; IMvis = visual memory index; Ia/c = attention concentration index; IMdg = delayed memory index; ns = not significant.

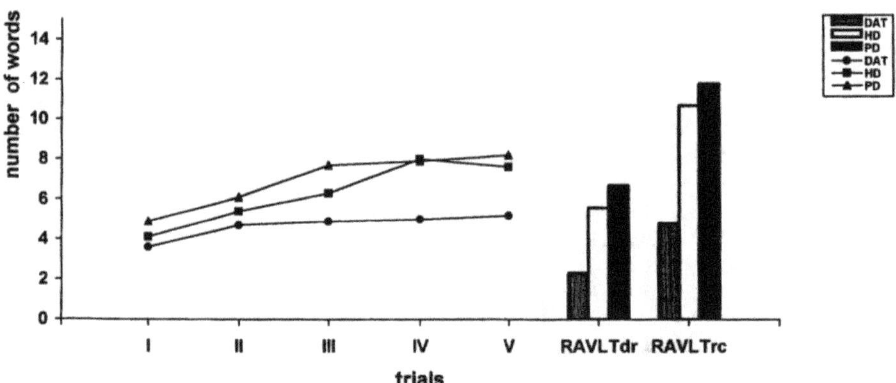

Figure 1. Performance on Rey-Auditory Verbal Learning Test (R-AVLT) across five learning trials, 30 minutes delay recall (dr), and recognition trials (rc).

previously learned words relative to PD and HD patients (Figure 1). One way ANOVA revealed a significant intergroup difference in terms of produced confabulations [$F_{(2,27)}$ = 14.3; $p < 0.001$] and in the number of perseverated words on recall trials [$F_{(2,27)}$ = 7.5; $p < 0.01$] post hoc Scheffé analysis suggested that the DAT group was predominant in confabulation production relative to HD and PD, while on recall trials the HD patients perseverated more than DAT and PD patients.

Significantly different 3-minutes [$F_{(2,27)}$ = 9.6; $p < 0.001$] and 45-minutes [$F_{(2,27)}$ = 11.4; $p < 0.001$] delayed recalls on the R-OCFT were found: the DAT group was significantly insufficient in comparison to the PD group on both tasks. The same pattern was obtained for semantic fluency [$F_{(2,27)}$ = 11.6; $p < 0.001$] and BNT [$F_{(2,27)}$ = 19.5; $p < 0.001$]: the DAT group was insufficient in comparison to the HD and PD groups. The DAT group was severely impaired on the copy trial of R-OCFT, compared to HD and PD patients' performance [$F_{(2,27)}$ = 8.0; $p < 0.001$]. The same pattern of insufficiency was obtained for the Hooper visual organization test [$F_{(2,27)}$ = 9.8; $p < 0.001$].

A significant intergroup difference was obtained for achieved number of categories [$F_{(2,27)}$ = 3.7; $p < 0.05$]) and number of perseverative errors [$F_{(2,27)}$ = 3.5; $p < 0.05$] on WCST, but post hoc tests only showed a dfference between the PD and DAT groups on these measures.

One way ANOVA revealed that the DAT group had significantly [$F_{(2,27)}$ = 4.5; $p < 0.05$] prolonged completion of TMT A compared to PD patients only, while on TMT B [$F_{(2,27)}$ = 11.8; $p < 0.001$], the disability in DAT was clearly distinct in both PD and HD groups.

The variables that differed between the studied groups of patients were classified into two groups: (a) first, the "attention/executive function" group included the WAIS-R subtest scores (arithmetic, picture completion, and digit symbol), WMS-R scores (attention/concentration index, visual span), WCST scores (number of categories and perseverative errors), and TMT A and B scores; and (b) second, the "memory" group was comprised of WAIS-R VIQ score, WMS-R scores (IM dg, visual and verbal paired associates), delayed recall and recognition scores on R-AVLT, and delayed recall score on R-OCFT and BNT scores. A step-wise discriminant function analysis was performed to assess the prediction of membership in the three groups (DAT, HD and PD) from the nine variables from the first group. A significant discrimination [$F_{(12,44)}$ = 7.7; $p < 0.001$] was obtained on the basis of six included variables (arithmetic, picture completion, digit symbol, visual span, WCST categories and TMT B score), so the 100% of patients with PD, 70% with HD and 90% with DAT were correctly classified. On these six predictor variables two discriminant functions were calculated with the combined $\chi^2(5) = 15.5$ (p < 0.01). The two discriminant functions accounted for 82% and 18% of the intergroup variability. The first function maximally discriminated PD and DAT patients, with the HD group falling between the two groups (Figure 2). The second discriminant function differed HD and PD groups on one side and DAT patients on another. Correlations of six predictor variables and the two discriminant functions suggest that the first could be defined as attention or "working memory" function and the second as executive function. For the second, "memory" group a step-wise discriminant function analysis was also performed using ten memory scores (see above) as predictors of membership in three groups of patients. On the basis of six variables (WAIS-R VIQ, verbal paired associates, delayed recall and recognition scores on RAVLT, and BNT scores) 90% of all the patients were correctly classified. Two discriminant functions were obtained with combined $\chi^2(5) = 24.16$ (p < 0.001). The two discriminant functions accounted for 72% and 28% of the between-group variability. The first function maximally separates DAT patients from the other two groups. The second discriminant function differs HD and DAT group from PD patients. Three predictors (verbal paired associates, delay recall on RAVLT, and correct naming on BNT) have high account in the first discriminant function which appears to tap episodic memory functions. The second discriminant function has its main contribution from VIQ and number of correct naming with phonemic clue, and appear to represent general verbal semantic knowledge.

DISCUSSION

The results of the MMSE items analysis in this study indicate the existence of qualitative differences in cognitive impairment among the DAT, HD and demented PD patients,

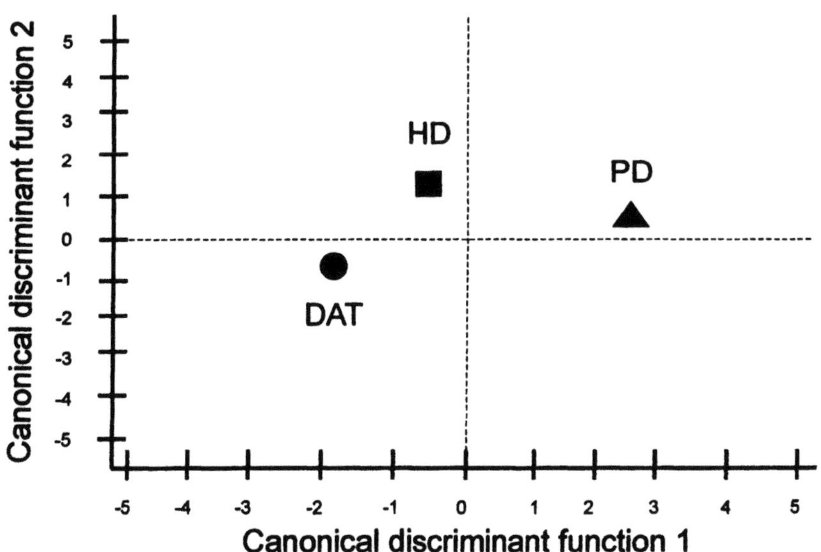

Figure 2. Plot of the three groups' (DAT, HD, and PD) centroides on two canonical discriminant functions derived from six scores from "attention/executive" function group.

who were otherwise matched according to the global MMSE scores, even in the early stages of dementing illness. An insufficiency on the date and place orientation, as well as short delay items, was specific for the DAT group, while repetition and praxis items were specific for the HD group. Brandt et al. (1988) have shown that the distinct pattern of cognitive impairment evidenced with a relatively simple, standardized test (memory and attention/conceptual tracking items from MMSE) are sufficiently robust to classify patients with DAT and HD with 84% accuracy. However, Mayeux et al. (1983), using modified MMSE in patients with DAT, HD and PD, failed to find evidence for differential neuropsychological deficits. Although our results suggest that differences between these groups of demented patients can be identified even with a brief mental status examination test, they should be taken cautiously due to the small number of included patients.

DAT patients were also distinctly impaired on the episodic memory task for verbal and visual modality, on the cued learning task (visual and verbal paired associates) and on semantic memory. It is worth mentioning that a deficient general verbal semantic knowledge was evident early in the course of DAT and HD. The study on DAT patients showed a significant impairment on tests which depend upon the integrity of semantic knowledge compared to HD subjects, whose poor performance on episodic and semantic memory tasks has been associated with a general retrieval deficit (Hodges et al., 1990). Also, the DAT patients in our study generated more intrusions and false recognition on learning tasks. Performance on the Brown Peterson task (another task for short-term memory) was impaired in HD, DAT and demented PD patients, but not in PD without dementia (Beatty, 1992). Our results did not show a difference in the digit span task (WMS-R) between studied groups, but for the visual span capacity a clear sensitivity was revealed, indicating that DAT subjects were impaired even in the early stages of dementia.

A significant sensitivity in the HD group was registered for the visual episodic memory task (free and cued recall). Further, a deficient and unstable rate of improvement across successive learning trials and greater perseverative rate was observed in our HD

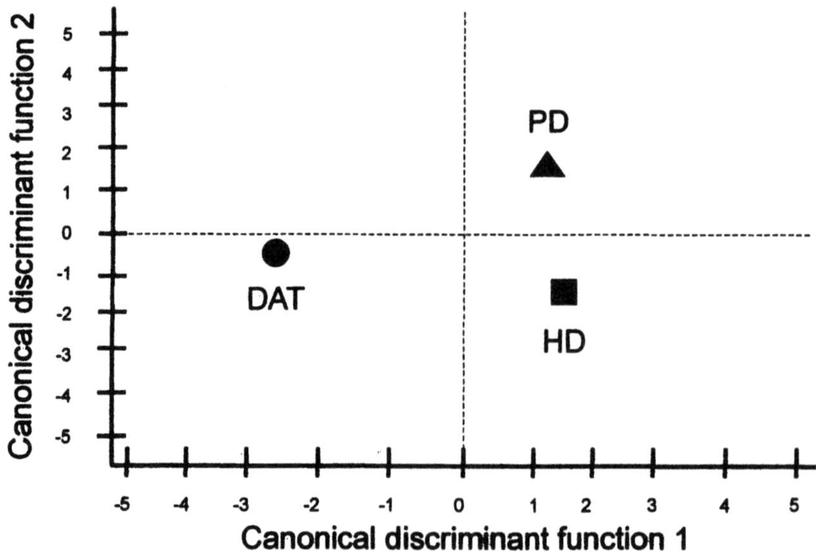

Figure 3. Plot of the three groups' (DAT, HD, and PD) centroides on two canonical discriminant functions derived from six scores from "memory" group.

group with mild dementia, which is in accordance to previously published data (Massman et al., 1990). Recognition was still well preserved, confirming the suggestion of mild encoding impairment, preserved storage and free recall deficits in HD subjects (Pillon et al., 1993). A distinct, insufficient performance was also observed on attention/concentration abilities in our HD group.

Executive deficits, as well as visuospatial disabilities were present in all three groups, especially in our mildly demented DAT patients. The PD group showed difficulties only on visuomotor tracking performance and, interestingly enough, was slightly insufficient in comparison to the HD group on global executive measuring, when various tests were considered. Mohr et al. (1990) reported visuospatial function deficits in DAT, demented PD patients, and even in high-functioning PD subjects early in the course of the disease. The PD group was superior to DAT and HD patients on attention or working memory measures.

In conclusion, even in the early stages of DAT, HD and PD with dementia, and despite equal scores on the MMSE, it seems possible to define specific measures that give acceptable discrimination of the patterns of cognitive deficits associated with these three entities.

REFERENCES

Albeit, M., Feldman, R.G., and Willis, A.L., 1974, The "subcortical dementia" of progressive supranuclear palsy. *J. Neurol. Neurosurg. Psychiatry* 3 7:121–13 0.

Beatty, W.W., 1992, Memory dysfunction in the subcortical dementias. In: *Memory functioning in dementia*, Backman, L., ed., Amsterdam, Elsevier, pp. 153–173.

Brandt, J., Folstein, S.E., and Folstein, M.F., 1988, Differential cognitive impairment in Alzheimer's disease and Huntingon's disease. Ann. Neurol. 23:555–561.

Brown, R.G., and Marsden, C.D., 1988, "Subcortical dementia": the neuropsychological evidence. *Neuroscience 25:363–387.*

Hodges, J.R., Salmon, D.P., and Butters, N., 1990, Differential impairment of semantic and episodic memory in Alzheimer's and Huntington's diseases: a controlled prospective study. *J. Neurol Neurosurg.Psychiatry 53:1089–1095.*

Massman, P.J., Delis, D.C., Butters, N., Levin, B.E., and Salmon, D.P., 1990, Are all subcortical dementias alike? Verbal learning and memory in Parkinson's and Huntington's disease patients. *J. Clin. Exp. Neuropsychol. 12:729–744.*

McKhann, G., Drachmann, D., Folstein, M., Katzman, R., Price, D., and Stadlan, E.M., 1984, Clinical diagnosis of Alzheimer's disease: report of the NINCDS-ADRDA criteria Work Group under the auspices of Department of Health and Human Services Task Force on Alzheimer's disease. *Neurology* 34:939–944.

Mohr, E., Litvan, I., Williams, J., Fedio, P., and Chase, T., 1990, Selective deficits in Alzheimer and parkinsonian dementia: visuospatial function. *Can. J. Neurol. Sci.* 17:292–297.

Pillon, B., Dewee, B., Agid, Y., and Dubois, B., 1993, Explicit memory in Alzheimer's, Huntington's and Parkinson's diseases. *Arch. Neurol.* 50:374–379.

Shoulson, I., and Fahn, S., 1979, Huntington's disease: clinical care and evaluation. *Neurology 29:1–3.* PSS, 1994, Statistical package for social sciences, version 6. Chicago, SPSS.

54

RECALL OF YTZHAK RABIN'S ASSASSINATION BY DEMENTED PEOPLE

T. A. Treves, S. Klimowitzky, R. Verchovsky, and A. D. Korczyn

Department of Neurology
Tel Aviv Medical Center
Sackler Faculty of Medicine
Tel Aviv University

INTRODUCTION

Patients with Alzheimer's disease (AD) suffer from decline of memory, which may be more pronounced for anterograde than retrograde events. The deficits refer mostly to biographical and public events (Lezak, 1995; Greene and Hodges, 1996). Nevertheless, it is likely that repetition of information may prevent forgetting. The historical importance of Prime Minister Ytzhak Rabin's assassination in 1995 prompted us to ask whether such an event, which was repetitively covered by the media, is retained by demented patients.

METHODS

We included in this study consecutive patients examined at our Memory Disorders Clinic in the first months of 1996, provided that their memory decline started prior to November 1995. They were required to respond to questions related to Ytzhak Rabin's death and to political personalities murdered in other countries. Dementia and AD were diagnosed by the DSM-IV and the NINCDS-ADRDA criteria (APA, 1994; McKahnn et al., 1984). Only patients with probable AD (n = 40) were included. Controls were also requested to respond to the same questions. The controls (n = 41), who were patients' caregivers, generally the spouses, had been presumably equally exposed to the public broadcasts and were of similar educational background. Patients with memory decline, but who did not fulfill criteria for dementia (subjective memory complaints, SMC, n = 37), were interviewed in a similar way. The questions were asked approximately 6 months (mean = 6.2 months, SD = 1.2) after the assassination. The subjects were also graded according to the Clinical Dementia Rating scale [(CDR), Hughes et al., 1982]. In the frame of neuropsychological assessment,

Progress in Alzheimer's and Parkinson's Diseases
edited by Fisher *et al.*, Plenum Press, New York, 1998.

all the patients underwent a minimental status examination [(MMSE), Folstein et al., 1975]. The answers given by the patients were compared to those obtained from the controls, using the χ^2 test. The probability of forgetting Ytzhak Rabin's name, or what happened to him, were assessed using logistic regression model wherein the age, gender, schooling level, and cognitive status (MMSE) were included as independent variables.

RESULTS

The patients' characteristics are summarized in Table 1. Sixteen patients (40%), but none of the non-demented subjects, could not recall Rabin's name. When reminded, only 3 patients, but none of the controls or SMC, did not remember that the fact that Ytzhak Rabin was assassinated (Table 2). Thus, this question did not differentiate between demented and non-demented subjects. Conversely, none of the AD patients and only 2 controls and 6 SMC subjects recalled the weekday of the event (Table 2). All the controls and SMC subjects, but only 52% of AD patients, knew the nationality of the murderer ($\chi^2 = 19$, p < .001). AD patients commonly failed to answer questions related to the assassination of Presidents Sadat, Kennedy, Lincoln or Prime Minister Indira Gandhi, while most of the patients and controls did not remember the name of Olof Palme (Table 2). Answers given by SMC subjects were similar to those obtained from controls, except for the name of India's Prime Minister for which correct answers were significantly (χ^2, p < .05) more commonly given by the controls than by SMC subjects (Table 2).

Among patients, incorrect answers to "who was the previous prime minister" were associated with lower MMSE scores and older age [OR = .6 (CI: .4–.8), p = .0002 and OR = 1.3 (CI: –1.1–1.6), p = .004] but not by the other variables included in the model. In these terms, "what happened to Ytzhak Rabin" could not be analyzed because there were too few incorrect answers.

DISCUSSION

Although relatively few demented patients could recall the name of the previous Israeli Prime Minister, almost all recalled that he was assassinated. However, they could not recall details of the event. The fact that they could remember what happened to Ytzhak

Table 1. Sample population characteristics

	AD* n = 40	SMC* n = 37	Controls n = 41
Males/females**	15/25	26/11	22/19
Age [mean (SD), in years]**	74 (6.7)	71.5 (8.8)	69.2 (7.7)
Schooling [mean (SD), in years]	11 (4)	12 (3)	11 (3)
MMSE [mean (SD)]**	19 (7.3)	28.7 (1.2)	—
CDR (median)**	1	.5	0
Duration of memory decline [mean (SD) in years]	3.6 (2)	5 (4)	—
Time elapsed since Rabin's death to interview [mean (SD) in months]	6.1 (1.3)	6.1 (1.2)	6.5 (1)

*AD = Alzheimer's disease, SMC = people with subjective memory complaints only.
**Variables for which there were statistically significant differences between the groups [Pearson χ^2 for gender (df = 3, p = .02), ANOVA for age (F = 4.6, df = 2, p = .01) and MMSE (F = 61, df = 1, p < .001), median test for CDR].

Table 2. Frequency of answers to questions related to public events (correct/incorrect)

	AD (n = 40)	SMC (n = 37)	Controls (n = 41)
Name of present prime minister (Peres)*	26/14	37/0	41/0
Name of previous prime minister (Rabin)*	24/16	37/0	41/0
What happened to Ytzhak Rabin	36/3	37/0	41/0
Rabin's death			
-day of the week (Saturday)	0/40	6/31	2/39
-day of the month (4th)*	1/39	11/26	16/25
-month (November)*	4/36	18/19	18/23
-year (1995)*	8/32	28/9	34/7
-place (Kings of Israel Square)*	19/21	36/2	39/2
Murderer's			
-name*	9/30	32/5	40/0
-age*	26/14	37/0	41/0
-nationality*	21/19	37/0	41/0
-profession*	21/19	36/1	41/0
-University's name*	19/21	36/1	40/1
-present residence*	27/13	37/0	41/0
Name of Egypt's murdered President (Sadat)*	12/28	32/5	40/1
Names of murdered U.S. Presidents			
-Kennedy*	12/28	34/3	41/0
-Lincoln*	10/30	16/21	30/11
Name of Sweden's murdered Prime Minister (Palme)	1/39	3/34	5/36
Name of India's murdered Prime Minister (Gandhi)*	9/31	20/17	33/8

*Items for which the differences in the answers obtained from AD patients were significantly different from those obtained from the other groups (χ^2 test, p < .001).

Rabin could have been surprising, since it related to an event that had occurred after the onset of dementia. It is possible that rehearsal of the information, and/or emotional factors associated with the assassination, played a role in this retention. It is likely that major historical events with superimposed emotional elements can be retained by demented patients, although they fail to register or retrieve significant details of the events. Patients might have retained Ytzhak Rabin's murder, rather than the other events, which had occurred prior to the development of dementia, because it was relatively recent. Although time elapsed since acquisition of information and age have been shown to affect biographical memory (Greene and Hodges, 1996), these variables were not found to affect the event of interest of the present study. However, most of the patients were examined at about same time after the event.

REFERENCES

American Psychiatric Association (APA), 1984, Diagnostic and Statistical Manual of Mental Disorders, Fourth Edition (DSM-IV), American Psychiatric Press, Washington, DC.

McKahnn, G., Drachman, D., Folstein, M., et al., 1984, Clinical diagnosis of Alzheimer's disease: report of NINCDS-ADRDA, *Neurology* 34:939–944.

Folstein, M.F., Folstein, S.E., and McHugh, P.R., Mini-mental state: a practical method for grading the cognitive state of patients for the clinician, *J. Psychiatr. Res.* 12:189–198.

Greene J.D.W., Hodges J.R., The fractionation of remote memory. Evidence from a longitudinal study of dementia of Alzheimer type, *Brain* 119:129–142.

Hughes C.P., Berg L., Danziger W.L., Coben L.A., Martin R.L., A new clinical scale for the staging of dementia, *Brit. J. Psychiatry* 140:566–572.

Deutsch Lezak M., 1995, Neuropsychological Assessment, Oxford University Press, New York.

55

STUDY OF DEMENTIA IN CHINA

Xianhao Xu, Hong Guo, Bin Qin, Hua Zhang, Xiangyu Zeng, Dantao Peng,
Xiuyun Wang, Hong Sun, Shiguang Wen, Yun Jiang, Baolin Li,
Fengzhen Pang, and Hong Wang

Department of Neurology
Beijing Hospital
Beijing 100730, People's Republic of China

INTRODUCTION

The incidence and prevalence of dementia have been reported to be lower in Eastern than in Western countries. In dementia, the incidence and prevalence of vascular dementia (VD) is higher than that of Alzheimer's dementia in Eastern than in Western countries. This has been attributed to a lower carrier of apolipoprotein Apo E4 gene in the total population in the East than in the West, even in patients with Parkinson's disease and dementia compared to those without dementia (Siest et al., 1995; Strittmatter et al., 1993; Xu et al., 1995). Treatment is quite different in the various dementias (Xu et al., 1997).

The purpose of this study was to examine the reality of the aforementioned phenomena, and to explore the possible mechanisms.

MATERIALS AND METHODS

A nationwide epidemiological study of dementia (including vascular and Alzheimer's dementia), cerebral vascular disorders and hypertension in China was conducted.

A two-phase procedure was adopted: using Mini-Mental State Examination (MMSE) to screen out the potentially demented elderly people, then followed by a clinical evaluation examined by neurologists with the cognitive part in Geriatric Mental State Examination (GMS) and diagnosed by neurologists with DSM-III diagnostic criteria for dementia and Dementia Differential Diagnostic Schedule (DDDS) (Kua, 1992; Shen et al., 1994).

RESULTS

The incidence and mortality rate of dementia was 5.34% (13/812/3) and 3.48% (86/825/3) respectively according to the data from the Beijing area in 1986. The prevalence of dementia in Northern China, Beijing area (3.9%, 35/906) was significantly higher than that in Middle China, Shanghai (2.18%, 33/1515) ($\chi^2 = 5.55$, P < 0.05) and Southern China, Zunyi City (1.73%, 20/1159) ($\chi^2 = 8.48$, P < 0.01), but there was no significant difference between the latter two cities ($\chi^2 = 0.66$, P > 0.05).

The prevalence of vascular dementia in the Beijing area (2.65%, 24/906) was significantly higher than that in Shanghai (0.26%, 4/1515; $\chi^2 = 27.03$, P < 0.01) and Zunyi City (0.09%, 1/1159; $\chi^2 = 271.41$, P < 0.001), but there was no significant difference between the latter two cities ($\chi^2 = 1.11$, P > 0.2).

The prevalence of hypertension in Beijing (32.12%, 291/906) was significantly higher than that in Zunyi City (17.52%, 203/1159; $\chi^2 = 32.0$, P < 0.001). According to the statistics in the Beijing area, the prevalence of dementia in the elderly with hypertension (8.25%, 24/291) is significantly higher than that in elderly without hypertension (1.46%, 9/615; $\chi^2 = 23.55$, P < 0.001).

There is no statistically significant difference of different ε genes of Apo E among normal controls (NC), Parkinson's disease control group (PD), and Parkinson's disease with dementia (PDD) (Table 3).

DISCUSSION

Aging and Dementia Is Progressing around the World

The population of aged people is rapidly increasing. By the year 2050 it will become a big problem (Table 1). Dementia will become one of the most prominent problems (Table 2).

The Prevalence of Dementia Is Lower in China Than in the West

During the 18–20th centuries, owing to the rapid decrease of mortality over the age of 45, the percentage of elderly people in total population has been rapidly increasing (Table 1). The incidence and prevalence of dementia is increasing with aging (Table 2). Dementia in elderly people has been increasingly growing and has became one of the most remarkable problems all over the world. During 1900–1980, due to the life expectancy increase around 50% in advanced countries, the elderly people now comprise 20–40% of the total population. The incidence of dementia in elderly over age of 65 is 4.5% and 9% in Japan and United States, respectively.

Table 1. The percentage of elderly people in total population in 2050

	Of and over (%)	
	65 years	80 years
China	35.0	22.0
Germany	36.2	21.6
France	34.0	20.0
Canada	33.0	19.7
Japan	33.1	17.0
United States	29.0	16.0
United Kingdom	28.7	15.5
Italy	31.0	15.2

Table 2. Increasing prevalence
of dementia by aging

Age groups (years)	Prevalence	(%)
60–64	3/1619	0.19
65–69	8/1445	0.55
70–74	6/108	0.55
75–79	7/624	1.12
80 and up	15/397	3.78
Total	39/5172	0.75

The prevalence of dementia reported in Shanghai is 2.18% (33/1515); it is much lower than that in Western countries.

The Increased Prevalence of Vascular Dementia in China May Be Related to Increased Prevalence of Cerebrovascular Diseases and Hypertension, and High Daily Intake of Sodium Chloride

The prevalence of dementia in Western countries is around 4–6% for the elderly over age of 65. It is increasing with aging, and it has increased to 91.42% over the age of 80. Vascular dementia in Western countries is significantly lower than that in eastern countries. It may be related to a variety of causes including genetics, but is very complex.

Our data reveal that the prevalence of dementia is decreasing from northern to southern China, and the prevalence of cerebrovascular diseases and hypertension, and daily intake of sodium chloride also decrease from northern to southern China. It is suggested that the increased prevalence of vascular dementia in China may be related to increased prevalence of cerebrovascular diseases and hypertension, and high daily intake of sodium chloride.

The Relation between Apo E4 Gene and Dementia Has to Be Further Explored

Patients with severe dementia usually can survive for around 5 years. The necessity and load of society for those patients has sharply increased, due to rapid industrialization. Therefore the investigation of (environmental and genetic) risk factors, early diagnosis and prevention of dementia, reasonable care for patients with dementia, and decreasing the load of family and society have become one of the most critical problems in geriatrics.

In 1989, Shimano reported that senile dementia is closely related to Apo E. Two years later Apo E was proven to exist in senile plaques and neurofibrillary tangles in the brain of patients with Alzheimer's disease (Siest et al., 1995). In 1993, Strittmatter et al. proposed that Apo E4 allele is closely related to the late-onset familial Alzheimer's disease (Strittmatter et al., 1993). More recently, most observations have concentrated on the correlation between Alzheimer's disease and Apo E genotypes and phenotypes, and a consensus has been reached that Apo E4 is one of the risk factors. Our data do not show a difference in Apo E4 between the general normal population and Parkinson's disease patients with dementia (Table 3). This may be related to the fact that our sample size was too small. Anyway the relation between Apo E4 gene and dementia has not been proven by our data. It needs to be further explored.

Table 3. Distribution of different genotypes of Apo E

	NC n = 88		PD n = 17		PDD n = 26	
¦Å4	5	2.84	0	0	1	1.92
¦Å3	168	95.46	33	97.06	51	98.08
¦Å2	3	1.70	1	2.94	0	0
E4/4	1	1.14	0	0	0	0
E3/4	3	3.41	0	0	1	
E2/4	0	0	0	0	0	0
E3/3	82	93.18	16	94.12	25	0
E2/3	2	2.27	1	5.88	0	0
E2/2	0	0	0	0	0	0

*Normal Control (NC), Parkinson's Disease Control (PD), and Parkinson's disease with Dementia (PDD).

CONCLUSION

The prevalence of dementia, vascular dementia and hypertension are higher in northern China than that in southern China. The prevalence of dementia in the elderly with hypertension is significantly higher than that without hypertension. The higher prevalence of dementia in northern China may be related to the higher prevalence of cerebrovascular diseases and hypertension, and higher daily intake of sodium chloride in northern China than in southern China.

ACKNOWLEDGMENT

This work was partly supported by a Research Grant from the Ministry of Health, the People's Republic of China, Grant No. 96-906-05-07.

REFERENCES

Kua E.H., 1992, A community study of mental disorders in elderly Singaporean Chinese using the GMS-AGECAT package, *Aust. N. Z. J. Psychiatry* 26:502.

Shen Y.-C., Chen C.H., Li S.R. et al., 1994, Epidemiology of age-related dementia in China. *J. Hong Kong Coll. Psychiatry* 4:17.

Siest G., Pillot T., Regis-Bailly A. et al., 1995 Apolipoprotein E: An important gene and protein to follow in laboratory medicine, *Clin. Chem.* 41:1068.

Strittmatter W.J., Saunders A.M., Schmechel D. et al., 1993, Apolipoprotein E: high-avidity binding to beta-amyloid and increased frequency of type 4 allele late-onset family Alzheimer's disease, *Proc. Natl. Acad. Sci. USA* 90:1977.

Xu X.-H., Guo H., Zhang H. et al., 1995, Apolipoprotein E and Geriatrics, with special reference to Alzheimer's Disease, *Chin. J. Neuroimmunol. Neurol.* 2:239.

Xu X.-H. and Sun H., 1997, Advances in Treatment of Alzheimer's Disease, *Chin. J. Neuroimmunol. Neurol.* 4:60.

56

GENETIC ASPECTS OF PARKINSON'S DISEASE

Yoshikuni Mizuno, Hiroto Matsumine, Nobutaka Hattori,
Satoe Matsubayashi, Tomonori Kobayashi, Asako Yoritaka, and Mei Wang

Department of Neurology
Juntendo University School of Medicine
Tokyo, Japan

INTRODUCTION

Parkinson's disease (PD) is characterized by tremor, rigidity, bradykinesia, and loss of postural reflex clinically and degeneration of pigmented neurons in the substantia nigra and the locus coeruleus pathologically. It has been postulated that the nigral cell death is initiated by the interaction of genetic predisposition and environmental or endogenous nigral neurotoxins (Jenner et al., 1992). Although most of the patients with PD are sporadic cases, a small group of patients have affected members in their families. In these familial cases, a molecular genetic approach is very important to find a primary cause of nigral cell death in respective families. In addition, information obtained in the studies on familial PD will give us a clue to explore the etiology and pathogenesis of more common sporadic PD. Recently, the genes for two familial forms of parkinsonism have been mapped to the specific chromosome regions and in one of them, what appears to be the causative gene was identified. In this chapter, we will discuss recent progress in the genetics of PD.

AUTOSOMAL DOMINANT LEWY BODY-POSITIVE PARKINSON'S DISEASE

Golbe et al. (1990, 1996) reported a large kindred with autosomal dominant PD of Italian descent; 60 persons were affected in 5 generations. Clinical features were similar to more common sporadic PD, however, the age of onset was younger (45.6 ± 13.5 years, range 20–85) and the disease duration (onset to death) was shorter (9.2 ± 4.9 years, range, 2–20); in addition, dementia of highly variable severity developed in many patients, and resting tremor was seen in 58% which was less frequent than in the sporadic PD. No clear anticipation was noted. Postmortem examination in two patients revealed severe neuronal loss in the substantia nigra with Lewy bodies in the remaining neurons. The locus coeruleus, dorsal motor nucleus of the vagus, and nucleus basalis of Meynert also showed mild to moderate cell loss with Lewy bodies. Polymeropoulos et al. (1996) mapped the gene for this family to chromosome 4q21–q23. This is the first autosomal dominant familial PD in which the gene locus was identified. In this chromosomal location, the gene for α-synuclein has been mapped to 4q21–22 (Chen et al., 1995; Spilantini et al., 1995). Using this gene as a candidate, Polymeropoulos et al. (1997) identified what appears to be the causative gene for this autosomal dominant familial PD; all the affected members studied showed guanine to adenine mutation at base pair 209 causing alanine to threonine amino acid substitution at position 53.

α-Synuclein is a protein identified by the screening of the cDNA library prepared from the electric organ of torpedo (Maroteaux et al., 1988). It is a neuron specific protein localized in the presynaptic nerve terminals and in the nucleus (Maroteaux & Scheller, 1991). In the central nervous system, it is expressed in the cerebral cortex (2nd, 3rd, and 5th layers), olfactory bulb, amygdaloid nucleus, hippocampus, striatum, substantia nigra, raphe, and the cerebellar granular layer; the expression is more prominent in the cerebral cortical areas than the basal ganglia structures (Maroteaux & Scheller,, 1991). Interestingly, α-synuclein was found to be a non-amyloid component of the senile plaque (Iwai et al., 1995), and it may play a role in the pathogenesis of Alzheimer's disease.

AUTOSOMAL RECESSIVE LEWY BODY-NEGATIVE FAMILIAL PARKINSONISM

Autosomal recessive Lewy-body negative parkinsonism is a distinct clinical and genetic entity. This entity was first described by Yamamura et al. (1973). They reported 16 patients (13 familial in 5 unrelated families and 3 sporadic cases); clinical features of 11 patients from the initial 4 families are essentially identical; only in one of those 11 patients, the disease started at age 42; in the remaining 10 patients the initial symptoms appeared between 17 and 28 years; female preponderance was noted (M:F = 1:10); all the patients showed tremor, rigidity, bradykinesia, and postural instability; spontaneous diurnal fluctuations were seen in all. Dementia and autonomic failures are not the clinical features. Consanguineous marriage was seen in two families; and none of the parents of the affected patients had parkinsonism indicating autosomal recessive mode of inheritance. The progression was slow.

Recently, Ishikawa and Tsuji (1996) reported 17 patients (5 men, 12 women) in Niigata district, a northern part of Japan facing the Japan Sea. The age of onset was between 20 and 43; in only one exceptional patient the disease started at age 43. Clinical features are essentially similar to those reported by Yamamura et al. (1996). Progression was very slow. One of their patients who had the onset of the disease at age 11 lived until 67 years of the age (Takahashi et al., 1994) and our patient lived 38 years after the onset at age 24. Postmortem examination revealed loss of nigral neurons in the pars compacta of the substantia nigra and gliosis, but no Lewy bodies or neurofibrillary tangles were seen in the remaining neurons (Takahashi et al., 1994; Mori et al., submitted). As no Lewy bodies were found in this type of familial cases, it appears to be inappropriate to call this form as familial PD; therefore, we use the term familial "parkinsonism". But they do respond to levodopa quite well and they show selective degeneration of the pigmented neurons. This is a good model to study genetically to find a clue to the mechanism of nigral cell death.

Recently, we mapped the gene for this autosomal recessive parkinsonism to chromosome 6q25.2–27 at a very close region to *sod 2* locus (Matsumine et al., 1997). While we were working on the genetic association study on sporadic as well as familial PD, we were lucky enough to encounter a family in which all the affected members showed a complete segregation with a novel polymorphic mutation of Mn SOD gene (*sod 2*). This polymorphic mutation was located in the mitochondrial targeting sequence of *sod 2* (Shimoda-Matsubayashi et al., 1996). The coding region for mature Mn SOD protein did not contain specific mutations; therefore, *sod 2* does not appear to be the causative gene; using nearby microsatellite markers, we were able to map the gene to the long arm of chromosome 6 (Matsumine et al., 1997).

CLINICAL PHENOTYPES OF FAMILIAL PARKINSONISM

There are numbers of families with parkinsonism in which the gene loci have not been identified. As clinical phenotypes differ considerably, it appears likely that there are many different genetic loci which are responsible for nigral degeneration. These familial cases are summarized in Table 1. Familial PD and parkinsonism can be classified according to the presence or absence of Lewy bodies in the first line, and then according to the mode of inheritance. But autosomal recessive Lewy body-positive type must be very rare. To our knowledge, no well documented such families have been reported in the literature.

Table 1. Clinical phenotypes of familial Parkinson's disease and parkinsonism

Classification	Reference
Lewy body-positive	
Autosomal dominant	
Young onset 4q-linked	Golbe et al., 1992, 96;
	Polymeropoulos et al., 1996, 97
Late onset without demenia, typical	Wszolek et al., 1995
Late onset with dementia	Denson & Wszolek, 1995
Late onset with amyotrophy	Denson & Wszolek, 1995
Early onset with visual symptoms	Golbe et al., 1994
With depression and hypoventilation	Perry et al., 1990;
	Bhatia et al., 1993
Young onset with dementia	Inose et al., 1988
With Lewy body, NFT, & senile plaques	Denson & Wszolek, 1995
Lewy body unknown	
Autosomal dominant	
With anticipation	Waters & Miller, 1994;
	Markopoulou et al., 1995;
	Morrison et al., 1996
Early onset with dystonia	Dobyns et al., 1993
Lewy body-negative	
Autosomal dominant	
Late onset	Nukada et al., 1978
Early onset	Dwork et al., 1993
Autosomal recessive	
Early onset 6q-linked	Yamamura et al., 1973;
	Ishikawa et al., 1996;
	Matsumine et al., 1997

GENETIC PREDISPOSITION IN SPORADIC PARKINSON'S DISEASE

As endogenous or exogenous neurotoxins may be involved in the pathogenesis of PD (Naoi et al., 1996), genetic polymorphisms of enzymes regulating the metabolism of those compounds have extensively been studied to find genetic risk factors for PD. Some of the representative studies are summarized in Table 2. CYP2D6 is a hepatic enzyme responsible for the metabolism of debrisoquine, spartein, and MPTP; five mutant alleles (A, B, C, D, and L) have been identified (Johansson et al., 1993; Whilhelmsen et al., 1997), and A to D alleles are poor metabolizers while the L type is a hyper-extensive metabolizer allele (Johansson et al., 1993). As shown in Table 2, controversies exist in the results (Agúndez et al., 1995; Akhmedova et al., 1995; Armstrong et al., 1992; Diederich et al., 1996; Sandy et al., 1996; Smith et al., 1992), but poor metabolizers are slightly more represented among PD patients than the controls. Tsuneoka et al. (1993) reported that the L allele was more frequent among PD patients. CYP1A1 is another hepatic enzyme regulating the activation of benzopyrene and aromatic hydrocarbons; recently Takakubo et al. (1996) reported that homozygosity of this mutant allele was more frequent among PD patients, but the relationship between this mutation and the enzyme activity is not known.

Catechol-*O*-methyl transferase (COMT) is an enzyme regulating the *O*-methylation of catechol compounds. Mutation from high activity (COMT^H) to low activity (COMT^L) is determined by a single amino acid substitution of valine at the 108 position to methionine, and the frequency of COMT^L was reported not to be increased among Caucasian PD patients (Hoda et al., 1996). However, among Japanese, homozygosity of COMT^L was reported to be

Table 2. Genetic predisposition in sporadic Parkinson's disease

	No. of patients		Genotype distribution	
Authors	PD/cont	PD/cont (%)	PD/cont (%)	PD/cont (%)
CYP2D6				
Smith et al., 1992	229/720	61/64 (w/w)	28/31 (w/m)	12/5 (m/m)*
Armstrong et al., 1992	53/72	57/63 (w/w)	38/18 (w/B)*	
Sandy et al., 1996				
Onset > 51	100/137	68/60 (w/w)	26/33 (w/m)	6/7 (m/m)
Diederich et al., 1996				
Total	52/71	67/65 (w/w)	31/26 (w/B)	4/7 (B/B)
Onset < 40	13/71	65/67 (w/w)	30/26 (w/B)	5/7 (w/B)
Onset > 50	28/71	58/67 (w/w)	38/26 (w/B)	4/7 (w/B)
Agúndez et al., 1995				
Onset < 50	33/150	52/73 (w/w)*	46/17 (w/B)	3/0 (B/C)
Onset > 50	90/150	76/73 (w/w)	16/17 (w/B)	1/3 (B/B)
Akhmedova et al. 1995				
Total	80/70	68/79 (w/w)	32/20 (w/B)	0/1 (B/B)
Akineto-rigido-tremor	38/70	58/79 (w/w)	42/20 (w/B)*	0/1 (B/B)
Tasuneoka et al., 1993	63/91	63/85 (w/w)	23/13 (w/L)*	11/2 (L/L)*
CYP1A1				
Takakubo et al., 1995	126/176	51/65 (w/w)	35/32 (w/m)	14/4 (m/m)*
COMT				
Hoda et al., 1996	139/173	23/23 (H/H)	70/88 (H/L)	27/26 (L/L)
Kunugi et al., 1997	109/153	42/48 (H/H)	43/46 (H/L)	15/9 (L/L)*
Yoritaka et., 1997	176/156	57/44 (H/H)	35/49 (H/L)*	8/6 (L/L)

w: wild, m: mutant, B: B allele, C: C allele, L: L allele, H: COMTH, L: COMTL, *: Statistical significance

more frequent among PD patients (Kunugi et al., 1997). According to our results, the heterozygotes of COMT^H and COMT^L was less frequent among PD (Yoritaka et al., 1997).

Genes for monoamine oxidase (MAO) A (Hotamisligil et al., 1994; Nanko et al., 1996), MAOB (Ho et al., 1995; Kurth et al., 1993; Morimoto et al., 1995; Nanko et al., 1996), and D2 dopamine receptor (Nanko et al., 1994; Higuchi et al., 1995; Planté-Bordeneuve et al., 1997) have also been studied, however, the results are controversial. We reported that *SOD 2*-targeting sequence mutation from valine to alanine was more frequent among PD patients (Shimoda-Matsubayashi et al., 1996). Association between PD and genes for tyrosine hydroxylase (Planté-Bordeneuve et al., 1994), D3 and D4 dopamine receptors (Higuchi et al., 1995; Nanko et al., 1994), dopamine transporters (Higuchi et al., 1995; Nanko et al., 1994), apolipoprotein A (Koller et al., 1995; Whitehead et al., 1996)), glutathione S-transferase (Stroombergen et al., 1996; Tison et al., 1994), and nitric oxide synthase (Kurth et al., 1997) have all been excluded. Thus more extensive studies appear to be necessary to find genetic risk factors for PD; a question may arise whether or not such association studies are really rewarding to elucidate the etiology and pathogenesis of PD.

ACKNOWLEDGMENTS

This study was supported in part by a Grant-in-Aid for Scientific Research on Priority Areas and by a Grant-in-Aid for Neuroscience Research from the Ministry of Education, Science and Culture, Japan, Grant-in-Aid for intractable Disorders from Ministry of Health and Welfare, Japan, and by a "Center of Excellence" Grant from the National Parkinson Foundation, Miami.

REFERENCES

Agúndez, J.A.G., Jiménez-Jiménez, F.J., Luengo, A., Bernal, M.L., Molina, J.A., Ayuso, L., Vázquez, A., Parra, J., Duarte, J., Coria, F., Ladero, J.M., Alvarez, J.C., and Benítez, J., 1995, Association between the oxidative polymorphism and early onset of Parkinson's disease, *Clin. Pharmacol. Ther.* 57:291–298.

Akhmedova, S.N., Pushnova, E.A., Yakimovsky, A.F., Avtonomov, V.V., and Schwartz, E.I., 1995, Frequency of a specific cytochrome P4502D6B(CYP2D6B) mutant allele in clinically differentiated groups of patients with Parkinson's disease, *Biochem. Mol. Med.* 54:88–90.

Armstrong, M., Daly, A.K., Cholerton S, Bateman DN, and Idle JR., 1992, Mutant debrisoquine hydroxylation genes in Parkinson's disease, *Lancet* 339:1017–1018.

Bhatia, K.P., Daniel, S.E., and Marsden, C.D., 1993, Familial parkinsonism with depression: a clinicopathological study, *Ann. Neurol.* 34:842–847.

Chen, X., Silva, H.A.R, Pettenati, M.J., Rao, P.N, St George-Hyslop, P., Roses, A.D, Xia, Y., Horsburgh, K., Uéda, K., and Saitoh, T., 1995, The human NACP/a-synuclein gene: chromosome assignment to 4q21.3-q22 and *TaqI* RFLP analysis, *Genomics* 26:425–427.

Denson, M. and Wszolek, Z.K., 1995, Familial parkinsonism: our experience and review, *Parkinsonism Related Disord.* 1:35–46.

Diederich, N., Hilger, C., Goetz, C.G., Keipes, M., Hentges, F., Vieregge, P, and Metz, H., 1996, Genetic variability of the CYP 2D6 gene is not a risk factor for sporadic Parkinson's disease, *Ann. Neurol.* 40:463–465.

Dobyns, W.B., Ozelius, L.J., Kramer, P.L., Brashear, A., Farlow, M.R., Perry, T.R., Walsh, L.E, Kasarskis, E.J., Bultler, I.J, and Breakfield, X.O., 1993, Rapid-onset dystonia-parkinsonism, *Neurology* 43:2596–2602.

Dwork, A.J., Balmaceda, C., Fazzini, E.A, MacCollin, M., Côté, L, and Fahn, S., 1993, Dominantly inherited, early-onset parkinsonism: neuropathology of a new form, *Neurology* 43:69–74.

Golbe, L.I., Di Iorio, G., Bonavita, V., Miller, D.C., and Duvoisin, R.C., 1990, A large kindred with autosomal dominant Parkinson's disease, *Ann. Neurol.* 27:276–282.

Golbe, L.I., Lazzarini, A.M., Schwarz, K.O., Mark M.H, Dickson, D.W., and Duvoisin, R.C., 1994, Autosomal dominant parkinsonism with benign course and typical Lewy-body pathology, *Neurology* 43:2222–2227.

Golbe, L.I., Di Iorio, G., Sanges, G., Lazzarini, A.M., La Sala, S., Bonavita, V., and Duvoisin, R.C., 1996. Clinical genetic analysis of Parkinson's disease in the Contursi Kindred, *Ann. Neurol.* 40:767–775.

Higuchi, S., Muramatsu, T., Arai, H., Hayashida, M., Sasaki, H., and Trojanowski, J.Q., 1995, Polymorphisms of dopamine receptor and transporter genes and Parkinson's disease, *J. Neural. Transm. [P-D Sect]* 10:107–113.

Ho, S.L., Kapadí, A.L., Ramsden, D.B., and Williams, A.C., 1995, An allelic association study of monoamine oxidase B in Parkinson's disease, *Ann. Neurol.* 37:403–405.

Hoda, F., Nicholl, D., Bennett, P., Arranz, M., Aitchison, K.J., Al-Chalabi, A., Kunugi, H., Vallada, H., Leigh, P.N., Chaudhuri, K.R., and Collier, D.A., 1996, No association between Parkinson's disease and low-activity alleles of catechol *O*-methyltransferase, *Biochem. Biophys. Res. Commun* 228:780–784.

Hotamisligil, G.S, Girmen, A.S, Fink, J.S., Tivol, E., Shalish, C., Tfofatter, J., Baenziger, J., Diamond, S., Markham, C., Sullivan, J., Growdon, J., and Breakefield, X.O., 1994, Hereditary variations in monoamine oxidase as a risk factor for Parkinson's disease, *Mov. Disord.* 9:305–310.

Inose, T., Miyakawa, M., Miyakawa, K., Mizushima, S., Oyanagi, S., and Ando, S., 1988, Clinical and neuropathological study of a familial case of juvenile parkinsonism, *Jpn. J. Psychiatry. Neurol.* 42:265–276.

Ishikawa, A. and Tsuji, S., 1996, Clinical analysis of 17 patients in 12 Japanese families with autosomal-recessive type juvenile parkinsonism. *Neurology* 47:160–169.

Iwai, A., Masliah, E., Yoshimoto, M., Ge, N., Flanagan, L., Silva, R., Kittel, A., and Saitoh, T., 1995, The precursor protein of non-Ab component of Alzheimer's disease amyloid is a presynaptic protein of the central nervous system, *Neuron* 14:467–475.

Jakes, R., Spillantini, M.G., and Goedert, M., 1994, Identification of two distinct synucleins from human brain, *FEBS Lett.* 345:27–32.

Jenner, P., Schapira, A.H., and Marsden, C.D., 1992, New insights into the cause of Parkinson's disease, *Neurology* 42:2241–2250.

Johansson, I., Lundqvist, E., Bertilsson, L., Dahl, M.L., Sjöoqvist, F., and Ingelman-Sundberg, M., 1993, Inherited amplification of an active gene in the cytochrome P450 CYP2D locus as a cause of ultra-rapid metabolism of debrisoquine, *Proc. Natl. Acad. Sci. USA* 90:11825–11829.

Koller, W.C., Glatt, S.L., Hubble, J.P., Paolo, A., Tröster, A.I., Handler, M.S., Horvar, R.T., Martin, C., Schmidt, K. Karst, A., Wijsman, E.M., Yu C.E., and Schellenberg, G.D., 1995, Apolipoprotein E Genotypes in Parkinson's disease with and without dementia, *Ann. Neurol.* 37:242–245.

Kunugi, H., Nanko, S., Ueki, A., Otsuka, E., Hattori, M., Hoda, F., Vallada, H.P., Arranz, M.J., and Collier, D.A., 1997, High and low activity alleles of catechol-*O*-methyltransferase gene: ethnic difference and possible association with Parkinson's disease, *Neurosci. Lett.* 221:202–204.

Kurth, J.H., Kurth, M.C., Poduslo, S.E., and Schwankhaus, J.D., 1993, Association of a monoamine oxidase B allele with Parkinson's disease. *Ann. Neurol.* 33:368–372.

Kurth, J.H., Eggers-Sedlet, B., Lieberman, A.N., and Kurth, M.C., 1997, Nitric oxide synthase gene polymorphisms and Parkinson's disease, *Neurology* 48: A183 (abstract).

Markopoulou, K., Wszoke, Z.K, and Pfeiffer, R.F., 1995, A Greek-American kindred with autosomal dominant, levodopa-responsive parkinsonism and anticipation. *Ann. Neurol.* 38:373–378.

Maroteaux, L., Campanelli, J.T., and Scheller, R.H., 1988, Synuclein: a neuron-specific protein localized to the nucleus and presynaptic nerve terminal. *J. Neurosci.* 8: 2804–2815.

Maroteaux, L., Scheller, R.H., 1991, The rat brain synucleins; family of proteins transiently associated with neuronal membrane. *Mol. Brain Res.* 11:335–343.

Matsumine, H., Saito, M., Shimoda-Matsubayashi, S., Tanaka, H., Ishikawa, A., Nakagawa-Hattori, Y., Yokochi, M., Kobayashi, T., Igarashi, S., Takano, H., Sanpei, K., Koike, R., Mori, H., Kondo, T,, Mizutani, Y., Schaffer, A.A., Yamamura, Y., Nakamura, S, Kuzuhara, S, Tsuji, S, and Mizuno, Y., 1997, Localization of a gene for autosomal recessive form of juvenile parkinsonism (AR-JP) to chromosome 6q25.2–27, *Am. J. Hum. Genet.* 60:588–596

Morimoto, Y., Murayama, N., Kuwano, A., Kondo, I., Yamashita, Y., and Mizuno, Y., 1995, Association analysis of a polymorphism of the monoamine oxidase B gene with Parkinson's disease in a Japanese population. *Amer. J. Med. Genet.* 60:570–572.

Morrison, P.J., Dogwin-Austin, R.B., and Raeburn, J.A., 1996, Familial autosomal dominant dopa responsive Parkinson's disease in three living generations showing extreme anticipation and childhood onset. *J. Med. Genet.* 33:504–506.

Nanko, S., Ueki, A., and Hattori, M., 1996, No association between Parkinson's disease and monoamine oxidase A and B gene polymorphisms. *Neurosci. Lett.* 204:125–127.

Nanko, S., Ueki, A., Hattori, M., Dai, X.Y., Sasaki, T., Fukuda, R., Ikeda, K., and Kazamatsuri, H., 1994, No allelic association between Parkinson's disease and dopamine D2, D3, and D4 receptor gene polymorphisms. *Am. J. Med. Genet.* 54:361–364.

Naoi, M., Maruyama, W., Dostert, P., Hashizume, Y., Nakahara, D., Takahashi, T., and Ota, M., 1996, Dopamine-derived endogenous 1(R),2(N)-dimethyl-6,7-dihydroxy-1,2,3,4-tetrahydroisoquinoline,N-methyl-(R)-salsolinol, induced parkinsonism in rat: biochemical, pathological and behavioral studies. *Brain Res.* 709:285–295.

Nukada, H., Kowa, H., Saito, T., Tasaki, Y., and Miura, S., 1978, A big family of paralysis agitans. *Rinshoushinnkeigaku* 18:627–634.

Perry, T.L., Wright, J.M., Berry, K., Hansen, S., and Perry, T.L., Jr., 1990, Dominantly inherited apathy, central hypoventilation, and Parkinson's syndrome: clinical, biochemical, and neuropathologic studies of 2 new cases. *Neurology* 40:1882–1887.

Planté-Bordeneuve, V., Davis, M.B., Maraganore, D.M., Marsden, C.D., and Harding, A.E., 1994, Tyrosine hydroxylase polymorphisms in Familial and sporadic Parkinson's disease, *Mov. Disord.* 9:337–339.

Planté-Bordeneuve, V., Taussig, D., Thomas, F., Said, G., Wood, N.W., Marsden, C.D., and Harding, A.E., 1997, Evaluation of four candidate genes encoding proteins of the dopamine pathway in familial and sporadic Parkinson's disease: evidence for association of a DRD2 allele, *Neurology* 48:1589–1593.

Polymeropoulos, M.H., Higgins, J.J., Golbe, L.I., Johnson, W.G., Ide, S.E., Iorio, G.D., Sanges, G., Stenroos, E.S., Pho, L.T., Schaffer, A.A., Lazzarini, A.M., Nussbaum, R.L., and Duvoisin, R.C., 1996, Mapping of a gene for Parkinson's disease to chromosome 4q21-q23, *Science* 274:1197–1199.

Polymeropoulos, M.H., Lavedan, C., Leroy, E., Ide, S.E., Dehejia, A., Pike, A.D.B., Root, H., Rubenstein, J., Boyer, R., Stenroos, E.S., Chandrasekharappa, S., Athanassiadou, A., Papapetropoulos, T., Johnson, W.G., Lazzarini, A.M., Duvoisin, R.C., Di Iorio, G., Golbe, L.I., and Nussbaum, R.L., 1997, Mutation in the a-synuclein gene identified in families with Parkinson's disease, *Science* 276:2045–2047.

Sandy, M.S., Armstrong, M., Tanner, C.M., Daly, A.K., Di Monte, D.A., Langston, J.W., and Idle, J.R., 1996, CYP2D6 allelic frequencies in young-onset Parkinson's disease, *Neurology* 47:225–230.

Shimoda-Matsubayashi, S., Matsumine, H., Kobayashi, T., Nakagawa-Hattori ,Y., Shimizu, Y., and Mizuno, Y., 1996, Structural dimorphism in the mitochondrial targeting sequence in the human MnSOD gene. A predictive evidence for conformational change to influence mitochondrial transport and a study of allelic association in Parkinson's disease, *Biochem. Biophys. Res. Commun.* 226:561–565.

Smith, C.A., Gough, A.C., Leigh, P.N., Summers, B.A., Harding, A.E., Maranganore, D.M., Sturman, S.G., Schapira, A.V., Williams, A.C., Spurr, N.K., and Wolf, C.R., 1992, Debrisoquine hydroxylase gene polymorphism and susceptibility to Parkinson's disease. *Lancet* 339:1375–1377.

Spillantini, M.G., Diavane, A., Goedert, and M., 1995, Assignment of human a-synuclein (SNCA) and b-synuclein (SNCB) genes to chromosomes 4q21 and 5q35, *Genomics* 27:379–381.

Stroombergen, M.C.M.J., Waring, R.H., Bennett, P., and Williams, A.C., 1996, Determination of the GSTM1 gene deletion frequency in Parkinson's disease by allele specific PCR. *Parkinsonism Related. Disord.* 2:151–154.

Takahashi, H., Ohama, E., Suzuki, S., Horikawa, Y., Ishikawa, A., Morita, T., Tsuji, S., and Ikuta, F., 1994, Familial juvenile parkinsonism: clinical and pathologic study in a family, *Neurology* 44:437–441.

Takakubo, F., Yamamoto, M., Ogawa, N., Yamashita, Y., Mizuno, Y., and Kondo, I., 1996, Genetic association between cytochrome P4501A1 gene and susceptibility to Parkinson's disease, *J. Neural. Transm.* 103:843–849.

Tison, F., Coutelle, C., Henry, P., and Cassaigne, A., 1994, Gluathione S-transferase (Class m) phenotype in Parkinson's disease. *Mov. Disord.* 9:117–118.

Tsuneoka, Y., Matsuo, Y., Iwahashi, K., Takeuchi, H., and Ichikawa, Y., 1993, A novel cytochrome P-450IID6 gene associated with Parkinson's disease. *J. Biochem.* 114:263–266.

Waters, C.H. and Miller, C.A., 1994, Autosomal-dominant Lewy body parkinsonism in a four-generation family, *Ann. Neurol.* 35:59–64.

Whilhelmsen, K., Mirel, D., Marder, K., Bernstein, M., Naini, A., Leal, S.M., Cote, L.J., Tang, M.-X., Freye,r G., Graziano, J., and Mayeux, R., 1997, Is there a genetic susceptibility locus for Parkinson's disease on chromosome 22q13? *Ann. Neurol.* 41:813–817.

Whitehead, A.S., Bertrandy, S., Finnan, F., Butler, A, Smith, G.D, and Ben-Shlomo, Y., 1996, Frequency of the apolipoprotein E epsilon 4 allele in a case-control study of early onset Parkinson's disease, *J. Neurol. Neurosurg. Psychiatry* 61:347–351.

Wszolek, Z.K., Pfeiffer, B., Fulgham, J.R., Parisi, J.E., Thompson, B.M., Uitti, R.J., Calne, D.B., and Pfeiffer, R.F., 1995, Weatern Nebraska family (family D) with autosomal dominant parkinsonism, *Neurology* 45:502–505.

Yamamura, Y., Sobue, I., Ando, K., Iida, M., Yanagi, T., and Kono, C., 1973, Paralysis agitans of early onset with marked diurnal fluctuation of symptoms, *Neurology* 23:239–244.

Yoritaka, A., Hattori, N., Yoshino, H., and Mizuno, Y., 1998, Catechol-O-methyltransferase genotype and susceptibility to Parkinson's disease in Japan, *J. Neural. Transm.* (in press)

57

A CHROMOSOME 6q-LINKED PARKINSONISM

Hiroto Matsumine,[1] Masaaki Saito,[2] Atsushi Ishikawa,[3] Yasuhiro Yamamura,[4] Shoji Tsuji,[2] and Yoshikuni Mizuno[1]

[1]Department of Neurology
Juntendo University School of Medicine
2-1-1 Hongo, Bunkyo-ku, 113 Tokyo, Japan
[2]Department of Neurology
Brain Research Institute
Niigata University
Niigata, Japan
[3]Department of Neurology
Nishi-Ojiya National Hospital
Niigata, Japan
[4]Institute of Health Science
Hiroshima University School of Medicine
Hiroshima, Japan

INTRODUCTION

Molecular mechanism of specific neuronal loss in the central nervous system is one of the challenging questions to be answered. A primary abnormality observed in Parkinson's disease (PD) is the selective degeneration of dopaminergic neurons in the substantia nigra pars compacta (SNPC). Although a complex multifactorial mechanism has been proposed as the cause of this disease, the exact pathogenic mechanism of this disease is unknown.

We present here a genetic model of parkinsonism with selective degeneration of the neurons in the substantia nigra and provide the evidence that this abnormality is linked to a single genetic locus on chromosome 6q25.2–27 that flanks the manganese superoxide dismutase gene. This is a clear indication of an idea that a single etiologic mechanism, which is genetically determined, can provoke specific neuron death in the substantia nigra.

Characteristics of the Autosomal Recessive Form of Levodopa-Responsive Parkinsonism

In the analyses of familial parkinsonism, Lewy body-positive neurodegeneration in the SNPC and a slowly progressive course of levodopa-responsive parkinsonism without

Progress in Alzheimer's and Parkinson's Diseases
edited by Fisher *et al.*, Plenum Press, New York, 1998.

accompaniment of disturbances of other neural systems are the major criteria for the definition of a typical parkinsonian phenotype. Unfortunately, multiplex families which present such phenotype have rarely been reported.

Most cases of autosomal dominant parkinsonism show Lewy-body pathology (Golbe et al., 1990). However, clinical features of these cases are heterogeneous and do not show a typical parkinosonian phenotype, but frequently accompany dementia of moderate to severe degree with aggressive course and poor levodopa response. On the other hand, there is a benign levodopa-responsive parkinsonism with autosomal recessive inheritance, which constitutes a characteristically uniform and distinctive clinicopathological entity (Yamamura et al., 1973; Ishikawa and Tsuji, 1996).

The clinical pictures almost uniformly seen in this disease is an insidious onset of parkinsonism at the age before around 40 (ranging from 8 to 43 with the peak incidence of onset at the age from 20 to 29 years-old), slow and protracted course, superb response to levodopa, frequent occurrence of dopa-induced dyskinesia and wearing-off phenomenon, absence of dementia and a rare occurence of autonomic dysfunctions. Other characteristic clinical features include diurnal fluctuation of symptoms due to sleep benefit, hypreactive tendon reflex, and mild foot dystonia.

This disease was first reported in Japan as "paralysis agitance of early-onset with marked diurnal fluctuation of symptoms" (PEDF) (Yamamura et al., 1973). Subsequently, Ishikawa and Tsuji found a total of 12 families originating in a small geographic area of Japan and designated this disease as "autosomal recessive juvenile parkinsonsism" (ARJP; MIM#600116). Pathological findings are essentially similar between ARJP and PEDF, showing selective degeneration of neurons with severe gliosis in the SNPC without Lewy body formation and much milder neuron loss in the locus ceruleus (Yamamura et al., 1993; Takahashi et al., 1994). Extensive reduction of tyrosine hydroxylase activity in nigrostriatal system in the brains from the patients was observed (Kondo et al., 1990; Matsumine et al., 1997), indicating that this disease is a syndrome of a parkinsonism resulting from selective destruction of the nigrostriatal dopamine system.

Allelic Segregation of Polymorphism in Manganese Superoxide Dismutase (MnSOD) Gene to Autosomal Recessive Juvenile Parkinsonism (ARJP)

MnSOD is an intramitochondrial enzyme that scavenges superoxide anions which are generated from the mitochondrial respiratory chain. MnSOD is not constitutively expressed but is inducible by superoxide anions, and does not exhibit product inhibition (Hassan, 1996). MnSOD activity is reported to be increased in the substantia nigra in idiopathic PD (Saggu et al., 1989). Together with the fact that mitochondrial respiration is impaired in idiopathic PD (Mizuno et al., 1989; Shapira et al., 1989), an important role of MnSOD was suggested in the mechanism of nigral degeneration in this disease.

Using primers designed from the human cDNA sequence encompassing presumptive exons 1 and 2 , which we predicted from the reported genomic structure of rat SOD2 gene, we were able to obtain a human genomic fragment (450 bp length) for the mitochondrial targeting sequence of the MnSOD gene(Shimoda-Matsubayashi et al., 1996). Nucleotide sequence analyses of the PCR product revealed that the genomic structure coding for the mitochondrial targeting sequence consisted of two exons and one intron in-between as expected from the rat genomic structure. Further analysis of the sequences of PCR products from control samples revealed a polymorphic mutation of C to T transition which substitutes alanine for valine at position –9 of the mitochondrial targeting sequence. We converted this nucleotide substitution to fluorescence-based PCR-SSCP and performed genetic segregation analysis in familial parkinsonism.

One family (family 101) presenting juvenile levodopa-responsive parkinsonism showed a perfect co-segregation of this biallelic intragenic polymorphism to the disease (Matsumine et al., 1997). In this family, four of six siblings were affected and born to normal parents. The phenotypically normal mother was heterozygous for the –9 alanine and –9 valine alleles, whereas all three of the affected children were homozygous for the –9 alanine allele and the two unaffected siblings were heterozygous. Through analysis of 248 normal Japanese chromosomes, we already found that the allele frequencies of –9 alanine and –9 valine in a normal population were 0.113 and 0.887, respectively. Thus there was a perfect cosegregation of the rare allele (–9Ala) with the disease in this family. The highest pairwise lod scores of 1.34 were obtained at the MnSOD gene (q = 0). The genotype in each member was confirmed by direct nucleotide sequence analysis of the PCR product. (Figure 1).

To confirm this segregation, we genotyped 6 microsatellite markers (D6S255, D6S411, D6S305, D6S253, D6S264 and D6S297) which are located in the vicinity of SOD2 gene (Matsumine et al., 1997). As shown in Figure 1, the markers including D6S255, D6S411, D6S305, and D6S253 revealed ultimate co-segregation with the disease with an obligatory recombination at D6S264 in an affected individual (a subject 7 in Fig. 1). The highest multipoint lod scores of 1.70 were obtained at the locus covered by

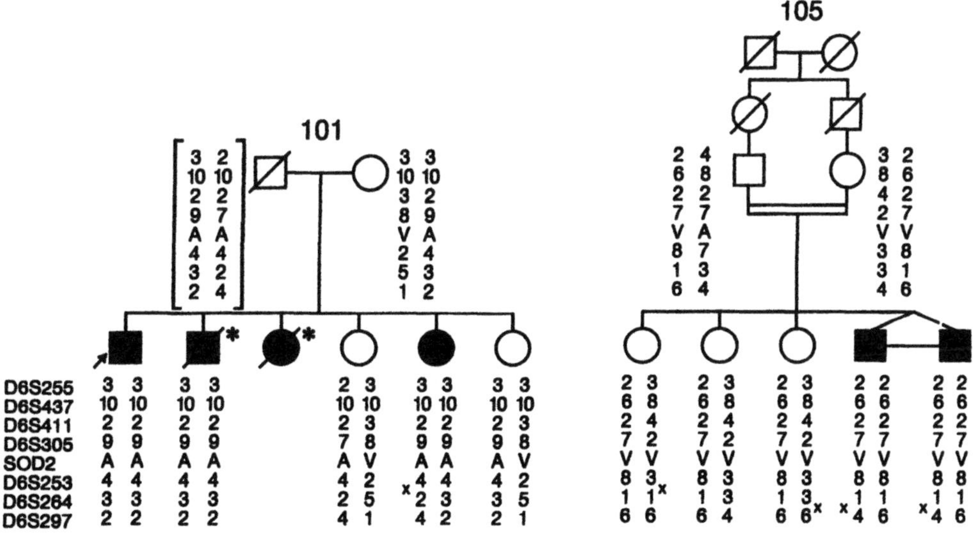

Figure 1. Haplotype analyses of family 101 and family 105. In family 101, determination of allotypes of the intragenic marker of the MnSOD gene and its flanking markers showed a clear homozygous segregation of the haplotype (3–10–2–9–A–4–3–2) to the disease. Autopsy studies and the measurement of tyrosine hydroxylase activity in the brains were performed in the two affected individuals (individual 4 and 5) who were marked with an asterisk (*) (Matsumine et al., 1997). SOD2 indicates the MnSOD gene. Polymorphism of the mitochondrial targeting sequence of the MnSOD gene is indicated as A for –9 Alanine allele and as V for –9 Valine allele (see Text). In family 105, an A/V polymorphism of MnSOD gene was not informative enough to detect the segregation. However, the markers flanking this gene were informative enough to detect the homozygous segregation of the haplotype (2–6–2–7–V–8–1–6) with a recombination event at D6S297. Inferred haplotypes are shown in brackets. x indicates the recombination point, which has been determined by genetic information including allele frequencies and the genetic distance of the markers.

the D6S305, D6S411 and MnSOD gene, which were 0 cM apart from each other. The clinical, biochemical and neuropathologic features of this family were similar to those of ARJP (MIM#600116).

The usage of these microsatellite markers increased the sensitivity to detect the segregation, resulting in the identification of another family of juvenile parkinsonism showing a clear homozygous segregation of the haplotype to the disease (family 105) (Figure 1).

The Linkage of ARJP to Chromosome 6q25.2–27

Following the identification of the haplotypic segregation of the disease and its suggestive linkage to chromosome 6q25.2–27, we extended our analysis to include 11 families which Ishikawa and Tsuji (1996) have diagnosed as ARJP (Matsumine et al., 1997). For this analysis, we used 10 microsatellite markers (D6S311, D6S441, D6S255, D6S415, D6S437, D6S411, D6S305, D6S253, D6S264 and D6S297), which encompasses a 35 cM region of the long arm of chromosome 6q24–27. The maximum pairwise cumulative lod scores in a total of 13 AR-JP families, which include family 101 and 105, were 7.26 and 7.71 at D6S305 (theta = 0.03) and D6S253 (theta = 0.02), respectively. Additional markers in this region also gave positive scores, including D6S411 (z = 4.44, theta = 0.05) and SOD2 (z = 1.69, theta = 0.0). We found no evidence for locus heterogeneity among our AR-JP families and confirmed locus homogeneity by testing with the HOMOG program. Multipoint linkage analysis by the Linkage and Fastlink programs indicated that the AR-JP gene was most likely located in the interval between D6S437 and D6S264 with the highest maximal lodscore of 9.44 obtained 0.9 cM telomeric to D6S253. Multipoint likelihood calculations by homozygosity mapping with the MAPMAKER/HOMOZ program gave us the highest maximal lod-score of 14.1 at 2 cM telomeric to D6S253 by the analysis using 6S311, D6S411, D6S415, D6S305, D6S253, D6S264, and D6S297. Haplotype analysis also showed co-segregation between the chromosome 6q markers and the AR-JP phenotype. Obligatory recombination events for the telomeric border of the AR-JP region were observed at D6S264 in two families, and that for the centromeric border was observed at D6S437 in one family, thus defining the critical chromosomal region for AR-JP between D6S437 and D6S264, which are 17 cM apart (Fig. 2). We therefore mapped the AR-JP gene in an interval of 17 cM between D6S437 and D6S264 on chromosome 6q25.2–27, which includes the MnSOD gene.

No linkage disequilibrium nor any commonly shared haplotype for AR-JP chromosomes was observed with the markers used in this study. Either the presence of multiple

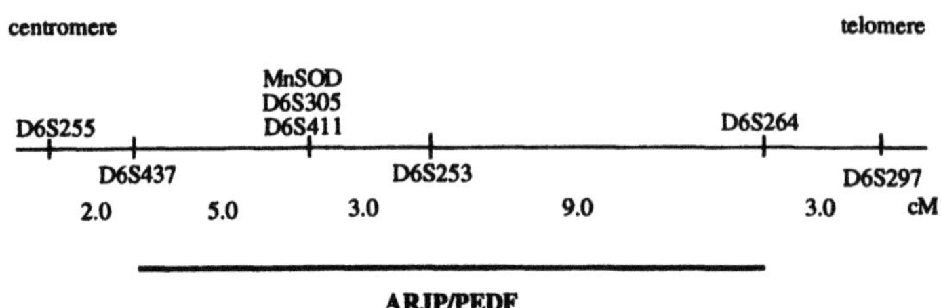

Figure 2. The critical interval region for ARJP locus and map positions of the MnSOD gene and microsatellite markers. Seven microsatellite markers (D6S255, D6S437, D6S411, D6S305, D6S253, D6S264, and D6S297) that span the MnSOD gene were used for the segregation analysis in addition to the MnSOD gene polymorphism. The most likely location for the ARJP locus on chromosome 6q is given. The genetic distances between the markers are shown in cM (Kosambi).

independent mutations in the causative gene or the decay of allelic disequilibrium due to a long period of evolution of the chromosomal region around the AR-JP gene is suggested.

Detailed nucleotide sequence analyses of all the exons and the splicing junctions of MnSOD gene were performed in the affected individuals from each pedigree, which revealed any disease-specific mutations (Matsumine et al., 1997).

Paralysis Agitance of Early-Onset with Marked Diurnal Fluctuation of Symptoms (PEDF) Is Linked to the ARJP Locus

PEDF was first reported by Yamamura in 1973 as an early-onset parkinsonism with a possible recessive inheritance and the characteristic accompaniment of diurnal fluctuation of the symptoms, which he attributed to the result of transient but ameliorating effect of sleep (sleep benefit) (Yamamura et al., 1973). Overall clinical and pathologic features of PEDF are similar to that of ARJP (Yamamura et al., 1993, 1996; Ishikawa and Tsuji, 1996). However, unlike ARJP, the ancestors of PEDF families were distributed widely throughout Japan, and about a half of them (8 in 17 families) had no parental consanguinity. The linkage analysis of 17 families, in which 4 families were described in the original paper (Yamamura et al., 1973) revealed the evidence of genetic linkage to the same genetic region which was found to be linked to ARJP, giving cumulative maximal multipoint lod score of 14.17 at the region 1.0 cM telomeric to D6S305 (Matsumine et al., 1997). An admixture test for heterogeneity gave an alpha score of 1.00, supporting the hypothesis for genetic homogeneity. The gene for PEDF was thus mapped to the same locus for ARJP, indicating that PEDF and ARJP is a genetically identical disease.

CONCLUSION

In this report, a genetic model of parkinsonism with selective degeneration of the neurons in the substantia nigra was presented. Furthermore, we have provided evidence that this abnormality is linked to a single genetic locus on chromosome 6q25.2–27.

So far, MPTP-induced parkinsonism has been a model for selective destruction of dopamine neurons in the SNPC (Langston et al., 1982). We here provide an important idea that a selective death of dopamine cells within the substantia nigra could also be caused by a single genetic mechanism. The delineation of the function of the ARJP gene will therefore elucidate why only nigral neurons are degenerated in this disease and how the survival of nigral dopamine neurons are maintained.

The main criticism of ARJP/PEDF as a model for idiopathic PD, which has also been addressed to MPTP-induced parkinsonism, is the absence of Lewy body formation and the lack of widespread involvement of other neural systems, which have been present in the brains of patients dying with PD. However, our demonstration of the monogenic mechanism as the cause of parkinsonism with selective nigral degeneration indicates that there is a specific molecular mechanism to govern the survival of nigral dopamine cells. Thus the elucidation of this mechanism will provide us an important clue to identify the etiologic mechanism of PD. Furthermore, analysis of the mechanism of cell death by a loss of function mutation of the ARJP gene will lead us to the development of a new restorative therapy to protect dopamine cells in the substantia nigra. Further mapping analysis to reduce the size of the ARJP locus is necessary to clone the ARJP gene and is now in progress in our laboratories.

ACKNOWLEDGMENTS

We thank all of the family members who kindly agreed to provide us with research samples. It is also a pleasure to acknowledge the contribution to the present work by Drs. T. Kondo, H. Mori, Y. Sugita, N. Hattori, S. Matsubayashi, T. Kobayashi, Y. Hattori and Ms. Y. Shimizu (Department of Neurology, Juntendo University School of Medicine), Drs. H. Tanaka (Department of Neurology, Brain Research Institute, Niigata University), A. Schäffer (National Human Genome Research Institute National Institute of Health), M. Yokochi (Department of Neurology, Tokyo Metropolitan Ebara Hospital), Y. Mizutani (Deaprtment of Clinical Pathology, Tokyo Metropolitan Matsuzawa Hospital), S. Nakamura(The third department of Internal Medicine, Hiroshima University School of Medicine), and S. Kuzuhara (Department of Neurology, Mie University School of Medicine). This work was supported in part by a Grant-in-Aid for Scientific Research on Priority Areas, a Grant-in-Aid for Neuroscience Research, and a Grant-in-Aid for Creative Basic Research (Human Genome Program) from Ministry of Education, Science, and Culture, Japan, a Grant-in-Aid for Neurodegenerative Disorders from Ministry of Health and Welfare, Japan, Special coordination funds from the Japanese Science and Technology Agency, a Grant from the Uehara Memorial Foundation, and from the National Parkinson Foundation, Miami.

REFERENCES

Golbe, L.I., DiIorio, G., Bonavita, V., Miller, D.C., and Duvoisin, R.C.., 1990, *Ann. Neurol.* 27:276.

Hassan , H.M.., 1988, *Free. Radic. Biol. Med.* 5: 377–385.

Ishikawa, A., and Tsuji, S., 1996, *Neurology* 47:160–166.

Kondo, T., Sugita, H., Mizutani, H., and Mizuno, Y., 1990, *Mov. Disord.* 5 (Suppl): 29.

Langston, J.W., Ballard, P., Tetrud, J.W., and Irwin, I., 1982, *Science* 219:979–80.

Matsumine, H., Saito, M., Shimoda-Matsubayashi, S., et al., 1997, *Am. J. Hum. Genet.* 60:588–596.

Matsumine, H, Yamamura, Y, Kuzuhara, S., et al., 1997, *Neurology* 48:A394. (Abstract in 49th Annual meeting of American academy of neurology, April 17, 1997, Boston, MA).

Mizuno, Y, Ohta, S, Tanaka, M, Takamiya, S, Suzuki, K, Sato, T, Oya, H, Ozawa, T, and Kagawa, Y. , 1989, *Biochem. Biophys. Res. Commun.* 163: 1450–1455.

Saggu H, Cooksey J, Dexter D, Wells FR, Lees A, Jenner P, Marsden CD., 1989, *J. Neurochem.* 53: 692–697.

Schapira, A.H.V., Cooper, J.M., Dexter, D., Jenner, P., Clark, J.B., and Marsden, C,D,.., 1989, *Lancet 1:* 1269

Shimoda-Matsubayashi, S., Matsumine, H., Kobayashi, T., Nakagawa-Hattori, Y., Shimizu, Y., and Mizuno, Y.., 1996, *Biochem. Biophys. Research. Comm.* 226:561–565.

Takahashi, H. et al., 1994, *Neurology* 44:437–441.

Yamamura, Y., Sobue, I., Ando, K., Iida, M., Yanagi, T., and Kondo, C., 1973, *Neurology* 23:239–244.

Yamamura, Y., Arihiro, K., Kohriyama, T., and Nakamura, S., 1993, *Clin Neurol.* (Tokyo) (Abstract in English) 33:491–496.

Yamamura, Y. et al., 1996, In: *The Basal Ganglia V,* Ohye, C. et al.), Plenum, New York, pp 485–489.

58

CYTOKINES IN PARKINSON'S DISEASE

Toshiharu Nagatsu[1,2] and Makio Mogi[1,2]

[1]Institute Institute for Comprehensive Medical Science
School of Medicine
Fujita Health University
Toyoake 470-11, Japan
[2]Department of Pharmacology
School of Dentistry
Aichi-Gakuin University
Nagoya 466, Japan

INTRODUCTION

Cytokines are proteins or glycoproteins produced by leukocytes and other types of cells, and are involved in chemical communication between cells in immune response. An association of altered immune responsiveness with neurodegenerative disorders has recently been suggested. In Parkinson's disease (PD), the nigro-striatal dopaminergic neurons specifically degenerate due to unknown causes (Temlett, 1996). Neurochemical imbalances in the substantia nigra and striatum in PD might result in some compensatory mechanisms that modify the chronic neurodegenerative process in PD, including the changes in cytokines, neurotrophins, and cell death-related proteins. Although the pathogenesis of PD remains enigmatic, apotosis, i.e. programmed cell death, might be involved in the degeneration of the nigro-striatal dopaminergic neurons in PD. The key role of cytokines, neurotrophins, and apoptosis-related proteins in the regulation of cell death has recently been outlined. Therefore, we have investigated changes in cytokines, neurotrophins, and apoptosis-related proteins in the brain (striatum) and ventricular cerebrospinal fluid (VCSF) and lumber CSF (LCSF) from parkinsonian patients (Mogi et al., 1989, 1994a, b; 1995a, b, c; 1996a, b, c).

MATERIALS AND METHODS

Control human brains from patients without neurological diseases and parkinsonian brains were obtained in autopsy. They were age- and sex-matched with the patients. Postmortem times were from 3 to 21 hours. The striatum (caudate nucleus and putamen) and cerebral cortex were dissected and stored frozen at –80°C. Brain tissues were homogenized with 0.32 M sucrose containing protease inhibitors (100 μM phenylmethylsulfonylfluoride; 50 μg/ml each of leupeptine, pepstatin and antipain). The following cytokines, neurotrophins, and apoptosis-related proteins were measured by enzyme immunoassays (EIAs): tumor necrosis factor-α (TNF-α), interleukin-1β (IL-1β), IL-2, IL-4, IL-6, epidermal growth factor (EGF), transforming growth factor α (TGF-α), basic fibroblast growth factor (bFGF), TGF-β1, bcl-2, soluble Fas (sFas), and β2-microglobulin (β2-MG). The immunoreagents and the immunoassay systems were similar to those described previously for the EIA of tyrosine hydroxylase (Mogi et al., 1984, 1988). Samples of VCSF were obtained during ventriculography prior to operation from patients with PD and with juvenile parkinsonism (JP). The control group consisted of patients with non-parkinsonian neurological diseases (NPD); idiopathic tremor, dystonia torticollis, Huntington's disease, cerebral palsy, and brachial tremor after vascular accident, who underwent stereotaxic surgery. The LCSF was obtained through lumbar puncture from control patients without neurological diseases who were operated under lumbar anesthesia. Consent was obtained from each patient.

Protein concentration was estimated by the method of Bradford (1976) with bovine serum albumin as a standard.

Table 1. Cytokines, neurotrophins, and apoptosis-related proteins in the brain in Parkinson's disease (PD) and controls

	Controls		PD	
protein	striatum	cerebral cortex	striatum	cerebral cortex
Cytokines and neurotrophins (pg/mg protein)				
TNF-α	6.7 ± 3.5	23.6 ± 10.4	52.7 ± 15.3**	13.9 ± 8.0
IL-1β	4.9 ± 0.8	2.3 ± 0.3	17.1 ± 5.0*	4.4 ± 1.2
Il-2	0.80 ± 0.15	0.00	15.3 ± 7.1*	0.89 ± 0.89
IL-6	2.2 ± 0.9	5.9 ± 2.4	23.4 ± 9.1*	45.1 ± 36.0
EGF	23.9 ± 6.7	62.7 ± 24.7	90.2 ± 29.7*	74.4 ± 5.1
TGF-α	0.9 ± 0.9	2.9 ± 2.9	42.1 ± 20.2*	15.7 ± 6.1
bFGF	2.72 ± 0.17	3.33 ± 0.32	2.75 ± 0.24	4.21 ± 0.47
TGF-β1	46.5 ± 17.5	73.8 ± 36.3	138 ± 42*	106 ± 39
apoptosis-related proteins				
bcl-2 (U/mg protein)	13.4 ± 0.9	13.0 ± 1.7	23.2 ± 1.6**	15.3 ± 8.9
sFAs (pg/mg protein)	52.9 ± 4.0	55.0 ± 4.0	131 ± 21**	71.5 ± 9.4
β2MG (ng/mg protein)	58.8 ± 16.5	30.3 ± 9.5	131 ± 21**	44.4 ± 7.4

Each value represents the mean ± SEM.
Significantly different from controls, *p<0.05, **p<0.01.

RESULTS

Cytokines, Neurotrophins, and Apotosis-Related Proteins in Parkinsonian Brain

We measured the following cytokines, neurotrophins, and apotosis-related proteins in the striatum (putamen and caudate nucleus) and cerebral cortex in controls and PD: TNF-α, IL-1β, IL-2, IL-6, EGF, TGF-α, bFGF, TGF-β1, bcl-2, sFas, and β2MG (Table 1). All the cytokines, neurotrophins, and apoptosis-related proteins except bFGF were elevated specifically in the striatum, but not in the cerebral cortex, in PD. Our preliminary data also indicate that interferon (IFN)-γ level was increased in the striatum in PD.

Cytokines, Neurotrophins, and Apoptosis-Related Proteins in VCSF and LCSF in PD and JP

We measured the levels of TNF-α, IL-1β, IL-2, IL-4, IL-6, EGF, TGF-α, TGF-β1, in VCSF from patients with PD and control patients with NPD (Table 2). The levels of IL-

Table 2. Cytokines, neurotrophins, and apoptosis-related proteins in ventricular cerebrospinal fluid (VCSF) and lumbar CSF in Parkinson's disease (PD), juvenile parkinsonism (JP), non-parkinsonian neurological diseases (NPD), and controls (C)

	VCSF			LCSF	
	NPD	JP	PD	C	PD
Cytokines and neurotrophins (pg/ml)					
TNF-α				22.3 ± 9.5	96.3 ± 9.1**
IL-1β	0.40 ± 0.07	1.16 ± 0.41*	0.56 ± 0.28	<0.1	
IL-2	11.9 ± 2.5	24.5 ± 6.4*	18.0 ± 1.3*	<1.5	
IL-4	1.78 ± 1.20	9.52 ± 4.74*	4.05 ± 1.29	<1.0	
IL-6	1.11 ± 0.14	0.96 ± 0.33	1.71 ± 0.24*	<0.7	
EGF	25.2 ± 13.6	48.6 ± 30.2	46.8 ± 27.1	<0.5	
TGF-α	11.6 ± 4.5	36.6 ± 13.1*	22.1 ± 6.9	0.36 ± 0.07	
TGF-β1	114 ± 10		211 ± 19**		
Apoptosis-related proteins					
bcl-2 (U/ml)	<5		<5	<5	<5
sFas (pg/ml)	<16		<16	<16	<16

Each value represents the mean ± SEM.
Significantly different fron controls, *p<0.05, **p<0.01.

1β, IL-2, IL-4, IL-6, and TGF-α in VCSF were elevated in JP or PD. The EGF levels were also higher in JP or PD, but were not significantly higher than those in control patients with NPD.

Cytokine levels in LCSF were very low compared with those in VCSF. Only TNF-α level was significantly detected in LCSF in both controls and parkinsonian patients, and was increased in PD.

Relationship between the Levels of Cytokines and Apoptosis-Related Proteins in the Brain in PD

There are significantly positive correlations between the levels of bcl-2 and those of sFas, IL-1β or IL-2. The levels of sFas are also positively correlated with those of IL-1β, IL-6, TNF-α, or β2MG.

DISCUSSION

Our results suggest that up-regulation of cytokines, neurotrophins, and apoptosis-related proteins may be involved in the pathogenesis of neurodegeneration in PD. The up-regulation of cytokines was seen neither in control striatum nor in parkinsonian cerebral cortex, indicating that these elevations in cytokines are topographically specific in the parkinsonian striatum.

Cytokines act as growth and/or differentiation factors of cells in the brain (Sternberg, 1989). Since cytokines are pleiotropic, they may play a role either in a compensatory response as neuroprotective factors or in producing cell death as neurotoxic factors, in the pathophysiology of PD.

The increase in cytokines as neurotrophins in the striatum in PD may be a compensatory response following neuronal death of the nigro-striatal dopaminergic neurons. IL-1β, a cytokine known to act synergistically with TNF-α, may stimulate astrocyte proliferation in vivo as a trophic factor (Giulian et al., 1985). As neurodegeneration in the brain progresses in PD, several neurotrophic factors may be produced probably for compensatory function. IL-1β, TNF-α, EGF, and FGF were reported to enhance nerve growth factor (NGF) production by astrocytes (Lindholm et al., 1987; Yoshida and Gage, 1991). Marked increases in the contents of IL-1β, IL-2, IL-3, IL-6 and TNF-α were also observed in the hippocampal formation in Alzheimer's disease (Wood et al., 1993).

The results also suggest that an immune response may occur in the nigro-striatal regions of parkinsonian brain. It has been suggested that patients with idiopathic PD have altered function of the immune system (Fiszer et al., 1991). The expression of major histocompatibility complex-I (MHC-I) on the glial cells may be associated with an increase in β2-microglobulin (β2-MG) that is one component of MHC-I. β2-MG level was increased in the striatum in PD. Therefore, the expression of MHC-I antigens may also be elevated in the parkinsonian brain. MHC-I antigens in the brain may become the target for cytolytic T lymphocytes, and may lead to cellular destruction. It has not been reported that MHC-I antigens are positive in the parkinsonian brain. However, reactive microglial cells were reported to produce MHC-II antigen in the substantia nigra of the brain from patients with PD or Alzheimer's disease (McGeer et al., 1988). TNF-α was demonstrated to be produced at the site of neural injury in multiple sclerosis (Hoffman et al., 1989) to modulate MHC-I (Mauerhoff et al., 1988); Benveniste et al., 1989), and to lead to the increase of β2-MG. The induction of MHC-I antigen/β2-MG may render brain cells competent to initiate immune reactions and may therefore contribute to both immunoprotective and immunopathological responses in the parkinsonian brain.

All cytokines and neurotrophins were found to be increased both in the striatum and in VCSF or LCSF. One exception is β2-MG which is increased in the striatum (Mogi et al., 1995a) but is decreased in LCSF (Mogi et al., 1989). We cannot explain the discrepancy in the changes in β2-MG contents in the parkinsonian striatum and in LCSF. This problem remains to be further elucidated.

An importent question is the origin of the increased cytokines in PD. Microglial cells which are activated cells of the macrophage lineage, astrocytes, neurons, or vascular endothelial cells can produce cytokines. Microglial cells and astrocytes are thought to be the most probable candidates to produce cytokines.

Another question is the specificity of the changes in cytokines in the striatum in PD. In a preliminary study we have found that the β2-MG and TNF-α contents in the striatum from patients with Huntinton's disease or striatonigral degeneration, which are characterized by the degeneration of neurons in the striatum, were similar to those of control subjects. Thus, the elevated levels of cytokines in the striatum may be specific for PD. However, more detailed study is needed, since without appropriate controls the significance of the increased cytokine levels is extremely limited.

Cytokines have both neurotrophic and neurotoxic functions, and are considered to be closely related to apoptosis. The content of bcl-2 protein capable of blocking or delaying apoptosis was shown to be increased in the striatum from patients with PD. Expression of bcl-2 protein has also been reported in the brain from patients with PD (Mochizuki et al., 1996). The Fas antigen/APO-1 is a cell-surface receptor belonging to the nerve growth factor family of apoptosis-signaling molecules (Nagata and Goldstein, 1995). A human Fas messenger RNA variant encodes sFas molecule lacking the transmembrane domain because of the deletion of an exon encoding this region (Cheng et al., 1994). Though we have no direct evidence which connects the elevation of cytokines with the increase of bcl-2 and sFas in the brain from patients with PD, sFas expression is significantly correlated with the levels of IL-1β, IL-6, and bcl-2. Since both bcl-2 and sFas are related to apoptosis (Itoh et al., 1993), the apoptosis reaction may be involved in the pathogenesis of PD.

In conclusion, the increment of cytokines in the brain in PD may the factors in the degeneration of dopaminergic neurons in PD.

ACKNOWLEDGMENTS

We gratefully acknowledge the collaboration in this work with M. Harada (Matsumoto Dental College, Shiojiri, Japan), A. Togari (School of Dentistry, Aichi-Gakuin University, Nagoya, Japan), H. Narabayashi, Y. Mizuno, T. Kondo (Juntendo University, Tokyo, Japan), and P. Riederer (Würzburg University, Würzburg, Germany). This work is supported by Grants-in-Aid for Scientific Research from the Ministry of Education, Science, Sports and Culture of Japan (to T. Nagatsu) and by the Grant for the Research Committee of CNS Degenerative Diseases, the Ministry of Health and Welfare of Japan (to T. Nagatsu).

REFERENCES

Benveniste, E.N., Sparacio, S.M., and Bethea, J.R., 1989, Tumor necrosis factor-α enhances interferon-ä mediated class II antigen expression on astrocytes, *J. Immunol.* 25:209–219.

Bradford, M.M., 1976, A rapid and sensitive method for the quantitation of microgram quantities of protein utilizing the principle of protein-dye binding, *Anal. Biochem.* 72:248–254.

Cheng, J., Zhou, T., Liu, C., Shapiro, J.P., Brauer, M.J., Kiefer, M.C., Barr, P.J., and Mountz, J.D., 1994, Protection from Fas-mediated apoptosis by a soluble form of the Fas molecule, *Science* 263:1759–1762.

Fiszer, U., Piotrowska, K., Korlak, J., and Czlonkowska, A., 1991, The immunological status in Parkinson's disease, *Med. Lab. Sci.* 48:196–200.

Giulian, D. and Lachman, L.B., 1985, Interleukin-1 stimulation of astroglial proliferation after brain injuty, *Science* 228 : 497–499.

Hoffman, F.M., Hinton, D.R., Johnson, K., and Merrill, J.E., 1989, Tumor necrosis factor identified in multiple sclerosis brain, *J. Exp. Med.* 170:607–612.

Itoh, N., Tsujimoto, Y., and Nagata, S., 1993, Effect of bcl-2 on Fas antigen-mediated cell death, *J. Immunol.* 151:621–627.

Lindfolm, D., Heumann, R., Meyer, M., and Thoenen, H., 1987, Interleukin-1 regulates synthesis of nerve growth factor in non-neuronal cells of rat sciatic nerve, *Nature* 330:658–659.

Mauerhoff, T., Pujol-Borrell, R., Mirakian, R., and Bottazzo, G.F., 1988, Differential expression and regulation of major histocompatibility complex (MHC) products in neural and glial cells of the human fetal brain, *J. Neuroimmunol.* 18:271–289.

McGeer, P.L., Itagaki, S., Boyes, B.E., and McGeer, E.G., 1988, Reactive microglia are positive for HLA-DR in the substatia nigra of Parkinson's and Alzheimer's disease brains, *Neurology* 38:1285–1291.

Mochizuki, H., Goto, K., Mori, H., and Mizuno, Y., 1996, Histochemical detection of apoptosis in Parkinson's disease, *J. Neurol. Sci.* 137:120–123.

Mogi, M., Kojima, K., and Nagatsu, T., 1984, Detection of inactive or less active forms of tyrosine hydroxylase in human adrenals by a sandwich enzyme immunoassay, *Anal. Biochem.* 138:123–132.

Mogi, M., Harada, M., Kiuchi, K., Kojima, K., Kondo, T., Narabayashi, H., Rausch, D., Riederer, P., Jellinger, K., and Nagatsu, T., 1988, Homospecific activity (activity per enzyme protein) of tyrosine hydroxylase increases in Parkinsonian brain, *J. Neural Transm.* 72:77–82.

Mogi, M., Harada, M., Kojima, K., Adachi, T., Narabayashi, H., Fujita, K., Naoi, M., and Nagatsu, T., 1989, β2-Microglobulin decrease in cerebrospinal fluid in parkinsonian patients, *Neurosci. Lett.* 104: 41–246.

Mogi, M., Harada, M., Riederer, P., Narabayashi, H., Fujita, K., and Nagatsu, T., 1994a, Tumor necrosis factor-α (TNF-α) increases both in the brain and in the cerebrospinal fluid from parkinsonian patients, *Neurosci. Lett.* 165:208–210.

Mogi, M., Harada, M., Kondo, T., Riederer, P., Inagaki, H., Minami, M., and Nagatsu, T., 1994b, Interleukin-1β, interleukin-6, epidermal growth factor and transforming growth factor-α are elevated in the brain from parkinsonian patients, *Neurosci. Lett.* 180:47–150.

Mogi, M., Harada, M., Kondo, T., Riederer, P., and Nagatsu, T., 1995a, Brain 2-microglobulin levels are elevated in the striatum in Parkinson's disease, *J. Neural. Transm.* [P-D Sect] 9:87–92.

Mogi, M., Harada, M., Kondo, T., Narabayashi, H, Riederer, P., and Nagatsu, T., 1995b, Transforming growth factor-β1 levels are elevated in the striatum and in ventricular cerebrospinal fluid in Parkinson's disease, *Neurosci. Lett.* 193:129–132.

Mogi, M., Harada, M., Narabayashi, H, Inagaki, H., Minami, M., and Nagatsu, T., 1995c, Interleukin (IL)-1β, IL-2, IL-6, and transforming growth factor-α levels are elevated in ventricular cerebrospinal fluid of juvenile parkinsonism and Parkinson's disease, *Neurosci. Lett.* 211:13–16.

Mogi, M., Harada, M., Kondo, T., Narabayashi, H, Riederer, P., and Nagatsu, T., 1996a, Interleukin-2 but not basic fibroblast growth factor is elevated in parkinsonian brain, *J. Neural Transm.* 103:1077–1081.

Mogi, M., Harada, M., Kondo, T., Mizuno, Y., Riederer, P., and Nagatsu, T., 1996b, bcl-2 Protein is increased in the brain from parkinsonian patients, *Neurosci. Lett.* 215:137–139.

Mogi, M., Harada, M., Kondo, T., Mizuno, Y., Riederer, P., and Nagatsu, T., 1996c, The soluble form of Fas molecule is elevated in parkinsonian brain tissues, *Neurosci. Lett.* 220:195–198.

Nagata, S. and Goldstein, P., 1995, The Fas death factor, *Science 267:1449–1456.*

Sternberg, E.M., 1989, Monokines, lymphokines and the brain, Year Immunol. 5:205–217.

Temlett, J.A., 1996, Parkinson's disease : biology and etiology, *Curr. Opi. Neurol.* 9 :303–307.

Wood, J.A., Wood, P.L., Ryan, R., Graff-Radford, N.R., Pilapil, C., Robitaille, Y., and Quirion, R., 1993, Cytokine induces in Alzheimer's temporal cortex : no changes in mature IL-1β or IL-1RA but increases in the associated acute phase proteins IL-6, α2-macroglobulin and C-reactive protein, *Brain Res.* 629:245–252.

Yoshida, K. and Gage, F.H., 1991, Fibroblast growth factors stimulate nerve growth factor synthesis and secretion by astrocytes, *Brain Res.* 538:118–126.

59

N-METHYL(*R*)SALSOLINOL AND (*R*)SALSOLINOL *N*-METHYLTRANSFERASE AS POSSIBLE PATHOGENIC FACTORS IN PARKINSON'S DISEASE

Makoto Naoi[1] and Wakako Maruyama[2]

[1]Department of Biosciences
Nagoya Institute of Technology
Gokiso-cho, Showa-ku, Nagoya 466, Japan
[2]Laboratory of Biochemistry and Metabolism
Department of Basic Gerontology
National Institute for Longevity Sciences
Obu 474, Japan

INTRODUCTION

Parkinson's disease (PD) is characterized by the selective degeneration of dopamine (DA) neurons in the pars compacta of the substantia nigra. Recent results suggest that apoptosis may be a major feature of the cell death (Mochizuki et al., 1996). The apoptotic process is known to be initiated by oxidative stress, energy crisis or perturbation of calcium homeostasis. In addition, endogenous and xenobiotic neurotoxins were reported to initiate the apoptotic process. A potent dopaminergic neurotoxin, 1-methyl-4-phenylpyridinium ion (MPP$^+$), an oxidation product of 1-methyl-4-phenyl-1,2,3,6-tetrahydropyridine (MPTP), was reported to induce apoptosis in cultured cerebellar granule neurons (Dipasquale et al., 1991) and in pheochromocytoma PC12 cells (Mutoh et al., 1994).

As an endogenous neurotoxin candidate, we propose 1(*R*),2(*N*)-dimethyl-6,7-dihydroxy-1,2,3,4-tetrahydroisoquinoline [N-methyl(R)salsolinol, NM(R)Sal] (Naoi et al., 1997). In human brain 1(*R*)-methyl-6,7-dihydroxy-1,2,3,4-tetrahydroisoquinoline [(*R*)salsolinol, (*R*)Sal] is enantio-selectively synthesized from DA and acetaldehyde by a novel enzyme (Naoi et al., 1996a) and *N*-methylated by an *N*-methyltransferase (Maruyama et al., 1992), as shown in Figure 1.

The selective neurotoxicity of *N*M(*R*)Sal has been confirmed by *in vivo* experiments. Injection of *N*M(*R*)Sal into the striatum induced parkinsonism in rats, whereas the (*S*)en-

Progress in Alzheimer's and Parkinson's Diseases
edited by Fisher *et al.*, Plenum Press, New York, 1998.

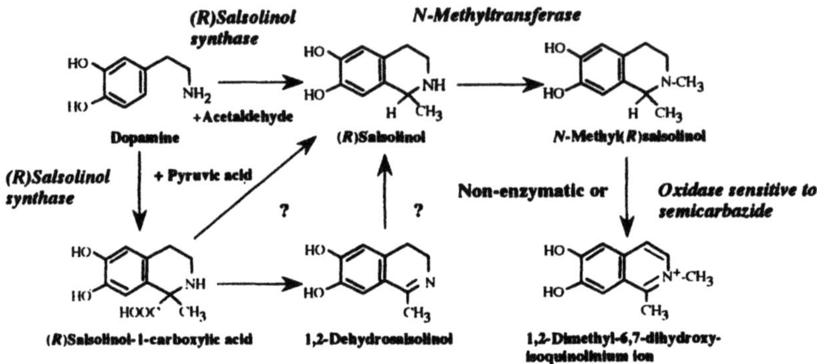

Figure 1. Metabolism pathway of NM(R)Sal and its derivatives in the human brain.

antiomer of NMSal, (R)- and (S)Sal, 6,7-dihydroxy-1,2,3,4-tetrahydroisoquinoline (norsalsolinol), N-methylnorsalsolinol did not (Naoi et al., 1996b). In the substantia nigra DA neurons were selectively depleted without necrotic tissue reaction, suggesting that the cell death may be apoptotic.

This review presents the results indicating the possible involvement of NM(R)Sal to the pathogenesis of PD. The effects of NM(R)Sal and structurally-related compounds on DNA were examined, and only NM(R)Sal was found to induce DNA damage in dopaminergic neuroblastoma SH-SY5Y cells (Maruyama et al., 1997b). NM(R)Sal was found to increase significantly in the cerebrospinal fluid from parkinsonian patients (Maruyama et al., 1996a). The biochemical mechanism underlying the increase was studied by analyses of enzymes related to the metabolism of NM(R)Sal in the lymphocytes. A neutral N-methyltransferase specific for (R)Sal was confirmed to increase in PD lymphocytes. The involvement of NM(R)Sal to the pathogenesis of PD is discussed.

Apoptosis Induced by NM(R)Sal

SH-SY5Y cells were incubated with NM(R)Sal and other isoquinolines, and DNA damage was assessed by a single cell gel electrophoresis (comet) assay (Östling and Johanson, 1984). The cells were mixed with low-melting agarose, subjected to alkaline lysis, then to electrophoresis. After neutralization, DNA was stained with 4',6-diamidino-2-phenylindole.

The typical comet image of the apoptotic cells was observed after incubation with NM(R)Sal. In the cells incubated with NM(R)Sal this took the form of a "head" and a migrated "tail" composed of DNA fragmented into smaller size and broken ends. The migration distance of DNA from the comet head to the tip of the tail was significantly larger in the NM(R)Sal-treated cells than in control samples.

Figure 2 shows the histogram of the migration distance of DNA in the cells treated with (R)- and (S)enantiomers of Sal and NMSal, and DMDHIQ$^+$. The mean head-tail distances of control and cells incubated with (R)- and (S)Sal or DMDHIQ$^+$ were distributed between 10 to 20 μm (mean ± SD, 11.2 ± 0.02 μm), which is consistent with intact nuclei with undamaged DNA. On the other hand, those of the cells incubated with NM(R)Sal were larger than 45 μm. A tail-length of 45 μm or larger was taken to indicate extensive apoptosis. With 1 mM NM(R)Sal almost all the cells showed the DNA damage and with 100 μM about 5 % of the total cells were estimated to be positive for DNA damage. NM(S)Sal was less potent in inducing DNA damage and at 1 mM only about 10% cells were positive.

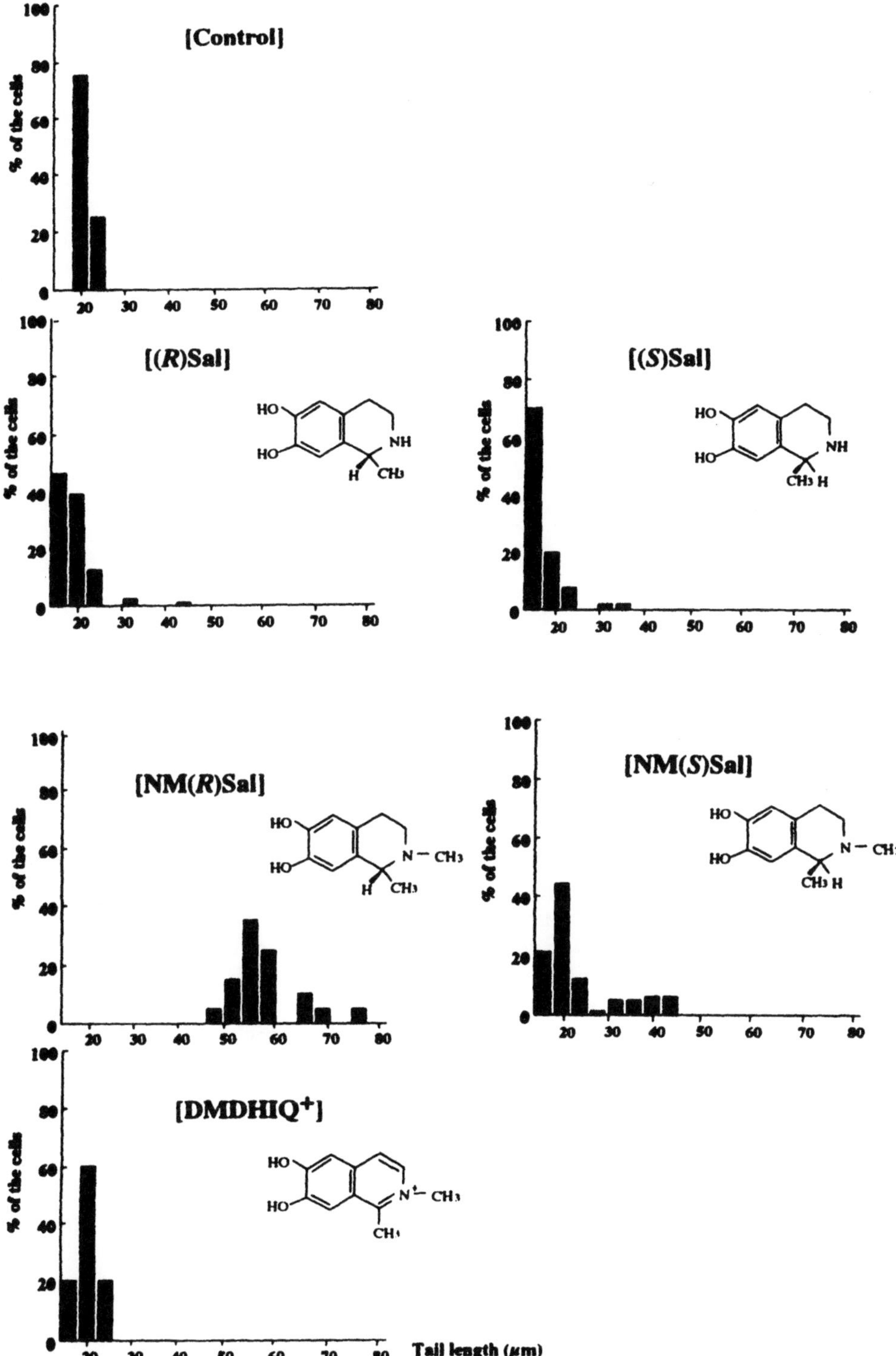

Figure 2. Frequency distribution of DNA migration distance in SH-SY5Y cells incubated with catechol isoquinolines. The cells were incubated at 37°C for 3 hours with 1 mM concentrations of the (R)- and (S)-enantiomers of Sal and NMSal, DMDHIQ⁺, or without isoquinolines as a control. The migration distance was measured as described in the text. The distribution of the cells with DNA image of a given migration distance was expressed as the percentage of the total 200 cells. Each column represents the mean value of four experiments.

A protein synthesis inhibitor, cycloheximide, reduced occurrence of the DNA damage. Anti-oxidants and anti-oxidative enzymes protected the cells from the DNA damage. With 0.5 mM NM(R)Sal about 18% cells showed typical comet images of DNA damage, and pre-treatment with catalase, reduced glutathione, deprenyl or semicarbazide significantly reduced the DNA damage. On the other hand, superoxide dismutase did not prevent the DNA damage.

The nature of DNA damage by NM(R)Sal was confirmed by morphological observation. After incubation with NM(R)Sal, some of the cells showed morphological features typical for apoptosis; condensation of chromatin materials and also "apoptotic" bodies. The TdT (terminal deoxynucleotidyl transferase)-mediated dUTP-biotin nick-end labeling (TUNEL) method was applied to detect 3'-OH ends of increased small nucleosomal units. Positive staining was detected in the cells incubated with NM(R)Sal, while in control cells such morphological changes were not detected.

Apoptosis is an active intracellular death process involving a chain of events, which may be initiated by various physiological and pathological factors. Inhibition of mitochondrial respiratory chain complex I in PC12 cells by MPP^+ and rotenone (Hartley et al., 1994) was reported to induce apoptosis. In our experiments, reduced glutathione and catalase could prevent DNA damage by scavenging of hydroxyl radicals produced from NM(R)Sal oxidation (Maruyama et al., 1995). This result suggests that apoptosis may be initiated by oxidative stress.

Increase of NM(R)Sal in Parkinsonian CSF

Lumbar CSF samples from 16 newly-diagnosed and untreated parkinsonian patients and from 29 control subjects without neurological disorders were used for the analysis NM(R)Sal was detected in CSF from control and patients with PD, whereas another enantiomer, NM(S)Sal, was under detection limit (< 0.01 nM). NM(R)Sal concentration in the control group was not affected by age from 22 to 76 years (r = 0.141) or by sex [male; 4.39 ± 1.73 nM, female; 4.89 ± 2.79 nM (mean ± SD)]. Figure 3 shows the distribution of NM(R)Sal levels in control and PD patients. NM(R)Sal concentrations in PD patients were significantly higher than in control. In control (27 out of 29), NM(R)Sal level was lower than 6 nM. On the other hand, in PD patients (12 out of 16) the level was higher than 6 nM. The mean of NM(R)Sal concentration was significantly higher in PD patients than

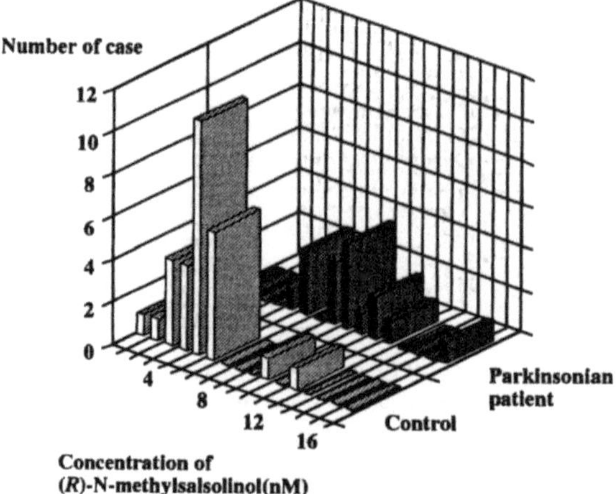

Figure 3. Concentration of NM(R)Sal in the CSF of control and parkinsonian patients (PD). The amounts of NM(R)Sal were plotted against the age of the patients. In most of PD patients the concentration was higher than 6 nM.

that in control: 8.32 ± 2.89 nM *versus* 4.53 ± 2.08 nM ($p < 0.0001$). These results suggest that the biosynthesis of *N*M(*R*)Sal may be determined by some endogenous factors, such as activity of enzymes related to the synthesis and catabolism of catechol isoquinolines.

Enantio-Specific Biosynthesis of *N*M(*R*)Sal in the Brain

Our data on the analyses of human brain and CSF suggest that the (*R*)enantiomers of Sal and *N*MSal are synthesized enzymatically *in situ*. Recently we purified an enzyme catalyzing condensation of DA with acetaldehyde to generate (*R*)Sal directly (Naoi et al., 1996a). The (*R*)salsolinol synthase catalyzes the condensation of DA with acetaldehyde, pyruvic acid or formaldehyde into (*R*)Sal, (*R*)Sal-1-carboxylic acid or norsalsolinol. This enzyme uses DA as the only amine substrate, and neither *N*-methyldopamine (epinine), adrenaline, noradrenaline, nor L-DOPA was a substrate. This enzyme is localized in the cytosol and purified to about 2 000 times with a molecular weight of 34.3 ± 8.3 kDa.

In human brain the activity of two types of *N*-methyltransferase with different optimal pH were detected, using (*R*)Sal as a substrate and S-adenosyl-L-methionine as a methyl donor. The neutral N-methyltransferase with the optimal pH around 7 was found to be specific for (*R*)Sal, whereas neither (*S*)Sal nor norsalsolinol was a substrate. The substrate specificity and localization in the brain suggest that this enzyme is different from the hitherto-reported *N*-methyltransferase. The purification of an *N*-methyltransferase is now in progress.

*N*M(*R*)Sal is oxidized into 1,2-dimethyl-6,7-dihydroxyisoquinolinium ion (DMDHIQ$^+$) enzymatically (Naoi et al., 1995a) and non-enzymatically (Maruyama et al., 1995). The oxidase is not mitochondrial monoamine oxidase, but sensitive to semicarbazide and localized in cytosol. At present it is not clear whether this *N*M(*R*)Sal oxidase is the same as semicarbazide-sensitive amine oxidase detected in the periphery.

Table 1 summarizes the distribution of *N*M(*R*)Sal and related isoquinolines in human brain regions. (*R*)Sal was found to be distributed ubiquitously, which may be due to the fact that the activity of a (*R*)salsolinol synthase is virtually the same in all brain regions. *N*M(*R*)Sal accumulates in the nigro-striatal system selectively, which may be due to the high activity of an *N*-methyltransferase and its uptake by a DA transport system (Takahashi et al., 1994). DMDHIQ$^+$ was detected only in the substantia nigra and not in other

Table 1. Distribution of dopamine, (*R*)Sal, *N*M(*R*)Sal
and DMDHIQ$^+$ in normal human brain regions

Dopamine (nmol/g wet weight)	Concentration in the brain regions (pmol/g wet weight)		
	(*R*)Sal	*N*M(*R*)Sal	DMDHIQ$^+$
Frontal cortex 0.73 ± 0.78	134 ± 125	N.D. (< 10)	N.D. (< 100)
Caudate 26.4 ± 19.0*	73.3 ± 79.9	5.7 ± 88.3	N.D. (< 100)
Putamen 20.7 ± 11.9*	37.8 ± 23.0	110 ± 126*	N.D. (< 100)
Substantia nigra 3.5 ± 2.7	94.5 ± 78.7	76.6 ± 23.0	254 ± 59.0*

Dopamine, (*R*)Sal, and *N*M(*R*)Sal were analyzed by HPLC with multi-ECD and (*R*)- and (*S*)-enantiomers were separated using a β-cyclodextrin-bonded column. DMDHIQ$^+$ was analyzed by HPLC with fluorometric detection.
Each value represents the mean ± SD of duplicate measurements of 10 samples.
*p < 0.01 compared with the concentration in the frontal cortex by ANOVA.
N.D.: not detected.

brain regions, which may be ascribed to its binding to neuromelanin (Naoi et al., 1994). These results clearly demonstrate the selective accumulation of NM(R)Sal and DMDHIQ$^+$ in the nigro-striatal system.

Increased Activity of a Neutral N-Methyltransferase in Parkinsonian Lymphocytes

The increase in NM(R)Sal in parkinsonian CSF was suggested to be due to the abnormality in its synthesis or catabolism. To prove this hypothesis, the activity of a (R)salsolinol synthase, (R)salsolinol N-methyltransferase and N-methyl(R)salsolinol oxidase, were examined in the lymphocytes. The results are summarized in Table 2. The (R)salsolinol synthase was not detected in lymphocytes. The activity of N-methyl(R)salsolinol oxidase was the same in lymphocytes from PD patients and control. Also in lymphocytes as in the brain, two species of N-methyltransferase activity with different optimal pH were detected by use of (R)Sal as a substrate. The activity of a neutral N-methyltransferase was found to increase significantly in PD lymphocytes, whereas the activity of another N-methyltransferase with the optimal pH around 8 did not change. Kinetics of a neutral (R)salsolinol N-methyltransferase show that the values of the Michaelis constant for (R)Sal were almost the same; 183.6 ± 52.1 μM and 232.9 ± 37.8 μM for control and parkinsonian patients, respectively. However, the maximal velocity increased in parkinsonian patients; 1478.8 ± 165.5 *versus* 16.49 ± 2.98 pmol/min/mg protein. The results suggest that quantitative, but not qualitative, changes may occur in the enzyme. Further studies are required for the characterization of the changes in the enzyme.

Relevance to Parkinson's Disease

In Parkinson's disease DA neurons in the substantia nigra are irreversibly and progressively degenerated over a long duration. If a neurotoxin is involved in the selective cell death, it should be synthesized and accumulated in or around DA neurons. The accumulation of NM(R)Sal was confirmed in the nigro-striatal system (Maruyama et al., 1997a). Our data from an animal PD model and cultured cells suggest that NM(R)Sal is a potent neurotoxin which induces apoptosis selectively in DA neurons. The analysis of CSF demonstrates the increase in PD, which may be due to the increased synthesis by a neutral N-methyltransferase. N-Methylation and oxidation of (R)Sal may account for the specific-

Table 2. Activity of enzymes related to the metabolism of NM(R)Sal in lymphocytes

Enzyme	Enzymatic activity (pmol/min/mg protein)	
	Parkinsonian patients	Controls
(R)Salsolinol synthase	N.D.	N.D.
Neutral N-methyltransferase*	100.2 ± 81.8**	18.9 ± 15.0**
Alkaline N-methyltransferase*	41.8 ± 17.3	25.0 ± 23.0
N-methyl(R)salsolinol oxidase	2.15 ± 2.43	1.38 ± 2.23

*N-methyltransferase activity was measured at pH 7.0 or 8.0 using (R)Sal as a substrate.
**statistically significant; $p < 0.0001$
N.D.: not detected.

ity to DA neurons and also the potency as a neurotoxin. Only *N*M(*R*)Sal was found to be transported into SH-SY5Y cells by a DA transport system, and the potent cytotoxicity of DMDHIQ⁺ was confirmed by an Alamar Blue assay (Takahashi et al., 1997).

Apoptosis was induced by *N*M(*R*)Sal (Maruyama et al., 1997b), and this is the first report on the induction of apoptosis by an endogenous neurotoxin. The DNA damage was found to be enantio-specific, suggesting that an enzyme can distinguish the (*R*)-configuration and may initiate the cell death program. Studies to identify the enzyme and the intracellular process are on the way.

Our data demonstrate that at present *N*M(*R*)Sal is the most possible neurotoxin candidate to elicit PD in humans. The selective increase in the activity of a neutral (*R*)salsolinol *N*-methyltransferase suggests that a genetic factor regulating the enzyme synthesis may be an endogenous factor involved in the pathogenesis of PD. Future molecular studies on this enzyme will bring us new insight into the pathogenesis of Parkinson's disease.

ACKNOWLEDGMENTS

This work was supported by a Grant-In-Aid for Scientific Research on Priority Areas, and a grant from the Ministry of Education, Science and Culture, Japan.

REFERENCES

Dipasquale B., Marini A.M. and Youle R.J., 1991, Apoptosis and DNA degradation induced by 1-methyl-4-phenylpyridinium in neurons. *Biochem. Biophys. Res. Commun.* 181:1442–1448.

Hartley A., Stone J.M., Heronm C., Cooper J.M., and Shapira A.H.V., 1994, Complex I inhibitors induce dose-dependent apoptosis in PC12 cells: Relevance to Parkinson's disease. *J. Neurochem.* 63:1987–1990.

Maruyama W., Nakahara D., Ota M., Takahashi T., Takahashi A., Nagatsu T. and Naoi M., 1992, N-Methylation of dopamine-derived 6,7-dihydroxy-1,2,3,4-tetrahydroisoquinoline, (*R*)-salsolinol, in rat brains: *In vivo* microdialysis study. *J. Neurochem.* 59:395–400.

Maruyama W., Dostert P., Matsubara K. and Naoi M., 1995, N-Methyl(*R*)salsolinol produces hydroxyl radicals: Involvement to neurotoxicity. *Free Radic. Biol. Med.*19:67–75.

Maruyama W., Abe T., Tohgi H., Dostert P. and Naoi M., 1996a, A dopaminergic neurotoxin, (*R*)-N-methylsalsolinol, increases in parkinsonian CSF. *Ann. Neurol.* 40:119–122.

Maruyama W., Sobue G., Matsubara K., Hashizume Y., Dostert P. and Naoi M., 1997a, A dopaminergic neurotoxin, 1(*R*),2(*N*)-dimethyl-6,7-dihydroxy-1,2,3,4-tetrahydroisoquinoline, and its oxidation product, 1,2(*N*)-dimethyl-6,7-dihydroxyisoquinolinium ion, accumulate in the nigro-striatal system in the human brain. *Neurosci. Lett.* 223:61–64.

Maruyama W., Naoi M., Kasamatsu T., Hashizume Y., Takahashi T., Kohda K. and Dostert P., 1997b, An endogenous dopaminergic neurotoxin, N-methyl(*R*)-salsolinol, induces DNA damage in human dopaminergic neuroblastoma SH-SY5Y cells. *J. Neurochem.*, in press.

Mochizuki H., Goto G., Mori H., and Mizuno Y., 1996, Histochemical detection of apoptosis in Parkinson's disease. *J. Neurol. Sci.* 137:120–123.

Mutoh T., Tokuda A., Marini A. M. and Fujiki, N., 1994, 1-Methyl-4-phenylpyridinium kills differentiated PC12 cells with a concomitant change in protein phosphorylation. *Brain Res.* 661:51–55.

Naoi M, Maruyama W, Dostert P., 1994, Binding of 1,2(N)-dimethyl-6,7-dihydroxyisoquinolinium ion to melanin: effects of ferrous and ferric ion on the binding. *Neurosci. Lett.* 171:9–12.

Naoi M., Maruyama W., Zhang Y. H., Takahashi T., Deng Y. and Dostert P., 1995a, Enzymatic oxidation of the dopaminergic neurotoxin, 1(*R*), 2(N)-dimethyl-6,7-dihydroxy-1,2,3,4-tetrahydroisoquinoline, into 1,2-dimethyl-6,7-dihydroxyisoquinolinium ion. *Life Sci.* 57:1061–1066.

Naoi M., Maruyama W., Dostert P., Kohda K. and Kaiya T. (1996a) A novel enzyme enantio-selectively synthesizes (*R*)salsolinol, a precursor of a dopaminergic neurotoxin, *N*-methyl (*R*)salsolinol. *Neurosci. Lett.* 212:183–186.

Naoi M., Maruyama W., Dostert P., Hashizume Y., Nakahara D., Takahashi T. and Ota M., 1996b, Dopamine-derived endogenous 1(*R*), 2(*N*)-dimethyl-6,7-dihydroxy-1,2,3,4-tetrahydroisoquinoline,N-methyl-(*R*)-salsolinol, induced parkinsonism in rat: Biochemical, pathological and behavioral studies. *Brain Res.* 709:285–295.

Naoi M., Maruyama W, Dostert P. and Hashizume Y., 1997, *N*-Methyl-(*R*)salsolinol as a dopaminergic neurotoxin: From an animal model to an early marker of Parkinson's disease. *J. Neural Transm. [Suppl.]* 50:89–105.

Östling O. and Johanson K.J., 1984, Microelectrophoretic study of radiation-induced DNA damage in individual mammalian cells. *Biochem. Biophys. Res. Commun.* 123:291–298.

Takahashi T., Deng Y., Maruyama W., Dostert P., Kawai M. and Naoi M., 1994, Uptake of a neurotoxin-candidate, (*R*)-1,2-dimethyl-6,7-dihydroxy-1,2,3,4-tetrahydroisoquinoline into human dopaminergic neuroblastoma SH-SY5Y cells by dopamine transport system. *J Neural Transm [GenSect]* 98:107–118.

Takahashi T., Maruyama W., Deng Y., Dostert P., Nakahara D., Niwa T., Ohta S. and Naoi M., 1997, Cytotoxicity of endogenous isoquinolines to human dopaminergic neuroblastoma SH-SY5Y cells. *J Neural Transm* 104, in press.

Wolvetang E.J., Johnson K.L., Knauer K., Ralph S.J. and Linnane A.W., 1994, Mitochondrial respiratory chain inhibitors induce apoptosis. *FEBS Lett.* 339:40–44.

60

ANTIOXIDANT AND CYTOPROTECTIVE PROPERTIES OF APOMORPHINE

Michael Gassen,[1] Aviva Gross,[2] and Moussa B. H. Youdim[2]

[1]Merck KGaA
Biomedical Research CNS
Darmstadt, Germany
[2]Department of Pharmacology
Eve Topf and National Parkinson's Foundation Centers
Bruce Rappaport Family Research Institute
Faculty of Medicine, Technion
P. O. Box 9649, Haifa 31096, Israel

INTRODUCTION

Neurodegenerative diseases like Parkinson's disease, Alzheimer's disease, and Huntington's disease are generally typified by highly specific patterns of cell death in characteristic regions of the brain, leading to the clinically distinguishable features of the respective disorders. Every mechanistic concept of the etiology of these diseases has to provide a biochemical basis for an understanding of the time course and the regioselectivity of neuronal death. A vast body of experimental evidence supports the importance of free radicals, iron, catecholamine oxidation, and neuromelanin for the nigro-striatal neurodegeneration which characterizes Parkinson's disease. The identification of endogenous 6-hydroxydopamine (6-OHDA) formed through iron catalyzed oxidation of dopamine, has strongly reinforced the concept of oxidative stress being a key factor in neurodegenerative diseases (Andrew et al., 1993). This finding raised serious questions about of the long term effects of the treatment in Parkinson's disease with drugs such as l-DOPA or the mixed type dopamine D1-D2-receptor agonist apomorphine on the progression of the disease. In this chapter we will present the latest findings about antioxidant effects of apomorphine, and will discuss the implications for the treatment of Parkinson's disease.

REACTIVE OXYGEN SPECIES IN NEURODEGENERATIVE DISEASES

Free oxygen radicals and other reactive oxygen species (ROS) are formed ubiquitously as side products of respiration from about 5–10% of the oxygen that we breath

Progress in Alzheimer's and Parkinson's Diseases
edited by Fisher *et al.*, Plenum Press, New York, 1998.

(Stadtman, 1993). Normally, they are rapidly deactivated by highly efficient scavenging systems before they can cause any damage. Pathological conditions (e.g. inflammation, toxic stress, reperfusion after ischemia) or tissue aging lead to increased formation of ROS and decreased scavenging capacity in the cell. Here, ROS can cause widespread structural damage to unsaturated membrane lipids, to proteins or DNA, leading eventually to cell death. The reaction between ROS and polyunsaturated fatty acids leads to the generation of aldehydic breakdown products, many of which are toxic by themselves. As these species have a much longer half life than ROS, they can spread by diffusion and exert their effects remote from the site of primary radical damage (Yoritaka et al., 1996; Esterbauer 1980).

Iron, like ions of other transition metals that occur in different oxidation states under physiological conditions (e.g. copper), can form reactive hydroxyl radicals (HO$^{\cdot}$) from hydrogen peroxide (H_2O_2) and superoxide ($O_2^{\cdot-}$) by Fenton-type reactions. There is strong histological evidence supporting an involvement of iron in the development and/or progression of neurodegenerative disease; a marked increase in the concentration of iron in the affected brain areas has been confirmed for Parkinson's disease, Huntington's disease, supranuclear palsy, multisystem atrophy as well as Alzheimer's disease (Gerlach et al., 1994). The late stage of Parkinson's disease is characterized by the accumulation of iron in the substantia nigra (pars compacta) of the affected brains (Sofic et al., 1991). This obviously occurs in parallel to the progression of the disease, as in the early phases, iron content and distribution in parkinsonian brains is normal as compared with non-symptomatic controls (Riederer et al., 1992).

CATECHOLAMINE TOXICITY: FREE RADICAL, AND MITOCHONDRIAL MECHANISMS

What are the factors that render the dopaminergic neurons of the substantia nigra more vulnerable to reactive oxygen species than other neuronal populations? To answer this question, it is important to consider the specific chemical and biochemical properties of dopamine and its metabolites. There is significant evidence that catecholamines interfere with cellular oxygen metabolism at several points: 1) Catecholamine metabolism by monoamine oxidases leads to the formation of H_2O_2, which can be converted into more reactive hydroxyl radicals through the interaction with ferrous iron (Fe^{2+}); 2) Catecholamines can be autooxidized to generate $O_2^{\cdot-}$, H_2O_2, and reactive quinones and semiquinone radicals as intermediates with neuromelanin as the end product; and 3) Catecholamines and their catechol metabolites as well as neuromelanin are excellent iron chelators, which can form stable complexes especially with ferric iron (Fe^{3+}). Thus, they contribute to maintain the low molecular weight iron pool that is able to participate in redox chemistry, e.g. in the Fenton reaction. Neuromelanin selectively binds ferric iron and is able to reduce it, releasing Fe^{2+} back into the cytosol (Ben Shachar et al., 1991b).

The reaction between H_2O_2, iron and dopamine, as it was demonstrated *in vitro* (Jellinger et al., 1996), may be a source of endogenous 6-OHDA formation. This dopaminergic neurotoxin has originally been regarded as of synthetic origin only, but was recently discovered in urine samples of Parkinson's disease patients (Andrew et al, 1993). These mechanisms can be of high relevance, as the relatively high concentrations of iron in the striatum are even more increased after Parkinson's disease (Dexter et al., 1992). Iron dependent mechanisms and ROS may also contribute to the toxicity of 6-OHDA, which has been shown to liberate iron from ferritin (Monteiro et al., 1989) and to increase the availability of Fe^{2+} for the Fenton reaction. Such a mechanism could explain the finding that the iron chelator desferrioxamine provides protection against brain lesions induced by 6-OHDA injections in rats (Ben Shachar et al., 1991a).

Catecholamines like dopamine (Ben Shachar et al., 1995) and 6-OHDA (Glinka et al., 1996) are strong reversible inhibitors of complexes I and IV of the mitochondrial respirator chain with IC_{50} values in the 10 μM range. The nature of the interaction between the mitochondrial enzymes and catecholamines is not clear, but it does not seem to be free radical dependent. However, the reversible interference of catecholamines with cellular respiration may be an additional free radical forming process.

ANTIOXIDANT PROPERTIES OF APOMORPHINE

During the last few years, the mixed type dopamine D_1-D_2-receptor agonist apomorphine has frequently replaced L-DOPA in the therapy for late stage Parkinson's disease (Gancher et al., 1995). The serious gastrointestinal side effects that originally prevented a widespread use of apomorphine, can be controlled by coadministration of the peripherally acting dopamine receptor antagonist domperidone (for a review see Lees, 1993).

However, the discovery that catecholamines can be cytotoxic has raised the question of the long term effects of treatment in Parkinson's disease with drugs like L-DOPA or apomorphine. Catecholamines can be both pro- and antioxidants. The radical scavenging effect of catechols has been established with dopamine = norepinephrine > dihydroxyphenylacetic acid > homovanillic acid (Liu and Mori 1993). We investigated the pro- and antioxidant properties of dopamine and apomorphine, as these two compounds are most relevant in Parkinson's disease.

APOMORPHINE AND DOPAMINE PROTECT ISOLATED BRAIN MITOCHONDRIA FROM OXIDATIVE STRESS

A major source of ROS is cellular respiration, e.g. by the mitochondrial respiratory chain. Due to the short half life of radical species, they will cause damage mainly close to the site where they are formed. For this reason, free radical biochemistry can be easily studied in isolated mitochondria. We examined the effect of dopamine and apomorphine on the formation of thiobarbituric acid reactive substances (TBARS) from radical induced lipid and DNA oxidation. Incubation of rat brain mitochondria with ascorbic acid (50 μM) and $FeSO_4$ (1–10 μM) leads to a rapid increase of TBARS formation which slows down after 2 h (see Fig. 1). This effect can be almost completely abolished by addition of 0.6 μM apomorphine (Gassen et al., 1996). The addition of 0.3 μM apomorphine, approximately the EC_{50} for 2.5 μM Fe^{2+}, slows down the formation of free radical products. The concentration of apomorphine required for an effective protection depends on the Fe^{2+} concentration (see Table 1). Oxidation of apomorphine, which eventually leads to a dark melanin-like polymer, was monitored by photometric determination of the strong chromophor of the oxidation products at $\lambda = 619$ nm. Autoxidation of apomorphine is slow in the presence of 50 μM ascorbic acid, but markedly accelerated in the presence of mitochondria reflecting the protection of mitochondrial lipids. Kinetic experiments revealed a negative correlation between apomorphine oxidation and TBARS formation. The former reaction occurs at a high rate during early incubation, completely suppressing TBARS. When apomorphine oxidation slows down later on, increasing amounts of TBARS are generated in the system (data not shown).

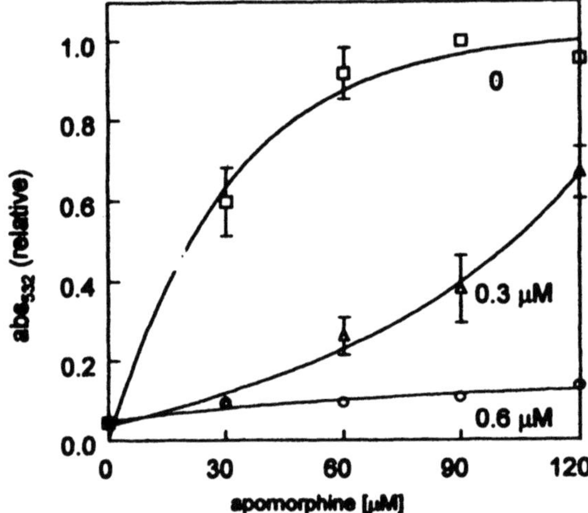

Figure 1. Time course of thiobarbituric acid reactive substances formation in the presence of 50 µM ascorbic acid and 5.0 µM $FeSO_4$. Controls (squares) with no apomorphine, 0.3 µM (triangles) and 0.6 µM (circles). Statistical analysis (n =3): Control: r = 0.998, P < 0.005; 0.3 µM apomorphine: r = 0.997, P < 0.005; 0.6 µM apomorphine: r = 0.992, P < 0.01.

Dopamine also showed antioxidant properties in the rat brain mitochondrial system, although it was not quite as effective (Table 1). On the basis of these data, iron chelation by dopamine may be a major contribution to the observed inhibition of TBARS formation. This can be ruled out for apomorphine, as apomorphine provides complete inhibition at concentrations much lower than the Fe^{2+}-concentration. Apomorphine also protects against oxidation of proteins. ROS induce cysteine-cysteine and tyrosine-tyrosine cross links and react with proline, arginine, lysine, and threonine leading to the formation of new keto- and aldehyde-functional groups (Stadtman, 1993). In order to detect these, we labeled the carbonyl groups with the specific reagent 2,4-dinitrophenylhydrazine. We found that forcing conditions (250 µM Fe^{2+}, 15 mM ascorbic acid) were needed to induce a threefold increase of protein carbonyls in the mitochondrial proteins. This effect could be reduced by 50% in the presence of 100 µM apomorphine.

APOMORPHINE PROTECTS PHEOCHROMOCYTOMA (PC12) CELLS AGAINST H_2O_2 AND 6-OHDA

A key question that remains concerns the balance between possible catecholamine toxicity and possible beneficial effects due to antioxidation. We looked at this problem in

Table 1. Inhibition of ascorbate/iron induced lipid peroxidation by apomorphine, dopamine, and desferrioxamine (Gassen et al., 1996)

FeSO_4 (µM)[a]	Apomorphine		Dopamine	Desferrioxamine
	2.5	5.0	2.5	2.5
IC_{50} [µM][b]	0.28 ± 0.02	0.61 ± 0.02	6.59 ± 0.2	0.78 ± 0.04
Max. inhib.[c] [%]	92 ± 1	93 ± 2	93 ± 1	75 ± 1
Hill coefficient 2[d]	1.7 ± 0.1	4 ± 0.3	1.0 ± 0.1	0.9 ± 0.15

a) Concentration of ascorbate was 50 µM in all cases.
b) Obtained from regression data (mean ± SE, n = 6).
c) Maximum inhibition as determined from a triplicate experiment (mean ± SEM).
d) Apparent values (mean ± SE, n = 5), as obtained from the slope of the cooperativity plot (Hill plot), log [apomorphine] versus log $(I/(I_{max} + I)$.

PC12 cell culture, a well established system to study apoptotic and necrotic cell death (Vimard et al., 1996). Oxidative stress can be induced by various agents like H_2O_2, organic hydroperoxides, or 6-OHDA.

We treated PC12 cells with H_2O_2 and 6-OHDA and observed cell death in a concentration dependent manner within 24 h. There was no significant difference of the sensitivity between cells that were grown in medium containing 15% serum (1/3 fetal calf serum, 2/3 horse serum) and those that had been differentiated for six days with additional 100

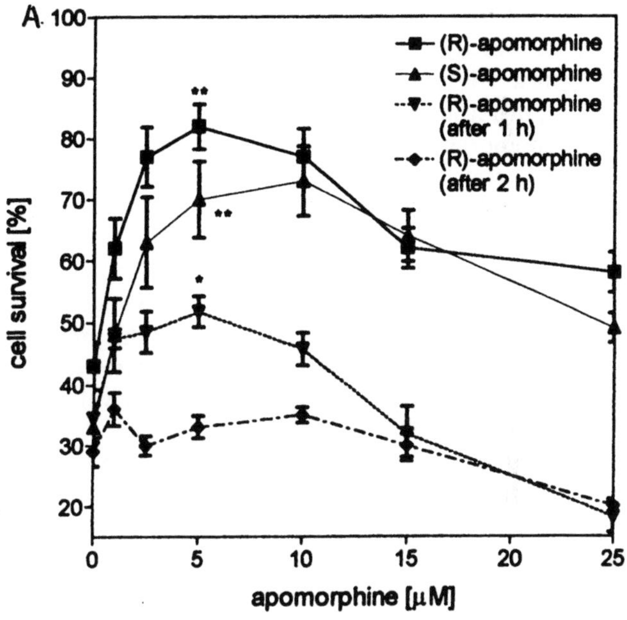

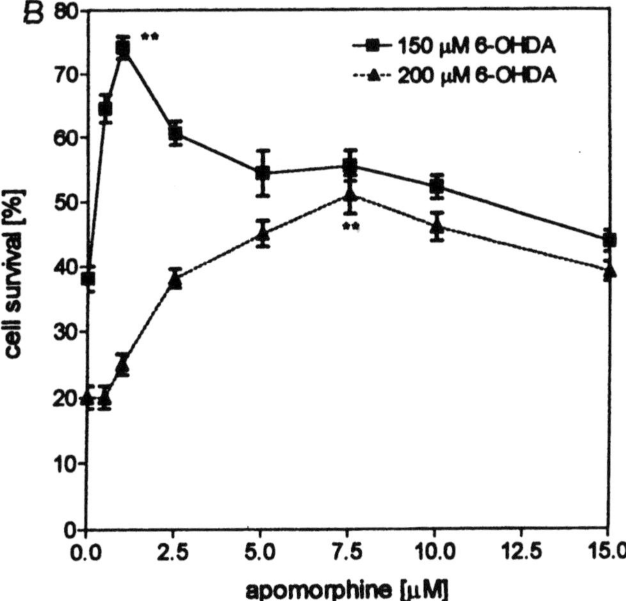

Figure 2. 0.6 mM H_2O_2 (a) and 6-OHDA (b) toxicity in PC12 cell culture and protection by apomorphine. a: Cell viability was assayed with MTT 24 h later and expressed as percent of controls (Data ± S.E.M., n = 8). The difference between (R)- and (S)-apomorphine in Fig. 2a is not significant (two-way-ANOVA: p = 0.08).

µg/ml 7S-NGF (Liu and Mori, 1993), if all the NGF had been washed out prior to the experiment. Although it takes 24 h to observe maximum cell death, only two hours exposure to the toxic agent is sufficient to induce full damage. The viability of the cells has been alternatively measured by counting cells after trypan blue exclusion or by measurement of metabolic conversion of the tetrazole MTT into a colored formazane derivative. Both methods produced equivalent results and we used the faster MTT-procedure for routine experiments.

Exact EC_{50} values were obtained: 400 µM for H_2O_2 and 150 µM for 6-OHDA were necessary to kill 50% of the cultured cells. In this system, dopamine and apomorphine were tested for their ability to protect PC12 cells from the oxidative insults. At the same time, the toxicity can be monitored to obtain information about the therapeutic window of the agents. We found, that apomorphine and dopamine, although they are both catecholamines, differ markedly in their toxicity and in their potency to protect the cells against H_2O_2. Apomorphine is by far more efficient as an antioxidant; only 5 µM improve the rate of survival from 50% to 85% in the presence of 400 µM H_2O_2. The same concentration of dopamine does not provide any significant protection; as much as 125 µM of dopamine are required to obtain the same effect. The toxicity of apomorphine, however, is much higher with an ED_{50} = 50 µM, than that of dopamine, which unlike 6-OHDA, does not lead to any significant cell degeneration at concentrations below 250 µM. Any protection against H_2O_2 by apomorphine depended on the presence of the drug during the insult. Preincubation with apomorphine and washout prior to H_2O_2 addition or addition of H_2O_2 one hour after the toxin did not improve the survival, as compared with controls treated only with the oxidant.

Apomorphine but not dopamine was able to provide protection against 6-OHDA insults. The survival rate after 150 µM 6-OHDA (EC_{50}) was improved to 70% with only 1 µM apomorphine. This is the first example for attentuation of the toxicity of 6-OHDA by a catecholamine in cell culture. As the catecholamines dopamine and apomorphine are widely used in the treatment of Parkinson's disease, it is of interest to investigate further the influence of these agents on the biochemical processes involved in the progression of neurodegeneration. We found that apomorphine is a representative of a catecholamine with pronounced antioxidant effects, although problems might arise due to its narrow therapeutic window. However, we consider this study also as an incentive for the design of novel, less toxic catecholaminergic dopamine receptor agonists with antioxidant properties.

ACKNOWLEDGMENTS

The authors acknowledge the support of the Goldings Parkinson Fund (Technion, Haifa, Israel), and the National Parkinson Foundation (USA). MG thanks the Minerva Foundation (Heidelberg, Germany) for his postdoctoral fellowship. We also wish to thank Ms. Bilha Pinchasi for experimental support.

REFERENCES

Andrew, R., Watson, D.G., Best, S.A., Midgley, J.M., Wenlong, H., and Petty, R.K., 1993, The determination of hydroxydopamines and other trace amines in the urine of parkinsonian patients and normal controls. *Neurochem. Res.* 18:1175–1177.

Ben Shachar, D., Eshel, G., Finberg, J.P., and Youdim, M.B., 1991a, The iron chelator desferrioxamine (Desferal) retards 6-hydroxydopamine-induced degeneration of nigrostriatal dopamine neurons. *J. Neurochem.* 56: 1441–1444.

Ben Shachar, D., Riederer, P., and Youdim, M.B., 1991b, Iron-melanin interaction and lipid peroxidation: implications for Parkinson's disease. *J. Neurochem.* 57:1609–1614.

Ben Shachar, D., Zuk, R., and Glinka, Y., 1995, Dopan-fine neurotoxicity: inhibition of mitochondrial respiration. *J. Neurochem.* 64:718–723.

Dexter, D.T., Jenner, P., Schapira, A.H., and Marsden, C.D., 1992, Alterations in levels of iron, ferritin, and other trace metals in neurodegenerative diseases affecting the basal ganglia. The Royal Kings and Queens Parkinson's Disease Research Group. *Ann. Neurol.* 32 (Suppl.):S94–100.

Esterbauer, H., 1980, Aldehydes of lipid peroxidation. In: *Free radicals, peroxidation, and cancer.* D.C.H. McBrien and T.F. Slater (Eds.), Academic Press, London, pp. 101–122,

Gancher, S.T., Nutt, J.G., and Woodward, W.R., 1995, Apomorphine infusional therapy in Parkinson's disease: clinical utility and lack of tolerance. *Mov. Disord.* 10:37–43.

Gassen, M., Glinka, Y., Pinchasi, B., and Youdim, M.B., 1996, Apomorphine is a highly potent free radical scavenger in rat brain mitochondrial fraction. *Eur. J. Pharrnacol.* 308:219–225.

Gerlach, M., Ben Shachar, D., Riederer, P., and Youdim, M.B., 1994, Altered brain metabolism of iron as a cause of neurodegenerative diseases? *J. Neurochem.* 63:793–807.

Glinka, Y., Tipton, K.F., and Youdim, M.B., 1996, Nature of inhibition of mitochondrial respiratory complex I by 6-hydroxydopamine. *J. Neurochem.* 66:2004–2010.

Jellinger, K., Linert, L., Kienzl, E., Herlinger, E., Youdim, M.B., Ben Shachar, D., and Riederer, P., 1996, Chemical evidence for 6-hydroxydopamine to be an endogenous toxic factor in the pathogenesis of Parkinson's disease iron-melanin interaction and lipid peroxidation: implications for Parkinson's disease. *J. Neural. Transm.* 57(Suppl):1609–1614.

Lees, A.J., 1993, Dopamine agonists in Parkinson's disease: a look at apomorphine. *Fundam. Clin. Pharmacol.* 7:121–128.

Liu, J., and Mori, A., 1993, Monoamine metabolism provides an antioxidant defense in the brain against oxidant- and free radical-induced damage. *Arch. Biochem. Biophys.* 302:118–127.

Monteiro, H.P., Winterbourn, C.C., Mytilineou, C., and Danias, P., 1989, 6-hydroxydopamine releases iron from ferritin and promotes ferritin-dependent lipid peroxidation 6 hydroxydopamine toxicity to dopamine neurons in culture: potentiation by the addition of superoxide dismutase and N-acetylcysteine. *Biochem. Pharmacol.* 38:1872–1875.

Riederer, P., Dirr, A., Goetz, M., Sofic, E., Jellinger, K., and Youdim, M.B., 1992, Distribution of iron in different brain regions and subcellular compartments in Parkinson's disease. *Ann. Neurol.* 32 (Suppl):S101–4.

Sofic, E., Paulus, W., Jellinger, K., Riederer, P., and Youdim, M.B., 1991, Selective increase of iron in substantia nigra zona compacta of parkinsonian brains. *J. Neurochem.* 56:978–982.

Stadtman, E.R., 1993, Oxidation of free amino acids and amino acid residues in proteins by radiolysis and by metal-catalyzed reactions. *Annu. Rev. Biochem.* 62:797–821.

Vimard, F., Nouvelot, A., and Duval, D., 1996, Cytotoxic effects of an oxidative stress on neuronal-like pheochromocytoma cells (PC 12). *Biochem. Pharmacol.* 51:1389–1395.

Yoritaka, A., Hattori, N., Uchida, K., Tanaka, M., Stadtman, E.R., and Mizuno, Y,. 1996, Immunohistochemical detection of 4-hydroxynonenal protein adducts in Parkinson disease. *Proc. Natl. Acad. Sci.* USA 93:2696–2701.

61

TOXICITY OF 1BnTIQ, ENDOGENOUS AMINE IN THE BRAIN, IN MESENCEPHALIC SLICE CULTURE

Yaichiro Kotake,[1] Masaki Sakurai,[2] Ichiro Kanazawa,[2] Shigeru Ohta[3]

[1]Faculty of Pharmaceutical Sciences
[2]and Faculty of Medicine
University of Tokyo, 7-3-1 Hongo
Bunkyo-ku, Tokyo 113, Japan
[3]Institute of Pharmaceutical Sciences
Hiroshima University School of Medicine
1-2-3 Kasumi, Minami-ku, Hiroshima 734, Japan

INTRODUCTION

1,2,3,4-Tetrahydroisoquinoline (TIQ) and 1-methyl-1,2,3,4-tetrahydroisoquinoline (IMETIQ) (Figure 1), which are endogenous substances in the brain of both parkinsonian patients and control subjects, are considered to be parkinsonism-inducing and preventing agents, respectively (Kohno et al., 1986; Ohta et al., 1987; Tasaki et al., 1991). We recently reported the existence of 1-benzyl-1,2,3,4-tetrahydroisoquinoline (1BnTIQ) in human CSF and mouse brain (Figure 1), and proposed that 1BnTIQ is biosynthesized from 2-phenylethylamine and phenylacetaldehyde, which is a metabolite of 2-phenylethylamine generated by MAO-B (Figure 2) (Kotake et al., 1995). We showed that the 1BnTIQ content in CSF of parkinsonian patients is higher than that of patients with other neurological diseases (Figure 3) (Kotake et al., 1995). Further, repeated administration of this compound induced parkinsonism in monkey and mouse (Kotake et al., 1995; Kotake et al., 1996). Though these TIQ derivatives appear to play an important role in Parkinson's disease, the mechanisms of their pharmacological effects remain unknown.

In this study, we have employed the organotypic slice co-culture technique to investigate the toxicity of 1BnTIQ in the rat ventral mesencephalon and striatum. This culture system best mimics the *in vivo* condition among the many culture systems available, and preserves the basic structural organization of the tissue (Gähwiler, 1988; Ostergaard et al., 1990). It is possible to prepare co-cultures of different brain regions utilizing this method. We focused on the mesencephalon and striatum, since they are of interest from the view-

Progress in Alzheimer's and Parkinson's Diseases
edited by Fisher *et al.*, Plenum Press, New York, 1998.

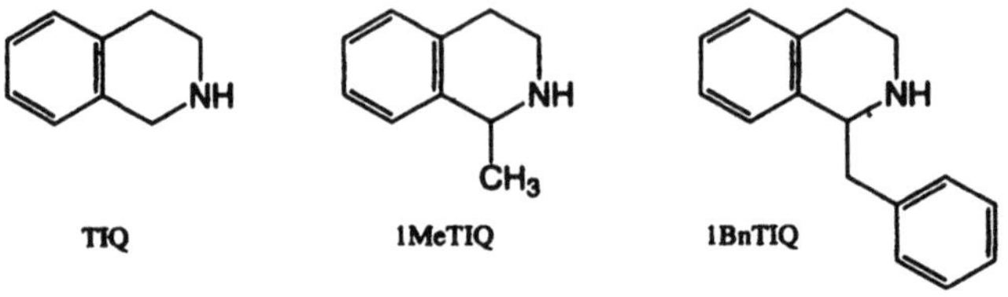

Figure 1. Structures of TIQ derivatives.

point of the function of the dopaminergic neurons and its relationship to dopaminergic neurodegenerative diseases, such as Parkinson's disease.

MATERIALS AND METHODS

1BnTIQ and Other Reagents

1BnTIQ for assay was synthesized according to the method described previously. NADH, sodium pyruvate, perchloric acid, ascorbic acid, semicarbazide hydrochloride and isoproterenol hydrochloride was purchased from Wako Pure Chemical Industry Ltd. (Tokyo, Japan). Dopamine hydrochloride was purchased from Tokyo Kasei (Tokyo, Japan). EDTA·4Na was purchased from Dojin (Kumamoto, Japan).

Organotypic Slice Co-Culture

Ventral mesencephalic slices were prepared from E16 Wistar rats. Forebrain of newborn rats was cut into 400-μm-thick slices with Microslicer, and the striatum was separated. Mesencephalic and striatal slices were put on a dish consisting of collagen coated membrane at a separation of 500 μm. DMEM/F-12 was employed as the culture medium.

Measurement of LDH Activity in the Medium

The activity of lactate dehydrogenase (LDH) in the medium was measured at intervals as an index of cell death, to determine the time course of cell death in this organo-

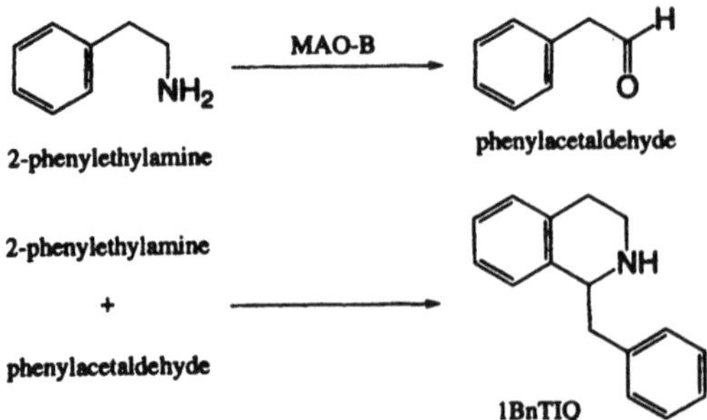

Figure 2. Proposed biosynthetic pathway of 1BnTIQ.

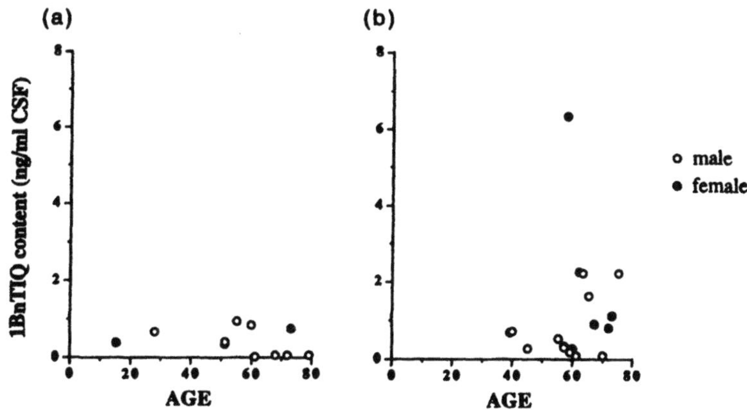

Figure 3. 1BnTIQ content in parkinsonian CSF. (a) Neurological control. (b) Parkinsonian.

typic culture system. The medium was added in the presence of NADH and sodium pyruvate, and the decrease of absorbance at 340 nm was measured. After exposure of the slices to 1BnTIQ, LDH activity in the media was determined on day 0, day 4, day 7 and day 9.

Measurement of Dopamine Content in Mesencephalic Slice

The slices were cultured for about 10 days, then 1BnTIQ was supplemented in the medium for 24 h or 7 days. Mesencephalic and striatal slices were separated, and each mesensephalic slice was homogenized by the use of a sonifier with 0.4 M perchloric acid containing 0.05% (wt/vol) EDTA·4Na 0.05% (wt/vol) ascorbic acid, and 0.02% (wt/vol) semicarbazide hydrochloride. The homogenate was centrifuged (20,000 g for 15 min at 4°C). Isoproterenol was added to the supernatant as an internal standard, and the solution was filtered through a 0.45 μm pore disposable filter (Millipore, Tokyo, Japan). Dopamine content was assayed by high-performance liquid chromatography with an electrochemical detector (HPLC-ECD). The detection voltage of ECD was +700 mV.

RESULTS

LDH activity in the medium was about 5 mU/well at the beginning of the culture, and was gradually decreased as time passed (Figure 4). After about 10 days, the activity become constant at about 1 mU/well, when ventral mesencephalic slices were exposed to 1BnTIQ for 24 h, their dopamine content decreased in a dose-dependent manner; at 100 μm, the dopamine content was about 10 % of that in the control (Table 1). After contact of the slices with 1BnTIQ for 7 days, dopamine content was further decreased; it fell to about 20 % of that in the control, in slices exposed to 10 μm 1BnTIQ (data not shown), and to an undetectable level in those exposed to 10 μm 1BnTIQ. Dopamine content in the control was also slightly decreased.

At 100 μm 1BnTIQ, LDH activities in the media on day 4 and day 7 were significantly higher than in the control (data not shown), when each measurement value was normalized with respect to the average of the control values measured at the same time.

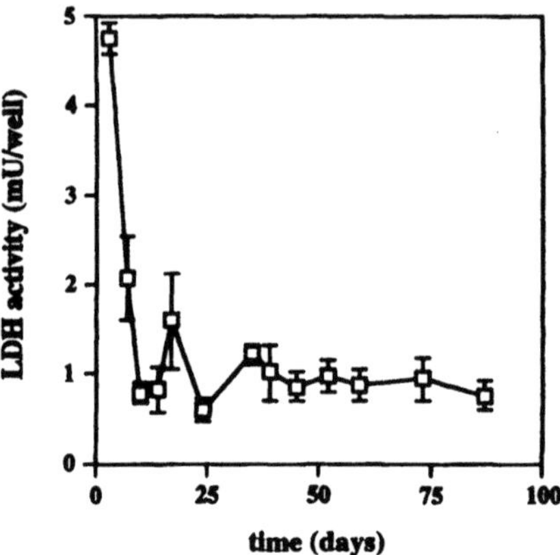

Figure 4. Time course of LDH activity in the medium of organotypic slice culture.

DISCUSSION

Organotypic slice culture has been extensively used in immunohistochemical and electrophysiological studies (Ostergaard et al., 1990; Steensen et al., 1995), but generally not in biochemical studies. Here, we employed it to examine the time courses of LDH activity in the medium and dopamine content in mesencephalic slices. LDH activity in the medium was initially high, but decreased progressively to a plateau by about 10 days (Figure 4). By this time, neuronal network formation is supposed to be completed. This time should be a suitable one at which to evaluate the effect of 1BnTIQ on the formed synaptic connections.

Exposure to 1BnTIQ for 24 h or 7 days caused a dose-dependent decrease in the dopamine content of mesencephalic slices (Table 1). This may have two possible causes. One is a functional deterioration of dopaminergic neurons, and the other is inhibition of tyrosine hydroxylase by 1 BnNTIQ. The former seems more likely in view of the very slow decrease of dopamine content. This view is supported by the data of LDH activity in the media. Thus, we suggest that prolonged exposure to low concentrations of 1IBnNTIQ may induce a decrease of dopamine content followed by cell death, and may play an important role in the pathogenesis of Parkinson's disease. Similar studies with slices of other brain regions may show whether or not 1BnTIQ is specifically toxic to nigrostriatal dopaminergic neurons. We are also planning an immunohistochemical study of tyrosine hydroxylase.

Table 1. Effect of 1BnTIQ on dopamine content in ventral mesencephalic slices

	Dopamine content (pmol/mg protein)	
Contact time	24 hr	7 days
Control	237.3 ± 54.1	177.6 ± 31.7
30 µM 1 BnTIQ	83.7 ± 33.4	42.1 ± 9.4
100 µM 1BnTIQ	27.1 ± 4.6	N.D.

The slices were exposed to 1BnTIQ from about 10 days after the start of culture.
N.D.: not detected

REFERENCES

Gähwiler, B.H., 1988, Organotypic cultures of neural tissue, *Trends Neurosci.* 11: 484-489.

Kohno, M., Ohta, S., and Hirobe, M., 1986, Tetrahydroisoquinoline and 1-methyl tetrahydroisoquinoline as novel endogenous amines in rat brain. *Biochem. Biophys. Res. Commun.* 140:448–454.

Kotake, Y., Tasaki, Y., Makino, Y., Ohta, S., and Hirobe, M., 1995, 1-Benzyl-1,2,3,4-tetrahydro- isoquinoline as a parkinsonism-inducing agent: a novel endogenous amine in mouse brain and parkinsonian CSF, *J. Neurochem.* 65:2633–2638.

Kotake, Y., Yoshida, M., Ogawa, M., Tasaki, Y., Hirobe, M., and Ohta, S., 1996, Chronic administration of 1-benzyl-1,2,3,4-tetrahydroisoquinoline, an endogenous amine in the brain, induces parkinsonism in a primate, *Neurosci. Lett.* 217:69–71.

Ohta, S., Kohno, M., Makino, Y., Tachikawa, O., and Hirobe, M. 1987, Tetrahydroisoquinoline and 1-methyltetrahydroisoquinoline are present in the human brain: relation to Parkinson's disease, *Biomed. Res.* 8:453–456.

Ostergaard, K., Schou, J.P., and Zimmer, J., 1990, Rat ventral mesencephalon grown as organotypic slice cultures and co-cultured with striatum, hippocampus, and cerebellum, *Exp. Brain Res.* 82:547–565.

Steensen, B.H., Nedergaard, S., Ostergaard, K., and Lambert, J.D.C., 1995, Electrophysiological characterization of dopaminergic and non-dopaminergic neurones in organotypic slice cultures of the rat ventral mesencephalon, *Exp. Brain Res.* 106:205–214.

Tasaki, Y., Makino, Y., Ohta, S., and Hirobe M., 1991, 1-Methyl-1,2,3,4 tetrahydroisoquinoline, decreasing in 1-methyl-4-phenyl-1,2,3,6-tetrahydropyridine-treated mouse, prevents parkinsonism-like behavior abnormalities, *J. Neurochem.* 57:1940–1943.

62

DOPAMINERGIC RESPONSIVENESS OF HYPOKINESIA BUT NOT OF RIGIDITY AND TREMOR IS REDUCED IN FLUCTUATING PARKINSON'S DISEASE*

Jan Roth, Evžen Růžička, Irena Svobodová, Robert Jech, and Petr Mečiř

Clinic of Neurology
Charles University
Prague, Czech Republic

SUMMARY

Motor fluctuations and dyskinesias (FD) complicate advanced stages of Parkinson's Disease (PD). Although L-DOPA may play a key role in the development of FD, it is unclear whether motor symptoms remain equally sensitive to dopaminergic therapy in advanced stages of PD. We studied the effects of Apomorphine (APO), a potent dopamine agonist drug. We examined 17 patients without FD (non-FD group) and 19 patients presenting FD (FD group). The patients were examined twice, before and after APO (0.05 mg/kg s.c.). Motor status was tested using the Columbia University Rating Scale (CURS). Total CURS score and subscores for tremor, rigidity and hypokinesia were compared between both groups. The duration of L-DOPA therapy was significantly longer in FD than in non-FD group. Before APO, significantly higher CURS scores and subscores were found in FD than in non-FD patients. After APO, in both groups, significant improvements of total CURS scores and subscores were observed. However, hypokinesia remained significantly worse in FD than in non-FD patients whereas rigidity and tremor did not differ between both groups after APO. Our results confirm the notoriously known fact that FD correlate with the duration of L-DOPA treatment in PD patients. More interestingly, it seems that there is a common denominator between FD and reduced dopaminergic responsiveness of hypokinesia in PD. Thus, the difference between the reactivity to APO of tremor and rigidity on one hand and of hypokinesia on the other hand, may reflect modified pathophysiology of main PD symptoms in fluctuating compared to non-fluctuating PD.

* The study was supported by a grant from the Czech Ministry of Health Care (reg.No IGA MZ 3572-3).

Progress in Alzheimer's and Parkinson's Diseases
edited by Fisher *et al.*, Plenum Press, New York, 1998.

INTRODUCTION

The major Parkinson's disease (PD) signs—tremor, rigidity, and hypokinesia—are known to be related to a striatal dopamine deficit, however their pathophysiological mechanisms have not been entirely understood yet. In addition, in advanced stages of PD, motor fluctuations and dyskinesias (FD) can occur. FD are triggered by the administration of L-DOPA or dopamine agonist drugs but their appearance is dependent upon the severity of the degeneration of dopaminergic neurons and upon changes at postsynaptic receptors. Long-term intermittent dopaminergic treatment increased the risk of developing FD (Chase et al., 1990). Non-dopaminergic neurotransmitter dysbalance within the basal ganglia (BG) may also considerably influence late PD stages (Agid et al., 1987). To assess the dependency of tremor, rigidity, and hypokinesia on dopamine deficit, and possible differences between patients with early and advanced PD we studied the effects of Apomorphine (APO), a potent and short acting direct agonist of D1 and D2 dopamine receptors with effects comparable to dopamine (Cotzias et al., 1970; Gancher et al., 1990; Colosimo, 1996).

PATIENTS AND METHODS

We examined 36 PD patients divided in two age-matched groups. NonFD group consisted of 17 patients without FD, 11 males, 6 females, mean age 60.0 yrs (SD = 7.1), duration of PD 5.3 yrs (3.5), Hoehn & Yahr stage 2.13 (0.83), duration of L-DOPA therapy 2.3 yrs (2.8). In the FD group there were 19 patients with FD, 13 males, 6 females, mean age 58.3 yrs (7.8), PD duration 12.8 yrs (5.5), Hoehn & Yahr stage 3.4 (0.5), duration of L-DOPA therapy 9.2 yrs (4.6). The presence of FD was based on patients' historical information and verified during a standardized examination.

Domperidone (20 mg t.i.d.) was given to the patients during 48 hours prior to the testing to avoid adverse peripheral effects of APO. After a 12 hours withdrawal from all dopaminergic drugs, APO was administered (0.05 mg/kg of body weight s.c.).

Motor state was examined by means of the Columbia University Rating Scale (CURS) (maximum disability score, 100, maximum subscores for tremor, rigidity, hypokinesia, 16 points each). The score was assessed immediately before and 20 min. after APO. CURS total score and subscores for tremor, rigidity, and hypokinesia were compared with respect to pre- and post-APO state and between FD and non-FD patient groups using paired and unpaired t-tests, respectively.

RESULTS

Significant differences between FD and non-FD group were found regarding the duration of PD (p < 0.001), Hoehn & Yahr stage (p < 0.001), and duration of L-DOPA therapy (p < 0.001). After APO administration, CURS scores and subscores for tremor, rigidity, and hypokinesia significantly decreased compared to pre-treatment results in both FD and non-FD patients (see Table 1).

Comparing both patients' groups, before APO, CURS total score and subscores for rigidity and hypokinesia were significantly higher in FD than in non-FD patients. The tremor subscore was not different in FD compared to non-FD patients. After APO, CURS

Table 1

	CURS I	CURS II	T I	T II	R I	R II	H I	H II
Non-FD	17.80	9.00***	2.87	0.33**	3.73	1.67***	3.13	1.47**
	{1.78}	{1.30}	{0.66}	{0.15}	{0.39}	{0.34}	{0.45}	{0.32}
FD	44.81	19.33***	3.48	0.48**	7.86	2.76***	9.24	3.52***
	{3.30}	{2.13}	{0.84}	{0.20}	{0.62}	{0.51}	{0.58}	{0.50}
Non-FD/FD	###	###	ns	ns	###	ns	###	##

Values are group means and {SEM: standard error of the measurement}
Non-FD: 17 PD patients without fluctuations or dyskinesias
FD: 19 PD patients with fluctuations or dyskinesias
CURS: Columbia University Rating Scale total score
T: CURS subscore for tremor
R: CURS subscore for rigidity
H: CURS subscore for hypokinesia
I: test result before APO administration
II: test result after APO administration
Statistics: Comparison between test results I and II: **$p < 0.01$; ***$p < 0.001$; non-FD/FD: comparison between
FD and non-FD patients: ##$p < 0.01$; ###$p < 0.001$; ns: non-significant.

total score and subscore for hypokinesia were significantly higher in FD than in non-FD patients while subscores for tremor and rigidity did not differ between both patient groups.

DISCUSSION

As far as FD are known to be late complications of PD, it is not surprising that patients with FD presented with longer duration of the disease and of L-DOPA treatment, as well as with more severe clinical signs of PD. APO produced a marked improvement of motor scores in both patients' groups, with or without FD. More interestingly, the comparison between FD and non-FD patients showed that after APO, hypokinesia remained significantly worse in FD than in non-FD patients whereas rigidity did not differ between both groups anymore.

Hypokinesia is considered to be one of the "pure" dopaminergic signs of PD directly resulting from the striatal dopamine deficit (Jankovic, 1987). The dopamine deficit produces, in turn, disinhibition of GABA-ergic output of the BG and increased inhibition of thalamocortical neurons involved in movement initiation and execution (Hallett, 1993). Presumably akinesia (impaired movement initiation) in PD depends on disinhibition of an indirect pathway connecting putamen with the internal segment of globus pallidus via external pallidum and subthalamic nucleus. Bradykinesia (slowness of movement) is produced by decreased activation of a direct pathway (Albin, 1995; DeLong et al., 1993; Hallett, 1993). After dopaminergic stimulation of striatal D1 and D2 type receptors, the activation of both direct and indirect pathways is normalized. Good initial response of hypokinesia to dopaminergic treatment is thus considered as a hallmark of PD (Jankovic, 1987). On the other hand, tremor and rigidity are presumably produced by a release or inhibition of brain and spinal cord reflex mechanisms (Delwaide et al., 1988; DeLong et al., 1993; Jankovic, 1987). These signs respond less well to L-DOPA (Jankovic, 1987; Albin, 1995). Consequently, the above results seem to be somewhat paradoxical. In patients with advanced PD and late motor complications (FD), after dopaminergic stimulation, rigidity decreased to a level similar to that found in non-fluctuating patients. This may in fact signify the preservation of the effect of dopaminergic stimulation to cerebral and spinal tonogenic mechanisms even in the late stages of PD. On the contrary, the relative persistence of hypokinesia after APO supports previous assumptions of the role for a complex neurotransmitter imbalance within the BG-thalamocortical motor circuit in late PD patients (Agid et al., 1987). In these patients, non-dopaminergic lesions in the striatal downstream may intervene and counteract the effects of dopaminergic stimulation. Moreover, the non-dopaminergic lesions may, in combination with pre- and postsynaptic changes within the nigrostriatal pathway, contribute to the late motor complications of PD.

REFERENCES

Agid, Y., Javoy-Agid, F., Ruberg, M., 1987, Biochemistry of neurotransmitters in Parkinson's disease: In: *Movement Disorders*, Marsden, C.D., Fahn, S., eds., New York and London, Butterworth's:166–231.

Albin, R.L., 1995, The pathophysiology of Chorea/Ballism and Parkinsonism. *Parkinsonism and Related Disorders*, 1: 3–11.

Chase, T.N., Fabbrini, G., Juncos, J.L., Mouradian, M.M., 1990, Motor response complications with chronic levodopa therapy. In: *Advances in Neurology 53*, Streifler, M.B. et al.., eds., Raven Press, New York: 377–381

Colosimo, C., 1996, Motor response to acute dopaminergic challenge with apomorphine and levodopa in Parkinson's Disease: implications for the pathogenesis of the on-off phenomenon. *J. Neurol. Neurosurg. Psychiatry,* 61: 634–637.

Cotzias, G.C., Papavasiliou, P.S., Fehling, C., Kaufman,B., Mena, I., 1970, Similarities between neurologic effects of L-DOPA and of apomorphine. *N. Engl. J. Med.* 1: 31–33.

DeLong,M.R., 1990, Primate models of movement disorders of basal ganglia origin. *Trends Neurosci.* 13: 281–285.

DeLong, M.R., Wichmann,T., 1993, Basal Ganglia-Thalamocortical Circuits in Parkinsonian Signs. *Clin. Neurosci.* 1:18–26.

Delwaide, P.J., Gonce, M., 1988, Pathophysiology of Parkinson's Signs. Parkinson's. In: *Disease and Movement Disorders,* Jankovic, J., Tolosa, E., eds., Urban and Schwarzenberg: 1–15.

Gancher, S.T., Woddward, W.R., Gliessman, P., Boucher, B., Nutt, J.G., 1990, The short duration response to apomorphine: implications for the mechanism of dopaminergic effects in parkinsonism. *Ann. Neurol.* 27: 660–665.

Hallet, M., Physiology of basal ganglia disorders: An overview, 1993, *Can. J. Neurol. Sci.* 20:177–183

Jankovic, J., 1987, Pathophysiology and Clinical Assessment of Motor Symptoms in Parkinson's Disease. In: *Handbook of Parkinson's Disease*, Koller, W.C., ed., Marcel Dekker Inc.: 99–126.

63

MOTOR FLUCTUATION AND LEVODOPA ABSORPTION

Miho Murata and Ichiro Kanazawa

Department of Neurology
School of Medicine
University of Tokyo
Tokyo, Japan

INTRODUCTION

Levodopa is the most effective and reliable drug for Parkinson's disease. Levodopa therapy, however, generally produces motor fluctuation such as wearing-off, on-off, or deterioration of levodopa effects. "Wearing-off" is the most frequently encountered motor fluctuation. Candidate factors for the development of wearing-off are: 1) change in the peripheral pharmacokinetics; 2) decrease in striatal dopamine storage; and 3) modification of post synaptic receptors. The peripheral pharmacokinetics of levodopa is considered an important contributory factor to wearing-off because wearing-off appears to be correlated temporally with falling levodopa levels in the peripheral circulation. In this respect, we reported that long-term levodopa (with dopa decarboxylase inhibitor; DCI) administration not only reduced the dopamine storage capacity of the striatum and the "supersensitive response" of dopamine receptors but accelerated levodopa absorption from the gut in intact rats (Murata and Kanazawa, 1993). We speculate, therefore, that the acceleration of levodopa absorption of could account for the development of wearing-off.

We evaluated here the effects of the chronic administration of levodopa on: 1) the peripheral pharmacokinetics and the development of wearing-off; 2) the development of on-off or deterioration of levodopa effect, which are usually seen in later phase of the therapy; and 3) the senile-onset parkinsonian patients (aging effect on the development of wearing-off).

MATERIALS AND METHODS

Fifty-five patients with idiopathic Parkinson's disease (63.0 ± 10.2 years [mean ± standard deviation]) consented to participate in this study after the full disclosure of its purposes, risks, and potential benefits. They were divided into two groups; the "stable" group (n = 32) and the "wearing-off" group (n = 23).

Progress in Alzheimer's and Parkinson's Diseases
edited by Fisher *et al.*, Plenum Press, New York, 1998.

L-dopa Test

The methodology of the L-dopa test has been previously reported (Murata et al, 1996). Briefly, after overnight withholding of medication and food, the patients received an oral dose of levodopa (100 mg) plus benserazide (25 mg) at 8:00 AM on the test day. Venous blood samples were obtained 7 times before and until 4 hours after drug administration for measurements of the plasma levodopa concentrations. The concentration of levodopa was assayed by an HPLC-ECD (Neurochem; ESA, Bedford, Massachusetts). In addition, the L-dopa test was given twice over 2 to 4 years to five of the patients who agreed to a second test. For the analysis of later phase phenomenon, 6 patients who had experienced "wearing-off" for more than 7 years were added to the test.

RESULTS

Duration of Levodopa Therapy and Peripheral Pharmacokinetics

Long-term levodopa therapy significantly increased the values of Cmax and AUC and decreased the values of Tmax and T1/2. Furthermore, the amount of daily levodopa dose significantly increased Cmax and decreased T1/2. The duration of disease, however, did not affect the peripheral pharmacokinetics (Table 1).

"Stable" and "Wearing-off" Group

The "wearing-off" group had a significantly higher Cmax and AUC, and a significantly shorter Tmax and T1/2 than the "stable" group (Table 2). The pattern of time-concentration curve of the "wearing-off" group was obviously steeper than that of the "stable" group (Figure 1).

Table 1. Correlation between clinical characteristics and pharmacokinetics

	Cmax	Tmax	T1/2	AUC
Age at test	NS	NS	NS	NS
Age at onset	$p < 0.05$	NS	NS	NS
Duration of disease	NS	NS	NS	NS
Duration of dopa therapy	$p < 0.001$	$p < 0.05$	$p < 0.05$	$p < 0.05$
Dose/day	$p < 0.01$	NS	$p < 0.05$	NS

Table 2. Comparison between stable and wearing-off group

	Stable	Wearing-off	p
Age at test	64.7 ± 11.7	60.6 ± 7.6	NS
Age at onset	54.8 ± 8.3	46.6 ± 8.3	0.005
Duration of disease (years)	8.5 ± 4.6	13.3 ± 6.8	0.001
Duration of dopa therapy (years)	4.1 ± 3.3	9.2 ± 3.3	0.005
Dose/day (mg)	350 ± 139	526 ± 168	0.001
Cmax (nmol/ml)	6.56 ± 2.26	12.02 ± 5.86	0.001
Tmax (min)	73.8 ± 45.8	33.0 ± 27.7	0.001
T1/2 (min)	76.2 ± 35.3	52.2 ± 7.7	0.02
AUC (nmol,hr/ml)	13.1 ± 4.5	17.1 ± 5.7	0.05

Mean ± SD.

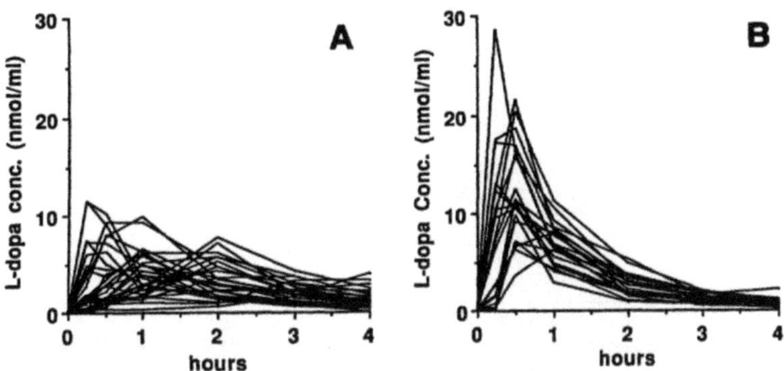

Figure 1. Time-concentration curve of plasma levodopa. A: "stable" group, B: "wearing-off" group. The pattern of the "wearing-off" group is obviously steeper than that of the "stable" group.

Longitudinal Monitoring

On the second test 4 of the 5 patients, who received the test twice, had a higher Cmax and AUC, and a shorter Tmax and T1/2 (Figure 2). In these four patients, "wearing-off" appeared or became more severe during the interval between tests.

The Relation between Levodopa Pharmacokinetics and the Phase of Wearing-off

The patients in the later phase (who suffered wearing-off for more than 7 years) had a different pattern of levodopa pharmacokinetics; i.e. lower Cmax and longer Tmax and T1/2 (Figure 3).

Wearing-off and Aging

In the middle-age onset (40 < < 60 year old) group, long-term levodopa therapy resulted in a very steep levodopa time-concentration curve (as shown above). In contrast, in

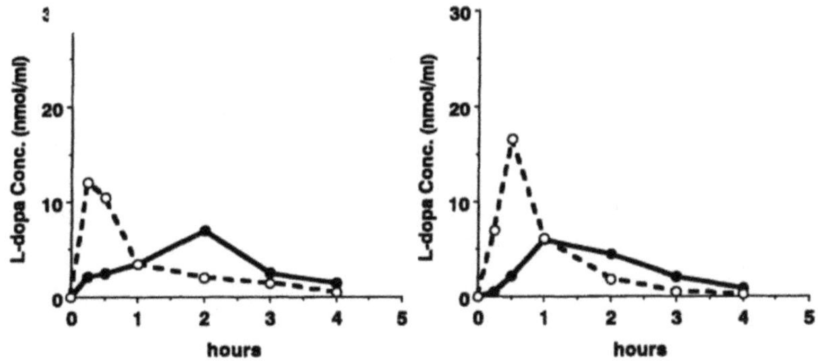

Figure 2. Longitudinal monitoring of a representative case. Straight line: the 1st test, dotted line: the 2nd test. The pattern of the 2nd test is steeper than the 1st test. The patient developed "wearing-off" during the interval between the test.

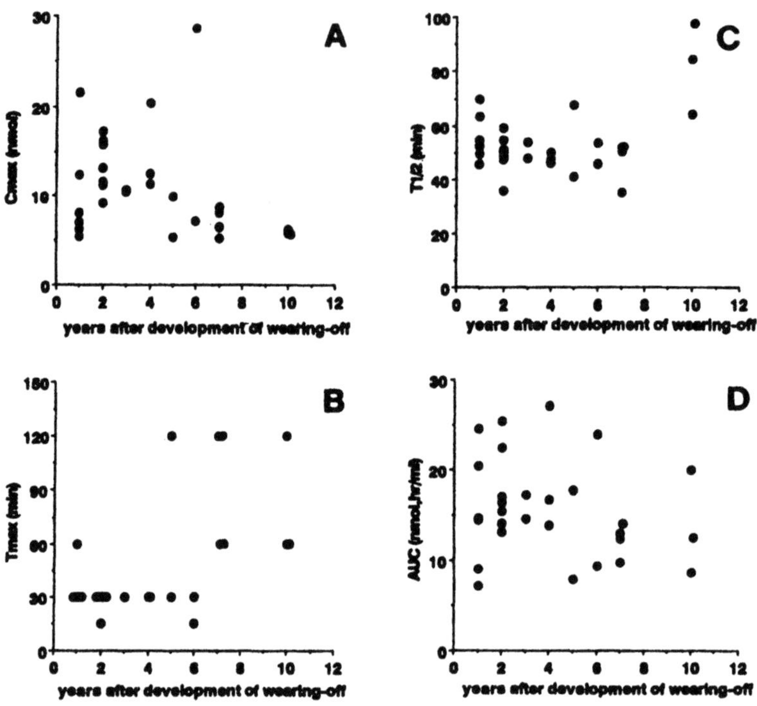

Figure 3. Correlation between pharmacokinetic factors and the duration of wearing-off. A: Cmax, B: Tmax, C: T1/2, D: AUC, Later phase patients (duration of "wearing-off" > 7 years) tended to lower Cmax and longer Tmax values.

the senile onset (> 60 years old) group the dose pattern did not change even after long-term levodopa therapy (Figure 4).

DISCUSSION

Levodopa Absorption and Wearing-off

Long term levodopa therapy clearly affects peripheral pharmacokinetic features. It is reasonable to suppose that these changes of pharmacokinetic features are due to the changes in absorption or metabolism of levodopa. Decreased metabolism of levodopa can explain the increase of Cmax and AUC but cannot explain the shortening of Tmax and T1/2. Increased absorption, however, can explain the increase of Cmax and AUC and the shortening of Tmax. If the system of absorption is saturable, increased absorption can explain also the shortening of T1/2. Furthermore, intravenous administration showed that the distribution and elimination of levodopa was not changed after long-term levodopa therapy (Fabbrini et al, 1987). Based on these facts, our findings suggest that long term oral levodopa administration affects the absorption of the drug by accelerating its absorption. We suppose that long-term levodopa therapy induces the transporter of LNAA (Large Neutral Amino Acid) system, which mediates levodopa absorption from the gut. The experiments to show the induction of this system are now under way.

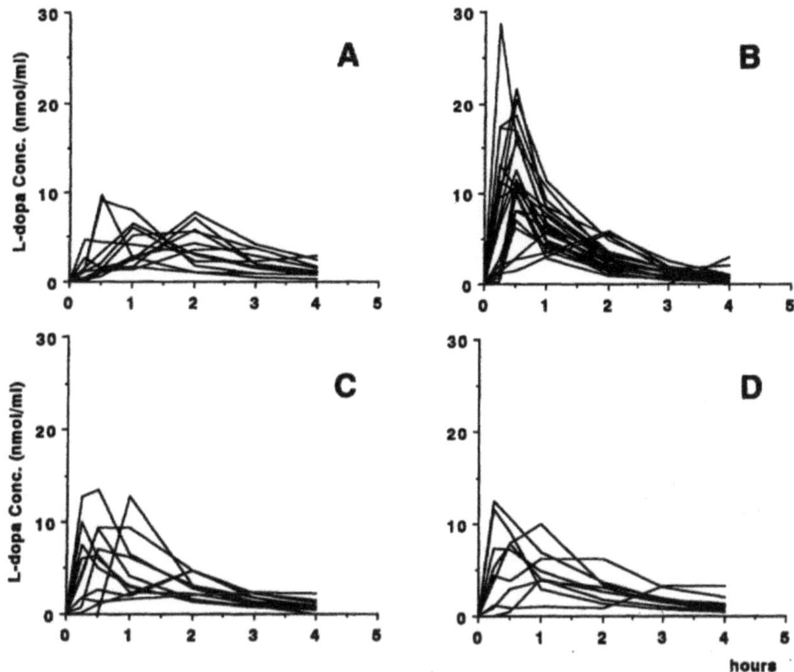

Figure 4. Aging effect on the development of wearing-off. A) Middle-age onset, levodopa therapy < 5 years (short-term group). B) Middle-age onset, levodopa therapy > 5 years (long-term group. C) Senile onset, levodopa therapy < 5 years (short-term group). D) Senile onset, levodopa therapy > 5 years (long-term group). In the middle-age onset group, the pattern of long-term group is obviously steeper than that of short-term group (A,B). In the senile onset group, the pattern does not change even after long-term therapy (C,D).

The "wearing-off" group showed an obviously steep pattern of levodopa pharmacokinetics. The shorter half time of plasma levodopa would shorten the duration of the response, i.e. the condition known as "wearing-off". Our results showed that the changes in peripheral pharmacokinetics of levodopa contributed to the wearing-off.

Longitudinal monitoring showed that long-term levodopa therapy undoubtedly changed levodopa pharmacokinetics during the development of wearing-off in the individual patient.

Later Phase Motor Fluctuation

Within 5 years after the development of wearing-off, the effective time was shortened and the motor fluctuation was highly predictable ("wearing-off"). In later phases, the time before the appearance of levodopa's effect after dosing was lengthened and the effect of levodopa weakened. Furthermore, the motor fluctuation became unpredictable ("on-off"). These changes of clinical features suggest that peripheral pharmacokinetics change in the course of "wearing-off". To clarify this point, we studied the relation between levodopa pharmacokinetics and the course of "wearing-off". The results are consistent with the clinical features. Some studies (Contin et al., 1993; Gancher et al., 1987) claimed that there were no difference between "stable" and "wearing-off" patients in levodopa pharmacokinetics after oral levodopa administration. It is probable that these studies involved the later phase patients who showed unpredictable motor fluctuation. Furthermore, we showed that levodopa dose as well as the duration of levodopa therapy affect pharmacokinetics. In Japan, the usual daily dose of levodopa (+ DCI) is rather small (300–400 mg) so that patients in Japan may exhibit the late phase phenomena, such as on-off, later and to a lesser extent than that seen in North American and European countries.

Aging and "Wearing-off"

In senile onset parkinsonian patients, the frequency of the "wearing-off" phenomenon was much less than in the middle-age onset group. In our study, the frequency of wearing-off in the middle-age (40 ≤ < 60 year-old) onset group and in the senile onset (≥ 60 year-old) group was 74.4% and 11.1%, respectively. We showed, in the senile onset group that pharmacokinetic changes seen in the middle-age onset group did not appear even after long-term levodopa therapy. This difference of the pattern of levodopa pharmacokinetics in the two groups suggests that the senile onset group hardly develops "wearing-off", even after long-term levodopa therapy.

All these results suggest that peripheral pharmacokinetics of levodopa contribute to the various motor fluctuations in Parkinson's disease as a result of alterations in absorption.

REFERENCES

Contin, M., Riva, R., Martinelli, P., Cortelli, P., Albani, F., and Baruzzi, A., 1993, Pharmacodynamic modeling of oral levodopa: clinical application in Parkinson's disease. *Neurology* 43:367–371.

Fabbrini, G., Juncos, J., Mouradian, M.M., Serrati, C., and Chase, T., 1987, Levodopa pharmacokinetic mechanisms and motor fluctuations in Parkinson's disease. *Ann. Neurol.* 21: 370–376.

Gancher, S.T., Nutt, J.G., and Woodward, W.R., 1987, Peripheral pharmacokinetics of levodopa in untreated, stable, and fluctuating parkinsonian patients. *Neurology* 37: 940–944.

Murata, M. and Kanazawa, I., 1993, Repeated L-DOPA administration reduces the ability of dopamine storage and abolishes the supersensitivity of dopamine receptors in the striatum of intact rats. *Neurosci. Res.* 16:15–23.

Murata, M., Mizusawa, H., Yamanouchi, H. and Kanazawa, I., 1996, Chronic levodopa therapy enhances dopa absorption: contribution of wearing-off. *J. Neural. Transm.* 103: 1177–1185.

64

THE RATIONALE FOR DEVELOPMENT OF CHOLINERGIC THERAPIES IN AD

Albert Enz[1] and Paul T. Francis[2]

[1]Research Nervous System
Novartis Pharma Ltd.
Basel, Switzerland
[2]Dementia Research Laboratory
Division of Biochemistry and Molecular Biology
United Medical and Dental Schools of Guy's and St. Thomas' Hospitals
    (UMDS)
London, United Kingdom

NEUROTRANSMITTER CHANGES IN AD

Biochemical investigation of the brains of AD patients uncovered substantial deficits in the enzyme responsible for the synthesis of acetylcholine (ACh), choline acetyltransferase (ChAT) in the neocortex (Bowen et al., 1976). Subsequent discoveries of reduced choline uptake, acetylcholine release and loss of cholinergic perikarya from the nucleus basalis of Meynert confirmed a substantial presynaptic cholinergic deficit in AD. These studies, together with the emerging role of acetylcholine in learning and memory (Drachman and Leavitt, 1974) led to the proposal that degeneration of basal forebrain cholinergic neurones with attendant loss of cholinergic neurotransmission in the cerebral cortex and other areas contributed significantly to the cognitive deficits seen in AD (Bartus et al., 1982).

Studies of cholinergic receptors have shown a reduction in the number of nicotinic receptors (Whitehouse et al., 1988), some of which are considered to be located on cholinergic terminals, with relative preservation of postsynaptic muscarinic receptors (Nordberg et al., 1992). However, there is some evidence for a disruption of the coupling between the muscarinic M_1 receptor, G-proteins and second messenger systems (Warpman et al., 1993).

A biochemical study of biopsy tissue from AD patients indicated selective neurotransmitter pathology within 3.5 years after the onset of symptoms (Francis et al., 1993). Thus, presynaptic markers of the cholinergic system were uniformly reduced while only some noradrenergic markers were affected. There were no alterations in markers for dopamine, GABA or somatostatin. Reductions in choline acetyltransferase and ACh synthesis in AD correlate strongly with the degree of cognitive impairment see (Francis et al., 1993). None of the other changes correlated with dementia.

On the basis of the above evidence cholinergic varicosities are probably lost from the neocortex at an early stage of the disease, however there are other parameters that correlate with measures of cognitive decline. Thus, cortical pyramidal neurone and synapse loss, neurofibrillary tangle counts and a modest reduction in glutamate concentration all correlate with dementia rating (see Francis et al., 1993). These findings clearly indicate that pyramidal neurones and their transmitter, glutamate play a major role in the cognitive symptoms of AD. It is also necessary to consider how alterations in other neurotransmitter systems influence pyramidal neurone activity. The presence of muscarinic and nicotinic receptors upon such cells makes it reasonable to propose that one of the actions of cholinomimetic drugs in the AD brain is to increase the activity of glutamatergic neurones (Chessell et al., 1995). This contention is supported by evidence obtained from electrophysiological studies of the effect of cholinomimetics on human and rat pyramidal neurones *ex vivo* (McCormick and Prince, 1985; Halliwell, 1986) and microdialysis studies in rats (Dijk et al., 1995). The profound reduction in glutamatergic neurotransmission as a result of loss of other pyramidal neurones and cholinergic innervation will clearly lead to pyramidal hypoactivity compounded by maintained levels of inhibition by GABAergic neurones. Therefore, in addition to the deleterious effects of neurone loss and tangle formation, it may be hypothesised that there is a change in the balance of neurotransmission in the AD brain favouring lower neuronal activity. This may be reflected in the hypometabolism seen in AD patients with imaging techniques, although a component of this is also likely to be due to atrophy (Najlerahim and Bowen, 1988). Likewise, it is of interest that regional cerebral blood flow may be increased in AD patients by acetylcholinesterase inhibitors such as physostigmine (Gustafson et al., 1987; Geaney et al., 1990).

NEUROTRANSMISSION AND PATHOLOGY

Observations by Nitsch and colleagues that activation of muscarinic and other phospholipase C linked receptors favours non-amyloidogenic processing of amyloid precursor protein (APP) (Nitsch,1996) suggests that cholinomimetics being developed for symptomatic treatment may have a serendipitous effect on the continuing emergence of pathology by reducing the production of â-amyloid. Little data has yet been reported regarding the potential beneficial effects of cholinomimetic drugs either by increasing APP or reducing â-amyloid production in AD patients. Other studies have shown that the phosphorylation of tau, believed to be an important step in the formation of tangles, may also be reduced by activation of the phospholipase C second messenger system (Davis et al., 1995). If these neurotransmitter-protein interactions occur in the AD brain, it is not inconceivable that the change in balance of neurotransmission proposed to occur in the AD brain may contribute to neurodegeneration in selectively vulnerable regions. Therefore, since they act against these processes, cholinomimetics may slow disease progression.

CHOLINOMIMETIC APPROACHES TO AD

There are a number of approaches to the treatment of the cholinergic deficit in AD, ACh replacement with precursor (choline or lecithin), the inhibition of acetylcholine esterase (AChE) or use of non-selective muscarinic agonists. More recent studies have used selective muscarinic agonists and antagonists, nicotinic agonist or improved AChE inhibitors. More speculative approaches include administration of trophic factors (such as nerve growth factor) and the transplantation of ACh-rich fetal tissue grafts. However, the most well-developed approach is the use of AChE inhibitors.

PRECLINICAL STUDIES OF AChE INHIBITION

The first cholinomimetic compound, tacrine an AChE inhibitor, underwent clinical trials and was subsequently approved for use in some, but not all, countries. Problems of modest therapeutic efficacy and potential serious adverse side effects have limited the use of this compound. The modest success of tacrine may be due to a number of factors including the onset of side effects at or before 30% acetylcholinesterase inhibition thereby limiting tolerability (Becker et al., 1991) and continuing pathological changes in non-cholinergic neurones (above) (Francis et al., 1993).

Newer AChE inhibitors are emerging with better preclinical profiles than tacrine and these include donepezil, metrifonate, galanthamine and ENA 713. All have distinct intrinsic properties regarding mode of inhibitory action, enzyme selectivity and metabolism. All of these compounds are available or in late phase III of clinical trials.

Mode of Inhibitory Action

AChE inhibitors can be divided into three classes, based on their mode of inhibition, reversable (e.g. tacrine, galanthamine and donepezil), pseudo-irreversable (e.g. physostigmine and ENA 713) and irreversable (metrifonate following conversion to its active form, dichlorvos). In the case of reversable inhibition the compound competes with the natural substrate (ACh) for the active site of the enzyme and in general such compounds have a relatively short duration of action. Pseudo-irreversable inhibitors mimic the substrate by interacting with the active site but are characterised by a much slower hydrolysis of the resulting covalent bond. This feature typically gives such compounds a long-lasting action. Irreversable inhibition is as the name implies permanent and requires new enzyme synthesis for restoration of activity. The mode of action defines, in general, the relative size and frequency of drug dosage.

Drug Metabolism

The size and frequency of drug dosage also has implications for drug metabolism if metabolites are toxic and large amounts of compound have to be processed. This point is best illustrated by reference to tacrine and ENA 713. The apparent inhibitory constant for AChE by tacrine is in the nM range yet the human dose is very much higher, this discrepancy may indicate rapid drug metabolism and contribute to the observed elevation of liver enzymes. In contrast, ENA 713 is decomposed by its action at the target enzyme, AChE, leading to a phenolic cleavage product which is rapidly excreted via the kidney following suphate conjugation (Enz and Floersheim, 1992). This may be the explaination for the lack of organ toxicity observed with ENA 713.

Brain Selectivity

Adverse effects due to peripheral cholinergic stimulation as a consequence of AChE inhibition can be overcome by targeting the inhibitors to central compartments. Compounds

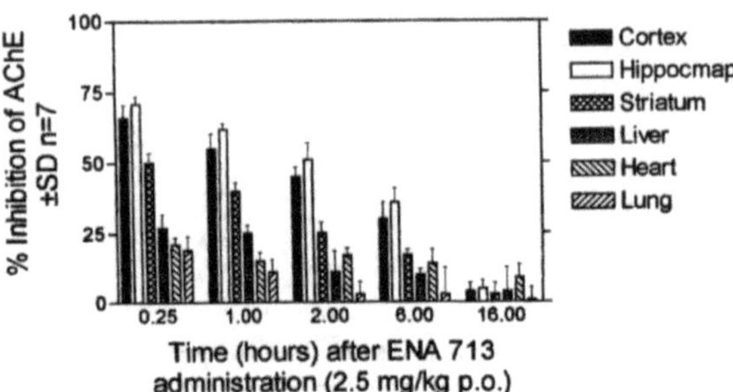

Figure 1. Time dependent inhibition of AChE by ENA 713 following a single oral dose in rat brain and peripheral organs. Enzyme activity was determined in the presence of etopropazine to exclude peripheral AChE activity (Enz et al., 1993).

that easily penetrate the blood-brain barrier interact with their target enzyme, resulting in an inhibited enzyme over a long period of time will fulfil such criteria. ENA 713 a highly lipophilic compound is a good example. This compound exerts AChE inhibition in the rat brain after few minutes following oral administration which last for more than 6 hours. On the other hand the enzyme in peripheral organs are only marginal inhibited. As a consequence ENA 713 has no effect on cardiovascular parameters at doses where the AChE activity in brain regions are blocked about 70–80%. In addition, this drug inhibited the AChE in cortex and hippocampus more potent when compared to other regions such as striatum and pons/medulla (Figure 1) (Enz et al., 1993). Since cortex and hippocampus are the main regions affected in AD this drug may have improved therapeutic benefit in this disease.

Molecular Forms

That AChE exists in different molecular forms on the basis of their solubility characteristics and sedimentation velocities, has been known for some time (Massoulie and Bon,1982) and, although the significance of these different forms is not yet clear, their tissue distribution is thought to reflect specific physiological functions. Total AChE levels and the distribution of the molecular forms varies from region to region in the human brain, the most abundant form being the globular tetrameric G4 form. The monomeric G1 form is also present in the brain but to a lesser extent. During ageing, and to a greater extent in AD, the levels of the G4 form of AChE decreases, whereas no change for the G1 form was observed.

In *in vitro* studies with isolated G1 and G4 forms of AChE from post-mortem human AD brain samples the inhibitory effects of ENA 713 was compared to those of physostigmine, heptylphysostigmine and tacrine. In summary, while physostigmine and tacrine inhibited the G1 and G4 forms equally well as expressed by their near unity of the ratio of the IC50's G4/G1, a clear difference was found for ENA 713 and heptylphysostigmine (Figure 2). Such a preferential inhibition of the G1 form has several important implications for the potential therapeutic use of ENA 713. The membrane-bound form G4 is probably located presynaptically at cholinergic nerve endings and may be directly involved in the regulation of ACh transmission. It seems therefore that the loss of G4 represents a selective depletion of the membrane pool, possibly reflecting the state of degeneration of cholinergic terminals in AD. On the other hand, the activity of the G1 form, reflecting ACh degradation unrelated to release remains unchanged. A preferential inhibition of the G1 form of AChE could be beneficial in situations of cholinergic hypofunction.

The brain-selective and long-lasting AChE inhibition by ENA 713, as a consequence of the mechanism of enzyme inhibition, reported in rodents has been confirmed in clinical

Figure 2. Pooled fractions containing G1 and G4 from AD brains were incubated with various AChE inhibitors and the remaining AChE activity determined. The IC_{50} values were calculated by linear regression of the log concentration versus % inhibition. Values represent means ± SD from at least 7 individual experiments.

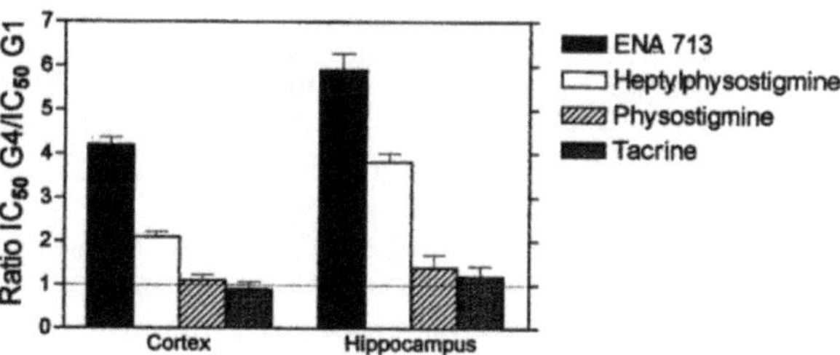

studies. Furthermore, the absence of peripheral organ toxicity in animals, resulting from a frugal drug metabolism by the target enzyme, is also borne out in humans. Therefore the preclinical results obtained in animals with ENA 713 appear to accurately predict for results in human clinical studies.

CONCLUSIONS

Biochemical studies have identified loss of cholinergic innervation of the cortex in AD accompanied by loss and dysfunction of cholinoceptive glutamatergic pyramidal neurones. These features are the strongest correlates of dementia in the disorder and provide a rational therapeutic target. Cholinomimetics are beginin to be licenced for the sympotomatic treatment of AD with AChE inhibitors in the forefront. From preclinical studies, ENA 713, one of the newer generation of AChE inhibitors, appears to have a long-lasting mode of action and to be brain and brain region selective and to be metabolised by the target enzyme. It is possible that such compounds, in addition to improving cognitive dysfunction, may have unexpected benefits in terms of slowing disease progression in AD.

REFERENCES

Bartus, R. T., Dean, R. L., Beer, B., and Lippa, A. S.,1982, The cholinergic hypothesis of geriatric memory dysfunction. *Science* 217:408–417.

Becker, R. E., Moriearty, P., and Unni, L.,1991, The second generation of cholinesterase inhibitors: clinical and pharmacological effects. In: *Cholinergic basis for Alzheimer Therapy*, R. E. Becker and E. Giacobini., eds., Boston: Birkhauser, p. 263–296.

Bowen, D. M., Smith, C. B., White, P., and Davison, A. N., 1976, Neurotransmitter related enzymes and indices of hypoxia in senile dementia and other abiotrophies. *Brain* 99:459–496.

Chessell, I. P., Francis, P. T., and Bowen, D. M., 1995, Changes in cortical nicotinic acetylcholine receptor numbers following unilateral destruction of pyramidal neurones by intrastriatal volkensin injection. *Neurodegeneration* 4:415–424.

Davis, D. R., Brion, J., Gallo, J., Hanger, D. P., Ladhani, K., Lewis, C., Miller, C.C.J., Rupniak, T., Smith, C., and Anderton, B. H., 1995, The phosphorylation state of the microtubule- associated protein tau as affected by glutamate, colchicine and α-amyloid in primary rat cortical neuronal cultures. *Biochem. J.* 309:941–949.

Dijk, S. N., Francis, P. T., Stratmann, G. C., and Bowen, D. M., 1995, Cholinomimetics increase glutamate outflow by an action on the corticostriatal pathway: Implications for Alzheimer's disease. *J. Neurochem.* 65:2165–2169.

Drachman, D. A. and Leavitt, J., 1974, Human memory and the cholinergic system. *Arch. Neurol.* 30:113–121.

Enz, A., Amstutz, R., Boddeke, H., Gmelin, G., and Malnowky, J., 1993, Brain selective inhibition of acetylcholinesterase: a novel approach to therapy for Alzheimer's disease. In: *Cholinergic Function and Dysfunction*, C. Cuello, ed., Amsterdam: Elsevier, p. 431–438.

Enz, A. and Floersheim, P., 1992, Cholinesterase inhibitors: an overview of their mechanisms of action. In: *Alzheimer's disease: From Molecular Biology to Therapy*, R. Becker and E. Giacobini, eds.,. Boston: Birkhaeuser, p. 211–215.

Francis, P. T., Sims, N. R., Procter, A. W., and Bowen, D. M.,1993, Cortical pyramidal neurone loss may cause glutamatergic hypoactivity and cognitive impairment in Alzheimer's disease: investigative and therapeutic perspectives. *J. Neurochem.* 60:1589–1604,

Geaney, D. P., Soper, N., Shepstone, B. J., and Cowen, P. J.,1990, Effect of central cholinergic stimulation on regional cerebral blood flow in Alzheimer's disease. *Lancet* 335:1484–1487.

Gustafson, L., Edvinsson, L., Dahlgren, N., Hagberg, B., Risberg, J., Rosen, I., and Ferno, H., 1987, Intravenous physostigmine treatment of Alzheimer's disease evaluated by psychometric testing, regional cerebral blood flow (rCBF) measurement, and EEG. *Psychopharmacology* 93:31–35.

Halliwell, J. V.,1986, M-Current in human neocortical neurones. *Neurosci. Lett.* 67:1–6.

Massoulie, J. and Bon, S.,1982, The molecular forms of cholinesterase and anticholinesterase in vertibrates. *Ann. Rev. Neurosci.* 5:57–106.

McCormick, D. A. and Prince, D. A.,1985, Two types of muscarinic responses to acetycholine in mammalian cortical neurones. *Proc. Natl. Acad. Sci. USA.* 82:6344–6348.

Najlerahim, A. and Bowen, D. M.,1988, Biochemical measurements in Alzheimer's disease reveal a necessity for improved neuroimaging techniques to study metabolism. *Biochem. J.* 251:305–308.

Nitsch, R. M.,1996, From acetylcholine to amyloid: neurotransmitters and the pathology of Alzheimer's disease. *Neurodegeneration* 5:477–482.

Nordberg, A., Alafuzoff, I., and Winblad, B.,1992, Nicotinic and muscarinic subtypes in the human brain: changes with aging and dementia. *J. Neurosci. Res.* 31:103–111.

Warpman, U., Alafuzoff, I., and Nordberg, A.,1993, Coupling of muscarinic receptors to GTP proteins in postmortem human brain—alterations in Alzheimer's disease. *Neurosci. Lett.* 150:39–43.

Whitehouse, P. J., Martion, A. M., Marcus, K. A., and Zweig, R. M.,1988, Reductions in acetylcholine and nicotine binding in several degenerative diseases. *Arch. Neurol.* 45:722–724.

DEMENTIA WITH LEWY BODIES

A New Avenue for Research into Neurobiological Mechanisms of Consciousness?

Robert H. Perry,[1] Matthew Walker,[2] and Elaine K. Perry[2]

[1]Department of Neuropathology
[2]MRC Neurochemical Pathology Unit
Newcastle General Hospital
Westgate Road, Newcastle upon Tyne, NE4 6BE

CONSCIOUSNESS, MENTAL DISORDERS, AND DEGENERATIVE DISEASES OF THE BRAIN

The term consciousness is generally applied medically with reference to the level of consciousness apparent to the observer—awake or comatose/unrousable with varying degrees between, or with reference to general anaesthesia. Far less consideration has been given, in the past, to the subjective experience of conscious awareness. However, consciousness is rapidly emerging as a subject of intense scientific enquiry. Innumerable books have been published within the last decade and international meetings are becoming abundant.

There are still those who consider the subject to be beyond the realms of current scientific methods, based on the view that conscious awareness is an entirely subjective experience and that such mind-brain connections cannot be bridged using current scientific paradigms. However many subjective aspects of experience have been provided with valuable scientific explanations. Increasing numbers of neuroscientists consider that new insights will emerge by applying contemporary 'tools' such as neuroimaging, analysis of the neurophysiology of sleep-wake consciousness, the neuropsychology and physiology of object perception, neural network modelling and neuropharmacology or by examining advances in the fields of mental disorder. (Delacour, 1997; Perry and Perry, 1996; Turner and Knapp, 1995; Hesslow, 1994).

Some of the most prevalent diseases affecting various aspects of consciousness are summarized in Table 1. Although a unitary definition of consciousness has defied agreement, exploring cerebral correlates of disturbances in particular aspects of conscious experience in distinct disease entities is likely to be worthwhile. Of the disorders listed in

Progress in Alzheimer's and Parkinson's Diseases
edited by Fisher *et al.*, Plenum Press, New York, 1998.

Table 1. Some alterations in consciousness in common mental disorders

Disorder	Positive symptoms	Negative symptoms
Alzheimer's disease	delusions, hallucinations (some patients)	loss of explicit, more than implicit short term (and eventually longterm) memory, cognitive impairment, ultimate loss of self identity
Autism	extraordinary abilities to attend to, process and retain information in a narrow focus, creativity	inability to distinguish 'mind' as it relates to self and nonself
Dementia with Lewy bodies	visual hallucinations, delusions	attentional deficits, 'absences', loss of consciousness, fluctuating cognitive impairment
Depression	delusions	loss of self value and initiative
Fronto-temporal lobe dementia	delusions	loss of self awareness and social awareness, judgement, foresight and executive functions
Mania	delusions	
Parkinson's disease	visual hallucinations	cognitive impairment, frontal lobe deficits, lack of mental (and motor) 'drive'
Schizophrenia	auditory hallucinations, hyperattention, experiences of thought control/insertion	cognitive impairment, social and other forms of inertia/withdrawal

The list is not intended to be exhaustive either in terms of disease types or relevant mental symptoms.
The terms positive and negative are used as they are applied in symptom classification in schizophrenia.
For a description of DLB symptoms see McKeith et al., 1992 and 1996; for evidence of retention of implicit as opposed to explicit memory in AD, see e.g. Scott et al., 1991, Postle et al., 1996, Hirono et al., 1997.

Table 1, the most dramatic advances in understanding brain mechanisms have emerged, in the last 2 or 3 decades, in degenerative conditions associated with dementia—Alzheimer's disease, Parkinson's disease, Dementia with Lewy bodies and Frontotemporal lobe dementia, for example. Research in the other disorders—schizophrenia, autism, depression or manic depressive illness has progressed to a greater or lesser extent in terms of psychological theory, cognitive and pharmacotherapy and neuroimaging although consensus on neuronal systems or mechanisms has not yet been reached.

DISTINCT FEATURES OF DEMENTIA WITH LEWY BODIES (DLB)

Dementia with Lewy bodies (DLB) has recently been recognized as a disease entity distinct in many respects from Alzheimer's and Parkinson's disease (Perry et al., 1997), with newly formulated clinical criteria and pathological guidelines (McKeith et al., 1996 reproduced in Tables 2 and 3). Ultimate classification of DLB, or subgroups, will depend on new research initiatives (clinical, psychological, pathological, molecular, genetic, neurochemical, therapeutic, epidemiological) as these relate to Alzheimer's and Parkinson's diseases. In the interim, observations supporting the distinct categorization of DLB are summarized in Table 4. There are however areas of overlap such as the occurrence of typical Alzheimer type pathology (including tangles) in some DLB cases, a degree of overlap in cortical Lewy body density between DLB and PD, similarities in some but not all extrapyramidal symptoms and reports that hallucinations as in DLB may be experienced much more frequently than previously recognized in PD. But for the purposes of this article, it is the unique cluster of clinical features that involve alterations in consciousness that is of interest.

Table 2. Consensus criteria for the clinical diagnosis of probable and possible DLB[a]

1. The central feature required for a diagnosis of DLB is progressive cognitive decline of sufficient magnitude to interfere with normal social or occupational function. Prominent or persistent memory impairment may not necessarily occur in early stages but is usually evident with progression. Deficits on tests of attention and of frontal-subcortical skills and visuospatial ability may be especially prominent.
2. Two of the following core features are essential for a diagnosis of probable DLB, and one is essential for possible DLB:
   a. Fluctuating cognition with pronounced variations in attention and alertness
   b. Recurrent visual hallucinations that are typically well formed and detailed
   c. Spontaneous motor features of parkinsonism
3. Features supportive of the diagnosis are:
   a. Repeated falls
   b. Syncope
   c. Transient loss of consciousness
   d. Neuroleptic sensitivity
   e. Systematized delusions
   f. Hallucinations in other modalities
4. A diagnosis of DLB is less likely in the presence of:
   a. Stroke disease, evident as focal neurologic signs or on brain imaging
   b. Evidence on physical examination and investigation of any physical illness or other brain disorder sufficient to account for the clinical picture

[a]From McKeith et al., 1996.

Table 3. Pathologic features associated with DLB (McKeith et al., 1996)

Essential for diagnosis of DLB
  Lewy bodies
Associated but not essential
  Lewy-related neurites
  Plaques (all morphologic types)
  Neurofibrillary tangles
  Regional neuronal loss—especially brainstem (substantia nigra and locus coeruleus) and nucleus basalis of Meynert
  Microvacuolation (spongiform change) and synapse loss
  Neurochemical abnormalities and neurotransmitter deficits

Table 4. Distinguishing features of dementia with Lewy bodies

Clinical	Much higher incidence of visual hallucinations compared to AD and to lesser extent PD
	More attentional deficits than in AD
	Fluctuating cognitive impairment, rarely seen in AD
	Absences or transient loss of consciousness/syncope (may be associated with falling)
	Extrapyramidal symptoms distinct from PD include less tremor, less need for and response to levodopa and more myoclonus
Neuropathological	Less neocortical Alzheimer type pathology than in classical AD, including variable ß-amyloidosis and few or no tangles in most cases
	More cortical Lewy bodies than in most cases of PD
	Variable substantia nigra neuron loss ranging from mild to typical of PD
Genetic	Increased frequency of ApoE ε4 allele, as in AD but not PD
Neurochemical	More extensive neocortical and less extensive archicortical cholinergic deficits than in AD
	Striatal cholinergic and dopaminergic deficits (only the latter shared with PD but to a lesser extent and affecting caudate to a greater extent)
Neuroimaging	Dopamine transporter loss, not seen in AD, equal in caudate and putamen, contrasting with PD where putamen is most affected
	Hypometabolism in occipital primary and association visual cortex, not evident in AD
Drug response	Much greater susceptibility to adverse effects of neuroleptics (D2 antagonists) than in AD (preliminary evidence) more positive response to cholinesterase inhibitors especially, non-cognitive symptoms

For relevant references see recent proceedings of the first workshop on Dementia with Lewy bodies, edited Perry R et al., 1996, also Klatka et al., 1996 and Louis et al., 1997; neuroimaging data on the dopamine transporter are from Donnemiller et al., 1977 and unpublished (Katona, Costa, Walker et al) and metabolic imaging refers to Albin et al., 1996.

Consciousness is affected in DLB both in terms of intensity and content (for discussion of these two components, see Baars, 1993). Negative features include: fluctuations in the level of conscious awareness; absences—when the patient appears awake but unaware of the surroundings; or unresponsive to external stimul, and transient or chronic loss of consciousness which can have serious consequences.

Positive features include the high incidence of hallucinations (>80% of patients) which are usually visual but can include other sensory modalities and prevalence of delusions which are reported to be more prevalent and persistent than in AD, perhaps on account of accompanying hallucinations (Ballard et al., 1995, 1996). Some of these features are considered in terms of possible biological mechanisms affected in the disease (Table 5) with a view to highlighting opportunities for more focused research in this area.

VISUAL HALLUCINATIONS, NEUROCHEMICAL PATHOLOGY, AND RELATED PSYCHOPHARMACOLOGY

As proposed elsewhere (Perry and Perry, 1995), the visual hallucinations experienced in DLB are more typical of those occurring as a result of cholinergic muscarinic receptor blockade than those induced by manipulations of other specific cerebral neurotransmitter function. Visions induced by scopolamine or atropine include integrated images of people or animals (as in DLB) whereas those induced by 5-HT$_2$ receptor agonists (e.g. LSD), monoamine release (eg mescaline), NMDA receptor antagonists (eg ketamine or PCP) are generally of a different type. A recent literature survey (BIDS, 1993–7) included reports of visual hallucinations associated with a variety of chemical agents (Table 6), amongst which anti-muscarinics were the most commonly reported. Consistent with this psychopharmacological evidence, in DLB patients experiencing hallucinations cortical cholinergic activity is lower compared to non-hallucinating patients and in the neocortex activity is lower in DLB compared in AD (Perry et al., 1994) in which this symptom is less frequent (20% compared to 80% in DLB).

Table 5. Possible neuronal mechanisms in symptoms involving consciousness in DLB

Symptom	Potential correlates
Visual hallucinations	Impaired neocortical cholinergic transmission
	Relative monoaminergic hyperactivity
	Modulation of GABA synaptic plasticity
	Disruption of brainstem nuclear groups controlling REM sleep
Transient loss of consciousness	Brainstem nuclear group pathology, e.g., pedunculopontine cholinergic projections to thalamus
	Noradrenergic locus coeruleus neuron loss
	Autonomic dysfunction
	Nicotinic receptor reductions (brainstem and/or cortex)
Chronic loss of consciousness	Basal ganglia pathology
	Brainstem pathology
Fluctuating cognitive function	Disruption of rhythmic brainstem nuclear group switching controlling sleep/wake, non REM/REM sleep cycles
	Transient compensatory responses to degenerating cortical input
Delusions	Hypoactivity of dorsal raphé neurons
	Intrinsic neuronal loss related to Lewy body formation in archicortical regions
Attentional deficits	Cortical cholinergic hypoactivity
	Brainstem reticular or thalamic dysfunction

Table 6. Neurochemicals implicated in hallucinations (visual)

Induced by		Relieved by
DA	levodopa	neuroleptics (typical/atypical, D2/D3 antagomists)
ACh	anti-muscarinics (e.g. atropine)	cholinesterase inhibitors
GABA	GABA benzodiazepine site (e.g. lorazepam, zolpidem)	
	ethanol/baclofen withdrawal	
GLU	NMDA antagonists (ketamine, PCP)	
HIS	H_2antagonist (famotidine)	
	H_1antagonist (cyclizine)	
OPIOID	agonists/withdrawal	
5-HT	5-HT$_{2/1C}$agonists	5-HT$_2$antagonists (mianserin)

Summary of literature search, BIDS, 1993–7; see also Perry and Perry, 1995.

Similar types of hallucination do occur in patients with Parkinson's disease treated with Levodopa although a hyperactive dopaminergic influence is difficult to reconcile with degeneration of nigrostriatal neurons, apparent to a greater or lesser extent in most DLB cases. The Charles Bonnet syndrome, occurring in individuals with visual defects such as cataract, involves very similar types of visual imagery as in DLB. Whilst the mechanism in this condition is not established, it is of interest that in animals deprived of visual input experimentally there is a selective loss of GABA as opposed to other types of synapses in the visual cortex (Marty et al., 1997). A reduction in inhibitory GABA control could release normally suppressed network interactions based eg on past memory. This could account for the familiarity of the imagery (contrasting with the novelty reported with agents interfering with eg. noradrenergic or 5-HT systems). Since excitation of GABA neurons, promoting inhibitory tone, is one of the central actions of cortical acetyl-choline it would be worth exploring cortical GABA indices in DLB. However there is a complicating factor in autopsy tissue—the presynaptic GABA marker glutamate decar-boxylase is sensitive to terminal coma or reduced conscious awareness, probably for the same reason, sensory deprivation, that affects GABA synaptic plasticity.

Cortical acetylcholine is widely implicated in attentional processes (Everitt and Rob-bins, 1997) and, as reviewed by Wenk (1997), particularly in "the control of shifting atten-tion to potentially relevant and brief sensory stimuli that predict a biologically relevant event". It is likely that attentional deficits in DLB relate to extensive neocortical cholinergic deficits. This correlate has not yet been quantified nor has it been established if relationships exist between attentional deficits or 'absences' (see below) and hallucinations.

DISTURBANCES IN THE LEVEL OF CONSCIOUSNESS

Transient disturbances in the level of consciousness, occurring at an early stage of DLB appear from the observers point of view, as "absences" during which patient, while not unconscious or asleep, is out of touch with outside stimuli. The eyes are usually open, and stare ahead in blank fashion, the patient does not respond to external stimuli—auditory, tactile (pain, heat, or cold) or visual. The superficial features of the patient may lead the ob-server to conclude that the patient is having a type of fit or non-motor convulsion. The pa-tient does not undergo uni or bilateral repetitive/convulsive limb movements or other features typical of classical epilepsy eg. the tongue is not bitten, and there are no clonic or tonic movements. The time course of such events may last from seconds, minutes, or hours—occasionally longer. Post or pre event EEG recordings have not demonstrated background activity of a standard epileptiform nature, though often requested in the belief that the episode is epileptic in origin. During and after these episodes, blood pressure and pulse are normal. They are not obviously precipitated by specific events and frequently occur with the patient in a sitting or recumbent position. Myocardial infarction, often suspected by nursing or medical stff, is not demonstrable on ECG recording or related laboratory tests (cardiac enzymes). After such episodes the patient is unaware of what has happened.

Later, usually in the terminal phases of the disease chronic loss of consciousness can occur, often precipitated by neuroleptic administration (McKeith et al., 1992). The patient appears relatively inaccessible, and cognitive and behavioural function is markedly decreased. There is hypokinesia and the patients are usually confined to bed. Spontaneous movements are decreased, spontaneous conversation and interactions are decreased or absent. Plantar responses are usually flexor and extrapyramidal features such as stiffness and limb rigidity may be noted. There is also facial hypokinesia. Patients may show some fluctuation in this state but rarely if ever return to their previous level of performance and death usually ensues.

The cause or causes of these acute or chronic reductions in the level of conscious awareness in DLB are unknown. Although non central cardiovascular pathology is unlikely, autonomic (sympathetic or parasympathetic) dysregulation cannot be excluded. Carotid sinus syndrome has recently been identified in a large proportion of DLB but not Alzheimer patients (R. Kenny et al., unpublished observations). Autonomic function is regulated centrally not only in the brainstem but also in areas o the cerebral cortex (Hugdahl, 1996) which are affected in DLB. Precipitation of an unconscious state in DLB by typical (but not atypical) neuroleptic medication implicates D2 receptors in the basal ganglia. The basal ganglia are already compromized in the disease as a result of nigrostriatal dopaminergic degeneration. If similar clinical features are not evident in Parkinson's disease in which such degeneration is more extensive, this would imply basal ganglia pathology distinct to DLB such as intrinsic striatal abnormalities (Table 4).

Since the 1960's, it has been customary to relate mechanisms of brain stem activation to arousal. As reductions of, or fluctuations in, the level of conscious awareness occur more frequently in DLB compared to AD it is unlikely that the noradrenergic locus coeruleus is primarily involved since this is equally affected in both diseases (Perry et al., 1990). Similarly the raphé neurons are severely affected by tangles in AD, also by Lewy bodies in DLB and there is unlikely to be a major difference in neuronal degeneration between the two disorders. There may however be distinctions between the disorders based on the involvement of the brainstem cholinergic nuclear groups (CH5 and CH6, pedunculopontine and dorsolateral tegmental nuclei). These neurons are spared in AD but reduced in Parkinson's disease and remain to the evaluated in DLB.

Over 80% of the thalamic inputs from the brainstem are cholinergic and there are significant reductions in thalamic, particularly reticular nucleus choline acetyltransferase in DLB (Perry et al., in press). This nucleus has been proposed as a physiological substrate of selective attention (Mitrofanis and Guillery, 1993). Loss of cholinergic input to the reticular nucleus in DLB may reflect CH5 or 6 neurodegeneration or, since the thalamus also receives a cholinergic input from the forebrain cholinergic nuclear group (Heckers et al., 1992), it may as is the cortex reflect degenerative changes in the forebrain nuclei. Thalamic cholinergic deficits in DLB thus need to be investigated for clinical correlates as do other thalamic components in relation to variations in consciousness level.

The non-specific thalamus relays many of the highly specific efferents of the midbrain reticular formation (MRF) stimulation to widespread areas of the cortex (Schebeil,

1980). It is the collage of "gatelets" in the nucleus reticularis which close down high-frequency oscillations by generating synchronous activity in the circuits looping between the thalamus and cortex. The interplay of these excitatory and inhibitory systems produces complex patterns of activation in the cortex, gate opening allowing information flow to a cortical area, generating high frequency, desynchronised activity (Steriade and Llinas, 1988; Steriade et al., 1991). If this "gate" is dysfunctional in DLB, as initial findings on cholinergic thalamic activities suggest, then perhaps it is free to swing open and closed, resulting in fluctuating cortical activity, manifest as transient clouding of consciousness. Whilst the midbrain reticular formation may be the first accumulation site for a wide variety of stimulating fields in the nervous system whose role is to filter, sensor and coherently order those inputs in terms of their saliency to the organisms immediate concerns (Newman and Baars, 1993), a second rudimentary "sort" point is the thalamic reticular nucleus. This provides the basic circuitry by which the cortex itself is able to regulate the flow of incoming information. At this level decisions about saliency involve not simple questions of danger or novelty, but the intentional focusing of awareness as a function of prior experience, present requirements, and future goals, all of which appear to be compromized in DLB, in times of clouding of consciousness.

A third pathway, outside of the thalamus, regulating cortical activiation is the nucleus basalis. Acetylcholine-mediated activation of the cortex is important for expression of desynchronised EEG patterns (low voltage, mixed high frequencies characteristic of waking and REM sleep). Transmitter levels at the cortical surface are elevated during waking and REM sleep, compared to non REM sleep (Jasper and Tessier, 1971). Reduced cortical acetylcholine levels produced by excititoxic lesions of the caudal basal forebrain in rats result in enhanced slow-wave activity in the neocortical EEG during waking and REM sleep (Reikinen et al., 1990). Intracortical grafts of fetal basal forebrain tissue rich in cholinergic cells restore the behavioural modulation of cortical acetylcholine release and result in a return of normal waking EEG patterns (Vanderwolf et al., 1990). Cortical cholinergic deficits in DLB have already been implicated in hallucinations (see above) but there is no reason why reductions in arousal level or transient losses of consciousness could now also be related to this neurochemical pathology.

IS ANAESTHESIA RELEVANT?

Further clues regarding mechanisms worth investigating in relation to conscious level may be gleaned from the field of anaesthesia. Muscarinic antagonists eg scopolamine have been employed to induce "twighlight sleep" where the patient is conscious but unaware. While apparently awake, the patient has no awareness of or recall of current events. Scopolamine antagonises muscarinic receptors which (particularly the M_1 subtype) predominate in forebrain including cortical areas. Its effect is consistent with the notion that cortical acetylcholine governs the stream of conscious awareness (Perry and Perry, 1995), increasing doses leading from relative increases in the 'noise' (reduced signal: noise ratio) level eg confusion and hallucinations to lack of signal (loss of conscious awareness) and ultimately coma. The effects of general eg volatile anaesthetics such as halothane are distinct in reducing arousal and inducing sleep. Interestingly, recent research on the effect of such volatile anaesthetic chemicals on transmitter gated ionic receptors indicates that they interact most potently with the central nicotinic ($\alpha_4\beta_2$) cholinergic channel and it is suggested this may be a common mechanism of action in general anaesthesia (Violet et al., 1997; Flood et al., 1997).

Nicotinic receptors of this type which bind nicotine with high affinity are widely distributed in human brain but concentrated in thalamic nuclei such as the lateral geniculate which relays visual stimuli (reviewed Court and Perry, 1995). Although thalamic (^{3}H) nicotine binding is not affected in DLB (Spurden et al unpublished) there is a substantial loss from the brainstem substantia nigra (Perry et al., 1995), which may be relevant to alterations in conscious level and also reductions nicotine binding in various neocortical areas in DLB (Perry et al., 1990).

IS THE DREAMING BRAIN A RELEVANT MODEL?

"Every night of our lives, when our brains automatically enter a fascinating phase of sleep called REM (for rapid eye movement) our minds become quite flagrantly psychotic. We see things that aren't there (we hallucinate), believe things that could not possibly be true (we are deluded), become confused about times, places and persons (we are disoriented), experience intense and wildly fluctuating emotion (we are affectively labile) and then conveniently forget the whole thing (we are amnesic). The fact that the nocturnal madness of our dreams is not only normal but probably even essential to our health should not deflect our attention from two important conclusions. The first is that, by any standard of assessment, we are temporarily out of our minds, and the second is that this temporary psychosis is caused by the physical changes in our brains in REM sleep" (Hobson JA, 1996).

Enough is known of the mechanisms of REM sleep (see eg Hobson, 1988), which is associated with the most vivid and bizarre type of dreaming, to provide a fertile area for speculation into the nature of psychopathology associated with degeneration in neuronal nuclear groups, especially in the brainstem. Sleep is characterized neurophysiologically by a gradual diminution in the firing of locus coeruleus and raphé neurons which reach a state of inactivity during the onset of REM. The onset of REM is also characterized by burst firing of the cholinergic but not other neurons in the brainstem which contribute to the characteristic pedunculo-geniculate-occipital (PGO) waves. Electrophysiological indices such as cortical EEG patterns of desynchronization during REM resemble those during normal wakefulness (Pare and Llinas, 1995). The brain/mind is an extraordinarily active state driven principally by internally generated neurophysiological patterns.

Neurotoxic lesions in cat of the cholinergic mesopontine region by kainic acid cause extensive loss of cholinergic neurons paralleled by loss of REM sleep, decreases in PGO spiking and absent or decreased neck muscle atonia. PGO spiking rate and amount of REM sleep remaining are negatively correlated with number of remaining cholinergic cells and not with noradrenergic neurons. There is also extensive pharmacological evidence of cholinergic mediation of REM sleep. Muscarinic agonists and acetylcholinesterase inhibitors cause increased cortical activation during waking followed by a decrease in REM latency and an increase in REM duration (Jones, 1991). Since pontine cholinergic nuclei also increase firing rate during the awake state (Steriade and McCarley, 1990), the question arises as to how increased activity in these nuclei results in two such distinctly different states of consciousness, waking and REM sleep. The answer is believed to lie in other brainstem nuclei, namely the locus coeruleus suggesting a reripricol interaction between cholinergic and catecholamine cell groups during sleep and wakefulness (Hobson and Baghdogan, 1986). This interesting interplay is highlighted by eserine pharmacological challenges in experimental animals. Eserine peripherally causes increased acetylcholine levels and waking behaviour, but if monoamines are previously depleted and the eserine treatment is repeated REM sleep behaviour, not waking is evident (Karczmar et al., 1970). Suppression of REM related events such as PGO waves and muscle atonia during waking may thus be the result of monoaminergic influences on cholinergic mesopontine neurons. Lack of activity of monoaminergic systems during REM sleep may allow disinhibition of the cholinergic neurons responsible for mediation of REM-related events.

Many other neuronal pathways are involved (eg the loss of histaminergic neuronal activity) during the entire sleep cycle and much remains to be characterized in relation the complexity of REM neurophysiologically. Nevertheless the pathology of brainstem cholinergic neurons in conjunction with locus coeruleus and raphé neurons in DLB deserves to be analysed in relation to symptoms affecting conscious awareness, discussed above, and also in relation to delusions which occur in around 50% of patients with both DLB and AD.

Delusions being characterized by an unshakeable belief in the reality of their component ideation (contrasting with hallucinations in DLB which involve degrees of insight either during or after the experience) are perhaps not far removed from the experience of dreaming. Psychosis, not specifically delusions but likely to include delusions, in AD has been related to loss of raphé neurons and of cortical 5-HT (Zubenko et al., 1991; Forstl et al., 1994). The action of 5-HT, which its primarily inhibitory, may be to prevent neurons from firing in response to currently irrelevant stimuli. In REM, when 5-HT release is abolished and perhaps also in diseases with raphé pathology, this process of censorship is lifted. It would be worth relating raphé pathology and cortical 5-HT pre and post synaptic activities to the incidence of delusions in such diseases as DLB.

If wake/sleep or non REM/REM switch mechanisms are disrupted in DLB, these could account for fluctuations in cognition which is one of the diagnostic features of DLB (Table 2). Variations in cognitive performance are measurable on tests of mental function such as MMSE or MTS which include short and long term memory ability and other aspects of information processing. Their time course varies from hours, days or weeks with days to weeks being most common. Periods of remission to normal or near normal function clearly distinguish DLB from typical AD. Identifying mechanisms involved in such 'cycling' carries the reward of identifying potential therapeutic strategies.

CONCLUSION

DLB is a particularly fascinating disorder on account of specific changes in both the content and level of consciousness that are part of the core symptomatology. In contrast to other diseases affecting consciousness such as schizophrenia, there are clearly identifiable neuropathological and neurochemical abnormalities that can be related to the extent and severity of symptoms. Although categorizing these symptoms in terms of consciousness treads on philosophical grounds, there are areas ripe for neurobiological investigation. These include the mechanisms of hallucinations, absences in conscious awareness and fluctuations in cognition. Preliminary notions such as the relation between neocortical cholinergic deficiency and visual hallucinations or between brainstem cholinergic projections and loss of consciousness could be pursued using chemical imaging and by monitoring the effects of cholinotherapy which is now prescribed in AD. There are already reports that cholinesterase inhibitors control hallucinations in AD and PD (Cummings and Kaufer, 1996; Hutchinson and Fazzini, 1996; Schmidt et al., in press).

In AD, the evidence of a loss of explicit as opposed to implicit memory (Table 1) suggests that important correlates of conscious awareness itself may emerge from examining neuronal pathways affected in this disorder. Arguments supporting a key role of the thalamus, particularly thalamic intralaminar nuclei in subjective awareness (Bogen, 1995;

Newman, 1995) suggest that neuropathology and neurochemistry of thalamic neuronal nuclei would be worth examining in this context. In both AD and DLB, the complexity of clinical symptoms and of neuronal pathways affected is, to say the least, challenging to any correlative exercise. Nevertheless, one of the most consistent neurochemical abnormalities in both AD and DLB is in the cholinergic neurotransmitter system projecting from the forebrain to the cortex. The way in which this transmitter signal globally modulates cortical function, providing at least one possible mechanism for the 'binding' phenomenon of conscious awareness, is worth considering. As suggested by Woolf (1991): "The connectional patterns involving cholinergic cells mandate greater significance to system properties of the network rather than to properties of individual cells".

The advent of new centrally active cholinergic drugs (cholinesterase inhibitors, muscarinic and nicotinic agonists) provides an exciting opportunity to explore therapeutic outcome in dementia not only in terms of cognitive enhancement, but also in relation to some of the more subtle aspects of conscious experience identified in disorders such as DLB (eg. level of arousal, hallucinations, delusion and perhaps also REM patterns). Human conscious experience, as a core component of self identity and fulfilment, deserves a central position in any research programme aimed at identifying mechanisms, management and therapeutic outcome of diseases such as DLB affecting the quality of life in the elderly.

ACKNOWLEDGMENTS

The authors are indebted to Clive Ballard, Evelyn Jaros, Dean Spurden, Rose Anne Kenny and Rose Goodchild for stimulating ideas on this topic and to Lorraine Hood, Tracey Nicholl and Anne Nicholson for manuscript and table preparation.

REFERENCES

Albin, R.L., Minoshima, S., D'Amato, C.J., Frey, K.A., Kuhl, D.A., and Sima, A.A.F., 1996, Fluorodeoxyglucose positron emission tomography in diffuse Lewy body disease. *Neurology* 47:462–466.

Baars, B.J., 1993, How does a serial integrated and very limited stream of consciousness emerge from a nervous system that is mostly unconscious, distributed, parallel and of enormous capacity? In: *Experimental and theoretical studies of consciousness*, Broch, G., and Marsh, J., eds, New York. Wiley.

Ballard, C., Lowery, K., and Harrison, R., 1996, Noncognitive symptoms in Lewy body dementia. In: *Dementia with Lewy bodies*, Perry, R.H., McKeith, I.G., and Perry, E.K., eds, Cambridge. Univ. Press, Cambridge, 67–84.

Ballard, C.G., Saad, K., Patel, A., Gahir, M., Solis, M., Coope, B., and Wilcock, G., 1995, The prevalence and phenomenology of psychotic symptoms in dementia sufferers. *Int. J. Geriatr. Psychiatry.* 10:477–486.

Bogen, J.E., 1995, On the neurophysiology of consciousness: 1. An overview, *Consciousness Cogn.* 4:52–62.

Court, J.A., and Perry, E.K., 1995, Nicotinic receptor distribution in the CNS, In: Stone, T.W., ed, CNS neurotransmitters and neuromodulators - acetylcholine, CRC Press. Boca Raton. pp85–104.

Cummings, J.L., and Kaufer, D., 1996, Neuropsychiatric aspects of Alzheimer's disease: The cholinergic hypothesis revisited. *Neurology.* 47:876–883.

Delacour, J., 1997, Neurobiology of consciousness. *Behav. Brain. Res.* 85:127–141.

Donnemiller, E., Heilman, J., Wenning, G.K., Berger, W., Decristoforo, C., Moncayo, R., Poewe, W., and Ransmayr, G., 1997, Brain perfusion scintigraphy with ^{99m}TC-HMPAO or ^{99m}TC-ECD and ^{123}I-ß-CIT single-photon-emission tomography in dementia of the Alzheimer-type and diffuse Lewy body disease. *Eur. J. Nucl. Med.* 24:320–325.

Everitt, B.J., and Robbins, T.W., 1997, Central cholinergic systems and cognition. *Annu. Rev. Psychol.* 48:649–684.

Flood, P., Ramirez – Latorre, J., and Role, L., 1997, $\alpha_4\beta_2$ Neuronal nicotinic acetylcholine receptors in the central nervous system are inhibited by isoflurane and propofol, but $\alpha7$ - type nicotinic acetylcholine receptors are unaffected. *Anesthesiology.* 86:859–865.

Forstl, H., Burns, A., Levy, R., and Cairns, C., 1994, Neuropathologic correlates of psychotic phenomena in confirmed Alzheimer's disease. *J. Psychiatr.* 165:53–59.

Heckers, S., Geula, C., and Mesulam, M.M., 1992, Cholinergic innervation of the human thalamus: dual origin and differential nuclear distribution. *J. Comp. Neurol.* 325:68–82.

Hesslow, G., 1994, Will neuroscience explain consciousness? *J. Theoret. Biol.* 17:29–39.

Hobson, J.R., 1988, The Dreaming Brain. Penguin Books, Cox and Wyman Ltd, Reading.

Hobson, J.A., Lydic, R., and Baghdogan, H.A., 1986, Evolving concepts of sleep cycle generation: from brain centres to neuronal populations. *Science.* 189:55–58.

Hobson, J.A., 1996, How the brain goes out of its mind. *Endeavour.* 20(2):86–9.

Hugdahl, K., 1996, Cognitive influences on human antonomic nervous system. *Curr. Opin. Neurobiol.* 6:252–258.

Hutchinson, M., and Fazzini, E., 1996, Cholinesterase inhibition in Parkinson's disease. *J. Neurol. Neurosurg. Psychiat.* 61:324–325.

Jasper, H.H., and Tessier, J., 1971, Acetylcholine liberation from cerebral cortex during paradoxical (REM) sleep. *Science.* 172:601–602.

Jones, B.E., 1999, Paradoxical sleep and its chemical/structural substrates in the brain. *Neurosci.* 40:637–656.

Jones, B.E., and Webster, H.H., 1988, Neurotoxic lesions of dorsolateral pontomesencephalic tegmentum-cholinergic cell area in the cat. I. Effects upon the cholinergic innervation of the brain. *Brain Res.* 451:13–32.

Jones, B.E., and Webster, H.H., 1988, Neurotoxic lesions of dorsolateral pontomesencephalic tegmentum-cholinergic cell area in the cat. II. Effects upon sleep-waking states. *Brain Res.* 458:285–302.

Karczmar, A.G., Longo, V.G., and Scoti de Carolis, A., 1970, A pharmacological model of paradoxical sleep: the role of cholinergic and monoaminergic systems. *Physiol. Behav.* 5:175–182.

Klatka, L.A., Louis, E.D., and Schiffer, R.B., 1996, Psychiatric features in diffuse Lewy body disease: a clinico pathologic study using Alzheimer's disease and Parkinson's disease comparison groups. *Neurology.* 47:1148–1152.

Louis, E.D., Klatka, L.A., Liv, Y., and Fahn, S., 1997, Comparison of extrapyramidal features in 31 pathologically confirmed cases of diffuse Lewy body disease and 34 pathologically confirmed cases of Parkinson's disease. *Neurology.* 48:376–380.

McKeith, I.G., Perry, R.H., Fairbairn, A.F., Jabeen, S., and Perry, E.K., 1992, Operational criteria for senile dementia of Lewy body type (SDLT). *Psychol. Med.* 22:911–922.

McKeith, I.G., Galasko, D., Kosaka, K., Perry, E.K., Dickson, D.W., Hansen, L.A., Salmon, D.P., Lowe, J., Mirra, S.S., Byrne, E.J., Lennox, G., Quinn, N.P., Edwardson, J.A., Ince, P.G., Bergeron, C., Burns, A., Miller, B.L., Lovestone, S., Collerton, D., Jansen, E.N., Ballard, C., de Vos, R.A., Wilcock, G.K., Jellinger, K.A., and Perry, R.H., 1996, Consensus guidelines for the clinical and pathologic diagnosis of dementia with Lewy bodies (DLB). *Neurology.* 47:113–1124.

McKeith, I.G., Perry, R.H., Fairbairn, A.F, and Perry, E.K., 1992, Neuroleptic sensitivity in patients with senile dementia of Lewy body type. *Brit. Med. J.* 305:673–678.

Marty, S., de Penha Berzaghi, M., and Berninger, B., 1997, Neurotrophins and activity dependant plasticity of cortical interneurons. *Trends. Neurosci.* 20:198–202.

Mitrofanis, J., and Guillery, R.W., 1993, New views of the thalamic reticular nucleus in the adult and developing brain. *Trends. Neurosci.* 13:1719–1729.

Newman, J., and Baars, B.J., 1993, A neural attentional model for access to consciousness. A global workspace perspective. *Concepts Neurosci.* 4:255–290.

Pare, D., and Llinas, R., 1995, Conscious and pre-conscious processes as seen from the stand point of sleep-waking cycle neurophysiology. *Neuropsychologia* 33:1155–1168.

Perry, E.K., and Perry, R.H., 1995, Acetycholine and hallucinations, disease-related compared to drug-induced alterations in human consciousness. *Brain and Cognition* 28:240–258.

Perry, E.K., and Perry, R.H., 1996, Altered consciousness and transmitter signalling in Lewy body dementia. In: *Dementia with Lewy bodies*, Perry, R.H., McKeith, I.G., Perry, E.K., eds, pp. 397–413, Cambridge. Univ. Press, Cambridge.

Perry, E.K., Smith, C.J., Court, J.A., and Perry, R.H., 1990, Cholinergic nicotinic and muscarinic receptors in dementia of Alzheimer, Parkinson and Lewy body types. *J Neural. Transm.* 27:149–158.

Perry, E.K., Haroutunian, V., Davis, K.L., Levy, R., Lantos, P., Eagger, S., Honavar, M., Dean, A., Griffiths, M., McKeith, I.G., and Perry. R.H., 1994, Neocortical cholinergic activities differentiate Lewy body dementia from classical Alzheimer's disease. *Neuroreport* 55:1454–1456.

Perry, E.K., Morris, C.M., Court. J.A., Cheng, A., Fairbairn, A., McKeith, I.G., Irving, D., Brown, A., and Perry, R.H., 1995, Alteration in nicotine binding sites in Parkinson's disease, Lewy body dementia and Alzheimer's disease: possible index of early neuropathology. *Neuroscience* 64:385–395.

Perry, R.H., Irving, D., Blessed, G., Fairbairn, A., and Perry, E.K., 1990, Senile dementia of Lewy body type: a clinically and neuropathologically distinct form of Lewy body dementia in the elderly. *J. Neurol. Sci.* 95:119–135.

Perry, R.H., McKeith, I.G., and Perry, E.K., 1997, Lewy body dementia: clinical, pathological and neurochemical interconnections. *J. Neural. Trans. PD and Dementia Sect.* Suppl 4, in press.

Postle, B.R., Corkin, S., and Growdon, J.H., 1996, Intact implicit memory for novel patterns in Alzheimer's disease. *Learn. Mem.* 3:305–312.

Reikinen, P., Sirvio, J., Hannila, T., Miettinen, R., and Riekkinen, P., 1990, Effects of quisqualic acid nucleus basalis lesioning on cortical EEG, passive avoidance and water maze performance. *Brain. Res. Bull.* 24:839–842.

Sarter, M., and Bruno, J.P., 1997, Cognitive functions of cortical acetylcholine: towards a unifying hypothesis. *Brain. Res. Revs.* 23:28–46.

Schebeil, A.B., 1980, Anatomical and physiological substrates of arousal: a view from the bridge. In: *Reticular formation revisited*, Hobson, J.A., and Brazier, M.A., eds, New York: Raven Press,, pp. 55–66.

Schmidt, B.H., Fanelli, R.J., and van der Staay, F.J., Preclinical pharmacology of metrifonate: an overview (this book).

Scott, L.C., Wright, G.K., Rai, G.S., Exton-Smith, A.N., and Gardiner, J.M., 1991, Further evidence of preserved memory function in Alzheimer's disease. *Int. J. Geriatr. Psychiat.* 6:583–588.

Steriade, M., and Llinas, R.R., 1988, The functional states of the thalamus and the associated neuronal interplay. *Physiol. Rev.* 68:649–742.

Steriade, M., and McCarley, R.W., 1990, Brainstem control of wakefulness and sleep. Plenum, New York.

Steriade, M., Curro Dossi, D., Pare, D., and Oakson, G., 1991, Fast oscillations (20–40Hz) in the thalamocortical systems and their potentiation by mesopontine cholinergic nuclei in the cat. *Proc. Nat. Acad. Sci.* USA. 88:4396–4400.

Tokimasa, A., and Yamadori, A., 1997, Procedural memory in patients with mild Alzheimer's disease. *Dement. Geriatr. Cogn. Disord.* 8:210–216.

Newman, J., 1995, Thalamic contributions to attention and consciousness. Consciousness and Cognition. 4:172–93.

Turner, B.H., and Knapp, M.E., 1995, Consciousness a neurobiological approach. *Integr. Physiol. Behav. Sci..* 30:151–156.

Vanderwoolf, C.H., Fine, A., and Cooley, R.K., 1990, Intracortical grafts of embryonic basal forebrain tissue restore low voltage fast activity in rats with basal forebrain lesions. *Exp. Brain. Res.* 81:426–432.

Violet, J.M., Downie, D.L., Nakinsa, R.C., Lieb, W.R., and Franks, N.P., 1997, Differential sensitivities of mammalian neuronal and muscle nicotinic acetylcholine receptors to general anaesthetics. *Anesthesiology.* 86:866–874.

Wenk, G.L., 1997, The nucleus basalis magnocellularis cholinergic system. One hundred years of progress. *Neurobiol. Learn. Mem.* 67:85–95.

Woolf, N.C., 1991, Cholinergic systems in mammalian brain and spinal cord. *Progr. Neurobiol.* 37:475–524.

Zubenko, G.S., Moossy, J., Martinez, J., Rao, G., Claassen, D., Rosen, J., and Kopp, U., 1991, Neuropathologic and neurochemical correlates of psychosis in primary dementia. *Arch. Neurol.* 48:619–624.

66

NICOTINIC RECEPTORS AS A NEW TARGET FOR TREATMENT OF ALZHEIMER'S DISEASE

Agneta Nordberg, Anne-Lie Svensson, Ulrika Warpman, Linda Bud,
Amelia Marutle, Hui Miao, Olga Gorbounova, Ivan Bednar,
Ewa Hellström-Lindahl, and Xiao Zhang

Department of Clincal Neuroscience and Family Medicine
Division of Nicotine Research, Karolinska Institutet
Huddinge University Hospital
S-141 86, Huddinge, Sweden

INTRODUCTION

The neuronal nicotinic acetylcholine receptors (nAChRs) show rich abundance in human brain. Three nAChR binding sites with super-high, high and low affinities have been identified using nicotinic agonists with different receptor affinity (Nordberg et al. 1988, Warpman and Nordberg 1995). Molecular biology studies have identified eight nAChR subunits ($\alpha2$-$\alpha9$, $\beta2$-$\beta4$) in rodent brain and seven nAChR subunits ($\alpha3$-$\alpha5$, $\alpha7$, $\beta2$-$\beta4$) in human brain (Sargent et al. 1993). Different combinations of α and β subunits can form different nAChR subtypes in pentaineric structures which upon activation elicit varying physiological and pharmacological effects (McGee and Role 1995, Zhang and Nordberg 1995). The $\alpha4\beta2$ nAChR subtype is considered to be the most common in rodent brain (Flores et al. 1992). Whether this is also the case in human brain has to be proven. It has recently been suggested that the presynaptic modulation of transmitter release may represent a major function of the nAChRs (McGee et al. 1995, Wonnacott 1997). The nAChRs may play a modulatory role for several neurotransmitters in brain (Figure 1). It is quite possible that the nAChRs can be tuned regarding channel opening time, agonists sensitivity and densitization properties to fulfil the requirements for a certain neurotransmitter and brain region. Figure 1 shows some examples of transmitters that appear to be regulated by presynaptic nAChRs. The nAChR subunits may differ between different regions of the brain as well as transmitter systems. Thus the presynaptic nAChR regulating dopamine release appears to contain the $\alpha4$ subunit (Wonnacott 1997), while the $\alpha7$ nAChR subunit seem to facilitate the release of glutamate (Gray et al. 1996) (Figure 1). The occurence of more than one nAChR subtype presynaptically might be possible and is therefore an important issue to explore when focusing on drug development.

Progress in Alzheimer's and Parkinson's Diseases
edited by Fisher *et al.*, Plenum Press, New York, 1998.

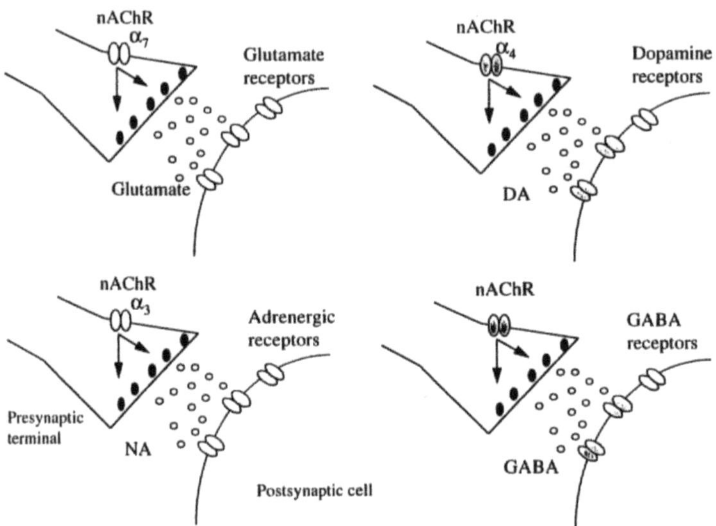

Figure 1. Schematic drawing of the presynaptic modulation of glutamate, dopamine, noradrenaline, and GABA release by nicotinic receptor subtypes in brain.

NICOTINIC RECEPTOR CHANGES IN ALZHEIMER BRAINS

The human nAChRs are important for cognitive processes in human brain (Sahakian et al. 1989, Warburton et al. 1994). Studies of AD patients with positron emission tomography (PET) have also shown marked deficits in nicotinic receptors early in the course of the disease which are related to cognitive functions (Nordberg et al. 1995). Both the α4 and α7 nAChR subunits have been suggested to play an important role in cognitive functions (Albuquerque et al. 1997). The nicotinic receptors are markedly reduced in cortical regions of patients with Alzheimer's disease (AD) (Nordberg and Winblad 1986). A selective loss has been measured in the α4β2 nAChRs when using the nicotinic agonists epibatidine and ABT-418 as receptor ligands (Warpman and Nordberg 1995).

Chromosomal aberrations appear to be a significant risk factor for developing AD. For the late onset form of AD the apolipoprotein E (APOE) ε-4 allele on chromosome 19 is associated with an increased risk of developing AD (Corder et al. 1994). We found by PET no difference in cerebral glucose metabolism in AD patients with different APOE genotype (Corder et al. 1997). Similarly, no difference in nicotinic receptors or other cholinergic parameters was measured in the temporal cortex of autopsy AD brains with differing APOE genotype (Svensson et al. submitted) despite a greater deposition of β-amyloids and neurofibrillary tangles in APOE ε4 carriers (Ohm et al. 1995, Polvikoski et al. 1995). Others have reported a more pronounced loss in cholinergic activity in AD brains of APOE ε4 compared to ε3 carriers (Poirier et al. 1994, Soininen et al. 1995). Recent studies in autopsy brain tissue from AD patients with 670/671 APP mutation (the Swedish mutation) indicate a more pronounced deficits in nAChRs losses in the cortical brain regions in comparsion with subjects with sporadic AD (Marutle et al. submitted). No strict correlation could however be observed between nicotinic receptor losses, neuritic plaques and neurofibrillary tangles suggesting that the processes may not be intimately coupled (Marutle et al. submitted).

NICOTINIC RECEPTOR CHANGES IN ALZHEIMER LYMPHOCYTES

Human lymphocytes express similar nAChRs subunits as found in human brain (α3,α4, α5, α7, β2, β4) but not the (α5 and β3 subunits. A significant reduction in the levels of α3, α4, β2 and β4 subunits was observed in lymphocytes from AD patients while the level of α7 was significantly increased compared to controls (Hellström-Lindahl et al. 1997). Ongoing studies will reveal whether AD subjects with chromosomal aberrations differ in their nAChRs on lymphocytes in comparison with sporadic AD cases.

EFFECT OF NICOTINIC AGONISTS ON NICOTINIC RECEPTORS

The reports on the beneficial effects of acute doses of nicotine on AD (Newhouse et al. 1994) prompted further studies on the underlying mechanisms for the long-term effects of nicotinic agonists on nAChRs in brain. Chronic exposure to nicotine is known to upregulate the nicotinic receptors in brain of rodents and man. Is it possible to restore cholinergic function in AD brains by long-term treatment with nicotinic agonists? Based upon studies in transfected α4β2 MIO cells the nicotine-induced upregulation seem to occur through postranslational mechanisms probably reflecting an altered receptor turnover (Peng et al. 1994, Zhang et al. 1994). Chronic treatment with nicotinic agonists indicates that the upregulation of the α4β2 nAChRs in M10 cells is influenced by the affinity of the nicotinic agonist and they are also more readily upregulated than the α3 nAChR subunits expessed in SH-SY5Y neuroblastoma cells (Warpman et al. submitted). The findings indicate a difference in effect of nicotinic agonists on α4 and α3 nAChRs. A further understanding of the underlying mechanisms for this differences, e.g. rate of resensitization, conformational state changes, are of importance in the attempts to design selective nicotinic agonists useful in the treatment of AD.

INTERACTION WITH ALLOSTERIC SITE ON THE NICOTINIC RECEPTORS

The cholinesterase inhibitors are the first drugs used in clinical practice for treatment of cognitive disorders in AD patients. Long-term treatment with the cholinesterase inhibitor tacrine restores the nicotinic receptors in cortical brain regions of AD patients as measured by PET (Nordberg et al. 1992, 1996). Chronic treatment with tacrine in transfected α4β2 MIO cells causes an dose-dependently both increase and decrease in the number of nAChRs (Svensson and Nordberg 1996). Tacrine thereby seem to interact with two sites on the nAChR. An activation of a non-competitive allosteric site (Albuquerque et al. 1997) occurs at clinical relevant concentration of tacrine and leads to an increase in number of nicotinic receptors (Svensson et al. 1996). Interestingly, various cholinesterase inhibitors may differ following chronic treatment in their effect on nicotinic receptors (Figure 2). Tacrine and galanthamine seem to interact with both the allosteric activator site and the ACh binding site. Other cholinesterase inhibitors such as E2020 and NXX-066 most probably interfere solely with the nAChR allosteric activator site (Svensson and Nordberg 1997) (Figure 2). The interaction via the allosteric site might be of special clinical importance for outcome of treatment effects and suggest al-

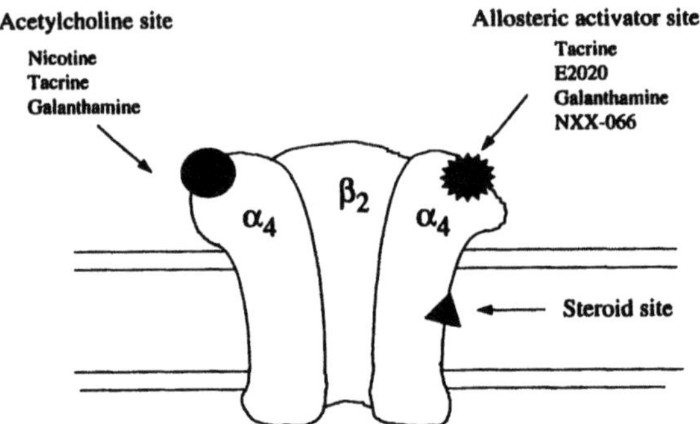

Figure 2. Putative binding sites for nicotine and cholinesterase inhibitors on the α4β2 nicotinic receptor.

ternative ways of activating of the nAChRs than directly via the nicotine binding site (Figure 2).

NEUROPROTECTION AND NICOTINIC RECEPTORS

In vivo and *in vitro* studies suggest an involvement of nAChRs in neuroprotective mechanisms exterted by nicotinic agonists. Nicotine has been shown to block glutamate induced neurotoxicity in cells and the effect can be inhibited by mecamylamine (Akaike et al. 1994). Similarly, ABT-418 has been shown to prevent glutamate neurotoxicity in cortical primary cell cultures (Donnelly-Roberts et al. 1996). The effect is assumed to be mediated via the α7 nAChRs subtype since the effect is blocked by α-bungarotoxin (Donnelly-Roberts et al. 1996). Interestingly it has recently been shown that nicotine *in vitro* can inhibit amyloid formation (Salmon et al. 1996). We are presently using a test system where the effects of nicotinic receptor stimulation on β-amyloid and glutamate induced neurotoxicity is studied measuring MTT (mitochondrial activity) or LDH activity (cell death) (Figure 3). The possible cognitive and neuroprotective effects of estrogen in AD patients has recently been discussed (Wickelgren 1997). Since a steroid site is known to be present on the nAChR (Figure 2) we are investigating whether estrogen can exert neuroprotective effects via nAChRs. In preliminary studies we have observed that nicotine (10^{-5}–10^{-4} M) in PC 12 cells can prevent the reduction in MMT conversion induced by 7 days of treatment with 10^{-8} M Aβ (25–35). Interestingly, also tacrine at clinical relevant concentrations seems to be able to inhibit β-amyloid toxicity in PC 12 cells.

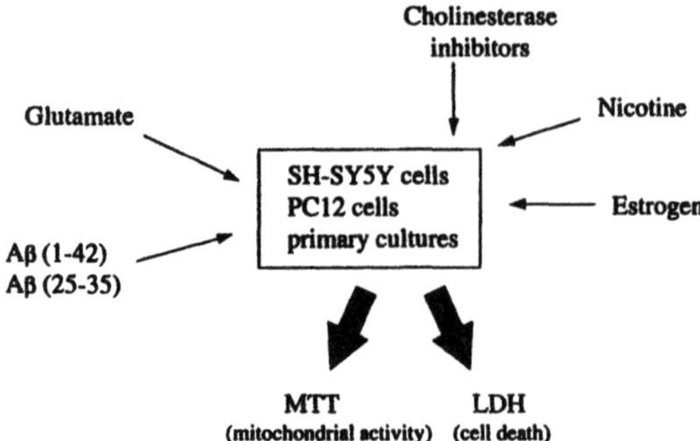

Figure 3. Experimental system for testing of neuroprotective effects of nicotine, cholinesterase inhibitors, and estrogen on glutamate and β-amyloid toxicity.

The underlying mechanisms for these interactions with the nAChRs are presently under investigation.

CONCLUSIONS

The nAChRs are involved in cognitive processes in brain. AD patients show early in the course of the disease significant losses of nAChRs. Therapeutic strategies aiming to improve nAChRs seem to be a promising approach. At present relative few of the nAChRs subtypes have been identified and pharmacologically tested in human brain. A further understanding of the functional characteristics for nAChRs subtypes will be essential for providing novel nicotinic agonists with modulatory function and possible neuroprotective properties in AD brains.

ACKNOWLEDGMENTS

This study was supported by grants from the Swedish Medical Research Council (05817), Loo and Hans Osterman's foundation, KI foundations, Stiftelsen för Gamla Tjänarinnor, Swedish Match.

REFERENCES

Akaike, A., Tamura, Y., Yokota, T., Shimohama, S., and Kimura, J., 1994, Nicotine-induced protection of cultured cortical neurons against N-methyl-D-aspartate receptor-mediated glutamate cytotoxicity. *Brain Res.* 644:181–187.

Albuquerque, E.X., Manickavasagom, A., Pereira, E.F.R., Castro, N.G., Schrattenholz, A., Barbosa, C.T.F., Bonfante-Carbarcas, R., Aracava, Y., Eisenberg, H.M., and Maelicke A., 1997, Properties of neuronal nicotinic acetylcholine receptors: pharmacological characterization and modulation of synpatic function. *J. Pharmacol. Exp. Ther.* 280:1117–1136.

Corder, E.H., Jelic, V., Basun, H., Lannfelt, L., Valind, S., Winblad, B., and Nordberg, A., 1997, No difference in cerebral glucose metabolism in Alzheimer patients with differing apolipoprotein E genotype. *Arch. Neurol.* 54:273–277.

Corder, E.H., Saunders A.M., and Strittmatter W.J. et al., 1993, Gene dose of apolipoprotein E type 4 allele and the risk of Alzheimer's disease in late onset families. *Science* 261:921–923.

Donnelly-Roberts, D.L., Xue, I.C., Americ, S.P., and Sullivan, J.P., 1996, *In vitro* neuroprotective properties of the novel cholinergic channel activator (ChCA), ABT-418. *Brain Res.* 719:36–44.

Flores, C.M., Rogers, S.W., Pabreza L.A., Wolfe B.B., and Keller, K.J., 1992, A subtype of nicotinic cholinergic receptor in brain is composed of α4 and β2 subunits and is upregulated by chronic nicotine treatment. *Mol. Pharmacol.* 41:31–37.

Gray S., Rajan A.S., Radcliffe K.A., Yakehiro M., and Dani J.A., 1996, Hippocampal synaptic transmission enhanced by low concentrations of nicotine. *Nature* 383:713–716.

Hellström-Lindahl E., Zhang X., and Nordberg A., Expression of nicotinic receptor subunit mRNAs in lymhocytes from normal and Alzheimer patients. *Alzheimer's Research*, in press.

McGehee, D.S., Heath M.J.S., Gelber S., Deway P., and Role L.W., 1995, Nicotine enhancement of fast excitatory synaptic transmission in CNS by presynaptic receptors. *Science* 269:1692–1696.

McGehee, D.S., and Role, L.W., 1995, Physiological diversity of nicotinic acetylcholine receptors expressed by vertebrate neurons. *Ann. Rev. Physiol.* 57:521–546.

Newhouse, P.A., Potter, A., Corwin, J., and Lenox, R., 1994, Modeling of the nicotinic receptor loss in dementia using the nicotinic antagonist mecamylamine: Effects on human cognitive functioning. *Drug Dev. Res.* 31:71–79.

Nordberg, A., Adem, A., Hardy J. and Winblad B., 1988, Change in nicotinic receptor subtypes in temporal cortex of Alzheimer brains. *Neurosci. Lett.* 86:317–321.

Nordberg, A., Lilja, A., Lundqvist, H., Hartvig, P., Amberla, K., Viitanen, M., Warpman, U., Johansson, M., Hellström-Lindahl, E., Bjurling, P., Fasth, K.J., Långström, B., and Winblad, B., 1992, Tacrine restores cholinergic nicotinic receptors and glucose metabolism in Alzheimer patients as visualized by positron emission tomography. *Neurobiol. Aging* 13:747–758.

Nordberg, A., Lundqvist, H., Hartvig, P., Andersson, J., Johansson, M., Hellström-Lindahl, E. and Långström, B., 1997, Imaging of nicotinic and muscarinic receptors in Alzheimer's disease:effect of tacrine treatment. *Dement. Geriatr. Cogn. Disord.* 8:78–84.

Nordberg, A., Lundqvist, H., Hartvig, P., Lilja, A., and Långström, B., 1995, Kinetic analysis of regional (S)(-)[11] c-nicotine binding in normal and Alzheimer brains- *in vivo* assessment using positron emission tomography. *Alzheimer Dis. Assoc. Disord.* 9:21–27.

Nordberg, A., and Winblad, B., 1986, Reduced number of ^{3}H-nicotine and ^{3}H-acetylcholine binding sites in the frontal cortex of Alzheimer brains. *Neurosci. Lett.* 72:115–119.

Ohm, T.G., Kirca, M., Bohl, J., Scharnagl, H., Gross, W., and März, W., 1995, Apolipoprotein E polymorphism influences not only cerebral plaque load but also Alzheimer-type neurofibrillary tangle formation. *Neuroscience* 66:583–587.

Poirier, J., Delisle, M.C., Quirion, R., Aubert, I., Farlow, M., Lahiri, D., Hui, S., Bertrand, P., Nalbantoglu, J., Gilfix, B.M., and Gauthier, S., 1995, Apolipoprotein E4 allele as a predictor of cholinergic deficit and treatment outcome in Alzheimer disease. *Proc. Natl. Acad. Sci.* 92:12260–12264.

Peng, X., Gerzanich, V., Anand, R., Whiting, P., and Lindstrom, J., 1994, Nicotine-induced increase in neuronal nicotinic receptors results from a decrease in the rate of receptor turnover. *Mol. Pharmacol.* 46:523–530.

Polvikoski, T., Sulkava, R., Haltia, M., Kainulainen, K., Vourio, A., Verkkoniemi, A., Niinisto, L., Halonen, P., and Kontula, K., 1995, Apolipoprotein E, dementia and cortical deposition of β-amyloid protein. *N. Engl. J. Med.* 333:1242–1247.

Sargent, P.B., 1993, The diversity of neuronal nicotinic acetylcholine receptors. *Ann. Rev. Neurosci.* 16:403–433.

Sahakian, B., Jones, G., Levy, R., Gray, J., and Warburton, D., 1989, The effects of nicotine on attention, information processing, and short-term memory in patients with dementia of Alzheimer's type. *Br. J. Psychiatry* 154:797–800.

Salmon, A.R., Marcinowski, K.J., Friedland, R.P., and Zagorski, M.G., 1996, Nicotine inhibits amyloid formation by the β-peptide. *Biochemistry* 35:13568–13578.

Soininen, H., Kosunen, O., Helisalmi, S., Mannermaa, A., Paljärvi, L., Talasniemi, S., Ryynänen M., and Riekkinen, Sr. P., 1995, A severe loss of choline acetyltransferase in the frontal cortex of Alzheimer patients carrying apolipoprotein ε4 allele. *Neurosci. Lett.* 187:79–82.

Svensson, A-L., and Nordberg, A., 1997, Interaction of tacrine, galanthamine, NXX-066 and E2020 with neuronal α4β2 nicotinic receptors expressed in fibroblast cells. In: *Alzheimer's Disease: Biology, Diagnosis and Therapeutics*, K. Iqbal, B. Winblad, T. Nishimura, M. Takeda, H.M. Wisniewski, eds., John Wiley & Sons, Chichester, pp. 751–756.

Svensson, A-L., and Nordberg, A., 1996, Tacrine interacts with an allosteric activator site on α4β2 nAChRs in M10 cells. *NeuroReport* 7:2201–2205.

Warburton, D.M., Rusted, J.M., and Fowler, J., 1992, A comparison of the attentional and consolidation hypotheses for the facilitation of memory by nicotine. *Psychopharmacology* 108:443–447.

Warpman, U., and Nordberg, A., 1995, Epibatidine and ABT 418 reveal selective losses of α4β2 nicotinic receptors in Alzheimer brains. *NeuroReport* 6:2419–2423.

Wickelgren, I., 1997, Estrogen stakes claim to cognition. *Science* 276:675–678.

Wonnacott, S., 1997, Presynaptic nicotinic ACh receptors. *TINS* 20:92–98.

Zhang, X., Gong, Z-H., Hellström-Lindahl, E., and Nordberg, A., 1994, Regulation of α4β2 nicotinic acetylcholine receptors in M10 cells following treatment with nicotinic agents. *NeuroReport* 6:313–317.

Zhang, X., and Nordberg, A., Characterization of nicotinic acetylcholine receptors in brain. In: *Brain Imaging of Nicotine and Tobacco Smoking*, E.F. Domino, ed., NPP Books, Ann Arbor, pp. 59–71.

67

S 12024-2, A COGNITIVE ENHANCER, INTERACTS WITH NICOTINIC NEUROTRANSMISSION

Jean M. Lépagnol, Philippe Morain, Jean-Yves A. Thomas, Murielle Méen, Marianne Rodriguez, and Pierre J. Lestage

Department of Cerebral Pathology
Institut de Recherche Servier
125, Chemin de Ronde
78290, Croissy-sur-Seine, France

INTRODUCTION

S 12024-2 (R,S methyl-1 (morpholinyl-2 methoxy)-8 tetrahydro-1,2,3,4 quinoline) was selected in a new chemical series as a potent *in vivo* facilitatory compound on brain noradrenergic neurotransmission (Lépagnol and Lestage, 1994). Indeed, after i.p. or oral administration in rodents, S 12024-2 dose-dependently enhanced both the yohimbine-induced mortality or norepinephrine (NE)-induced seizures and inhibited the sedation induced by xylazine, a centrally acting $\alpha 2$ agonist. However, neurochemical studies clearly demonstrated that S 12024-2 was devoid of any classical mechanism of action with regards to noradrenergic neurotransmission (adrenoreceptors binding, NE reuptake inhibition, IMAO, ICOMT, ...). In contrast, S 12024-2 was able to increase the *in vitro* K^+-induced NE release, notably in hypothalamic slices. This effect was in good agreement with the *in vivo* regional brain distribution of [^{3}H]-S 12024-2 which was preferentially observed in hypothalamic vasopressinergic nuclei (PVN, SON). Moreover, S 12024-2 strongly prevented the time-dependent natural forgetting in the episodic social memory test in the rat, a form of memory in rodents which was demonstrated as being linked to both noradrenergic (Griffin and Taylor, 1995) and vasopressinergic (Bluthe and Dantzer, 1992) neurotransmitter systems. The cognition enhancing effects of S 12024-2 were prevented by the administration of a vasopressinergic antagonist or alleviated in vasopressin deficient Brattleboro rats (Lépagnol and Lestage, 1994). However, S 12024-2 failed to bind either V1 or V2 receptors. Interestingly, the NE stimulating effects of S 12024-2 were more pronounced with the racemate compared with both isomers named S 14706-1 and S 14707-1. Present studies were aimed in order to determine whether as noradrenergic stimulating effects, the cognitive effects of S 12024-2 were of greater potency compared with the isomers of the compound.

Moreover, in a phase IIb clinical study of 3 months duration in Alzheimer's patients, S 12024-2 exerted beneficial effects and slowed down the progression of the disease. These effects were significantly observed in moderate cases (MMS 14–18). Furthermore, S 12024-2 was more active in patients with the ApoE-ε4 allele (Amouyel et al., 1996).

By taking into consideration 1) the hypothalamic positive interactions between nicotinic and noradrenergic (Matta et al., 1993), nicotinic and vasopressinergic (Faiman et al., 1988; Larose et al., 1988) and finally, vasopressinergic and noradrenergic neurotransmissions (Leibowitz et al., 1990; Shioda et Nakai, 1992), 2) the recent observation regarding the dramatic decrease in nicotinic receptors in Alzheimer's brain, particularly in patients with the ApoE-ε4 allele (Poirier et al., 1994), 3) the chemical structure of S 12024-2, the present studies were performed in order to determine an eventual interaction of S 12024-2 with nicotinic receptors. For this purpose, electrophysiological experiments were performed using Xenopus oocytes expressing the α7 subunit of human nicotinic receptor, one of the major subclasses in the brain (Séguéla et al., 1993), notably in limbic and thalamic areas (Williams et al., 1994). Furthermore, nicotinic effects of S 12024-2 were studied in a recently reported model of nicotine-dependent wet-dog shakes induced by kainic acid in the rat (Shytle et al., 1995).

MATERIALS AND METHODS

Behavioral Studies

The protocols and the procedures were approved by the Ethical Animal Care and Use Commitee of the Institut de Recherches Internationales Servier. Male OFA rats (200–250 g body weight; Iffa credo, France) and male Wistar rats (280–320 g body weight; Iffa Credo, France) were used in the passive avoidance test and in the social memory test, respectively. They were maintained in the animal house facilities during at least 6 days before the experiment under standardized conditions (light-dark cycle 12h/12h—light on from 7 a.m. to 7 p.m.) with food and water *ad libidum*. Similar housing conditions were applied on the days of experiments except that animals were housed individually and reduced illumination was used during both the learning and recall phases of the memory tests.

Passive Avoidance Test

The one trial step-through passive avoidance test was performed by using a two-compartment (30×30×32 cm) apparatus. The black compartment, connected to a foot-shock generator by the grid floor, and the white, illuminated by a 20 W daylight lamp, were separated by an automatically driven guillotine-type door. The acquisition trial consisted of placing the rat in the white compartment, opening the door after 60 s, shutting the door as soon as four legs of the rat had entered the dark compartment, delivering a 0.6 mA-3s scrambled foot shock, leaving the rat for 30 s after the shock delivery and then, removing the animal from the apparatus. The retention test was conducted 24 h later and consisted of placing the rat in the white compartment and measuring the time before the rat entered the dark compartment, up to a maximum of 300 s (retention latency of the passive avoidance response). Under these experimental conditions, the mean latency of control rats was of 270–300 s. In contrast, treatment with scopolamine HBr (1 mg/kg i.p.), 30 min before the acquisition trial, induced a pronounced amnesia as shown by a dramatic decrease of retention latency. Treated rats received S 12024-2 or its isomers 60 min before both the acquisition and retention trials.

Social Memory Test

An unfamiliar juvenile rat (26–31 days old) was placed in the home cage of an adult rat for 5 min. The time spent (T1) by the adult rat investigating the juvenile (nosing, sniffing, close following) was recorded (videocamera system) and expressed the social recognition behavior. The adult rat was again exposed for a second 5 min exposure presentation to the same juvenile 120 min later and the investigation time was recorded (T2). Previous studies clearly demonstrated a significant decrease (40 to 50s) of investigatory behaviour (T2–T1) for a shorter interval (less than 30 min) between the 2 exposures to the same juvenile congener. In contrast, no significant difference could be observed for a 120 min interval and expressed the loss of social memory performances. Under these experimental conditions, treated rats received S 12024-2 or its isomers immediately after the first exposure to the juvenile.

Kainate-Induced Wet-Dog Shakes (WDS)

Rats were given kainic acid KA (12 mg/kg s.c.) then individually observed during 10 min in order to determine the total number of WDS. Treated rats received a nicotinic agonist by s.c. route 15 min before KA. In the interaction studies using mecamylamine (5 mg/kg s.c.), the nicotinic antagonist was also injected 15 min before KA.

Electrophysiological Studies

Molecular Cloning of Human α7 Subunit of Nicotinic Receptor (α7-nAChR). The template cDNA strand was synthesized from 1 µg of total RNA of SKNSH-SY5Y cells using Superscript II (Stratagene), then subjected to PCR amplification (primers sense 5′GACTCAACATGCGCTGCTCG3′ and antisense 5′TCCGTCGTAATGTGCGGTG3′) using Pfu polymerase (Stratagene). Amplification was carried out by 35 cycles at 94°C for 1 min, 55°C for 1 min and 72°C for 3 min, followed by one extension step at 72°C for 5 min. The expected 1614 base pair fragment was isolated from low melting temperature agarose and cloned into pCR-Script SK vector (Stratagene) in order to obtain the recombinant plasmid pSK/α7. The subcloned insert was sequenced on both strands by automated sequencing. The plasmid PSK/α7 was linearized at the 3′ end with restriction enzyme STU I and RNA was synthesized *in vitro* using Ampliscribe T7 transcription kit (Tebu).

Xenopus Oocyte Preparation. Female *Xenopus laevis* frogs (CNRS Montpellier, France) were anesthetized in ice-cold water, and a section of one ovary was removed surgically then placed in Barth's solution (NaCl 88 mM, KCl 1 mM, $MgSO_4$ 0.8 mM, $Ca(NO_3)_2$ 0.3 mM, $CaCl_2$ 0.4 mM, Tris 7.5 mM, $NaHCO_3$ 2.4 mM, gentamycine 100 µg/ml, pH 7.6). Each isolated oocyte was injected with 70 ng of the human α7 mRNA in 70 nl), then incubated at 19°C in Barth's solution for at least 3 days.

Recording Conditions and Experimental Protocols

Nicotine-induced currents were recorded using standard two-electrode voltage clamp system (Axoclamp 2A, Axon instruments, USA). The electrodes (ref. GC120F-10, Clark instruments) were filled with 3 M KCl and the holding potential was −60 mV. The oocyte was placed in a 50 μl microchamber then normally superfused at 3 ml/min flow rate with OR2 medium consisting of (mM): NaCl (82.5), KCl (2.5), Na_2HPO_4 (1), $MgSO_4$ (1), $CaCl_2$ (2), HEPES (5), pH 7.4. For the rapid application of nicotine during 20 s every 10 min, the flow rate was adjusted to 10 ml/min. In experiments of pharmacological interaction, the compound was applied at a normal flow rate during 3 min, before nicotine administration.

RESULTS

Mnemocognitive Effects of S 12024-2 or Its Isomers S 14706-1 and S 14707-1

Scopolamine-Induced Amnesia in the Passive Avoidance Test in OFA Rat. From 0.25 to 25 mg/kg, S 12024-2 inhibited the scopolamine-induced amnesia in the passive avoidance test. The dose-effect was an inverted U shape, a characteristic of cognition enhancers. The cognitive effect of S 12024-2 was significant from 0.75 mg/kg dose and an almost complete inhibition of amnesia was obtained at 2.5 mg/kg (Figure 1). In contrast, under the same range of doses, no significant preventive effect could be observed with both isomers and the mean retention latency remained of lower magnitude compared with S 12024-2.

Social Memory Test in Wistar Rat

In the range of tested doses (0.25 to 7.5 mg/kg), S 12024-2 significantly prevented the time-dependent forgetting in the episodic social memory test. As in the passive avoidance test, the dose-effect was of inverted U shape and a complete inhibition of amnesia

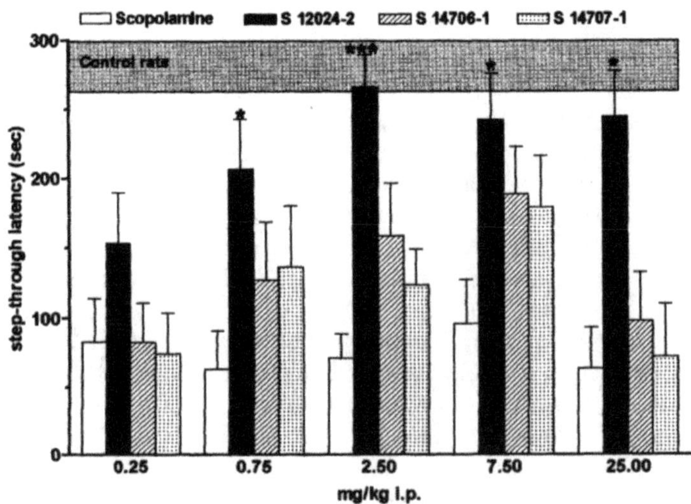

Figure 1. Comparative effects of S 12024-2 and its isomers, S 14706-1 and S 14707-1, on scopolamine-induced amnesia in the passive avoidance test in the rat. Values are mean ± s.e.m. retention latencies measured 24 h after learning trial. Shaded area indicates the range of retention latency in normal rats. Scopolamine HBr treatment (1 mg/kg i.p.) was performed 30 min before learning trial, and i.p. treatment with S 12024-2 or its isomers was performed 60 min before both learning and retention trials. Statistical analysis with ANOVA and log-rank test: *p ≤ 0.05, *** p ≤ 0.001 vs scopolamine-treated group.

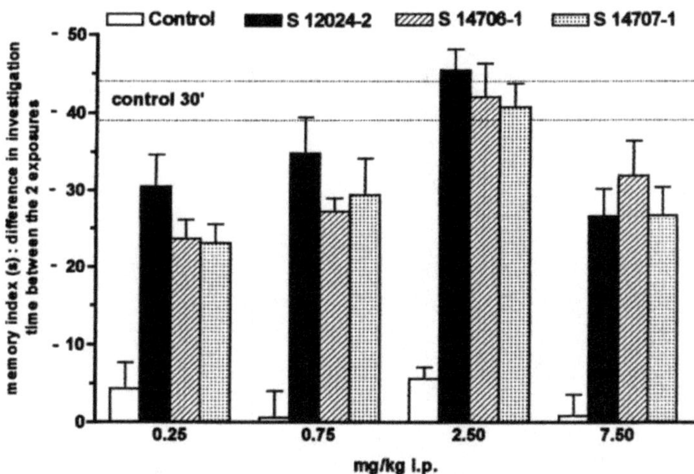

Figure 2. Comparative effects of S 12024-2 and its isomers, S 14706-1 and S 14707-1, on time-dependent forgetting in the social memory test in the rat. Values are mean ± s.e.m. difference in exploration time (memory index) between the two exposures to a same juvenile (inter-exposure delay = 120 min). Dashed lines delineate the range of memory index in non-amnesic rats (inter-exposure delay = 30 min). i.p. treatment with S 12024-2 or its isomers was performed immediately after the first exposure. Statistical analysis with ANOVA indicate a significant effect for all treatments (p ≤ 0.001).

could be observed at 2.5 mg/kg. Consequently, the memory index of 2.5 mg/kg treated animals when using a 120 min interval between the two exposures was of a similar value compared with control non-amnesic rats (30 min interval between exposures). For all tested doses, the cognitive effects of S 12024-2 were not significantly different from those of both isomers (Figure 2).

Nicotinic Interactions of S 12024-2

In Vitro Nicotinic Interaction of S 12024-2 on Human α7-nAChR. From 1 to 300 μM, nicotine induced a concentration-dependent activation of α7-nAChR. By using normalized current amplitudes to the maximal response (100 μM), the EC50 value was 42 μM (Hill coefficient = 1.5). Consequently, all the following experiments were realized using 30 μM nicotine. Under these experimental conditions, the activating effect of nicotine could be prevented by a pre-application of mecamylamine. S 12024-2 (1 to 100 μM) failed to activate the α7-nACh receptor but inhibited in a concentration-dependent manner the nicotine-induced current (IC50 = 9 μM) (Figure 3-left). Surprisingly, similar effects were observed with lobeline (IC50 = 7.1 μM) or GTS21 (IC50 = 7.5 μM), two well-described nicotinic agonists which applied alone, did not activate the receptor as observed with S 12024-2. Furthermore, the inhibitory effects of S 12024-2 were of greater potency compared with both isomers, S 14706-1 (IC50 = 16.1 μM) and S 14707-1 (IC50 = 13.2 μM) (Figure 3-left). Moreover, the antagonism of nicotine-induced current by S 12024-2 was of a non-competitive nature (Figure 3-right) and similar results were observed with lobeline (data not shown).

Kainate-induced WDS in Wistar Rat

S 12024-2 markedly prevented the kainate-induced WDS in the rat. The effect was dose-dependent and a pronounced inhibition could be obtained at 22.5 mg/kg (20.7 ± 2.6

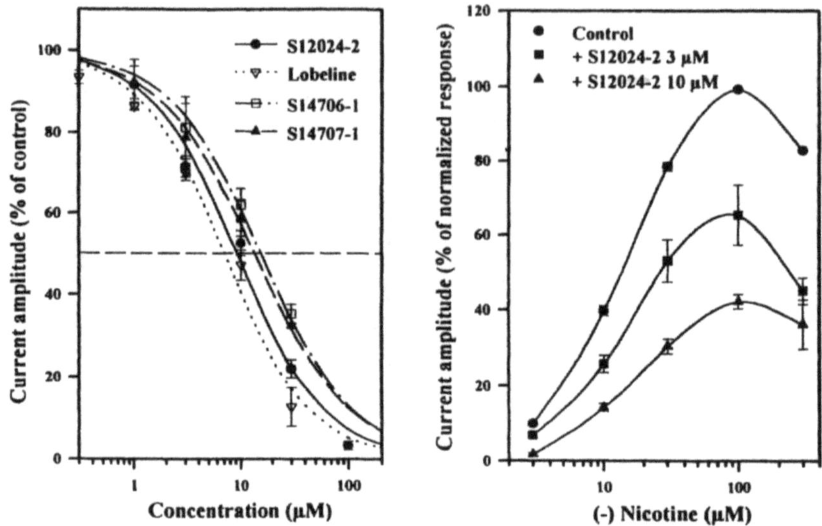

Figure 3. Inhibitory effect of S 12024-2 on nicotine-induced current in *Xenopus* oocytes expressing human α7-nAChR (holding potential = –60 mV). 3a. Comparative inhibitory effects of S 12024-2, its isomers and lobeline on nicotine (30 μM)-induced current. 3b. Non-competitive antagonistic effect of S 12024-2.

and 4.3 ± 2.6 WDS/10 min in control and treated groups, respectively). A similar efficacy was observed with nicotine (1 mg/kg) or lobeline (30 mg/kg). When mecamylamine (5 mg/kg) was administered conjointly with S 12024-2, a significant inhibition of the protective effect of S 12024-2 was obtained (20.6, 0.8 and 12.8 WDS/10 min for control, S 12024-2 and mecamylamine + S 12024-2 groups, respectively). In contrast, the inhibitory effects of nicotine on kainate-induced WDS were potentiated by mecamylamine (11.3 ± 2.8 and 4.8 ± 2.7 WDS/10 min for nicotine and nicotine + mecamylamine groups, respectively) whereas the nicotinic antagonist failed to influence the effect of kainate when administered alone.

DISCUSSION

Present studies clearly demonstrated that S 12024-2 was a potent cognition enhancer and could modulate brain nicotonic neurotransmission. In the mnemocognitive experiments, conducted using episodic memory tasks, S 12024-2 was able to prevent both the scopolamine-induced amnesia and time-dependent natural forgetting. These beneficial effects were obtained in the same range of doses and under and inverted U shape, a characteristic of promnesic compounds acting notably on cholinergic neurotransmission (Gamzu, 1985). The efficacy of S 12024-2 in both passive avoidance and social memory test are in agreement with an interaction of the compound with brain nicotinic (Levin, 1992) and indirectly, vasopressinergic (Dantzer et al., 1987; Laczi et al., 1984) pathways. Indeed, both neurotransmitters were demonstrated as being intimately linked (Faiman et al., 1988; Larose et al., 1988) and able to increase the attentional processing (Snel et al., 1987; Warburton, 1992).

Furthermore, S 12024-2 exerted significantly (passive avoidance) or slightly (social memory) greater cognitive effects compared with its isomers. These results favour a complex mechanism of action of the racemate compound, notably on nicotinic neurotransmission. Indeed, it could be hypothesized that S 12024-2 and/or its isomers could interact with many nicotinic receptor subtypes which in the brain are composed of a large diversity of molecular entities (Vidal and Changeux, 1996; Williams et al., 1994). In such an hypothesis, the greater (2–3 fold) potency of S 12024-2 in the passive avoidance test could be related with its better (2 fold) affinity for $\alpha 7$ nACh receptor, compared with its isomers. Comparative studies on other nicotinic subtypes are currently in progress.

Surprisingly, the present studies have shown that S 12024-2 and other nicotinic agonists (lobeline, GTS21) could inhibit in a concentration-dependent manner, the nicotine-induced current on $\alpha 7$ nAChR as recently demonstrated for GTS21 (Briggs et al., 1995), a potent cognition enhancer (Arendash et al., 1995). It must be mentioned that lobeline was described as a nonclassic nicotinic compound which is able to inhibit the nicotine-induced dopamine release and paradoxically enhance cognitive performances (Williams et al., 1994) without eliciting dependence potential (Stolerman and Shoaib, 1991) as demonstrated for S 12024-2 (Yanagita et al., 1994). Similarly, GTS21 was shown to act both as a partial agonist and a non-competitive blocker depending on the subtypes of nicotinic receptors (Williams et al., 1994) as presently demonstrated with S 12024-2 on $\alpha 7$ nAChR. The mechanism of inhibition induced by S 12024-2 or other "agonists" on $\alpha 7$ nAChR remains unclear and could be explained by a competitive interaction with nicotine, a blockade of the receptor channel or a stabilization of the receptor in a desensitized state. Furthermore, potential differences in the pharmacological responses to nicotinic agonists between the native heteromeric and the artificially expressed homomeric receptors cannot be ruled out (Anand et al., 1993). Nevertheless, present *in vivo* experiments on nicotine-dependent WDS induced by kainate (Shytle et al., 1995), favour a functional agonistic interaction of S 12024-2 with nicotinic neurotransmission. Furthermore, they clearly indicated that a full, albeit non-selective, nicotinic antagonist such as mecamylamine, could influence the effects of nicotine and S 12024-2 in diametrically opposed directions. Such a difference is in agreement with the "antagonistic" effect of S 12024-2 on $\alpha 7$ nicotine-induced current. Furthermore, present results with some atypical nicotinic agonists suggest it may be possible to dissociate the different effects of nicotine on brain functions.

In conclusion, the present studies have clearly demonstrated that S 12024-2, a potent cognition enhancer, acts by interacting with brain nicotinic neurotransmission. These results are in agreement with those of clinical studies on S 12024-2. Indeed, even after a short 3 months treatment duration, S 12024-2 exerted beneficial effects in moderate Alzheimer's patients in which a dramatic decrease in nicotinic receptors has been reported and more especially, in patients possessing ApoE-$\varepsilon 4$ allele, a risk factor of AD, notably associated with a more pronounced decrease in nicotinic receptors (Poirier et al., 1994). Further studies are needed in order to fully define the mechanism by which S 12024-2 could interact with nicotinic neurotransmitter systems, in particular regarding the receptor subtypes. Nevertheless, the present studies favour nicotinic compounds as promising therapeutic agents for the treatment of cognitive deficits associated with age-related neurodegenerative diseases such as Alzheimer's disease.

REFERENCES

Amouyel, P., Neuman, E., Dillemann, L., Richard, F., Barrandon, S., Lepagnol, J., and Guez. D., 1996, Characterization of the apolipoprotein E genotypes in a European multicenter trial on Alzheimer's disease with the S-12024-2 (memory enhancer), *Neurology.* 46(2, Suppl.):14.003.

Anand, R., Peng, X., and Lindstrom, J., 1993, Homomeric and native α7 acetylcholine receptors exhibit remarkably similar but non-identical pharmacological properties, suggesting that the native receptor is a heteromeric protein complex, *FEBS Lett.* 327:241–246.

Arendash, G.W., Sengstock, G.J., Sanberg, P.R., and Kem, W.R., 1995, Improved learning and memory in aged rats with chronic administration of the nicotinic receptor agonist GTS-21, *Brain Res.* 674:252–253.

Bluthe, R., and Dantzer, R., 1992, Chronic intracerebral infusions of vasopressin and vasopressin antagonist modulate social recognition in rat, *Brain Res.* 572:261–264.

Briggs, C.A., McKenna, D.G., and Piattoni-Kaplan, M., 1995, Human α7 nicotinic acetylcholine receptor responses to novel ligands, *Neuropharmacology* 34:583–590.

Dantzer, R., Bluthe, R.M., Koob, G.F., and Le Moal, M., 1987, Modulation of social memory in male rats by neurohypophyseal peptides, *Psychopharmacology.* 91:363–368.

Faiman, C.P., De Erausquin, G.A., and Baratti, C.M., 1988, Vasopressin modulates the activity of nicotinic cholinergic mechanisms during memory retrieval in mice, *Behav. Neural Biol.* 50:112–119.

Gamzu, E., 1985, Animal behavioral models in the discovery of compounds to treat memory dysfunction, *Ann. N.Y. Acad. Sci.* 444:370–393.

Griffin, M.G., and Taylor, G.T., 1995, Norepinephrine modulation of social memory: evidence for a time-dependent functional recovery of behavior, *Behav. Neurosci.* 109:466–473.

Laczi, F., Gaffori, O., Fekete, M., De Kloet, E.R., and De Wied, D., 1984, Levels of arginin-vasopressin in cerebrospinal fluid during passive avoidance behavior in rats, *Life Sci.* 34:2385–2391.

Larose, P., Ong, H., Januszewicz, P., Cantin, M., and Du Souich, P., 1988, Characterization of the effect of nicotine on vasopressin and atrial natriuretic factor in the rabbit, *J. Pharmacol. Exp. Ther.* 244:1093–1097.

Leibowitz, S.F., Eidelman, D., Suh, J.S., Diaz, S., and Sladek, C.D., 1990, Mapping study of noradrenergic stimulation of vasopressin release, *Exp. Neurol.* 110:298–305.

Lépagnol, J.M., and Lestage, P., 1994, Memory-enhancing effects of S 12024. Involvement of vasopressinergic neurotransmission, *3rd Int. Springfield Symp. Adv. Alzheimer Ther.* P.29.

Levin, E.D., 1992, nicotinic systems and cognitive function, *Psychopharmacology* 108:417–431.

Matta, S.G., Foster, C.A., and Sharp, B.M., 1993, Nicotine stimulates the expression of cFos protein in the parvocellular paraventricular nucleus and brainstem catecholaminergic regions, *Endocrinology.* 132:2149–2156.

Poirier, J., Aubert, I., Bertrand, P., Quirion, R., Gauthier, S., and Nalbantoglu, J., 1994, Apolipoprotein E4 and cholinergic dysfunction in Alzheimer's disease, *in. Alzheimer disease: therapeutic strategies*, E. Giacobini,, and R. Becker, eds, *Birkhäuser*, 72–78.

Séguéla, P., Wadiche, J., Dineley-Miller, K., Dani, J.A., and Patrick, J.W., 1993, Molecular cloning, functional properties, and distribution of rat brain α7: a nicotinic cation channel highly permeable to calcium, *J. Neurosci.* 13:596–604.

Shioda, S., and Nakai, Y., 1992, Noradrenergic innervation of vasopressin-containing neurons in the rat hypothalamic supraoptic nucleus, *Neurosci. Lett.* 140:215–218.

Shytle, R.D., Borlongan, C.V., and Sanberg, P.R., 1995, Nicotine blocks kainic acid-induced wet dog shakes in rats, *Neuropsychopharmacology.* 13:261–264.

Snel, J., Taylor, J., and Wegman, M., 1987, Does DGAVP influence memory, attention and mood in young healthy men?, *Psychopharmacology.* 92:224–228.

Stolerman, I.P., and Shoaib, M., 1991, The neurobiology of nicotine addiction, *Trends Pharmacol. Sci.* 12:467–473.

Vidal, C., and Changeux, J-P., 1996, Neuronal nicotinic acetylcholine receptors in the brain, *News Physiol. Sci.* 11:202–208.

Warburton, D.M., 1992, Nicotine as a cognitive enhancer, *Prog. Neuro-Psychopharmacol. & Biol-Psychiat.* 16:181–219.

Williams, M., Sullivan, J.P., and Arneric, S.P., 1994, Neuronal nicotinic acetylcholine receptors, *Drugs News Perspect.* 7:205–223.

Yanagita, T., Wasaka, Y., Detolle-Sarbach, S., and Guez, D., 1994, S 12024-2 shows no dependence potential in rats, *Can. J. Physiol. Pharmacol.* 72(1 Suppl.):366.

68

LEWY BODY INFLUENCE ON TACRINE EFFICACY

Florence Lebert,[1] Lydie Souliez,[2] Florence Pasquier,[1] and Henri Petit[1]

[1]Memory Unit
Centre Hospitalier Universitaire and Faculté de Médecine
Hôpital Roger Salengro 59037
Lille, France
[2]Faculté de Psychologie
Lille III, France

INTRODUCTION

A great variability in response has been found in trials of cholinesterase inhibitors in Alzheimer's disease (AD). Simple characteristics such as age, sex, duration and severity of the illness have not been identified as predictors of tacrine responsiveness. Although Apo E4 AD patients might be at a greater risk for a non efficacy of tacrine, some Apo E4 AD patients were responders in the results of Poirier et al (1995). The findings require replication. The selection of patients for treatment with tacrine used the National Institute of Neurological and Communicative Disorders and Stroke-Alzheimer's disease and Related Association criteria (NINCDS-ADRDA) (McKhann et al., 1984) in all the studies. With these criteria 10–20% of patients with an alternative cause of dementia could have been included (Dewan & Gupta, 1992). Another confounding factor is the heterogeneity of the AD neuropathology. Galasko et al (1994), looking at 137 patients fulfilling the NINCDS-ADRDA criteria for probable or possible AD, reported 24% of cases who had cortical Lewy bodies. The low activity of the choline acetyltransferase in brains of AD-Lewy Body Variance (LBV) patients suggested that AD-LBV patients could be high responders to tacrine (Perry et al., 1994). Moreover, Levy et al (1994) reported the brain examination of 3 tacrine "responders" who, at necropsy, had mixed Alzheimer's and Lewy body pathology. Today several different therapeutic agents can be prescribed in AD, and criteria to predict tacrine responsiveness are necessary. The aim of this study was to compare the neuropsychological qualitative and quantitative efficacy of tacrine between AD-nonLBV and AD-LBV patients, in consecutive mild or moderate AD patients followed in the Lille memory unit.

Progress in Alzheimer's and Parkinson's Diseases
edited by Fisher *et al.*, Plenum Press, New York, 1998.

PATIENTS AND METHODS

Consecutive outpatients with diagnostic evidence of probable AD (NINCDS-ADRDA criteria), compiled during cognitive assessment with the CERAD battery (Morris et al., 1989), were included in this study. MMSE was between 10 and 24 inclusive at the time of study entry. Exclusion criteria included: evidence of other psychiatric or neurologic disorders (especially, frontotemporal dementia, drug misuse); delirium episode during the study; neuroleptics or anticholinergic agents used during and within 3 months of entry into the study; serotonin reuptake inhibitors and benzodiazepines when the dosage was not stable for one month prior to the study or modified during the study; and conditions increasing risks from tacrine (peptic ulcer, cardiac conductions abnormalities...).

LBV was diagnosed using McKeith criteria (1992). At entry into the study, tacrine was given at a dose of 40 mg/day during 6 weeks. Capsules were administered four times a day, half an hour before meals. During the next 6 weeks, the patients were treated with 80 mg/day and afterwards with 120 mg/day. Patients were assessed at baseline and post 120 mg/day of tacrine for 2 weeks. A patient was considered a "responder" if there was an increase on the DRS total score.

Non parametrical tests (Wilcoxon matched pair test, Mann & Whitney test) were run using Statview 4.0 for Macintosh.

RESULTS

Thirty nine patients were included. Their mean age was 74.9 years (SD = 6.2), their mean duration of the disease was 3 years (SD = .9), and their mean MMSE was 19.6 (SD = 5.1). Twenty patients were in agreement with AD-nonLBV, 19 with AD-LBV criteria. These 2 groups of patients did not differ in sex ratio, mean age, age at onset, MMSE and DRS scores at baseline. Descriptive analysis showed 2 groups of patients: one with an increase in the total DRS score, the "responders" (n = 22, mean DRS baseline = 107.0 ± 16.6, mean DRS follow-up = 112.9 ± 16.9), and the other with a decrease in the total DRS score, the "nonresponders" (n = 17, mean DRS baseline = 100.3 ± 19.1, mean DRS follow-up = 83.7 ± 24.4) (Table 1). These 2 groups were not different for age, sex, duration of the disease, MMS and DRS scores at baseline. DRS follow-up differed significantly between the "nonresponders" and the "responders" patients (U = −3.62; p = .0003). The AD-LBV/AD-nonLBV ratio did not differ among the "nonresponder" and "responder" groups. However, cognitive improvement was not observed on the same subtests in the 2 groups (AD-nonLBV/AD-LBV. In the AD-LBV group performance was improved on digit span (−1.96; p = .05); and on verbal initiation (−1.95; p = .05); in the AD-nonLBV group performance was improved on similarities (−2.85; p = .004).

DISCUSSION

These results are in agreement with the reported frequency of tacrine improvement (Eagger and Harvey, 1995). In the literature, reported improvement of neurospychological performance is highly variable. Specific effects on memory or attention may remain undetected in tasks which fail to separate the modalities. However, a positive effect of tacrine has been reported on attention using a specific neuropsychological battery, test of simple and choise reaction time (Sahakian et al., 1993). An improvement on digit span and trail

Table 1. Characteristics and statistical comparison of neuropsychological performances of responder and nonresponder patients

	Responders (N = 22)	Nonresponders (N = 17)	Total (N = 39)
Mean age (SD)	74.8 (4.7)	73.4 (8.8)	74.9 (6.2)
Mean duration of disease (SD)**	2.9 (0.8)	3.2 (0.9)	3.0 (0.9)
Men/women	10/11	4/14	14/25
Mean MMSE (SD)	21.3 (4.7)	17.5 (4.5)	19.6 (5.1)
n of AD-LBV	11	8	19
DRS at baseline	107.0 (16.6)	100.3 (19.1)	
DRS follow up	112.9 (16.9)	83.7 (24.4)*	

n = number of patients; SD = standard deviation; MMSE = mini mental state examination; DRS = dementia rating scale; AD-LBV = Lewy body variant of Alzheimer's disease.
*p = .0003 (U = −3.62).
**In years.

making test has been reported after a single dose of 50mg of tacrine in responding patients in a small open study (Alhainen et al., 1993). The authors suggested that tacrine improves attention and frontal functions rather than mnemonic functions. Moreover, tacrine could have a positive effect on the digit span in long term treatment (Amberla et al., 1993). However, in all these studies, criteria of LBV were never defined. The cholinergic system is involved in the control of attentional processes (Lawrence and Sahakian, 1995). AD-LBV has a dramatic cholinergic deficit (Perry et al., 1994) and attentional functions are impaired earlier (McKeith et al., 1996) than memory in AD-LBV. In this study, tacrine appears to have efficacy in AD-LBV but not only in them, which confirms the results of Wilcock et al (1994). An improvement with tacrine does not appear more frequently on AD-LBV than on AD-nonLBV, but is qualitatively different. Tacrine improves the concept subtest of DRS (similarities) only in the AD-nonLBV group, in agreement with our preliminary results (Lebert et al 1996). The non significant effect of tacrine on memory items cannot exclude efficacy on memory, since the DRS only assesses free recall. Improvement on attention is especially observed in AD-LBV. According to these results, usual batteries such as ADAS-Cog should be completed for attentional and frontal lobe dysfunction assessments. Another interest of this study is to show the importance of distinguishing between subtypes of AD in the assessment of treatment effects.

REFERENCES

Alhainen, K. and Riekkinen, P.J., 1993, Discrimination of Alzheimer patients responding to cholinesterase inhibitor therapy. *Acta Neurol. Scand.* (Suppl) 149:16–21.

Amberla, K., Nordberg, A., Vitanen, M. et al., 1993, Long term treatment with tacrine (THA) in Alzheimer's disease—evaluation of neuropsychological data. *Acta Neurol. Scand.* (suppl) 149:55–57.

Dewan, M.J., Gupta, S., 1992, Toward a definite diagnosis of Alzheimer's disease (Review). *Comp. Psychiatry* 33:282–290.

Eagger, S., Harvey, R.J., 1995, Tacrine and other anticholinesterase drugs in dementia. *Curr. Opin. Psychiatry* 8:264–267.

Galasko, D., Hansen, L.A., Katzman, R., et al., 1994, Clinical-neuropathological correlations in Alzheimer's disease and related dementias. *Arch. Neurol.* 51:888–895.

Laurence, A.D., Sahakia, B.J., 1995, Alzheimer disease, attention and the cholinergic system. *Alzheimer Dis. Assoc. Disord.* (Suppl 2) 9:43–49.

Lebert, F., Souliez, L., Pasquier, F., 1996, Tacrine and symptomatic treatment in SDLT. *In: "Dementia with Lewy bodies"*, Perry, E., ed, Cambridge: Cambridge University Press, pp. 439–448.

Levy, R., Eagger, S., Griffiths, M. et al., 1994, Lewy bodies and response to tacrine in Alzheimer's disease. *Lancet* 343:176.

Mattis, S., 1976, Mental status examination for organic mental syndrome in the elderly patients. In: *Geriatric Psychiatry: A handbook for psychiatrists and primary care physicians*. Bellak L., Karasu, T.B., eds., New York, NY, Grune & Stratton, 77–121.

McKhann G., Drachman, D., Folstein, M. et al., 1984, Clinical diagnosis of Alzheimer's disease: report of the NINCDS-ADRDA work group under the auspices of Department of Health and Human services Task force on Alzheimer's disease. *Neurology* 34:939–944.

Mc Keith, I.G., Perry, R;H., Fairburn, A.F. et al., 1992, Operational criteria for senile dementia of Lewy body type (SDLT). *Psychol. Med.* 22:911–922.

McKeith, I.G., Galasko, D., Kosaka, K. et al., 1996, Consensus guidelines for the clinical and pathologic diagnosis of dementia with Lewy bodies (DLB). *Neurology* 47:1113–1124.

Morris, J.C., Heyman, A., Mohs, R. et al., 1989, The Consortium to establish a Registrary for Alzheimer's disease (CERAD). Part I: Clinical and neuropsycholgical assessment of Alzheimer's disease. *Neurology* 39:1159–1165.

Perry, E.K., Haroutunian, V., Davis, K.L. et al., 1994, Neocortical cholinergic activities differentiate Lewy body dementia from classical Alzheimer's disease. *NeuroReport* 5: 747–749.

Poirier, J., Delisle, M.C., Gilfix, B.M. et al., 1995, Apolipoprotein E4 allele as a predictor of cholinergic deficits and treatment outcome in Alzheimer's disease. *Proc. Natl. Acad. Sci. USA* 92:12260–12264.

Sahakian, B.J., Owen, A.M., Morant, N.J. et al., 1993, Further analysis of the cognitive efects of tetrahydroaminoacridine (THA) in Alzheimer's disease: assessment of attentional and mnemonic function using CANTAB. *Psychopharmacology* 110:395–401.

Wilcock, G.K. and Scott, M.I., 1994, Tacrine for senile dementia of Alzheimer's or Lewy body type. *Lancet* 344:544.

69

TACRINE TREATMENT IN PARKINSON'S DISEASE DEMENTIA

A. E. Werber, S. Perlov, B. Mildorf, and J. M. Rabey

Department of Neurology
Assaf Harofe Medical Center, Zerifin
Sackler School of Medicine
Tel-Aviv University, Israel

INTRODUCTION

Patients with Parkinson's disease (PD) have a greater risk to develop dementia (PDD) compared to other individuals of the same age. PDD prevalence estimates vary between 11 to 41% according to different population based studies and PPD seems to be age related like Alzheimer's disease (AD) (Mayeux et al. 1992). Moreover, the neuropathologic changes found in PDD patients are AD-like with neurofibrillary tangles, senile plaques and decreased choline-acetyltransferase (ChAT) activity in cortex and hippocampus, concurrently with nigral degeneration and Lewy bodies (Braak, 1990). This cholinergic deficiency has been directly related to the cognitive decline in PDD patients (Nakano, 1984). For that reason, we hypothesized that Tacrine, a cholinesterase inhibitor reported as having a beneficial response in AD patients, might also improve the cognitive state of PDD patients . However, cholinergic drugs are generally not recommended in PD since they are regarded as potentially able to worsen the extrapyramidal signs (Duvoisin, 1967).

The present study was designed to find out whether Tacrine has any beneficial effect on cognitive performance of PDD patients, and if motor function is adversely affected by the drug.

METHODS

The study was conducted as a non blinded trial. Six PD patients suffering from cognitive deterioration were included in the study. PD had been diagnosed according to 2 of the following: rigidity, bradykinesia, tremor, postural disturbances. Dementia was diagnosed according to DSM-IV criteria (American Psychiatric Association 1994) years after

Progress in Alzheimer's and Parkinson's Diseases
edited by Fisher *et al.*, Plenum Press, New York, 1998.

Table 1. Patient characteristics

No. of patients	6
M/F	4/2
Age*	74 Y (62–82)
Duration of PD*	9.5 Y (5–14)
Hoehn & Yahr	4 pts. stage III, 2 pts. stage IV
L-DOPA treatment*	562.5 mg/day (375–750)
Other anti PD treatments	Amantadine (1 pt), Pergolide (1 pt)
	Promocriptine (1 pt), selegiline (1 pt)
Anti-depressants	Favoxil (1 pt), Anafranil (1 pt)
Anti-hallucinatory drugs	Clozapine (3 pts.)
Duration of dementia*	4 Y (3–5)
Baseline ADAS-cog*	39.3 (7.6-73)
Baseline MMSE*	15.7 (9–24)
Tacrine daily dosage*	100 mg/day (80–120)
Duration of tacrine treatment*	4 months (2–6)

*Mean (range)

PD developed. Mini-Mental-State-Examination (MMSE) equal to, or less than 24 was mandatory for inclusion (Folstein et al., 1975). Patients had no focal neurological signs or focal findings on brain CT scan. TSH , FT4 B12 VDRL and routine bloods including liver function tests were within the normal range. Patients had no history of previous neurological or psychiatric disorder other than PD. They had all been treated with L-DOPA and other anti-Parkinsonian medications except for anticholinergic drugs within the last year. Some of them received antidepressants as well. For patient characteristics see Table 1.

Tacrine was administered starting 10mg bid increasing gradually (tid; bid) toward 160mg/day. Titration lasted for 6 weeks. Most of our patients did not exceed 120 mg/day and some even failed to reach 100 mg/day. Therefore a maximal optimal daily dose was adjusted and maintained for each person according to individual compliance and tolerability to the drug.

Liver function was tested every two weeks during the titration period and once a month later on. Participants were evaluated for cognitive and emotional state at baseline and while receiving maximal Tacrine dose, by: MSE, ADAS-cog (Rosen et al., 1984) and Hamilton Depression Scale.

Patients were evaluated for their motor performance by the UPDRS and SPES motor scales (Fahn et al., 1987, Rabey et al., in press, respectively). Each patient was examined before and during Tacrine treatment (after achieving the maximal tolerable dose). Each examination consisted of 2 stages: first after 12 hours without medication (while "off"- last L-DOPA dose taken on the previous night), and 90 minutes after the first early morning L-DOPA dose had been taken (while "on").

For statistical analysis we used the two tailed Student's t-test.

RESULTS

The results of cognitive response to Tacrine measured by ADAS-cog and MMSE are shown in Figure 1. The mean values for pretreatment and maximal Tacrine dose are: ADAS-cog 39.4 ± 3 and 30.5 ± 23, respectively, MMSE 15.7 ± 9.7 and 18.5 ± 11.4, respectively. No statistical significance was found. One patient (PD1) responded to adjustment of individual maximal dose with a typical "U shape" dose/response curve (Figure 2).

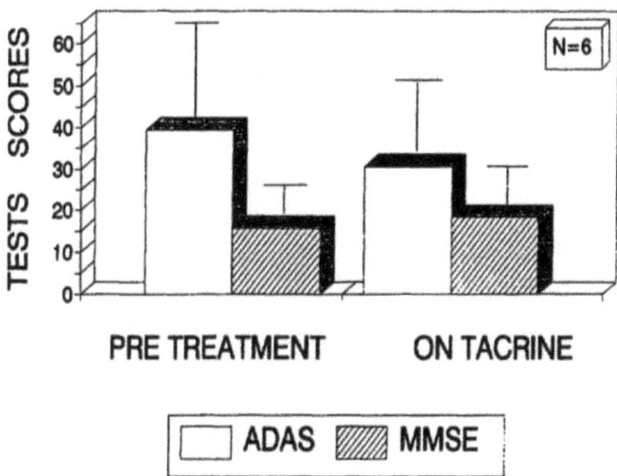

Figure 1. Cognitive response of PDD patients on tacrine optimal dose compared to baseline as measured by ADAS-cog and MMSE.

His pretreatment ADAS-cog was 23.9; on 80 mg/day ADAS-cog was 14; on 100 mg/day ADAS-cog deteriorated to 21. While getting back to 80 mg/day ADAS-cog improved to 10.3. The main side effects were: nausea (4 patients) and dizziness (2 patients).

The results of motor function measured by UPDRS and SPES are presented in Figures 3 and 4. The mean motor UPDRS values for pretreatment and maximal Tacrine dose while off L-DOPA were 50.2 ± 17.8 and 49.25 ± 19.6, respectively. The mean pretreatment and maximal dose SPES values were 18.5 ± 5.9 and 17.75 ± 6.4, respectively. The motor performance of patients 90 minutes after the first L-DOPA morning dose is shown in Figure 4. UPDRS values of pretreatment and on maximal Tacrine dose were 10 ± 3.1, and 12.25 ± 4.5, respectively; and 4.25 ± 1.25, 3.25 ± 2 for SPES. These results show clearly that Tacrine did not affect the motor performance while patients were off treatment and also did not alter the motor response to L-DOPA. Much to our surprise, one patient (PD2) markedly improved his motor performances under Tacrine treatment, as shown in Figure 5.

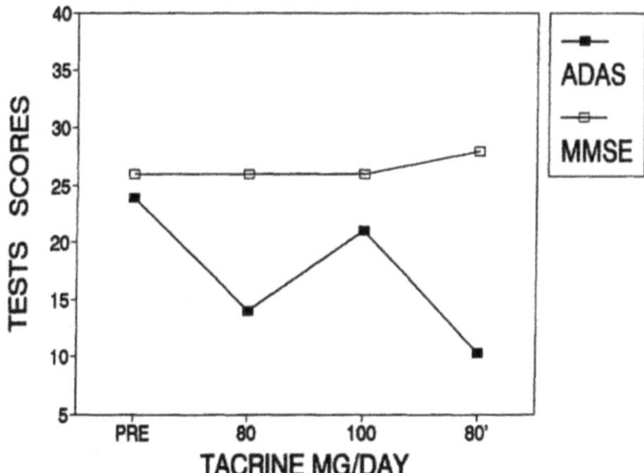

Figure 2. Dose response curve to tacrine, shows benefit at 80 mg/day over 100 mg/day, when rechallenged at 80 mg/day patient score improved again.

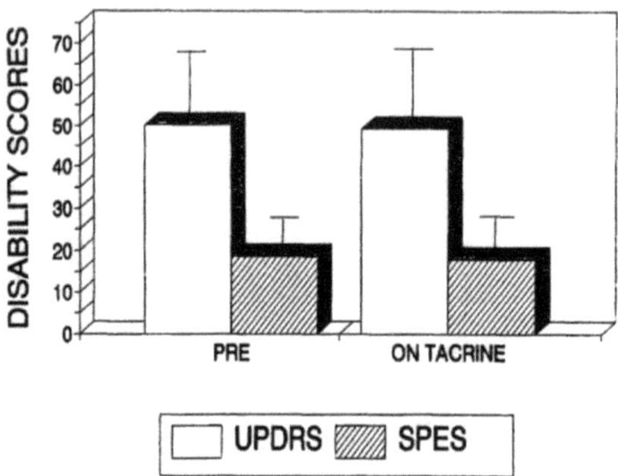

Figure 3. The motor response to tacrine while PDD patients "off" levodopa, measured by UPDRS and SPES. There is no change between baseline and on tacrine.

DISCUSSION

Brain levels of acetylcholine (ACh) and dopamine (DA) are highest in the neostriatum (Glowinski, 1990). Early clinical data showed that anti-muscarinic drugs were effective in treating the symptoms of PD (Duvoisin, 1967). This observation and others had led to the hypothesis that cholinergic and dopaminergic systems must maintain a " balance" in the normal neostriatum (Barbeau, 1962). This theory suggested that the dopaminergic activity in projection neurons has been mediated by cholinergic interneurons and that cholinergic treatment might worsen Parkinsonian symptomatology (Duvoisin, 1967).

During recent years, a bulk of information has emerged, suggesting a different view on the issue of ACh in PD. Glowinski has reported that ACh at physiological levels stimulates the release of DA from striatum via muscarinic heteroreceptors. It was also suggested that nicotinic receptors located at presynaptic endings on dopaminergic cells may play a

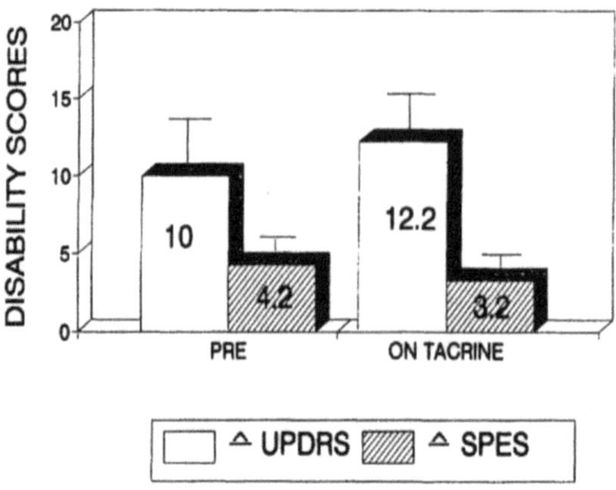

Figure 4. The best motor response to tacrine while PDD patients "on" levodopa as measured by UPDRS and SPES, with minimal change between baseline scoring and on tacrine.

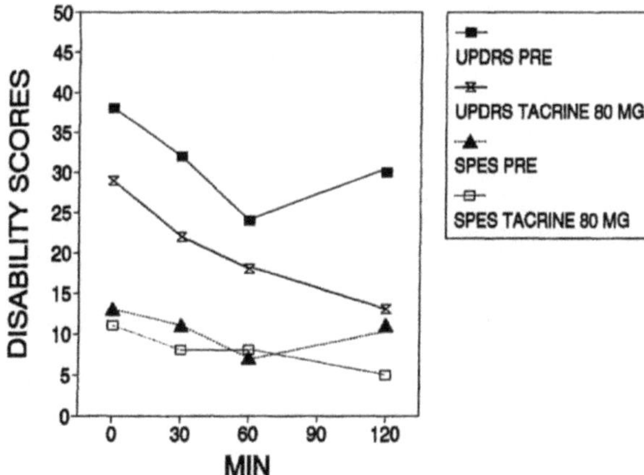

Figure 5. The best motor response in patient PDD2 shows a clear improvement in UPDRS and SPES scores on tacrine as compared to baseline.

similar role (Graybiel, 1983). Moreover, an additive effect between ACh and DA on neostriatal function by modulating ionic conductance, and probable involvement at the level of molecular events modulating GABAergic cells has also been reported (Westerink, 1989).These theories refute the old one and may explain the lack of motor deterioration observed in our Tacrine treated PD patients. Even more interesting is the fact that patient PD2 submitted to Tacrine, improved in both cognitive and motor performances.That patient may have suffered from Lewy body dementia (Wilcock, 1994).

The cognitive improvement in our PD patients,(though not statistically significant), resembles the results of Hutchison et al. in their recently published study (1996) and is supported by the work of Lloyd et al. (1997).

In summary, we conclude that there is a place for cholinergic therapy in PDD patients. However, a further large scale blinded trial is warranted in order to confirm our findings.

REFERENCES

American Psychiatric Association, 1994, Diagnostic and statistical manual of mental disorders. (DSM - IV). Washington DC: American Psychiatric Association.

Braak, H, 1990, Cognitive impairment in Parkinson's disease: amyloid plaques neurofirillary tangles and neuropil threads in the cerebral cortex. *J. Neurol. Trans.* (P-D sect) 2:45–57.

Duvoisin, R., 1967, Cholinergic-anticholinergic antagonism in Parkinsonism. *Arch. Neurol.* 17:124–135.

Fahn, S., Elton, R.L. and members of the UPDRS committee, 1987, In: *Recent Developments in Parkinson's disease,* Fahn, S.,Marsden, C.D. Calne, D.B. and Goldstein, M., eds, vol 2., McMillan Health Care Information, Florham Park, NJ, pp 153–163, 293–304.

Folstein, M., et al., 1975 , "Mini-mental state": A practical method for grading the cognitive state of patients for the clinician. *J. Psychiatr. Res.* 2:89–198.

Hutchinson, M et al., 1996, *J. Neurol. Neurosurg. Psychiatr.* (letter). 61:324–325.

Glowinski, J., 1990, Recent findings on dopaminergic transmission in the Basal Ganglia. In: *Advances in Neurology,* Vol. 53 Parkinson's Disease, New York, Raven Press, pp. 67–73.

Graybiel, A.M., 1983, Biochemical anatomy of the striatum. In: *Clinical Neuroanatomy.,* New York, Raven Press, pp. 427–504.

Lloyd, G.K. et al. The potential of a subtype-selective neuronal acetylcholine ion channel receptor (NACHR) agonist, SIB-1508Y, for the treatment of the cognitive, affective and motor dysfunction of Parkinson's disease. Presented at OHOLO 41st Conference Progress in Altzheimer's and Parkinson's diseases. Fourth International Conference, Eilat, Israel, May 1997.

Mayeux, R. et al., 1992, A population based investigation of Parkinson's disease with and without dementia: relationship to age and gender. *Arch. Neurol.* 49:492–497.

Nakano, I., 1984, Parkinson' s disease: neurone loss in the nucleus basalis without concomitant Alzheimer's disease. *Ann. Neurol.* 15:415–418.

Rabey, J.M. et al . Evaluation of the Short Parkinson's Evaluation Scale: A New Friendly Scale for the Evaluation of Parkinson's Disease in Clinical Drug Trials. *Clin. Neuropharmacol.,* in press.

Rosen, W.G. et al., 1984, A new rating scale for Alzheimer's disease. *Am. J. Psychiatry* 141: 1356–364.

Westerink, BHC, 1989, Brain microdyalisis fails to detect a dopamine-acetylcholine interaction in the Basal Ganglia. *Trends Pharmacol. Sci.* 40:262–263.

Wilcock GK, 1994, Tacrine for senile dementia of Alzheimer's or Lewy body type (letter). *Lancet* 344:544.

70

APP LOCALIZATION AND TRAFFICKING IN THE CENTRAL NERVOUS SYSTEM

J. D. Buxbaum,[1,2] A. Ikin,[1] Y. Luo,[1] J. Naslund,[1] S. Sabo,[1] B. Vincent,[1] T. Watanabe,[1] and P. Greengard[1]

[1]Laboratory of Molecular and Cellular Neuroscience and
   Zachary and Elizabeth M. Fisher Center
The Rockefeller University
1230 York Avenue, New York, New York 10021
[2]Laboratory of Molecular Neuroscience
Mount Sinai School of Medicine
Department of Psychiatry
One Gustave Levy Place, New York, New York 10029

INTRODUCTION

Aβ Accumulation Is a Causative Factor in at Least Some Forms of AD

One of the hallmarks of Alzheimer's disease (AD) pathology is amyloid plaque deposition in the brain (reviewed in Sisodia and Price, 1995). The amyloid plaque core consists primarily of a 4 kDa peptide known as β-amyloid or Aβ. Aβ is derived by proteolytic processing of a type I integral membrane protein, the amyloid Aβ protein precursor, or APP. Based on strong genetic and biochemical data (reviewed in Hardy and Duff, 1993), it is widely agreed that at least some forms of AD are caused by excess Aβ deposition in the brain, particularly excess Aβ of 42 or 43 amino acids in length (Aβ1-42/43). The genetic evidence includes the identification of five distinct mutations in APP, all of which cosegregate with rare forms of AD: four of these mutations have been shown to increase the levels of Aβ1-42/43. More recently, AD-associated mutations in the presenilin-1 and presenilin-2 genes have also been shown to cause increased levels of Aβ1-42/43 (e.g., Scheuner et al., 1996). Finally, it has been suggested that the AD-associated form of apolipoprotein E is involved in the accumulation of Aβ (e.g., Strittmatter et al., 1993; Strittmatter et al., 1993).

Amyloid Protein Precursor Processing

The amyloid Aβ protein precursor, or APP, is a membrane-spanning glycoprotein which is ubiquitously expressed in mammalian cells (reviewed in Sisodia and Price,

1995). Because proteolytic processing of APP results in the generation of Aβ, the processing and trafficking of APP have generated great interest. APP has been shown to undergo secretory cleavage in cultured cells. Secretory cleavage generally involves cleavage of APP within the Aβ domain to release the extracellular domain (APP$_s$) into the extracellular space. An unidentified enzyme called a-secretase is responsible for the cleavage of APP within the Aβ region. In various cells a very small minority of secreted APP molecules are cleaved at the amino terminal of the Aβ domain by an enzyme termed b-secretase. Both a-secretase and b-secretase cleavage are followed by further processing of the carboxy-terminal of APP which remains cell-associated. This processing involves cleavage at sites just carboxy-terminal to the Aβ domain by an enzyme called g-secretase. When g-secretase acts on the cell-associated carboxy-terminal remaining after b-secretase cleavage, Aβ is formed, while when g-secretase acts on the cell-associated carboxy-terminal remaining after a-secretase cleavage, a 3kD peptide called p3 is formed.

Aβ Formation in the Central Nervous System

With the brain being the major site of Aβ deposition and of Alzheimer pathology, several studies have been carried out to determine which cells in the brain are prominent producers of Aβ. Early studies demonstrated that human astrocytes, derived from postmortem samples, produce significant levels of Aβ (Busciglio et al., 1993). More recently, however, it has been shown that neurons, derived from rat cerebral cortex, generate more Aβ than do similarly derived astrocytes or microglia (LeBlanc et al., 1996). Furthermore, studies in which the Semlinki Forest virus (SFV) vector was used to introduce human APP into primary cultures derived from rat brain clearly demonstrate that hippocampal neurons expressing human APP are able to produce very significant levels of Aβ (Simons et al., 1996). These data together suggest that neurons are a primary source of Aβ formation in the nervous system. These same studies suggest that neurons are also a major source of APP$_s$. With neurons being a major source of Aβ and of APP$_s$ in the brain, the trafficking and processing of APP in these cells has generated considerable interest.

Aβ Formation Apparently Occurs Largely in the Endocytic Pathway

Detailed studies of the role of endocytosis in Aβ formation in non-neuronal cultured cell lines have been carried out. Some of those studies will be summarized here with the expectation that these results will ultimately prove relevant to neurons; studies with neuronal cells are summarized below. An NPXY motif, first identified as a sequence important for internalization of LDL receptors (Chen et al., 1990), is found in the cytoplasmic domain of APP. Deletion of YENPTY or truncation of the C-terminus of APP upstream of YENPTY results in increased secretion of secreted APP (APP$_s$) and p3, and increased levels of newly synthesized APP found at the cell surface of transfected CHO cells (Koo and Squazzo, 1994; Lai et al., 1995). Furthermore, APP truncated 15 residues upstream of NPTY is secreted 1.8-fold more efficiently in COS-1 cells than wild-type APP (De Strooper et al., 1993). In these experiments, Aβ secretion was significantly decreased compared to wild-type APP, and release of surface radiolabeled Aβ was nearly eliminated. Taken together, these data strongly support the hypothesis that, in cells expressing wild-type APP, Aβ can be generated in the endocytic pathway. Most recently, it has been shown that, in cultured CHO cells expressing wild-type APP (Squazzo and Koo, personal communication) and in primary neuronal cultures expressing wild-type APP (Beyreuther, personal communication), 80–85% of the Aβ is formed in the endocytic pathway.

One possibility that has been explored is that Aβ is generated by lysosomal enzymes following endocytosis. Intact APP and carboxy-terminal fragments of APP, including some containing the entire Aβ region, can be recovered from a subcellular fraction enriched in lysosomes. However, I-cell fibroblasts expressing severe lysosomal deficiency produce Aβ (Podlisny et al., Soc Neuro Sci Abs 19, 1276), suggesting that only a fraction of Aβ, at most, is a result of lysosomal degradation. Furthermore, the lysosomal cysteine proteaes inhibitor leupeptin does not affect secretion of Aβ or p3 in COS-1 cells (Busciglio et al., 1993) or of Aβ in 293 cells (Haass et al., 1993). Although there are some conflicting results with other lysosomal inhibitors, the data imply that generation of Aβ can occur in the endosomal/lysosomal system, but not in lysosomes. It is important to note that, in neurons, early endosomes are found in the cell periphery, while lysosomes are found in the cell body. One implication of this is that Aβ formation in neurons may occur in axonal and/or dendritic compartments.

APP LOCALIZATION AND TRAFFICKING IN THE NERVOUS SYSTEM

Localization of APP in Neurons

Immunocytochemical studies of APP in cultured cells and in brain tissue reveal that a predominant fraction of APP is localized to the endoplasmic reticulum and the Golgi apparatus (Caporaso et al., 1994; Tomimoto et al., 1995). The localization of APP to biosynthetic organelles can be explained in part by the very high rate of synthesis and turnover of this protein. In synaptic and axonal compartments, APP is apparently concentrated in large vesicular organelles, as determined by immunoelectron microscopic analyses (Caporaso et al., 1994; Tomimoto et al., 1995).

Anterograde Transport of APP within Neurons

In neurons, transmembrane proteins like APP are transported along defined pathways, making use of specific organelles. APP undergoes fast axonal transport to the nerve terminal in both peripheral and central neurons (Koo et al., 1990; Morin et al., 1993). It is likely that APP is carried to the nerve terminal in carrier vesicles or multivesicular bodies (MVB). What is not fully known is which of the distinct carrier vesicle classes, associated with specific kinesin-family (KIF) members, is involved in the anterograde transport of APP. Recently, an antisense oligonucleotide directed against a region of kinesin heavy chain was injected into the optic tract and the effects on APP transport studied (Amaratunga et al., 1995). In these studies, APP transport was inhibited, as was the transport of synaptophysin, synaptotagmin, and SV2.

Insertion of APP into the Nerve-Terminal Plasma Membrane

After anterograde axonal transport, APP can be inserted into the presynaptic plasma membrane (Simons et al., 1995; Yamazaki et al., 1995). It is unknown whether the insertion of APP into the synaptic plasma membrane involves the known pathways of constitutive and/or regulated exocytosis. It has recently been shown that soluble APP (APP$_s$) can be released at central synapses (G. Thinakaran, J. D. Buxbaum, J. O'Callahan, and S. S. Sisodia, unpublished observation). In these experiments, [^{35}S]methionine was injected onto the entorhinal cortex of rats and, after six hours, radiolabeled intact APP, secreted APP, and carboxy-terminal fragments of APP were precipitated from the projection fields in the hippocampus. Radiolabeled intact APP, secreted APP, and carboxy-terminal fragments were all found in the nerve terminal fraction. These experiments are consistent with the possibility that soluble APP is generated at the synapse.

Endocytosis of APP from the Nerve-Terminal Plasma Membrane

Clathrin-coated vesicles purified from PC12 cells are enriched in full-length, mature APP and carboxy-terminal fragments (CTFs) resulting from secretory cleavage (Nordstedt et al., 1993). APP colocalizes with fluid phase markers and endocytic tracers in neurons and in C6 glioma cells (Refolo et al., 1995; Yamazaki et al., 1995). Evidence that full-length APP is endocytosed was obtained from surface labeling of APP in transfected CHO cells and in neurons (Yamazaki et al., 1995). Surface iodination and immunoprecipitation revealed that cell surface APP, at least in nonneuronal cells, is a precursor to Aβ (Koo and Squazzo, 1994). This observation was confirmed when it was shown that potassium depletion, which inhibits internalization through coated pits, decreases APP internalization and Aβ release.

Retrograde Transport of APP to Somatodendritic Compartments in Neurons

From the early endosomes in nerve terminals, APP can be transported retrogradely (Simons et al., 1995; Yamazaki et al., 1995), likely via carrier vesicles or multi-vesicular bodies. Again, it is not known which retrograde transport pathways are involved. The retrogradely transported APP can then be directed to late endosomes and lysosomes, or can be inserted into the plasma membrane of the somatodentritic compartment (Simons et al., 1995; Yamazaki et al., 1995). From this compartment, APP may again be internalized via clathrin-coated vesicles (CCV) and early endosomes, and either reinserted into the plasma membrane or transferred to lysosomes (Koo et al., 1996; Yamazaki et al., 1996).

Knowledge Gap

The above review underscores important gaps in our understanding of APP trafficking and processing in neurons. We know that APP can undergo fast axonal transport, and we know that it can be inserted in the nerve terminal plasma membrane. We also know that APP undergoes retrograde transport and can subsequently be inserted into the somatodendritic plasma membrane. However, there is a surprising lack of knowledge concerning the trafficking of APP in neurons. For example, we do not know fully which membrane trafficking pathways are involved in the anterograde transport, retrograde transport, exocytosis or endocytosis of APP. This is particularly striking because, as mentioned above, neurons appear to be a primary source of Aβ, and the insertion of APP into the plasma membrane, followed by endocytosis, appears to be an important step in Aβ formation. For an understanding of APP pathogenesis, it is therefore imperative to understand precisely the components of membrane trafficking involved in APP movement within axons, nerve terminals and dendrites. Furthermore, without such knowledge, the functional importance of APP trafficking and processing in neurons may remain elusive.

RESULTS

APP Is Not Enriched in Small Synaptic Vesicles

As a step towards identifying the pathways involved in APP trafficking in the nerve terminal, conventionally purified small synaptic vesicles were prepared (Ikin et al., 1966). Immunoblotting of 50 μg of total protein from each fraction showed no enrichment of APP in conventionally purified small synaptic vesicles, although there was a small amount of APP immunoreactivity in the purified synaptic vesicles.

In order to localize APP and synaptophysin within this vesicle preparation, immunolabeling of frozen ultrathin sections was carried out using either anti-synaptophysin or anti-APP (369) antibodies (Ikin et al., 1966). Immunolabeling with anti-synaptophysin antibodies demonstrated that the vast majority of the vesicles contained synaptophysin, as expected. In contrast, only very few structures contained APP. The paucity of profiles which were immunoreactive for APP is consistent with the results of immunoblotting, and presumably represents trace amounts of contaminating vesicles of unknown origin. Thus, these results indicate that APP is virtually absent from small synaptic vesicles.

Immunoisolation of Synaptic Organelles

To further characterize APP-containing organelles in the synapse, we chose a two-step procedure to isolate synaptic organelles (Ikin et al., 1966). First, synaptosomes were prepared using a combination of differential centrifugation and Ficoll-density gradient centrifugation. This procedure yields a fraction that is highly enriched in nerve terminals with associated dendritic structures, with only low levels of contamination by soma-derived organelles, myelin or mitochondria. Second, these purified nerve terminals were lysed by osmotic shock to release internal organelles, followed by immunoisolation of organelles using methacrylate beads coated with antibodies directed against synaptophysin, synaptobrevin or rab5a.

Comparison of the vesicular organelles immunoisolated with rab5 and synaptophysin revealed significant differences. The synaptophysin immunoisolates contained mostly small synaptic vesicles (< 60 nm in diameter). Rab5 immunoisolates contained significant levels of a variety of distinct vesicles, including small synaptic vesicles, large unilamellar vesicles, large bilamellar vesicles, and multivesicular bodies. The preponderance of organelles in rab5 immunoisolates consisted of small synaptic vesicles (74.2%) and large unilamellar vesicles (17.3%), with large bilamellar vesicles (7.4%) and multivesicular bodies (1.1%) constituting a minor portion of the profiles; synaptophysin immunoisolates consisted of small synaptic vesicles (91.3%), with large unilamellar vesicles (4.6%) and large bilamellar vesicles (4.0%) constituting a minor portion of the profiles. Therefore, the rab5 immunoisolates contain approximately four times the levels of large unilamellar vesicles, and twice as many bilamellar vesicles, when compared to synaptophysin immunoisolates. Whereas the small synaptic vesicles in rab5 immunoisolates were heavily immunoreactive with anti-synaptophysin, the large unilamellar vesicles, bilamellar vesicles and multi-vesicular bodies showed little or no such immunoreactivity.

APP Is Dramatically Enriched in Rab5 Immunoisolates Derived from Synapses

The levels of APP were determined in vesicular organelles immunoisolated from nerve terminal preparations (Ikin et al., 1966). Since the immunoisolates contained significant amounts of added immunoglobulins, synaptophysin content, rather than total protein, was used as a basis for comparing the various preparations. Samples of each immunoisolate, containing equivalent amounts of synaptophysin, were subjected to immunoblotting with an antibody (369) raised against a peptide corresponding to the cytoplasmic domain of APP or an antibody (3129) raised against a peptide corresponding to the Aβ domain of APP. High levels of APP were observed in the rab5 immunoisolates, but not in the synaptobrevin or synaptophysin immunoisolates. Quantitative immunoblotting for APP and synaptophysin indicated that the APP/synaptophysin ratio was ten-fold higher in Rab5-immunoisolates than in synaptophysin immunoisolates. Control immunoisolates, prepared using irrelevant antibodies or antibody-free beads, contained levels of APP and synaptophysin that were below the levels of detection of the assay system.

To confirm that the vesicular organelles present in rab5 immunoisolates from nerve terminal preparations were of neuronal origin, rab5 immunoisolates from the rat pheochromocytoma (PC12) cell line were prepared (Ikin et al., 1966). These organelles were enriched in APP, when compared to synaptophysin immunoisolates.

Lysed nerve terminal preparations were also used to estimate the proportion of total APP which could be depleted by the rab5 immunobeads (Ikin et al., 1966). For this purpose, samples of lysates were incubated with varying amounts of immobilized anti-rab5 antibodies, followed by centrifugation and immunoblotting. Replicate samples were used to determine total APP content. With the highest amount of anti-rab5 immunobeads used, ca. 70% of the total APP could be immunodepleted.

APP Processing in Cell Free Systems

One interesting possibility is that the APP-containing synaptic organelles contain components of the machinery for the proteolysis of APP into Aβ and/or APP$_s$. This can be addressed by reconstituting the metabolism of intact APP in purified organelles and/or by assaying for proteolytic activity associated with the purified organelles. We have recently been able to reconstitute the formation of Aβ, from intact transmembrane APP, in a cell-free system (Desdouits et al., 1996), and hence feel that such a reconstitution procedure can be developed for purified organelles. In our recent studies we used a Balch homogenizer to prepare cracked cells, and were able to reconstitute Aβ formation in this system. The reconstituted Aβ formation was temperature dependent and required ATP. Introduction of protein kinase C (PKC) into the cell-free system induced a pronounced inhibition of Aβ formation, similar to what is observed in intact cells upon stimulation of PKC. A protein phosphatase counteracting the action of PKC on Aβ formation was identified as the calcium/calmodulin activated protein phosphatase calcineurin (see Buxbaum et al., this volume). We are currently using the cell-free system to identify the molecular pathways involved in Aβ formation and to determine whether isolated organelles contain sufficient machinery for the generation of Aβ.

Fe65 and APP Localization and Trafficking

It is important to elucidate the mechanisms involved in the trafficking of APP. Since only the cytoplasmic tail of APP is expected to be exposed to the cytoplasm, it seems possible that proteins which interact with the cytoplasmic domain of APP can regulate its localization and/or trafficking. We are studying several proteins which interact with the cytoplasmic domain of APP, including proteins identified by biochemical methods or by the yeast 2-hybrid system. These proteins, which include the protein Fe65, may be important in the trafficking of APP in neurons.

Rat Fe65 (rFe65), was cloned by its homology to retroviral integrases. Database searches revealed that it contains two tandem PI (for phosphotyrosine interaction), or PTB (for phosphotyrosine binding), domains and a WW domain, all of which are involved in protein-protein interactions (Bork and Margolis, 1995). The PI domain binds to proteins containing an NPxY motif. The WW domain binds proteins that contain the sequence PPxY. By screening a human brain cDNA library using the two-hybrid system with the rFe65 PI as bait, three clones were identified: the first was a fragment of APP, the second was a fragment of APP fused to a segment of a repeat sequence, and the third was a fragment of APLP1 (Fiore et al., 1995). Based on the overlap of the three fragments and on the specificity of other PI domains, it is likely that rFe65 recognizes the NPTY sequence in the APP cytoplasmic tail; it is possible that, if the WW domain is interacting with a third protein, Fe65 links APP with that third protein in a ternary complex.

Several lines of evidence suggest that the interaction between APP and Fe65 is physiologically relevant. First, both rFe65 PI domains fused to GST associate with in vitro transcribed and translated APP (Fiore et al., 1995). In addition, the rFe65 PI domain-GST fusion protein interacts with APP in PC12 cell extracts. Finally, the interaction appears to occur in vivo since APP and rFe65 co-immunoprecipitate from cell lysates with antibodies to WW domain of rFe65 or with antibodies to APP (Zambrano et al., 1997).

Two human Fe65 homologs, hFe65L (Guenette et al., 1996) and hFe65 (Bressler et al., 1996), were recently cloned. They bind to the C-terminus of APP and co-immunoprecipitate both APP and the major APP CTF from various cells. hFe65L interacts with APP and APLP2 but not APLP1. The consensus sequences for the WW domain, both PI domains, and the retroviral integrase domain are conserved in the human homologs: hFe65L is 51% identical to rat Fe65 and hFe65 is 95% identical to rat Fe65; another human clone, hFe65L2, identified from cDNA fragments, is 59% identical to rat Fe65. In contrast to the relatively brain-specific expression of rat Fe65 (Fiore et al., 1995) and human Fe65, hFe65L mRNA has been found in all tissues tested.

CONCLUSIONS

APP-containing vesicular organelles obtained by immunoisolation from purified synaptosomes of rat brain have been characterized. The use of synaptosomes has made it possible to study the distribution of APP in organelles derived from nerve terminals without significant contamination by trafficking organelles from other sources. APP was highly enriched in rab5-containing vesicles, but virtually absent from synaptophysin- or synaptobrevin-containing vesicles. This indicates that APP is found in novel vesicular organelles distinct from the well-characterized recycling pathways for small synaptic vesicles and for large dense-core vesicles. It is now of interest to further purify and characterize the APP containing vesicles. Characterizing these organelles in Alzheimer, as compared to control brains may be of great importance. It will also be of interest to determine the role rab5 and rab5-associated organelles have in APP trafficking, localization and processing. Finally, cytoplasmic proteins, such as Fe65, may be important in the localization and trafficking of APP. Further characterization of such proteins may shed light on these processes.

ACKNOWLEDGMENTS

This work was supported by grants from the National Institute on Aging (PG), the American Health Assistance Foundation (JDB), and the Alzheimer Association (JDB).

REFERENCES

Amaratunga, A., Leeman, S. E, Kosik K. S. and. Fine, R. E , 1995, *J Neurochem,* 64:2374–6.

Bork, P. and Margolis, B. 1995, *Cell* 80:693–4.

Bressler, S. L., Gray, M D, Sopher, B L , Hu, Q., Hearn, M. G., Pham, D. G, Dinolus, M. B., Fukuchi, K., Sisodia, S., Miller, M. A , and Martin, G. M., 1996, *Hum. Mol. Genet.* 5:1589–98.

Busciglio, J.,. Gabuzda, D. H , Matsudaira, P. and Yankner, B.A., 1993, *Proc. Natl. Acad. Sci.* USA 90:2092–6.

Caporaso, G. L., Takei, K., Gandy, S. E.,. Matteoli, M,. Mundigl, O., Greengard, P. and De Camilli, P., 1994, *J. Neurosci.*

Chen, W. J., Goldstein, J. L and Brown, M. S., 1990, *J. Biol. Chem.* 265:3116–23.

De Strooper, B., Umans, L., Van Leuven, F. and Van Den Berghe, H., 1993, *J. Cell. Biol.* 121:295–304.

Desdouits, F., Buxbaum, J. D., Desdouits-Magnen, J., Narin, A. and Greengard, P., 1996, *J. Biol. Chem.* 271:24670–4.

Fiore, F., Zambrano, N., Minopoli, G., Donini, V., Duilio, A. and Russo, T., 1995, *J. Biol. Chem.* 270:30853–6.

Guenette, S. Y., Chen, J., Jondro, P. D. and Tanzi, R. E., 1996, *Proc. Natl. Acad. Sci.* USA 23:10832–7.

Haass, C., Hung, A. Y., Schlossmacher, M. G., Teplow, D. B. and Selkoe, D. J., 1993, J. Biol. Chem. 268: 3021–4.

Hardy, J. and Duff, K., 1993, *Ann. Med.* 25:437–40.

Ikin, A., Annaert, W. G., Takei, K., De Camilli, P., Jahn, R., Greengard, P. and Buxbaum, J. D., 1996, *J. Biol. Chem.* 271:31783–6.

Koo, E. H., Sisodia, S. S., Archer, D. R., Martin, L. J., Weidemann, A., Beyreuther, K., Fischer P.C., Masters, L. and Price, D. L., 1990, *Proc. Natl. Acad. Sci.* USA 87:1561–5.

Koo, E. H. and Squazzo, S. L., 1994, J. Biol. Chem. 269:17386–9.

Koo, E. H., Squazzo, S. L., Selkoe, D.J. and Koo, C. H., 1996, *J. Cell. Sci.* 109:991–8.

Lai, A., Sisodia, S. S. and Trowbridge, I. S., 1995, *J. Biol. Chem.* 270:3565–73.

LeBlanc, A. C., Xue, R. and Gambetti, P., 1996, J. Neurochem. 66:2300–10.

Morin, P. J., Abraham, C. R., Amaratunga, A., Johnson, R. J., Huber, G., Sandell, J. H. and Fine, R. E., 1993, *J. Neurochem.* 61:464–73.

Nordstedt, C., Caporaso, G. L., Thyberg, J., Gandy, S. E. and Greengard, P., 1993, *J. Biol. Chem.* 268: 608–12.

Refolo, L. M., Sambamurti, K., Efthimiopoulos, S., Pappolla, M. A. and Robakis, N. K., 1995, *J. Neurosci. Res.* 40:694–706.

Scheuner, D., Eckman, C., Jensen, M., Song, X., Citron, M., Suzuki, N., Bird, T. D., Hardy, J., Hutton, M., Kukull, W., Larson, E., Levy-Lahad, E., Viitanen, M., Peskind, E., Poorkaj, P., Schellenberg, G., Tanzi, R., Wasco, W., Lannfelt, L., Selkoe, D. and Younkin, S., 1996, *Nature Med.* 2:864–70.

Simons, M., de Strooper, B., Multhaup, G., Tienari, P. J., Dotti, C. G. and Beyreuther, K., 1996, *J. Neurosci.* 16, 899–908.

Simons, M., Ikonen, E., Tienari, P. J., Cid-Arregui, A., Monning, U., Beyreuther, K. and Dotti, C. G., 1995; *J. Neurosci. Res.* 41:121–8.

Sisodia, S. S. and. Price, D. L, 1995, *Faseb J.* 9:366–70.

Strittmatter, W. J., Saunders, A. M., Schmechel, D., Pericak-Vance, M., Enghild, J., Salvesen, G. S. and Roses, A. D., 1993, *Proc. Natl. Acad. Sci.*USA 90:1977–91.

Strittmatter, W. J., Weisgraber, K. H., Huang, D. Y. Dong, L. M., Salvesen, G. S., Pericak-Vance, M., Schmechel, D., Saunders, A. M., Goldgaber, D. and Roses, A. D., 1993, *Proc. Natl. Acad .Sci.* USA 90: 8098–12.

Tomimoto, H., Akiguchi, I., Wakita, H., Nakamura, S. and Kimura, J., 1995, *Brain Res.* 672:187–95.

Yamazaki, T., Selkoe, D. J. and Koo, E. H., 1995, *J. Cell. Biol.* 129:431–42.

Yamazaki, T., Koo, E. H. and Selkoe, D. J., 1996, *J. Cell. Sci.* 109:999–1088.

Zambrano, N., Buxbaum, J. D., Minopoli, G., Fiore, F., De Candia, P., De Renzis, S., Faraonio, R., Sabo, S., Cheetham, J., Sudol, M. and Russo, T., 1997, *J. Biol. Chem.* 272:6399–405.

71

THE CHOLINERGIC BUT NOT THE SEROTONERGIC PHENOTYPE OF A NEW NEURONAL CELL LINE IS SENSITIVE TO β-AMYLOID-INDUCED TOXICITY

Ole F. Olesen, Lone Fjord-Larsen, and Jens D. Mikkelsen

Department of Neurobiology
H. Lundbeck A/S, Ottiliavej 9
2500 Copenhagen-Valby, Denmark

INTRODUCTION

The extracellular deposition of insoluble senile plaques constitute one of the neuropathological hallmarks of Alzheimer's disease. Senile plaques are complex structures that consist of the 39–43 amino acids amyloid β (Aβ) peptide as well as a large number of other components, including heparan sulphate proteoglycan (Snow et al., 1988), α_1-antichymotrypsin (Abraham et al., 1988), apolipoprotein E (Namba et al., 1991), and non-amyloid-β component (NAC) (Ueda et al., 1993). Senile plaques are frequently surrounded by dystrophic neurites and typically associated with areas of selective neuronal loss. This has led to the proposal that highly concentrated Aβ may be harmful to neurons and have a direct effect on the neurodegeneration observed in AD.

Many studies have shown that Aβ is toxic in vitro when added directly to neuronal cell cultures (Yankner et al., 1990; Koh et al., 1990; Pike et al., 1993). The neurotoxicity of Aβ is located in the sequence between amino acid residues 25 and 35 [Aβ(25-35)] and a decapeptide encompassing this region induces neuronal cell death equally potent to that induced by full length Aβ(1-40) (Yankner et al., 1990). The exact mechanism by which Aβ exerts its effect is debatable, but ageing and the formation of fibrillar aggregates seems to increase toxicity (Pike et al., 1993; Simmons et al., 1994).

In the present study, we have tested the neurotoxic effect of Aβ on a newly established cell line termed RN46A (White et al., 1994). To establish this cell line, dissociated embryonic day 13 rat medullary raphe cells were infected with a retrovirus encoding the temperature-sensitive mutant of the SV40 large T antigen. This yielded a cell line that proliferates at 33°C, whereas a shift in cultivation temperature to 39°C halts proliferation and

Progress in Alzheimer's and Parkinson's Diseases
edited by Fisher *et al.*, Plenum Press, New York, 1998.

induces differentiation. Low levels of serotonin are expressed at 33°C in the undifferentiated RN46A cells, but during differentiation at 39°C in the presence of BDNF, the expression is strongly upregulated thus yielding a serotonergic phenotype (White et al., 1994). However, if BDNF is substituted with CNTF during differentiation, the serotonin immunoreactivity is lost and replaced by an expression of choline acetyltransferase (ChAT), thus yielding a cholinergic phenotype (Rudge et al., 1996). This unique property makes the cell line ideal for studying the toxic effect of Aβ on neurons with a common precursor background, but different phenotypes.

MATERIALS AND METHODS

Materials

Different batches of Aβ(1-42) peptides were synthesized by Bachem (CH) or Shaefer-N (DK). Aβ(25-35) was purchased from Bachem (CH), Sigma (USA) or Schaefer-N (DK). Peptides were dissolved in phosphate buffered saline (pH 7.4) 2 h prior to application.

Cell Cultures

PC-12 Cells. Rat PC12 pheochromocytoma cells were grown in Dulbecco's modified Eagle's medium (DMEM) containing 1% penicillin-streptomycin, 5% fetal calf serum and 10% horse serum in a humidified incubator with 5% CO_2.

RN46A cells were grown at 33°C in 1:1 solution of Ham's F12/DMEM supplemented with 10% fetal calf serum, 1% penicillin-streptomycin and 250 µg/ml G418. For differentiation, RN46A cells were transferred to 39°C and cultivated for 8 days in B16 medium supplemented with 1% penicillin-streptomycin, 1% L-glutamine, 20 nM progesterone, 100 µM putrescine, 60 nM transferrin and 600 nM insulin. BDNF or CNTF was added to a final concentration of 25 ng/ml or 40 ng/ml respectively. 40 mM KCl was added after 4 days cultivation at 39°C.

Primary Cortical Cell Culture. Wistar rat fetuses were removed at gestation day 16 (E16). The cortices were dissected free and a single cell suspension established by treatment with 0.25% trypsin (GIBCO) followed by 100 µg/ml deoxyribonuclease type I (Sigma). Cells were plated at 500 cells/mm^2 in basal Eagle's medium (BME) supplemented with 6 g/l glucose (Sigma), 5% heat inactivated horse serum (GIBCO), 1% (v/v) N2 additives, 2 mM L-glutamine (GIBCO) and 0.25% (v/v) penicillin-streptomycin (GIBCO). The cells were kept in a 5% CO_2 humidified environment at 37°C and used after 8 days in culture.

Toxicity Assay

Cells were plated on 96-wells plates in 100 µl of the appropriate medium. After 24 h, either full length Aβ(1-42) or Aβ(25-35) peptide was added and incubation continued for 24 h, unless specifically indicated otherwise. Following incubation, MTT reduction was measured using a commercially available assay according to the manufacturer's instructions (Boehringer). Assay values obtained by vehicle alone were defined as 100%. For experiments involving the measurement of cell proliferation by MTS reduction, the Celltiter 96 cell proliferation assay kit (Promega) was used according to the manufacturer's instructions.

RESULTS

Aβ Specifically Inhibits MTT Reduction in Non-Differentiated RN46A Cells

The sensitivity of RN46A cells to Aβ(25-35) was assessed and compared with primary cortical neurons and PC12 cells by monitoring MTT or MTS reduction following a single application of Aβ(25-35). Virtually no effect on MTT reduction was observed with concentrations of Aβ at 10 nM or less, but higher concentrations led to an inhibition of MTT reduction that became more pronounced up to 10 μM (Fig. 1A). At this concentration, all three cell types exhibited a decreased MTT reduction. PC12 cells were found to be the most sensitive with up to 60% inhibition of MTT reduction upon exposure to 10 μM Aβ. The effect on primary cortical neurons was similar with a MTT reduction that decreased to approximately 55% of control upon exposure to 10 μM Aβ. The RN46A cells had a slightly lower sensitivity, as 24 h incubation with 10 μM Aβ resulted in a 30% inhibition of MTT reduction.

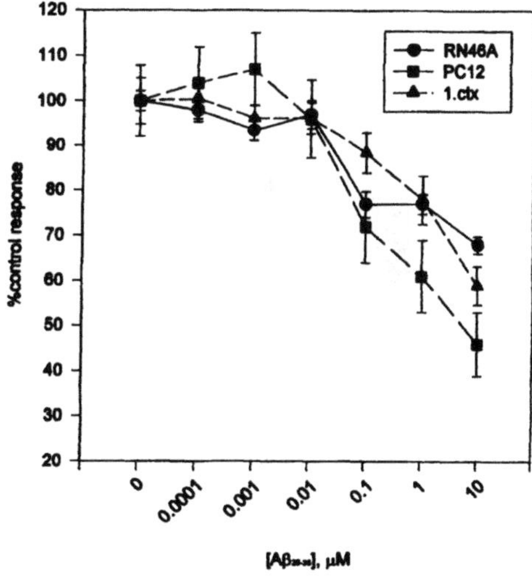

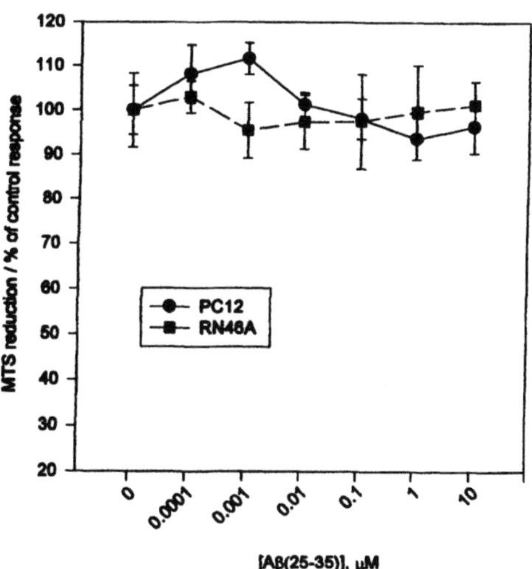

Figure 1. A: Sensitivity of rat primary cortical cultures, PC12 cells and undifferentiated RN46A cells to Aβ(25-35) mediated inhibition of MTT reduction. Inhibition of MTT reduction is expressed as % of control response. Each data point represents the arithmetic mean ± SD of eight replicates. One experiment of a series of three is shown. B: Sensitivity of PC12 cells and undifferentiated RN46A cells to Aβ(25-35) mediated inhibition of MTS reduction. Inhibition of MTS reduction is expressed as % of control response. Each data point represents the arithmetic mean ± SD of eight replicates. One experiment of a series of three is shown.

Next, we compared the effect of Aβ(25-35) on MTS reduction in undifferentiated RN46A cells. Previous reports have demonstrated that Aβ specifically inhibts the cellular reduction of MTT whereas the reduction of MTS is largely unaffected in PC12 cells (Shearman et al., 1995). We confirmed these observations with RN46A cells (Fig. 1B). Whereas high concentrations of Aβ inhibited MTT reduction in PC12 as well as RN46A cells, no significant effect of Aβ on MTS reduction was observed in either PC12 or RN46A cells.

Aβ(25-35) Is Equally Potent as Aβ(1-42)

Previous reports have demonstrated that Aβ(25-35) is equally potent as Aβ(1-42) in inhibiting MTT reduction in various cell lines. We confirmed this in RN46A cells. At 0.1, 1 and 10 µM, both Aβ(25-35) and Aβ(1-42) resulted in a similar and significant inhibition of MTT reduction after 24 h incubation (Fig. 2A).

Doubling the incubation time of undifferentiated RN46A cells with Aβ(25-35) from 24 h to 48 h affected the inhibition of MTT reduction modestly (Fig. 2B). Slightly higher inhibition was observed after prolonged incubation. However, extending the incubation time even longer (up to 96 h) had no effect (not shown).

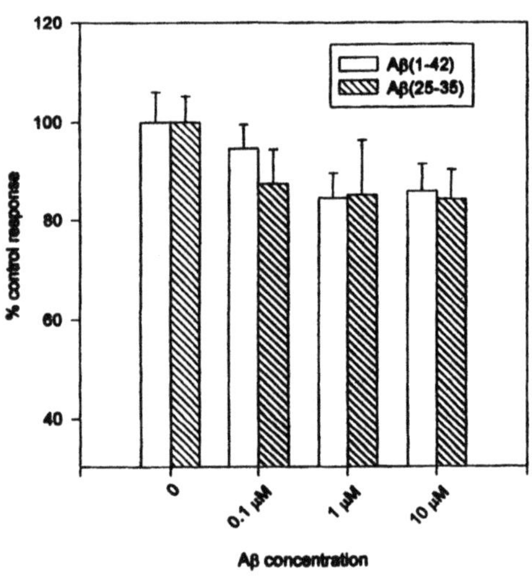

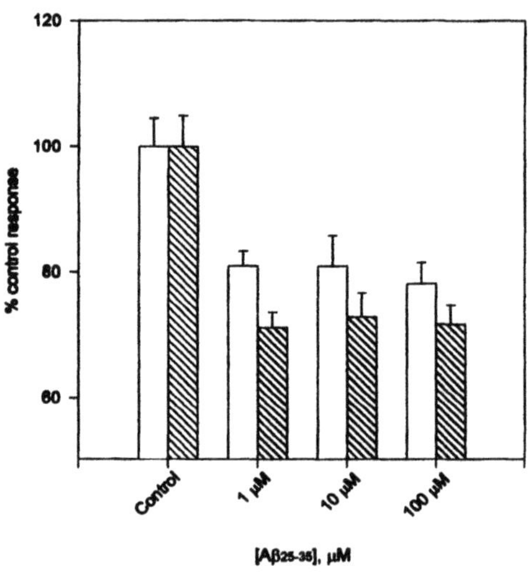

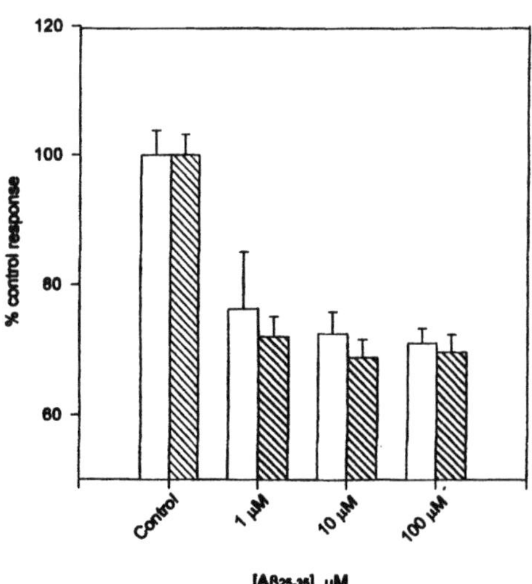

Figure 2. A: Comparison of the neurotoxic effect of Aβ(25-35) and Aβ(1-42) on undifferentiated RN46A cells. RN46A cells were incubated with the indicated concentrations of Aβ peptide for 24 h, whereupon MTT reduction was measured. B: Effect of prolonged incubation with Aβ(25-35). Undifferentiated RN46A cells were incubated with Aβ(25-35) for 24 h (open columns) or 48 h (filled columns) whereupon MTT reduction was measured. C: Effect of cell density. Undifferentiated RN46A cells were plated at 2000 cells/well (open columns) or 16000 cells/well and exposed to Aβ for 24 h whereupon MTT reduction was measured.

The effect of cell density was tested by plating undifferentiated RN46A cells at low density (2000 cells/well) or high density (16000 cells/well), followed by incubation with Aβ for 24 h. As can be seen in Fig. 2C, Aβ(25–35) inhibited MTT reduction to a similar extent in RN46A cells at high and low density.

The Effects of CNTF and BDNF on Aβ Induced Toxicity

Differentiation of RN46A cells can result in either a serotonergic or cholinergic phenotype, depending on the treatment during differentiation. Treatment with BDNF will upregulate the expression of serotonin, thus resulting in a serotonergic phenotype, whereas treatment with CNTF will halt the production of serotonin, induce the expression of ChAT and thus result in a cholinergic phenotype (Rudge et al., 1996).

The effect of CNTF and BDNF on Aβ induced toxicity was estimated in both differentiated and undifferentiated RN46A cells. As shown in Fig. 3A, the presence of BDNF or CNTF had no effect on Aβ sensitivity in undifferentiated cells. Similar to our findings

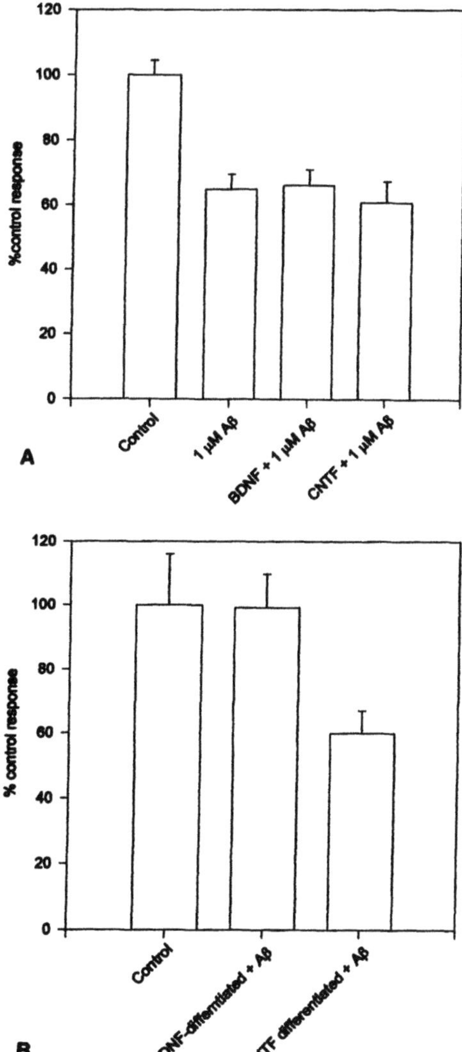

Figure 3. A: Effect of BDNF and CNTF on undifferentiated RN46A cells. RN46A cells were cultivated for 8 days in the presense of vehicle alone (1 μM Aβ), BDNF (BDNF + 1 μM Aβ) or CNTF (CNTF + 1 μM Aβ) and exposed to 1 μM Aβ whereupon MTT reduction was measured. B: Effect of BDNF and CNTF in differentiated RN46A cells. RN46A cells were differentiated for 8 days in the presence of either BDNF or CNTF and subsequently exposed to 1 μM Aβ for 24 h before MTT reduction was measured.

above, the addition of Aβ(25-35) inhibited the MTT reduction in cells to approximately 70% of control level. Undifferentiated cells that were cultivated in the presence of either CNTF or BDNF for up to 8 days prior to Aβ application showed an MTT reduction indistinguishable from cells that had been treated with vehicle alone.

In differentiated cells, however, CNTF and BDNF had distinct but opposite effects on Aβ induced toxicity (Fig. 3B). Differentiation by CNTF to a cholinergic phenotype resulted in a cell population where MTT metabolism could be inhibited by up to 45% following exposure to 10 μM Aβ(25-35). Contrary to this, the differentiation of RN46A cells by BDNF to a serotonergic phenotype yielded a cell population that was unaffected by Aβ. Incubation of the cells with concentrations of Aβ(25-35) up to 10 μM induced no detectable decrease in MTT reduction. These results thus indicate that the cholinergic phenotype of RN46A cells is highly susceptible to Aβ induced toxicity whereas the serotonergic phenotype is unaffected.

DISCUSSION

In this report we examined the effect of Aβ on the reduction of the tetrazolium salts MTT and MTS by undifferentiated as well as differentiated RN46A cells. MTT and MTS are substrates for intracellular and plasma membrane oxidoreductases and have been widely used to measure reductions of cell redox activity, which is demonstrated to be an early indicator of Aβ-mediated cell death (Shearman et al., 1994).

We found that Aβ(25-35) or Aβ(1-42) had a moderate but significant effect in undifferentiated RN46A cells, resulting in a 25–30% decrease in MTT reduction. In similar experiments, the metabolism of another tetrazolium salt, MTS (Owen's reagent), was not affected by Aβ. This observation is in accordance with Hertel et al. (1996), who found that the metabolism of tetrazolium salts like XTT, MTS and WST-1, that all form soluble formazan products, were unaffected by Aβ. Contrary to MTS that forms a soluble formazan product upon reduction, MTT forms intracellular crystals. The formation of such crystals may render RN46A cells more more vulnerable to the toxic effect of Aβ. In that case, the intracellular formation of neurofibrillary tangles, one of the pathological hallmarks of Alzheimer's disease, may have a similar effect, rendering the affected neurons vulnerable to Aβ toxicity.

We found that differentiation of RN46A cells strongly affected their response to Aβ. Differentiation of RN46A cells with BDNF protected against Aβ neurotoxicity. No inhibition of MTT reduction upon treatment with Aβ was observed in BDNF differentiated cells. Contrary to this, differentiation with CNTF resulted in a cell population that was highly sensitive to Aβ. Treating CNTF differentiated cells with Aβ resulted in approximately 50% decrease in MTT reduction. This indicates that the serotonergic phenotype protects cells against Aβ neurotoxicity, whereas a cholinergic phenotype renders the cells more vulnerable.

Various reports have recently indicated that Aβ may have specific effects on different populations of neurons in vitro (Kasa et al., 1993; Pike et al., 1995) and in vivo (Harkany et al., 1995). In this paper we show that cells with a common origin can be differently affected by Aβ depending on their phenotype being serotonergic or cholinergic. Further investigations into the differential sensitivity of various neuronal cell types to Aβ will be valuable for understanding the pathogenesis of AD and designing specific compound for its treatment.

ACKNOWLEDGMENT

We thank Dr. S. R. Whittemore for providing the RN46A cell line.

REFERENCES

Abraham, C.R., Selkoe, D.J., and Potter, H., 1988, Immunochemical identification of the serine inhibitor α-antichymotrypsin in the brain amyloid deposits of Alzheimer's disease. *Cell* 52: 487–501.

Harkany, T., De Jong, G.I., Soos, K., Penke, B., Luiten, P.G.M., and Gulya, K., 1995, β-amyloid affects cholinergic but not parvalbumin-containing neurons in the septal complex of the rat. *Brain Res.* 698: 270–274.

Hertel C., Hauser N., Schubenel R., Seilheimer B., and Kemp, J.A., 1996, amyloid-induced cell toxicity: Enhancedment of 3-(4,5-dimethylthiazol-2yl)-2,5-diphenyltetrazolium bromide-dependent cell death. *J. Neurochem.* 67:272–276.

Kasa, P., Pakaski, M., and Penke, B., 1993, Synthetic human β-amyloid has selective vulnerable effects on different types of neurons. *Adv. Biosci.* 87: 311–312

Koh, J., Yang, L.L., and Cotman, C.W., 1990, β amyloid protein increases the vulnerability of cultured cortical neurons to excitotoxic damage, *Brain Res.* 533: 315–320.

Namba, Y., Tomonaga, M., Kawasaki, H., Otomo, E., and Ikeda, K., 1991, Apolipoprotein E immunoreactivity in cerebral amyloid deposits and neurofibrillary tangles in Alzheimer's disease and kuru plaque amyloid in Creutzfeldt-Jakob disease. *Brain Res.* 541:163–166

Pike, C.J., Burdick, D., Walencewicz, A.J., Glabe, C.G., and Cotman, C.W., 1993, Neurodegeneration induced by β-amyloid peptides in vitro: the role of peptide assembly state. *J. Neurosci.* 13:1676–1687.

Pike, C.J., and Cotman, C.W., 1993, Cultured GABA-immunoreactive neurons are resistant to toxicity induced by β-amyloid. *Neuroscience* 56: 269–274

Rudge, J.S., Eaton ,M.J., Mather, P., Lindsay, R.M.., and Whittemore, S.R., 1996, CNTF induces raphe neuronal precursors to switch from a serotonergic to a cholinergic phenotype in vitro. *Mol.. Cell. Neurosci.* 3: 204 221.

Shearman, M.S., Ragan, C.I., and Iversen, L.L., 1994, Inhibition of PC12 cell redox activity is a specific, early indicator of mechanism of β-amyloid-mediated cell death. *Proc. Natl. Acad. Sci., USA* 91:1470–1474.

Shearman, M.S., Hawtin ,S.R., and Tailor, V.J., 1995, The intracellular component of cellular 3- (4,5-dimethylthiazol-2-yl)-2,5-Diphenyltetrazolium bromide (MTT) reduction is specifically inhibited by β-amyloid peptides. *J. Neurochem.* 65:218–227.

Simmons, L.K., May ,P.C., Tomaselli, K.J., Rydel, R.E., Fuson, K.S., Brigham, E.F., Wright, S., Lieberburg, I.,Becker, G.W., Brems D.N., Li ,W.Y. , 1994, Secondary structure of amyloid β peptide correlates with neurotoxic activity in vitro. *Mol. Pharmacol.* 45:373–379.

Snow, A.D., Mar, H., Nochlin, D., Kimata, K., Kato, M., Suzuki, S., Hassell, J., and Wright, T.N., 1988, The presence of heparan sulfate proteoglycans in the neuritic plaques and congophilic angiopathy in Alzheimer's disease. *Am. J. Pathol.* 133: 456–463.

White, L.A., Eaton, M.J., Castro, M.C., Klose, K.J., Globus, M.Y., Shaw, G., and Whittemore, S.R. , 1994, Distinct regulatory pathways control neurofilament expression and neurotansmitter synthesis in immortalized serotonergic neurons. *J. Neurosci.*14: 6744–6753.

Ueda, K., Fukushima, H., Masliah, E., Xia, Y., Iwai, A., Yoshimoto, M., Otero, D.A.C., Kondo, J., Ihara, Y., and Saitoh, T (1993) Molecular cloning of cDNA encoding an unrecognized component of amyloid in Alzheimer disease. *Proc. Natl. Acad. Sci. USA* 90:11282–11286, 1990.

Yankner, B.A., Duffy, L.K., and Kirschner, D.A., 1990, Neurotrophic and neurotoxic effects of amyloid β protein: reversal by tachykinin neuropeptides. *Science* 25:279–282.

72

THE MOLECULAR BASIS UNDERLYING THE DISCRETE ACTIVATION OF SIGNAL TRANSDUCTION PATHWAYS BY SELECTIVE MUSCARINIC AGONISTS

Relevance to Treatment of Alzheimer's Disease

E. Heldman,[1] Z. Pittel,[1] R. Haring,[1] N. Eshhar,[1] R. Levy,[2] Z. Vogel,[2] D. Marciano,[1] Y. Kloog,[3] and A. Fisher[1]

[1]Israel Institute for Biological Research
Ness-Ziona, Israel
[2]Weizmann Institute
Rehovot, Israel
[3]Tel-Aviv University
Tel-Aviv, Israel

INTRODUCTION

Selective muscarinic agonists that are directed at the m1 muscarinic acetylcholine receptor (M1 mAChR) have been suggested as a rational treatment of Alzheimer's disease (AD) (Fisher and Barak, 1995). Such muscarinic receptor agonists may activate a variety of transduction pathways, some of which are beneficial while others may be deleterious to AD. For example, activation of M1 mAChR increases phosphoinositide (PI) hydrolysis, arachidonic acid release, elevates intracellular calcium, increases the nonamyloidogenic processing of beta-amyloid precursor protein (APP), mediates tau dephosphorylation, induces formation of neurites and increases adenylate cyclase (AC) activity (Fisher and Barak, 1995; Haring et al., 1995; Heldman et al., 1996; Pittel et al., 1996). While most of these biochemical responses are considered to be beneficial for alleviating AD pathology, activation of AC may be deleterious, since mRNA of Gs, that mediates activation of AC, is elevated in AD brain (Harrison et al., 1991). Several muscarinic agonists that were synthesized in our laboratory activate preferentially distinct transduction pathways that lead to desirable effects, without affecting significantly AC activity (Fisher and Barak, 1995; Gurwitz et al., 1994). This chapter describes studies aimed at elucidating the mechanism

Progress in Alzheimer's and Parkinson's Diseases
edited by Fisher *et al.*, Plenum Press, New York, 1998.

which dictate the selectivity of these agonists. In addition, this chapter reports results of studies designed to identify transduction pathways that mediate the non-amyloidogenic APP processing induced by m1 agonists (Fisher, 1997).

RESULTS AND DISCUSSION

Mechanisms of Agonist Selectivity

Two types of selective activation of muscarinic receptors by agonists were addressed in the present study: 1) selectivity at the level of signal transduction, where selective agonists activate preferentially discrete signal transduction pathways; and 2) selectivity at the level of receptor subtypes, where selective agonists preferentially activate a distinct receptor subtype. To study the mechanism of these types of selectivity, we employed Chinese Hamster Ovary (CHO) cells which were stably transfected with cDNA encoding the human M1 mAChR (hm1 cells) and M3 mAChR (hm3 cells). Carbachol (CCh), a non-selective muscarinic receptor agonist, activates PI hydrolysis, as well as AC, similarly in hm1 and in hm3 cells (Heldman et al., 1996). On the other hand, two m1 agonists, McN-A-343, and AF102B (Fisher and Heldman, 1990) activate hm1 cells more potently than hm3 cells (Fig. 1) in regard to both PI hydrolysis and AC activity. In addition, these selective agonists activate PI hydrolysis to a greater extent than AC in both cell lines (Fig. 1). These experiments demonstrate both types of selectivity, at the level of the receptor subtypes, and at the level of the signal transduction. Differences in binding affinities of these agonists between the two receptor subtypes cannot be responsible for the two types of selectivity, since selective compounds show similar affinities to M1 mAChR and M3 mAChR as well as to other muscarinic receptor subtypes (for data regarding affinities of McN-A-343 to mAChR see Heldman et al., 1996 and results for AF102B are described in Fig. 2). The Ki values derived from competition experiments with ^{3}H-N-methylscopolamine (described in Fig. 2) for AF102B, as was measured in CHO cells stably transfected with the relevant human receptors, are 20, 13, 18, 11 μM for M1, M2, M3 and M4 mAChR, respectively.

We examined the possibility that differences between the receptor reserves for PI hydrolysis versus AC, which may affect the degree of the degree of the response of each of these functions to non-efficacious agonists, play a role in determining the above mentioned types of agonist selectivity. For this purpose we induced receptor down-regulation

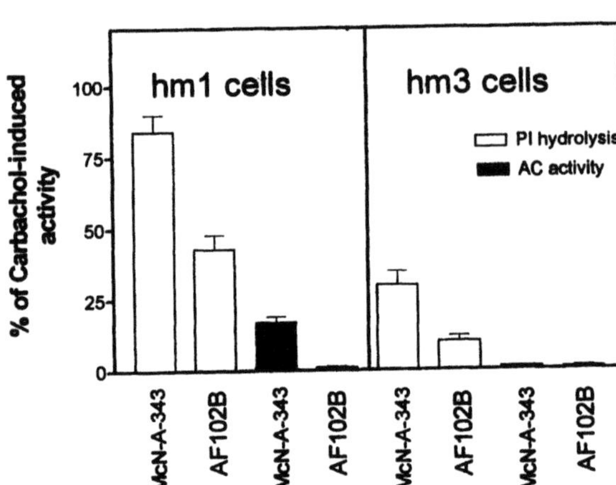

Figure 1. Activation of phosphoinositide (PI) hydrolysis and adenylate cyclase (AC) in hm1 and hm3 CHO cells by McN-A-343 and AF102B. Cells were simulated with either McN-A-343 (1mM) or AF102B (1mM) for 20 min. The activity obtained with each of these agonists was compared to that obtained with 1mM carbachol (considered as 100%).

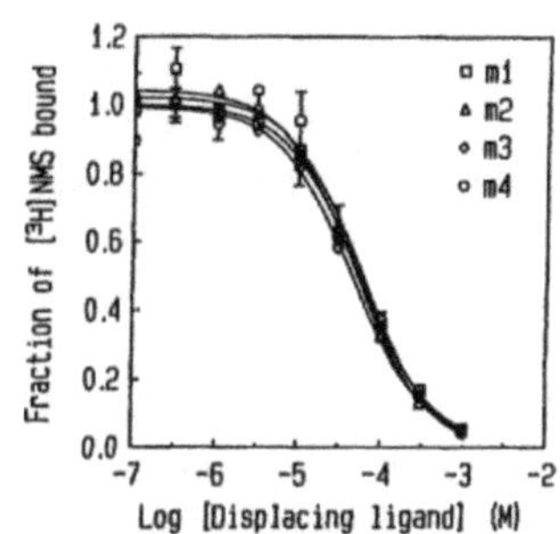

Figure 2. Competition curves for AF102B in CHO cell lines, each expressing one of the mAChR subtypes. CHO cells were incubated for one hour in presence of 1nM [³H]NMS and various concentrations of AF102B. Bound [³H]NMS was determined at the end of the incubation.

in hm1 cells by a prolonged incubation with CCh and then measured the degree of the activation of PI hydrolysis and AC activity in the receptor down-regulated cells and compared them to the initial response to carbachol, obtained in cells in which receptor down-regulation was not induced (defined as 100%). We found that down-regulating the receptors to 20% of their original value reduced CCh-induced AC to 10% of its initial value, whereas CCh-induced PI hydrolysis was only reduced to 55% of its initial value (Heldman et al., 1996). These results suggest the existence of higher amounts of spare receptors for PI hydrolysis than for AC.

Corroboration to this conclusion came from experiments with atropine, where higher concentrations of the antagonist were needed to inhibit CCh-induced PI hydrolysis as compared to those needed to inhibit CCh-induced AC activity (Heldman et al., 1996). However, there were no differences in the pattern of the inhibitions of each of these biochemical responses between hm1 cells and hm3 cells. Similar results were obtained with receptor alkylation where partial alkylation of the receptors by acetylethylcholine aziridinium ion reduced CCh-induced activation of AC more than CCh-induced PI hydrolysis (Heldman et al., 1996). Yet, both of these biochemical functions (PI hydrolysis and AC activity) were reduced similarly in hm1 and hm3 cells (Heldman et al., 1996). Thus functional selectivity, exhibited at the level of the signal transduction (preferential activation of PI hydrolysis versus AC activity by selective agonists), is a result of the existence of higher amounts of spare receptors for PI hydrolysis than for AC activity in both hm1 and hm3 cells. However, agonist selectivity at the level of the receptor subtype cannot be attributed to differences in receptor reserve, since hm1 cells and hm3 cells contain similar amounts of spare receptors for each of the above mentioned biochemical responses.

Thus, the selectivity at the level of the receptor subtype must be related to a different mechanism. We postulate that upon agonist binding, the transition of the receptor to its active conformational state is more efficient for M1 mAChR than for the M3 mAChR. Thus, non-efficacious agonists activate more efficiently hm1 cells than hm3 cells, a tendency that was found for all partial muscarinic receptor agonists which we examined so far. Evidence for the hypothesis that differences in the transition from the inactive to the active state between M1 and M3 mAChR is responsible for the preferential activation of the M1 mAChR, comes from binding experiments in which we demonstrated two affinity states for hm1 cells and only one apparent affinity state for hm3 cells (Heldman et al., 1996).

In summary, it seems that in order to obtain selective activation of m1 mAChR receptors, partial M1 agonists (which show functional selectivity) should be preferred over full agonists, which activate all the transduction pathways and all receptor subtypes in a non-discriminative manner. This feature of partial agonists might be important for the treatment of AD as the functional selectivities of partial agonist may prevent adverse side effects that are characteristic of non-selective full agonists.

IDENTIFICATION OF TRANSDUCTION PATHWAYS THAT MEDIATE BETWEEN THE M1 mAChR AND NON-AMYLOIDOGENIC APP PROCESSING

An important response of M1 mAChR to receptor agonists, in the context of its relevance to the treatment of AD, is the nonamyloidogenic APP processing (Nitsch et al., 1992; Buxbaum et al., 1992). We previously demonstrated that the m1 selective agonist, AF102B, activates non-amyloidogenic APP processing (Haring et al., 1995). We also showed that pre-treatment of the cells with nerve growth factor (NGF) augments synergistically the effect of AF102B on APP processing (Haring et al., 1995). This synergism between growth factors and selective m1 agonists may have clinical relevance, as functionally selective agonists are partial agonists in their nature and elevating their beneficial activity may increase their efficacy in the treatment of AD without causing adverse side effects. Here we describe experiments aimed at identifying the signal trnsduction pathways that mediate the synergism between AF102B and NGF in regard to the activation of the non-amyloidogenic APP processing.

The experiments were performed with PC12 cells that were stably transfected with cDNA encoding the M1 mAChR (PC12M1 cells). We found that in addition to NGF, basic fibroblast growth factor (bFGF) also enhances the muscarinic response. These findings suggest that the transduction pathways of several receptor tyrosine kinases (RTK) cross-react with those that mediate between M1 mAChR and APP processing. We attempted to identify convergence points between these transduction pathways and to examine how activation of both pathways (muscarinic-associated and RTK-associated) affect the magnitude of the response at tentative convergence points. The *ras* protein, which has been reported to be activated by both muscarinic agonists and RTK agonists, may be a candidate for such a convergence point. Inhibition of *ras* activation by 25 µM of s-*trans*, *trans* farnesyl thiosalicilate (FTS) partially reduced APP secretion induced by CCh (Fig. 3). These results suggest that the *ras* protein is involved in the muscarinic agonist-induced APP processing but that alternative pathways may operate in parallel to the *ras*-dependent pathway.

Corroboration of our conclusion that *ras* is involved in muscarinic agonist-induced APP processing comes from experiments with COS-7 cells which were transiently co-transfected with m1AChR and dominant negative *ras* (N17*ras*). In these cells, unlike in control cells that were transfected with m1AChR alone, CCh did not evoke APP secretion (Fig. 4). Another signaling that may be involved in muscarinic agonist-induced APP processing is a protein kinase C (PKC)-dependent pathway. Indeed, the specific PKC inhibitor, GF109203X (2µM) partially inhibited CCh-induced APP secretion (Fig. 3). When FTS and GF10P203X were added together, CCh-induced APP secretion was almost completely abolished. However, another PKC inhibitor, K252a (2µM), did not inhibit CCh-induced

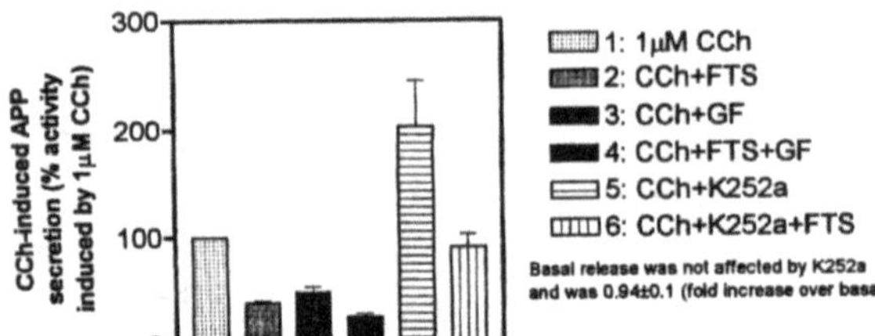

Figure 3. Effect of inhibitors of *ras* and PKC on APP secretion from PC12M1 cells. APP secretion induced by 1µM CCh was measured during one hour in absence (100%) or presence of the inhibitors.

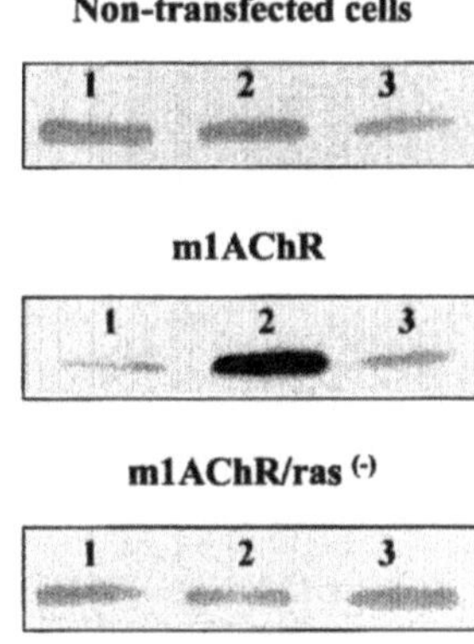

Figure 4. Immunoblots of APP in the growth medium of COS-7 cells transiently transfected with cDNA that encode the m1AChR together or without cDNA that encode dominant-negative *ras* (N17*ras*). APP was measured in the medium 1 h after stimulation with 1 mM carbachol in the absence, and presence of 10 µM atropine sulfate.

Figure 5. Phosphorylated myelin basic protein (MBP) by immonoprecipitated MAPK following activation of PC12M1 cells with muscarinic agonists and K252a. Phosphorylated proteins were visualized by autoradiography following incubation of MAPK and MBP with [^{32}P]ATP.

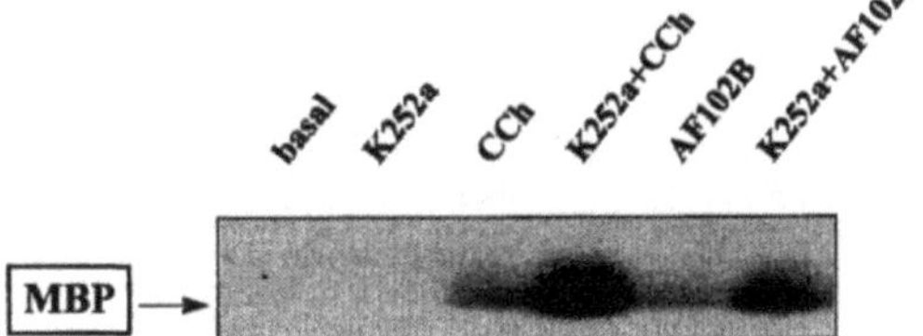

APP processing, but rather significantly enhanced it (Fig. 3). Moreover, K252a reversed the inhibitory effect of FTS (Fig. 3). We concluded that K252a has an additional site of action that bypasses both PKC and *ras* and thereby lifts the inhibition of CCh-induced APP secretion by FTS. From Fig. 5 it is apparent that K252a enhances the muscarinic agonist-induced activation of MAPK. These results suggest that activation of MAPK may play an important role in regulating non-amyloidogenic APP processing and that MAPK could be a target for growth factors-like drugs that together with partial muscarinic agonists induce synergistic beneficial effect. Thus, K252a, or similar compounds, may be used in conjunction with a partial muscarinic agonist in order to enhance the beneficial effects of partial muscarinic agonists. Our results also suggest that endogenous growth factors and exogenous m1 agonists may operate in concert and enhance APP processing, which could be beneficial in the treatment of AD (*re* also Fisher, 1997).

REFERENCES

Buxbaum, J.D., Masaki, O., Chen, H.I., Pinkas-Kramarski, R., Jaffe, E.A., Gandy, S.E., and Greengard. P., 1992, Cholinergic agonists and interleukin 1 regulate processing and secretion of the Alzheimer β/A4 amyloid protein precursor. *Proc. Natl. Acad. Sci. USA.* 92:10075–10078.

Fisher, A., 1997, Muscarinic agonists for the treatment of Alzheimer's disease: progress and perspectives. *Exp. Opin. Invest. Drugs.* 6(10):1395–1411.

Fisher, A., and Barak, D., 1994, Progress and perspectives in new muscarinic agonists. *Drug News & Perspectives.* 7:453–464.

Gurwitz, D., Haring, R., Heldman, E., Fraser, C.M., Manor, D., and Fisher, A., 1994, Discrete activation of transduction pathways associated with acetylcholine m1 receptor by several muscarinic lignads. *Eur. J. Pharmacol.* 267:21–31.

Haring, R., Gurwitz, D., Barg, J., Pinkas-Kramarski, R., Heldman, E., Pittel, Z., Wengier, A., Meshulam, H., Marciano, D., Karton, Y., and Fisher, A., 1994, Amyloid precursor protien secretion via muscarinic receptors: reduced desensitization using the M1-selective agonist AF102B. *Biochem. Biophys. Res. Comm.* 203:652–658.

Haring, R., Gurwitz, D., Barg, J., Pinkas-Kramarski, R., Heldman, E., Pittel, Z., Danenberg, H.D., Wengier, A., Meshulam, H., Marciano, D., Karton, Y., and Fisher, A., 1995, NGF promotes amyloid precursor protein via muscarinic receptor activation. *Biochem. Biophys. Res. Comm.* 213:15–23.

Harrison, P.J., Barton, A.J.L., McDonald, D., and Pearson, R.C.A., 1991, Alzheimer's disease: specific increse in a G protein subunit (Gsa)mRNA in hippocampal and cortical neurons. *Mol. Brain Res.* 10:71–81.

Heldman, E., Barg, J., Fisher, A., Levy, R., Pittel, Z., Zimlichman, R., Kushnir, M., and Vogel, Z., 1996, Pharmacological basis for functional selectivity of partial muscarinic receptor agonists. *Eur. J. Pharmacol.* 297:283–291.

Pittel, Z., Heldman, E., Barg, J., Haring, R., and Fisher, A., 1996, Muscarinic control of amyloid precursor protein secretion in rat cerebral cortex and cerebellum. *Brain Res.* 742:299–304.

Nitsch, R.M., Slack, B.E., Wurtman, R.J., and Growdon, J.H., 1992, Release of Alzheimer amyloid precursor derivatives stimulated by activation of muscarinic acetylcholine receptors. *Science.* 258:304–307.

Sadot, W., Gurwitz, D., Barg, J., Behar, L., Ginzburg, I. and Fisher A., Activation of m1-muscarinic acetylcholine receptor regulates TAU phosphorylation in transfected PC12 cells. *J. Neurochem.* 66:877–880, 1996.

73

MUSCARINIC MODULATION OF β-AMYLOID PRECURSOR PROTEIN (βAPP) PROCESSING IN VITRO AND IN VIVO

Zipora Pittel,[1] Nomi Eshhar,[1] Eliahu Heldman,[1] Michal Sapir,[1] Rachel Haring,[1] Moshe Kushnir,[2] and Abraham Fisher[1]

[1]Israel Institute for Biological Research
Ness-Ziona, Israel
[2]Kaplan Hospital
Rehovot, Israel

INTRODUCTION

Amyloid β peptide (Aβ) accumulation in distinct brain regions is an early event in the progression of Alzheimer's disease (AD). Increase in specific isoforms of Aβ production and/or aggregation appears concomitantly with several mutations. These include: 1) β-amyloid precursor protein (βAPP) mutations (Citron et al., 1992; Haass et al., 1994); 2) apolipoprotein E4 (apoE4) polymorphism (Corder et al., 1993); 3) presenilin 1 mutations (Scheuner et al., 1996); and 4) presenilin 2 mutations (Scheuner et al., 1996). The increased levels of Aβ may cause neurotoxicity and consequently lead to an inflammatory process which results in formation of extracellular plaques. The precursor of Aβ, β-amyloid precursor protein (βAPP), may be cleaved by the proteolytic enzymes β and γ secretase to yield amyloidogenic products or by α-secretase which cleaves βAPP within the βA sequence and thereby prevents Aβ formation. The result of α-secretase cleavage is the release of soluble βAPP (βAPPs) to the extracellular milieu, the non-amyloidogenic products. βAPPs is constitutively secreted in the brain into extracellular fluids like the cerebrospinal fluid (CSF). The synthesis and processing of βAPP was shown to be regulated by several neurotransmitters. Acetylcholine (ACh), which is significantly decreased in AD may mediate βAPP processing via muscarinic acetylcholine receptors (mAChR). In this regard, m1 mAChR mediate βAPPs processing (Nitsch et. al., 1992 & Pittel et al., 1996). Noradrenaline and serotonin were also shown to affect βAPPs secretion (Wallace & Haroutunian, 1993). In this study we tested the involvement of ACh in regulating βAPPs secretion *in vivo, ex vivo* and in primary cell cultures.

Progress in Alzheimer's and Parkinson's Diseases
edited by Fisher *et al.*, Plenum Press, New York, 1998.

RESULTS AND DISCUSSION

Increased βAPPs Secretion Mediated by M1 mAChR

Activation of m1 mAChR by m1 agonists results in an increase in the non-amyloidogenic processing of βAPP as evident by an increased level of secreted βAPPs. This was shown in cultured cells like HK293-M1 and HK293-M3 cells (Nitsch et al., 1992); in Chinese hamster ovary cells stably transfected with human m1 or m3 mAChR (Buxbaum et al., 1994); and in pheochromocytoma cells stably transfected with rat m1 mAChR (PC12M1) (Haring et al., 1994). βAPP processing in brain is also increased following activation of m1 mAChR. AF102B, a selective M1 muscarinic agonist (Fisher et al., 1991) activated βAPPs secretion from slices of the cerebral cortex, a brain region rich in M1 mAChR and failed to activate APPs secretion from slices of the cerebellum, a brain region rich in M2 mAChR (Table 1). Carbachol (CCh), a non-selective agonist showed a weaker response (Table 1) than AF102B in stimulating APPs secretion from cerebrocortical slices (Pittel et al., 1996). Similar results were found with WAL2014, a predominantly m1 agonist in the same preparation (Farber et al., 1995). In rat hippocampal and cortical primary cell cultures, CCh and AF102B, both increased APPs levels (Table 2). This stimulatory effect was blocked by pirenzepine, an m1 antagonist. It seems that in different systems such as cell lines, primary cell cultures and cortical brain slices, the m1 mAChR modulate secretion of βAPPs and increase the non-amyloidogenic cleavage and thereby indirectly decrease the formation of βA.

Table 1. CCh- and AF102B-stimulated βAPPs secretion from rat cerebrocortical and cerebellar slices

	βAPPs secretion (fold stimulation over basal)							
	Carbachol				AF102B			
Brain region	10^{-6} M	10^{-5} M	10^{-4} M	10^{-3} M	10^{-6} M	10^{-5} M	10^{-4} M	10^{-3} M
Cortex	1.0 ± 0.1	1.38 ± 0.15	1.5 ± 0.26	$2.00 \pm 0.38^*$	$2.13 \pm 0.3^*$	1.75 ± 0.32	$1.58 \pm 0.15^*$	$1.82 \pm 0.28^*$
Cerebellum	—	1.07 ± 0.15	2.1 ± 0.57	$2.37 \pm 0.27^*$	—	1.35 ± 0.42	0.97 ± 0.18	1.45 ± 0.37

$^*p < 0.05$.
Data were normalized according to the control values (obtained in absence of muscarinic agonist) for each experiment. Data presented as means ± SEM of 3–6 experiments each performed in duplicate.

Table 2. CCh- and AF102B-stimulated βAPPs secretion
from rat hippocampal and cortical primary cell cultures

	βAPPs secretion (fold stimulation over basal)			
	Carbachol		AF102B	
Brain region	10^{-4} M	10^{-4} M + gallamine, 50 μM	10^{-4} M	10^{-4} M + gallamine, 50 μM
Cortex	2.0 ± 0.50	4.9 ± 0.8	3.8 ± 0.90	8.0 ± 2.7
Hippocampus	2.2 ± 0.47	NT	2.6 ± 0.04	NT

Data were normalized according to control values (obtained in absence of muscarinic agonist) for each experiment. Data presented as means ± SEM of 2–3 experiments performed in duplicate.
NT = Not tested.

Decreased βAPPs Levels in the Hippocampus and the CSF following Activation of mAChR *in Vivo*

Physostigmine, a cholinesterase inhibitor was administered peripherally to rats (0.25 mg/kg; intramuscular; im). One hour after injection, animals were sacrificed by decapitation and the hippocampi were dissected out. The level of βAPPs was measured in the supernatant of the homogenate (following centrifugation at 100,000×g/4°C) by immunoblot technique using the monoclonal antibody 22C11. A significant decrease (44%) in released βAPP was observed in the hippocampi of physostigmine-treated rats as compared to saline-treated rats (Table 3). Similarly, when oxotremorine (1mg/kg; intarperitonal; ip), a putative m2 muscarinic agonist (Pittel et al., 1990) was administered, a significant decrease (51%) in released βAPPs levels was observed as compared to saline-treated rats (Table 3). Thus, in both cases when mAChR was activated either directly by oxotremorine or indirectly by ACh, following an increase due to acetylcholinesterase inhibition by physostigmine, the result was a decrease in the released βAPPs levels. A reduction in βAPPs and Aβ peptides was also reported after tacrine treatment in cell cultures (Lahiri et al., 1992 and 1994). Wallace and his colleagues (1993a) showed that when synaptic ACh level was decreased mRNA levels of βAPP were increased. These results may suggest the involvement of inhibitory mAChR in the regulation of βAPP. To further examine this possibility we studied the effect of gallamine, an m2 antagonist (Michel et al., 1990) and also an allosteric modulator of mAChR (Lee et al., 1992), on CCh- and AF102B-induced βAPP secretion in primary rat cultures. We found that in cortical and hippocampal primary cultures gallamine potentiates CCh- and AF102B-induced βAPP release (Table 2). These data support the notion that inhibitory mAChR may be involved in the modulation of βAPP. A similar tendency of decrease, as was already found in the brain, in released βAPPs levels was found also when βAPPs was measured in the CSF one hour after administering physostigmine (0.25 mg/kg; im) or oxotremorine (1 mg/kg; ip). We observed a significant decrease of 28 and 34% in βAPPs levels in the CSF by physostigmine and oxotremorine, respectively. These effects were blocked by scopolamine (1 mg/kg, ip, 15 minutes prior to the cholinergic treatment) indicating that mAChR are involved in the modulation of βAPP processing (Table 3). In studies using physostigmine or phenserine, similar results of reduced βAPPs levels in the CSF were reported (Haroutunian et al., 1997).

Lesion of Hippocampal Cholinergic Pathways by the Cholinotoxin AF64A

Additional evidence for the involvement of the cholinergic system in βAPP processing arise from experiments where the cholinergic system was lesioned by the cholinotoxin

Table 3. βAPPs levels in rat hippocampi and in CSF after administration of physostigmine (0.25 mg/kg, im) or oxotremorine (1 mg/kg, ip) with or without scopolamine (1 mg/kg, ip, 15 min prior to muscarinic treatment)

Treatment	βAPPs secretion (% of saline-treated rats)	
	Hippocampus	CSF
Physostigmine	56 ± 8*	72 ± 6*
Physostigmine + scopolamine	–	107 ± 10
Oxotremorine	49 ± 6*	67 ± 7*
Oxotremorine + scopolamine	–	101 ± 5

*$p < 0.01$.
Data presented as percent of saline-treated rats (calculated for each experiment) and expressed as means ± SEM of 5–9 animals. Each experiment was performed in duplicate.

AF64A. ACh levels were chronically reduced in rat hippocampus after administering AF64A (Pittel et al., 1989) to rat (3 nmoles/2 µl/side, bilateral *icv* injection). Released βAPPs levels were measured in the hippocampi (as detailed above) one week and one month after the lesion and the data were compared to those determined in saline-treated rats. We found that when the hippocampal cholinergic neurons were impaired, a significant decrease of 20 and 18% in secreted βAPPs was detected one week and one month, respectively, after a single AF64A dosing as compared to saline-treated rats. These data suggest that also in this case, when ACh level is chronically reduced, the result is a reduced βAPP processing.

In conclusion our data suggest that endogenous levels of ACh may be involved in the regulation of non-amyloidogenic βAPP processing. The dual action of ACh seems to be mediated by various subtypes of mAChR. We suggest that activation of stimulatory mAChR (e.g. m1 mAChR) (Pittel et al., 1990) potentiates non-amyloidogenic cleavage of βAPP while activation of inhibitory mAChR (m2 mAChR), through a synaptic decrease of ACh, mediates reduction of βAPPs. Finally, these data indicate that m1 agonists may be beneficial in AD by decreasing Aβ formation.

REFERENCES

Buxbaum, J. D., Ruefli, A. A., Parker, C. A., Cypess, A.M. and Greengard, P., 1994, Calcium regulates processing of the Alzheimer amyloid protein precursor in a protein kinase C-independent manner, *Proc. Natl. Acad. Sci. USA* 91:4489–4493.

Citron, M., Oltersdorf, T., Haass, C., McConlogue, L., Hung, A.Y., Sebert, P., Vigo-Pelfrey, C., Lieeberburg, I. and Selkoe, D.J., 1992, Mutation of the β-amyloid precursor protein in familial Alzheimer's disease increases β-protein production, *Nature* 360:672–674.

Corder, E.H., Sauders, A. M., Strittmatter, W.J., Schmechel, D.E., Gaskell, P.C., Small, G.W., Roses, A.D., Haines, J.L., Pericak-Vance, M.A., 1993, Gene dose of apolipoprotein E type 4 allele and he risk of Alzheimer's disease in late onset families, *Science* 261, 921–923.

Farber, S.A., Nitsch, R.M., Schulz, J.G., and Wurtman, R.J., 1995, Regulated secretion of β-amyloid precursor protein in rat brain, *J. Neurosci.* 15:7442–7451.

Fisher, A., Brandeis, R., Karton, Y., Pittel, Z., Gurwitz, D., Haring, R., Sapir, S., Levy, A. and Heldman, E., 1991, (±)-cis-2-Methyl-spiro(1,3-oxathiolane-5,3') quinuclidine, an M1 selective cholinergic agonist, attenuates cognitive dysfunction in an animal model of Alzheimer's disease, *J. Pharmacol. Exp. Ther.* 257:392–403.

Haass, C., Hung, A.Y., Selkoe, D.J., Teplow, D.B., 1994, Mutations associated with a locus for familial Alzheimer's disease result in alternative processing of amyloid β-protein precursor, *J. Biol. Chem.* 269:17741–17748.

Haring, R., Gurwitz, D., Barg, J., Pinkas-Kramarski, R., Heldman, E., Pittel, Z., Wengier, A., Meshulam, H., Marciano, D., Karton, Y. and Fisher, A., 1994, Amyloid precursor protein secretion via muscarinic receptors: reduced desensitization using the M1-selective agonist AF102B, *Biochem. Biophys. Res. Commun.* 203: 652–658.

Haroutunian, V., Grieg, N., Pei, X.-F-., Utsuki, T., Gluck, R., Davis, K.L., and Wallace, W.C., 1997, Pharmacological modulation of Alzheimer's β-amyloid precursor protein levels in the CSF of rats with forebrain cholinergic lesions, *Brain Res. Mol. Brain Res.* 46: 161–168.

Lahiri, D.K., Nall, C., and Farlow, M., 1992, The cholinergic agonist carbachol reduces intracellular beta-amyloid precursor protein in PC12 and C6 cells, *Biochem Int.*. 28:853–860.

Lahiri, D.K., Lewis, S., and Farlow, M., 1994, Tacrine alters the secretion of the beta-amyloid precursor protein in cell lines, *J. Neurosci. Res.* 37:777–787.

Lee N.H., Hu J. and El-Fakahany EE., 1992, Modulation by certain Lahiri, D.K., Lewis, S., and Farlow, M., 1994, Tacrine alters the secretion conserved aspartate residues of the allosteric interaction of gallamine at the m1 muscarinic receptor, *J. Pharmacol. Exp. Ther.* 262:312–316.

Michel, A.D., Delmendo, R.E., Lopez, M. and Whiting, R.L., 1990, On the interaction of gallamine with muscarinic receptor subtypes, *Eur. J. Pharmacol.* 182:335–345.

Nitsch, R.M., Slack, B.E., Wurtman, R.J. and Growdon, J.H., 1992, Release of Alzheimer amyloid precursor derivatives stimulated by activation of muscarinic acetylcholine receptors, *Science* 258:304–307.

Pittel, Z., Fisher, A. and Heldman, E., 1989, Cholinotoxicity induced by ethylcholine aziridinium ion after intracarotid and intracerebroventricular administration, *Life Sci,* 44:1437–1448.

Pittel, Z., Heldman, E., Rubinstein, R., Cohen., S., 1990, distinct muscarinic receptor subtypes differentially modulate acetylcholine release from corticocerebral synaptosomes, *J. Neurochem.* 55:665–672.

Pittel, Z., Heldman, E., Barg, J., Haring, R., and Fisher, A., 1996, Muscarinic Control of amyloid precursor protein secretion in rat cerebral cortex and cerebellum, *Brain Res.* 742:299–304.

Scheuner, D., Eckman, C., Jensen, M., Song, X., Citron, M., Suzuki, N., Bird, T.D., Hardy, J., Hutton, M., Kukull, W., Larson, E., Levy-Lahad, E., Vititanen,M., Peskind, E., Poorkaj, P., Schellenberg, G., Tanzi, R., Wasco, W., Lannfelt, L., Selkoe, D., and Younkin, S., 1996, Secreted amyloid peptide β-protein similar to that in the senile plaques of Alzheimer's disease is increased in vivo by the presenilin 1 and 2 and APP mutations linked to familial Alzheimer's disease, *Nature Med.* 2:864–870.

Wallace, W.C., Ahlers, S.T., Gotlib, J., Bragin, V., Sugar, J., Gluck, R., Shea, P.A., Davis, K.L. and Haroutunian, V., 1993a, Amyloid precursor protein in the cerebral cortex is rapidly and persistently induced by loss of subchronical innovation, *Proc. Natl. Acad. Sci. USA* 90:8712–8716.

Wallace, W.C. and Haroutunian, V., 1993, Using the subcortically lesioned rat cortex to understand the physiological role of amyloid precursor protein, *Behav. Brain Res.* 57: 99–206.

74

M1 MUSCARINIC AGONISTS: FROM TREATMENT TOWARD DELAYING PROGRESSION OF ALZHEIMER'S DISEASE

Abraham Fisher, Rachel Haring, Zipora Pittel, Nomi Eshhar, Yishai Karton, Rachel Brandeis, Haim Meshulam, Daniella Marciano, and Eliahu Heldman

Israel Institute for Biological Research
Ness-Ziona, Israel

INTRODUCTION

Alzheimer's disease (AD) is characterized, *inter alia*, by synaptic loss, neurofibrillary tangles, amyloid plaques containing the β-amyloid peptide (Aβ), and degeneration of cholinergic neurons that ascend from the basal forebrain to cortical and hippocampal areas (reviewed by Court and Perry, 1991). A presynaptic cholinergic hypofunction, as one of the major neuronal events in AD, is reflected, *inter alia*, in reduced levels of acetylcholine (ACh), acetylcholinesterase (AChE) and choline acetyltransferase (ChAT). As a result of neuronal degeneration, the density of presynaptic M2 muscarinic receptors (mAChR) is significantly decreased in AD, yet post-synaptic M1 mAChR are relatively unchanged in AD (review by Court and Perry, 1991) (*vide infra* for further discussion). Degeneration of cholinergic neurons in AD is presumably a principal cause of the dementia. The "cholinergic hypothesis" in AD implies that a cholinergic replacement therapy might be beneficial in alleviating some of the cognitive dysfunctions in this disorder (Court and Perry, 1991). Highly selective m1 agonists, producing cellular excitation, should be beneficial in AD, regardless of the extent of degeneration of presynaptic cholinergic projections to the frontal cortex or hippocampus. This represents the most relevant approach of cholinergic treatment due to the role of M1 mAChRs in memory and learning processing (Fisher and Barak, 1994, Fisher, 1997). The present overview is an attempt to address some of these findings and to propose an unifying hypotheses regarding m1 selective agonists aimed at treatment and therapy of AD.

mAChR SUBTYPES AS A TARGET FOR NOVEL TREATMENTS IN AD

Five structurally different human mAChR subtypes (m1-m5) genes have been cloned and expressed in suitable cell systems (reviewed by Hulme et al., 1990). The five

Progress in Alzheimer's and Parkinson's Diseases
edited by Fisher *et al.*, Plenum Press, New York, 1998.

mAChR subtypes belong to the family of cell surface receptors coupled to guanosine-triphosphate-binding proteins (G-proteins). When expressed in mammalian cells, these mAChR subtypes mediate a variety of signal transduction pathways (Hulme et al., 1990). The plethora of signal transduction pathways and responses mediated by the mAChR subtypes, in general and by each subtype, in particular, provides a broad potential for chemical inventiveness of muscarinic agonists (Fisher and Barak, 1994).

NEW MUSCARINIC AGONISTS

A number of selective M1 agonists have been reported. These agonists are in fact functionally selective compounds, showing the highest activity towards M1 mAChR (reviews: Fisher and Barak, 1994; Fisher 1997). These compounds are partial agonists, at least in some of the standard assays. The functional selectivity observed *in vitro* for the M1 mAChR by the new putative m1 agonists is reflected *in vivo* by a reduced side-effect profile in the peripheral and/or the central nervous system (Fisher and Barak, 1994). In general, selectivity among all the compounds reported has been achieved by a reduced functional activity at M2 or M3 mAChR while maintaining a modest degree of agonistic activity at M1 mAChR. By using some compounds from the *AF series* an attempt is made to overview some preclinical properties of m1 muscarinic agonists with relevance to AD treatment.

DISTINCT ACTIVATION OF M1 mAChR-MEDIATED SIGNAL TRANSDUCTION

The *AF series* compounds are full agonists when assayed for elevating $[Ca^{2+}]i$ in Chinese hamster ovary (CHO) cells stably transfected with cloned M1 mAChR. In CHO and in rat pheochromocytoma (PC12) cells stably transfected with M1 mAChR (PC12M1) [*re* Pinkas-Kramarski et al., 1992], AF102B and AF150(S) are partial agonists, while AF150, AF151, and AF151(S) are full agonists in stimulating phosphoinositide (PI) hydrolysis or arachidonic acid release. Yet, all these compounds behave as antagonists when compared with carbachol (CCh) in elevating cAMP levels (Fisher and Barak, 1994; Gurwitz et al., 1994). These data imply that selective muscarinic ligands may activate distinct sets of G-proteins and that drug selectivity may extend beyond the ligand recognition site (Gurwitz et al., 1994). No reports on distinct signal tranductions have been published with the other putative m1 agonists. It can be implied that some of these should have a similar profile to the *AF series*.

NEUROTROPHIC-LIKE EFFECTS OF MUSCARINIC AGONISTS

Neurite outgrowth was observed for oxotremorine and CCh in PC12M1 cells, and this effect was synergistic with nerve growth factor (NGF) (Pinkas-Kramarski et al., 1992). AF102B and AF150(S) induced only minimal neurite outgrowth, the effect was strongly synergistic with NGF and was atropine-sensitive (Fisher and Barak 1994; Gurwitz et al., 1995). The M1 mAChR-associated biochemical signals responsible for this synergistic response in PC12M1 cells did not seem to involve changes in either PI hydrolysis or cAMP levels (Pinkas-Kramarski et al., 1992; Gurwitz et al., 1995). Studies by Mount et al., (1994) show that cerebellar Purkinje cell survival is under the trophic control of ACh, acting *via* M1 mAChR. Similar results were reported for the *AF series* (Alberch et al., 1995). These m1 agonists elicited dose-dependent increases of survival of diverse populations of cultured primary CNS neurons (*e.g.* Purkinje and striatal neurons). NGF potentiated the trophic action of low agonist concentrations (Alberch et al., 1995). Thus m1 selective muscarinic agonists may be capable of promoting neurotrophic responses in brain neurons, as well. The complete mechanism underlying neurotrophic-like effects by these m1 muscarinic agonists, which is dependent on the presence of NGF, remains yet to be elucidated. Receptor coupling to phospholipase C and/or arachidonic acid release may underlie these actions (Alberch et al., 1995). It can be deduced that these m1 agonists exert neurotrophic activities in conjunction with some signal(s) mediated in part *via* NGF receptors (Fisher et al., 1997). Some of the neurotrophic-like effects induced by such agonists may involve increased release of APPs following activation of m1AChR (*vide infra*). Notably, the secreted forms of APPs, are known to regulate neurite outgrowth and to promote neuronal survival (Mattson, 1994). No data on neurotrophic-like effect were published with the other putative m1 agonists. It can be implied that some of these agonists should have a similar profile to the *AF series*.

M1 mAChR-STIMULATED APPS

Mismetabolism of amyloid precursor proteins (APP) may induce AD (Mattson, 1994). Recent studies indicate that some apparently different neuropathological damages in the AD brain may be linked. In particular, a relation between the formation of Aβ peptide and amyloid plaques, and the loss of cholinergic function in AD brains was reported (Nitsch et al., 1992). As originally demonstrated by Nitsch et al., (1992) and later by other labs (Buxbaum et al., 1992; Lahiri et al., 1992; Haring et al., 1994; Eckols et al., 1995), cholinergic stimulation of M1 mAChRs can increase cleavage of APP in the middle of its β-amyloid region. This cleavage produces the secreted, non-amyloidogenic APP (APPs), preventing the formation of Aβ peptide. The secretion is thought to be mediated by an, as yet, unidentified protease(s) designated α-secretase. Increased secretion of APP by cells treated with cholinergic agonists results in decreased synthesis of Aβ (Hung et al., 1993; Wolf et al., 1995), a major component of the amyloid plaques.

Stimulation of M1 mAChR by AF102B in PC12M1 cells enhances secretion of amyloid precursor protein (APPs) to the culture medium, and lowers the level of membrane associated APPs (Haring et al., 1994). The enhanced APPs secretion induced by AF102B is potentiated by NGF and blocked by atropine (Haring et al., 1995). AF102B, AF150(S) (Fisher, unpublished data) and other m1 selective agonists like xanomeline (Eckols et al., 1995), WAL-2014 (Stransky et al., 1995), or non-selective agonists like CI-979 (Emmerling et al., 1997). These agents also increase APPs release from CHO cell cultures. Increased APPs secretion by CCh or AF102B from rat cortical slices was also reported (Pittel et al., 1996). WAL 2014, an m1 functionally selective agonist, showed a similar profile to AF102B in cortical slices. In this study, however, CCh increased APPs only in presence of an m2 antagonist (gallamine), suggesting that activation of M2 mAChR suppresses APPs formation (Farber et al., 1995). If activation of M2 mAChR suppresses APPs release, this can have a major impact on the development of subtype selective muscarinic agonists. The more selective the agonist is for M1 mAChR, the better chances it should have to modulate APP processing in the brain (*re* also Farber et al., 1995; Muller et al., 1997).

In vivo studies in rats have shown that the levels of APPs in the cerebrospinal fluid (CSF) can be regulated by pharmacological manipulation of the cholinergic system. In naive rats certain cholinesterase inhibitors or AF102B reduced APPs in the CSF (Haroutunian et al., this book).

Very few reports suggests that m1 selective agonists may have a role in affecting APP processing in AD. In a small clinical trial it was found that AF102B, but not physostigmine or hydroxychloroquine, reduced the level of Aβ in the CSF from AD patients treated for 4 weeks with one of the 3 compounds (Nitsch, this book). Of the 12 patients receiving AF102B, seven showed at least a 20% reduction in Aβ levels in the CSF. These preliminary results, once corroborated in larger studies, may indicate that m1 agonists have an important role also in affecting Aβ levels in AD patients. Lack of an effect on APP processing by physostigmine may point towards a major role of specificity of an mAChR subtype in APP processing [i.e. M1 (and M3) mAChR]. An increased synaptic concentration of ACh, due to AChE inhibition, may not be sufficient to decrease Aβ level. ACh is an agonist for all mAChR subtypes, but activation of M2 and M4 mAChRs may cancel M1 mAChR-induced effects on APP processing (Muller et al., 1997).

M1 mAChR-DEPHOSPHORYLATION OF *TAU* PROTEINS

Tau microtubule-associated protein is neuronal specific, and its expression is necessary for neurite outgrowth. Hyperphosphorylated *tau* proteins are the principal fibrous component of the neurofibrillary tangle pathology in AD (reviewed by Goedert, 1993). Stimulation of M1 mAChR in PC12M1 cells with CCh or AF102B decreased *tau* phosphorylation as indicated by specific *tau* monoclonal antibodies which recognize phosphorylation-dependent epitopes and by alkaline phosphatase treatment (Sadot et al., 1996). In addition, a synergistic effect on *tau* phosphorylation was found between treatments with these muscarinic agonists and NGF (Sadot et al., 1996). No reports on *tau* dephosphorylation were published with the other putative m1 agonists. It can be implied that some of these agonists should have a similar profile to the *AF series*.

STUDIES IN ANIMAL MODELS

Some of the m1 agonists, including the *AF series*, were tested in a variety of such animal models (reviewed by Fisher and Barak, 1994). Thus, AF102B, AF150(S) and some of its congeners restored memory and learning deficits in a variety of animal models, which mimic cholinergic deficits reported in AD, without producing adverse central and peripheral side-effects at effective doses and showing a relatively wide safety margin.

Recent studies suggest that the extent of brain cholinergic degeneration in AD is most pronounced in patients who are homozygous for the E4 allele of apolipoprotein E (apoE) (Roses, 1994). This led to the suggestion that apoE plays a specifically important role in brain cholinergic function and that the E4 allele of apoE (apoE4), which is a major AD risk factor, may be a predictor of the extent of cholinergic dysfunction and of the efficacy of cholinergic therapy in this disease (Poirier et al., 1995). Animal model studies along these lines revealed that apoE-deficient (knockout) mice are cognitively impaired and that their memory deficit is associated with distinct dysfunction of basal forebrain cholinergic neurons (Gordon et al., 1995; Chapman and Michaelson, in press). Treatment of apoE-deficient mice with AF150(S) for three weeks completely abolished their working memory impairments in a Morris Water Maze. Furthermore, this cognitive improvement was associated with a parallel increase of brain ChAT and AChE levels, and in the recovery of these cholinergic markers back to control levels. These findings show that apoE deficiency-related cognitive and cholinergic deficits can be ameliorated by the m1 selective agonist AF150(S). This provides a unique value for m1 agonists in the treatment of AD (Fisher et al., 1997).

CLINICAL STUDIES

It is beyond the scope of this paper to summarize in detail clinical studies with m1 agonists, since the information available is incomplete, preliminary or undisclosed, and most of the clinical studies are still ongoing. Very few clinical results with m1 functionally selective agonists have already been reported (reviewed by Fisher, 1997). Muscarinic agonists that have reached already some phases of clinical trials include at least: AF102B, xanomeline, SB-202026, WAL-2014 YM-796 and Lu 25-109. milameline (CI-979), a non-selective muscarinic agonist, is also presently in clinical trials (Fisher, 1997).

DISCUSSION AND FUTURE PERSPECTIVES

An effective therapy for AD is to treat the cognitive disorders of AD patients. Originally the cholinergic approach was aimed only at treating the symptoms of AD, such as memory loss and cognitive dysfunctions. Such effective treatment strategies could provide patients with some improved cognitive functions in the early and moderate stages of the disease. However, without knowing the etiology of AD, the recent data with m1 muscarinic agonists indicate that also some aspects of therapeutic solutions can be identified within such compounds.

Following interaction with the M1 mAChR, selective responses are presumably achieved when the agonist-mAChR complex activates only *certain* G-proteins, which in turn activate *distinct* signal transduction pathways. The *AF series* compounds exhibit such an activity. It is expected that similar select activities will be shown with some other m1 selective agonists. The notion of *"ligand-mediated selective signaling"* (Gurwitz et al., 1994), *e.g.*, activation of only distinct G-protein subset(s) (but not Gs), might be of clinical significance, since altered signal transduction *via* Gs might be relevant in the pathophysiology of AD (Harrison et al., 1991). As a hypothesis we can suggest that the desired M1- or m1-selective agonists for the treatment of AD, should not stimulate adenylyl cyclase via M1 mAChR, but should still activate PI hydrolysis (Fisher and Barak., 1994; Gurwitz et al., 1994). In case this hypothesis is valid, it can raise serious questions as to the long term use in AD patients of some highly efficacious muscarinic agonists which can activate all M1 mAChR-mediated signal transductions in a promiscuous way including the M1 mAChR coupling with Gs, leading eventually to an increased cAMP level in the brain. The same caution should be given to AChE inhibitors in a long term treatment in AD since in such a scenario elevated ACh levels, due to AChE inhibition, can again enhance brain cAMP levels.

What might be some potential consequences of increased cAMP due to M1 (and M3) mAChR activation? In AD M2 mAChR are reduced (Court and Perry, 1991). Less stimulation of M2 mAChR by ACh would reduce Gi activation, the G-protein which mediates inhibition of adenylate cyclase. This could lead to elevated cAMP levels, which could activate cAMP-dependent protein kinase (protein kinase A). Protein kinase A, about one third of which is associated with microtubule-associated proteins, can overphosphorylate *tau* proteins (reviewed by Jope, 1996). Thus it is possible that a combined loss of ACh-induced presynaptic signalling, due to decreased ACh release and reduced M2 mAChR, together with post-synaptic activation of M1 (and M3 mAChR)-mediated elevation in cAMP [by a very potent agonist (e.g. a full m1 agonist) or increase in ACh levels (due to inhibition of AChE)] contribute to activated kinases which progressively can elevate hyperphosphorylated *tau* (also reviewed by Jope, 1996).

The above findings may be linked with the enhanced secretion of APPs following stimulation of M1 mAChR by the *AF series* compounds and other functionally m1 selective agonists. Thus activation of M1 mAChR leads to opposite effects on APPs secretion and Aβ production Consequently, M1 (or m1) agonists may be of value in preventing amyloid formation by selectively promoting the "α-secretase" processing pathway in AD, suggested originally by Nitsch et al., (1992) and later by others (Buxbaum et al., 1992; Lahiri et al., 1992; Hung et al., 1993; Haring et al., 1994; Eckols et al., 1995; Farber et al., 1995; Wolf et al., 1995; Pittel et al., 1996; Emmerling et al., 1997; Muller et al., 1997). Based on our results (Pittel et al., 1996) and data reported from other labs (Farber et al., 1995; Muller et al., 1997) it can be deduced that m1 selective agonists may alter APP processing in cortex and hippocampus where M1 (and M3) mAChRs are abundant.

Recent studies show that activation of mAChR in cultured cerebellar neurons (Yan et al., 1996) and of M1 mAChR inhibits apoptosis in PC12M1 cells (Lindenboim et al., 1995). This is an additional and important value of m1 agonists emphasizing again that activation of M1 mAChRs is therefore a most viable strategy to delay progression of AD.

Neurotrophic-like effects of M1 mAChR stimulation can promote regeneration or cell rescue and therefore, slow down degeneration (Fisher, 1997). If such effects will be demonstrated *in vivo*, these might have important clinical relevance and may constitute a novel treatment for AD. Notably, NGF does not cross the blood-brain barrier. A more practical approach would involve modulation of the function of endogenous NGF (and perhaps other neurotrophines) by a synergistic agent such as an M1 (or m1) agonist.

The decreased phosphorylation of *tau* protein via M1 mAChR deserves special attention. This suggests for the first time a linkage between the muscarinic signal transduction system(s) and the neuronal cytoskeleton, *via* regulation of phosphorylation of *tau* microtubule-associated protein (Sadot et al., 1996). Moreover, these studies propose a possible correlation between the cholinergic deficiency and *tau* hyperphosphorylation in AD. It can be speculated that activation of M1 mAChRs might provide a novel treatment strategy for AD by modifying *tau* processing in the brain and perhaps delaying the formation and accumulation of overphosphorylated *tau*. Thus M1 (or m1) agonists, in addition to the expected use as a cholinergic replacement strategy, might have a more important and complex role and be of unique value in delaying the progression of AD.

A UNIFYING HYPOTHESIS OF M1 AGONISTS REGARDING AD TREATMENT AND THERAPY

A cholinergic hypofunction in AD may lead to formation of β-amyloids which might impair the coupling of mAChR with G-proteins (Jope, 1996; Kelly et al., 1996). This uncoupling leads to decreased signal transduction, a reduction in levels of trophic secreted amyloid precursor proteins (APPs) and generation of more Aβ. Aβ can also suppress ACh synthesis and release, aggravating further the cholinergic deficiency (Abe et al., 1994; Hoshi et al., 1997). This "viscious cycle", due to lack of ACh in early stages of the disease, may be prevented by m1 selective agonists that, unlike AChE inhibitors, are less limited by the extent of degeneration of presynaptic cholinergic projections in AD (*re* also reservations raised above regarding AChE inhibitors). Based upon the findings described in this review about m1 agonists, a *unifying hypothesis* for the treatment and delaying progress of AD with m1 muscarinic agonists can be proposed. It appears that activation of M1 mAChR is beneficially modulating certain molecules, risk factors and dysfunctions which are associated with AD. These include among other: certain G-proteins, amyloids, *tau*, ApoE, neurotrophins, presenilin-1 (for presenilin-1; Nitsch, personal communication). Interestingly, activation of m1 mAChR promotes also expression of the Egr gene family of transcription factors (Nitsch, personal communication). Although the relevance of some of these exciting new findings in AD remains yet to be elucidated, m1 agonists may represent the next generation of therapies in AD, due to the positive role of M1 mAChR on most of the identified culprits and risk factors in AD. Long term use of m1 agonists in early stage AD patients and/or other populations at risk may provide the value of this strategy in treatment and in delaying the onset or progression of AD. As a future goal, clinical studies can be envisaged to determine whether preventive strategies with m1 agonists, which may decrease Aß and prevent *tau* overphosphorylation, reduce the risk of getting AD, delay its onset, and/or slow its clinical progressive course.

REFERENCES

Abe, E., Casamenti, F., Giovannelli, L., Scali, C. and Pepeu G., 1994, Administration of amyloid beta- peptides into the medial septum of rats decreases acetylcholine release from hippocampus *in vivo*. *Brain Res.* 636:162–164.

Alberch, J., Gurwitz, D., Fisher, A., and Mount H.T.S., 1995, Novel muscarinic M1receptor agonists promote survival of CNS neurons in primary cell culture. *Soc. Neurosci.* Abst. 21:2040.

Buxbaum, J.D., Oishi, M., Chen, H.I., Pinkas-Kramarski, R., Jaffe, E.A., Grandy, S.E. and Greengard, P., 1992, Cholinergic agonists and interleukin 1 regulate processing and secretion of the Alzheimer β/A4 amyloid protein precursor. *Proc. Natl. Acad. Sci.* USA. 89:10075–10078.

Chapman, S., and Michaelson, D.M., Impairments of cholinergic but not of nigrostriatal dopaminergic projections in apolipoprotein E deficient mice. *J. Neurochem.*, in press.

Court, J.A., and Perry, E.K., 1991, Dementia: the neurochemical basis of putative transmitter orientated therapy. *Pharmacol. Ther.* 52: 423–443.

Eckols, K., Bymaster, F.P., Mitch, C.H., Shannon, H.E., Ward, Y.S., Delapp, N.W., 1995, The muscarinic M1 agonist xanomeline increases soluble amyloid precursor protein release from CHO m1 cells. *Life Sci.* 57:1183–1190.

Emmerling, M.R., Schwarz, R.D., Spiegel, and Collahan, M.J., 1997, New perspectives on developing muscarinic agonists for treating Azheimer's disease. *Alzheimer's Dis.* 2[4].

Farber, S.A., Nitsch, R.M., Schulz, J.G., and Wurtman, R.J., 1995, Regulated secretion of β-amyloid precursor protein in rat brain. *J. Neurosci.*15:7442–7451.

Fisher, A., and Barak, D., 1994, Progress and perspectives in new muscarinic agonists. *Drug News & Perspectives* 7:453–464.

Fisher, A, 1997, Muscarinic agonists for the treatment of Alzheimer's disease: progress and perspectives. *Exp.Opin. Invest. Drugs* 6:1395–1411.

Fisher, A., Brandeis, R., Chapman, S., Pittel, Z., Michaelson D.M., M1 muscarinic agonist treatment reverses cognitive and cholinergic impairments of apolipoprotein E-deficient mice. *J. Neurochem.*, in press.

Goedert, M., 1993, Tau protein and the neurofibrillary pathology of Alzheimer's disease. *Trends Neurosci.* 16:460–465.

Gordon, I., Grauer, E., Genis, I., Sehayek, E., and Michaelson, D.M., 1995, Memory deficits and cholinergic impairments in apolipoprotein E-deficient mice. *Neurosci. Lett.* 199:1–4.

Gurwitz, D., Haring, R., Heldman, E., Fraser, M.C., Maor, C.M., and Fisher, A., 1994, Discrete activation of transduction pathways associated with acetylcholine m1 receptor by several muscarinic ligands. *Eur. J. Pharmacol. (Mol. Pharmacol.)* 267:21–31.

Gurwitz, D., Haring, R., Heldman, E., Pinkas-Kramarski, R., Stein, R., and Fisher, A., 1995, NGF- dependent neurotrophic-like effects of AF102B, an M1muscarinic agonist, in PC12M1 cells. *NeuroReport* 6:485–488.

Haring, R., Gurwitz, D., Barg, J., Pinkas-Kramarski, R., Heldman, E., Pittel, Z., Wengier, A., Meshulam, H., Marciano, D., Karton, Y., and Fisher, A., 1994, Amyloid precursor protein secretion via muscarinic receptors: Reduced desensitization using the M1-selective agonist AF102B. *Biochem. Biophys. Res. Comm.* 203:652–658.

Haring, R., Gurwitz, D., Barg, J., Pinkas-Kramarski, R., Heldman, E., Pittel, Z., Danenberg, H.D., Wengier, A., Meshulam, H., Marciano, D., Karton, Y. and Fisher, A., 1995, NGF promotes amyloid protein secretion via muscarinic receptor activation. *Biochem. Biophys. Res. Comm.* 213:15–23.

Harrison, P.J., Barton, A. J.L., McDonald, B., and Pearson, R.C.A., 1991, Alzheimer's disease: specific increases in a G-protein subunit (Gsα) mRN in hippocampal and cortical neurons. *Mol. Brain Res.*10:71–81.

Hoshi, M., Takashima, A., Murayama, M., Yasutake, K., Yoshida, N., Ishiguro, K., Hoshino, T., and Imahori, K., 1997, Nontoxic amyloid β peptide$_{1-42}$ suppresses acetylcholine synthesis. *J. Biol. Chem.* 272:2038–2041.

Hulme, E.C., Birdsall, N.J.M., and Buckley, N.J., 1990, Muscarinic receptor subtypes. *Ann. Rev. Pharmacol. Toxicol.* 30:633–673.

Hung, A.Y., Haass, C., Nitsch, R.T., Qiu, W.O., Citron, M., Wurtman, R.J., Growdon, J.M., and Selkoe, D.J., 1993, Activation of protein kinase C inhibits cellular production of the amyloid β-protein. *J. Biol. Chem.* 268:22959–22962.

Jope, R.S., 1996, Cholinergic muscarinic receptor signalling by phosphoinositides signal transduction system in Alzheimer's disease. *Alzheimer's Dis. Rev.*1:2–14.

Kelly, J.F., Furukawa, K., Barger, S.W., Rengen, M.R., Mark, R.J., Blanc, E.M., Roth, G.S., and Mattson, M.P., 1996, Amyloid β-peptide disrupts carbachol-induced muscarinic cholinergic signal transduction in cortical neurons. *Proc. Natl. Acad. Sci.* 96:6753–6758.

Lahiri, D.K., Nall, C., and Farlow, M.R., 1992, The cholinergic agonist carbachol reduces intracellular β- amyloid precursor protein in PC12 and C6 cells. *Biochem. Int.* 28:853–860.

Lindenboim, L., Pinkas-Kramarski, R., Sokolovsky, M., and Stein, R., 1995, Activation of muscarinic receptors inhibits apoptosis in PC12M1 cells. *J. Neurochem.* 64:2491–2499.

Mattson, M.P., 1994, Secreted forms of beta-amyloid precursor proteins modulate dendrite outgrowth and calcium responses to glutamate in cultured embryonic hippocampal neurons. *J. Neurobiol.* 25:439–450.

Mount, H.T.J., Dreyfus, C.F., and Black, I.B., 1994, Muscarinic stimulation promotes cultured Purkinje cell survival: A role for acetylcholine in cerebellar development? *J. Neurochem.* 63:2065–2073.

Muller, D.M., Mendla, K., and Farber, S.A., 1997, Muscarinic M1 receptor agonists increase the secretion of the amyloid precursor protein ectodomain. *Life Sci.* 60:985–991.

Nitsch, R.N., Slack, B.E., Wurtman, R.J., and Growdon, J.H., 1992, Release of Alzheimer amyloid precursor derivatives stimulated by activation of muscarinic acetylcholine receptors. *Science.* 258:304–307.

Pinkas-Kramarski, R., Stein, R., Lindenboim, L., and Sokolovsky, M., 1992, Growth factor-like effects mediated by muscarinic receptors in PC12M1 cells. *J. Neurochem.* 59:2158–2166.

Pittel, Z., Heldman, E., Barg, J., Haring, R., and Fisher, A., 1996, Muscarinic control of amyloid precursor protein secretion in rat cerbral cortex and cerebellum. *Brain Res.* 742:299–304.

Poirier, J., Delisle, M.-C., Quirion, R., Auberts, I., Farlowm M., Hui, S., Bertrand, P., Nalbantoglu, J., and Grefix, B.M., 1995, Apolipoprotein E4 allele as a predictor of cholinergic deficits and treatment outcome in Alzheimer disease. *Proc. Natl. Acad. Sci.* 92:12260–12264.

Roses, A.D., 1994, Apolipoprotein E affects the rate of Alzheimer disease expression: beta-amyloid burden is of secondary consequence dependent on APOE genotype and duration of disease. *J. Neuropathol. Exp. Neurol.* 53:429–437.

Sadot, E., Gurwitz, D., Barg, J.,Behar, L., Ginzburg, I., and Fisher, A., 1966, Activation of m1- muscarinic acetylcholine receptor regulates tau phophorylation in transfected PC12 cells. *J. Neurochem.* 66:877–880.

Stransky, W., Mendla, K.D., and Briem, H., 1995, WAL 2014 FU, an M1 agonist which influences APP secretion. 2nd Symp. Med. Chem. *Approaches to Alzheimer's Disease* (Aug 28–30, Strasbourg).

Wolf, B.A., Wertkin, A.M., Jolly, Y.C., Yasuda, R.P., Wolfe, B.B., Manning, D., Ravi, S., Williamson, J.R., and Lee, V.M.-Y., 1995, Muscarinic regulation of Alzheimer's disease amyloid precursor protein secretion and amyloid beta-protein production in human neuronal NT2N cells. *J. Biol. Chem.* 270:4916–4922.

Yan, G.M., Lin, S.Z., Irwin, R.P., and Paul, S.M., 1996, Activation of muscarinic cholinergic receptors blocks apoptosis of cultured cerebellar granule neurons. *Mol. Pharmacol.* 47:257.

75

CRYSTALLOGRAPHIC STUDIES ON COMPLEXES OF ACETYLCHOLINESTERASE WITH THE NATURAL CHOLINESTERASE INHIBITORS FASCICULIN AND HUPERZINE A

Israel Silman, Michal Harel, Mia Raves, and Joel L. Sussman

Departments of Neurobiology and Structural Biology
Weizmann Institute of Science
Rehovoth 76100, Israel

INTRODUCTION

Acetylcholinesterase (AChE) terminates synaptic transmission at cholinergic synapses by rapid hydrolysis of acetylcholine (ACh) (Quinn, 1987). Anticholinesterase agents are used in the treatment of various disorders (Taylor, 1990), and have been proposed as therapeutic agents for the management of Alzheimer's disease (Giacobini & Becker, 1991, 1994). Two such anti- cholinesterase agents, both of which act as reversible inhibitors of AChE, have been licensed by the FDA: tacrine (Gauthier & Gauthier, 1991), under the trade name Cognex, and, more recently, E2020 (Sugimoto *et al.*, 1992), under the trade name Aricept. Several other anticholinesterase agents are at advanced stages of clinical evaluation. The active site of AChE contains a catalytic subsite, and a so-called 'anionic' subsite, which binds the quaternary group of ACh (Quinn, 1987). A second, 'peripheral' anionic site is so named since it is distant from the active site (Taylor & Lappi, 1975). Bisquaternary inhibitors of AChE derive their enhanced potency, relative to homologous monoquaternary ligands (Main, 1976), from their ability to span these two 'anionic' sites, which are *ca.* 14 Å apart.

The 3D structure of *Torpedo* AChE (Sussman *et al.*, 1991) reveals that, like other serine hydrolases, it contains a catalytic triad. Unexpectedly, however, for such a rapid enzyme, the active site is located at the bottom of a deep and narrow cavity; this cavity was named the 'aromatic gorge', since >50% of its lining is composed of the rings of 14 conserved amino acids (Sussman *et al.*, 1991; Axelsen *et al.*, 1994).

X-ray crystallographic studies of complexes of AChE with drugs of pharmacological interest can reveal which amino acid residues are important for binding the drug, and where space might exist for modifying the drug itself, information crucial for structure-based drug design. Valuable information can also be achieved by site-directed mutagenesis (Harel *et al.*, 1992). In earlier studies (Harel *et al.*, 1993), we described the structures of complexes of *Torpedo* AChE (TcAChE) with three ligands of pharmacological interest: namely, edrophonium, a strong competitive AChE inhibitor (Wilson & Quan, 1958), whose pharmacological action is in the peripheral nervous system (Taylor, 1990); de-camethonium, a bisquaternary ligand which is both a neuromuscular blocker and a choli-nesterase inhibitor (Zaimis, 1976); and tacrine, already licensed as an anti-Alzheimer drug (see above), which is also a strong reversible inhibitor (Heilbronn, 1961). Modelling had predicted that the principal interaction of the quaternary group of ACh would be with Trp84, via electrostatic interaction with the π electrons of its indole ring (Sussman *et al.*, 1991), rather than with a cluster of acidic amino acids, as had been predicted previously (Nolte *et al.*, 1980); such an assignment was also supported by affinity labelling (Weise *et al.*, 1990). The crystallographic data fully confirmed this unexpected interaction (Harel *et al.*, 1993). Furthermore, they revealed a prominent role for others of the conserved aro-matic residues within the gorge. Thus the phenyl ring of Phe330 contributed substantially to the 'anionic' subsite of the active site, while the 'peripheral' anionic site, located at the top of the gorge, contained three aromatic residues, Tyr70, Tyr121 and Trp279. The inter-action of the two quaternary groups of decamethonium, located at the top and the bottom of the gorge, was primarily with these two sets of aromatic residues (Harel *et al.*, 1993).

In the following, we describe the structure of two additional TcAChE-ligand com-plexes recently solved in our laboratory: with fasciculin-II (FAS), a member of the three-finger polypeptide toxin family, which was isolated from mamba venom (Harel *et al.*, 1995); and with (−)-huperzine A (HupA), an alkaloid purified from a moss used in Chi-nese herbal medicine (Raves *et al.*, 1997).

RESULTS AND DISCUSSION

FAS-TcAChE Complex

The venoms of elapid snakes, including the Asian cobras and kraits, as well as the Afri-can mambas, contain a number of small proteins, containing 60–70 amino acids, which dis-play a broad spectrum of toxic activities (Harvey, 1991). Among the best studied are the α-neurotoxins of the venoms of the kraits and cobras, such as α-bungarotoxin, from the For-mosan krait, *Bungarus multicinctus,* which are potent and specific blockers of the nicotinic acetylcholine receptor (Changeux *et al., 1970*). Other toxins of this family have been shown to act as blockers of ion channels (Albrand *et al.*, 1995), muscarinic agonists (Ségalas *et al.*, 1995) and anticholinesterases (Cerveñansky *et al.*, 1991). Despite their diverse biological ac-tivities, they display substantial sequence and structural homology. X-ray and NMR studies show that the toxins share a common structural motif: a core, containing four disulfide bridges, from which three loops protrude, roughly like the fingers of a hand (le Du *et al.*, 1992). Accordingly, they are known as the three-fingered toxin family (Wonnacott & Dajas, 1994). Superposition of their structures reveals that, whereas the structure of the central core is conserved, the orientation of the fingers can vary considerably (Albrand *et al.*, 1995), sug-gesting that they serve as determinants of biological specificity. No three-dimensional struc-ture of a complex of a three-fingered toxin with its target was, however, available.

Whereas in previous cases, the AChE-ligand complex was obtained by soaking the ligand into crystals of the native enzyme, FAS is too large to permit such an approach. Ac-cordingly, orthorhombic crystals of the complex were obtained from a solution containing

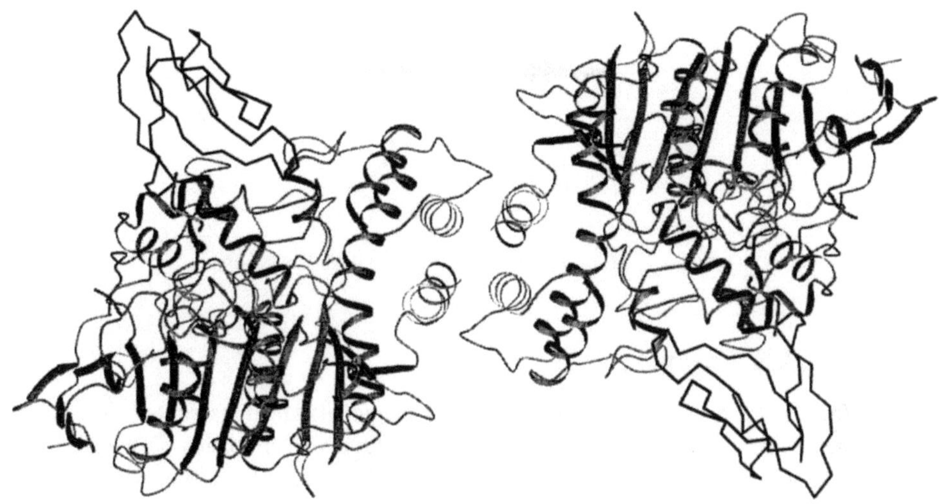

Figure 1. Stoichiometric complex of fasciculin-II (FAS) with TcAChE. Shown is a ribbon diagram of the biological dimer, in which the two subunits interact via a 4-helix bundle and a disulfide bridge (not shown). The two FAS molecules, displayed as a line trace, are positioned over the top of the gorge leading to the active site of each subunit.

stoichiometric (1:1) amounts of the purified TcAChE and of FAS purified from the venom of the green mamba (*Dendroaspis angusticeps*), and a data set was obtained which could be refined at 3.0 Å resolution. The structure indeed reveals a stoichiometric complex, with one FAS molecule bound to each subunit of the TcAChE dimer (Fig. 1). FAS is bound on the surface of the subunit, at the 'peripheral' anionic site, thus sealing the top of the narrow gorge leading to the active site. A similar structure was reported independently, by Bourne *et al.* (1995), for a complex of FAS with mouse recombinant AChE.

It has been noted previously that AChE has a large dipole moment (>1000 Debye), aligned approximately along the axis of the 'aromatic' gorge (Ripoll *et al.*, 1993; Porschke *et al.*, 1996). The field generated by this dipole might actually draw the positively charged substrate, ACh, down the gorge towards the active site. Similarly, FAS has its charges separated (dipole moment *ca.* 185 Debye), with most basic residues occurring in the first two fingers, which make intimate contact with TcAChE, and most acidic residues in the third finger. Visual inspection suggests that the two dipole moments are roughly aligned, and electrostatic calculations show that the angle between the dipole vectors is only 30°.

The high affinity of FAS for AChE can be attributed to many residues either unique to FAS or rare in other three-fingered toxins (Giles *et al.*, 1997), and to a remarkable surface complementarity, involving a large contact area (2000 Å²). This is substantially larger, for example, than the contact area between lysozyme and an antibody raised against it, 1700 Å², or between trypsin and bovine pancreatic trypsin inhibitor, 1400 Å² (Janin & Chothia, 1990). A most striking and rare interaction is a stacking of the side chains of Met33 in FAS and of Trp279 in *Torpedo* AChE. Mutation of this tryptophan residue to a nonaromatic residue decreases the affinity of FAS for AChE by over five orders of magnitude (Radic *et al.*, 1994), and its absence from the AChEs cloned so far from avian and invertebrate sources (e.g. Eichler *et al.*, 1994; Cousin *et al.*, 1996), as well as from butyrylcholinesterase BChE (Harel *et al.*, 1992), provides a clear structural explanation for their poor inhibition by FAS.

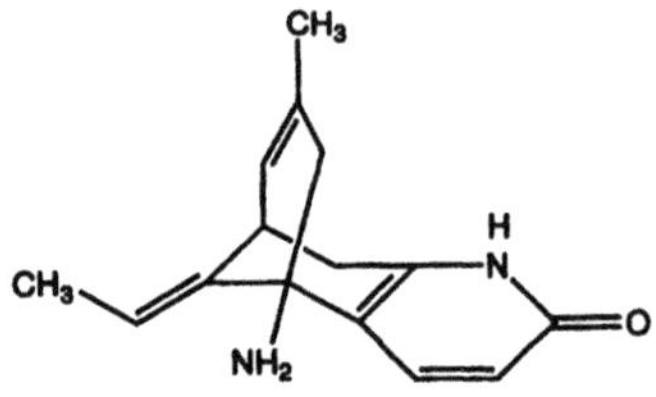

Figure 2. Molecular structure of (−)-huperzine A (HupA).

HupA-TcAChE Complex

(−)-Huperzine A (HupA, Fig. 2) is a nootropic alkaloid extracted from the club moss, *Huperzia serrata*, which has been used in China for centuries as a folk medicine (Liu *et al.*, 1986). HupA is a potent reversible inhibitor of AChE that lacks potentially complicating muscarinic effects (Kozikowski *et al.*, 1992). The existence of a natural AChE inhibitor, taken together with its unique pharmacological features and relative lack of toxicity (Laganière *et al.*, 1991), render HupA a particularly promising candidate for treatment of Alzheimer's disease. Indeed, studies on experimental animals reveal significant cognitive enhancement (Xiong *et al.*, 1995), and clinical trials in China have both established the safety of HupA, and provided preliminary evidence for significant effects on patients exhibiting dementia and memory disorders (Zhang *et al.*, 1991). The structure of HupA reveals no obvious similarity to that of ACh. In fact, a number of studies, utilising either computerised docking techniques and/or site-directed mutagenesis (Ashani *et al.*, 1994; Pang *et al.*, 1994; Saxena *et al.*, 1994), predicted various possible orientations of HupA within the active site of AChE. It seemed, therefore, desirable to solve the structure of a TcAChE-HupA complex by X-ray crystallography. It would thus be possible to establish that it indeed binds at the active-site and to determine its correct orientation, thus providing the basis for future structure-based drug design.

Soaking of HupA into native trigonal crystals of *Torpedo* AChE yielded a crystalline complex from which a data set was collected which could be refined to 2.5 Å resolution. Examination of a difference map for the complex, as compared to the native enzyme, clearly revealed a prominent electron density peak near the bottom of the 'aromatic gorge' with an outline resembling that of HupA. Indeed, excellent fitting of the molecule to the electron density was obtained.

The crystal structure of the HupA-TcAChE complex (Fig. 3) shows an unexpected orientation for the inhibitor, with surprisingly few strong direct interactions with protein residues to explain its high affinity. The principal interactions include: (a) a strong hydrogen bond (2.6 Å) of the carbonyl group of the ligand to Tyr130; (b) hydrogen bonds to water molecules within the active-site gorge which are, themselves, hydrogen-bonded to other waters or to side-chain and backbone atoms of the protein, notably to the carboxylic oxygens of Glu199 and to the hydroxyl oxygen of Tyr121; (c) interaction of the primary amino group of the ligand, which can be assume to be charged at the pH of the mother liquor, with the aromatic rings of Trp84 and Phe330; (d) an unusually short (3.0 Å) C-H·O bond between the ethylidene methyl group of HupA and the main-chain oxygen of His440; and (e) several hydrophobic contacts notably with the side chains and main-chain atoms of Trp84 and with residues Gly118 through Ser122.

Modelling Phe330 in the crystal structure as tyrosine, which is the corresponding residue in mammalian AChE, permits formation of a 3.3 Å hydrogen bond between the hydroxyl oxygen and the primary amino group of HupA. This extra hydrogen bond, in addition to π-cation interactions, may help to explain why HupA binds to mammalian AChE 5–10-fold more strongly than to TcAChE, and only weakly to BChE, which lacks an aromatic residue at this position (Ashani *et al.*, 1994).

It seems surprising that an inhibitor with a relatively high affinity for AChE—K_i *ca.* 6 nM for fetal bovine serum AChE, and 250 nM for TcAChE (Saxena *et al.*, 1994)—binds through so few direct contacts. Even though HupA has three potential hydrogen-bond donor and acceptor sites (Fig. 2), only one strong hydrogen bond is seen, between the pyridone oxygen and Tyr130. Analogous compounds with a methoxy replacing the oxygen show no inhibition at all (Kozikowski *et al.*, 1992). It is also of interest that the ring nitrogen is hydrogen-bonded to the protein via a water molecule, and hydrogen bonds between the NH_{3+} group and the protein are mediated through at least two waters. The aromatic rings of both Trp84 and Phe330 are near the primary amino group. However, the structure displays a large number of hydrophobic interactions: there are 11 contacts between a carbon atom of HupA and oxygen or nitrogen atoms of the protein, and 20 carbon-to-carbon contacts within 4.0 Å. Consequently, there does not appear to be much room for adding additional groups without causing clashes. Nevertheless, addition of a methyl group near the amide group of HupA leads to an 8-fold increase in affinity, probably due to extra hydrophobic contacts with Trp84 (Kozikowski *et al.*, 1996).

In summary, the crystal structure of the HupA-TcAChE complex reveals an unexpected orientation of the ligand within the active site, as well as unusual protein-ligand interactions. This information should be of value in the design and analysis of analogs of HupA with improved pharmacological characteristics.

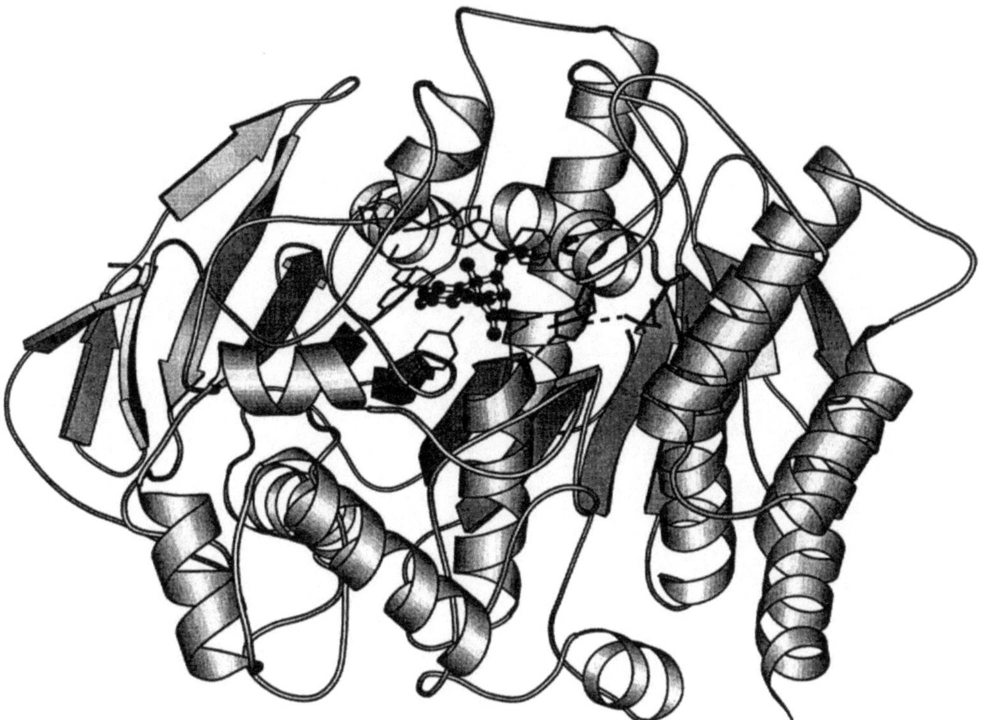

Figure 3A. Ribbon diagram of the HupA-TcAChE complex, showing the HupA molecule at the bottom of the active-site gorge.

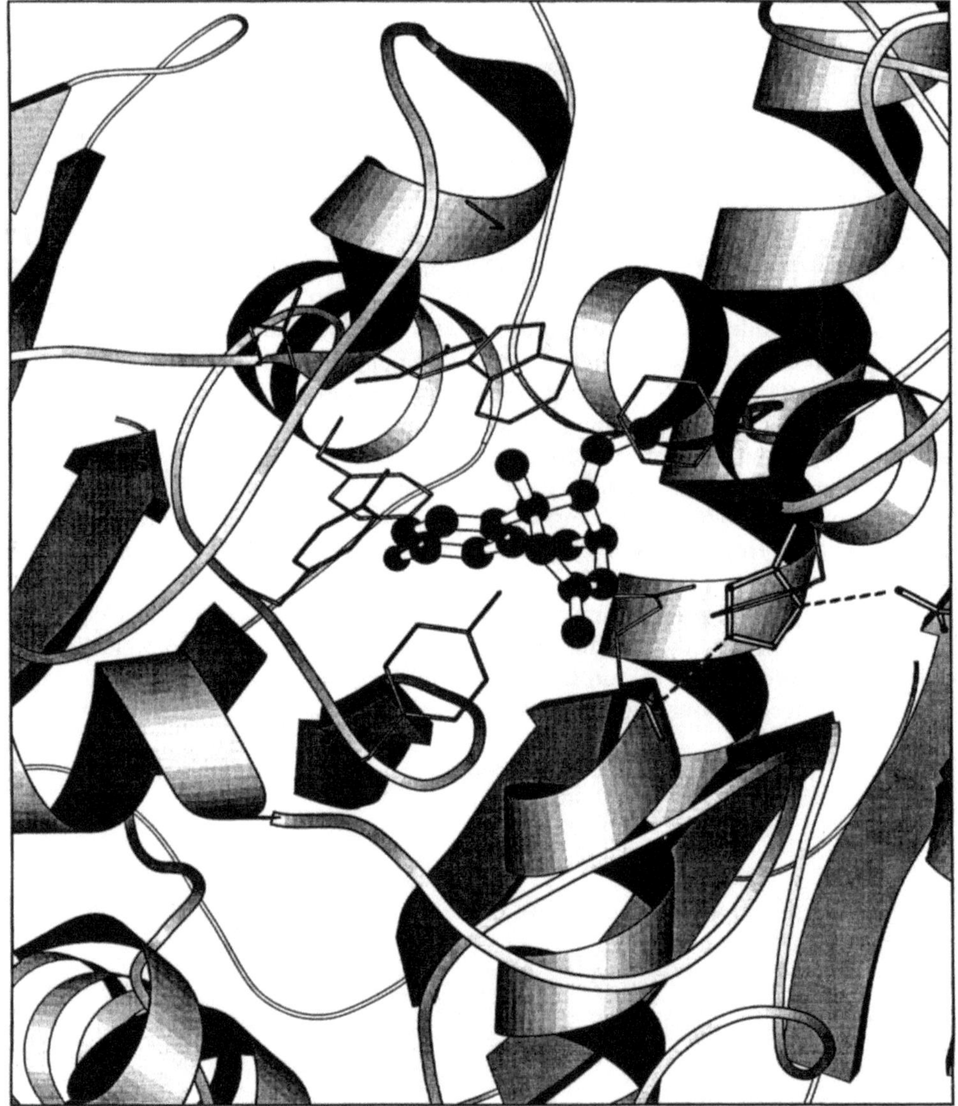

Figure 3B. Enlargement of the active site region, showing the catalytic triad to the right, and some of the aromatic residues surrounding the HupA molecule making contact.

ACKNOWLEDGMENTS

This research was supported by the U.S. Army Medical Research and Development Command, the Minerva Foundation, the Kimmelman Center for Biomolecular Structure and Assembly, and the Scientific Cooperation of the European Union with Third Mediterranean Countries through the Israeli Ministry of Science. I.S. is Bernstein-Mason Professor of Neurochemistry.

REFERENCES

Albrand, J.-P, Blackledge, M.J., Pascaud, F., Hollecker, M., and Marion, D., 1995, *Biochemistry* 34:5923–5937.

Ashani, Y., Grunwald, J., Kronman, C., Velan, B., and Shafferman, A., 1994, *Mol. Pharmacol.* 45:555–560.

Axelsen, P.H., Harel, M., Silman, I., and Sussman, J.L., 1994, *Protein Sci* 3:188–197.

Bourne, Y., Taylor, P., and Marchot, P., 1995, *Cell* 83:503–512.

Cerveñansky, C., Dajas, F., Harvey, A.L., and Karlsson, E., 1991, In: *SnakeToxins,* Harvey, A.L., ed., pp. 131–164, Pergamon, New York .

Changeux, J.-P., Kasai, M., and Lee, C.Y., 1970, *Proc. Natl. Acad. Sci. USA* 67:1241–1247.

Cousin, X., Bon, S., Duval, N., Massoulié, J., and Bon, C., 1996, *J. Biol. Chem.* 271:15099–15108.

Eichler, J., Anselmet, A., Sussman, J.L., Massoulié, J., and Silman, I., 1994, *Mol. Pharmacol.* 45:335–340.

Sugimoto, H., Tsuchiya, Y., Sugumi, H., Higurashi, K., Karibe, N., Imura, Y., Sasaki, A., Araki, S., Yamanishi, Y., and Yamatsu, K., 1992, *J. Med.Chem.* 35:4542–4548.

Gauthier, S., and Gauthier, L., 1991, In: *Cholinergic Basis for Alzheimer Therapy,* Giacobini, E., and Becker, R., eds., Birkhäuser, Boston, pp. 224–230.

Giacobini, E., and Becker, R., 1991, *Cholinergic Basis for Alzheimer Therapy*, Birkhäuser, Boston.

Giacobini, E., and Becker, R., 1994, *Alzheimer Disease: Therapeutic Strategies,* Birkhäuser, Boston.

Giles, K., Raves, M.L., Silman, I. , and Sussman, J.L., 1997, In: *Theoretical and Computational Methods in Genome Research,* Suhai, S., ed., Plenum Press, New York, in press.

Harel, M., Sussman, J.L., Krejci, E., Bon, S., Chanal, P., Massoulié, J., and Silman, I., 1992, *Proc. Natl. Acad. Sci. USA* **89**, 10827–10831.

Harel, M., Schalk, I., Ehret-Sabatier, L., Bouet, F., Goeldner, M., Hirth, C., Axelsen, P., Silman, I., and Sussman, J.L., 1993, *Proc. Natl. Acad Sci. USA* 90:9031–9035.

Harel, M., Kleywegt, G.J., Ravelli, R.B.G., Silman, I., and Sussman, J.L., 1995, *Structure* 3:1355–1366.

Harvey, A.L., 1991, *Snake Toxins*, Pergamon, New York.

Heilbronn, E., 1961, *Acta Chem. Scand* . 15:1386–1390.

Janin, J. , and Chothia, C., 1990, *J. Biol. Chem.* 265:16027–16030.

Kozikowski, A., Thiels, E., Tang, X.-C. , and Hanin, I., 1992, *Adv. Med. Chem.* 1:175–205.

Kozikowski, A.P., Campiani, G., Sun, L.-Q., Wang, S., Sega, A., Saxena, A., and Doctor, B.P., 1996, *J. Am. Chem. Soc.* 118:11357–11362.

Laganière, S., Corey, J., Tang, X.-C., Wülfert, E. , and Hanin, I., 1991, *Neuropharmacology* 30:763–768.

le Du, M.H., Marchot, P., Bougis, P.E., and Fontecilla-Camps, J.C., 1992, *J.Biol. Chem.* 267:22122–22130.

Liu, J.-S., Zhu, Y.-L., Yu, C.-M., Zhou, Y.-Z., Han, Y.-Y., Wu, F.-W., and Qi, B.-F., 1986, *Can. J. Chem.* 64, 837–839.

Main, A.R., 1976, In: *Biology of Cholinergic Function,* Goldberg, A.M., and Hanin, I., eds., pp. 269–353, Raven, New York.

Nolte, H.-J., Rosenberry, T.L., and Neumann, E., 1980, *Biochemistry* 19:3705–3711.

Pang, Y.-P. , and Kozikowski, A., 1994, *J. Computer-Aided Mol. Design* 8:669–681.

Porschke, D., Créminon, C., Cousin, X., Bon, C., Sussman, J., and Silman, I., 1996, *Biophys. J.* 70:1603–1608.

Quinn, D.M., 1987, *Chem. Revs.* 87:955–975.

Radic, Z., Durán, R., Vellom, D.C., Li, Y., Cerveñansky, C., and Taylor, P., 1994, *J. Biol. Chem.* 269:11233–11239.

Raves, M.L., Harel, M., Pang, Y.-P., Silman, I., Kozikowski, A.P., and Sussman, J .L., 1997, *Nature Struct. Biol.* 4:57–63.

Ripoll, D., Faerman, C., Axelsen, P., Silman, I. , and Sussman, J.L., 1993, *Proc. Natl. Acad. Sci. USA* 90:5128–5132.

Saxena, A., Qian, N., Kovach, I.M., Kozikowski, A.P., Pang, Y.P., Vellom, D.C., Radic, Z., Quinn, D., Taylor, P. , and Doctor, B.P., 1994, *Protein Sci.* 3:1770–1778.

Ségalas, I., Roumest, and , C., Zinn-Justin, C., Gilquin, B., Ménez, R., Ménez, A., and Toma, F., 1995, *Biochemistry* 34:1248–1260.

Silman, I., Harel, M., Eichler, J., Sussman, J.L., Anselmet, A. , and Massoulié, J., 1994, In: *Alzheimer Disease: Therapeutic Strategies,* Giacobini, E., and Becker, R., eds., pp. 88–92, Birkhäuser, Boston.

Sussman, J.L., Harel, M., Frolow, F., Oefner, C., Goldman, A., Toker, L., and Silman, I., 1991, *Science* 253:872–879.

Taylor, P., 1990, In: *The Pharmacological Basis of Therapeutics,* Gilman, A.G., Nies, A.S., Rall, T.W., and Taylor, P., eds., 5th Ed., Macmillan, New York, pp. 131–150.

Taylor, P. , and Lappi, S., 1975, *Biochemistry* 14:1989–1997.

Weise, C., Kreienkamp, H.-J., Raba, R., Pedak, A., Aaviksaar, A., and Hucho, F., 1990, *EMBO J* 9:3885–3888.

Wilson, I.B., and Quan, C., 1958, *Arch. Biochem. Biophys.* 73:131–143.

Wonnacott, S.M., and Dajas, F., 1994, *Trends Pharmacol. Sci.* 15:1–3.
Xiong, Z.Q. , and Tang, X.C., 1995, *Pharmacol. Biochem. Behav.* 51:415–419.
Zaimis, E. , and Head, S., 1976, *Handb. Exp. Pharmacol.* 42:365–420.
Zhang, R.W., Tang, X.C., Han, Y.Y., Sang, G.W., Zhang, Y.D., Ma, Y.X., Zhang, C.L. , and Yang, R.M., 1991, *Acta Pharmacol. Sinica* 12:250–252.

76

WHAT CAN BE LEARNED FROM THE USE OF HuAChE MUTANTS FOR EVALUATION OF POTENTIAL ALZHEIMER'S DRUGS

Avigdor Shafferman, Arie Ordentlich, Naomi Ariel, Dov Barak,
Chanoch Kronman, Tamar Bino, Moshe Leitner, Dino Marcus, Arie Lazar,
and Baruch Velan

Israel Institute for Biological Research
Ness-Ziona, 70450, Israel

INTRODUCTION

Senile dementia of the Alzheimer's type (SDAT) is characterised by loss of cholinergic neuronal markers like the enzymes choline acetyltransferase (ChAT) and acetylcholinesterase (AChE), in selected brain regions (Bierer et al., 1995). These indications of progressive depletion of cholinergic synapses led to the hypothesis that increasing the central nervous system (CNS) levels of acetylcholine (ACh), through inhibition of AChE, will improve cognition in SDAT (Court & Perry, 1991). This approach is theoretically preferable to other means of cholinergic augmentation since it may amplify the natural temporal pattern of ACh release, rather than globally stimulating the cholinergic system. Yet up to the present most of these agents show only mild to moderate ameliorating effects on memory deficits (Schneider & Tariot, 1994; Kan, 1992). To further optimize the therapeutic efficacy of these agents, a better understanding is needed of the structural features determining their interactions with AChE. The recent progress in the elucidation of structure-function characteristics of AChE, is therefore of considerable importance for these efforts.

The x-ray structure of AChE is characterized by a deep and narrow 'gorge', which penetrates halfway into the enzyme and contains the catalytic site at about 4Å from its base (Sussman et al., 1991). The specific functional roles of many residues in the active center gorge were recently elucidated by chemical affinity labelling (Weise et al., 1990), x-ray studies (Sussman et al., 1991; Harel et al., 1993, 1996), site directed mutagenesis and molecular modeling (Shafferman et al., 1992a,b; Ordentlich et al., 1993a, 1995, 1996; Barak et al., 1992, 1994, 1995; Vellom et al., 1993; Taylor & Radic, 1994; Radic et al., 1993).

Progress in Alzheimer's and Parkinson's Diseases
edited by Fisher *et al.*, Plenum Press, New York, 1998.

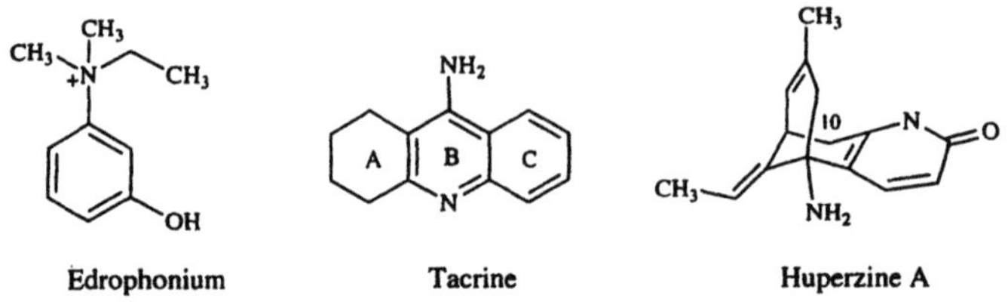

Figure 1. Chemical formulas of the anticholinesterase agents used in this study.

The x-ray structures of AChE and its complexes with inhibitors guided several recent attempts to design novel AChE inhibitors (Inoue et al., 1996; Cho et al., 1996). The underlying assumption in all these modeling experiments was that the solution structures of AChE - inhibitor complexes closely resemble those in the crystal. However recent findings, regarding the inhibition patterns of certain HuAChE mutants by peripheral site specific ligands, appear to indicate that this assumption might not be generally correct (Barak et al., 1995).

In the present study we explore the interactions of HuAChE with three lead structures for development of potential SDAT therapeutic agents, edrophonium, tacrine and huperzine A (Fig. 1) by methods of molecular biology, enzyme kinetics and modeling. We show that the functional architecture of the AChE active center, characterized in the past through studies with a variety of both covalent and noncovalent ligands, allows now to propose plausible molecular models of the enzyme-inhibitor complexes. Examination of these models, in view of the past SAR studies of the specific inhibitors and the available x-ray data, indicates that the solid state structural information may not always apply to these structures in solution and that a combination of structural and functional data is necessary to guide future structure-based design of novel AChE inhibitors.

RESULTS AND DISCUSSION

The Aromatic Active Center Residues Trp86, Tyr133, and Tyr337 Are Key Elements in Stabilizing of the Noncovalent Complexes of HuAChE

The role of residue Trp86 as the primary locus of interaction with positively charged moieties of active center ligands is well established (Sussman et al., 1991; Shafferman et al, 1992a; Ordentlich et al., 1995; Harel et al., 1996). Indeed, replacement of this residue by alanine resulted in a significant decrease in the inhibitory activity of all the three anticholinesterase agents tested toward the W86A enzyme as compared to the wild type HuAChE (Table 1, see also Fig. 2A, 3A, and 3C). Accommodation of the structurally different positively charged moieties, by the extended aromatic system of Trp86, takes place mainly through cation-π interaction (Ordentlich et al., 1995; Harel et al., 1996), but also via stacking with charged aromatic systems like that of tacrine (Harel et al., 1993). Multiple modes of interactions with the ligand are also exhibited by other aromatic residues in the active center gorge and in particular by the hydrophobic pocket residues Tyr133 and Tyr337. Examination of the specific roles of each of these residues delineates the binding properties of AChE active center and may account for the structural versatility of the anticholinesterase agents currently in clinical use or investigation (Brufani & Filocamo, 1996).

Table 1. Relative inhibition constants of HuAChE
and its mutants with active center ligands

HuAChE	Edrophonium	Tacrine	Huperzine
WT	1	1	1
Hydrophobic pocket			
W86F	54	74	103
W86A	(>64300)	18750	(>55555)
Y133A	1110	106	55
Y337A	8	0.075	272
Y337F	1	2	6
F338A	1	0.5	3
H-bond network			
Y133F	26	68	2
E202A	266	38	100
E202Q	18	6	8
E450A	4	6	0.3
Acyl pocket			
F295A	1	1	11
F297A	1	3	3
Peripheral site			
D74N	5	59	1
Y124A	2	0.5	1
W286A	1	1	4
Y341A	3	1	2

Distinct interaction modes with the different ligands are suggested also for residue Tyr133. The similar decrease in the inhibitory activity of tacrine toward the Y133F and the Y133A mutant enzymes, relative to the wild type HuAChE is due to the loss of a hydrogen-bond interaction of the Tyr133 hydroxyl group with the amino substituent of the ligand (Fig. 3A). In addition, interactions of residue Tyr133 with adjacent active center residues, were suggested to be essential in maintaining the functional architecture of the HuAChE (Ordentlich et al., 1995). Therefore its replacement may have also indirect effects on the enzyme affinity toward active center ligands as already shown in the case of

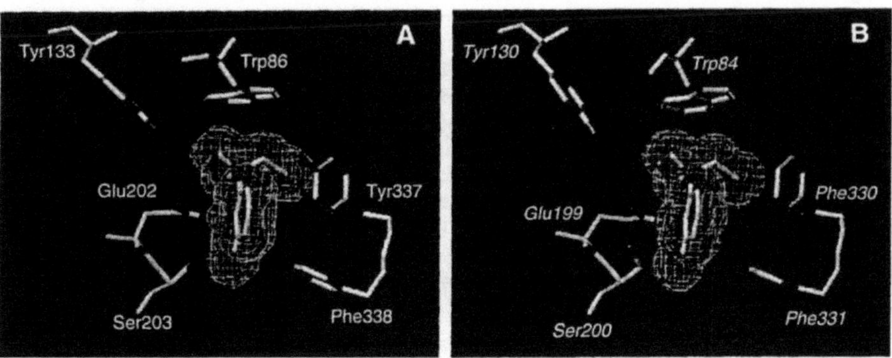

Figure 2. Models of edrophonium complexes with HuAChE and TcAChE. Only active center residues vicinal to edrophonium are shown. The molecular volume of edrophonium is displayed as a grid. A. HuAChE-edrophonium complex—constructed according to results from mutagenesis. B. TcAChE-edrophonium complex—coordinates taken from the x-ray structure published by Harel et al. (1993).

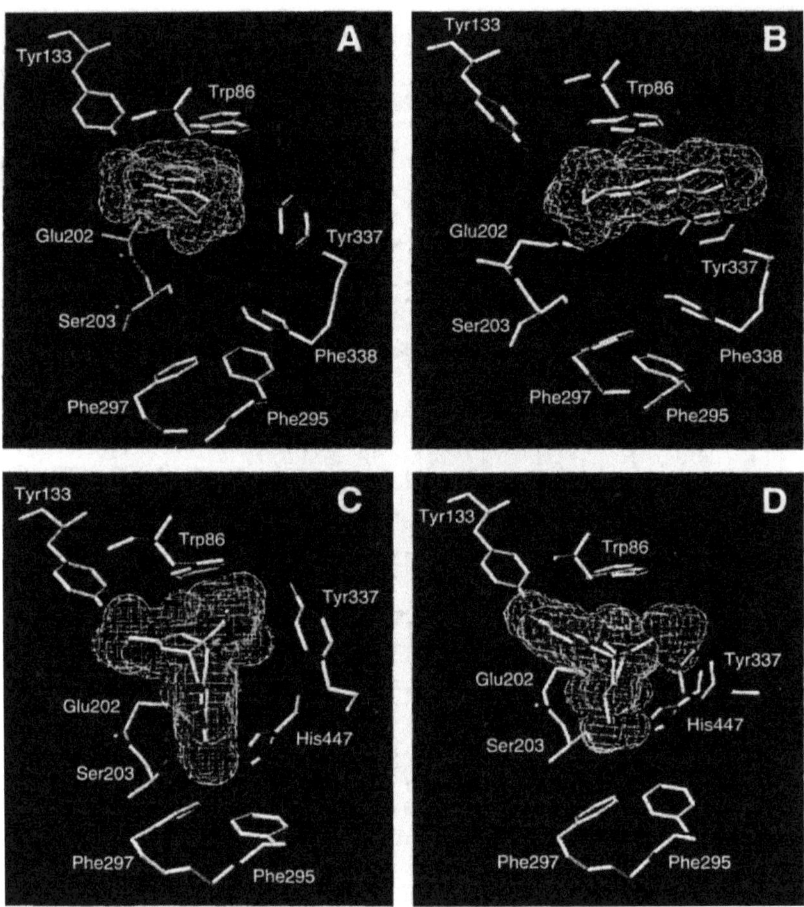

Figure 3. Molecular models of HuAChE complexes with tacrine and (–)-huperzine A. Only active center residues vicinal to the ligands are shown. The molecular volumes of the ligands are displayed as a grid. For each ligand, the model constructed according to results from mutagenesis, representing the HuAChE complex structure in solution, is compared to an analogous complex model built by docking the "crystallographic" orientation of the inhibitor, representing its structure in the solid. **A.** HuAChE-tacrine complex—constructed according to results from mutagenesis. The amine substituent of tacrine is within hydrogen-bond distance from Tyr133; there is no aromatic-aromatic interaction of the tetrahydroacridine moiety with Tyr337. **B.** HuAChE-tacrine complex—obtained by docking the "crystallographic" orientation of tacrine (in the corresponding TcAChE complex). The tetrahydroacridine moiety is stacked between the aromatic moieties of Trp86 and Tyr337; the amine substituent of tacrine is within hydrogen bond distance fron Tyr337; there is no interaction between tacrine and residue Tyr133. **C.** HuAChE-(–)-huperzine A complex—constructed according to results from mutagenesis. The ammonium substituent points toward the indole moiety of Trp86 but interacts also with Tyr337; the pyridone oxygen is within hydrogen bond distances from the catalytic residue Ser203; there is no polar interaction of huperzine A with residue Tyr133. **D.** HuAChE-(–)-huperzine A complex—obtained by docking the "crystallographic" orientation of (–)-huperzine A (in the corresponding TcAChE complex). The pyridone oxygen is within hydrogen bond distance from Tyr133; the ammonium substituent is nearly equidistant from the aromatic moieties of Trp86 and Tyr337.

edrophonium (Ordentlich et al., 1995). Similarly, the decrease in affinity of the Y133A toward huperzine A (2.4 kcal/mole), relative to both the wild type and the Y133F mutant HuAChE, is probably due to an indirect effect since the molecular model (see Fig. 3C) does not indicate a direct interaction of the aromatic moiety of Tyr133 with the ligand.

The contribution of the third constituent of the hydrophobic pocket, residue Tyr337, to the accommodation of active center ligands is less pronounced than that of either residue Trp86 or Tyr133. In the HuAChE complexes with tacrine, this aromatic moiety seems to present a minor *steric obstruction* to ligand binding, since the corresponding Ki value for the Y337A mutant enzyme was 11-fold *lower* than that for the wild type HuAChE. The most pronounced contribution of Tyr337 is in stabilization of the HuAChE- huperzine A complex, involving both the hydroxyl group and the aromatic moiety (see Table 1).

Residues Phe295 and Phe297 of the acyl pocket were shown to restrict the size of the inhibitor in the vicinity of the active site (Ordentlich et al., 1993a; Radic et al., 1993). The somewhat diminished inhibitory activity of huperzine A towards F295A and F297A mutant enzymes (20-fold and 5-fold respectively relative to the wild type enzyme), suggests a direct interaction of part of the ligand structure with the acyl pocket.

In conclusion, it appears that of the six aromatic residues adjacent to the active site, Trp86 and Tyr133 and to a lesser extent Tyr337, are the major participants in the stabilization of HuAChE complexes, irrespective of the ligand structure. Such ability of the hydrophobic pocket elements to accommodate structurally diverse ligands originates from the different modes of interaction exhibited by these residues, including polar (cation-π, hydrogen-bond) and nonpolar (aromatic -aromatic hydrophobic), as well as from their contribution to the stability of the functional architecture of the active center. The participation of residue Phe 338, also associated with the hydrophobic pocket, and of the acyl pocket residues Phe295, Phe297 is much less significant and is characterized mostly by nonspecific interactions.

The Role of the Active Center Acidic Residues in Stabilization of the Noncovalent Complexes of HuAChE

Residues Glu202 and Glu450, near the base of the gorge, were already shown to constitute part of an H-bond network which presumably maintains the functionally viable positioning of the Glu202 carboxylate (Ordentlich et al., 1995, 1996). This carboxylate group is adjacent to the positively charged moieties of most of the ligands, and could therefore be expected to participate in electrostatic stabilization of the HuAChE complexes. Replacement of Glu202 by glutamine is thought to partially eliminate this stabilization while maintaining the H-bond network, whereas replacement of this residue by alanine disrupts also the network (Table 1). The effects of these replacements on the inhibitory activities of the ligands indicates that both the charge and the positioning of Glu202 carboxylate are significant to the stabilization of the corresponding HuAChE complexes. Residue Glu450 is too remote for a direct interaction with the ligands (the C^δ– E450 is 9.72Å away from O^γ–S203) and the moderate effects of its replacement by alanine can be mostly attributed to the disruption of the H-bond network (Ordentlich et al., 1993b).

Residue Asp74 is located near the rim of the active center gorge and constitutes part of the PAS (Shafferman et al., 1992a; Barak et al., 1994). Its replacement by asparagine has a considerable effect on the inhibitory activity of tacrine as opposed to the effects on the corresponding activities of huperzine A and edrophonium. The reason for this puzzling reactivity pattern of the D74N HuAChE is not clear, since it cannot be explained by direct effects of residue Asp74 like electrostatic steering of the ligand at the gorge entrance (Zhou et al., 1996), or ligand binding to the PAS (Masson et al., 1997). The steering mechanism should have been similarly evident for all the positively charged ligands, whereas binding to the PAS should have involved other residues of this subsite.

The Complexes of Tacrine and Huperzine A with AChE in Solution May Be Different from Those Determined by X-Ray Crystallography

Results from site directed mutagenesis and enzyme inhibition studies identified the main interaction loci for the various ligands in the HuAChE active center and allowed for the construction of molecular models for the corresponding complexes. The model of HuAChE-edrophonium complex resembles closely the x-ray structure of the corresponding *Torpedo californica* AChE (TcAChE) adduct (Harel et al., 1993), supporting the notion that the structures of the active center regions of the two enzymes are quite similar (see Fig. 2). On the other hand, few of the specific ligand-enzyme interactions, evident in the crystallographic structures of TcAChE complexes with tacrine (Harel et al., 1993) and huperzine A (Raves et al., 1997), do not conform with the mutagenesis results reported here.

In the crystallographic structure of the TcAChE-tacrine complex, both residues Trp*84*(86)[*] and Phe*330* (Tyr337) seem to participate in ligand accommodation, through aromatic-aromatic interactions with the protonated acridinium moiety (see Fig. 3B for analogous model of the HuAChE-tacrine complex). However, replacement of Tyr337 by alanine *increased* the affinity of the resulting HuAChE enzyme toward tacrine, implying that the aromatic moiety at position 337 presents a *steric obstruction* to ligand binding rather than participating in stabilizing interactions. In addition, from the x-ray structure one could predict that if residue Phe*330*, in TcAChE, would have been replaced by tyrosine an additional hydrogen-bond would have been formed, with the amine substituent of tacrine (see Fig. 3B). In HuAChE, tyrosine is actually present at position 337*(330)* yet, its replacement by phenylalanine had only a marginal effect on enzyme affinity toward tacrine. Moreover, while removal of the hydroxyl group from position 133 of HuAChE results in a 68-fold decrease of the tacrine inhibitory activity toward the Y133F enzyme, the x-ray structure shows no direct involvement of residue Tyr*130*(133) in the accommodation of tacrine. The molecular model of the HuAChE-tacrine complex, proposed here, accounts for these findings and is also compatible with results of published SAR studies of tacrine analogues, with regard to effects of aromaticity of rings A and C (see Fig. 1) and of substitutions on the ring system and on the exocyclic nitrogen atom (Shustkie et al., 1989; Steinberg et al., 1975).

In the recently described structure of TcAChE-(−)-huperzine A complex (Raves et al., 1997), two principal protein-ligand interactions were pointed out: a) hydrogen-bond of the pyridone oxygen to the hydroxyl group of Tyr*130*(133); b) cation-π interaction of the protonated amino group of the ligand with the aromatic moieties of residues Trp*84*(86) and Phe*330*(Tyr337) (distances between the nitrogen and the centroids of the rings 4.8 and 4.7 Å respectively; Raves et al., 1997). In contrast with these observations, we find that: a) replacement of residue Tyr133 by phenylalanine has practically no effect on the affinity toward huperzine A, suggesting that in solution there is no hydrogen-bond between residue Tyr133 and the ligand; and b) the inhibitory activity of huperzine A toward W86A is over 55000-fold lower than that toward the wild type enzyme, whereas the corresponding ratio for the Y337F and Y337A mutant enzymes is only 43-fold. We note that the ratio of huperzine A Ki values for W86F/W86A (>500) is still much larger than the corresponding ratio of Y337F/Y337A.

As in the case of tacrine, the molecular model of the HuAChE complex with (−)-huperzine A, corresponds better to the experimental findings from mutagenesis studies than

---

[*] Amino acids and numbers refer to HuAChE, the numbers in italics refer to the positions of analogous residues in TcAChE according to the recommended nomenclature (Massoulie et al., 1992).

the crystal-like structure (Fig. 3C,D). This model is also consistent with published results of the SAR studies carried out with huperzine A analogues (for a partial compilation see Raves et al., 1997). In particular, the reported 8-fold increase in the inhibitory activity of the axial 10-methyl huperzine A (see Fig. 1), relative to the unsubstituted compound, can be explained by an interaction of the methyl group with the aromatic moiety of residue Tyr124*(121)*.

These inconsistencies, between the x-ray data for the TcAChE complexes and the mutagenesis data for the corresponding HuAChE complexes, may simply point to the actual differences in the structures of active center regions of the two enzymes. However, such explanation is difficult to reconcile with the following observations: a) the accommodation of edrophonium and decamethonium in HuAChE active center, suggested by the mutagenesis data, is very similar to that observed by x-ray crystallography in the corresponding TcAChE complexes (Harel et al., 1993; Barak et al., 1994); b) the only difference in the composition of the amino acids (over 30 residues), lining the AChE active center gorge, is phenylalanine at position *330*(337) of TcAChE instead of tyrosine in the mammalian AChE's; c) the recently reported crystallographic analyses of the fasciculin complexes with TcAChE and with the mammalian enzyme (mouse AChE), demonstrate the nearly equivalent molecular architectures of the active center regions for the two AChE's (Bourne et al., 1995; Harel et al., 1995); and d) the inhibition constants of (−)-huperzine A for the Y337F mutant of mouse AChE and for TcAChE were reported as 2.73×10^{-7} M and 1.85×10^{-7} M respectively (Saxena et al., 1994), which is consistent with an equivalent positioning/orientation of the ligand in the mouse and Torpedo AChE active centers. These values are also consistent with the huperzine A inhibition constant (1.30×10^{-7} M) reported here for the Y337F mutant HuAChE.

A more intriguing explanation of these inconsistencies between the x-ray data and the mutagenesis results is that the same ligand may be accommodated in different orientations when the AChE binding environment is modified by the protein transition from the crystal to solution. The relative stability of our model structures of the HuAChE complexes with tacrine and huperzine A, as compared to the corresponding models in which the ligands have been docked in their "crystallographic" orientations, shows only small differences (4.0 kcal/mole for tacrine and −4.9 kcal/mole for huperzine A). These minor energy differences, for such large molecular systems, indicate that both the "crystallographic" and the modelled orientations of the ligands are almost equally probable in these complexes. Therefore even minor changes in the relative mobility of active center gorge residues in the less rigid solution environment, may be sufficient to alter the equilibrium orientation of the ligand in the complex. In the crystalline state, the active center region of TcAChE appears to be relatively rigid, since it is nearly equivalent in all the x-ray structures of its complexes with various active center ligands (Sussman et al., 1991; Harel et al., 1993, 1996; Raves et al., 1997) . In addition, the crystallographic dimensions should preclude the access of ACh or larger ligands to the active site (Axelsen et al., 1994).

From the analysis presented above it appears that the structural diversity of AChE active center inhibitors may originate from two properties of the ligand binding environment: a) the versatility of interaction modes of aromatic residues lining the active center gorge and in particular of those comprising the hydrophobic subsite (Trp86, Tyr133 and to a lesser extent Tyr337); and b) enhanced flexibility of the AChE active center gorge in solution, as compared to the crystalline state. Future structure-based inhibitor design studies should take into account the possibility of differences between the structures of AChE complexes in the crystalline state and in solution. Since information regarding the complex structure in solution cannot be currently obtained from direct measurements, comprehensive characterization of the AChE-ligand complexes should rely on both, the x-ray methods and the combination of site directed mutagenesis and molecular modeling.

ACKNOWLEDGMENT

This work was supported by the US Army Research and Development Command, Contract DAMD 17-96-C-6088 to A.S.

REFERENCES

Axelsen, P. H., Harel, M., Silman I., and Sussman, J.L., 1994, Structure and dynamics of the active site gorge of acetylcholinesterase: Synergistic use of molecular dynamics simulation and x-ray crystallography. *Protein Sci.* 3:188–197.

Barak, D., Ariel, N., Velan, B., and Shafferman, A., 1992, Molecular models for human AChE and its phosphonylation products.In: *Multidisciplinary Approaches to Cholinesterase Functions*, A.Shafferman and B. Velan, eds, Plenum Publishing Corp., New York, pp 195–199.

Barak, D., Kronman, C., Ordentlich, A., Ariel, N., Bromberg, A., Marcus, D., Lazar, A., Velan, B., and Shafferman A., 1994, Acetylcholinesterase peripheral anionic site degeneracy conferred by amino acid arrays sharing a common core. *J.Biol.Chem.* 269:6296–6305.

Barak, D., Ordentlich, A., Bromberg, A., Kronman, C., Marcus, D., Lazar, A., Ariel, N., Velan, B., and Shafferman, A., 1995, Allosteric modulation of acetylcholinesterase activity by peripheral ligands involves conformational transition of the anionic subsite. *Biochemistry* 34:15444–15452.

Bierer, L.M., Haroutunian,V., Gabriel, S., Knott, P.J., Carlin, L.S., Purohit, D.P., Perl, D.P., Schmeider, J., Kanof, P. and, Davis, K.L., 1995, Neurochemical correlates of dementia severity in Alzheimer's disease: Relative importance of the cholinergic deficits. *J. Neurochem.* 64:749–760.

Bourne, Y., Taylor, P., and Marchot, P., 1995, Acetylcholinesterase inhibition by fasciculin: crystal structure of the complex. *Cell* 83:503–512.

Brufani, M., and Filocamo, L., 1996, Rational design of new acetylcholinesterase inhibitors. In: *Alzheimer Disease: From Molecular Biology to Therapy*, R. Becker and E.Giacobini, eds., Birkhaûser Boston , pp 171–177.

Cho, S.J., Garsia, M.L.S., Bier, J., and Tropsha, A., 1996, Structure-based alignment and comparative molecular fields analysis of acetylcholinesterase inhibitors. *J. Med. Chem.* 39:5064–5071.

Court, J.A., and Perry, E.K., 1991, Dementia:The neurochemical basis of putative transmitter oriented therapy. *Pharmacol. Ther.* 52:423–443.

Harel, M., Schalk, I., Ehret-Sabatier, L., Bouet, F., Goeldner, M., Hirth, C., Axelsen, P.H., Silman, I., and Sussman, J.L., 1993, Quaternary ligand binding to aromatic residues the active-sitè gorge of acetylcholinesterase. *Proc. Natl. Acad. Sci. U.S.A.* 90:9031–9035

Harel, M., Kleywegt, G.J., Ravelli, R.BG., Silman, I., and Sussman, J.L., 1995, Crystal structure of an acetylcholinesterase-fasciculin complex: interaction of a three-fingered toxin from snake venom with its target. *Structure* 3:1355–1366.

Harel, M., Quinn, D.M., Nair, H.K., Silman, I., and Sussman, J.L., 1996, The x-ray structure of a transition state analog complex reveals the molecular origins of the catalytic power and substrate specificity of acetylcholinesterase. *J. Am. Chem. Soc.* 118:2340–2346.

Inoue, A., Kawai, T., Wakita, M., Iimura, Y.,Sugimoto, H., and Kawakami, Y., 1996, The simulated binding of (±)-2,3-dihydro-5,6-dimethoxy-2-((1(phenylmethyl)-4-piperidinyl)methyl-1H-inden-1-onehydrochloride (E2020) and related inhibitors to free and acylated acetylcholinesterases and corresponding structure-activity analyses. *J. Med. Chem.* 39:4460- 4470.

Kan, J.P., 1992, Current and future approaches to therapy of Alzheimer's disease. *Eur. J. Med. Chem.* 27:565–570.

Masson, P., Legrand, P., Bartels, C.F., Froment, M.-T., Schopfer, L.M. and Lockridge, O., 1997, Role of aspartate 70 and tryptophan 82 in binding of succinyldithiocholine to human butyrylcholinesterase. *Biochemistry* 36:2266–2277 .

Massoulie, J., Sussman, J.L., Doctor, B.P., Soreq, H., Velan, B., Cygler, M., Rotundo, R.,Shafferman, A., Silman, I. and Taylor, P., 1992, Recommendations for nomenclature in cholinesterases, In: *Multidisciplinary Approaches to Cholinesterase Functions* (A. Shafferman and B. Velan eds.) Plenum Publishing Co., New York, pp 285–288.

Ordentlich, A., Barak, D., Kronman, C., Flashner, Y., Leitner,M., Segall, Y., Ariel, N., Cohen, S., Velan, B. and Shafferman, A., 1993a, Dissection of the human acetylcholinesterase active center, determinants of substrate specificity. *J. Biol. Chem.* 268:17083–1709.

Ordentlich, A., Kronman, C., Barak, D., Stein, D., Ariel, N., Marcus, D., Velan, B., and Shafferman, A., 1993b, Engineering resistance to 'aging' of phosphylated human acetylcholinesterase. *FEBS Lett.* 334:215–220.

Ordentlich, A., Barak, D., Kronman, C., Ariel, N., Segall, Y., Velan, B. and Shafferman, A, 1995, Contribution of aromatic moieties of tyrosine 133 and of the anionic subsite tryptophan 86 to catalytic efficiency and allosteric modulation of acetylcholinesterase. *J. Biol. Chem.* 270:2082–2091.

Ordentlich, A., Barak, D., Kronman, C., Ariel, N., Segall, Y., Velan, B. and Shafferman, A, 1996, The architecture of human acetylcholinesterase active center probed by interactions with selected organophosphate inhibitors. *J. Biol.Chem.* 271:11953–11962.

Radic, Z., Pickering, N.A., Vellom, D.C., Camp, S.and Taylor, P., 1993, Three distinct domains in the cholinesterase molecule confer selectivity for acetyl- and butyryl-cholinesterase inhibitors. *Biochemistry* 32:12074–12084 .

Raves, M., Harel, M., Pang, Y-P., Silman, I., Kozikowski , A.P., and Sussman, J.L., 1997, Structure of acetylcholinesterase complexed with the nootropic alkaloid, (-)-huperzine A. *Nature Struc. Biol.* 4:57–63.

Saxena, A., Qian, N., Kovach, I.M., Kozikowski, A.P., Pang, Y.P., Vellom, D.C., Radic, Z., Quinn, D., Taylor, P., and Doctor, B.P., 1994, Identification of amino acid residue involved in the binding of huperzine A to cholinesterases. *Prot. Sci.* 3:1770–1778 .

Schneider, L.S., and Tariot, P.N., 1994, Emerging drugs for Alzheimer's disease. *Medical Clinics of North America*, 78:911–934.

Shafferman, A., Velan, B., Ordentlich, A., Kronman, C., Grosfeld, H., Leitner, M., Flashner, Y., Cohen, S., Barak, D., and Ariel, N., 1992a, Substrate inhibition of acetylcholinesterase: residues involved in signal transduction from the surface to the active center. *EMBO J.* 11:3561–3568.

Shafferman, A., Kronman, C., Flashner, Y., Leitner, M., Grosfeld, H., Ordentlich, A., Gozes, Y., Cohen, S., Ariel, N., Barak, D., Harel, M., Silman, I., Sussman, J.L., and Velan, B., 1992b, Mutagenesis of acetylcholinesterase. Identification of residues involved in catalytic activity and in polypeptide folding. *J. Biol. Chem.* 267:17640–17648.

Shustke, G.M., Fierrat, F.A., Kapples, K.J., Cornfeld, M.L., Szewczak, M.R., Huger, F.P., Bores, G.M., Haroutunian, V., and Davis, K.L., 1989, 9-Amino-1,2,3,4-tetrahydroacridin-1-ols: Synthesis and evaluation as potential Alzheimer's disease therapeutics. *J. Med. Chem.* 32:1805–1812.

Steinberg, G.M., Mednick, M.L., Maddox, J., and Rice, R., 1975, A hydrophobic binding site in acetylcholinesterase. *J. Med. Chem.* 18:1056–1061.

Sussman, J.L., Harel, M., Frolow, F., Oefner, C., Goldman, A., and Silman, I., 1991, Atomic structure of acetylcholinesterase from *Torpedo californica*: a prototypic acetylcholine binding protein. *Science* 253:872–879.

Taylor, P., and Radic, Z., 1994, The cholinesterases: from genes to proteins. *Annu. Rev. Pharmacol. Toxicol.* 34:281–320.

Vellom, D.C., Radic, Z., Li, Y., Pickering, N.A.,Camp, S., and Taylor, P., 1993, Amino acid residues controlling acetylcholinesterase and butyrylcholinesterase specificity. *Biochemistry* 32:12–17.

Weise, C., Krienkamp, H.J., Raba, R., Aaviksaar, A., and Hucho, F., 1990, Anionic subsites of the acetylcholinesterase from Torpedo californica : affinity labelling with the cationic reagent N,N-dimethyl-2-phenyl-aziridinium. *EMBO J.* 9:3885–3888.

Zhou, H.-X., Briggs, J.M., and McCammon, J.A., 1996, A 240-fold electrostatic rate enhancement for acetylcholinesterase-substrate binding can be predicted by the potential within the active site.*J. Am. Chem. Soc.* 118:13069–13070.

CHOLINESTERASES IN NEUROGENESIS

Pharmacological and Transfection Studies of the Reaggregating Chick Retina

Paul G. Layer, Andrea Robitzki, Alexandra Mack, and Elmar Willbold

Darmstadt University of Technology
Department of Developmental Biology and Neurogenetics
Schnittspahnstrasse 3, D-64287 Darmstadt, Germany

INTRODUCTION

Developmental biology is fundamental to all biomedical research. The credo of developmental biologists is to study the simple state in order to understand the complex, the healthy to understand the diseased, and to follow growth in order to understand the final decay of biological systems. This applies particularly to the study of the most complex organ that has evolved, the human brain and its slow deterioration as observed in dementia. Following this principle, general studies on neurogenesis are a prerequisite for detecting defects in Alzheimer's disease.

A major part inflicted in the brains of Alzheimer patients is the nucleus of Meynert, presenting large numbers of pathological structures known as plaques and tangles. Physiologically, the cholinergic deficits of that brain part have been known for long. Irrespective of whether these cholinergic deficits are a primary cause for the disease or not, medical treatment of the disease—albeit often unsatisfactory—relies on the application of drugs that inhibit cholinesterases (see this volume). According to the cholinergic hypothesis, such treatment is supposed to ameliorate the deficits of cholinergic neurotransmission in the afflicted areas. A number of studies indicate that our knowledge about particular molecular forms and functions of cholinesterases in Alzheimer's disease is incomplete (reviews see Layer and Willbold, 1995; Layer, 1995). For instance, both classes of cholinesterases are typically changed in Alzheimer's disease; both acetylcholinesterase (AChE) and butyrylcholinesterase (BChE) are increased in the pathological structures, thereby presenting specific substrate and inhibitor properties (Mesulam et al., 1992; Wright et al., 1993). Since cholinesterases can exist in a large number of molecular forms (Massoulié and Bon, 1982), it was a significant finding that the small molecular forms prevail in Alzheimer's disease, similar to the situation as found in embryonic nervous tissue (Arendt

Progress in Alzheimer's and Parkinson's Diseases
edited by Fisher *et al.*, Plenum Press, New York, 1998.

et al., 1992). Recently, AChE has been reported to accelerate the assembly of β-amyloid into Alzheimer's fibrils in vitro (Inestrosa et al., 1996). Therefore, in order to understand the roles of cholinesterases in Alzheimer's disease, it seems appropriate to unravel the roles that cholinesterases play in the young embryo. Together with a number of other groups (see this volume), we have investigated novel roles of cholinesterases during neurogenesis of avian species. The results that are summarized here may very well shed new light on the significance of these enzymes in Alzheimer's disease.

Early steps of brain development involve the proliferation of neuroepithelial cells, their migration and local displacement, their differentiation, process formation and specific wiring. Cells not being integrated into the developing networks disappear by cell death. Major aspects of brain development are comparable within different brain subregions, and are very similar in the vertebrate hierarchy. Therefore, by studying e.g. the early zebrafish eye, one may well learn about principles that are as well relevant for the human cortex or cerebellum. The retina represents a particularly suited model to study the establishment of neural networks in general, since it is a fully wired neural network like other brain parts; thereby, the eye develops very early, the retina is easily accessible, and the retinal architecture is relatively simple. The retina consists of three nuclear layers containing the cell somata of a handful of major cell types, while their processes interconnect within two so-called plexiform layers. The light-perceiving cells are the photoreceptors; they are found in the outer nuclear layer. After transmission through several interneurons in the inner nuclear layer (horizontal, bipolar, amacrine cells), the ganglion cells located in the ganglion cell layer send a largely processed signal to the brain.

Acetylcholinesterase is not only found at cholinergic synapses, but rather both types of cholinesterases are most abundant in different tissues of the early vertebrate embryo, particularly so in the nervous system (Drews, 1975; Layer, 1983, 1990; Layer and Willbold, 1995). Interestingly, their appearance is coordinately regulated in time and space; they closely correlate with the change of neuroepithelial cells into a differentiated state. Thereby, BChE is transiently expressed, shortly preceding the much stronger expression of AChE. Due to its appearance in several stem cell systems, we have called BchE a "transmitotic marker", most likely having a role in the regulation of cell proliferation, differentiation and/or cell death. In contrast, AChE in neurons represents a very early sign of their postmitotic differentiation. AChE precedes the migration of neurons, or alternatively, their extension of long projection processes. In several in vitro systems, AChE indeed can alter neurite growth, as evidenced by specifically interfering with AChE (Layer et al., 1993; Jones et al., 1995; Karpel et al., 1996; Sritvatsan and Peretz, 1997); thereby, the enzymatic activity seems to be irrelevant. Complementing these observations, cholinesterases were found to share sequence homologies with the cell adhesion molecules neurotactin and glutactin from *Drosophila* (Barthalay et al., 1990; de la Escalera et al., 1990). Together with a number of other unrelated proteins, cholinesterases constitute a new family of "cholinesterase-like proteins" (review see Massoulié et al., 1993). A chimeric recombinant protein between neurotactin and the homologous sequence of *Torpedo* AChE indeed presented adhesive functions (Darboux et al., 1996).

All these general features of cholinesterases in the embryonic brain are well represented in the chicken retina. Therefore, the chicken retina presents a valuable model tissue to study both general neurogenesis and possible roles of cholinesterases thereby.

Retinospheroids as in Vitro Assay Systems of Retinogenesis

Another advantage of the retina as a model system relies on its regenerative ability. While this capacity is limited up to specific embryonic stages, it can be exploited to study retinogenesis and regeneration under in vitro conditions. Using eyes from six-day-old chick embryos, we isolate the neural retina and/or the anterior part around the lens consisting both of pigmented and non-pigmented cells. The tissues are then dissociated into isolated cells or into small cell clusters, respectively. After transfer of cells into rotation culture, two different types of histotypic structures—so-called *retinospheroids*—are generated. In a conventional reaggregation system (Moscona, 1956), dissociated cells from the entire retina are reaggregated to then form so-called *rosetted retinospheroids*. Thereby, single retinal cells from the central part of the eye gradually build up a spherical structure. Processes of cell-cell recognition, cell aggregation and to a certain degree sorting out and cell movement play crucial roles during the initial phases in this culture system. Cellular rosettes consisting of photoreceptor precursors are the typical structures in these rosetted spheroids. Concomitantly, cell numbers increase up to about day 4–5 in culture. Lateron, specific cell differentiation and the formation of nuclear and plexiform areas lead to highly developed retinal structures. Due to the fusion of several rosettes and their related „subunits", rosetted spheroids are complex composite structures. Nevertheless, they hold all constituents of an embryonic retina such as all three nuclear layers, the two plexiform layers and a variety of specific cell types. However, in one major aspect this system appears incomplete, since the orientation of the cell layers is reversed when compared with the normal in vivo situation (review in Layer and Willbold, 1993; 1994).

In addition, we have introduced another technique by including cells of the pigmented epithelium (Vollmer et al., 1984). In this case, cell aggregation and sorting out play only a minor role; more important is the onset of cell proliferation involving the induction of multipotent neuronal precursor cells by pigmented cells. In fact, the genesis of these *stratospheroids* is more comparable to normal retinogenesis. Multipotential neuroblasts first form a primitive neuroepithelium which then grows into the third dimension as well. Thereby, well-structured radial cell columns are formed which span the entire width of the stratospheroid. When a multitude of cell columns is composed together side-by-side, they establish all main layers and cell types of a retina. Their histological organization is much more pronounced than in rosetted spheroids, and their orientation of layers is correct. Accordingly, the photoreceptors are facing towards the outside medium, while the ganglion cells are found in the most internal layer.

Retinogenesis Quantified

It is important to realize that spheroids present a number of advantages when compared with other conventional culture techniques. In contrast to monolayer or explant cultures, in spheroids three-dimensional networks are re-established. As an outstanding feature of spheroid cultures, the development from isolated cells to mature and fully wired networks can be followed and/or manipulated. Thereby, the degree of final differentiation can come very close to the normal in vivo situation. Due to the availability of a large number of markers and procedures, their development can be qualitatively and quantitatively documented. These measurable parameters include cell numbers, spheroid volume, rates of cell proliferation and cell death. Also, the establishment of three nuclear layers and plexiform areas can be precisely followed, including differentiation of radial glia systems, photoreceptors, amacrine and other cell types. Once interconnected, the coupling of specific cell populations can be detected by fluorescence dyes. This list could be complemented by a number of measurable physiological parameters.

Thus, retinospheroid technology is not only ideal to analyse processes of genesis and regeneration of the vertebrate retina, but rather it can find wide applications as pharmacological, toxicological and molecular biology assay system. For most investigations presented here, we have predominantly used the rosetted spheroid system, since it is technically easier to handle.

RETINOSPHEROIDS APPLIED: CHOLINESTERASES INTERFERE WITH RETINOGENEIS IN VITRO

Pharmacological Intervention with Cholinesterase Expression

In an extended series of experiments using a selection of highly specific cholinesterase inhibitors, we have investigated the effects of pharmacological inhibition of both AChE and BChE on laminar histogenesis in retinospheroids (Layer et al., 1992; Willbold and Layer, 1994). In the presence of the specific BChE inhibitor iso-OMPA, the number of spheroids per dish was increased, while their average diameter was decreased by about 20%. The overall viability of the system was not affected. But the volume size of each spheroid was reduced to about 50%. Since the cell density appeared to be normal, this result indicates that the inhibited BChE led to a strong reduction of the average cell number in each spheroid. The small variance in spheroid diameters indicated that the cell number per spheroid is precisely balanced. As a corollary, the course of histotypical differentiation was significantly accelerated. By using an antibody to the cell recognition molecule F11 (Rathjen et al., 1987) it was possible to document that, as a consequence of BChE inhibition, both the organization of nuclear cell layers and of plexiform-like (neuropil) areas is temporally advanced by at least two days in comparison to untreated samples (Fig. 1). Along with it, AChE is almost fully diminished in these neuropil areas. Moreover, the normally pronounced release of AChE into the supernatant is almost entirely reduced (Layer et al., 1992). These results indicate that BChE plays a role in regulating cell proliferation. Most likely, in the presence of the BChE inhibitor, the formation of specific cell types from their precursor cells is inhibited, while the remaining population enters more quickly stages of advanced differentiation. A detailed investigation of the inflicted cell types is still missing (see also below). Based on these results, we suggested that inhibition of BChE may change the cell lineage of a retina, and, as a consequence, then affects laminar histogenesis of coherent neural networks in vitro.

Intervention with Cholinesterase Expression by Transfection Studies

To further analyse these observations on a molecular level, we have started transfection studies on retinospheroids, allowing to overexpress AChE, or alternatively, to suppress BChE. To this end, appropriate pSVK3 eukaryotic-prokaryotic shuttle expression vectors were constructed (Robitzki et al., 1997a, b). In a first approach, we have inserted 577 base pairs (bp) of the 5′-upstream region plus 106 bp of the coding sequence of the rabbit BChE gene (Chatonnet et al., 1991) in reverse orientation; for controls, the sense vector was also created. This antisense BChE vector was introduced by calcium phosphate-mediated transfection into both rosetted and stratospheroids during their first days of reaggregation (Robitzki et al., 1997a). Thus, the transfected cells after having integrated the vector will produce their own antisense-5′-BChE mRNA, enabling them to suppress the endogenously expressed BChE in the system. Although the entire chicken BChE gene sequence is not yet available, it is clear that the chicken and rabbit sequences are homologous enough to achieve a pronounced inhibition of transcription and translation. In

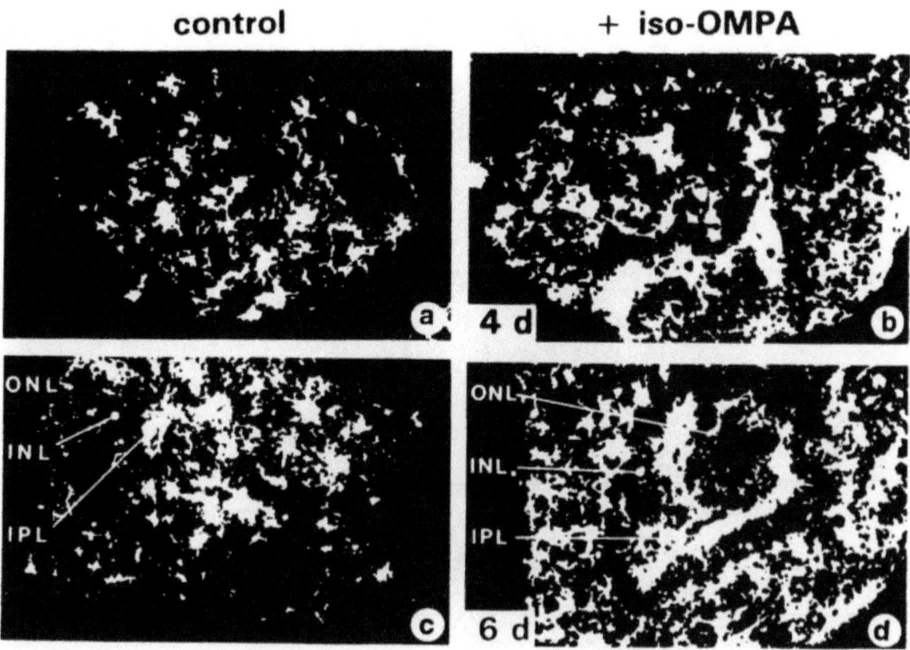

Figure 1. The BChE inhibitor iso-OMPA accelerates differentiation within inner plexiform-like (IPL) areas of retinospheroids. Iso-OMPA treated (b, d) and control retinospheroids (a, c) were stained with the fibre-specific antibody F11 after 4 days (a, b), and 6 days in culture (c, d), respectively. After 4 days in culture, only in iso-OMPA-treated retinospheroids the IPL-areas are already clearly visible. After 6 days in culture, differences are even more pronounced. Bar = 100 μm (from Willbold and Layer, 1994).

both spheroid systems, antisense-5'-BChE transcripts decreased the steady state mRNA level of BChE and the translation of BChE protein. As a corollary, this antisense treatment inhibited proliferation and accelerated histogenesis in both cellular systems. Diminished proliferation was determined by the size of spheroids and by BrdU uptake studies. As shown in Fig. 2, antisense-transfected rosetted spheroids remain smaller, similar to what was detected in the iso-OMPA experiment (see above). Most interestingly, antisense-transfected stratospheroids show not only a smaller total size, but the number of pigmented cells is drastically reduced. Moreover, the laminar histogenesis of rosetted spheroids was accelerated. This was established by the formation of radial glia and plexiform layers, as monitored immunocytochemically using vimentin- and F11-antibodies, respectively. These data fully support the pharmacological inhibition data as described above. Furthermore, transfection of spheroids with this antisense-5'-BChE vector not only resulted in a down-regulation of BChE expression, but also strongly increased chicken AChE transcripts, protein and enzyme activity. This is further evidence that suppression of BChE shifts the system into a more differentiated state with more cells becoming postmitotic, thereby expressing AChE. How AChE is regulated by BChE remains an open question.

AChE Affects Neurogenesis by a Non-Enzymatic Mechanism

As an alternative and more direct way of AChE overexpression, we transfected retinospheroids with another expression vector, into which a cDNA construct encoding for the entire rabbit AChE gene (Jbilo et al., 1994) had been inserted in sense orientation (Ro-

control   antisense-5′BChE

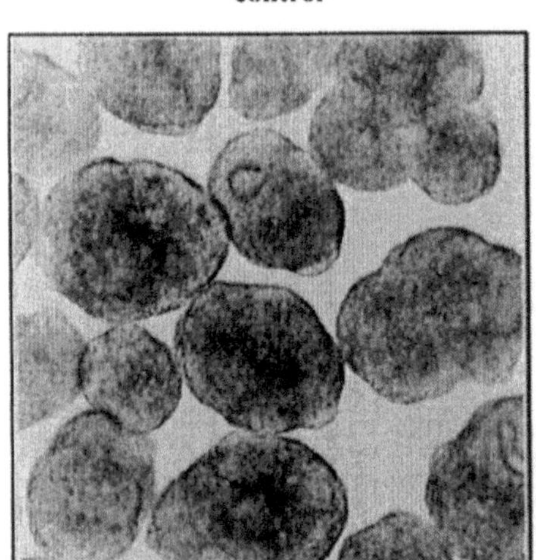
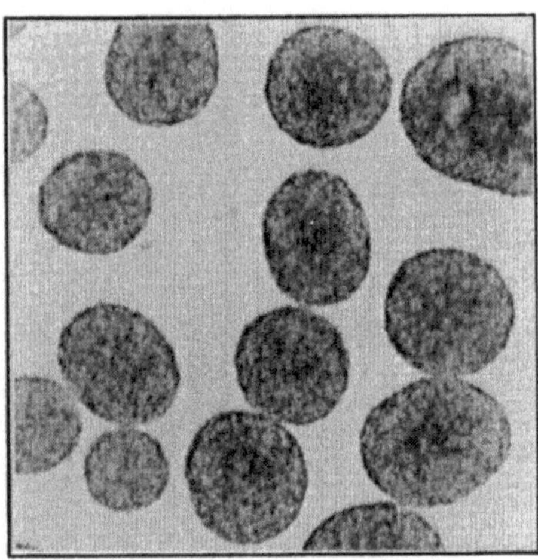

Stratospheroids (div 2)
control   antisense-5′BChE

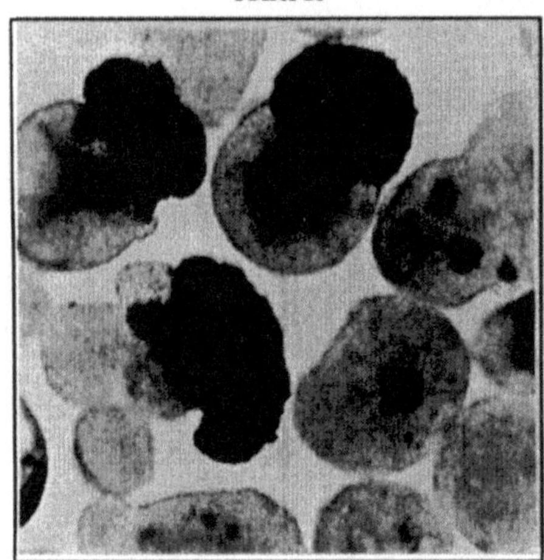
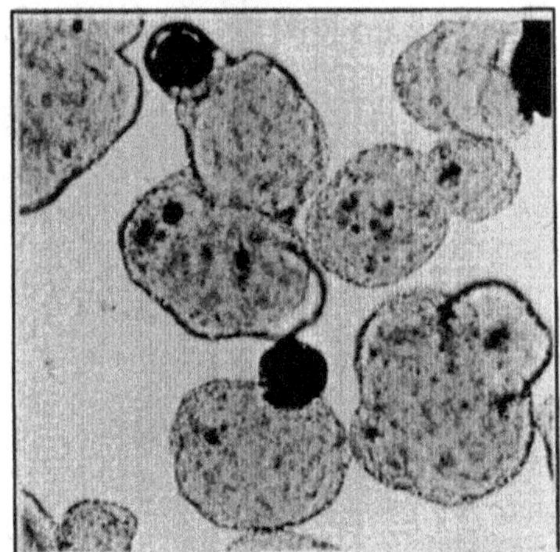

Figure 2. Structure of rosetted and stratospheroids is affected by antisense-5′-BChE transfection. Rosetted (upper) and stratospheroids (lower) were arrested at 2 days in vitro (div) and transfected with the sense (control) and antisense 5′-BChE vector; their morphology 48h after transfection is documented by brightfield microscopy. Note different shapes of both types of spheroids; stratospheroids have black clusters of retinal pigmented epithelium. The average diameter of antisense-5′-BChE-transfected rosetted spheroids is only about 50–60% of control spheroids, indicating a strong inhibition of cell proliferation by the antisense transcripts. In stratospheroids, a strong inhibition—particularly of RPE proliferation is evident. Bar = 200 μm (from Robitzki et al., 1997a).

bitzki et al., 1997b). As detected on the mRNA level, the introduced rabbit AChE is indeed heterologously overexpressed in chicken retinospheroids. Remarkably, this is also accompanied by a strong increase of endogenous chicken AChE protein, while the total AChE activity is only slightly increased. This minor increase in AChE activity is due to the overproduction of chicken enzyme, as shown by species specific inhibition studies using fasciculin (Marchot et al., 1995). Obviously, the total AChE activity in spheroids is post-translationally regulated. Again, the advantages of spheroid systems were exploited

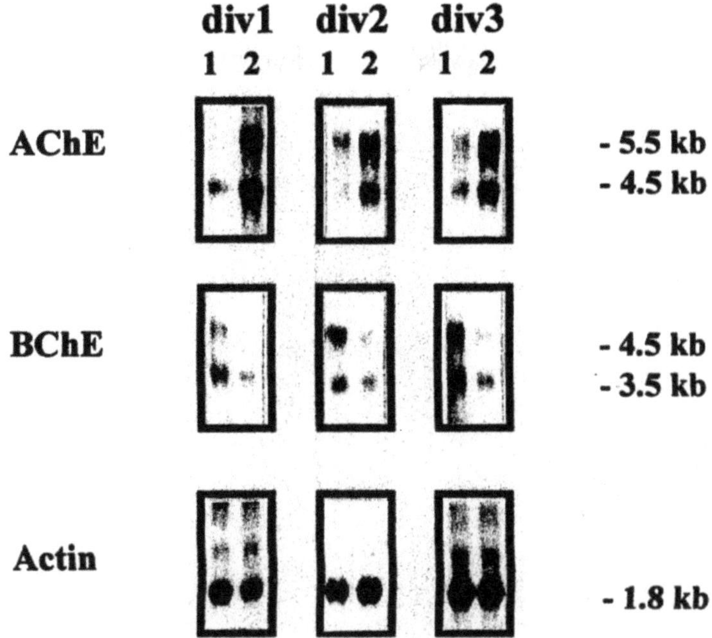

Figure 3. Upregulation of AChE transcripts in antisense-5′-BChE transfected spheroids. Northern blotting analysis of rosetted spheroids arrested at days in vitro (div) 1, 2 and 3 and transfected with a sense- (control; lanes 1) and an antisense 5′-BChE-pSVK3 expression vector (lanes 2). The hybridization of the poly(A)$^+$ RNA with a ^{32}P-labelled AChE cDNA (upper), a BChE cDNA (exon-2; middle) and a β-actin probe (lower) is documented. Note that mRNA of BChE is down-regulated in antisense-manipulated spheroids (middle, cf. lanes 1 and 2); as a corollary, AChE transcripts are strongly upregulated (upper); note a 4.5-kb and an embryonic 5.5-kb mRNA for AChE. Further explanations see text (from Robitzki et al., 1997b).

by following their morphological and histological appearance after their transfection. It could be shown that a higher concentration of AChE protein (as a consequence of either AChE overexpression or BChE suppression) is associated with an advanced degree of tissue differentiation, as detected by immunostaining for the cytoskeletal protein vimentin. Since the activity of AChE was only slightly increased, this supports the notion that such morphogenetic effects of AChE are due to non-enzymatic mechanisms, as first shown by us (Layer et al., 1993) and a number of other groups (refs., see Introduction).

CONCLUSION: EMBRYOLOGY AND DEMENTIA

A major objective of this study was to underline the necessity of developmental studies in order to better understand why an adult brain deteriorates. This study strongly supports the notion that embryonic cholinesterases are involved in regulating processes of cell proliferation and cell differentiation in the early embryonic chick retina. Some of these functions are likely to be unrelated to the esteratic activity of cholinesterases. Therefore, in the immature brain cholinesterases seem to have important functions irrespective of their later synaptic role(s). Together with recent data from several independent studies, this notion gains more and more experimental support (e.g. see Soreq et al., this book). Does such an embryological approach give us new insights into the problem of Alzheimer's disease?

We suggest that the changed expression and localization of cholinesterases in Alzheimer's disease could reflect the activation of a "neoembryonic" restorative program (see Layer, 1995). Accordingly, cholinesterases in Alzheimer's diesease could be involved in the regulation of cell survival and cell death in the aging brain, and possibly also in restorative neuritic (re)growth. If such views of cholinesterases in Alzheimer's diesease could be experimentally further substantiated, then new therapeutic approaches could be envisaged.

ACKNOWLEDGMENTS

We thank Dr. A. Chatonnet (Montpellier) for the gift of AChE and BChE cDNA's and Dr. K. Tsim (Hongkong) for the 3D10 antibody. We acknowledge the expert technical assistance by R. Alber, U. Hoppe and S. Haase. This work was supported by grants from the Deutsche Forschungsgemeinschaft (DFG, SFB 269/A2 and B3).

REFERENCES

Arendt, T., Brückner, M.K., Lange, M., and Bigl, V., 1992, Changes in acetylcholinesterase and butyrylcholinesterase in Alzheimer's disease resemble embryonic development - a study of molecular forms. *Neurochem. Int.* 21:381–396.

Barthalay, Y., Hipeau-Jacquotte, R., de la Escalera, S., Jimenéz, F., and Piovant, M. 1990, *Drosophila* neurotactin mediates heterophilic cell adhesion. *EMBO J.* 9:3603–3609.

Chatonnet, A., Lorca, T., Barakat, A., and Jbilo, O., 1991, Structure of rabbit butyrylcholinesterase gene deduced from genomic clones and from cDNA with introns. *Cell. Mol. Neurobiol.* 11:119–130.

Darboux, I., Barthalay, Y., Piovant, M., and Hipeau-Jacquotte, R., 1996, The structure-function relationships in *Drosophila* neurotactin show that cholinesterasic domains may have adhesive properties. *EMBO J.* 15:4835–4843.

De la Escalera, S., Bockamp, E.O., Moya, F., Piovant, M., and Jiménez, F., 1990, Characterization and gene cloning of neurotactin, a *Drosophila* transmembrane protein related to cholinesterases. *EMBO J.* 9:3593–3601.

Drews, U., 1975, Cholinesterase in embryonic development. *Prog. Histochem. Cytochem.* 7:1–53.

Inestrosa, N.C., Alvarez, A., Pérez, C.A., Moreno, R.D., Vicente, M., Linker, C., Casanueva, O.I., Soto, C., and Garrido, J., 1996, Acetylcholinesterase accelerates assembly of amyloid-β-peptides into Alzheimer's fibrils: possible role of the periberal site of the enzyme. *Neuron* 16:881–891.

Jbilo, O., L'Hermite, Y., Talesa, V., Toutant, J.-P., and Chatonnet, A., 1994, Acetylcholinesterase and butyrylcholinesterase expression in adult rabbit tissues and during development. *Eur. J. Biochem.* 225:115–124.

Jones, S.A., Holmes, C., Budd, T.C., and Greenfield, S.A., 1995, The effect of acetylcholinesterase on outgrowth of dopaminergic neurons in organotypic slice culture of rat mid-brain. *Cell Tissue Res.* 279:323–330.

Karpel, R., Sternfeld, M., Ginzberg, D., Guhl, E., Graessmann, A. and Soreq, H., 1996, Overexpression of alternative human acetylcholinesterase modulates process extensions in cultured glioma cells. *J. Neurochem.* 66:114–123.

Layer, P.G., 1983, Comparative localization of acetylcholinesterase and pseudocholinesterase during morphogenesis of the chick brain. *Proc. Natl. Acad. Sci. USA* 80:6413–6417.

Layer, P.G., 1990, Cholinesterases preceding major tracts in vertebrate neurogenesis. *BioEssays* 12:415–420.

Layer, P.G., Weikert, T., and Willbold, E., 1992, Chicken retinospheroids as developmental and toxicological in vitro models: acetylcholinesterase is regulated by its own and by butyrylcholinesterase activity. *Cell Tissue Res.* 268:409–418.

Layer, P.G., and Willbold, E., 1993, Histogenesis of the avian retina in reaggregation culture: from dissociated single cells to laminar neuronal networks. *Int. Rev. Cytol.* 146:1–47.

Layer, P.G., Weikert, T., and Alber, R., 1993. Cholinesterases regulate neurite growth in chick nerve cells in vitro by means of a non-enzymatic mechanism. *Cell Tissue Res.* 273:219–226.

Layer, P.G., and Willbold, E., 1994, Regeneration of the avian retina by retinospheroid technology. *Prog. Ret. Res.* 13:197–229.

Layer, P.G., 1995, Nonclassical roles of cholinesterases in the embryonic brain and possible links to Alzheimer disease. *Alzheimer Dis. Assoc. Disord.* 9:29–36.

Layer, P.G. and Willbold, E., 1995, Novel functions of cholinesterases in development, physiology and disease. *Prog. Histochem. Cytochem.* 29:1–94.

Marchot, P., Camp, S., Radic, Z., Bougis, P.E., and Taylor, P., 1995, Structural determinants of fasciculin specificity for acetylcholinesterase. In: *Enzymes of the cholinesterase family,* Quinn, D.M., Balasubramanian, A.S., Doctor, B.P., and Taylor, P. eds., Plenum Press, New York, pp 197–202.

Massoulié, J., and Bon, S., 1982, The molecular forms of cholinesterase and acetylcholinesterase in vertebrates. *Ann. Rev. Neurosci.* 5:57–106.

Massoulié, J., Pezzementi, L., Bon, S., Krejci, E., and Vallette, F.M., 1993, Molecular and cellular biology of cholinesterases. *Progr. Neurobiol.* 41: 31–91.

Mesulam, M., Carson, K., Price, B., and Geula, C., 1992, Cholinesterases in the amyloid angiopathy of Alzheimer's disease. *Ann. Neurol.* 31:565–569.

Moscona, A.A., 1956, Development of heterotypic combinations of dissociated embryonic chick cells. *Proc. Soc. Exp. Biol. Med.* 292:410–416.

Rathjen, F.G., Wolff, J.M., Frank, R., Bonhoeffer, F., and Rutishauser, U., 1987, Membrane glycoproteins involved in neurite fasciculation. *J. Cell. Biol.* 104:343–353.

Robitzki, A., Mack, A., Chatonnet, A., and Layer, P.G., 1997a, Transfection of reaggregating embryonic retinal cells with an antisense-5'DNA butyrylcholinesterase expression vector inhibits proliferation and alters morphogenesis. *J. Neurochem.,* in press.

Robitzki, A., Mack, A., Hoppe, U., Chatonnet, A., and Layer, P.G., 1997b, Regulation of cholinesterase gene expression affects neuronal differentiation as revealed by transfection studies on reaggregating embryonic chicken retinal cells. *Eur. J. Neurosci.,* in press.

Srivatsan M., and Peretz, B., 1997, Acetylcholinesterase promotes regeneration of neurites in cultured adult neurons of *Aplysia. Neuroscience* 77:921–931.

Vollmer, G., Layer, P.G., and Gierer, A., 1984, Reaggregation of embryonic chick retina cells: pigment epithelial cells induce a high order of stratification. *Neurosci. Lett.* 48:191–196.

Willbold, E., and Layer, P.G., 1994. Butyrylcholinesterase regulates laminar retinogenesis of the chick embryo in vitro. *Eur. J. Cell Biol.* 64:192–199.

Wright, C.I., Geula, C., and Mesulam, M.M., 1993, Protease inhibitors and indoleamines selectively inhibit cholinesterases in the histopathologic structures of Alzheimer disease. *Neurobiology* 90:683–686.

78

THE NON-CATALYTIC ROLE AND COMPLEX MANAGEMENT OF ACETYLCHOLINESTERASE IN THE MAMMALIAN BRAIN CALL FOR RNA-BASED THERAPIES

Hermona Soreq and Shlomo Seidman

Department of Biological Chemistry
The Life Sciences Institute
The Hebrew University of Jerusalem
Jerusalem 91904, Israel

THE CHOLINERGIC THEORY OF ALZHEIMER'S DISEASE

The cholinergic theory of Alzheimer's disease (Coyle, Price, and DeLong, 1983) suggests that the selective loss of cholinergic neurons in Alzheimer's disease results in a relative deficit of acetylcholine in specific regions of the brain that mediate learning and memory functions and require acetylcholine to do so. The primary approach to treating Alzheimer's disease has therefore aimed to augment the cholinergic system. Reduced levels of acetylcholine in the brains of Alzheimer's patients leaves a relative excess of acetylcholinesterase, the enzyme responsible for terminating nerve impulses during normal brain activity by disposing of used acetylcholine (Soreq and Zakut, 1993). A relative excess of acetylcholinesterase accentuates the growing cholinergic deficit by further reducing the availability of acetylcholine. The most successful strategy to date for reinforcing cholinergic neurotransmission in Alzheimer's patients is pharmacological inhibition of acetylcholinesterase. Indeed, the only currently approved drugs for Alzheimer's disease are potent acetylcholinesterase inhibitors (Winker, 1994).

CURRENTLY APPROVED DRUGS TO TREAT ALZHEIMER'S DISEASE

Tacrine, the first and most well-characterized acetylcholinesterase inhibitor used for treating Alzheimer's disease offers limited palliative relief to 30–50% of mild-moderately

Progress in Alzheimer's and Parkinson's Diseases
edited by Fisher *et al.*, Plenum Press, New York, 1998.

affected Alzheimer's patients for up to 6 months (Winker, 1994). The positive, albeit partial, success of Tacrine attests to the utility of the cholinergic theory and the potential value of improved anticholinesterase treatment for Alzheimer's disease. Another approved drug, E-2020 (Aricept) has been reported to follow the same mode of action as Tacrine but at lower doses (Rogers et al., 1996). A number of other compounds are under development for inhibition of acetylcholinesterase (Johansson and Nordberg, 1993). All of these are aimed at blocking the fully folded protein from degrading acetylcholine.

ARE CURRENT ALZHEIMER'S DRUGS SATISFACTORY?

Acetylcholinesterase, attached to red blood cells, and a prominent acetylcholinesterase analog, butyrylcholinesterase (Soreq and Zakut, 1993), act to scavenge acetylcholinesterase inhibitors before they get to the brain. This explains why anti-acetylcholinesterase therapies for Alzheimer's disease require high doses of drug and may be the reason for the side-effects resulting from systemic drug administration. Tacrine, for example, has been associated with liver damage and blood disorders in some patients (Johansson and Nordberg, 1993). These considerations alone justify efforts to develop a new generation of anti-acetylcholinesterase drugs displaying increased target specificity, improved efficacy and reduced side-effects. Although newer inhibitors such as E-2020 having greater specificity for acetylcholinesterase provide for lower doses (Rogers et al., 1996), they are not likely to completely overcome the problem of cross-reactivity with butyrylcholinesterase, given the high degree of similarity between the two proteins (Loewenstein-Lichtenstein et al., 1996). Moreover, liver function, red blood cell counts, and natural variations in the genes encoding both acetylcholinesterase and butyrylcholinesterase will determine both the quantity and quality of the drug scavenging potential among individual patients. Several mutations in the butyrylcholinesterase gene already have been suggested to create a genetic predisposition for adverse responses to anticholinesterases (Loewenstein-Lichtenstein et al., 1995). This implies that even in the best case scenario for acetylcholinesterase inhibitor-based therapies, various elements must be considered in designing individualized dosage regimens on a patient-by-patient basis. Moreover, acetylcholinesterase inhibitors do not address recently discovered non-acetylcholine-degrading functions of acetylcholinesterase that may be important in the progression of Alzheimer's disease.

ACETYLCHOLINESTERASE HAS OTHER FUNCTIONS IN THE BRAIN

In addition to its role in regulating cholinergic neurotransmission, acetylcholinesterase appears to be involved in growth-regulating processes affecting neurons (Layer and Willbold, 1995; Small et al., 1995; Jones et al. 1995). This biological activity of acetylcholinesterase is independent of the protein's ability to breakdown acetylcholine and likely operates through cell-cell interactions (Sternfeld et al., 1997). Several laboratories have demonstrated that even inactivated forms of the protein may promote intensive neurites outgrowth in cultured neurons (Layer and Willbold, 1995; Small et al., 1995; Jones et al., 1995). The existence of acetylcholinesterase activities that affect neuronal development but that do not depend on the breakdown of acetylcholine suggests that excesses of acetylcholinesterase in the brain could themselves contribute to neurodegenerative processes.

THE ACETYLCHOLINESTERASE PROTEIN AS A BRAIN DAMAGE INDUCER IN ALZHEIMER'S DISEASE

The discovery of a secondary role for acetylcholinesterase in neurite growth is particularly significant in view of the fact that abnormal neurite projections are a characteristic feature of the Alzheimer's brain, as are abnormal deposits of acetylcholinesterase at sites of senile plaque formation—the principal histopathological hallmark of Alzheimer's disease (Mesulam and Geula, 1990). In the test tube, acetylcholinesterase was shown to mediate the aggregation of β-amyloid protein, the major component of Alzheimer's disease plaques (Inestrosa et al., 1996). This activity was unaffected by some potent acetylcholinesterase inhibitors (Inestrosa et al., 1996). In genetically manipulated mice, excess acetylcholinesterase in cholinergic brain cells promotes an adult-onset, progressive deterioration in learning and memory (Beeri et al., 1995) which is associated with an abnormal cessation of growth among a particular subset of neuritic dendrites (Beeri et al., 1997). The neurodeterioration observed in these mice is strikingly reminiscent of that observed in Alzheimer's disease patients. Thus, emerging evidence suggests that acetylcholinesterase may play a role in the etiology of Alzheimer's disease that goes beyond the scope of the cholinergic theory and may explain the overall disappointing performance of acetylcholinesterase inhibitors in providing effective long-term relief for Alzheimer's patients.

ACETYLCHOLINESTERASE INHIBITORS ACTIVATE A FEEDBACK LOOP THAT MIGHT CONTRIBUTE TO ACETYLCHOLINESTERASE-PROMOTED BRAIN DAMAGE

If acetylcholine-independent effects of acetylcholinesterase play a role in the etiology of Alzheimer's disease, acetylcholinesterase inhibitors could be expected to provide partial relief from symptoms, but cannot be expected to retard direct contributions of the protein to the progressive brain damage characterizing the disease. Recent findings demonstrated dramatically elevated levels of acetylcholinesterase RNA and protein in rodent brains exposed to acetylcholinesterase inhibitors like pyridostigmine (Friedman et al., 1996 - unpublished results). These observations suggest that current anticholinesterase treatments for Alzheimer's disease may actually aggravate the contribution of acetylcholinesterase to the disease process by activating a feedback loop that leads to a response of increased synthesis of the protein under conditions of inhibition. Although continued administration of the inhibitory drug will mask the added acetylcholine-degrading activity, it will not necessarily prevent the potentially disastrous effects of excess acetylcholinesterase protein on neuronal outgrowth. In that case, feedback loops, and the role of acetylcholinesterase as a catalytically inert, but morphogenetically active polypeptide must be seriously weighed in the development of new Alzheimer's drugs. Moreover, drugs which inhibit acetylcholinesterase, regardless of their inhibition of the catalytic activity, may not affect the accumulation of ever increasing levels of the protein with the negative results described here-above accumulating as well.

ANTISENSE OLIGONUCLEOTIDES OFFER A VIABLE ALTERNATIVE

Antisense oligonucleotides offer a viable alternative for specifically arresting the production, in addition to the biochemical activity, of acetylcholinesterase in cells and tissues.

This technology is based on disrupting the pathway leading to acetylcholinesterase biosynthesis by administration of very low doses of short, chemically synthesized DNA chains of antisense oligonucleotides (Grifman et al., 1997). These oligonucleotides are uniquely targeted against the mRNA encoding acetylcholinesterase rather than the ultimate gene product (i.e. the protein). Therefore, the molecular target of these antisense oligonucleotides exists in relatively low abundance. Moreover, antisense oligonucleotides against acetylcholinesterase neither interact with butyrylcholinesterase nor suppress butyrylcholinesterase gene expression. Hence, antisense acetylcholinesterase oligonucleotides should work to effectively suppress acetylcholinesterase production at low doses without the side effects associated with Tacrine and related cholinergic drugs for Alzheimer's disease. By preventing the production of protein, rather than simply blocking the breakdown of acetylcholine, antisense-based therapies would act against the non-catalytic contribution of acetylcholinesterase as well. Since it is targeting the messenger RNA, antisense oligonucleotides may avoid triggering the feedback loop acting to raise acetylcholinesterase levels in brain. Preliminary experiments have shown antisense oligonucleotides targeted against acetylcholinesterase mRNA to be biologically active in several experimental systems (Grifman and Soreq, 1997).

TRANSGENIC ANIMAL MODEL APPROPRIATE FOR TESTING NEW ALZHEIMER'S DRUGS

Since mice do not naturally develop a disease displaying the cholinergic impairments characterizing human dementia, and β-amyloid transgenic mice do not reconstitute the cholinergic imbalance characteristic of Alzheimer's disease, it was decided to generate a novel transgenic mouse model for Alzheimer's disease (Beeri et al., 1995). These genetically engineered mice overproduce human acetylcholinesterase in their cholinergic brain cells. It was predicted that excess acetylcholinesterase in brain cells should promote symptoms similar to those associated with Alzheimer's disease. Subsequent results showed that the ACHE transgenic mice display age-dependent defects in neurite outgrowth (Beeri et al., 1997) and a corresponding deterioration in cognitive performance as measured by a standardized swimming test for spatial learning and memory (Beeri et al., 1995; Beeri et al., 1997). Since the excess acetylcholinesterase in the brains of these mice is derived from human DNA, it is potentially susceptible to antisense oligonucleotides or to the yet more sophisticated family of antisense oriented RNA chains with catalytically active ribozyme activity targeted against the human acetylcholinesterase mRNA and capable of degrading it (Birikh et al., 1997). These transgenic mice, therefore, offer an unparalleled animal system with which to test the ability of anti-acetylcholinesterase antisense technology to relieve some of the impaired cognitive function from which Alzheimer's disease patients suffer. Also, since the time-course of the pseudo-disease condition in transgenic mice is well characterized, it is possible to use these animals to search systematically for molecular markers preceding and accompanying deterioration. Finally, they afford the unique opportunity to test the efficacy of treatments initiated at pre-symptomatic stage, which opens new roads to the development of urgently needed methods for early detection and treatment of Alzheimer's disease.

ACKNOWLEDGMENTS

The authors are grateful to F. Eckstein, R. Beeri, A. Friedman, D. Kaufer, M. Sternfeld and M. Grifman for their contributions towards this research, which is being supported by Ester Neurosciences, a Medica-IPC company.

REFERENCES

Beeri, R., Andres, C., Lev-Lehman, E., Timberg, R., Huberman, T., Shani, M. and Soreq, H, 1995, Transgenic expression of human acetylcholinesterase induces progressive cognitive deterioration in mice. *Curr. Biol.* 5:1063–1071.

Beeri, R., LeNovere, N., Mervis, R., Huberman, T., Grauer, E., Changeux, J.P. and Soreq, H., 1997, Enhanced hemicholinium binding and attenuated dendrite branching in cognitively impaired ACHE-transgenic mice. *J. Neurochem.*, in press.

Birikh, K., Berlin, U.A., Soreq, H. and Eckstein, F. ,1997, Probing accessible sites for ribozymes on human acetylcholinesterase RNA. *RNA* 4:429–437.

Coyle, J.T., Price, D.L. and DeLong, M.R., 1983, Alzheimer's diseaes: A disorder of cortical cholinergic innervation. *Science* 219:1184–1190.

Friedman, A., Kaufer-Nachum, D., Shemer, J., Hendler, I., Soreq, H. and Tur-Kaspa, I., 1996, Pyridostigmine brain penetration under stress enhances neuronal excitability and induces early immediate transcriptional response. *Nature Med.* 2:1382–1385.

Grifman, M., Lev-Lehman, E., Ginzberg, D., Eckstein, F., Zakut, H. and Soreq, H., 1997, Potential antisense oligonucleotide therapies for neurodegenerative diseases. M. Strauss and J.A. Barranger, Eds. *Concepts in Gene Ther*Grifman, M. and Soreq, H., 1997, Differentiation intensifies the susceptibility of phaeochromocytoma cells to antisense oligodeoxynucleotide-dependent suppression of acetylcholinesterase activity. *Antisense Res. Nucleic Acids Drug Dev,*. in press.

Grifman, M. Ginzberg, D. and Soreq, H., 1997, Antisense oligodeoxynucleotide-dependent suppression of acetylcholinesterase expression reduces process extension from primary mammalian neurons. In: *Progress in Alzheimer's and Parkinson's Diseases: Recent Advances.* Fisher, A., Yoshida, M. and Hanin, I., eds., Plenum Press, New York, in press.

Inestrosa, N.C., Alvarez, A., Perez, C.A., Moreno, R.D., Vicente, M., Linker, C., Casanueva, O.I., Soto, C. and Garrido, J., 1996, Acetylcholinesterase accelerates assembly of amyloid β-amyloid peptides into Alzheimer's fibrils: Possible role of the peripheral site of the enzyme. *Neuron* 16:881–891.

Johansson, I.M. and Nordberg, A., 1993, Pharmacokinetic studies of cholinesterase inhibitors. *Acta Neurol. Scad. Suppl.* 149:22–25.

Jones, S.A., Holmes, C., Budd, T.C. and Greednfield, S.A, 1995, The effect of acetylcholinesterase on outgrowth of dopaminergic neurons in organotypic slice culture of rat mid brain. *Cell Tissue Res.* 279:323–330.

Layer, P.G. and Willbold, E., 1995, Novel functions of cholinesterases in development, physiology and disease. Prog. Histochem. *Cytochemistry* 29:1–99.

Loewenstein-Lichtenstein, Y., Glick, D., Gluzman, N., Sternfeld, M., Zakut, H. and Soreq, H., 1996, Overlapping drug interaction sites of human butyrylcholinesterase dissected by site-directed mutagenesis. *Mol. Pharmacol.* 50:1423–1431.

Loewenstein-Lichtenstein, Y., Schwarz, M., Glick, D., Norgaard-Pederson, B., Zakut, H. and Soreq, H., 1995, Genetic predisposition to adverse consequences of anti-cholinesterases in "atypical" BCHE carriers. *Nature Med.* 1:1082–1085.

Mesulam, M.M. and Geula, C., 1990, Shifting patterns of cortical cholinesterases in Alzheimer's disease: Implications for treatment, diagnosis and pathogenesis. *Adv. Neurol.* 51:235–240.

Rogers, S.L., Friedhoff, L.T., Apter, J.T., Richter, R.W., Hartford, J.T., Walshe, T.M, Baumel, B., Linden, R.D., Kinney, F.C., Doody, R.S., Borison, R.L., Ahem, G.L., 1996, The efficacy and safety of Donepezil in patients with Alzheimers disease: results of a US multicentre, randomized, double blind, placebo controlled trial. *Dementia* 7:293–303.

Small, D.H., Reed, G., Whitefield, B. and Neurcombe, V., 1995, Cholinergic regulation of neurite outgrowth from isolated chick sympathetic neurons in culture. *J. Neurosci.* 15:144–151.

Soreq, H. and Zakut, H., 1993, *Human Cholinesterases and anticholinesterases.* Academic Press, San Diego, p. 300.

Sternfeld, Meira, Ming, Guo-li, Song, Hong-jun, Sela, Keren, Soreq, Hermona and Poo, Mu-ming, 1997, Acetylcholinesterase exerts a C-terminus specific, non-catalytic nerve growth promoting activity. Submitted for publication.

Winker, M.A.,1994, Tacrine for Alzheimer's disease; which patient, what dose? *JAMA* 271: 1023–1024.

79

ANTISENSE OLIGODEOXYNUCLEOTIDE DEPENDENT SUPPRESSION OF ACETYLCHOLINESTERASE EXPRESSION REDUCES PROCESS EXTENSION FROM PRIMARY MAMMALIAN NEURONS

Mirta Grifman, Dalia Ginzberg, and Hermona Soreq

The Department of Biological Chemistry
The Institute of Life Sciences
The Hebrew University of Jerusalem
91904, Jerusalem, Israel

INTRODUCTION

The only currently approved drugs for Alzheimer's disease (AD) are potent blockers of acetylcholinesterase (AChE) activity (Knapp et al., 1994). However, several lines of evidence suggest novel, non-catalytic morphogenic properties of AChE in process extension (Small et al., 1995; Layer and Willbold, 1995; Jones et al., 1995; Darboux et al., 1996; Sternfeld et al., 1997) and amyloid fibril formation (Inestrosa et al., 1996). This calls for the development of alternative approaches in which both AChE protein synthesis and enzymatic activity would be suppressed, such as the "antisense" technology (Grifman et al., 1997). To this end, we have designed seven synthetic 3'-phosphorothioated oligonucleotides (AS-ODNs) targeted towards AChEmRNA and tested their AChE suppression efficacies on the rat neuroendocrine pheochromocytoma cell line, PC12. Two of these AS-ODNs suppressed the catalytic activity of AChE in nerve growth factor (NGF) -treated PC12 cells by 25–35%, significantly more than the parallel suppression by control ODNs (Grifman and Soreq, 1997). To study the involvement of AChE in neurite outgrowth and differentiation of primary neurons, we added these two AS-ODNs to primary neuronal cultures from embryonic (E14) mouse whole brain.

MATERIALS AND METHODS

Primary mouse neuronal cultures were prepared from embryonic (E14) mouse (Balb/C) whole brains. Brains were removed and cells mechanically dissociated with a

Progress in Alzheimer's and Parkinson's Diseases
edited by Fisher *et al.*, Plenum Press, New York, 1998.

drawn Pasteur pipette. Cells were plated in serum-free medium (2.5×10^6 cells/ml) in 24-well (1 ml per well) Costar (Cambridge) culture dishes coated successively with poly-L-ornithine and culture medium containing 10% fetal calf serum (Weiss et al., 1986). Cultures grown for 24hr at 37°C, 5% CO_2 were treated with synthetic 20-mer terminally phosphorothioated oligonucleotides (Ehrlich et al., 1994) complementary to either ACHE exon 2 (AS1) or exon 5 (AS5). The inverse sequence of AS1 (inv1) was used for control. After 24 hr growth, cells were stained using May-Grunwald stain (Sigma) followed by Gurr's improved Giemsa stain (BDH). Cell viability was tested using a two-color fluorescence assay that measures the intracellular activity of all esterases and depends on plasma membrane integrity (LIVE/DEAD® EUKOLIGHT™ viability/ cytotoxicity kit (Molecular probes)). Enzymatic conversion of the cell permeable, non-fluorescent dye Calcein by ubiquitous esterases in viable cells renders an intensely fluorescent green form of Calcein. This product is retained within viable cells, producing an intense green fluorescence (about 530 μm). A second dye, Ethidium Homodimer, was used to identify dead cells, since it penetrates only through damaged membranes. In the cell it binds to nucleic acids, producing a bright red fluorescence (>600 μm).

RESULTS

The mouse ACHE gene includes 6 exons and 4 introns, and gives rise to two alternative mRNAs in mouse primary neuronal cultures, the "brain and muscle" ACHE mRNA which includes exons 1–4 and 6 and the "readthrough" ACHE mRNA which includes exons 1–4, pseudointron 4 which in certain tissues operates as an exon (Karpel et al., 1994) and exon 5. AS1 and AS5 were designed to hybridize with specific domains in exon 2 and exon 5, respectively. Therefore AS1 can potentially lead to destruction of both ACHE mRNAs, whereas AS5 can only interact with the "readthrough" mRNA or with the pre-splicing AChE mRNA precursor. Cells grown for 24hr in serum-free medium on "serum-coated" dishes were treated with these antisense oligos, complementary to two alternative 3'-exons in the ACHE gene (AS1 or AS5) or with an oligo oriented in an inverse 3'→5' orientation (Inv1), for control. Both AS1 and AS5 treatments but not Inv1 induced the appearance of multilayered cell aggregates and suppressed neurite outgrowth (Fig. 1). The effect appeared earlier with increasing doses of the oligos, indicating dose dependence (Fig. 1). Aggregated cells with decreased number of neurite extensions remained viable as assessed by a two-color fluorescence cell viability/cytotoxicity assay (Fig. 2). Cytochemical staining revealed a reduction of AChE activity within cholinoceptive neurons in the cell cultures treated with these AS-ODNs (Fig. 3), suppression which has been confirmed by electron microscopy (Fig. 4). These oligonucleotide-induced phenotypic changes suggest AChE involvement in neuronal growth and differentiation. Furthermore, our findings demonstrate susceptibility of mammalian neurons to limitation of neurite extension by low concentrations of AS-ODNs, suggesting the use of these synthetic molecules or corresponding ribozyme agents (Birikh et al., 1997) to suppress AChE levels and prevent abnormal process extension in the patients with neurodegenerative diseases associated with such pathologies.

CONCLUSIONS

Two oligonucleotides targetted at the ACHE gene, but not an inverse control sequence, caused neuronal aggregation and suppressed process extension, at the concentration range of 0.1 μM–0.5 μM. The time of initiation of this morphogenic effect was

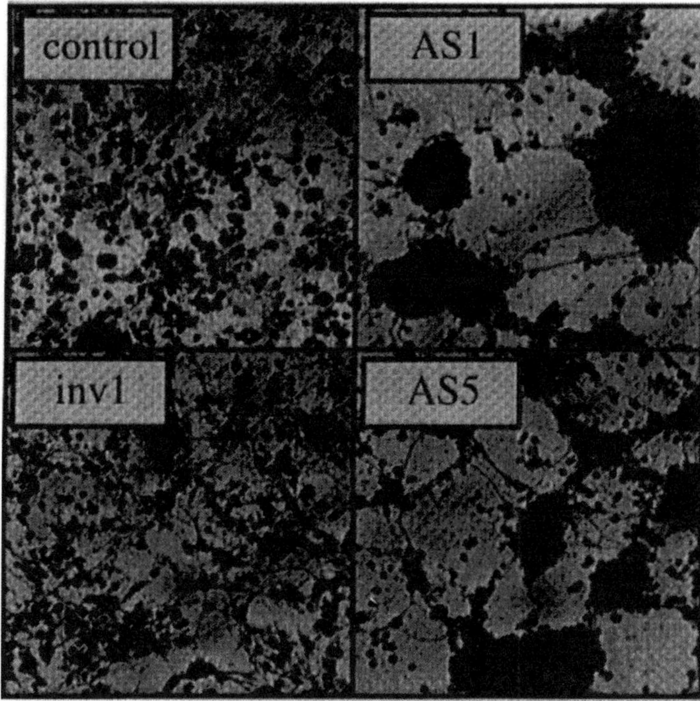

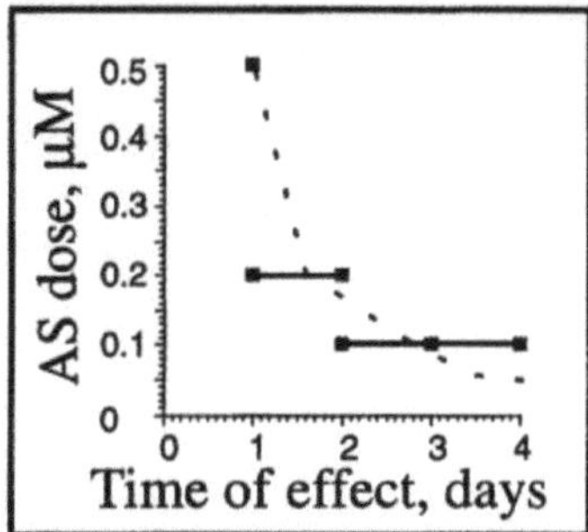

Figure 1. Both AS1 and AS5 exert dose-dependent morphogenic effects. **A.** The morphogenic effect. Cells were grown and treated for 24 hr with 0.5 mM of either AS1, AS5 or inv1 and stained with May-Grunwald stain followed by Gurr's improved Giemsa stain as described under Materials and Methods. After staining the cells optic microscopy was performed with a Zeiss inverted microscope, magnification X160. Note that while untreated or inv1 treated cells formed monolayers of single neurons with thin extensions, cells treated with either AS1 or AS5 were re-organized in multicellular, multilayered aggregates connected by few thick processes. **B.** Dose-dependence of morphogenic changes. Cell cultures treated with increasing concentrations (0.1–5.0 µM) of AS1 were monitored for 5 days and the day on which aggregation was first observed was noted. At the highest concentration of 5.0 µM oligonucleotide, cytotoxicity was observed, cells detached from the dishes and died. Presented are cumulative data from 6 experiments.

inversely related to the oligonucleotide concentration, being as short as 24 hr for 0.5 µM oligo. The aggregation effect does not affect cell viability. Cytochemical staining revealed reduced ChE activity in AS1 treated cultures as detected both by light and electron microscopy. Both the similar morphogenic effect and the reduced *in situ* activity staining with two distinct oligonucleotides targetted at the same gene suggest an antis-

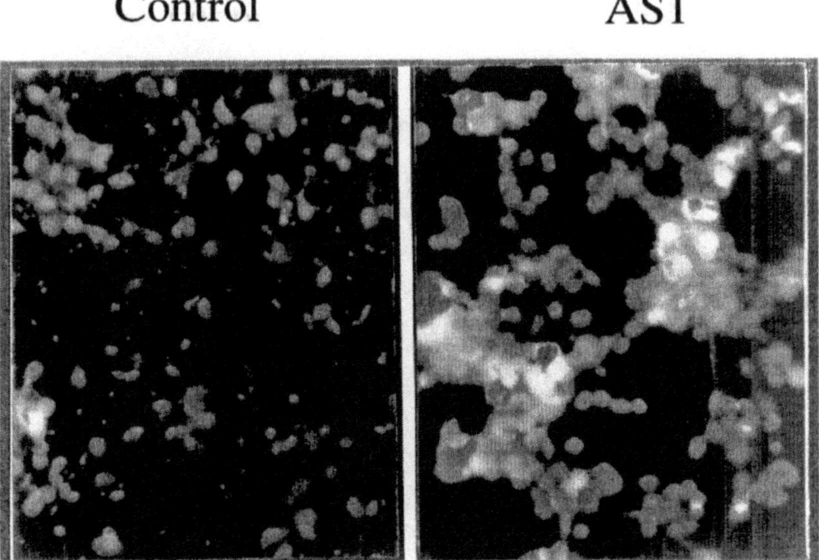

Figure 2. Aggregated cells in AS1 treated cultures are viable. The viability of neuronal primary cultures that displayed the cytomorphological effect following 24 hr growth in the presence of 0.5 μM AS1 was assayed with a viability/cytotoxicity kit. Fluorescence microscopy was performed with a Zeiss Axioplan microscope equipped with ×40 Achroplan lens, a HC100 camera and a FITC/Texas red 485/578 double excitation filter. Magnification ×400. Note that the aggregated cells in AS-mE2 treated cultures remained viable.

ense mechanism.Moreover, the outcome of this AS-ODN treatment is reciprocal to the excessive process extension induced in rat glia by AChE overexpression (Karpel et al., 1996). Therefore, these findings indicate involvement of AChE in neurite outgrowth and suggest the use of AS-ODNs to suppress both the cholinergic imbalance associated with relatively high AChE catalytic activity and the damage caused by excessive process extension.

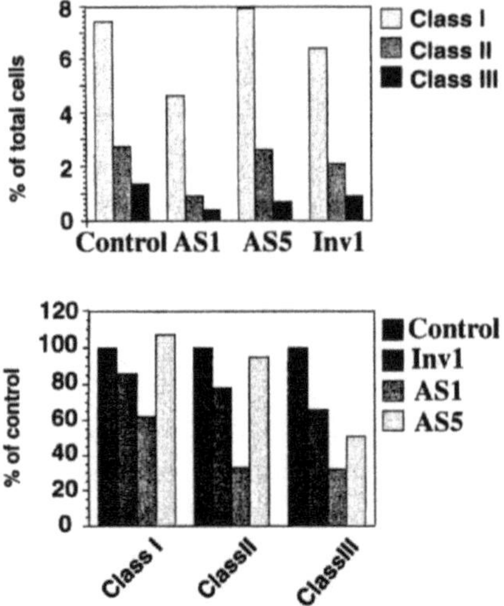

Figure 3. Antisense ACHE treatment reduces ChE levels in neuronal cultures. Neuronal cell cultures were treated for 24 hr with no oligonucleotide (Control), or with 0.5 μM of the noted oligomers (AS1 or Inv1). Cells were then stained for AChE activity overnight at 4°C with no prior fixation, (Seidman *et al.*, 1995). Stained cells in 20 different microscope fields for each preparation (magnification ×1000), were classified by the intensity of staining. Each field contained approximately 250 neurons. Stained neurons (approximately 5–7% of total) included, class I (light brown stain in cell body), class II (more intense staining particulay around the cell body) and class III (very intense, dark brown stain reaching into neuronal extensions). Note that within all classes, staining was considerably lower in AS1 treated cells but not in those treated with Inv1, suggesting an antisense mechanism.

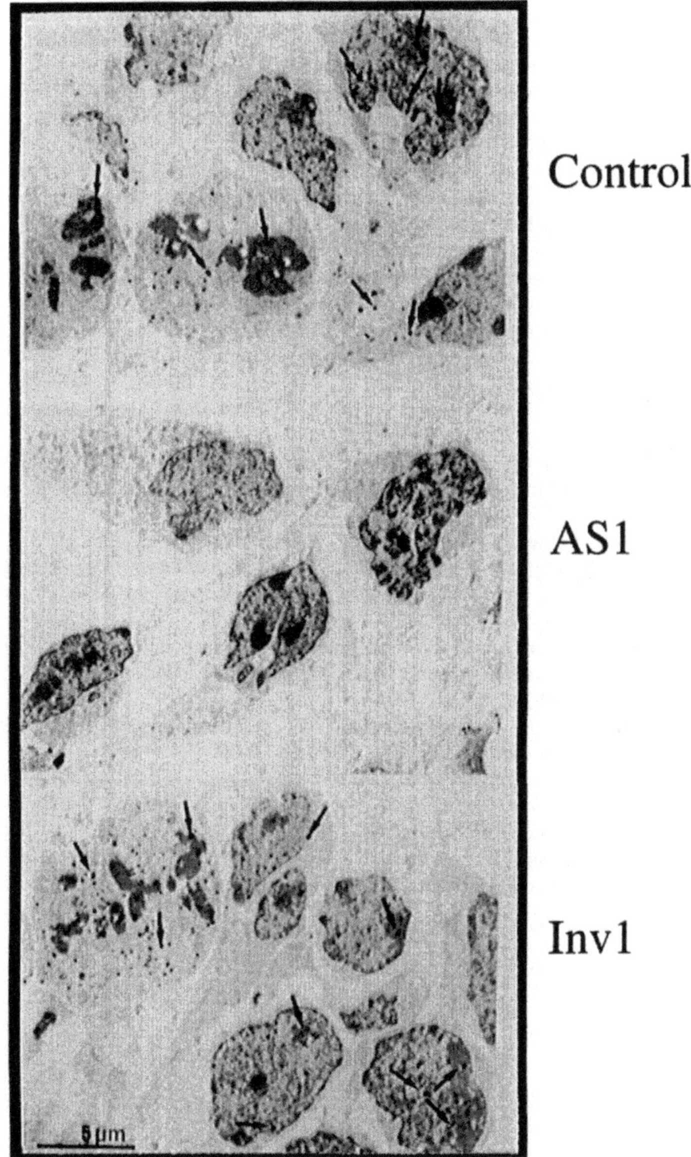

Figure 4. Antisense suppression of AChE activity visualized by electron microscopy. Neuronal cell cultures were treated for 24 hr with no oligonucleotide (Control), or with 0.5 μM of the noted oligomers (AS1 or Inv1). Cells were then fixed for 30 min in 4% paraformaldehyde and lightly stained for AChE activity for 4 hours at room temperature and analyzed by transmission electron microscopy as detailed elsewhere, (Seidman *et al.*, 1995). Arrows denote crystal reaction products of acetylthiocholine hydrolysis. Note absence of enzyme reaction products in neurons treated with AS1.

REFERENCES

Birikh, K., Berlin, U.A., Soreq, H. and Eckstein, F., 1997, Probing accessible sites for ribozymes on human acetylcholinesterase RNA. *RNA* 4:429–437.
Darboux, I., Barthalay, Y., Piovant, M. and Hipeau-Jacquotte, R., 1996, The structure-function relationships in *Drosophila* neurotactin shows that cholinesterasic domains may have adhesive properties. *EMBO J.* 15:4835–4843.

Ehrlich, G., Patinkin, D., Ginzberg, D., Zakut, H., Eckstein, F. and Soreq, H., 1994, Use of partially phosphorothioated "antisense" oligodeoxynucleotides for sequence-dependent modulation of hematopoiesis in culture. *Antisense Research and Development* 4:173–183.

Grifman, M. and Soreq, H., 1997, Differentiation intensifies the susceptibility of phaeochromocytoma cells to antisense oligodeoxynucleotide-dependent suppression of acetylcholinesterase activity. *Antisense and Nucl. Acid. Res. and Dev.*, in press

Grifman, M., Lev-Lehman, E., Ginzberg, D., Eckstein, F., Zakut, H. and Soreq, H., 1997, Potential antisense oligonucleotide therapies for neurodegenerative diseases. In: *Concepts in Gene Therapy*,. Strauss, M. and Barranger, J.A., eds., Walter de Gruyter & Co., Berlin.

Inestrosa, N.C., Alvarez, A., Perez, C.A., Moreno, R.D., Vicente, M., Linker, C., Casanueva, O.I., Soto, C. and Garrido, J., 1996, Acetylcholinesterase accelerates assembly of amyloid-beta-peptides into Alzheimer's fibrils: possible role of the peripheral site of the enzyme. *Neuron* 16:881–891.

Jones, S.A., Holmes, C., Budd, T.C. and Greenfield, S.A. 1995. The effect of acetylcholinesterase on outgrowth of dopaminergic neurons in organotypic slice culture of rat midbrain. *Cell Tissue Res.* 279:323–330.

Karpel, R., Ben Aziz-Aloya R., Sternfeld, M., Ehrlich, G., Ginzberg, D., Tarroni, P., Clementi, F., Zakut, H. and Soreq, H., 1994, Expression of three alternative acetylcholinesterase messenger RNAs in human tumor cell lines of different tissue origins. *Exp. Cell. Res.* 210:268–277.

Karpel, R., Sternfeld, M., Ginzberg, D., Guhl, E., Graessmann, A. and Soreq, H., 1996, Overexpression of alternative human acetylcholinesterase forms modulates process extensions in cultured glioma cells. *J. Neurochem.* 66:114–123.

Knapp, M.J., Knopman, D.S., Solomon, P.R., Pendlebury, W.W., Davis, C.S. and Gracon, S.I., 1994, A 30-week randomized controlled trial of high-dose tacrine in patients with Alzheimer's disease. *JAMA* 271:985–991.

Layer, P.G. and Willbold, E., 1995, Novel functions of cholinesterases in development, physiology and disease. Prog. Histochem. Cytochem. 29:1–99.

Seidman, S., Sternfeld, M., Ben Aziz-Aloya, R., Timberg, R., Kaufer-Nachum, D. and Soreq, H., 1995, Synaptic and epidermal accumulations of human acetylcholinesterase is encoded by alternative 3'-terminal exons. *Mol. Cell. Biol.* 15:2993–3002.

Small, D. H., Reed, G., Whitefield, B. and Nurcombe, V., 1995, Cholinergic regulation of neurite outgrowth from isolated chick sympathetic neurons in culture. *J. Neurosci.* 15:144–151.

Sternfeld, M., Seidman, S., Beeri, R. and Soreq, H., 1997, Catalytic and non-catalytic acetylcholinesterase functions implied from transgenic ACHE expression in vertebrates. In: *Neurotransmitter Release and Uptake*, S. Pogun, ed.., Springer-Verlag, Berlin, in press.

Weiss, S., Pin, J. P., Sebben, M., Kemp, D. E., Sladeczek, F., Gabrion, J. and Bockaert, J., 1986, Synaptogenesis of cultured striatal neurons in serum free medium: a morphological and biochemical study. *Proc. Natl. Acad. Sci. USA.* 83:2238–2242.

80

TACRINE REDUCES THE SECRETION OF SOLUBLE AMYLOID BETA-PEPTIDES IN A NEUROBLASTOMA CELL LINE

Debomoy K. Lahiri* and Martin R. Farlow

Institute of Psychiatric Research
Departments of Psychiatry and Neurology
791 Union Drive, Indiana
University School of Medicine
Indianapolis, Indiana 46202

INTRODUCTION

One of the major hallmarks of Alzheimer's disease is the deposition of the 39–43 amino acid residue (Mw ~4 kDa) amyloid beta-peptide as a major constituent of extracellular plaques which are detected in certain areas of the brain (Selkoe, 1997). This peptide is synthesized as part of the larger 110–120 kDa amyloid beta-protein precursor which is a type I integral membrane glycoprotein with a large N-terminal extracellular domain, a single transmembrane domain and a short cytoplasmic tail. The Aβ sequence spans portions of the extracellular and transmembrane domains of βAPP. Secreted derivatives arise after cleavage of βAPP at three different sites which are close to the transmembrane domain (Selkoe, 1997). The cleavage by (α-secretase occurs within the Aβ sequence after residue 16 and does not contribute to amyloid fon-nation. Other cleavage sites by enzymes referred to as 'β'- and 'γ'-secretase, occur at the amino- and carboxyl-ends of Aβ, respectively, resulting in secretion of soluble βAPP and Aβ, some forms of which are potentially amyloidogenic. The identification and characterization of the βAPP secretases are currently progressing in several laboratories. The pathological relevance of these proteolytic currently progressing in several laboratories. The pathological relevance of these proteolytic processes lies in the fact that at least five mutations in βAPP, all located in or near the Aβ domain, were identified in families with early onset of familial Alzheimer's disease

---

* Corresponding author.

Progress in Alzheimer's and Parkinson's Diseases
edited by Fisher *et al.*, Plenum Press, New York, 1998.

(Hisama and Schllenberg, 1996; Selkoe, 1997). Recently a correlation among memory deficits, Aβ elevation and amyloid plaques has been demonstrated in transgenic mice overexpressing βAPP containing one of these mutations (Hsiao et al., 1996). Different factors and agents that regulate amyloid depositions are central to understanding cerebrovascular depositions of Aβ in AD (Checler, 1995).

By using the cell culture technique we investigated whether the secretion of Aβ can be regulated by tacrine. In clinical use tacrine may improve memory and cognitive functions in some AD subjects (Farlow et al., 1992). We have previously demonstrated that normal levels of secretion of soluble βAPP derivatives into conditioned media were severely inhibited by treating cells with tacrine (Lahiri et al., 1994). Here we have analyzed the levels of different forms of soluble amyloid beta-peptides, such as the short form which ends at the 40th residue (Aβ40) and the long form which ends at the 42nd residue (AB42), in the conditioned medium of human neuroblastoma cells (SK-N-SH) that were treated with tacrine. We first observed that these cells could indeed secrete measurable levels of Aβ in the medium. Treating cells with tacrine reduced the levels of soluble Aβ and the reduction in levels of Aβ was observed as early as 4 hours (h) after treatment with the drug. For example, as compared to the untreated cells, the treatment with tacrine resulted in a 10–30% reduction in levels of Aβ depending upon the period of treatment. Possible toxic effects were assayed by the LDH assay which is a means of measuring the membrane integrity as a function of the amount of cytoplasmic LDH released into the medium. Under our conditions no detectable change was observed in the release of LDH between control and tacrine-treated samples. All these data taken together suggest that treatment with tacrine reduced the levels of soluble βAPP and Aβ, whose concentrations are critical *in vivo* in the formation of amyloid aggregates.

MATERIALS AND METHODS

Materials

Tacrine was bought from the Sigma Chemical Company (MD). Fetal bovine serum (FBS), horse serum and minimal essential medium (MEM) were purchased from Gibco/BRL (MD). The rest of the chemicals were of the molecular biology grade.

Cells and culture conditions: The human neuroblastoma cell line (SK-N-SH) was obtained from American Type Culture Collection (MD) and cultured in 60 mm tissue culture plates in MEM containing 10% FBS as described previously (Lahiri et al., 1994). Untransfected (such as with βAPP cDNA) cells were used throughout this study.

Treatment of Cells with Tacrine

SK-N-SH cells were cultured in 60 mm plates in the regular medium to confluence (5–7×10^6). Before adding the drug, the cells were fed with low serum (0.5% FBS)- containing media (LSM). The cells were then incubated either in the presence of a vehicle control or tacrine (10 μg/ml). Following incubation for different periods of time as indicated in Table 1, the conditioned medium from each plate was collected and clarified at 800 g for 8 minutes. For the purpose of control experiment, an equivalent concentration of vehicle (DMSO) was used which was finally less than 0.05% in media.

The experiment which had a control with 3 plates and tacrine with 3 plates was performed in a duplicate set with a total number of 12 plates. For each treatment, the

Table 1. Assay of the release of Aβ40 and Aβ42 in the conditioned medium from a neuroblastoma cell line

Time (hours)	A840 (C) (fmol/ nV)	A840 M (fmol/ ml)	A342 (C) (fmol/ m/)	A1342 M (fmol/ M/)
0	0	0	0	0
4	18.09	12.93	−0.03	−0.53
8	30.94	19.96	0.70	0.21
12	56.72	37.53	1.73	11.49
16	67.00	45.38	3.37	2.04
24	90.83	55.96	4.07	2.98
36	76.69	6.66	3.06	−0.03
48	63.92	5.42	3.09	0.07
72	19.67	5.91	1.20	0.14

SK-N-SH cells were cultured in the presence of either a vehicle control (C) or tacrine (T) and an equivalent amount of the conditioned medium was assayed for the level of and Aβ40 and Aβ42 species at various time period as indicated. The assay was performed using the Sandwich ELISA method. The values are expressed as mean minus zero hour.

neuroblastoma cells were first gown to confluence in the regular medium, then at the day of the experiment each treatment was initiated (zero time point) by feeding cells with 3 ml of LSM. For each successive time point, 0.25 ml of the conditioned medium was collected from each of the 3 plates and transferred to a tube. The pooled conditioned medium (0.75 ml) from each of the duplicate set was analyzed for subsequent experiments such as LDH assay, and ELISA for measuring levels of Aβ. Each of these assays were performed in duplicate. For detecting soluble βAPP, western blot was performed.

Assay of LDH

The measurement of released LDH in the conditioned medium was performed using reagents from the Sigma Company. The assay is based on the reduction of NAD by the action of LDH. The resulting reduced NAD (NADH) is utilized in the stoichiometric conversion of a: tetrazolium dye. The final colored compound is measured spectrophotometrically. If the cells are lysed prior to assaying the medium, an increase or decrease in cell number results in a concomitant change in the amount of substrate converted. This indicates the degree of inhibition of cell growth (cytotoxicity) caused by the test material. If cell-free aliquots of medium from cultures given different treatments are assayed, the amount of LDH activity can be used as an indicator of relative cell viability as a function of membrane integrity.

Assay of Soluble Forms of Aβ

The ELISA for measuring levels of Aβ in the conditioned medium was performed in collaboration with Dr. S. Younkin as briefly described below (Suzuki et al., 1994). The antibody BAN50 (against Aβ 1−16) was used to capture both Aβ40 and Aβ42 species from the conditioned medium while antibody βA27 (specific for Aβ40) and antibody BC05 (specific for Aβ42) was used to detect these Aβ forms, respectively using the sandwich ELISA system. The levels of Aβ were expressed in femtomols (fmol) per ml as deduced from the appropriate standard curve run in parallel with the assay.

RESULTS

Effect of Tacrine on the Secretion of LDH into the Conditioned Media of Cells

We have measured the toxic effects of the drug *in vitro* by counting the viable cells after staining with a vital dye. Additionally, we have also employed the lactate dehydrogenase assay which is a means of measuring either the number of cells via total cytoplasmic LDH or membrane integrity as a function of the amount of cytoplasmic LDH released into the medium. To determine the integrity of the cell membrane during the treatment of cells with tacrine, we measured the level of LDH in the conditioned medium from both untreated control and tacrine-treated cells under the same conditions. The measurement of LDH in control cells indicated that there was no detectable level of enzyme released in the conditioned medium of cultured cells collected at 4 h, 8 h and 12 h of treatment (Fig. 1). But from 16h onward, the percent of LDH release started increasing from 4.25% (at 16 h) to 71–75% and 88.5% at 24 h and 48 h, respectively. Beyond this period, the level of LDH started to drop because of a concomitant decrease in cell viability as measured by the trypan blue exclusion method. These data indicate that even the control cells have started leaking LDH after overnight culturing under our conditions. This could be due to growing the cells in low serum-

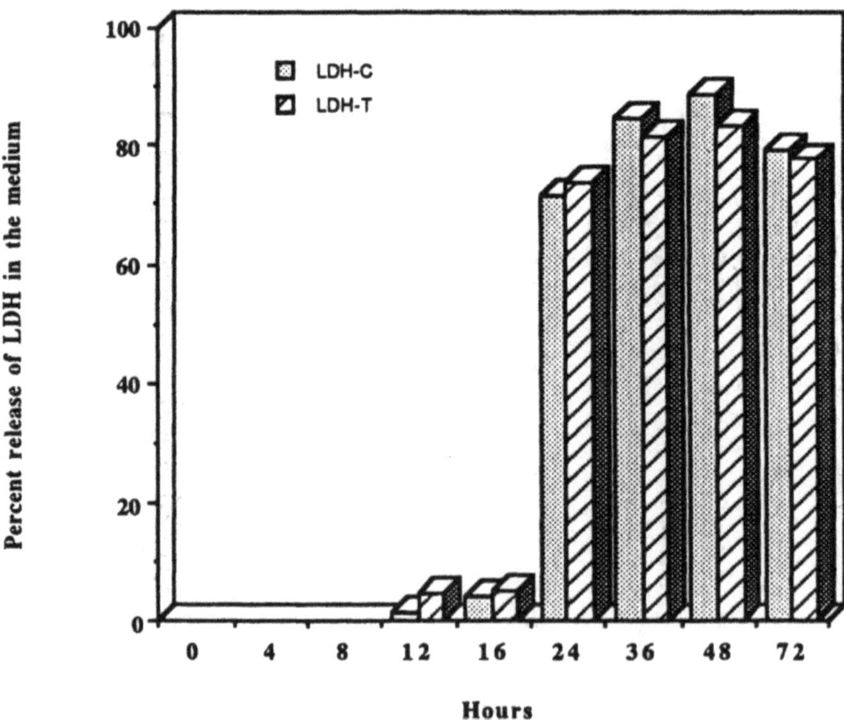

Figure 1. Measurement of the release of LDH in the conditioned medium from a neuroblastoma cell line. SK-N-SH cells were cultured in the presence of either a vehicle control (C) or tacrine (T) and an equivalent amount of the conditioned medium was assayed for the activity of LDH at various time period as indicated in the figure. The maximum activity of LDH was assigned as 100% release, which was then used to calculate the corresponding percent release of LDH at different time period of the treatment.

containing medium (starvation). Like the control cells, treatment with tacrine in these cells did not result in any significant release of LDH at 4h and 8h. There was about 5% release at 12h and 16h in tacrine-treated cells (Fig. 1). Although there was a slight increase in LDH release in tacrine-treated cells from the controls at 12h to 24h, overall the membrane integrity of cells was not very different between control and tacrine-treated cells.

Effect of Tacrine on the Secretion of AB into the Conditioned Media of Cells

We have investigated the effects of tacrine on the secretion of soluble Aβ into the conditioned medium. Since the level of Aβ in the media was very low, we were unable to measure the levels of Aβ by either the immunoblotting or immunoprecipitation method. Recently, we have been successful in assaying the levels of soluble Aβ peptides by the sandwich ELISA method as developed by Dr. Younkin's group (Suzuki et al., 1994). The same condition medium, as that used for LDH, was assayed for the levels of the short and the long form of Aβ, respectively. In the untreated cells, Aβ40 could be detected as early as 4h of treatment (18 fmol). The level of Aβ started increasing over time to 67 fmol at 16h and the level attained a maximum of 90 fmol at 24 h (Table 1). After that period of time the level of Aβ40 started dropping from its peak value, probably due to loss of cells as explained earlier for the LDH assay. Under the same conditions when the cells were cultured in the presence of tacrine, there was a decrease in the levels of Aβ40 at all time periods measured. A comparative study indicates that there was about a 30% decrease in the release of Aβ40 in the conditioned medium of tacrine-treated than control cultures.

The level of Aβ42 was independently measured in the same conditioned medium from these cells. However, the basal level of Aβ42 release was found to be approximately 20 to 25-fold less than that of Aβ40 at a given time point in control cells. For example, the level of Aβ42 that could be detected in the conditioned medium from control cells at 12h was 1.73 fmol which gradually increased over time to a maximum of 4 fmol at 24h. The release of Aβ42 was substantially inhibited in the conditioned medium of the tacrine-treated cultures at all time periods studied (Table 1).

DISCUSSION

In this report we have performed a time course experiment to study the secretion of Aβ in tacrine-treated cultures. For this, SK-N-SH cells were cultured either in the presence of the vehicle control or tacrine for 48 hours and samples of conditioned media from each plate were analyzed at regular intervals for the release of LDH as a function of membrane integrity and levels of Aβ. We observed that there was a sharp decrease of secreted Aβ in media from tacrine-treated cells at the period of time when there was a minimum damage of cell membrane as compared to control cells under the conditions used here. However, the experiments with a more sensitive assay to detect cell death such as MTT (3-[4,5-dimethylthiazol-2-yl]-2,5-diphenyl tetrazolium bromide) reduction assay, and TUNEL (terminal deoxynucleotidyl transferase dUTP nick end labeling) staining method to see if tacrine initiates cell death are in progress. Previously we reported that the inhibitory effect of tacrine on the secretion of soluble βAPP was observed after addition of the drug in a variety of cell lines (Lahiri et al., 1994). Prolonged treatment of the drug did not reduce the secretion proportionately. Tacrine may not be as effective over a longer period of time as over a shorter period of time because of the toxic effect on the cell. The treatment of cells with tacrine might also reduce the synthesis of βAPP. Although the treatment of cells with tacrine resulted in a decrease in the levels of soluble βAPP across cell lines, we consistently observed more of a decrease in the neuronal cell type such as SH-SY-5Y and PC12 cells. Immunoblots with KPI specific antibodies suggested that the 100- and 95 kDa bands correspond to soluble derivatives from KPI-containing and KPI-lacking forms of βAPP, respectively (data not shown). To confirm that the proteins detected by mAb22C11 were secreted βAPP and not due to only a βAPP-related homologue such as APLP-2, we have performed similar immunoblot analyses using mAb6E10 and results were very similar with mAb6E10, indicating that the drug-mediated change was specific for βAPP (data not shown). We are currently analyzing the carboxyl terminal fragments detected in the cell lysates using mAb4G8 (against Aβ 17-25) and the anti-C terminal (against βAPP 643-695) antibodies.

AD is characterized by a severe loss of presynaptic cholinergic neurons in nucleus basalis and their projections to the cerebral cortices and decreased levels of acetylcholine and choline acetyl transferase in the cortex (Becker et al., 1996; Lamy, 1994). The inhibition of cholinergic activity in the central nervous system in patients with AD correlates with decline in scores on dementia rating scales. Currently, cholinesterase inhibition is the most widely studied and developed approach for treating symptoms of AD. It should be mentioned here that the concentration of tacrine used here is much higher than that used clinically. Although the catalytic properties and the role of acetylcholinesterase in synaptic transmission are well established, non-catalytic functions of the enzyme are poorly understood. For example, it is possible that tacrine may bind to different sites of the same enzyme, one responsible for its anti-catalytic activity, the other for its anti-βAPP releasing function. The mechanism by which tacrine influences the secretion of βAPP and Aβ is not completely understood. From the IC50 values, it is noted that it has some overlapping acetylcholinesterase (AChE) and butyrylcholinesterase (BChE) inhibitory activity at higher concentrations (Greig et al., 1995). It is possible that the effect of tacrine on the secretion of βAPP may not be due to its effect on the enzyme itself rather the effect of the drug may be due to its lysosomotropic action because of its high pKa (~9.2) (Dell'Antone et al., 1995; Lahiri and Farlow, 1996). We have recently shown that as compared to the untreated neuroblastoma, the treatment of cells with physostigmine resulted in no change in levels of secreted βAPP in the conditioned medium (Lahiri and Farlow, 1996). The difference in action of tacrine and other anticholinesterases on the processing of βAPP in cell lines may also be due either to the selectivity for BChE over AChE or the instability of the drugs. Our results suggest that non-catalytic functions of cholinesterase inhibitors can be utilized to alter the metabolism of βAPP which might in turn affect the process of deposition of Aβ, a key component of the cerebrovascular amyloid detected in AD.

ACKNOWLEDGMENTS

These studies were supported by grants from NIH. We sincerely thank Drs. S. Younkin, L. Younkin and C. Eckman (Mayo Clinic, Jacksonville, FL) for fruitful discussion and performing the Aβ sandwich ELISA.

REFERENCES

Becker, R., Giacobini, E., and Robert, P., 1996, Alzheimer's Disease: Molecular Biology to Therapy. Birkhauser, Boston.

Checler, F., 1995, Processing of the β-amyloid precursor protein and its regulation in Alzheirmr's disease. *J. Neurochem.* 65:1431–1444.

Dell'Antone, P., Bragadin, M., and Zatta, P., 1995, Anticholinesterase drugs: tacrine but not physostigmine, accumulates in acidic compartments of the cells. *Biochim.Biophys. Acta* 1270:137–141.

Farlow, M., Gracon, S.I., Hershey, L.A., Lewis, K.W., Sadowsky, C.H., and Dolan-Ureno, J., 1992, A controlled trial of tacrine in Alzheimer's disease. *J. Am. Med. Assoc.*268:2523–2529.

Greig, N.H., Pei, X.-F., Soncrant, T.T., Ingram, D.K., and Brossi, A., 1995, Phenserine and ring C hetero-analogues: drug candidates for the treatment of Alzheimer's disease. *Med. Res. Revs.* 15:3–31.

Hisama, F.M., and Schllenberg, G.D., 1996, Progress in molecular genetics of Alzheimer's disease. *Neuroscient.* 2:3–6.

Hsiao, K., Chapman, P., Nilsen, S., Eckman, C., Harigaya, Y, Younkin, S., Yang, F., and Cole, G., 1996, Correlative memory deficits, Aβ elevation, and amyloid plaques in transgenic mice. *Science* 274:99–102.

Lahiri, D.K., Lewis, S., and Farlow, M.R., 1994, Tacrine alters the processing of beta amyloid precursor protein in different cell lines. *J. Neurosci. Res.* 37:777–787.

Lahiri, D.K., and Farlow, M.R., 1996, Differential effect of tacrine and physostigmine on the secretion of the beta-amyloid precursor protein in cell lines. *J. Mol. Neurosci.* 7:41–49.

Lamy, P. P., 1994, The role of cholinestemse-inhibitors in Alzheimer's disease. *CNS Drugs* 2:146–165.

Selkoe, D.J., 1997, Alzheimer's disease: genotypes, phenotype, and treatment. *Science* 275:630–631.

Suzuki, N., Cheung, T.T., Cai, X.D., Odaka, A., Otvos, L. Jr., Eckman, C., Golde, T.E., and Younkin, S.G., 1994, An increased percentage of long amyloid beta protein secreted by familial amyloid beta protein precursor (beta APP717) mutants. *Science* 264:1336–1340.

81

CHOLINESTERASE INHIBITORS FOR ALZHEIMER'S DISEASE THERAPY

Do They Work?

Ezio Giacobini

HUG, Belle-Idée
Department of Geriatrics
University Hospitals of Geneva
Route de Mon-Idée
CH-1226 Thonex
Geneva, Switzerland

CHOLINESTERASE INHIBITORS: DO THEY WORK? HOW DO THEY WORK? IS THERE A DIFFERENCE?

Cholinesterase inhibitors (ChEI) presently in clinical trials for the treatment of Alzheimer's disease (AD) in Japan, USA and Europe include more than a dozen drugs, most of which have already advanced to clinical phase III and two (tacrine and donepezil) are registered in the USA and Europe (Giacobini, 1996). It is likely that in the next two-year period (1997–1999) at least three other ChEI will be registered world wide. The second generation of ChEI, in order to replace tacrine, will have to fulfill specific requirements (Giacobini, 1996). After analyzing the results emerging from clinical trials, the first question to be answered is: do ChEI work in the AD patient, and if so, how do they work? A second question is: are there major differences among various compounds with regard to efficacy, percentage of treatable patients and side effects? These two fundamental questions can be partially answered by comparing recent clinical data (Table 1).

Table 1 compares the effect of five ChEI on the ADAS-cog test using ITT (intention to treat) criteria. The duration of these trials varied between 12 and 26 weeks. Based on the data reported in these studies, the answer to the first question is affirmative. All five ChEI produce statistically significant improvements evaluated with scales of standardized and internationally validated measures of both cognitive and non-cognitive function. Cognitive items have been most widely used in these investigations. One first observation is the similarity in size of cognitive effect for all five drugs when expressed as a difference

Progress in Alzheimer's and Parkinson's Diseases
edited by Fisher *et al.*, Plenum Press, New York, 1998.

Table 1. Comparison of the effect of five cholinesterase inhibitors on ADAS-cog test (ITT)

Drug (ref.)	Dose (mg/day)	Duration of study (weeks)	Treatment difference (from) Placebo*	Baseline**	Improved patients (percent)	Drop-out (percent)	Side effects (percent)
Tacrine (1)	120–160	24	2–3.8	0.8–2.8	30–50	50–73	40–58
Eptastigm. (2)	45	25	4.7	1.8	30	12	35
Donepezil (3)	5–10	26	2.7–3	0.7–1	25	25	13
ENA 713 (4)	6–12	26	4.9	0.75	31	27–17	28
Metrifon. (5) (6)	30–60	12–26	2.6–3	0.75–0.5	35	2–21	2–12

ADAS-cog = AD Assessment Scale-cognitive subscale. ITT = intention to treat. * Study endpoint vs. placebo. ** = study end point vs. baseline. Drugs: Tacrine (THA), Eptastigmine, Donepezil (E 2020), ENA 713, Metrifonate.
Ref. 1: Farlow et al. (1992) and Knapp et al. (1994).
Ref. 2: Canal and Imbimbo, (1996) and Imbimbo (1996).
Ref. 3: Roger and Friedhoff (1996).
Ref. 4: Anand et al. (1996).
Ref. 5: Becker et al. (1996 a,b)
Ref. 6: Morris et al. (1997).

between drug- and placebo-treated patients. Maximal differences in ADAS-cog between drug- and placebo-treated patients average aproximately 4 points (ADAS.cog) and an average difference of 1.4 points is seen at the study end point.

Differences at the study end point vary from a gain of 0.5 points (metrifonate high dose) to a maximum of 2.8 (tacrine high dose). Does this similarity in cognitive effect suggest a ceiling value of aproximately-5 ADAS-cog points average for ChEI at mild to moderate stages of the disease? Or does it suggest that some drugs may have not been tested at their full capacity? For tacrine, the high percentage of drop-outs and side-effects seem to indicate a limit in ChE inhibition as well as in drug effect. For other drugs (e.g.metrifonate and donepezil), in spite of a dosage producing higher ChE inhibition (up to 80%), severity of side effects does not seem to represent a limiting factor. The percentage of improved patients varies from 25% (donepezil, high dose) to 50% (tacrine, high dose) with an average of 34%. This indicates that approximately one third of treated patients show a positive response to ChEI.While this is not an impressive figure it may still improve significantly if the percent treatable patients could be increased to 80–90% by using ChEI with less severe side-effects.

Analyzing the available six months data it is possible to observe that in general patients treated with the active compound change little cognitively from baseline at the beginning treatment. As an example in a US study with ENA 713, patients administered placebo for 26 weeks deteriorated over 4 points on the ADAS-cog compared to only 0.3 in patients given 6–12 mg/day of the drug (Anand et al., 1996). The difference seen after six months between placebo-treated and drug treated groups seems to depend more on the difference in the rate of cognitive deterioration of the placebo group (2–4 points) than on a real improvement. This interpretation suggests an effect of the drug contrasting deterioration and protecting the patient rather than a symptomatic effect. This putative protective effect could be primary and structural, leading to an improvement of cholinergic function as reflected by the cognitive improvement measured by ADAS-cog, or be a secondary effect. Tacrine, and donepezil, on the other hand, seem to show a real initial improvement (2–3 points) as compared to the placebo group. This effect may last from 4 to 24 weeks, depending on the dose (Farlow et al., 1992; Knapp et al. 1994; Roger and Friedhoff, 1996). It remains to be demonstrated whether or not this improvement depends on a real difference in drug effects.

Table 2. Relation between percent ChE inhibition and effect on ADAS-cog or CGIC

Drug (ref.)	Dose (mg/day)	Steady state (% inhibition)	Optimal (% inhibition)	Correlation ChEI/ADAS-cog or CGIC
Physostigm. (1)	3–16	40–60 (BuChE)	30–40	U-shaped
Eptastigm. (2)	30–60	13–54 (AChE)	30–35	U-shaped
Metrifonate (3)	30	35–75 (AChE)	65–80	U-shaped
Donepezil (4)	5	64 (AChE)	60	linear
Tacrine (5)	160	40 (BuChE) 60 (AChE)	30	linear

ADAS-cog = AD Assessment Scale - cognitive subscale. CGIC = Clinician Global Impression of Change.
Drugs: Physostigmine, Eptastigmine, Metrifonate, Donepezil (E2020), Tacrine (THA).
Ref. 1: Thal et al. (1983).
Ref. 2: Imbimbo and Lucchelli (1994) and Canal and Imbimbo (1996).
Ref. 3: Becker et al. (1990).
Ref. 4: Roger and Friedhoff (1996).
Ref. 5: Farlow et al. (1992), Knapp et al. (1991) and Knapp et al. (1994).

As indicated by studies of longer duration (up to 24 months; Becker et al., 1996 and Table 2) it is possible to maintain the difference between placebo- and drug-treated subjects beyond the present six months limit for a period up to 12 months. This represents a significant gain for both patient and caregiver. ChEI could differ from one another with respect to duration of effect. In comparing results of clinical trials and different drugs one should take into consideration the fact that studies may differ one from another, depending on differences in selection criteria, age of subjects, severity of disease, concomitant illnesses, variable instruments of assessment and side effect evaluation. In addition to these variables, in order to evaluate differences in effect between drugs one has to take into consideration the rate of deterioration of the placebo-exposed group which is compared with the treatment-group. This rate of deterioration seems to be highly variable (1–4 points at 24 weeks) among different studies. Also, by using "completers" instead of ITT, the analysis could produce somewhat higher effects.

Thus, clinical studies are not entirely comparable and conclusions at this stage can only be indicative. Given these limitations, the immediate next goal to be achieved for a ChEI would be to enhance the effect up to 6–8 ADAS-cog points and to a 0.6–0.7 point gain on CIBIC (Clinical Interview-Based Impression of Change) during a six months treatment period. At least 50% of this effect should be maintained for 12 months, the number of drop-out patients should be no higher than 10%, and the level of side effects very low. Is this an achievable goal?

WHAT MAKES THE DIFFERENCE BETWEEN VARIOUS ChEI?

The relation between percent of peripheral ChE inhibition and cognitive (ADAS-cog) or global impression of change rated by the clinician (CGIC) effect is a relevant factor which is reported in Table 3. The data presented in Table 3 support the pharmacological knowledge that brain ChE inhibition relates directly to an improvement of functional ACh levels. This relationship might vary quantitatively for each drug and each compound may produce various levels of cognitive improvement and therapeutic effect (Giacobini et al., 1988, 1995; Giacobini, 1996). This hypothesis is in agreement with pharmacological data in animals (Mattio et al., 1986; Giacobini et al., 1989) and in humans (Giacobini et al., 1988). The level of peripheral enzyme inhibition which has been

Table 3. Long-term cognitive effects of tacrine and eptastigmine on Alzheimer's Disease progression

Reference	Daily dose (mg)	Test	Difference between treatment and baseline****	
			at 11–15 months	at 17–24 months
Amberla et al. 1993	80–160	Buschke	no change	–
Wilcock et al. 1994	80	MMSE, CAMCOG, ADAS	no change	–
Eagger et al. 1994	50–150	AMTS*	no change	–
Solomon et al. 1996	160	ADAS-Cog	no change	2.8
Knopman et al. 1996	80–120	NHP**		delay
Imbimbo et al. 1997***	30	ADAS-Cog		6.4
		MMSE		3.9
		IADL		4.8

AMTS* = Abbreviated Mental Test Score
NHP** = Nursing Home Placement
*** = Eptastigmine, IADL = Instrumental Activity of Daily Living.
**** = Study endpoint vs baseline

measured in the patient (AChE activity in erythrocites or plasma BuChE activity) producing a difference on the cognitive test varies between 30% and 80% depending on kinetic and pharmacological characteristics of the compound (Table 3). For some drugs (see donepezil and metrifonate) the achievable level of ChE inhibition can be as high as 90%. As predicted by pharmacological and behavioral data, there is a clear correlation between ChE inhibition (or drug plasma concentration) and cognitive effect (Giacobini et al., 1989; Giacobini and Cuadra, 1994). Drugs producing mild cholinergic side effects even at high dosage and a high level of brain ChE inhibition may be tested in the patient within their full range of therapeutic potential. For some ChEI (physostigmine, eptastigmine and metrifonate) the relation between ChE inhibition and cognitive effect is inversely-U shaped, while for others (such as tacrine, ENA 713 and donepezil) this relation seems to be linear. The U-shaped form can be explained by the fact that by increasing the dose of the inhibitor one obtains progressively increasing efficacy until adverse effects do not become a limiting factor.

Another reason for the U-shaped curve is the specific inhibition kinetic of the inhibitor- and the substrate- induced saturation effect of ChEs. The level of ACh brain elevation varies according to brain ChE inhibition (Giacobini, 1994, 1995, 1996). With increased brain concentrations of ACh, substrate inhibition of enzyme activity becomes a phenomenon of particular importance. It is observed in brain tissue *in vitro* and is probably present also *in vivo* (Giacobini, 1994). Plotting velocity of enzymatic reaction against substrate (ACh) concentration, a bell-shaped curve with a defined peak in the case of AChE activity (brain and erythrocytes) and a sigmoid curve in the case of BuChE activity (serum) are observed. Thus, AChE is inhibited by a large excess of ACh such as it can be produced by a high inhibition of brain AChE in AD affected patients. The substrate elevation has the effect of decreasing the catalytic potency of the enzyme and subsequently its pharmacological and therapeutical effect. From this relationship it can be predicted that a high ChE inhibition reached rapidly in time during treatment (rapid passage of the drug into the brain and fast accumulation in CNS) will not further increase efficacy but only augment CNS dependent side effects (drowsiness, nausea, vomit etc). It should be an advantage to use a slow-release type of ChEI inhibiting both brain enzymes (AChE and BuChE) at a slow pace in order to reach gradually steady-state levels of brain ACh. Such a procedure may also lower the risk of cholinergic receptor downregulation and enzyme induction.

Indeed, there is an excellent agreement between clinical and animal data for both physostigmine and tacrine with regard to dose/behavioral effects relationships. Rupniak et al. (1990) using two primate models (rhesus monkeys) found that both tacrine and physostigmine improved visual recognition memory significantly. Both drugs showed a clear inverse U-shaped relationship with a maximal effect at around 0.001–0.02 mg/kg i.m. for physostigmine and 0.8–1 mg/kg for tacrine. Lower or higher doses did not improve performance but only increase side effects. Central cholinergic side effects which may develop early in the treatment are not related directly to brain AChE inhibition but mainly to rapid elevation of ACh levels (Giacobini, 1994, 1995). Peripheral side-effects may also occur depending on a rapid redistribution of the drug (or its metabolites) between non-CNS (peripheral organs and muscles) and CNS compartments. A combination of pharmacokinetic and pharmacodynamic effects of the drug such as down -regulation of muscarinic and nicotinic receptors and decreased ChE inhibition due to new enzyme synthesis, may be responsible for the tolerance to therapeutic effect seen in experimental animals and patients treated with ChEI for 24 weeks or longer.

Last but not a least problem of ChEI therapy is the early identification of those patients most likely to benefit from therapy. Correlation of therapy effectivness to genetic risk factors (APOE-allele) represents a first attempt in this direction. Choosing the proper responder to cholinomimetics and selecting patients at earlier stages of the disease at which to start medication may be crucial for the success of the therapy.

CONCLUSIONS: THE FUTURE OF AD THERAPY

Cholinesterase inhibitors are presently the drugs of choice for AD. In less than ten years, starting from non-specific first generation drugs such as physostigmine a second generation of more selective and less toxic molecules has been developed. The data from clinical trials suggest that optimization of effect and maintainance of clinical gains for one year or more are possible. Further progress will depend on our knowledge of pharmacodynamic effects of long-term treatment. Cholinesterase inhibitors, particularly second generation (post-physo and post-tacrine compounds), affect cortical as well as sub-cortical neurotransmitters other than ACh (Giacobini, 1996). Their effects on NE and DA are of particular clinical interest. A newly demonstrated feature of ChEI is their ability to enhance the release of non-amyloidogenic soluble derivatives of APP in vitro and in vivo and possibly to slow down formation of amyloidogenic compounds in brain (Mori et al., 1995). This process might also slow down cognitive deterioration of the patient as indicated by the analysis of recent clinical data (Table 3). Cholinomimetic alternatives other than ChE inhibition are being explored. Drugs most investigated are those showing direct stimulation of postsynaptic M1 and M3 muscarinic receptors or nicotinic agonists of alpha-2-beta-4 receptors. This attractive line of cholinergic therapy has not yet produced convincing results mainly depending on gastrointestinal and cardiac side effects.

Depending on the success of ChEI one can see potential indications for applications to different stages of AD such as: 1) preclinical presymptomatic stages in at risk-individuals with MCI (minimal cognitive impairment); 2) early AD patients with manifested symptoms (CDR 0.5–1), presently the most treated group; and 3) late AD (CDR2) patients with behavioral symptoms. Combination of ChEI with muscarinic or nicotinic agonists or with beta-A4 processers or APP-releasers and estrogens represent another valid alternative, particularly in the case of development of tolerance to ChEI monotreatment.

ACKNOWLEDGMENT

The author thanks Christine Mesmer for typing and editing the manuscript.

REFERENCES

Amberla, K., Nordberg, A., Viitanen, M., and Winblad B., 1993, Long-term treatment with tacrine (THA) in Alzheimer disease evaluation of neuropsychological data. *Acta.Neurol.Scand: Suppl.*149: 55–57.

Anand, R., Hartman, R.D., and Hayes , P.E., 1996, An overview of the development of SDZ ENA 713, a brain selective cholinesterase inhibitor. *In: Alzheimer Disease: From Molecular Biology to Therapy.* Becker, R. and Giacobini, E., eds., Boston: Birkhäuser. pp 239–243.

Becker, R., Colliver, J., and Elbe, R.,1990, Effects of Metrifonate, a long-acting cholinesterase inhibitor *Drug Dev. Res.* 19:425–434.

Becker, R., Moriearty, P., and Unni, L., 1991, The second generation of cholinesterase inhibitors: Clinical and pharmacological effects *In: Cholinergic basis for Alzheimer Therapy,* Becker, R. and Giacobini, E. eds., Boston: Birkhäuser, pp 263–296.

Becker, R., Colliver, J.A., Markwell, S.J., Moriearty, P., Unni, L.K., and Vicari S.,1996, Double-blind, placebo-controlled study of metrifonate, an acetylcholinesterase inhibitor for Alzheimer disease. *Alz. Dis. Assoc. Dis.* 10:124–131.

Becker, R., Moriearty, P., Unni, L. and Vicari, S., 1996., Cholinesterase inhibitors as therapy in Alzheimer's disease: benefit to risk considerations in clinical application. *In: Alzheimer Disease:From Molecular Biology to Therapy,* Becker, R. and Giacobini, E., eds., Boston: Birkhäuser., pp 257–266.

Canal, I. and Imbimbo, B.P., 1996, Clinical trials and therapeutics: Relationship between pharmacodynamic activity and cognitive effects of eptastigmine in patients with Alzheimer's disease. *Clin. Pharm. Therap.* 15(12):49–59.

Eagger, S., Richards, M., and Levy, R., 1994, Long-term effects of tacrine in Alzheimers's disease: an open study. *Intern. J. Ger. Psych.* 9:643–647.

Farlow, M., Gracon, S.I., Hershey, L.A., Lewis, K.W., Sadowski, C.H., and Dolan-Ureno, J: A., 1992., Controlled trial of tacrine in Alzheimer's disease. *J. Am. Med. Assoc.* 268:2523–2529.

Giacobini, E., 1994, Cholinomimetic therapy of Alzheimer disease: does it slow down deterioration? *In: Recent Advances in the Treatment of Neurodegenerative Disorders and Cognitive Dysfunction,* Racagni, G., Brunello, N. and Langer, S.Z. Int. Acad. Biomed. Drug Res., New York: Karger, 7(23) pp 51–57.

Giacobini, E.,1995, Cholinesterase inhibitors: From preclinical studies to clinical efficacy in Alzheimer disease. *In: Enzymes of the cholinesterase family,* Quinn, D., Balasubramaniam, A.S., Doctor, B.P. and Taylor, P., New York: Plenum Press, pp 463–469.

Giacobini, E. 1996., Cholinesterase inhibitors do more than inhibit cholinesterase. *In : Alzheimer Disease: From Molecular Biology to Therapy,* Becker, R. and Giacobini, E., Boston: Birkhäuser, pp 187–204.

Giacobini, E., Becker, R., McIlhany, M. and Kumar, V., 1988, Interacerebroventricular administration of cholinergic drugs:preclinical trials and clinical experience in Alzheimer patients. *In: Current Research in Alzheimer Therapy,* Giacobini, E. and Becker, R., New York: Taylor and Francis, pp 113–122.

Giacobini, E. and Cuadra, G., 1994, Second and third generation cholinesterase inhibitors: From preclinical studies to clinical efficacy. *In: Alzheimer Disease: Therapeutic Strategies,* Giacobini, E. and Becker, R., eds., Boston: Birkhäuser, pp. 155–171.

Giacobini, E., DeSarno, P., Clark, B. and McIlhany, M., 1989, The cholinergic receptor system of the human brain - Neurochemical and pharmacological aspects in aging and Alzheimer. *In: Progress in Brain Research,* Nordberg, A., Fuxe, K. and Holmstedt, B., Amsterdam: Elsevier, pp 335–343.

Imbimbo, B.P.,1996, Eptastigmine: A cholinergic approach to the treatment of Alzheimer's disease. *In: Alzheimer Disease: From Molecular Biology to Therapy,* Becker, R. and Giacobini, E.. Boston: Birkhäuser

Imbimbo, B.P. and Lucchelli, P.E., 1994, A pharmacodynamic strategy to optimize the clinical response to eptastigmine. In: *Alzheimer Disease: Therapeutic Strategies,* Becker, R. and Giacobini, E., Boston: Birkhäuser, pp 223–230.

Imbimbo, B.P., Perini, M.Verdelli, G. and Troetel, W.M., 1997, *XVth World Congress of Neurology,* Buenos Aires, Sept., Abstr. 125.

Knapp, S.,Wardlow, M.L., Albert, W., Wazters. D., and Thal, J., 1991, Correlation between plasma physostigmine concentrations and percentage of acetylcholinesterase inhibition over time after controlled release of physostigmine in volunteer subjects. *Drug Metab. Disp.* 19 (12):400–404.

Knapp, M.J., Knopman, D.S., Solomon, P.R., 1994, A 30 week randomized controlled trial of high-dose tacrine in patients with Alzheimer's disease. *J. Am. Med. Assoc. 271:*985–991.

Knopman, D., Schneider L., and Davis K., 1996, Long-term tacrine (Cognex) treatment:effects on nursing home placement and mortality. *Neurology* 47:166–177.

Mattio, T., McIlhany, M., Giacobini, E. and Hallak, M., 1986, The effects of physostigmine on acetylcholinesterase activity of CSF, plasma and brain. A comparison of intravenous and intraventricular administration in beagle dogs. *Neuropharmacology 25:*1167–1177.

Mori, F., Lai, C.C., Fusi, F. and Giacobini, E., 1995, Cholinesterase inhibitors increase secretion of APPs in rat brain cortex. *NeuroRep. 6*(4):633–636.

Morris, J., Cyrus, P., Orazem, J., Mas, J., Bieber, F., and Gulanski, B., 1997, Metrifonate: potential therapy for Alzheimer's Disease. *Am. Soc. Neurol. Mtg.*, Boston, Abstr. 155.

Roger, S.L., and Friedhoff, T., 1996, The efficacy and safety of Donepezil in patients with Alzheimer's disease: Results of a US multicentre, randomized, double-blind, placebo-controlled trial. *Dementia 7:*293–30.

Rupniak, N.M.J., Field, M.J., Samson, N.A., Steventon , M.J. and Iversen, S.D. ,1990, Direct comparison of cognitive facilitation by physostigmine and tetrahydroaminoacridine in two primate models. *Neurobiol. Aging 11:*609–613.

Solomon, P.R., Knapp, M.J., Gracon, S.J., Groccia, M., and Pendlebury,W.W., 1996, Long-term tacrine treatment in patients with Alzheimer's disease. *Lancet* 348:275–276.

Thal, L., Fuld, P.A., Masur, D.M., and Sharpless, N.S., 1983, Oral physostigmine and lecithin improve memory in Alzheimer disease. *Ann. Neurol.* 13:491–496.

Wilcock, G.K., Scott, M., and Pearsall T, 1994, Long-term use of tacrine. *Lancet* 343:294.

82

THE PRECLINICAL PHARMACOLOGY OF METRIFONATE, A LONG-ACTING AND WELL TOLERATED CHOLINESTERASE INHIBITOR FOR ALZHEIMER THERAPY

Bernard H. Schmidt, Volker C. Hinz, and F. Josef van der Staay

CNS Research
Troponwerke GmbH & Co. KG
51063 Cologne, Federal Republic of Germany

INTRODUCTION

Progressive degeneration of the cholinergic system is nowadays well recognized as one of the most sensitive and specific hallmarks of Alzheimer's disease. Numerous approaches to overcome the cholinergic deficit and the resulting impairments in cognitive function have been investigated, including attempts to increase acetylcholine (ACh) synthesis by precursor therapy, replacement of ACh with muscarinic or nicotinic agonists, nerve growth factor therapy to stimulate the outgrowth of cholinergic neurones, and inhibition of ACh breakdown by cholinesterases (ChEs), such as acetyl- and butyryl-ChE. Most progress has been made with the last approach, thanks to the recent discovery of safe and well-tolerated, long-lasting and orally bioavailable ChE inhibitors.

One of these compounds is metrifonate [(O,O-dimethyl-2,2,2-trichloroethyl)-phosphonate]. Like many other ChE inhibitors, metrifonate was introduced as an insecticide (Lorenz et al., 1952). Only shortly thereafter (Cerf et al., 1960), the antihelminthic activity of metrifonate became apparent and the drug subsequently gained a reputation as a safe and efficient therapeutic agent against human Schistosoma haematobium infections (for review see Davis, 1991). In 1988, the possible use of metrifonate in Alzheimer therapy was suggested (Becker and Giacobini, 1988; Nordgren and Holmstedt, 1988). Metrifonate induces a long-lasting inhibition of ChE and has a good oral bioavailability, safety and tolerability. Moreover, it is not hepatotoxic, unlike the first generation ChE inhibitor, tacrine. In an open trial, Becker et al. (1990) provided preliminary clinical evidence that metrifonate has efficacy in Alzheimer patients. Since then, Bayer started to develop metrifonate for Alzheimer therapy; filing of a NDA is scheduled in the near future.

Progress in Alzheimer's and Parkinson's Diseases
edited by Fisher *et al.*, Plenum Press, New York, 1998.

The aim of this chapter is to review the preclinical pharmacology of metrifonate, with special emphasis on its unique mechanism of action, safety, and cognition-enhancing properties in animals.

METRIFONATE ACTS AS A PRODRUG

Of the ChE inhibitors under development as Alzheimer therapeutics, metrifonate is the only one which acts as a prodrug. In physiological fluids, it is slowly transformed non-enzymatically into the active metabolite, dimethyl dichlorovinyl-phosphate, DDVP. This hydrolytic transformation is base-catalyzed and occurs spontaneously in neutral-to-alkaline aqueous solutions (Nordgren and Holmstedt, 1988). Metrifonate is not a ChE inhibitor by itself; inhibition of ChE in vitro only occurs under conditions in which DDVP is formed (Hinz et al., 1996a).

In vitro experiments with rat brain ChE showed that inhibition of ChE by metrifonate develops slowly, in contrast to that elicited by the reference ChE inhibitor, tacrine (Figure 1). Whereas tacrine inhibits the enzyme virtually immediately and maintains this level of inhibition throughout a 30 min period, metrifonate after a delay of 2–5 min, inhibits the enzyme in a time-dependent way, and the effect is not maximal at the end of the 30 min observation time. Interestingly, ChE inhibition mediated by DDVP is also time-dependent and requires about 15 min to reach a maximum (Figure 1). It is probably this feature of metrifonate that it is a prodrug for a slow-acting metabolite, which determines its excellent safety and tolerability profile. This prevents an abrupt inhibition of ChE activity and the resulting strong fluctuation in extracellular ACh, and thereby helps the body to better adjust to the increased cholinergic tone.

The in vivo formation of DDVP has been demonstrated in various mammalian species including humans (Nordgren and Holmstedt, 1988; Villon et al., 1990). The amount of DDVP found in the plasma of schistosomiasis patients treated with a 10 mg/kg dose of metrifonate was in the range of 1–2% of the parent drug. The elimination kinetics of the metabolite paralleled those of metrifonate (elimination t1/2 2.3–3.3 hours). However, when administered directly, DDVP is very rapidly eliminated from the body with a half-life of about 13.5 min, mainly by renal excretion and degradation by plasma enzymes (Blair et al., 1975; Villon et al., 1990). Therefore, concentrations of DDVP sufficient to mediate therapeutically relevant inhibition of ChE are optimally achieved by administration of the "reservoir" prodrug, metrifonate. The pharmacologically active metabolite is not accumulated.

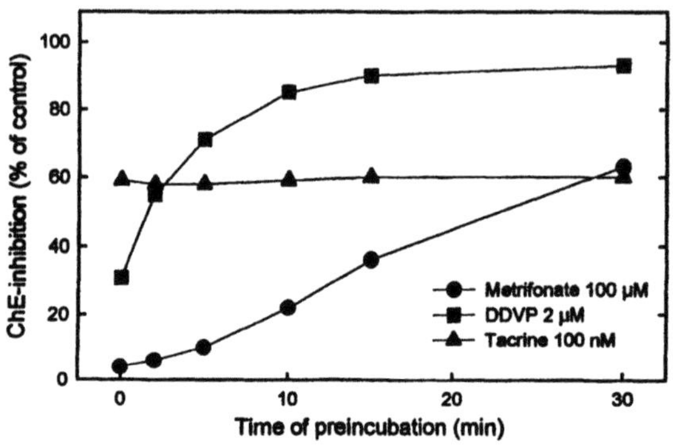

Figure 1. Effect of the preincubation time on ChE inhibition in vitro by metrifonate, DDVP, and tacrine. Selected concentrations of the drugs were preincubated with rat brain ChE for various times. The reaction was started by addition of 40 μM acetylthiocholine and was stopped after 6 min by addition of excess physostigmine (100 μM). Enzyme activity was determined photometrically at 412 nm. Results are expressed as percent of control ChE activity measured in the absence of inhibitors.

FACILITATION OF CHOLINERGIC NEUROTRANSMISSION

Metrifonate, administered orally or systemically to mice (Nordgren and Holmstedt, 1988), rats (Hallak and Giacobini, 1987; Hinz et al., 1996b), or rabbits (Kronforst-Collins et al., 1997a), mediates significant inhibition of brain ChE activity in a dose-dependent manner. As anticipated, metrifonate is less potent than DDVP. However, in vivo the parent compound is only 10-fold less potent than the active metabolite (Nordgren and Holmstedt, 1988; Hinz et al., 1996b), whereas in vitro it is 100-fold less potent than DDVP (Hinz et al., 1996a).

In parallel to ChE inhibition, metrifonate increases the extracellular levels of ACh in the cerebral cortex, as demonstrated in young adult rats (Mori et al., 1995; Scali et al., 1997). At a functional level, this leads to stimulation of local cerebral glucose utilization in a number of cortical and septohippocampal regions which are involved in cognitive function (Bassant et al., 1996), and to a desynchronization of neocortical EEG oscillations (Björklund et al., 1996). These effects of metrifonate are also seen in aged (Bassant et al., 1996; Björklund et al., 1996; Scali et al., 1997), and basal forebrain-lesioned rats (Itoh et al., 1997), in which metrifonate restores the age- or lesion-induced impairments in cholinergic transmission to the levels of young, intact controls.

Metrifonate appears to be slightly more potent in rats with a cholinergic deficit than in unimpaired controls. For instance, the ED50 value for orally administered metrifonate for ChE inhibition in the brain was 90 mg/kg in young adult controls but 60 mg/kg in aged rats (Hinz et al., 1996b), and equivalent doses of metrifonate were more effective in stimulating cortical ACh release and EEG activity in aged than in young adult rats (Scali et al., 1996; Björklund et al., 1996). Moreover, the effects of metrifonate on behavioural measures of cognitive functions were more consistent in aged or lesioned animals than in young, unimpaired animals, as summarized later in this chapter. The increased efficacy and potency of metrifonate in aged and lesioned animals may be linked to the initial competitive binding of DDVP to the catalytic site of ChE (Hinz et al., 1996a). From this, it can be anticipated that low endogenous levels of ACh favour the binding of the inhibitor, while high levels of the transmitter compete for DDVP binding according to the law of mass action. More studies are required to provide further evidence for this explanation, which suggests that ChE inhibitors which share their binding site on the enzyme with the natural ligand, ACh, preferentially target those brain areas that have defective cholinergic neurotransmission and spare those without cholinergic pathology.

LONG-LASTING INHIBITION OF ChE

As already mentioned, DDVP interacts with the substrate binding site of ChE (Hinz et al., 1996a). Initially, this interaction is competitive with the substrate, but within a few minutes the type of inhibition switches to non-competitive inhibition, due to covalent dimethyl-phosphorylation of the catalytic site. The resulting drug-enzyme complex is stable and no longer sensitive to the addition of excess substrate (Hinz et al., 1996a). However, during about the first 10 hours after the onset of inhibition, the enzyme is able to reactivate spontaneously (Reiner and Plestina, 1979), a process that can be accelerated by oximes (Moriearty and Becker, 1992).

After a single acute administration of metrifonate to rats (Reiner and Plestina, 1979; Hallak and Giacobini, 1987; Hinz et al., 1996b), mice (Nordgren and Holmstedt, 1988), or rabbits (Kolb and Schmidt, unpublished observations), ChE is rapidly inhibited. Most of this inhibition is reversed within 5 hours. But a small portion of the inhibition induced by metrifonate in vivo lasts for longer. The recovery of this component follows the kinetics of enzyme resynthesis (Reiner and Plestina, 1979).

Repeated administration of metrifonate to rats or rabbits accumulates the level of this long-lasting ChE inhibition and thereby decreases the fluctuations between the "peak" and "trough" ChE inhibition seen after each single dose. This effect continues until the level of long-lasting inhibition equals that of "peak" inhibition, a situation which is achieved after 15–20 single doses (Schmidt et al., 1997; Kronforst-Collins et al., 1997a). The level of ChE inhibition then remains stable despite continued treatment. Interestingly, this inhibition is not accompanied by a counterregulatory adaptation of the activity of choline-acetyltransferase, the ACh-synthesising enzyme, or in the number or affinity of muscarinic or nicotinic ACh receptors in the rat brain (Schmidt et al., 1997).

In all pharmacological studies performed to date, changes in brain ChE activity after treatment with metrifonate was accurately reflected by concomitant changes in erythrocyte ChE activity. This means that a convenient way to monitor the therapeutically envisaged changes in brain ChE activity during metrifonate treatment is to measure ChE activity in hemolyzed erythrocyte preparations, which are easy to obtain. This makes it possible to monitor not only loading and maintenance of inhibition, but also recovery after treatment cessation, because of a similar rate of recovery in brain and erythrocytes (Schmidt et al., 1997) in spite of the different underlying recovery mechanisms, i.e. neuronal enzyme resynthesis and hematopoesis, respectively.

In contrast, metrifonate does not cause long-lasting inhibition of plasma ChE activity (mainly butyryl-ChE) (Schmidt et al., 1997; Kronforst-Collins et al., 1997a,b). Consequently, plasma ChE activity is not a suitable surrogate parameter to monitor brain ChE activity.

SAFETY AND TOLERABILITY

Both metrifonate and DDVP have thoroughly been assessed for safety in pharmacological studies with laboratory animals. Both compounds are safe and well-tolerated over a wide dose range. Consistent with the mechanism of action and the very high selectivity of ChE as the drug target (Hinz et al., 1996c), the most frequent adverse effects in rats and mice are behavioral and physiological signs of cholinergic overstimulation, such as salivation, tremor, and hypothermia. Apart from these sensitive symptoms, diarrhea, piloerection, ptosis, flat body posture, gnawing, teeth chattering, difficulties in breathing, and clonic seizures are only occasionally observed after administration of high doses (Nordgren and Holmstedt, 1988; Blokland et al., 1995; Hinz et al., 1996c; Bassant et al., 1996). All symptoms were transient, with almost complete recovery occurring within 2 hours of drug administration. The oral threshold dose for adverse effects in young adult rats was 30 mg/kg for metrifonate, and 1 mg/kg for DDVP (Hinz et al., 1996c). Aged (19-month-old) rats were slightly more sensitive to metrifonate (Blokland et al., 1995), with an oral threshold dose for adverse effects of 10 mg/kg. This is consistent with the greater sensitivity of aged rats to ChE inhibition compared to young rats (Hinz et al., 1996a).

Mean arterial blood pressure or heart rate did not change significantly in young and aged rats treated i.p. with a dose of 80 mg/kg of metrifonate or 5 mg/kg of DDVP (Bassant et al., 1996). Neither the parent compound nor its active metabolite had analgetic or anticonvulsive effects in mice. They did not affect motor coordination or hexobarbital-induced anesthesia, or exhibit cataleptic potential in rats (Hinz et al., 1996c). However, at high doses both compounds reduced dose- dependently the convulsive threshold dose of pentylenetetrazole in mice (Hinz et al., 1996c) and caused slight hyperglycemia in rats (Bassant et al., 1996).

Compared to these symptoms observed after acute treatment with metrifonate, the incidence of adverse events is much lower following repeated administration of a high dose of 100 mg/kg p.o. to aged rats (Blokland et al., 1995). After only five doses, given at 24-hour intervals, the behavioral signs of cholinergic overstimulation were reduced by more than 50% compared to those observed after the first administration (Figure 2). This reduction was not paralleled by a concomitant decrease in the cognition-enhancing efficacy of metrifonate in these animals (Blokland et al., 1995). This finding indicates that the safety-efficacy profile of metrifonate improves with prolonged treatment. The reverse was found with tacrine given at a bioequivalent dose of 10 mg/kg, and the incidence of side effects even significantly increased by repeated administration of this dose (Figure 2).

COGNITION ENHANCEMENT

Numerous behavioral studies in animals have demonstrated that metrifonate stimulates cognitive behaviour in various paradigms. Metrifonate improved learning and memory of cognitively impaired aged, medial septal- and nucleus basalis-lesioned rats in the passive avoidance paradigm, the Morris water escape task, and the object recognition test (Blokland et al., 1995; van der Staay et al., 1996a; Riekkinen et al., 1996; Riekkinen et al., 1997a,b; Itoh et al., 1997; Scali et al., 1997). In the majority of these studies, metrifonate fully restored the performance of the animals to the levels of intact young control rats. In addition, the amnesic effects of scopolamine were partially prevented by metrifonate administration in rats, as demonstrated in the passive avoidance and water escape tests (Riekkinen et al., 1996; Itoh et al., 1997). Some studies have even indicated that metrifonate can improve the cognitive performance of normal young adult rats (van der Staay et al., 1996a,b), although this effect was not observed by others (Riekkinen et al., 1996; Scali et al., 1997).

The doses at which metrifonate is active cover a wide range and vary depending on the test paradigm. In general, the best effects were obtained with doses between 3 and 30 mg/kg, with two exceptions. First, a dose of 80 mg/kg was required to improve performance of aged rats in the object recognition test (Scali et al., 1997). Second, the initial ac-

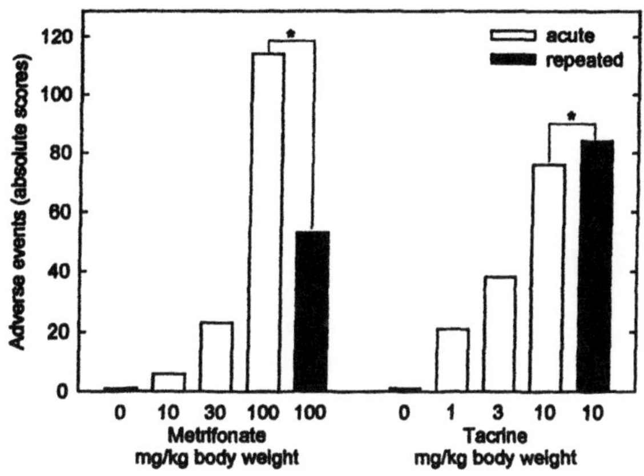

Figure 2. Effects of metrifonate and tacrine on behavioral symptoms in 19-month-old rats. Drugs were administered orally by gavage at the indicated doses either as a single acute dose (open bars) or as 5 repeated administrations given at 24-hour intervals (filled bars). Results shown are sum scores of the symptoms (salivation, tremor, diarrhoea, prone position and limb abduction) observed at eight observation times (every 15 min over a period of 2 hours). N = 6 per group, except for repeated administration of tacrine (N = 5). Asterisks indicate a significant difference (p < 0.05, t-test).

quisition in medial septal-lesioned rats was less sensitive to cognition improving effects of metrifonate than was reversal learning. While the reversal learning was improved at the low dose of 10 mg/kg p.o., the initial acquisition was facilitated at oral doses of 30–100 mg/kg (Riekkinen et al., 1996).

Special attention has been paid to the possible confounding effects of metrifonate in learning tasks. In particular, locomotor performance, swim speed, and the patterns of exploratory behavior have been analysed. It was concluded that metrifonate accelerates the acquisition of new information and facilitates memory retention (van der Staay et al., 1996b; Riekkinen et al., 1997b).

It should be added that in the learning and memory experiments summarized above metrifonate was given as short-term treatment for maximally 2 weeks, i.e. on an acute or subacute administration schedule. However, there are at least four studies in which metrifonate was administered subchronically, one of which was recently published (Kronforst-Collins et al., 1997a). In this study, aging rabbits were pretreated for 1 week with metrifonate at once-daily doses of 6, 12, or 24 mg/kg. Then the animals were trained on classical eye-blink conditioning for a further 5 weeks. The drug treatment was continued during behavioral testing. Metrifonate clearly improved the acquisition of the eye-blink response with 12 mg/kg being the most effective dose, whereas the higher dose of 24 mg/kg failed to cause significant improvement. However, in this study, each training session was started 15 min after drug administration and, although metrifonate was apparently well tolerated, the occurrence of subjective latent discomfort in the animals of the highest dose group could not be excluded. Therefore, a follow-up study was done in which training was given 6 hours after the daily dose of metrifonate. Now the dose of 24 mg/kg was as effective as the 12 mg/kg dose (Kronforst-Collins et al., 1997b). Two other studies with rats further confirmed that the cognition enhancing effects of metrifonate are well maintained upon long-term administration (unpublished results).

CONCLUSION

Metrifonate is a prodrug that is non-enzymatically and time dependently converted into a ChE inhibitor. The resulting enzyme inhibition improves cholinergic neurotransmission and cognitive performance by restoring the levels of ACh which are deficient as a result of aging and Alzheimer's disease. The stable binding of the active metabolite of metrifonate to the catalytic site of ChE allows for a titration of long-lasting enzyme inhibition which outlasts the presence of the drug in the body. Metrifonate is safe and well-tolerated in animals, and the incidence of behavioral or physiological signs of cholinergic overstimulation is greatly reduced upon repeated administration, thus broadening the therapeutic window and improving the safety-efficacy profile with time. These features warrant the development of metrifonate as a therapeutic agent for the cognitive disorders resulting from cholinergic denervation, such as Alzheimer's Disease.

REFERENCES

Bassant, M.H., Jazat-Poindessous, F., and Lamour, Y., 1996, Effects of metrifonate, a cholinesterase inhibitor, on local cerebral glucose utilization in young and aged rats. J. Cereb. Blood Flow Metab. 16:1014–1025.

Becker, R.E., Colliver, J., Elble, R., Feldman, E., Giacobini, E., Kumar, V., Markwell, S., Moriearty, P., Parks, R., Shillcutt, S.D., Unni, L., Vicari, S., Womack, C., and Zec, R.F., 1990, Effects of metrifonate, a long-acting cholinesterase inhibitor, in Alzheimer disease: Report of an open trial. Drug Dev. Res. 19:425–434.

Becker, R.E., and Giacobini, E., 1988, Mechanisms of cholinesterase inhibition in senile dementia of the Alzheimer type: Clinical, pharmacological, and therapeutic aspects. Drug Dev. Res. 12:163–195.

Björklund, M., Jäkälä, P., Schmidt, B., Riekkinen, M., Koivisto, E., and Riekkinen, P. Jr., 1996, An indirect cholinesterase inhibitor, metrifonate, increases neocortical EEG arousal in rats. NeuroReport 7:1097–1101.

Blair, D., Hoadley, E.C., and Hutson, D.H., 1975, The distribution of dichlorvos in the tissues of mammals after its inhalation or intravenous administration. Toxicol. Appl. Pharmacol. 31:243–253.

Blokland, A., Hinz, V., and Schmidt, B.H., 1995, Effects of metrifonate and tacrine in the spatial Morris task and modified Irwin test: Evaluation of the efficacy/safety profile in rats. Drug Dev. Res. 36:166–179.

Cerf, J., Lebrun, A., and Dierichx, J., 1962, A new approach to helminthiasis control: the use of an organophosphorous compound. Am. J. Trop. Med. Hyg. 11:514–517.

Davis, A., 1991, Metriphonate, In: Therapeutic Drugs, C. Dollery, ed., Churchill Livingstone, Edinburgh, Vol. 2:M164-M170.

Hallak, M., and Giacobini, E., 1987, A comparison of the effects of two inhibitors on brain cholinesterase. Neuropharmacology 26:521–530.

Hinz, V.C., Grewig, S., and Schmidt, B.H., 1996a, Metrifonate induces cholinesterase inhibition exclusively via slow release of dichlorvos. Neurochem. Res. 21:331–337.

Hinz, V.C., Grewig, S., and Schmidt, B.H., 1996b, Metrifonate and dichlorvos: Effects of a single oral administration on cholinesterase activity in rat brain and blood.Neurochem. Res. 21:339–345.

Hinz, V.C., Blokland, A., van der Staay, F.J., Gebert, I., Schuurman, T., and Schmidt, B.H., 1996c, Receptor interaction profile and CNS general pharmacology of metrifonate and its transformation product dichlorvos in rodents. Drug Dev. Res. 38:31–42.

Itoh, A., Nitta, A., Katono, Y., Usui, M., Naruhashi, K., Iida, R., Hasegawa, T., and Nabeshima, T., 1997, Effects of metrifonate on memory impairment and cholinergic dysfunction in rats. Eur. J. Pharmacol. 322:11–19.

Kronforst-Collins, M.A., Moriearty, P.L., Ralphs, M., Becker, R.E., Schmidt, B., Thompson, L. T., and Disterhoft, J.F., 1997a, Metrifonate treatment enhances acquisition of eyeblink conditioning in aging rabbits. Pharmacol. Biochem. Behav. 56:103–110.

Kronforst-Collins, M.A., Moriearty, P.L., Schmidt, B, and Disterhoft, J.F., 1997b, Metrifonate improves associative learning and retention in aging rabbits. Behav. Neurosci. in press.

Lorenz, W., Henglein, A., and Schrader, G., 1955, The new insecticide O,O-dimethyl-2,2,2-trichloro-1-hydroxyethylphosphonate. J. Am. Chem. Soc. 77:2554–2556.

Mori, F., Cuadra, G., and Giacobini, E., 1995, Metrifonate effects on acetylcholine and biogenic amines in rat cortex. Neurochem. Res. 20:1081–1088.

Moriearty, P.L., and Becker, R.E., 1992, Inhibition of human brain and RBC acetylcholinesterase (AChE) by heptylphysostigmine (HPTL). Meth. Find. Exp. Clin. Pharmacol. 14:615–621.

Nordgren, I., and Holmstedt, B., 1988, Metrifonate: A review, In: Current Research in Alzheimer Therapy, Giacobini, E. and. Becker, R.E, eds., Taylor and Francis, New York, 281–288.

Reiner, E., and Plestina, R., 1979, Regeneration of cholinesterase activities in humans and rats after inhibition by O,O-dimethyl-2,2,-dichlorovinyl phosphate.Toxicol. Appl. Pharmacol. 49:451–454.

Riekkinen, M., Schmidt, B., Kuitunen, J., and Riekkinen, P. Jr., 1997a, Effects of combined chronic nimodipine and acute metrifonate treatment on spatial and avoidance behavior. Eur. J. Pharmacol. 322:1–9.

Riekkinen, P. Jr., Schmidt, B., Stefanski, R., Kuitunen, J., and Riekkinen, M., 1996, Metrifonate improves spatial navigation and avoidance behavior in scopolamine-treated, medial septum-lesioned and aged rats. Eur. J. Pharmacol. 309:121–130.

Riekkinen, P. Jr., Schmidt, B., and Riekkinen, M., 1997b, Behavioral characterization of metrifonate-improved acquisition of spatial information in medial septum-lesioned rats. Eur. J. Pharmacol. 323:11–19.

Scali, C., Giovannini, M.G., Bartolini, L., Prosperi, C., Hinz, V., Schmidt, B., and Pepeu, G., 1997, Effect of metrifonate on extracellular brain acetylcholine and object recognition in aged rats. Eur. J. Pharmacol., in press.

Schmidt, B.H., Kolb, J., and Hinz, V.C., 1997, Loading and maintenance of long-lasting cholinesterase inhibition by repeated metrifonate administrationto rats.Abstract Book of the 6th World Congress of Biol. Psychiatry, Nice, June 1997, Abstract No. 638

van der Staay, F.J., Hinz, V.C., and Schmidt, B.H., 1996a, Effects of metrifonate on escape and avoidance learning in young and aged rats. Behav. Pharmacol. 7:56–64.

van der Staay, F.J., Hinz, V.C., and Schmidt, B.H., 1996b, Effects of metrifonate, its transformation product dichlorvos, and other organophosphorus and reference cholinesterase inhibitors on Morris water escape behavior in young-adult rats. J. Pharmacol. Exp. Ther. 278:697–708.

Villon, T., Aden Abdi, Y., Ericsson, Ö., Gustafsson, L.L., and Sjöqvist, F., 1990, Determination of metrifonate and dichlorvos in whole blood using gas chromatography and gas chromatography-mass spectrometry. J. Chromatogr. 529:309.

83

INCREASE IN CEREBRAL BLOOD FLOW AND GLUCOSE UTILIZATION IN BENEFICIAL EFFECT OF A CHOLINESTERASE INHIBITOR, ENA713 IN ALZHEIMER'S DISEASE

Marta Weinstock

Department of Pharmacology
School of Pharmacy
Hebrew University Hadassah Medical Centre
Ein Kerem, Jerusalem, Israel

INTRODUCTION

Alzheimer's disease (AD) of the sporadic type is a progressive degenerative disorder of unknown etiology, in which a number of potential risk factors have been identified. These include brain trauma, impaired cerebral circulation, and elevated plasma cortisol. Whatever the initial trigger, a reduction in glucose metabolism (GM) is consistently found in the posterior temporal and parietal regions of the cortex at a relatively early stage of the disease (Hoyer, 1992; Swerdlow et al., 1993). This is associated with decreased synaptic activity followed by neuronal loss, notably in the terminal fields of the cholinergic projection from the nucleus basalis of Meynert (nBM) (Vogels et al., 1990).

In the glycolytic breakdown of glucose, pyruvate dehydrogenase is responsible for the provision of the acetyl groups for energy production and of acetyl CoA for acetylcholine (ACh) synthesis. Patients with AD have higher pyruvate levels than controls in their cerebrospinal fluid, which are significantly correlated to the severity of dementia, testifying to an abnormality in glucose metabolism (Parnetti et al., 1995). This could be due to a primary abnormality in the activity of glycosolytic enzymes (Sheu et al., 1994), or to the expression of a functional down-regulation in a neuronal network in which energy demands have been regionally reduced by some other process. A recent study utilizing [^{18}F]-fluorodeoxyglucose for GM and [^{11}C] methionine accumulation for protein synthesis found a 45% decrease in glucose utilization in temporo-parietal regions which was correlated to dementia severity in subjects with AD, without any significant reduction in protein synthesis (Salmon et al., 1996). This showed that the decreased GM precedes, rather than results from the neurodegeneration. The reason for the abnormality in GM is not known but could partly result from a disturbance in CBF (see below) together with a reduction in insulin activity in the appropriate brain regions (Schwartz et al., 1989). As brain neurones are unable to synthesize or store glucose, they are dependent on its transport across the blood brain barrier by an insulin-dependent process. Any abnormality in the microcirculation can impede the absorption of nutrients from the circulation into brain tissue and hinder the removal of metabolic waste products, thereby compromising its homeostasis. Cerebral capillaries have been shown to be irregular, twisted and distorted in the brains of subjects with AD (De La Torre, 1994) and the deformities in the capillary lumen interfere with flow by increasing vessel resistance. The abnormalities in cerebral microvessels are probably responsible for the significant reduction in the number of GLUT 1 and GLUT 4 transporters in the endothelium, thereby further compromising cerebral GM (Simpson et al., 1994).

The cholinergic system arising from the nBM is responsible for the storage and retrieval of items in memory (Bartus et al., 1982) and its degeneration correlates well with the severity of cognitive and memory impairment in AD (Giacobini, 1990). Stimulation of this system, and that arising in the medial septal nucleus increases (Sato & Sato, 1992), while their destruction decreases cerebral blood flow (CBF) and glucose utilization in the cerebral cortex and hippocampus, respectively (Kiyosawa et al., 1989). These cholinergic neurones are particularly vulnerable to reductions in cerebral GM. This could explain their degeneration in subjects with AD, even when other neuronal systems still appear to be normal (Whitehouse et al., 1982). Recent studies indicate that the reduction in cholinergic transmission (measured by SPECT, with [^{123}I]iodobenzovesamicol) precedes actual neurone loss (measured by MRI) in subjects with AD (Kuhl et al., 1996). This could occur through a decrease in the availability of acetyl-CoA, because of the derangement of GM, or from a primary degeneration of the neurones from the nBM by an unknown cause. In the latter case, the changes in GM and CBF would be secondary to the reduction in cholinergic transmission. Irrespective of the initial pathology, it is clear that an impairment in CBF, GM or cholinergic activity can re-inforce each other causing further deficits in cognitive function.

The rate of progression of AD varies in different individuals but in some, deterioration becomes much more rapid at a certain stage (Helmes et al., 1995). This may be due to a combination of secondary events leading to the collapse of various systems. Thus, abnormalities in the oxidative GM can result in a decrease in ATP (Hoyer, 1992), and increase in lactic acid. The lactic acidosis can induce the release of Fe^{+++} ions from iron-binding proteins, which in turn, may promote the production of oxidative free-radicals (Rehncrona et al., 1989). The latter can produce cellular destruction by releasing glutamate, increasing cytosolic Ca^{++} ions, and causing lipid peroxidation and proteolysis (Davies & Goldberg, 1987). The cell damage releases mitogens from astroglial cells (Moonen et al., 1990), causing them to proliferate (Fredrickson, 1992). These reactive astrocytes express amyloid precursor protein (APP) which, in the presence of excess Ca^{++} ions, may be converted to 4-β-amyloid, the core substance of neural plaques. Evidence of a strong inflammatory response is also found in the brains of AD patients. This may result in autotoxic destruction of neurones, further aggravating the condition (McGeer & McGeer, 1995).

Traumatic brain injury commonly causes impairment of cognitive function and memory (Capruso & Levin, 1992) and is one of the possible causes of AD (Gentleman et al., 1993). Cerebral edema is an acute complication of brain injury and results from excess accumulation of water within the cells (Zauner & Bullock, 1995) and in the extracellular space (Lobato et al., 1988), because of a loss of the integrity of the blood brain barrier (Klatzo, 1967). The secondary brain damage following traumatic head injury is associated with acute vascular insufficiency, focal or global ischemia and delayed axotomy (Zauner & Bullock, 1995). Ischemia induced by arterial occlusion (Tanaka et al., 1994) or head trauma (Gorman et al., 1996) results in a longterm decrease in ACh and choline acetyl transferase levels in the cortex and hippocampus. Thus, the changes in cholinergic activity could be responsible for the cognitive and memory impairments induced by brain trauma.

The interrelationship between cholinergic activity, CBF and GM suggests that a therapeutic intervention to increase cholinergic transmission in hippocampal and cortical neurones could delay the decline in cognitive function if initiated at an early enough stage in the disease. Such a drug should also postpone the appearance of the later sequelae outlined above. ENA713 is an acetylcholinesterase inhibitor (AChEI), originally prepared in our laboratory (known as RA7, Weinstock et al., 1986) with a much wider safety margin and superior oral bioavailability to that of physostigmine or Tacrine (Enz et al., 1993; Weinstock et al., 1994). This drug has recently completed phase III clinical trials in patients with AD (Arnand et al., 1996). ENA713 reduced hippocampal cell loss and the release of reactive microglia (Tanaka et al., 1995) and prevented the decrease in ACh levels and muscarinic receptors following bilateral carotid occlusion in gerbils (Tanaka et al., 1994). It also dose-dependently decreased the rise in brain lactic acid and maintained ACh and ATP within normal limits after 60 min of ischemia in rats (Sadoshima et al., 1995). These data suggest that ENA713 may be able to reverse or prevent the decrements in cognitive function and the later sequelae arising from impairments in CBF and/or cerebral GM by maintaining cholinergic activity in the basal forebrain. We tested this hypothesis by measuring its effect on spatial memory in rats in which an impairment of cerebral GM was produced by intracerebroventricular (icv) injection of streptozotocin (STZ). We also assessed the effect of ENA713 on cerebral edema and impairment of reference memory in mice after closed head injury (CHI).

METHODS

Effect of ENA713 on Disruption of Spatial Memory by icv STZ

STZ was reported to disrupt glucose utilization in the temporal and parietal cortices and in the hippocampus after icv injection in rats (Duelli et al., 1994). In a preliminary experiment we found that STZ caused an impairment in spatial memory if injected bilaterally icv in young rats, 4 times at a dose of 2 mg/kg over a period of a week. The effect of ENA713, (1.5 mg/kg) injected sc once daily for 2 weeks, commencing immediately after STZ, was assessed on the memory impairment induced by icv STZ. This dose inhibited AChE in the rat cortex and hippocampus by $61 \pm 3\%$ and $57 \pm 2\%$, respectively. Drug treatment was continued after each exposure to the Morris water maze for testing of spatial memory, a week after the last STZ injection. Rats injected icv 4 times with STZ or artificial CSF and saline sc instead of ENA713 once daily, served as controls. The rats were exposed to the maze twice daily and the latency to find the hidden escape platform was measured (Morris, 1984). The position of the platform and entry point of the rat into the maze were changed every day.

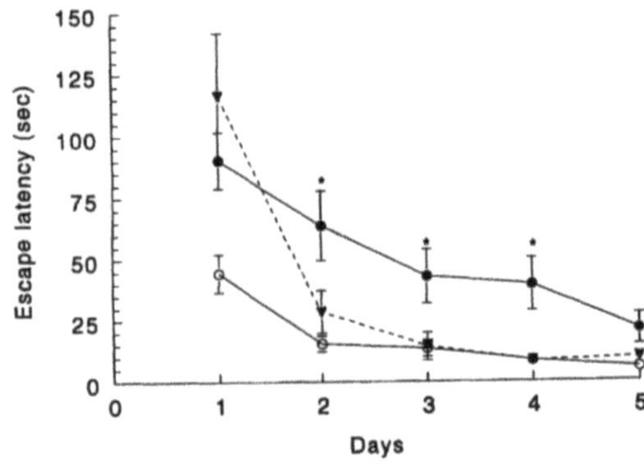

Figure 1. The effect of ENA713 on the impairment of spatial memory induced by icv injection of streptozotocin in rats. o–o icv CSF + saline sc. ●–● icv STZ + saline sc. ▼–▼ icv STZ + ENA713, 1.5 mg/kg sc. *Significantly different from other groups, p < 0.05.

Effect of ENA713 on Brain Edema and Memory Impairment Induced by CHI

CHI was induced in mice under ether anesthesia as previously described (Chen et al., 1996). In the first experiment the mice were divided into 4 groups of 8–10 animals and injected sc with saline, ENA713, (2 mg/kg) alone or in combination with scopolamine (0.2mg/kg or mecamylamine (2.5mg/kg), 5 min after CHI. Cerebral edema, which reaches its peak 24 hr after CHI (Chen et al., 1996), was determined by measuring the tissue water content in the injured brain (Shapira et al., 1988). In the second experiment, 48 mice were first given 3 trials per day for 5 consecutive days in the Morris water maze to establish baseline escape latencies. The location of the platform remained the same for all tests and the mice were released from the same starting point in the maze All the mice reached a stable performance with latencies ranging between 20–30 sec. After CHI they were divided randomly into 4 groups and injected with one of the 4 regimens as above. Post-injury testing commenced 24h after CHI and consisted of a session of 3 trials per day for 11 days.

RESULTS

STZ significantly impaired spatial memory as shown by the longer latencies taken by the rats to reach the goal platform during the first 4 days (p < 0.01) than those injected icv with artificial CSF (Fig. 1). ENA713 decreased escape latency of STZ-injected rats from the second day of testing to that of CSF-injected rats. These findings showed that ENA713 can prevent the spatial memory impairment in rats induced by a primary interference with cerebral GM.

Table 1. Effect of ENA713 on cerebral edema produced by CHI in the mouse

Treatment	Water content (%) ± sem
Sham injury	78.8 ± 0.3
CHI + saline (1 ml/kg)	83.9 ± 0.3*
CHI + ENA713 (2 mg/kg)	81.2 ± 0.5¶
CHI + ENA713 (2 mg/kg) + Scop. (0.2 mg/kg)	84.1 ± 0.4**
CHI + ENA713 (2 mg/kg) + Mec. (2.5 mg/kg)	82.9 ± 0.6**

Scop = scopolamine, Mec = mecamylamine. *significantly different from sham injury, p < 0.001; ¶significantly different from CHI saline, p < 0.01; **significantly different from ENA713, p < 0.05.

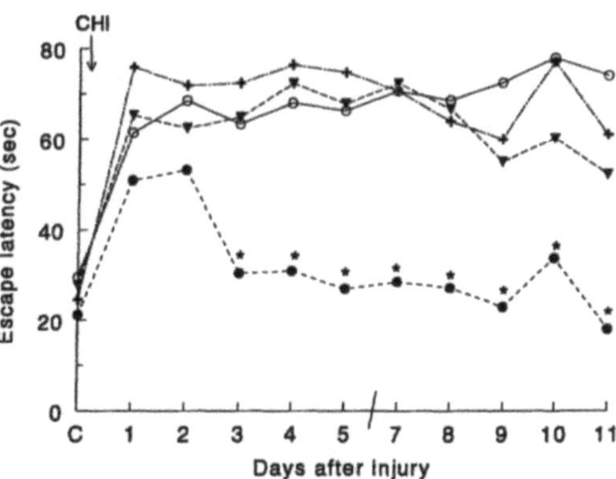

Figure 2. The effect of ENA713 on the impairment of reference memory induced by closed head injury in the mouse. o–o saline; •–• ENA713, 2 mg/kg; ▼–▼ ENA713, 2 mg/kg + scopolamine, 0.2 mg/kg; +–+ ENA713, 2 mg/kg + mecamylamine, 2.5 mg/kg.* Significantly different from other groups, p < 0.05.

CHI caused a marked increase in edema in the left contused hemisphere. This was reduced by about 50% by ENA713. This effect was completely prevented by simultaneous treatment with scopolamine or mecamylamine (Table 1). CHI resulted in a long-lasting deficit in reference memory since saline-treated mice failed to relearn the position of the platform throughout the 11 day testing period after injury. Mice given ENA713 regained their pre-injury latencies by the 3rd day after CHI (Fig. 2). This beneficial effect of ENA713 was also antagonized both by scopolamine and by mecamylamine.

CONCLUSIONS

The findings in the present study show that chronic treatment of rats with ENA713 can prevent the impairment of spatial memory induced by interference with cerebral glucose metabolism by icv STZ. It remains to be determined whether the drug also prevents the changes in GM or only the decreases in ACh levels associated with them. ENA713 given once only after acute CHI in mice significantly reduced the cerebral edema in the contused hemisphere and restored the impairment in reference memory. Both effects were abolished by simultaneous administration of ether a muscarinic or nicotinic receptor antagonist, indicating that they were mediated by increased cholinergic activity. Taken together with previous findings that ENA713 can prevent the reduction in cholinergic indices and reduce cell loss induced by global ischemia, the data suggest that the drug should be able to retard the development of cognitive impairment and the secondary sequelae of reduced GM and cerebral blood flow by maintaining cholinergic transmission in critical brain areas.

REFERENCES

Arnand, R., Gharabawi. G., and Enz, A., 1996, Efficacy and safety results of the early phase studies with Exelon™ (ENA 713) in Alzheimer's disease: an overview, *J. Drug Dev. Clin. Prac.* 8: 1–14.

Bartus, R.T., Dean, R.L., Beer, B., and Lypsa, A.S., 1982, The cholinergic hypothesis of geriatricmemory dysfunction, *Science* 217: 408–417.

Capruso, D.X., and Levin, H.S., 1992, Cognitive impairment following closed head injury, *Neurologic.Clin.* 10: 879–893.

Chen, Y., Constantini, S., Trembovler, V., Weinstock, M., and Shohami, E., 1996, An experimental model of closed head injury in mice: Pathophysiology, histopathology and cognitive deficits, *J. Neurotrauma* 13: 557–569.

Davies, K.J.A. and Goldberg, A.L., 1987, Oxygen radicals stimulate intracellular proteolysis and lipid peroxidation by independent mechanisms in erythrocytes, *J. Biol. Chem.* 262: 8220–8226.

De la Torre, J.C., 1994, Impaired brain microcirculation may trigger Alzheimer's disease, *Neurosci. Biobehav. Revs.* 18: 397–401.

Duelli, R., Schröck, G, Kuschinsky, W., and Hoyer, S., 1994, Intracerebroventricular injection of streptozotocin induces discrete local changes in cerebral glucose utilization in rats, *Int. J. Dev. Neurosci.* 12: 737–743.

Enz, A., Amstutz, R., Boddeke, H., Gmelin, G., and Malanowski, J., 1993, Brain selective inhibition of acetylcholinesterase: a novel approach to therapy for Alzheimer's disease, *Prog. Brain Res.* 98: 431–438.

Fredrickson, R.C., 1992, Astroglia in Alzheimer's disease, *Neurobiol. Aging* 13: 239–253.

Gentleman, S.M., Graham, D.I., and Robert, G.W., 1993, Molecular pathology of head trauma: Altered βAPP metabolism and the aetiology of Alzheimer's disease, *Progr. Brain Res.* 96: 237–246.

Giacobini, E., 1990, The cholinergic system in Alzheimer's disease. In: Aquilonius S-M, Gillberg P-G (eds) Cholinergic Neurotransmission: Functional and Clinical Aspects Progr. in: *Brain Res.* 84: Elsevier, Amsterdam, pp. 321–332.

Gorman, L.K., Fu, K., Hovda, D.A., Murray, M., and Traystman, R.J., 1996, Effects of traumatic brain injury on the cholinergic system in the rat, *J. Neurotrauma* 13: 457–463.

Helmes, E., Merskey, H., Fox, H., Fry, R.N., Bowler, J.V. and Hachinski, V.C., 1995, Patterns of deterioration in senile dementia of the Alzheimer type, *Arch. Neurol.* 52: 306–310.

Hoyer, S., 1992, Oxidative energy metabolism in Alzheimer brain. Studies in early-onset and late-onset cases, *Mol. Chem. Neuropathol.* 16: 207–224.

Kiyosawa, M., Baron, J-C., Hamel, E., Pappata, S., Duverger, D., Riche, D., Mazoyer, B., Naqurt, R.,and MacKenzie, E.T., 1989, Time course of unilateral lesions of the nucleus basalis of Meynert on glucose utilization by the cerebral cortex. Positron tomography in baboons, *Brain* 112: 435–455.

Klatzo, I., 1967, Neuropathological aspects of brain oedema, *J. Neuropath. Exp. Neurol.*26: 1–14.

Kuhl, D.E., Minoshima, S., Fessler, J.A., Frey, K.A., Foster, N.L., Ficaro, E.P., Wieland, D.M., and Koeppe, R.A., 1996, In vivo mapping of cholinergic terminals in normal aging, Alzheimer's disease, and Parkinson's disease, *Ann. Neurol.* 40: 399–410.

Lobato, R.D., Sarabia, R., Cordobes, F., Rivas, J.J., Adrados, A., 1988, Posttraumatic cerebral hemispheric swelling, *J. Neurosurg.* 68: 417–423.

McGeer, P.L. and McGeer, E.G., 1995, The inflammatory response system of brain: implications for therapy of Alzheimer and other neurodegenerative diseases, *Brain Res. Rev.* 21: 195–218.

Moonen, G., Rogister, B., Leprince, P., Rigo, J.M., Delree, P., Lefebvre, P.P. and Schoenen, J., 1990, Neuronoglial interactions and neuronal plasticity, *Prog. Brain Res.* 86: 63–73.

Morris, R., 1984, Developments of a water-maze procedure for studying spatial learning in the rat, *J. Neurosci. Methods* 11: 47–60.

Parnetti, L., Gaiti, A., Brunetti, M., Avellini, L., Polidori, C., Cecchetti, R., Palumbo, B. and Senin, U, 1994, Increased CSF pyruvate levels as a marker of impired energy metabolism in Alzheimer's disease, *J. Am. Geriatric Soc.* 43: 316–318.

Rehncrona, S., Hauge, H.N., and Siesjo, B.K., 1989, Enhancement of iron-catalyzed free radical formation by acidosis in brain homogenates: Difference in effect by lactic acid and CO_2, *J. Cereb. Blood Flow Metab.* 9: 65–70.

Sadoshima, S., Ibayashi, S., Fujii, K., Nagao, T., Sugimori, H. and Fujishima, M., 1995, Inhibition of acetylcholinesterase modulates the autoregulation of cerebral blood flow and attenuates ischemic brain metabolism in hypertensive rats, *J. Cereb. Blood Flow Metab.* 15: 845–851.

Salmon, E., Gregoire, M.C., Delfiore, G., Lemaire, C., Degueldre, C., Franck, G., and Comar, D., 1996, Combined study of cerebral glucose metabolism and [^{11}C] methionine accumulation in probable Alzheimer's disease using positron emission tomography, *J. Cereb. Blood Flow Metab.* 16: 399–408.

Sato, A. and Sato, Y., 1992, Regulation of regional cerebral blood flow by cholinergic fibers originating in the basal forebrain, *Neurosci. Res.* 14: 242–274.

Schwartz, M.W., Figlewicz, D.P., and Baskin, D.G., Woods, S.C., and Porte, D. Jr., 1992, Insulin in the brain: A hormonal regulator of energy balance, *Endocr. Rev.* 13:387–414.

Shapira, Y., Shohami, E., Sidi, A., Soffer, D., Freeman, S., and Cotev, S., 1988, Experimental closed head injury in rats: Mechanical, pathophysiologic and neurologic properties, *Crit. Care Med.* 16: 258–265.

Sheu, K.-F. R., Cooper, A.J.L., Koike, K., Koike, M., Lindsay, G., and Blass, J.P., 1994, Abnormality of the α- ketoglutarate dehydrogenase complex in fibroblasts from familial Alzheimer's disease, *Ann. Neurol.* 35: 312–318.

Simpson, I.A., Koteswara, R.C., Davies-Hill, T., Honer, W.G., and Davies, P., 1994, Decreased concentrations of GLUT1 and GLUT3 glucose transporters in the brains of patients with Alzheimer's disease, *Ann. Neurol.* 35: 546–551.

Swerdlow, R., Marcus, D.L., Landman, J., Kooby, D., Frey II, W., and Freedman, M.L., 1993, Brain glucose metabolism in Alzheimer's disease, *Am. J. Med. Sci.* 308: 141–144.

Tanaka, K., Mizukawa, K., Ogawa, N., and Mori, A., 1995, Post-ischemic administration of the acetylcholinesterase inhibitor ENA-713 prevents delayed neuronal death in the gerbil hippocampus, *Neurochem. Res* .20: 663–667.

Tanaka, K., Ogawa, N., Mizukawa, K., Asanuma, M., Kondo, Y., Nishibayashi, S., and Mori, A., 1994, Acetylcholinesterase inhibitor ENA-713 protects against ischemia-induced decrease in pre- and postsynaptic cholinergic indices in the gerbil brain following transient ischemia, *Neurochem. Res.* 19: 117–122.

Vogels, O.J.M., Broere, C.A.J., Ter Laak, H.J., Ten Donkelaar, H.J., Nieuwenhuys, R., and Schulte, B.P.M., 1990, Cell loss and shrinkage in the nucleus basalis Meynert complex in Alzheimer's disease, *Neurobiol. Aging* 11:3–13.

Weinstock, M., Razin, M., Chorev, M., and Enz, A., 1994, Pharmacological evaluation of phenyl-carbamates as CNS selective acetylcholinesterase inhibitors, *J. Neural. Transm.* s43:219–225.

Weinstock, M., Razin, M., Chorev, M., and Tashma, Z., 1986, Pharmacological activity of novel acetylcholinesterase agents of potential use in the treatment of Alzheimer's disease, in: *Advances in Behavioral Biology.* A. Fisher, I. Hanin, and C. Lachman (eds), Plenum Press: New York, 539–551.

Whitehouse, P.J., Price, D.L., Struble, R.G., Clark, A.W., Coyle, J.T., and DeLong, M.R., 1982, Alzheimer's disease and senile dementia; loss of neurons in the basal forebrain, *Science* 215:1237–1239.

Zauner, A. and Bullock, R., 1995, The role of excitatory amino acids in severe brain trauma: Opportunities for therapy: A review, *J. Neurotrauma,* 12:547–554.

84

QUATERNARY-LIPOPHILIC CARBAMATES WITH BLOOD BRAIN BARRIER PERMEABILITY AS POTENTIAL DRUGS FOR MEMORY IMPAIRMENT ASSOCIATED WITH CHOLINERGIC DEFICIENCY

Gabriel Amitai, Eliezer Rachaman, Rachel Adani, Ishai Rabinovitz, Rachel Brandeis, and Eliahu Heldman

Israel Institute for Biological Research
Ness Ziona 74100, Israel

INTRODUCTION

Cholinergic deficiency in the central nervous system is associated with cognitive impairment (Bartus et al, 1982, Fisher and Heldman, 1990, Wilson and Cook, 1994). In pathological conditions such as Alzheimer's disease (AD) cholinergic deficiency has been consistently observed in discrete brain regions such as the nucleus basalis of Meynert, cerebral cortex and the hippocampus (Sims, 1983; Tegliavini, 1984). Therefore, a rational approach for the treatment of such cognitive impairments would be to elevate the level of acetylcholine in brain. Cholinesterase (ChE) inhibitors such as the carbamates physostigmine (PHY) and ENA-713 have been clinically examined as potential treatments for AD, while tacrine (THA, Cognex) and E2020 (Aricept) have already been approved by the FDA for AD treatment. PHY displayed mild positive benefits (Millard and Broomfield, 1995), yet, its short half-life and relatively high acute toxicity could limit its clinical use. THA is indeed a long-acting reversible ChE inhibitor but its hepatotoxicity and peripheral side effects on the gastrointestinal system such as nausea and vomiting combined with its moderate efficacy only at high doses constitute its major disadvantages (O'Brien et al, 1991; Crimson, 1994). Pyridostigmine (PYR) is a reversible ChE inhibitor that is less toxic than PHY and has a longer duration of action than PHY. PYR serves as an effective drug for the treatment of myasthenia gravis (Pascuzzi, 1994). PYR is also used for the pretreatment against poisoning by organophosphorus insecticides and nerve agents (Millard, 1995). However, its quaternary positively charged pyridinium nitrogen limits its permeability into the CNS and confines its use only as a peripheral cholinomimetic drug. Earlier efforts were made to develop tertiary analogues of PYR but they displayed lower efficacy than PYR as AChE inhibitors (Arnal, 1990). The development of PYR derivatives that could cross the blood-brain barrier (BBB), will have longer duration of action and will also be less toxic than other AChE inhibitors that are currently evaluated for AD treatment, will provide a new series of cholinomimetics with improved efficacy and safety.

RESULTS AND DISCUSSION

Rationale and Synthesis of New ChE Inhibitors

The molecular design of the new ChE inhibitors related to the structure of PYR is based on the attachment of aliphatic chains of various lengths to the quaternary pyridinium nitrogen of PYR. Such alkyl chains conjugated to the PYR structure could introduce lipophilicity to the resulting new molecule. Based on the AChE protein structure and active-site topology (Sussman et al. 1991, Harel, 1993), we postulated that a long flexible alkyl chain coupled to the PYR basic structure will not affect significantly the overall inhibition potency of the carbamate. On the other hand, due to their increased lipophilicity these compounds may display improved permeability via biological membranes such as the BBB. These drugs could also have longer elimination kinetics from blood compared to that obtained for PYR. Aliphatic, alicyclic or mixed aliphatic/alicyclic chains could also serve as spacers or anchors for the attachment of functional groups that may further increase bioavailability in the CNS and improve the pharmacokinetic profile of the molecule. These functional groups may constitute specific carrier recognition factors for various transport mechanisms through biological barriers. As a demonstration for this novel concept we have chosen substituted and unsubstituted glucosyl moieties to be recog-

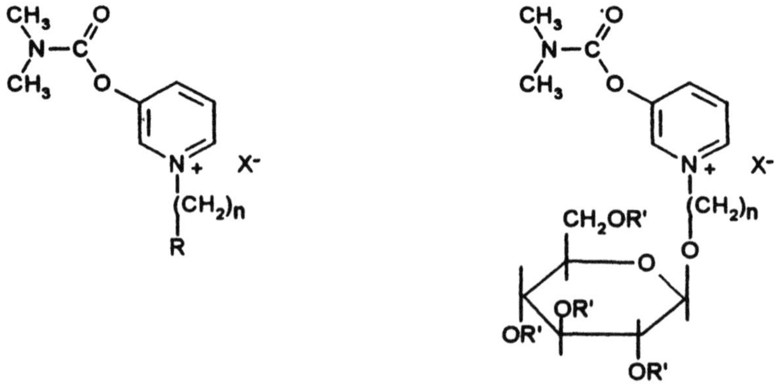

Group A Group B

n = 4-12
R = H, alkyl
X = Br-, Cl-, tartarate,
maleate, succinate etc.

R' = H, acetyl

Figure 1. Chemical structure of new PYR-X compounds.

Table 1. Distribution coefficients (k) of PYR-X compounds

Compound	PYR	PB	PH	POGA	PO	PD	PDOD
k (n-octanol/ PBS*)	0.009	0.021	0.149	0.275	1.680	10.816	97.250

*PBS-50mM phosphate pH=7.4

nized by the glucose transporter (Heldman et al., 1986). A series of 11 carbamates based on the structure of pyridostigmine (PYR-X) was synthesized and characterized by NMR, TLC and mass spectrometry. The chemical structure of the various alkyl chain analogs of pyridostigmine (Group A) and that of compounds with added glucosyl moiety (Group B) is shown in Figure 1.

Lipophilicity

The incorporation of alkyl chains at $(C_6\text{-}C_{12})$ to the basic structure of PYR renders some of these quaternary compounds more lipophilic as shown in Table 1. The addition of a tetraacetylglucosyl moiety at the end of the octyl (C8) spacer (POGA, Table 2) increases the polarity of the molecule (k=0.275) as compared to its simple alkyl analog PO (k=1.680). However, a sugar moiety may increase the bioavailability of the quaternary carbamate through cell membranes utilizing the glucose transporter.

Kinetics of AChE Inhibition

The kinetic parameters for inhibition of purified fetal bovine serum AChE (FBS-AChE) by these compounds are similar to those obtained for PYR (Table 2). Similar values were obtained with human AChE (not shown). Therefore, it is assumed that due to increased lipophilicity, central beneficial therapeutic effects are expected from the new PYR-X compounds, similarly to the beneficial effect of PYR in the PNS.

Table 2. Kinetic parameters for FBS-AChE inhibition by PYR-X compounds[*]

Compound[**]	K_I (M)	k' (min^{-1})	$t_{1/2}(k')$ (min)	k_a (min^{-1})	$t_{1/2}(k_a)$ (min)	k_i (M^{-1}m^{-1})
PYR	5.0×10^{-7}	0.15	5	0.016	43	3.0×10^{5}
PB (A, n=4)	8.8×10^{-6}	1.12	0.62	0.012	58	1.3×10^{5}
PH (A, n=6)	2.9×10^{-6}	0.14	5	0.016	43	4.8×10^{4}
PO (A, n=8)	1.8×10^{-5}	1.61	0.43	0.014	49	8.8×10^{4}
POGA (B,n=8)	2.3×10^{-5}	2.11	0.33	0.012	58	9.2×10^{4}
POG (B, n=8)	3.4×10^{-6}	0.23	3.0	0.012	58	1.5×10^{4}
PD (A, n=10)	3.4×10^{-7}	0.19	4	0.016	43	5.6×10^{5}
PDGA (B, n=10)	4.0×10^{-7}	0.19	3.6	0.011	63	4.7×10^{5}
PDG (B, n=10)	8.7×10^{-7}	0.09	7.7	0.006	110	1.0×10^{5}
PDOD (A, n=12)	2.0×10^{-6}	0.89	0.78	0.016	43	4.5×10^{5}
PDOGA (B, n=12)	3.6×10^{-7}	0.69	1	0.018	38	1.9×10^{6}
PDOG (B, n=12)	1.2×10^{-7}	0.31	2.2	0.059	12	2.6×10^{6}

[*]K_I is the dissociation constant for the reversible complex PYR-X/AChE, k' is the first order rate constant for carbamylation, k_a is the reactivation rate constant and k_i is the bimolecular rate constant. [**]The chemical structure of PYR-X compounds is shown in Figure 1, where A and B refer to groups A and B in Figure 1, n=number of methylenes, G=glucose and GA=tetraacetyl glucose

Table 3. Toxicity of PYR-X derivatives in mice and rats[*]

Compound	PYR[*]	PB	PH	PO[**]	POGA
LD$_{50}$ (mice, i.m.) mg/kg	2.13 (1.9-2.3)	1.74 (0.96-3.2)	6.51 (5.8-7.3)	37.58 (26.6-52.6)	1.34 (0.89-2.0)
POG	PD	PDGA[***]	PDG	PDOD	PDOGA
2.50 (1.7-3.7)	36.59 (25.5-52.5)	1.63 (0.74-3.56)	2.14 (1.9-2.4)	33.86 (26.5-43.2)	1.19 (0.85-1.67)

[*] LD$_{50}$ rat s.c. mg/kg 5.15 (4 - 6.6)
[**] LD$_{50}$ rat s.c. mg/kg 234.8 (139.7 - 394.4)
[***] LD$_{50}$ rat s.c. mg/kg 8.18 (4.51 - 14.84)

Acute Toxicity

Despite their similar inhibitory potency with AChE some of these carbamates are 16–18 fold less toxic than PYR in mice. The LD$_{50}$ values obtained for PO, PD and PDOD are 37.5, 36.6 and 33.9 mg/kg, im, respectively (Table 3). Moreover, PO (PYR-C$_8$) is 46 fold less toxic (LD$_{50}$ = 230mg/kg, sc) than PYR (5mg/kg, sc) in rats (see footnote in Table 3).

Pharmacodynamics

The long duration of action of the new compounds is demonstrated here with PO (Figure 2). Time-course of whole blood ChE activity was followed in rats following subcutaneous administration of 10 and 20 mg/kg of PO. Rat blood ChE inhibition in vivo by PO reaches its peak level within 15 minutes and sustained for 24 hours in a dose-dependent manner. Similar results were obtained with PD using the same dose levels in rats (not shown).

CNS Activity – Behavioral Studies

Central activity of PO was demonstrated by its ability to reverse scopolamine (SC)-induced impairment of memory retention in rats, using the passive avoidance test. As dem-

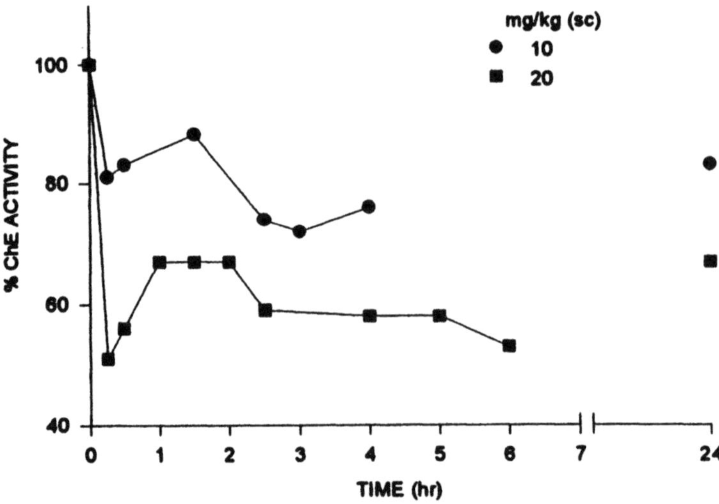

Figure 2. Time-Course of in vivo ChE inhibition by PO in rat blood.

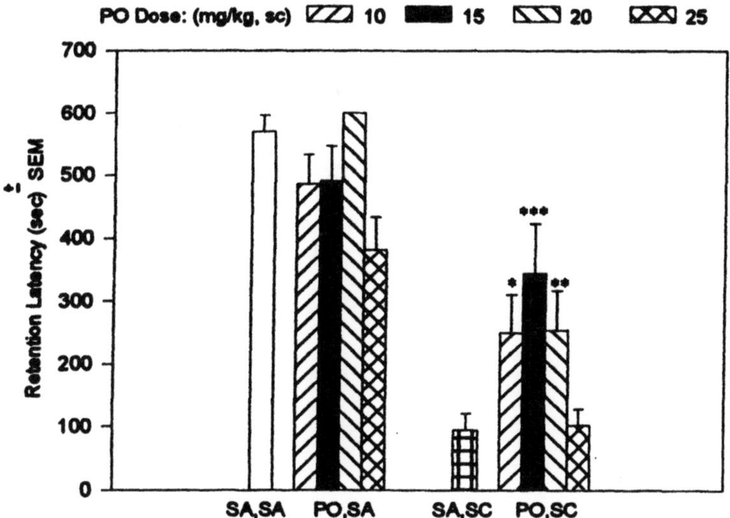

Figure 3. Retention latency of rats in the passive avoidance test - mean time for n=10 per group measured 24 hours post treatment with PO and scopolamine (SC) and initial test (SA=saline). *p<0.1, **p<0.05, ***p<0.02, compared to SA, SC according to Mann-Whitney-U-test.

onstrated in Figure 3, PO (injected subcutaneously, s.c.) partially reverses the impairment induced by SC in rats by significantly prolonging the retention latency (see PO, SC in Figure 3) as compared to SC-control treated animals (see SA, SC in Figure 3). PO by itself had only marginal effect on retention latency (except at 25 mg/kg, p<0.05) indicating its safety at a dose range of 10–20 mg/kg in rats.

Our results show that attachment of hydrophobic alkyl chains to PYR may provde centrally active non-toxic ChE inhibitors with long duration of action that alleviate cognitive impairments induced by cholinergic hypofunction.

REFERENCES

Arnal, F., Cote, L.J., Ginsburg, S., Lawrence G.D., Naini, A. and Sano, M., 1990, Studies on new centrally active and reversible acetylcholinesterase inhibitors. *Neurochem. Res.* 15:587–591.

Bartus, R.T., Dean, R.L., Beer, B. and Lippa, A.S., 1982, The cholinergic hypothesis of geriatric memory dysfunction. *Science* 217:408.

Crimson, M.L., 1994, Tacrine: first drug approved for Alzheimer's disease. *Ann. Pharmacother.* 28: 744–751.

Fisher, A. and Heldman, E., 1990, (±)-Cis-methyl spiro(1,3-oxathiolane-5,3') quinuclidine (AF102B): A new M1 agonist as a rational treatment strategy in Alzheimer's disease - An overview. In: *Basic, Clinical and Therapeutic Aspects of Alzheimer's and Parkinson's Disease.* Nagatsu, T., Fisher, A. and Yoshida, M., eds., Plenum Press, New York, vol. 2, pp. 309–319.

Harel, M., Schalk, I., Ehret-Sabatier, L., Bouet, F., Goldner, N., Hirth, C., Axelsen, P.H., Silman, I. and Sussman J.L., 1993, Quaternary ligand binding to aromatic residues in the active site gorge of acetylcholinesterase, *Proc. Natl. Acad. Sci. USA* 90:9031–9035.

Heldman, E., Ashani Y., Raveh, L. and Rachaman, E.S., 1986, Sugar conjugates of pyridinium aldoximes as antidotes against organophosphate poisoning. *Carbohydrate Res.* 151:337–347.

Millard, C.B. and Broomfield C.A., 1995, Anticholinesterases: Medical applications of neurochemical principles. *J. Neurochem.* 64:1909–1918.

O'Brien, J.T., Eagger, S. and Levy R., 1991, Effect of tetrahydro-aminoacridine on liver function in patients with Alzheimer's disease. *Age Aging* 20:129–131.

Pascuzzi, R.M., 1994, The history of myasthenia gravis. *Neurol. Clin.* 12:231–242.

Sims, N.R., Bowen, D.M., Allen, S.J., Smith, C.C.T., Neary D., Thomas, D.J. and Davison A.N., 1983, Presynaptic cholinergic dysfunction in patients with dementia. *J. Neurochem.* 40:03–509.

Sussman, J.L., Harel, M., Frulow, F., Oefner, C., Goldman, A., Toker, L., and Silman, I., 1991, Atomic Structure of acetylcholinesterase from Torpedo californica: A prototype acetylcholine binding protein. *Science* 253:872–879.

Tagliavini, F. and Pilleri, G., 1984, The basal nucleus of Meynert in cerebral aging and degenerative dementias. *Brain Pathol.* 1:181–218.

Wilson, W.J. and Cook, J.A., 1994, Cholinergic manipulations and passive avoidance in the rat: Effect on acquisition and recall. *Acta Neurobiol. Exp. Warsz.* 54:377–391.

85

CHARACTERIZATION OF C-10 SUBSTITUTED ANALOGUES OF HUPERZINE A AS INHIBITORS OF CHOLINESTERASES

Ashima Saxena,[1] Alan P. Kozikowski,[2] Shaomeng Wang,[2]
Giuseppe Campiani,[3] Qingjie Ding,[2] and B. P. Doctor[1]

[1]Division of Biochemistry
Walter Reed Army Institute of Research
Washington, DC 20307
[2]Georgetown University Medical Center
Institute for Cognitive and Computational Sciences
Washington, DC 20007
[3]Dipartimento Farmaco Chimico Tecnologico
Siena University
Siena, Italy

INTRODUCTION

Huperzine A is a potent and selective reversible inhibitor of mammalian acetylcholinesterase (AChE), the enzyme that catalyzes the hydrolysis of acetylcholine in the brain (Wang et al., 1986). *In vivo* studies have shown that huperzine A has the potential to improve memory in humans (Zhang et al., 1991), while *in vitro* studies indicate that it is superior to physostigmine and tacrine for the treatment of Alzheimer's disease (Wang et al., 1986). Due to the promise this drug holds for the palliative treatment of a disease that afflicts millions of individuals worldwide, several studies have explored the structure-activity relationships of this alkaloid (Ashani et al., 1992; Ashani et al., 1994; Saxena et al., 1994). Molecular modeling coupled with site-directed mutagenesis using mouse AChE mutants implicated Tyr337(*Phe330*) and mouse Trp86(*84*) in the binding of huperzine A to AChE (Ashani et al., 1994; Saxena et al., 1994). The X-ray crystal structure of the *Torpedo* AChE-huperzine A complex was recently resolved (Raves et al., 1997). In this structure, the interactions described were a major hydrogen bond between the carbonyl group of huperzine A and Tyr130 of AChE and a minor cation-π interaction between the primary nitrogen group of huperzine A and the aromatic rings of Trp84 and Phe330. However, the observed pharmacological data supports a major role for Y337(*F330*) in the binding and stereoselectivity of

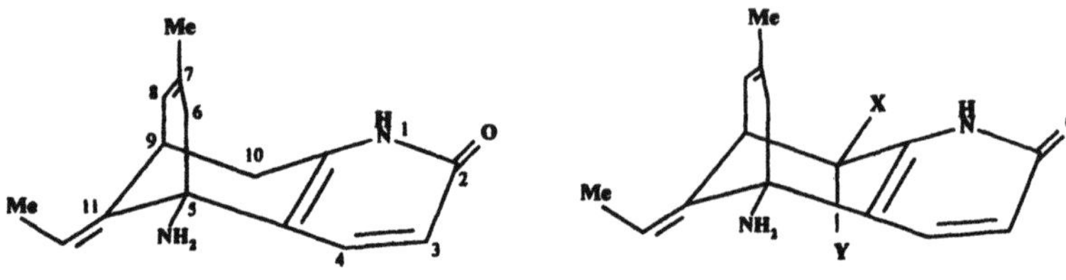

Huperzine A **Huperzine A Analogs**

8a. X=H Y=Me
8b. X=Me Y=H
8c. X=H Y=Et
8d. X=H Y=n-Pr
8e. X=Me Y=Me

Figure 1. Structures of huperzine A and its C-10 substituted analogues.

huperzine A for AChE. The superior inhibition properties of huperzine A have been attributed to the very slow dissociation ($t_{0.5}$ = 35 min) of the AChE-huperzine A complex in solution (Ashani et al., 1992). In an effort to discover more potent analogues of huperzine A, we chose to investigate the synthesis and biological activity of its C-10 substituted analogues.

Chemical Synthesis

The structures of huperzine A and its C-10 substituted analogues used in this study are shown in Figure 1, and the procedure for their synthesis has been described (Kozikowski et al., 1991a; Kozikowski et al., 1991b).

Biological Activity

The K_I values for the inhibition of fetal bovine serum (FBS) AChE by the various inhibitors were determined by the steady state method, as described (Ellman et al., 1961; Saxena et al., 1994). The K_I values for the inhibition of equine butyrylcholinesterase (BChE) by the various inhibitors were determined by analysis of kinetic data (Saxena et al., 1994). The results of the enzyme studies are summarized in Table 1.

As shown in Table 1, the C-10 axial methyl analogue of huperzine A appears about 8-fold more potent than (±)-huperzine A. The equatorial methyl analogue, on the other

Table 1. Inhibition of cholinesterases by huperzine A and its C-10 substituted analogues

	K_I^a (μM)		
Compound	FBS AChE	*Torpedo* AChE	Horse BChE
(±)-huperzine A	0.024	0.22	24
Axial methyl 8a	0.003	0.02	5.8
Equatorial methyl 8b	0.035	0.41	5.5
Ethyl 8c	2.04	14.7	>100
n-propyl 8d	>200	>100	>200
(±)-10,10-dimethylhuperzine A	0.017	0.11	9.5

[a] K_I is mean ± standard deviation; standard errors were all within 20% of the mean.

hand, is about 1.5-fold less active. The 10,10-dimethyl analogue is comparable in activity to huperzine A. Substitution of the methyl group at the C-10 position by bulkier groups such as ethyl and propyl, results in dramatic decreases in inhibitory activity, possibly due to severe steric hindrance of these substituents with the amino acid residues of the active site gorge. The data also show that the methyl analogues of huperzine A retain their high specificity for AChE compared to BChE, and, in fact, the axial methyl derivative shows a higher selectivity ratio of 2000-fold compared to the 1000-fold selectivity ratio of huperzine A. The selectivity of these inhibitors for AChE is important for the minimization of the peripheral effects of such agents in patients.

Molecular Modeling

To explain the kinetic data that revealed differences in the activity of the axial and equatorial methyl analogues, we carried out molecular modeling studies using *Torpedo* AChE. The X-ray crystal structures reported for edrophonium, tacrine, and decamethonium showed that they all included crystallographic waters in binding to the enzyme (Harel et al., 1993). Therefore, crystallographic waters were included in the model of *Torpedo* AChE-huperzine A, described previously (Kozikowski and Pang, 1993). The model showing the binding of huperzine A to *Torpedo* AChE obtained by docking, energy minimization, and molecular dynamics studies, is shown in Figure 2. The ammonium group of huperzine A forms hydrogen bonds with Asp72, Trp84, and Asn85 through two bridging water molecules. These two water molecules were present in the three X-ray crystal structures of AChE in complex with edrophonium, tacrine, and decamethonium (Harel et al., 1993). The ammonium group of huperzine A may also interact with the aromatic ring of Trp84 through a cation-π interaction. The lactam NH forms two hydrogen bonds with the hydroxyl oxygen of Tyr130 and the carboxyl group of Glu199. The lactam carbonyl group also forms two H-bonds with the hydroxyl group of Tyr130 and the main chain amide group of Leu124. The five aromatic residues, Trp84, Tyr121, Phe290, Phe330, and Phe331, and the two aliphatic residues, Ile439 and Ile444, of the enzyme are involved in hydrophobic interactions with huperzine A. The molecular modeling studies appear consistent with the X-ray crystal structure of *Torpedo* AChE-huperzine A complex reported recently (Raves et al., 1997).

Modeling of the C-10 methyl analogues of huperzine A into AChE showed that the presence of either one or two methyl groups at this position did not significantly affect the conformation of the enzyme or the binding of the analogues compared to huperzine A. The introduction of an axial ethyl group caused a slight conformational change to Trp84 and a significant conformational change to Glu199. However, substitution of methyl by an *n*-propyl group at the C-10 axial position caused significant alterations in the conformations of Trp84 and Glu199. For the C-10 dimethyl and equatorial methyl analogues, the equatorial methyl group was found to be in close contact with the main chain amide group of Gly117 and the carbonyl group of His440 and the side chains of Glu199 and His440. Since all these groups are hydrophilic in nature, the hydrophobic-hydrophilic contact is not beneficial to the overall binding energy. In contrast, the C-10 axial methyl group was found to interact with the hydrophobic side chains of Trp84 and Ile 444.

Taken together, the results of these modeling studies adequately explain the improved activity of the C-10 axial methyl derivative of huperzine A compared to the parent compound and its C-10 equatorial methyl counterpart. The C-10 equatorial methyl group is positioned in the polar and hydrophilic region of the enzyme, whereas the C-10 axial methyl group is positioned in the hydrophobic region of the enzyme. While the enzyme

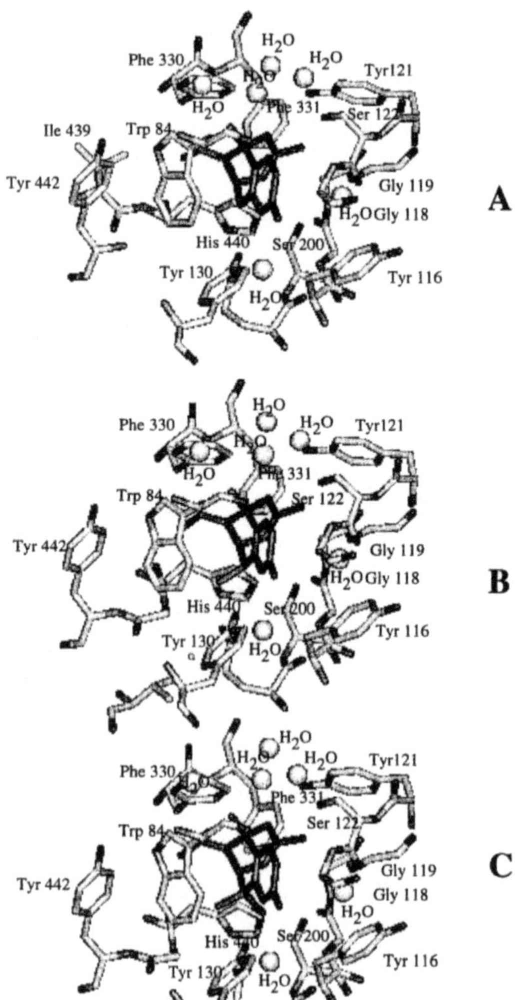

Figure 2. Molecular models showing huperzine A (panel A), its C-10 axial methyl analogue (panel B), and the 10,10-dimethyl analogue (panel C) in complex with *Torpedo* AChE.

can accommodate the methyl group in either region without causing significant conformational changes in the protein, only the axial methyl compound leads to favorable hydrophobic-hydrophobic interactions. These results suggest that larger alkyl groups at the C-10 axial position would further enhance such hydrophobic contacts. However, molecular modeling and enzyme inhibition studies show that the conformational energy penalty due to steric hindrance caused by these bulky groups overwhelms these favorable hydrophobic interactions, making these compounds poor inhibitors of AChE.

This work demonstrates that it is indeed possible to improve the potency of a compound derived from nature through a rather minor structural change. The study reveals the type of modification that imparts increased AChE inhibitory activity to the product, specifically, introducing a lipophilic substituent capable of providing additional hydrophobic contacts with the enzyme. Additionally, in view of the fact that the calculated Log P of the methyl analogue is 0.82 compared to 0.44 for huperzine A, the new analogue may exhibit an improved therapeutic profile through its increased ability to penetrate the blood brain barrier (Brewster et al., 1993).

REFERENCES

Ashani, Y., Peggins, J. O. III, and Doctor, B. P., 1992, Mechanism of inhibition of cholinesterases by huperzine A. *Biochem. Biophys. Res. Commun.* 184:719.

Ashani, Y., Grunwald, J., Kronman, C., Velan, B., and Shafferman, A., 1994, Role of Tyrosine 337 in the binding of huperzine A to the active site of human acetylcholinesterase. *Mol. Pharmacol.* 45:555.

Brewster, M. E., Pop, E., and Bodor, N., 1993, In: *Drug Design for Neuroscience,* Kozikowski, A. P., ed., Raven Press, New York.

Ellman, G. L., Courtney, D., Andres, V., and Featherstone, R. M., 1961, A new and rapid colorimetric determination of acetylcholinesterase activity. *Biochem. Pharmacol.* 1:88.

Harel, H., Schalk, I., Ehret-Sabatier, L., Bouet, F., Goeldner, M, Hirth, C., Axelsen, P. H., Silman, I., and Sussman, J. L., 1993, Quaternary ligand binding to aromatic residues in the active-site gorge of acetylcholinesterase. *Proc. Natl. Acad. Sci. USA* 90:9031.

Kozikowski, A. P., and Pang, Y. P., 1993, Topography of the huperzine A binding site in AChE: Ab initio docking of reversible inhibitors of AChE into the dynamic enzyme. In: *Trends in QSAR and Molecular Modeling '92,*. Wermuth, C. G., ed.; ESCOM. pp 422.

Kozikowski, A. P., Ding, Q., Saxena, A., and Doctor, B. P., 1996, Synthesis of (±)-10,10-dimethylhuperzine A - A huperzine A analogue possessing a slowere enzyme off-rate. *Bioorg. Med. Chem. Lett.* 6:259.

Kozikowski, A. P., Campiani, G., Sun, L.-Q., Wang, S., Saxena, A., and Doctor, B. P., 1996,. Identification of a more potent analogue of the naturally occurring alkaloid huperzine A. Predictive molecular modeling of its interaction with AChE. *J. Am. Chem. Soc.* 118:11357.

Raves, M. L., Harel, M., Pang, Y.-P., Silman, I., Kozikowski, A. P., and Sussman, J. L., 1997, Structure of acetylcholinesterase complexed with the nootropic alkaloid, (-)-huperzine A. *Nature Structural Biol.* 4,:57.

Saxena, A., Qian, N., Kovach, I. M., Kozikowski, A. P., Pang, Y. P., Vellom, D. C., Radic, Z., Quinn, D., Taylor, P., and Doctor, B. P., 1994, Identification of amino acid residues involved in the binding of huperzine A to cholinesterases. *Protein Sci.* 3:1770.

Wang, Y., Yie, D., and Tang, X., 1986, Anti-cholinesterase activity of huperzine A, *Acta Pharmacol. Sin.* 7:110.

Zhang, R.-W., Tang, X.-C., Han, Y.-Y., Sang, G.-W., Zhang, Y.-D., Ma, Y.-X., Zhang, C.-L., and Yang, R.-M., 1991, Drug evaluation of huperzine A in the treatment of senile memory disorders, *Acta Pharmacol. Sin.* 12:250.

86

FUNCTIONAL EFFECTS OF GDNF ON DOPAMINE NEURONS IN ANIMAL MODELS OF PARKINSON'S DISEASE

Alexander F. Hoffman,[1] Meleik A. Hebert,[1] Barry J. Hoffer,[1]
Zhiming Zhang,[2] Wayne A. Cass,[2] Don M. Gash,[2] and Greg A. Gerhardt[1]

[1]Departments of Pharmacology and Psychiatry
Neuroscience Training Program
and the Rocky Mountain Center for Sensor Technology
University of Colorado Health Sciences Center
Denver, Colorado 80262
[2]Department of Anatomy and Neurobiology
University of Kentucky
Lexington, Kentucky 40536

INTRODUCTION

Parkinson's disease (PD) is one of the most common neurological disorders of the elderly. It is characterized by a progressive degeneration of dopaminergic neurons of the substantia nigra (SN) with a subsequent loss of dopamine (DA) input to the striatum (Hornykiewicz and Kish, 1987; Graybiel et al., 1990). This loss leads to the cardinal symptoms of bradykinesia, rigidity, resting tremor, and akinesia seen in PD (Hornykiewicz and Kish, 1987) . Various clinical strategies have been employed in order to alleviate the symptoms of this disease, and can be grouped into two basic categories. The first involves the restoration of midbrain DA levels, either pharmacologically through drugs such as levodopa, or by transplantation of DA-producing cells into the striatum. The second approach attempts to normalize motor function by targeting downstream neuronal pathways that are affected by the loss of DA. These include surgical treatments such as the pallidotomy, as well as pharmacological treatment with anticholinergic drugs. The relative benefits and drawbacks of these approaches have been reviewed previously, and will not be discussed in this review (Iacono et al., 1994; Mizuno et al., 1995; Charles and Davis, 1996).

A more recent approach has focused on the use of neurotrophic factors that may specifically influence the function of midbrain DAergic neurons. Studies utilizing labeled

Progress in Alzheimer's and Parkinson's Diseases
edited by Fisher *et al.*, Plenum Press, New York, 1998.

tracers have revealed that damaged or diseased DA neurons, both in human PD and in animal models of the disease, may still retain some functional capacity for uptake and/or metabolism (Leenders et al., 1990). It has been proposed that these damaged neurons could be salvaged by the administration of the appropriate trophic factor(s). The utility of such factors rests in their ability to prevent further neuronal degeneration and to restore the functional capacity of diseased neurons (Lindsay et al., 1993). However, the number and identity of factors required to produce the optimal effects are still the subject of extensive research.

This review summarizes the effects of a novel peptide growth factor, glial cell line-derived neurotrophic factor (GDNF), in two animal models of PD. In both models, neurochemical and immunocytochemical markers suggest that GDNF produces profound effects on DA neurons within the SN. Despite significant behavioral improvements, striatal DA markers remain unaltered in these same animals, further highlighting the potential importance of extrastriatal DA systems in the treatment of PD (Chesselet and Delfs, 1996).

GDNF: A TROPHIC FACTOR FOR DA NEURONS

GDNF was first discovered in a conditioned media assay aimed at finding a neurotrophic factor for substantia nigra DA neurons (Lin et al., 1993, 1994). Initial studies demonstrated that the supernatant from the rat B49 glial cell line exerted potent and relatively specific trophic effects on embryonic midbrain DAergic cells in culture. These effects included maintenance of DA cell number and increases in cell size, neurite length and DA uptake. GDNF was purified as the protein responsible for the trophic actions.

The specificity of this peptide for DA neurons was determined in several assays *in vitro*. GDNF was shown to have an EC_{50} of 1.2 pM (36 pg/ml) for DA uptake, while high-affinity uptake of γ-aminobutyric acid (GABA) or serotonin was not affected by GDNF given at a concentration 30,000 times higher than the EC_{50} for DA uptake. In addition, GDNF was not seen to influence the density of astrocytes in DAergic cell cultures, nor was it seen to alter the content of glial fibrillary acidic protein (GFAP) in these cells (Lin et al., 1993). More recently, GDNF was also shown to promote the survival and neurite extension of cultured DA neurons damaged by the neurotoxin 1-methyl-4-phenylpyridinium (MPP+; Hou et al., 1996).

Cloning of GDNF suggests that this factor is a distant member of the transforming growth factor beta (TGFβ) superfamily. Recently, both a GDNF receptor and a related trophic factor which shares significant (42%) amino acid homology with GDNF, were described (Jing et al., 1996; Kotzbauer et al., 1996; Trupp et al., 1996). GDNF acts as a disulfide-bonded homodimer, each portion of the mature protein consists of 134 amino acid residues, with 93% identity between the human and rat sequences. The naturally occurring dimer has a molecular weight of 30kDa and is glycosylated. The mature human GDNF expressed in *Escherichia coli*, is not glycosylated but exhibits the same biological potency *in vitro* as the GDNF isolated from a natural source (Lapchak et al., 1996). The availability of large amounts of this recombinant human GDNF (rhGDNF) permitted the first characterization of the effects of this protein in intact animals . Intracranial administration of GDNF was found to enhance the function of midbrain DA neurons *in vivo*, both in normal rodents and in normal non-human primates (Hudson et al., 1995; Gash et al., 1995; Hebert et al., 1996). Thus, evidence from both *in vitro* and *in vivo* studies supports the hypothesis that GDNF acts as a potent and selective neurotrophic factor for midbrain DA neurons.

EFFECTS OF GDNF IN UNILATERALLY 6-HYDROXYDOPAMINE-LESIONED RATS

The potent effects of GDNF on normal midbrain DA neurons, both *in vivo* and *in vitro*, led to speculation that this growth factor could represent a "magic bullet" for the treatment of PD. The first test of the therapeutic potential of GDNF utilized a well-characterized rat model that reproduces the neurochemical deficits seen in PD. This model involves a unilateral injection of the catecholamine neurotoxin, 6-hydroxydopamine (6-OHDA), into the medial forebrain bundle (Ungerstedt and Arbuthnott 1970; Ungerstedt, 1971). Rats that have been unilaterally lesioned in this manner rotate contralaterally in response to systemic administration of low doses of apomorphine, a DA agonist. The magnitude of rotations is considered to accurately reflect the degree of DAergic degeneration (Ungerstedt and Arbuthnott, 1970; Marshall and Ungerstedt, 1977). All lesioned animals used in the studies reviewed here exhibited a stable rotation pattern and turned >300 times contralateral to the lesion after a low dose (0.05 mg/kg) of apomorphine. We have previously shown that such animals have a loss of striatal DA $\geq$ 95% and a DA depletion in the substantia nigra of about 70–75% (Hudson et al., 1993).

In the initial study, lesioned rats meeting the behavioral criteria received various doses (0.1–100µg) of rhGDNF or vehicle intranigrally (Hoffer et al., 1994). Following the 100µg GDNF administration, there was a rapid and long-lasting profound decrease in rotational behavior. No other dose of GDNF or vehicle produced significant changes in rotational behavior. The diminution in rotations was evident one week following GDNF treatment and remained at a significantly reduced level for five weeks. After five weeks, the animals were sacrificed, and neurotransmitters and metabolites were quantified in the striatum and the substantia nigra using HPLC-EC methods. In rats which received vehicle injections into the lesioned substantia nigra, there was a marked nigral DA depletion, similar to that which has been reported after 6-OHDA alone. In contrast, five weeks after animals received 100µg of GDNF, DA and DOPAC levels within the SN were restored to normal levels. GDNF treatment (100µg) had no significant effects on 5-HT and 5-HIAA levels within the striatum or SN. No changes in striatal DA, which was considerably reduced on the lesioned side ($\geq$ 99%), were produced by any dose of GDNF at the 5 week timepoint (Hoffer et al., 1994). These data demonstrate that intranigral injection of 100µg of GDNF elicits marked and long-lasting behavioral and neurochemical changes suggesting a reversal of 6-OHDA-induced DA depletion.

More recently, we have performed *in vivo* microdialysis studies of DA and its metabolites within the SN of GDNF-treated 6-OHDA-lesioned animals (Hoffman et al., 1997). In these experiments, lesioned animals received intranigral injections of rhGDNF (100 ig) or vehicle, and both rotational behavior and spontaneous locomotor behavior were assessed. GDNF-treated animals that showed a reduction in rotational behavior also manifested significant increases in spontaneous motor behaviors, whereas vehicle treated animals did not improve on either behavioral test. These changes were present one week and four weeks following treatment, although the enhancement of spontaneous activity was reduced at the later time point. Microdialysis studies in the SN were carried out at both the one and four week time points. The basal levels of DA metabolites, DOPAC and HVA, were greatly reduced in vehicle treated 6-OHDA-lesioned animals, relative to levels in normal rats. Similarly, stimulus-evoked DA release, produced by local delivery of potassium, d-amphetamine, or a combination of the two, was significantly reduced in 6-OHDA-lesioned rats. One week following GDNF treatment, the lesioned animals showed a slight but significant increase in nigral HVA levels, although stimulus-evoked DA release was not enhanced. In contrast, four weeks after GDNF treatment, there was a significant increase in d-amphetamine-induced DA overflow and an increase in the combined d-amphetamine/potassium-induced DA release. These studies confirm our previous findings that suggest a normalization of DA function within the SN occurs following GDNF administration in 6-OHDA-lesioned rats. However, although changes in DA function within the SN correlate with the behavioral effects at the four week time point, no change in DA function was seen at the *onset* of the behavioral changes. These findings suggest that other systems within the SN may play a role in producing some of the striking behavioral effects of GDNF in this model, at least at the earlier time points (Hoffman et al., 1997).

Taken together, these experiments using hemiparkinsonian rats suggest that GDNF produced an increase in DA and DA metabolite content within the SN without any apparent changes in these levels within the lesioned striatum. These data have also been supported by immunocytochemical studies that have suggested that, in lesioned rats, GDNF produces behavioral effects independent of changes in striatal DA function (Bowenkamp et al., 1995; Tseng et al., 1997). These neurochemical results, combined with the behavioral measurements, also support the hypothesis that DA levels in the substantia nigra may play a major role in apomorphine-induced rotational behavior (Robertson and Robertson, 1988, 1989; Hudson et al., 1993).

EFFECTS OF GDNF IN MPTP-LESIONED MONKEYS

Although crucial and informative, the initial studies involving GDNF treatment in 6-OHDA-lesioned rats are limited in their relevance to human PD. The rodent CNS differs significantly in numerous neuroanatomical and neurochemical parameters from the human. In contrast, nonhuman primates possess a central nervous system and behavioral repertoire much closer to the human than the rodent. In rhesus monkeys, a stable, hemiparkinsonian state can be produced by intracarotid infusion of the neurotoxin 1-methyl-4-phenyl-1,2,3,6-tetrahydropyridine (MPTP). In humans and nonhuman primates, MPTP produces neurochemical, neuropathological and behavioral effects that are similar to those found in idiopathic PD (Kurlan et al., 1991a,b; Langston et al., 1983, 1984). Thus, analogous to 6-OHDA-lesioned rats, the MPTP-lesioned monkey represents a useful paradigm in which novel therapies for PD can be investigated.

In these experiments, rhGDNF was administered to six lesioned monkeys, all of which manifested stable parkinsonian deficits for at least three months following MPTP treatment. GDNF was delivered by three different routes: two subjects received intranigral GDNF (150 µg), two intracaudate (450 µg), and two intracerbroventricular (ICV; 450 µg). Seven animals received a phosphate-buffered saline solution only, and served as controls. Pre and post-treatment behavioral measures were assessed using a nonhuman primate hemiparkinsonian rating scale (Ovadia et al., 1995). The results demonstrated that only the GDNF-treated animals showed significant improvements in motor behaviors, which were evident 2–4 weeks following drug treatment (Gash et al., 1996).

The ICV-treated animals were also assessed for the ability to respond to repeated dosing of GDNF. The sample size was increased by adding one additional animal to the 450µg treatment group and three animals which received 100µg of GDNF ICV. Each animal received three ICV injections spaced at least four weeks apart. In both of these dose groups, the effects of GDNF administration were very apparent by the third week following initial infusion. Three cardinal symptoms of PD, bradykinesia, rigidity, and postural instability, were significantly improved by ICV infusions of GDNF in MPTP-lesioned monkeys. In contrast, motor behaviors were not improved in the vehicle treated animals (Gash et al., 1996). Moreover, the only apparent side effect of this regimen was a transient weight loss, which normalized four weeks following treatment.

The intracaudate and intranigral injected animals were sacrificed four weeks after the first injection. Midbrains from these animals were processed for TH-immunoreactivity (TH-IR) and stereological cell counting. Cell size was measured for each TH-IR neuron counted. Within the SN, there was a trend towards increased TH-positive cells in GDNF-treated animals. This increase was not statistically significant, possibly owing to the variance on the lesioned side. However, neuronal size within the SN was found to be significantly larger in the GDNF recipients. From these data, it appears that GDNF is able to upregulate the expression of the TH enzyme within damaged nigral DA neurons.

Finally, tissue punches were taken from various midbrain structures of the ICV-treated monkeys for HPLC-EC determination of DA and its metabolites. Significant increases in DA were found in the SN, ventral tegmental area (VTA), and globus pallidus of the GDNF-treated animals. Similar to the results seen in the rat model, DA and its metabolites DOPAC and HVA were not altered in the striatum of the GDNF-treated animals. Thus, these data suggest that GDNF is able to increase midbrain DA levels within certain regions affected by the MPTP lesion (Gash et al., 1996).

Taken together, the findings from the MPTP-lesioned monkeys demonstrate that GDNF can partially restore DA levels within subregions of the basal ganglia, and can stimulate the function of surviving DA neurons. In addition, GDNF produces robust behavioral improvements in these animals, which persist for several weeks following single or repeated doses. All of these findings parallel the effects of GDNF administration in the 6-OHDA-lesioned rat model, further supporting the hypothesis that GDNF may be a useful therapy in PD.

SUMMARY AND FUTURE DIRECTIONS

Like many neurodegenerative diseases, PD represents a formidable challenge for patients, clinicians, and researchers. Although pharmacological treatment with dopamine agonists, anticholinergics, and MAO inhibitors can benefit most patients, these therapies also become less efficacious as the illness progresses. Transplantation strategies and other surgical approaches have also met with some clinical success, but many critical issues still remain with these newer techniques (Koutouzis et al., 1994; Kordower et al., 1997). It is possible that currently available treatments fail because they afford only symptomatic relief of PD, but do not reverse the ongoing degenerative process. Thus, it has been speculated that DA-selective neurotrophic factors may represent the best hope for a true "cure" for the disease, if these factors can slow or even partially reverse neuronal loss.

Although several novel proteins that target midbrain DA neurons have been described, GDNF can be distinguished by the following characteristics. First, in both the 6-OHDA-lesioned rat and in the MPTP-lesioned monkey, a single administration of GDNF is able to reverse behavioral deficits for several weeks following treatment (Hoffer et al., 1994; Gash et al. 1996; Hoffman et al., 1997). No other single factor, or combination of factors, has been reported to produce such long-lasting effects after a single dose. Secondly, in the animal models reviewed here, the effects of GDNF are apparent even when this factor is given weeks or months following the lesion. Thus, GDNF does not appear to be required at the time of the injury, although evidence exists for the neuroprotective effects of this protein as well (Opacka-Juffry et al., 1995; Winkler et al., 1996). Finally, and perhaps most striking, is the apparently selective effect of GDNF on "extrastriatal" DA systems. In unilaterally 6-OHDA-lesioned rats, neurochemical evidence from both whole tissue analyses and microdialysis studies suggests that DA is partially normalized within the SN, but not within the striatum, following GDNF treatment (Hoffer et al., 1994; Hoffman et al., 1997). Similarly, in MPTP-lesioned monkeys, DA levels are increased in the SN, globus pallidus, and VTA, but not within the caudate nucleus or putamen (Gash et al., 1996). These findings are further supported by changes in nigral, but not striatal, TH-like immunoreactive markers in these same animals (Bowenkamp et al., 1995; Gash et al., 1996). These effects on nigral DA, coupled with the striking behavioral effects observed, lead to two important questions for future studies. First, to what extent does DA release within the SN influence motor behaviors? We feel that the findings presented in this review should serve as an impetus to further explore this issue, which has received only limited attention in previous studies (Robertson and Robertson, 1988, 1989). In this regard, we concur with Chesselet and others who have also suggested that the role of DA outside of the striatum should continue to be investigated (Chesselet and Delfs, 1996; Levy et al., 1997). A second related question that must be addressed pertains to the possible effects of GDNF on nondopaminergic systems within the SN of these PD models. Given that the dose of GDNF utilized in the studies reviewed here is substantially higher than the EC_{50} for this factor on DA neurons *in vitro*, it cannot be assumed that all of the behavioral effects produced by GDNF occur via changes in DA systems. Specifically, GABAergic and glutamatergic systems are known to be important in controlling basal ganglia output, and the effects of GDNF on these systems in parkinsonian animals has yet to be addressed (Kish et al., 1987; Starr, 1995; Chase et al., 1996).

In summary, although the precise mechanism through which GDNF produces its effects in hemiparkinsonian animal models has yet to be elucidated, it appears that this neurotrophic factor may represent both a novel therapy for PD, as well as a valuable tool with which to explore basal ganglia function.

REFERENCES

Bowenkamp, K.E., Hoffman, A.F., Gerhardt, G.A., Henry, M.A., Biddle, P.T., Hoffer, B.J., and Granholm, A.C., 1995, Glial cell line-derived neurotrophic factor supports survival of injured midbrain dopaminergic neurons. *J, Comp. Neurol.* 355:479–489.

Charles, P.D. and Davis, T.L. ,1996, Drug therapy for Parkinson's disease. [Review] [22 refs]. *South. Med. J.,* 89:851–856.

Chase, T.N., Engber, T.M., and Mouradian, M.M. ,1996, Contribution of dopaminergic and glutamatergic mechanisms to the pathogenesis of motor response complications in Parkinson's disease. *Adv. Neurol.* 69:497–501.

Chesselet, M.F. and Delfs, J.M. ,1996, Basal ganglia and movement disorders-an update [Review]. *Trends in Neurosciences* 19:417–422.

Gash, D.M., Zhang, Z., Cass, W.A., Ovadia, A., Simmerman, L., Martin, D., Russell, D., Collins, F., Hoffer, B.J., and Gerhardt, G.A. ,1995, Morphological and functional effects of intranigrally administered GDNF in normal rhesus monkeys. *J. Comp. Neurol.* 363:345–358.

Gash, D.M., Zhang, Z., Ovadia, A., Cass, W.A., Yi, A., Simmerman, L., Russell, D., Martin, D., Lapchak, P.A., Collins, F., Hoffer, B.J., and Gerhardt, G.A. ,1996, Functional recovery in parkinsonian monkeys treated with GDNF. *Nature* 380:252–255.

Graybiel, A.M., Hirsch, E.C., and Agid, Y. ,1990, The nigrostriatal system in Parkinson's disease. [Review]. *Ad. Neurol.* 53:17–29.

Hebert, M.A., van Horne, C.G., Hoffer, B.J., and Gerhardt, G.A. ,1996, Functional effects of GDNF in normal rat striatum: Presynaptic studies using *in vivo* electrochemistry and microdialysis. *J. Pharmacol. Exp. Ther.* 279:1181–1190.

Hoffer, B.J., Hoffman, A., Bowenkamp, K., Huettl, P., Hudson, J., Martin, D., Lin, L.F., and Gerhardt, G.A., 1994, Glial cell line-derived neurotrophic factor reverses toxin-induced injury to midbrain dopaminergic neurons in vivo. *Neurosci. Lett.* 182:107–111.

Hoffman, A.F., C.G. van Horne, S. Eken, B.J. Hoffer, and G.A. Gerhardt, 1997, *In vivo* microdialysis studies of somatodendritic dopamine release in the rat substantia nigra: effects of unilateral 6-OHDA lesions and GDNF. Exp. Neurol. (In Press)

Hornykiewicz, O. and Kish, S.J., 1987, Biochemical pathophysiology of Parkinson's disease. *Ad. Neurol.* 45:19–34.

Hou, J.G., Lin, L.F., and Mytilineou, C. ,1996,Glial cell line-derived neurotrophic factor exerts neurotrophic effects on dopaminergic neurons in vitro and promotes their survival and regrowth after damage by 1-methyl-4-phenylpyridinium. *J. Neurochem.* 66:74–82.

Hudson, J., Granholm, A.C., Gerhardt, G.A., Henry, M.A., Hoffman, A., Biddle, P., Leela, N.S., Mackerlova, L., Lile, J.D., Collins, F., and et al ,1995, Glial cell line-derived neurotrophic factor augments midbrain dopaminergic circuits in vivo. *Brain Res. Bull.* 36:425–432.

Hudson, J.L., van Horne, C.G., Stromberg, I., Brock, S., Clayton, J., Masserano, J., Hoffer, B.J., and Gerhardt, G.A. ,1993, Correlation of apomorphine- and amphetamine-induced turning with nigrostriatal dopamine content in unilateral 6-hydroxydopamine lesioned rats. *Brain Res.* 626:167–174.

Iacono, R.P., Lonser, R.R., Mandybur, G., Morenski, J.D., Yamada, S., and Shima, F. ,1994, Stereotactic pallidotomy results for Parkinson's exceed those of fetal graft. [Review] [33 refs]. *Am. Surg.* 60:777–782.

Jing, S., Wen, D., Yu, Y., Holst, P.L., Luo, Y., Fang, M., Tamir, R., Antonio, L., Hu, Z., Cupples, R., Louis, J.C., Hu, S., Altrock, B.W., and Fox, G.M. ,1996, GDNF-induced activation of the ret protein tyrosine kinase is mediated by GDNFR-alpha, a novel receptor for GDNF. *Cell* 85:1113–1124.

Kish, S., Rajput, A., Gilbert, J., Rozdilsky, B., Chang, L.J., Shannak, K., and Hornykiewicz, O. ,1987, GABA-dopamine relationship in Parkinson's disease striatum. *Ad. Neurol.* 45:75–77.

Kordower, J.H., Goetz, C.G., Freeman, T.B., and Olanow, C.W. ,1997, Dopaminergic transplants in patients with Parkinson's disease: Neuroanatomical correlates of clinical recovery. *Exp. Neurol.* 144:41–46.

Kotzbauer, P.T., Lampe, P.A., Heuckeroth, R.O., Golden, J.P., Creedon, D.J., Johnson, E.M., and Milbrandt, J., 1996, Neurturin, a relative of glial-cell-line-derived neurotrophic factor. *Nature,* 384:467–470.

Koutouzis, T.K., Emerich, D.F., Borlongan, C.V., Freeman, T.B., Cahill, D.W., and Sanberg, P.R., 1994, Cell transplantation for central nervous system disorders. [Review] [275 refs]. *Crit. Rev. Neurobiol,* 8:125–162.

Kurlan, R., Kim, M.H., and Gash, D.M. ,1991a, Oral levodopa dose-response study in MPTP-induced hemiparkinsonian monkeys: assessment with a new rating scale for monkey parkinsonism. *Mov. Dis.* 6:111–118.

Kurlan, R., Kim, M.H., and Gash, D.M. ,1991b, The time course and magnitude of spontaneous recovery of parkinsonism produced by intracarotid administration of 1-methyl-4-phenyl-1,2,3,6-tetrahydropyridine to monkeys. *An. Neurol.* 29:677–679.

Langston, J.W., Ballard, P., Tetrud, J.W., and Irwin, I. ,1983, Chronic Parkinsonism in humans due to a product of meperidine-analog synthesis. *Science* 219:979–980.

Langston, J.W., Langston, E.B., and Irwin, I. ,1984, MPTP-induced parkinsonism in human and non-human primates--clinical and experimental aspects. *Acta Neurol. Scand. Suppl.* 100:49–54.

Lapchak, P.A., Miller, P.J., Jiao, S.S., Araujo, D.M., Hilt, D., and Collins, F. ,1996, Biology of glial cell line-derived neurotrophic factor (GDNF): Implications for the use of GDNF to treat Parkinson's disease. *Neurodegeneration* 5:197–205.

Leenders, K.L., Salmon, E.P., Tyrrell, P., Perani, D., Brooks, D.J., Sager, H., Jones, T., Marsden, C.D., and Frackowiak, R.S. ,1990, The nigrostriatal dopaminergic system assessed in vivo by positron emission tomography in healthy volunteer subjects and patients with Parkinson's disease. *Arch. Neurol.* 47:1290–1298.

Levy, R., Hazrati, L.N., Herrero, M.T., Vila, M., Hassani, O.K., Mouroux, M., Ruberg, M., Asensi, H., Agid, Y., Féger, J., Obeso, J.A., Parent, A., and Hirsch, E.C. ,1997, Re-evaluation of the functional anatomy of the basal ganglia in normal and parkinsonian states. *Neuroscience* 76:335–343.

Lin, L.F., Doherty, D.H., Lile, J.D., Bektesh, S., and Collins, F. ,1993, GDNF: a glial cell line-derived neurotrophic factor for midbrain dopaminergic neurons [see comments]. *Science* 260:1130–1132.

Lin, L.F., Zhang, T.J., Collins, F., and Armes, L.G. ,1994, Purification and initial characterization of rat B49 glial cell line-derived neurotrophic factor. *J. Neurochem.* 63:758–768.

Lindsay, R.M., Altar, C.A., Cedarbaum, J.M., Hyman, C., and Wiegand, S.J. ,1993, The therapeutic potential of neurotrophic factors in the treatment of Parkinson's disease. [Review]. *Exp. Neurol.* 124:103–118.

Marshall, J.F. and Ungerstedt, U. ,1977,Supersensitivity to apomorphine following destruction of the ascending dopamine neurons: quantification using the rotational model. *Eur.J.Pharmacol.* 41:361–367.

Mizuno, Y., Mori, H., and Kondo, T. ,1995, Parkinson's disease: from etiology to treatment. [Review] [139 refs]. *Internal Med.* 34:1045–1054.

Opacka-Juffry, J., Ashworth, S., Hume, S.P., Martin, D., Brooks, D.J., and Blunt, S.B. ,1995, GDNF protects against 6-OHDA nigrostriatal lesion: in vivo study with microdialysis and PET. *Neuroreport* 7:348–352.

Ovadia, A., Zhang, Z., and Gash, D.M. ,1995, Increased susceptibility to MPTP toxicity in middle-aged rhesus monkeys. *Neurobiol. Aging,* 16:931–937.

Robertson, G.S. and Robertson, H.A. ,1988, Evidence that the substantia nigra is a site of action for L-DOPA. *Neurosci. Lett.* 89:204–208.

Robertson, G.S. and Robertson, H.A. ,1989, Evidence that L-dopa-induced rotational behavior is dependent on both striatal and nigral mechanisms. *J. Neurosci.* 9:3326–3331.

Starr, M.S. ,1995,Glutamate/dopamine D1/D2 balance in the basal ganglia and its relevance to Parkinson's disease. [Review]. *Synapse* 19:264–293.

Trupp, M., Arenas, E., Fainzilber, M., Nilsson, A.S., Sieber, B.A., Grigoriou, M., Kilkenny, C., Salazar-Grueso, E., Pachnis, V., Arumae, U., and et al ,1996, Functional receptor for GDNF encoded by the c-ret proto-oncogene [see comments]. *Nature* 381:785–788.

Tseng, J.L., Baetge, E.E., Zurn, A.D., and Aebischer, P. ,1997, GDNF reduces drug-induced rotational behavior after medial forebrain bundle transection by a mechanism not involving striatal dopamine. *J. Neurosci.* 17:325–333.

Ungerstedt, U. ,1971, Postsynaptic supersensitivity after 6-hydroxy-dopamine induced degeneration of the nigrostriatal dopamine system. *Acta Physiol. Scand. Suppl.* 367:69–93.

Ungerstedt, U. and Arbuthnott, G.W. ,1970, Quantitative recording of rotational behavior in rats after 6-hydroxy-dopamine lesions of the nigrostriatal dopamine system. *Brain Res.* 24:485–493.

Winkler, C., Sauer, H., Lee, C.S., and Björklund, A. ,1996, Short-term GDNF treatment provides long-term rescue of lesioned nigral dopaminergic neurons in a rat model of Parkinson's disease. *J. Neurosci.* 16:7206–7215.

87

DEVELOPMENT AND USES OF SMALL MOLECULE LIGANDS OF TrkA RECEPTORS

Lynne LeSauteur,[1] Natalia Beglova,[2] Kalle Gehring,[2] and H. Uri Saragovi[1,3]

[1]Departments of Pharmacology and Therapeutics
[2]Department of Biochemistry
[3]Department of Oncology
McGill University, Montréal, Quebec
Canada H3G 1Y6

INTRODUCTION

Nerve Growth Factor (NGF), is a polypeptide that elicits widespread biological effects via interaction with a tyrosine kinase receptor termed TrkA (Kaplan et al., 1991). NGF a member of the neurotrophin (NT) family of growth factors is responsible for the survival, differentiation and maintenance of specific sensory, sympathetic and cholinergic neuronal populations (Levi-Montalcini, 1987). The NGF dependent cholinergic basal forebrain and septum neurons are areas implicated in memory and learning which are severely affected by neuronal loss in Alzheimer's disease (Hefti and Will, 1987). The neurotrophic hypothesis states that innervated tissues produce NTs which coordinate neuronal growth and programmed death during development (Purves et al., 1985). In adulthood NT levels stabilize at low levels thought to be sufficient to maintain the neuronal phenotype. While NT levels increase upon neuronal injury they do not attain levels found in development. It appears that the inability to rescue neurons from trauma or disease induced cell death may be due to inadequate NT production, because neuronal populations can be rescued by NGF treatment (Cuello et al., 1993) (Table 1). Agonistic small molecule TrkA ligands with improved pharmacological properties may be useful for the treatment of stroke or neurodegenerative diseases, or for treatment of neoplastic diseases (neuroblastoma, medulloblastoma, melanoma) that respond to neurotrophins. Herein, we describe the development and uses of artificial ligands of TrkA. These small molecule ligands are either structural mimics of NGF or structural mimics of anti-TrkA monoclonal antibodies (Figure 1).

NGF, The Endogenous TrkA Ligand

Almost fifty years ago NGF was discovered as a crucial factor mediating neuronal survival (Levi-Montalcini, 1987). The NTs (NGF, BDNF, NT-3 and NT-4\NT-5) signal cell sur-

Progress in Alzheimer's and Parkinson's Diseases
edited by Fisher *et al.*, Plenum Press, New York, 1998.

Table 1. The neurotrophic hypothesis

Tissue	NT synthesis	Biological role
Developing CNS	High	Selective target innervation
Mature CNS	Low	Phenotypic maintenance
Injury	Moderate	Attempt to rescue neurons*
Senescence	Very low	Apoptotic factors prevail

Neurotrophins play a role in CNS development and selection of functional connections. In the mature CNS neurotrophins maintain functional neurons and afford plasticity. Upon injury or neuronal senescence neurotrophin production is increased, likely in an attempt to prevent neuronal loss. Insufficient neurotrophin production or inappropriate delivery to injured sites results in no rescue. This is the therapeutic window where neurotrophic substances, especially small molecules, can be used.

vival, differentiation, growth cessation and apoptosis through two cell surface receptors, the Trks and p75 (Chao and Hempstead, 1995). Each NT has preference for a particular member of the Trk family (NGF/TrkA; BDNF/TrkB; NT-3/TrkC) which is thought to mediate most neurotrophic effects (Barbacid, 1994). All NTs bind p75 which is termed the common NT receptor. The function of p75 is largely undefined. In some cells (un)bound p75 plays a role in inducing apoptotic death, while in others it does not (Carter and Lewin, 1997).

NGF binds TrkA with high affinity causing receptor dimerization and activation of the tyrosine kinase domain of the receptor (Jing et al., 1992). Activation of the cytoplasmic tyrosine kinase leads to auto- and trans-phosphorylation of cytoplasmic tyrosine residues on TrkA. These phosphorylated tyrosines serve as recruitement sites for intracellular signaling molecules which lead to the activation of various signal transduction pathways, specific gene induction, and long term biological effects (Kaplan and Stephens, 1994).

The importance of the NGF\TrkA system is emphasized by recents knockout studies (Barbacid, 1994). Mice lacking either ligand or receptor display perinatal loss of dependent neurons including sensory and sympathetic neurons within the dorsal root ganglia. TrkA knockout mice also display a decrease in the cholinergic basal forebrain projections to the hippocampus and cortex. These findings demonstrate that TrkA is the primary mediator of the trophic actions of NGF *in vivo*.

Initial events of molecular recognition between NTs and their receptors, and the minimal structural or conformational factors which result in a multitude of receptor-mediated cellular responses are not well understood. The domains of NGF that bind to the receptor may be defined by the resolution of the three-dimensional structure of the molecule

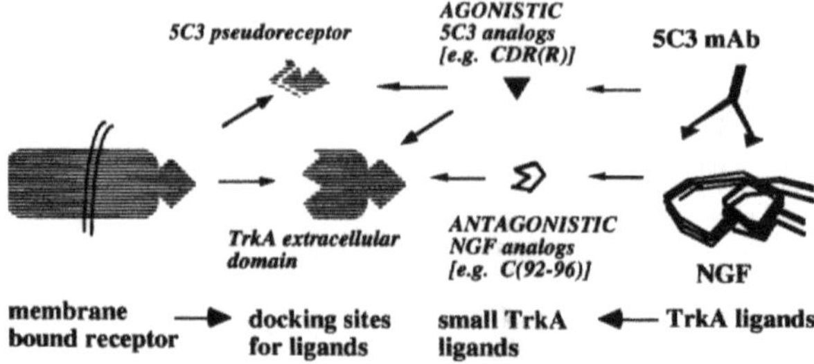

Figure 1. Overview and design of TrkA ligands.

(McDonald et al., 1991). NGF is a 26 kDa dimer whose interface encompasses about 1800 Å^2 and is mostly formed by antiparallel beta pleated sheets. The connecting beta-turns are solvent exposed and readily accessible for receptor interactions. All neurotrophins share striking sequence homology except in the beta-turn regions. While differences may be necessary for specific Trk receptor binding, common features may be required for all NTs to bind the shared low affinity p75 receptor.

Using mutagenesis and chimeric molecules, beta-turn A-A' of NGF has been shown to bind p75 and beta-turns A'-A" and C-D are important for TrkA recognition (Ibanez, 1995). Interestingly the amino-and carboxy terminus have also been shown to be important for binding TrkA (Kahle et al., 1992; Drinkwater et al., 1993).These results imply that terminal regions and beta-turns induce conformational changes leading to formation of a productive NGF-TrkA complex. Perhaps, binding of NGF to TrkA involves several contact points some of which may be more important for biological activity. Mutagenesis studies of TrkA implicate both immunoglobulin-like domains as well as leucine rich domains of the receptor in binding NGF (Windisch et al., 1995; Urfer et al., 1995; MacDonald and Meakin et al., 1996).

TrkA Ligand Development

Antagonistic NGF Mimics. We are interested in the identification of regions or subdomains which are responsible for the biological activity of large macromolecules, to generate small molecule mimics from these regions (Saragovi et al., 1991; 1992). Mimicking binding surfaces with rationally designed small molecules is feasible since many hormone\receptor interactions require only a small subset of side chains for tight binding and bioactivity (Livnah et al., 1996). Initial attempts to create biologically active analogs of NGF met with little success (Longo et al., 1990; Estenne-Bouhtou et al., 1996). Only a few studies of low molecular weight NGF analogs have been reported, and all are weak antagonists presumably because they do not structurally mimic NGF beta-turn regions.

Our approach consisted of constraining the analog conformation by cyclization of the peptides through cysteine disulfide bridges. Incorporation of cysteines in the appropriate position, with N-termini and C-termini capping, and other modifications to protect the molecule (LeSauteur et al., 1995) result in a cyclic more structured conformation after oxidation of the disulphide groups. Conformationally restricted peptides can be used for initial binding and functional studies as well as for structure-activity relationships. After the activity and the structure of the peptide analogs is understood, non-peptidic peptidomimetics can be synthesized by any number of organic approaches (Saragovi et al., 1992).

We made peptidic analogs of beta-turn regions of NGF (Table 2) as conformationally constrained beta-turn mimics (code C) by introducing cysteine residues not found in the original NGF sequences (LeSauteur et al., 1995). Identical sequences were also made as linear (code L) and random (code R) peptide controls that lack any conformational constrains. We tested these compounds in biological and binding assays. Biological assays were done *in vitro* using a PC12 cell line that responds to NGF or basic Fibroblast Growth Factor (bFGF) by differentiating and making long projections or neurites. We tested the NGF analogs for either enhancement or inhibition of differentiation function (Table 2 and Figure 2). The inset shows the PC12 cells in culture which are roundish and adherent. When these cells are cultured with NGF (top panels) or with bFGF (lower panels) they differentiate remarkably and make neurites. In the presence of some NGF analogs (e.g. C(92–96)) PC12 cells do not respond to NGF. However PC12 cells do differentiate in re-

Table 2. Sequence and bioactivity of NGF mimics and
control peptides

NGF analogue	NGF turn region	Inhibition of NGF function
C(32-35)	A'-A"	+
C(30-35)		+±
C(31-35)		+
L(28-36)		±
R(28-36)		±
C(92-96)	C-D	++++
C(92-97)		+++
L(91-99)		+
R(91-99)		±

Antagonistic bioactivity assessed as in Figure 2. Arbitrary units
relative to dosing of NGF from 0 ng/ml to 50 ng/ml (2 nM, optimal concentration).

sponse to bFGF in the presence of C(92–96), as expected, because the analog inhibits
NGF binding to TrkA but does not prevent basic FGF binding to its receptors (LeSauteur
et al., 1995).

The analogs were tested in binding competition assays using radiolabeled ^{125}I[NGF].
Binding assays were performed on a variety of cells expressing either TrkA, or TrkA and
p75 receptors (Table 3). A significant percent of ^{125}I[NGF] binding can be inhibited by cyclic NGF analogs. It is interesting that there are differences in the efficacy of inhibition of
^{125}I[NGF] binding by the NGF mimics when tested versus human receptor expressing cells

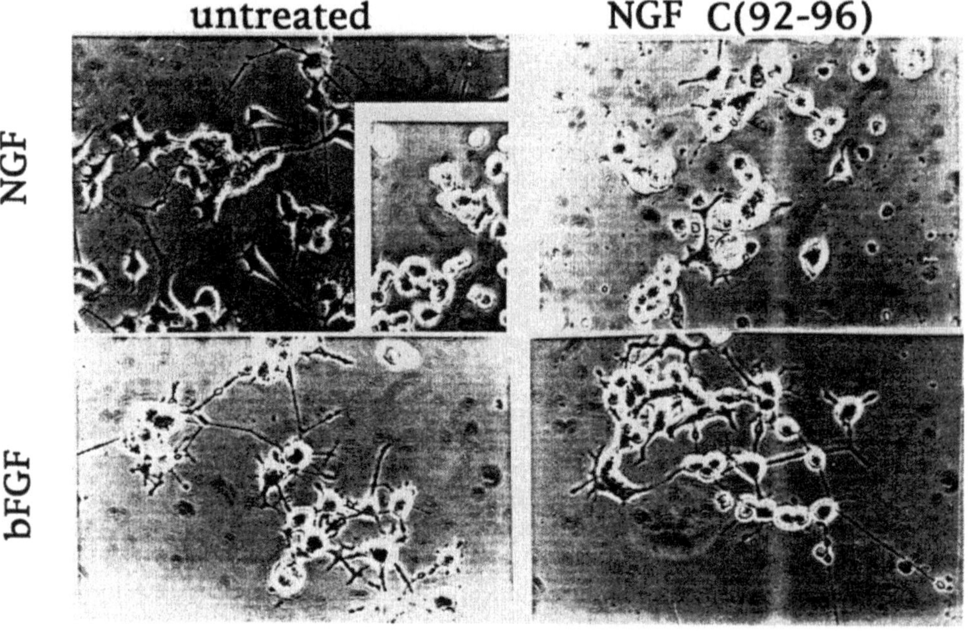

Figure 2. NGF analog C(92–96) specifically inhibits NGF mediated neurite outgrowth. NGF analogue C(92–96)
(10 µM) was co-cultured with NGF or bFGF each at 2 nM where indicated.

Table 3. ^{125}I[NGF] binding competition assays. NGF mimics block radiolabeled NGF from binding to the indicated receptor-expressing cells. Average ± 2 sem

| | % inhibition of ^{125}I[NGF] binding | |
Inhibitor	PC12 (TrkA+p75)	E25 cells (TrkA)
0.1 uM NGF	69.5 ± 4.5	93.3 ± 8.1
C(92-96)	86.4 ± 10.4	71.3 ± 13.5
C(92-97)	N.D.	64.9 ± 12.4
C(30-35)	N.D.	51.1 ± 0.7
C(32-35)	N.D.	30.7 ± 10.5
L(91-99)	11.4 ± 8.9	2.1 ± 0.05

(E25 cells) or rat receptor expressing cells (PC12 cells). Furthermore, peptides such as C(92–96) or a related analog with a different beta turn C(92–97) are quite efficient at inhibiting binding to human TrkA or TrkA and p^{75} co-expressed on the cell surface. These analogs are competitive antagonists as assessed by IC^{50}, direct binding and Scatchard plot analysis (not shown). The affinity of C(92–96) for human TrkA is on the order of 10^{-7}M (LeSauteur et al., 1995).

These data indicate that specific beta-turns are critical for TrkA binding and may confer receptor specificity, and that structural requirements for analog design are absolute since non-constrained linear analogs derived from the same regions had no activity. Overall, these results support the hypothesis that beta-turns are critical in NGF binding to its receptors and show that a large macromolecule can be reduced to small functional units if the native structure is retained. Structurally speaking, the C(92–96) peptide is a true mimic of the C-D beta-turn structure found in the NGF crystal, as shown by Nuclear Magnetic Resonance (NMR) analysis of the peptide (Figure 3). These data explain the basis for the TrkA binding activity of C(92–96), and structural information is being used to generate peptidomimetics of C(92–96).

Agonistic Anti-TrkA mAb. NGF induces dimerization of its receptor to induce signaling events, as shown for most growth factors (Heldin, 1995). Therefore, agonistic drugs must also possess the ability to dimerize receptors and\or induce receptor conformational changes leading to activation of the intracellular kinase activity. Antibodies are intrinsically symmetric dimeric molecules able to cause protein dimerization. However, not all antibodies against tyrosine kinase receptors are agonistic as would be expected if dimerization was the sole determinant. Several polyclonal antibodies are agonistic, however few mAb are agonistic. Presumably this is due to the fact that mAbs have one binding site which must induce the appropriate receptor conformational change as well as dimerization.

An agonistic polyclonal antibody against the rat TrkA receptor which caused activation of the signaling cascade has been reported (Clary et al., 1994). Thus it appears that oligomerization of TrkA by Ab-induced cross-linking is sufficient to produce the known cellular effects of NGF. Polyclonal antibodies are more likely to induce receptor dimerization because of multiple receptor docking sites. We have produced and characterized an agonistic mAb against human TrkA. This mAb called 5C3 mimics NGF structurally and functionally and binds in the NGF docking site on TrkA (LeSauteur et al., 1996a). Agonism is defined by early signals induced via TrkA receptors (activation of enzymatic

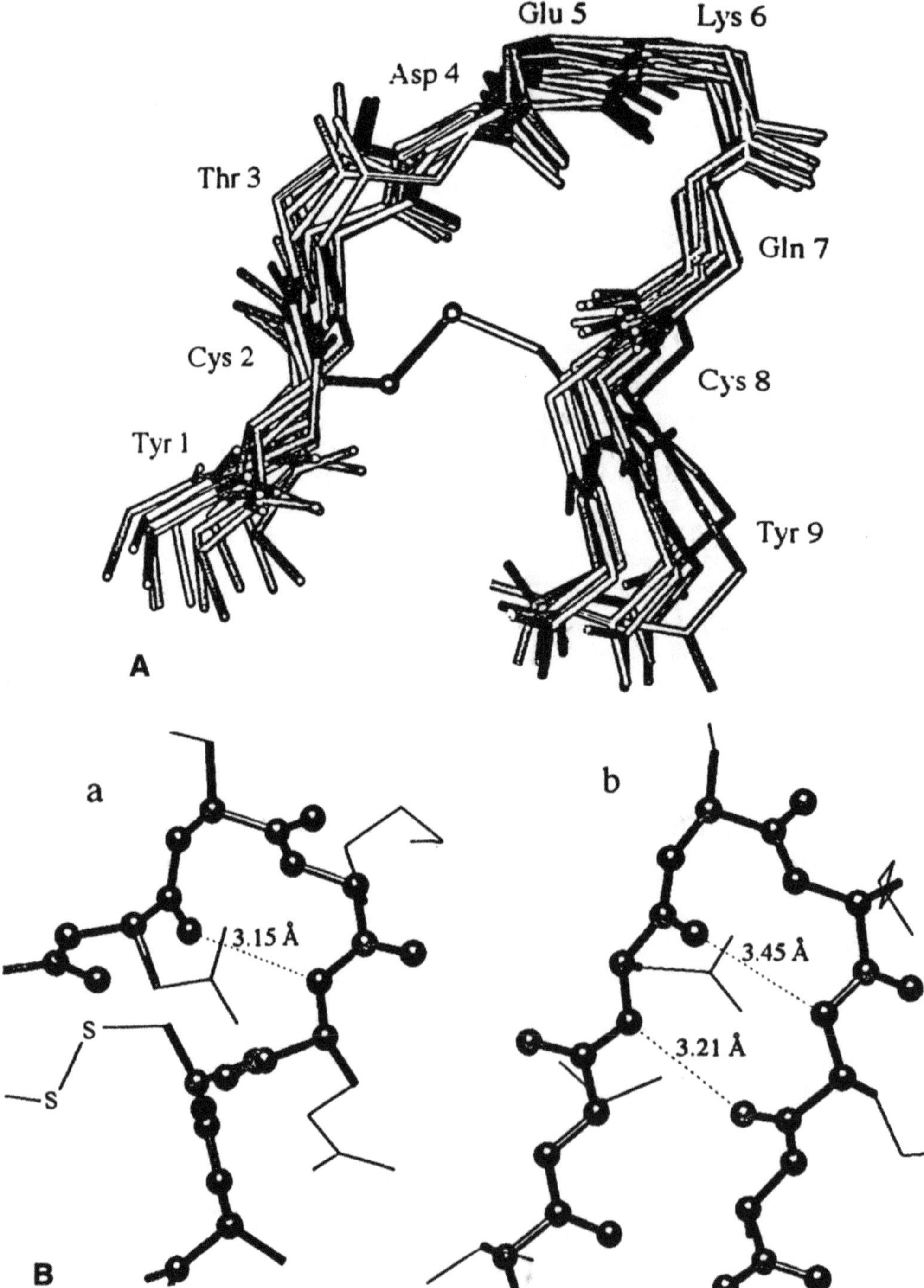

Figure 3. ^{3}H-NMR solution structure of C(92–96) mimic. (A) An ensemble of the lowest energy C(92–96) structures are shown. (B) Direct comparison of (a) C(92–96) peptide NMR structure, (b) C-D loop (residues 92–98) from the X-ray structure of mouse NGF. Strong similarities between the two structures can be seen not only in the backbones (solid filled) but also in the disposition of the sidechains (thin lines).

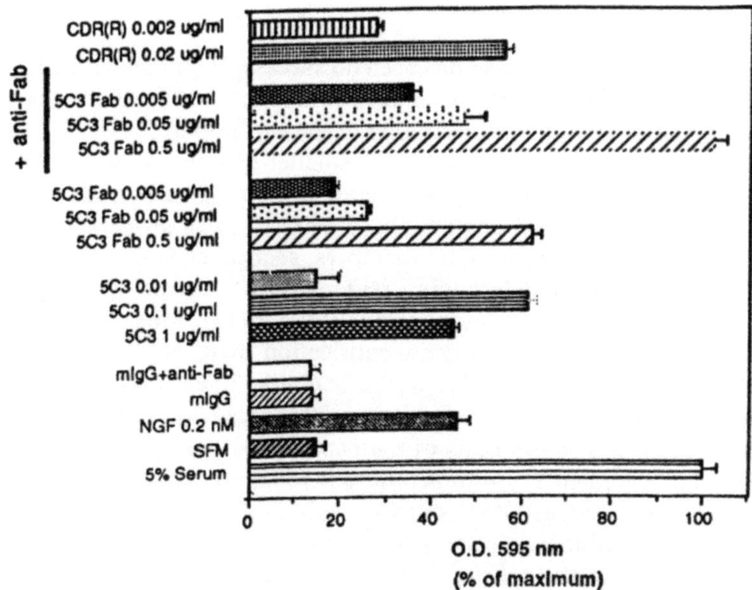

Figure 4. Survival of TrkA-expressing cells in Serum-free Media. Neuronal cells cultured in serum-free conditions (SFM) undergo apoptotic death. Protection from death (survival) is afforded by agonistic TrkA ligands. The indicated agents were added to the cells and cell viability was measured after 48 hours by the MTT assay. Proliferation was standardized to normal growth conditions (5% serum). NGF, mAb 5C3, 5C3 Fabs, and CDR(R) (recombinant 5C3 CDR analog) protect from apoptosis, but mouse IgG (control) does not.

activity, and tyrosine phosphorylation) (Kaplan and Stephens., 1994); and by long term signals (survival of neuronal cells in culture) (Figure 4) and neuronal differentiation (Table 4). The antibody is human TrkA specific so it does not induce the differentiation of rat PC12 cells. If PC12 cells are transfected and express human TrkA cDNA (6–2.4 cells), mAb 5C3 induces their full differentiation. As expected, NGF induces the differentiation of both wild type PC12 and 6–2.4 cells. Whether the dimeric nature of 5C3 is mandatory for agonistic signaling is unclear since Fab fragments of the antibody are also agonistic. These results illustrate that an artificial ligand specific for human TrkA can induce agonistic signaling.

Table 4. mAb 5C3 induces neurite outgrowth

| Cells | Neurite outgrowth | |
	mAb 5C3	NGF
PC12	–	+++
6-2.4	+++	+++

Rat PC12 cells (expressing rat TrkA) or PC12 cells transfected with human TrkA (6-2.4 cells, a kind gift of Dr. David Kaplan, Montréal Neurological Institute) were cultured for 48 hours with 2 nM NGF or mAb 5C3. Neurite outgrowth was scored. Both NGF and mAb 5C3 induce differentiation of 6-2.4 cells.

Agonistic Small Molecule Mimics

In spite of many attempts there has been no successful synthesis of small peptides displaying NGF biological activity. However such compounds are feasible as demonstrated by a peptide dimer shown to induce dimerization of the erythropoietin (EPO) receptor (Livnah et al., 1996). Therefore a peptide considerably smaller than the natural hormone can act as an agonist and induce the appropriate dimerization and biological response.

We reasoned that it would be possible to make analogs of the anti-TrkA mAb 5C3. In the case of mAbs and Ig superfamily members, sequences within the hypervariable region called complementarity determining regions (CDRs) make up most of the binding and bioactivity (Kabat, 1976; Saragovi et al., 1991; 1992). Most CDRs adopt beta-turn structures (Sibanda et al., 1989). After identification of relevant CDR sequences small peptide analogs can be synthesized. However, CDR-like linear peptide analogs are seldom bioactive because they do not adopt the appropriate (beta-turn) conformation in solution. Therefore, modelling and re-synthesis of the peptide analogs with constrains that restrict its conformation to a predicted type of beta-turn is required.

We have used the monoclonal antibody called 5C3 as a lead structure because it binds to the extracellular domain of human TrkA, has high affinity, and more importantly it is an agonist to TrkA (LeSauteur et al 1996a). We have reduced the size of mAb 5C3 to ~5 kDa and termed this molecule CDR(R). Synthesis of analogs of CDR(R) with minimal residues involved in interacting with TrkA are in progress. It may be possible to reduce the size of CDR(R) further to approximately 1,200 daltons while retaining agonistic function. Receptor specific, extracellular domain binding, small molecule agonists of TrkA should be very useful.

Diagnostic and Therapeutic Potential of Artificial TrkA Ligands

The *in vivo* targeting efficacy of these novel ligands: the C(92–96) NGF analog and mAb 5C3 was evaluated and compared (LeSauteur et al., 1996b). Both TrkA ligands were

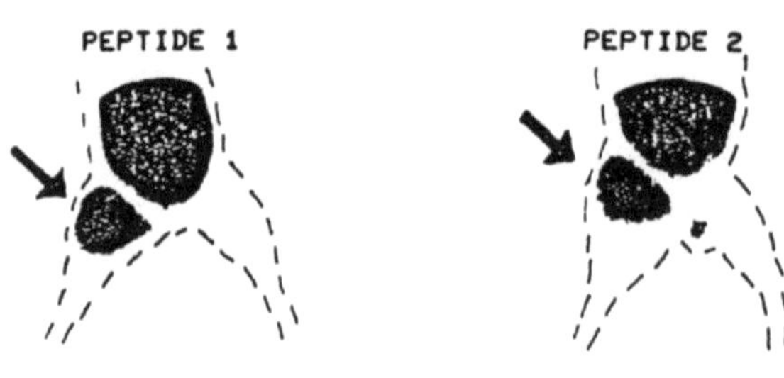

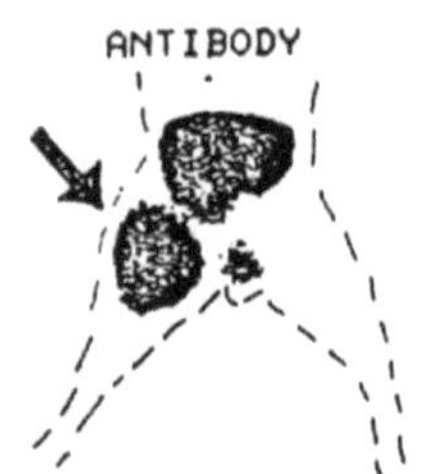

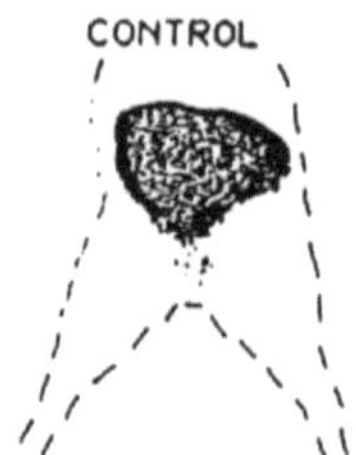

Figure 5. Efficient *in vivo* targeting of TrkA with small NGF mimics. Nude mice bearing TrkA expressing tumors in the right thigh were injected intraperitoneally with the following radioligands: NGF analogs ^{99m}Tc-[C(92–96)] (peptide 1 and 2); or with a high affinity anti-TrkA antibody ^{99m}Tc-[5C3] (antibody). Tumor targeting is indicated by arrows in the illustration depicting the profile of the mice. Label is present throughout the peritoneum (site of injection).

Table 5. Improved *in vivo* tumor targeting with small
molecule TrkA radioligands

	Tissue	T / nT ^{99m}Tc [5C3]	T / nT ^{99m}Tc [C(92-96)]
1	tumor	1	1
2	blood	13	26
3	muscle	20	28
4	heart	13	11
5	lung	7.3	8.5
6	liver	2.1	1.2
7	spleen	9.4	9.4

Biodistribution of ^{99m}Tc[TrkA ligands] in mice. T/nT: tumor to
non-tumor targeting ratio (standardized to the tumor). Biodistribution of radioligands was determined in the indicated tissues 28
hours after injection. Results are corrected for ^{99m}Tc decay, and
are expressed as mean values.

radiolabelled with technicium and used to image, *in vivo*, tumors expressing TrkA (Figure 5). Both radioligands specifically targeted TrkA expressing tumors. However, the kinetics of targeting, bioavailability and blood clearance of the NGF analog was better than mAb 5C3. Measurements of the radioactivity accumulated in the tumor versus other tissues (blood, skin, liver, etc) resolve the tumor to non-tumor targeting ratio. A high ratio means high delivery to the tumor. Table 5 shows a comparison of a monoclonal antibody of high affinity but large size (Kd 10^{-9} M; 150 kDa), versus C(92–96) NGF analog of lower affinity but much smaller size (Kd 10^{-7} M; 1 kDa). The C(92–96) NGF analog is a better targeting agent. For example blood targeting for the NGF mimic is 26 whereas the antibody is 13; muscle targeting is 28 vs. 20; etc (LeSauteur et al., 1996b). This study demonstrates that receptor specific small molecule analogs can be designed from large polypeptides and may be more useful than antibodies. In addition, we have shown that mAb 5C3 is a useful diagnostic and prognostic agent for human neuroblastoma (Kramer et al., 1996). MAb 5C3 may either kill tumors via complement fixation or by opsonization; or induce stop growth signals in NGF responsive tumors by terminal differentiation.

SUMMARY

Strategically, we aim to develop compounds as small peptidomimetics. We made peptidic NGF analogs using beta-turn regions of NGF as a model. NGF analog C(92–96) is an antagonist. We also have a lead monoclonal antibody which is agonistic to TrkA and has exclusive specificity for human receptors. Since antibodies are 150 kDa, we reduced the mAb to smaller peptides of 5 kDa called CDR(R) which retain agonistic activity (Figure 1). There remains an interesting pharmacological question. How is it possible that monovalent ligands such as CDR(R) activate the TrkA receptor? The possibility that these ligands behave as inverse antagonists (Milligan et al., 1995) is being explored. Combining these lead structures via chemical linkers may provide compounds with increased bioactivity.

These agents will be useful in the Central Nervous System (CNS) where agonists that promote neuronal survival, and enhance neuritogenesis may be therapeutics for neurodegenerative diseases (e.g. Alzheimer's disease), stroke, or trauma. However, for

CNS delivery it will be necessary that the compounds cross the blood-brain barrier, are protease resistant and ideally they should be less than ~600 daltons in size and orally bioavailable. Herein lies the challenge.

ACKNOWLEDGMENTS

We are grateful to S. Maliartchouk for discussions; and to N. Lavine for technical assistance. Supported by a grant of the Medical Research Council of Canada (MRC) to HUS. HUS received a Pharmaceutical Manufacturer's Association of Canada-MRC Scholar Award. LLS received a studentship from the MRC.

REFERENCES

Barbacid, M., 1994, The Trk family of neurotrophin receptors. *J. Neurobiol.* 25:1386.

Carter, B.D., and Lewin, G.R., 1997, Neurotrophins live or let die: does p75NTR decide? *Neuron* 18:187.

Chao, M.V., and Hempstead, B.L., 1995, p75 and trk: A two-receptor family of receptors. *Trends Neurosci.* 15:323.

Clary, D.O., Weskamp, G., Austin, L.R., and Reichardt, L.T, 1994, TrkA cross-linking mimics neuronal responses to nerve growth factor, *Mol. Biol. Cell* 5:549.

Cuello, A.C., Liberini, P., and Piccardo, P., 1993, Atrophy and regrowth of CNS forebrain neurons. In: Models of study and clinical relevance. Neuronal Cell Death and Repair. Cuello, A.C., ed., Elsevier Science Publishers.

Drinkwater, C.C., Barker, P.A., Suter, U., and Shooter, E.M., 1993, The carboxy terminus of nerve growth factor is required for biological activity. *J. Biol. Chem.* 268:23202.

Estenne-Bouhtou, G., Kullander, K., Karlsson, M., Ebendal, T., Hacksell, U., and Luthman, K., 1996, Design, synthesis, and tandem mass spectrometric sequencing and biological activity of NGF mimetics, *Int. J. Peptide Protein Res.* 48:337.

Hefti, F and Will, B., 1987, Nerve growth factor is a neurotrophic factor for forebrain cholinergic neurons; implications for Alzheimer's disease, *J. Neural Transm. Suppl.* 24:309.

Heldin, C.H., 1995, Dimerization of cell surface receptors in signal transduction, *Cell* 80:213.

Ibanez, C.F., 1995, Neurotrophic factors; from structure-function studies to designing effective therapeutics, *TIBTECH* 13:217.

Jing, S., Tapley, P., Barbacid, M., 1992, Nerve growth factor mediates signal transduction through Trk homodimer receptors, *Neuron* 9:1067.

Kabat, E.A., Structural concepts in Immunology and Immunochemistry, 1976, Holt, Reinhart and Winston, New York.

Kahle, P., Burton, L.E., Schmelzer, C.H., and Hertel, C., 1992, The amino terminus of nerve growth factor is involved in the interaction with the receptor tryosine kinase p140trkA. *J. Biol. Chem.* 267:22707.

Kaplan, D.R., and Stephens, R.M., 1994, Neurotrophin signal transduction by the Trk receptor, *J. Neurobiol.* 25:1404.

Kaplan , D.R., Hempstead, B.L., Martin-Zanca, D., Chao, M.V., Parada, L.F., 1991, The trk proto-oncogene product: a signal transducing receptor, *Nature* 350:158.

Kramer K., Gerald, W., LeSauteur, L., Saragovi, H.U., and Cheung, N-K.V., 1996, Prognostic value of trkA protein detection by monoclonal antibody 5C3 in Neuroblastoma, *Clin. Cancer. Res.* 8:1361.

LeSauteur, L., Cheung, N-K.V., Lisbona, R., and Saragovi, H.U., 1996b, Small molecule imaging of nerve growth factor receptors in-vivo, *Nature Biotechnology* 14:1120.

LeSauteur, L., Maliartchouk, S., Le Jeune, H., Quirion, R., and Saragovi, H.U., 1996a, Potent Human p140-TrkA agonists derived form an Anti-receptor monoclonal antibody, *J. Neurosci.* 16:1308.

LeSauteur, L., Wei, L., Gibbs, B., and Saragovi, H.U., 1995, Small peptide mimics of nerve growth factor bind TrkA receptors and affect biological responses, *J. Biol. Chem.* 270:6564

Levi-Montalcini, R., 1987, The nerve growth factor 35 years later, *Science* 237:1154.

Livnah, O., Stura, E.A., Johnson, D.L., Middleton, S.A., Mulcahy, L.S., Wrighton, N.C., Dower, W.J., Jolliffe, L.K., and Wilson, I.A., 1996, Functional mimicry of a protein hormone by a peptide agonist: The epo receptor complex at 2.8 Å. *Science* 273:464.

Longo, F.M., Vu, T.-K., and Mobley, W., 1990, The in-vitro biological effect of nerve growth factor is inhibited by synthetic peptides, *Cell Regul.* 1:189.

MacDonald, J.I.S., and Meakin, S.O., 1996, Deletions in the extracellular domain of rat TrkA lead to an altered differentiative phenotype in neurotrophin responsive cells, *Mol. Cell. Neurosci.* 7:371.

McDonald, N.Q., Lapatto, R., Murray-Rust, J., Gunning, J., Wlodawer, A., and Blundell, 1991, New protein fold revealed by a 2.3-Å resolution crystal structure of nerve growth factor, *Nature* 354:411.

Milligan, G., Bond, R.A., and Lee, M., 1995, Inverse agonism: pharmacological curiosity or potential therapeutic strategy? *TIPS* 16:10

Purves, D., Snider, W.D., Voyvodic, J.T., 1985, Trophic regulation of nerve cell morphology and innervation in the autonomic nervous system, *Nature* 366:123.

Saragovi, H.U., Fitzpatrick, D., Rakatabutr, A., Nakanishi, H., Kahn, M., and Greene, M.I., 1991, Design and synthesis of a mimetic from an antibody complementarity-determining region, *Science* 253:792.

Saragovi, H.U., Greene, MI., Chrusciel, R.A., and Kahn, M., 1992, Loops and secondary structure mimetics: development and applications in basic science and rational drug design. *Bio/technology* 10:773.

Sibanda, B.L., Blundell, T.L., and Thornton, J.M., 1989, Conformation of â-Hairpins in protein structure, *J. Mol. Biol.* 206:759.

Urfer, R., Tsoulfas, P., O'Connell, L., Shelton, D.L., Parada, L.F., and Presta, L.G., 1995, An immunoglobulin-like domain determines the specificity of neurotrophin receptors, *EMBO* 14:2795.

Windisch, J.M., Marksteiner, R., and Schneider, R., 1995, Nerve growth factor binding site on TrkA mapped to a single 24-amino acid leucine-rich motif, *J. Biol. Chem*:270:28133.

88

MOLECULAR CLONING, TRANSIENT EXPRESSION, AND NEUROTROPHIC EFFECT FOR DA NEURONS OF HUMAN BRAIN DERIVED NEUROTROPHIC FACTOR

Wang Jia-Zheng, Chen Qian, Yu Yun-Kai, and Fan Ming

Department of Neurobiology
Institute of Basic Medical Science
27 Tai Ping Road, Beijing, China, 100850

INTRODUCTION

Brain derived neurotrophic factor (BDNF) is a small, highly basic protein that was originally purified from pig brain, where it is present in concentrations of only a few µg/gm (Barde et al., 1982). It belongs to the nerve growth factor family of neurotrophins. The primary structure of BDNF is highly homologous to that of NGF. It shares ~55% seqence identity with NGF including six conserved cysteine residues which form three intramolecular disulfied bridges (Leirock et al., 1989). The distribution and biological activity of BDNF are unique. BDNF mRNA is localized principally in the CNS, and it is widely distributed through- out the brain. The biological activity of BDNF is distinctive. BDNF can support the survival of various kinds of sensory neurons originating from the neural crest and ectodermal placode and promote their development, growth and differentiation (Hofer et al., 1988). BDNF is also trophic for a variety of CNS neurons. In culture, BDNF supports the survival and axonal elongation of retinal ganglion cells (Thanes et al., 1989) and the survival of mesencephalic dopaminergic neurons (Hyman et al., 1991). BDNF increases the survival of rat septal cholinergic neurons and levels of their cholinergic enzymes (Alderson et al., 1990). BDNF neuroprotection against neuronal death has also been demonstrated. It ameliorates degeneration of mesencephlic dopaminergic neurons caused by 6-hydroxydopamine (6-OHDA) or 1-methyl 1,4-phenylpiperidinium (MPP^+) (Spina et al., 1992). These data, in turn, propose that BDNF might have the potential to become pharmaceutical agents in the treatment of neurodegenerative disease such as Alzheimer's disease or Parkinson's disease.

Progress in Alzheimer's and Parkinson's Diseases
edited by Fisher *et al.*, Plenum Press, New York, 1998.

MATERIAL AND METHODS

Materials

Reagents for polymerase chain reaction amplification were purchased from Perkin-Elmer Cetus; T_7 DNA sequencing™ kit was obtained from Phamacia; Lipofectin reagent, Dulbecco's Modified Eagle Medium (D-MEM) and Ham's F-12 Nutrient Mixture were purchased from GIBCO BRL; Prime-a-Gene Labeling System and all restriction enzymes were obtained from Promega; Insulin-transferrin-sodium selenite media supplement was obtained from sigma; *E.coli* JM103, *E.coli* DH5,COS7 cell line, bacteriophage M13mp18/19 and pCMV4 vector were provided by the laboratory. All other reagents were of AR grade.

Synthetic Oligonucleotides and DNA Amplification

The oligonucleotide primers were synthesized using an automatic DNA synthesizer. The upstream primer 5' CGGGTACCATGACCATCCTTTTCCT 3' contained a KpnI restriction site, while the downstream primer 5' CCGGATCCTATCTTCCCCTCTTAATG 3' contained a BamHI restriction site. We used fetal human brain genomic DNA as a template. The target sequence was amplified in a final reaction volume of 100μl, containing 1ug template DNA, 200μM each of dNTP mixture, 1μM each of the primers and 2.5 units of Ampli Taq DNA polymerase. Each cycle consisted of heat denaturation at 94 for 1 min, annealing at 60 for 1min and extension at 72 for 1.5min. The reaction was done for 35 cycles.

M13 Cloning and Sequencing

DNA fragments synthesized by PCR were digested and cloned between the KpnI and BamHI sites into M13mp18/19 RF DNA. *E.coli* JM103 was transformed and transformant was selected as described in Molecular Cloning. The single strand recombinant DNA was prepared and sequenced by using dideoxy termination method according to the instructions on the kit.

Construction of Expression Plasmid and Transfection into COS7 Cell

The entire 744bp human prepro-BDNF gene was excised from the recombinant M13mp18-preproBDNF plasmid by KpnI and XbaI digestion and cloned between the KpnI and XbaI sites in the pCMV4 vector. COS7 cells were maintained as stocks in DMEM supplemented with 10% fetal calf serum at 37°C with 5% CO_2. Using the lipofectin method 10μg of pCMV4-preproBDNF (carrying cytomegalovirus promoter) and pCMV4 vector were transfected, respectively, into 10^6 COS7 cells when the cells were 60% confluent. Five hours later, the normal growth medium containing 10% fetal calf serum was added and cells were incubated at 37°C for 24 hr, the medium was then replaced with serum free DMEM for 48 hr, the conditioned media were collected and stored at -70°C.

RNA Dot Hybridization and Biological Activity Assay

The probe of BDNF cDNA was labeled by $[\alpha\text{-}^{32}P]dATP$ through the Prime-α-Gene labeling system. Cells' total RNA was isolated by the acid guanidinium isothiocyanate-phenol-chloroform extraction procedure and identified by hybridization on slot blots. The biological activity of BDNF was detected using neurite outgrowth from E9 chicken dorsal root ganglion (DRG). The culture media was serum free DMEM containing 5g/ml insulin, 5g/ml human transferrin, and 5ng/ml sodium selenite. In the experiment,10% conditioned medium was added, and DRG was cultured at 37°C with 5% CO_2 for 24hr. The group containing 10ng/ml NGF was cultured as a positive control.

Ventral Mesencephalic Cell Culture and TH-Immunocytochemistry Assay

Ventral mesencephalic cells were prepared from fetal rat (Wistar, day15~16). These cells included the dopaminergic nuclei A8,A9 (substantia nigra) and A10 (ventral tegmental area) and were collected and dissociated in DMEM supplemented with 20% horse serum. After 16hr, the media were changed with serum free DMEM/F12 (1:1 v/v), containing 15mM Hepes, 2mM Gln, and saturated with N2. To three experimental groups were added 30% conditioned medium of pCMV4-preproBDNF transfected COS7 cells, and 30% conditioned medium of pCMV4 transfected COS7 cells and 50ng/ml NGF, respectively. After 8 days, TH-immunocytochemistry was used to selectively analyze the survival and differentiation of mesencephalic dopaminergic neurons.

RESULTS AND DISCUSSION

Cloning and Sequencing of Human BDNF Gene

Because of no intron in the sequence encoding the prepro-BDNF, mRNA isolation was not needed for reverse transcription. The PCR was performed to amplify the human prepro-BDNF gene directly by using human genomic DNA as a template. PCR products were analyzed by 1.2% agarose gel electrophoresis and the size was confirmed to be as predicted (about 0.75Kb) (Fig. 1). After digestion with two restriction enzymes (KpnI,

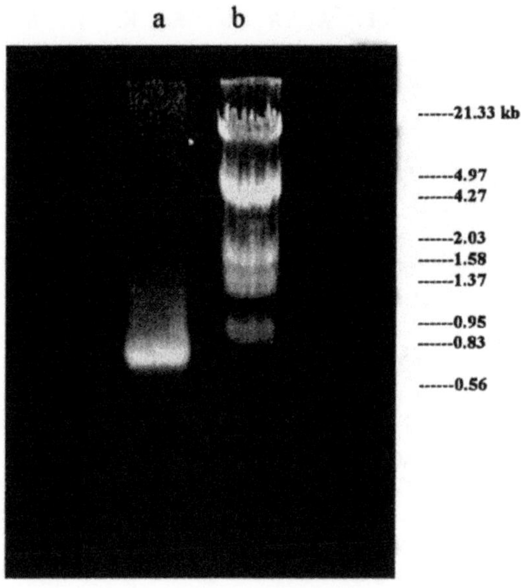

Figure 1. Electrophoresis of the PCR product. a) preproBDNF gene PCR product. b) λDNA/EcoRI+HindIII marker.

BamHI) and purification by electrophoresis, the PCR products were cloned into M13mp18/19 phage. The white bacteriophages were selected from the transformed *E.coli* JM103. The recombinant DNA was digested by KpnI+BamHI and ApaI restriction enzymes, respectively, giving the cut fragments with 0.74Kb and 0.51Kb. These results showed that the cloned DNA fragment was what we expected. DNA sequencing showed

```
ATG ACC ATC CTT TTC CTT ACT ATG GTT ATT TCA TAC TTT GGT TGC ATG AAG GCT GCC CCC   60
 M   T   I   L   F   L   T   M   V   I   S   Y   F   G   C   M   K   A   A   P    -119

ATG AAA GAA GCA AAC ATC CGA GGA CAA GGT GGC TTG GCC TAC CCA GGT GTG CGG ACC CAT   120
 M   K   E   A   N   I   R   G   Q   G   G   L   A   Y   P   G   V   R   T   H    -89

GGG ACT CTG GAG AGC GTG AAT GGG CCC AAG GCA GGT TCA AGA GGC TTG ACA TCA TTG GCT   180
 G   T   L   E   S   V   N   G   P   K   A   G   S   R   G   L   T   S   L   A    -69

GAC ACT TTC GAA CAC GTG ATA GAA GAG CTG TTG GAT GAG GAC CAG AAA GTT CGG CCC AAT   240
 D   T   F   E   H   V   I   E   E   L   L   D   E   D   Q   K   V   R   P   N    -49

GAA GAA AAC AAT AAG GAC GCA GAC TTG TAC ACG TCC AGG GTG ATG CTC AGT AGT CAA GTG   300
 E   E   N   N   K   D   A   D   L   Y   T   S   R   V   M   L   S   S   Q   V    -29

CCT TTG GAG CCT CCT CCT CTC TTT CTG CTG GAG GAA TAC AAA AAT TAG CTA GAT GCT GCA   360
 P   L   E   P   P   P   L   L   F   L   L   E   E   Y   K   N   Y   L   D   A   A  -9

AAC ATG TCC ATG AGG GTC CGG CGC CAC TCT GAC CCT GCC CGC CGA GGG GAG CTG AGC GTG   420
 N   M   S   M   R   V   R   R   H   S   D   P   A   R   R   G   E   L   S   V    12
                                ⇑
TGT GAC AGT ATT AGT GAG TGG GTA ACG GCG GCA GAC AAA AAG ACT GCA GTG GAC ATG TCG   480
 C   D   S   I   S   E   W   V   T   A   A   D   K   K   T   A   V   D   M   S    32

GGC GGG ACG GTC ACA GTC CTT GAA AAG GTC CCT GTA TCA AAA GGC CAA CTG AAG CAA TAC   540
 G   G   T   V   T   V   L   E   K   V   P   V   S   K   G   Q   L   K   Q   Y    52

TTC TAC GAG ACC AAG TGC AAT CCC ATG GGT TAC ACA AAA GAA GGC TGC AGG GGC ATA GAC   600
 F   Y   E   T   K   C   N   P   M   G   Y   T   K   E   G   C   R   G   I   D    72

AAA AGG CAT TGG AAC TCC CAG TGC CGA ACT ACC CAG TCG TAC GTG CGG GCC CTT ACC ATG   660
 K   R   H   W   N   S   Q   C   R   T   T   Q   S   Y   N   R   A   L   T   M    92

GAT AGC AAA AAG AGA ATT GGC TGG CGA TTC ATA AGG ATA GAC ACT TCT TGT GTA TGT ACA   720
 D   S   K   K   R   I   G   W   R   F   I   R   I   D   T   S   C   V   C   T    112

TTG ACC ATT AAG* AGG GGA AGA TAG                                                  744
 L   T   I   K   R   G   R                                                        120
```

(A)

Figure 2. Sequencing result of the full-length human BDNF gene. Sequence of cloned hpreproBDNF gene from ATG to TAG was identical with reference except for one nucleotide difference at position 732(A–G). The derived amino acid sequence is shown in the one-letter amino acid code, with numbering relative to the expected site of proteolytic processing of the precursor (arrow). The methionine and secretory signal sequence are underlined.

that the cloned human BDNF gene, 744bp-length from ATG to TAG, was identical to the reference (Jone et al., 1990), except for one nucleotide difference (position 732bp A-G) at the downstream primer caused by the usage of pig BDNF PCR primer. This alteration did not change the amino acid sequence (Fig. 2).

Transient Expression and Bioassay of Human BDNF Gene

The human prepro-BDNF fragment was removed by KpnI+XbaI digestion and was inserted into the pCMV4 vector. After being transformed into *E.coli* DH5 α, the recombinant DNA was isolated for identification by restriction mapping. Using lipofectin reagent, we successfully transfected COS7 cells with pCMV4-preproBDNF expression plasmid and pCMV4 control plasmid, respectively. Total RNA of transfected COS7 cells was isolated. Slot hybridization analysis showed that the human BDNF gene was transcribed by the CMV promoter (Fig. 3). The culture media containing the human rBDNF secreted by pCMV4-preproBDNF transfected COS7 cells promoted the neurite outgrowth of DRG from E9 chicken. In the controls, on the other hand, the culture media from pCMV4 transfected COS7 cells or from untransfected COS7 cells could not stimulate DRG neurite outgrowth. These experiments confirmed that the human prepro-BDNF gene which we have cloned could be translated and secreted by COS7 cells, and that the expressed protein has a neurotrophic activity.

Promotion of Dopaminergic Neuron Survival and Differentiation by Human BDNF

To assess dopaminergic neuron survival and to quantitate neurite growth in ventral mesencephallic cell cultures, TH-immunocytochemistry was performed. All cell cultures were maintained for 8 days. The results showed that the group containing human rBDNF secreted by transfected COS7 cells increased to a large extent the survival of dopaminergic cells with a significant increase in total TH-positive neurite length and area . Few TH-IR neurons survived in the other two groups (Fig. 4). These results indicated that BDNF is an important and necessary factor in the development and survival of dopaminergic neurons. These results were also in agreement with previous findings that NGF has no effect on the survival of dopamine neurons.

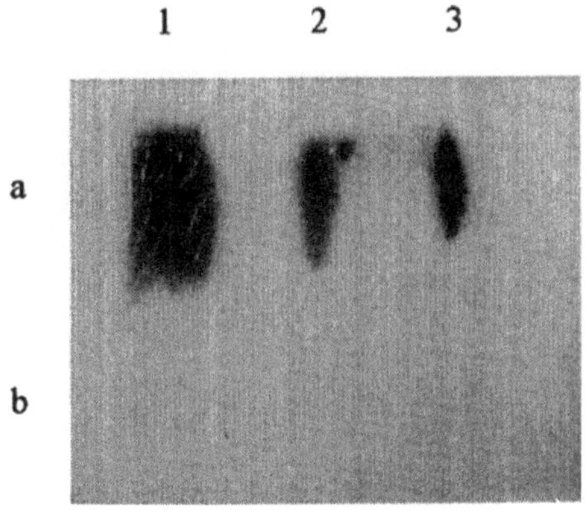

Figure 3. Slot hybridization of total RNA from transfected COS7 cells. a) The total RNA of pCMV4-hpreproBDNF transfected COS7 cells. b) The total RNA of pCMV4 transfected COS7 cells. 1~3, 15, 10, 5 μg RNA was added respectively.

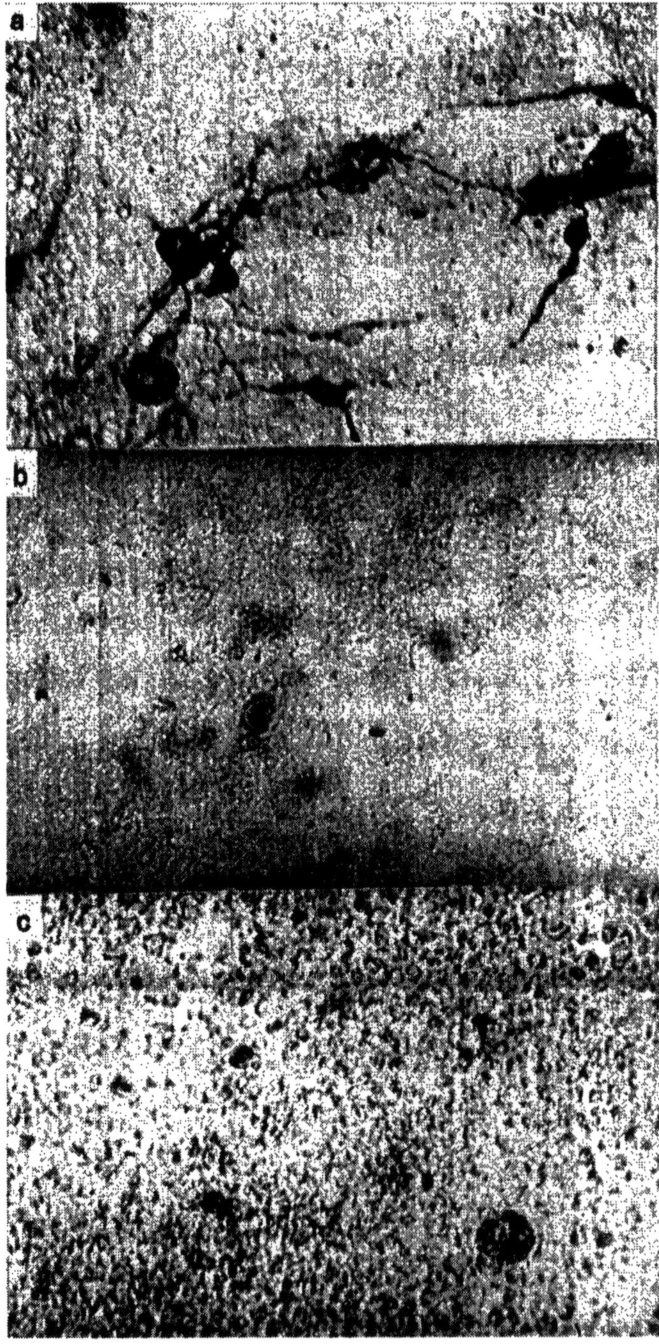

Figure 4. Immunocytochemical staining of DAergic neurons with TH antibody (x 400). Mesencephalic cultures were grown for 8 days with 30% pCMV4-preproBDNF transfected COS7 cells conditioned medium (a) 30% pCMV4 transfected COS7 cells conditioned medium (b) or 50ng/ml NGF (c) present for seven days starting from day 2 in vitro and then stained for TH.

CONCLUSION

A PCR product of a full-length human BDNF gene coding for its signal peptide and precursor was cloned and sequenced, and the transient expression of the gene was successfully performed in the COS7 cells. Its biological activity was tested by the stimulation of neurite outgrowth of E9 chicken DRG. The expressed human BDNF protein could promote the survival and differentiation of dopaminergic neurons in cultures of rat ventral mesencephalon. This work has laid a foundation for studying the role of human BDNF in the nervous system, and for gene therapy of some neurodegenerative diseases of the nervous system.

REFERENCES

Alderson, R.F., Alterman, A.L., Barde, Y.A., and Lindsay, R.M., 1990, Brain-derived neurotrophic factor increases survival and differentiated functions of rat septal cholinergic neurons in culture. *Neuron* 5:297.

Barde, Y.A., Edgar, D., Thoenen, H., 1982, Purification of a new neurotrophic factor from mammalian brain. *EMBO J.* 1:549.

Hofer, M.M., and Barade, Y.A., 1988, A neuronal mechanism for sensory gating during locomotion in a vertebrate. *Nature* 331:261.

Hyman, C., Hofer, M., Barde, Y.A., Juhasz, M., Yancopoulos, G.D., Squinoto, S., and Lindsay, R.M.,1991, BDNF is a neurotrophic factor for dopaminergic neurons of the substantia nigra. *Nature* 350:230.

Jones, K.R., and Reichardt, L.F., 1990, Molecular cloning of a human gene that is a member of the nerve growth factor family. *Proc. Natl. Acad. Sci.* USA 87:8060.

Leibrock, J., Lettspeich, F., Hohm, A., Hofer, M.,Hengerer, B.,Masiakowski, P.,Thoenen, H., and Barde, Y.A.,1989, Molecular cloning and expression of brain derived neurotrophic factor. *Nature* 41:149.

Spina, M.B., Squinto, S.P., Miller, J., Lindsay, R.M., and Hyman, C., 1992, Brain-derived neurotrophic factor protects dopamine neurons against 6-hydroxydopamine and N-methyl 1,4-phenylpyridinium ion toxicity: Involvement of the glutathione system. *J. Neurochem.* 59:99.

Thanes, S., Bahr, M., Barde, Y.A., and Vanselow, J., 1989, Survival and axonal elongation of adult rat retinal ganglion cells: *in vitro* effects of lesioned sciatic nerve and brain derived neurotrophic factor (BDNF). *Eur. J. Neurosci.* 1:19.

89

PREVENTIVE TREATMENT OF ALZHEIMER'S DISEASE

Peptide-Mediated Neuroprotection

Illana Gozes,[1] Ariane Davidson,[1] Michal Bachar,[1] Amos Bardea,[1] Orly Perl,[1] Sara Rubinraut,[2] Mati Fridkin,[2] Eliezer Giladi,[1] and Douglas E. Brenneman[3]

[1]Clinical Biochemistry, Sackler Medical School
Tel Aviv University
Tel Aviv, Israel
[2]Organic Chemistry
Weizmann Institute of Science
Rehovot, Israel
[3]Section on Developmental and Molecular Pharmacology
Laboratory of Developmental Neurobiology
NICHD, NIH
Bethesda, Maryland

INTRODUCTION

Stearyl-Nle^{17}-VIP (SNV) is a novel agonist of vasoactive intestinal peptide (VIP) exhibiting a 100-fold greater potency than the parent molecule and specificity for a receptor associated with neuronal survival. SNV protected neurons against the β-amyloid peptide, Alzheimer associated neurotoxicity *in vitro*, and against memory impairments induced by cholinergic deficiencies *in vivo*. To further test the breadth of neuroprotection offered by SNV, mice deficient in apolipoprotein E (apoE), a molecule associated with the etiology of Alzheimer's disease, served as a model to investigate the developmental effects of SNV. In comparison to control animals, the deficient mice exhibited: 1) reduced amounts of VIP mRNA; 2) decreased cholinergic activity (decreased activity of choline acetyl-transferase); 3) significant retardation in the acquisition of developmental milestones: forelimb placing behavior and cliff avoidance behavior; and 4) impairments in learning and memory. Daily injections of SNV to apoE-deficient new-born pups resulted in increased cholinergic activity and marked improvements in the acquisition of behavioral milestones, with peptide-treated animals developing as fast as control animals. Furthermore, SNV-treated apoE-deficient animals exhibited marked improvements in their learning abilities observed after cessation of peptide treatment. Specificity was demonstrated in that treatment with pituitary adenylate cyclase activating peptide (PACAP, a VIP-related peptide) produced only limited amelioration. The neuroprotective effects of VIP and its derivative VIP required the presence of glial cells in the culture. We have recently isolated a novel femtomolar-acting neuroprotective protein (with stress protein sequences) secreted from glial cells in the presence of VIP. The novel protein was named activity-dependent neurotrophic factor (ADNF) as it protected neurons from death mediated by electrical blockade. Neutralizing antibodies to ADNF indicated the existence of endogenous ADNF-like protein in the cerebral cortex, secreted in the presence of VIP. Thus, the protective effects of VIP and SNV may be mediated via endogenous glial derived molecules such as ADNF. SNV and ADNF may provide lead compounds in the design and synthesis of growth-factor-based Alzheimer's disease therapeutics. Furthermore, as certain genotypes of apolipoprotein E increase the probability of Alzheimer's disease, early counseling and preventive treatments may now offer an important route for therapeutics design.

VASOACTIVE INTESTINAL PEPTIDE (VIP)

The neuropeptide vasoactive intestinal peptide (VIP) has been implicated in the acquisition of learning and memory. Original studies have indicated that the expression of the VIP gene is markedly reduced with aging (Gozes et al., 1988) and parallel studies have shown that VIP is important in maintaining nerve cells alive when their electrical activity is blocked (Breneman et al., 1986). Antagonism of VIP activity with a specific VIP hybrid antagonist [neurotensin$_{6-11}$VIP$_{7-28}$ (Gozes et al., 1989; Gozes et al., 1991)] resulted in impairment of cognitive functions that could be partially ameliorated by co-treatment with VIP (Glowa et al., 1992). Similarly, reduced VIP expression in transgenic animals resulted in learning and memory dysfunction (Gozes et al., 1993). VIP affects neuronal capabilities not only in the mature nervous system, but also during development. Administration of the VIP hybrid antagonist during pregnancy resulted in severe microcephaly (Gressens et al., 1994), and chronic injection of VIP hybrid antagonist during postnatal development produced neuronal dystrophy (Hill et al., 1994), retardation in the acquisition of developmental milestones (Hill et al., 1991), and blockade of circadian rhythmicity (Gozes et al., 1995a). The involvement of VIP in multiple neurotrophic activities prompted the development of novel VIP derivatives with increased specificity, stability and biological availability.

stearyl-Nle^{17}-VIP (SNV)

We have recently developed a superactive VIP agonist, stearyl-Nle^{17}-VIP, [(SNV), (Gozes et al., 1994; Gozes et al., 1995a; Gozes et al., 1995b; Gozes et al., 1996a)], that promoted neuronal survival with a potency 100-fold greater than VIP (Gozes et al., 1995a). This new molecule contains two chemical modifications in VIP, the addition of an N-terminal long chain fatty acid and the substitution of the methionine in position 17 with norleucine (Nle). These changes confer stability, increased half-life and increased bioavailability. The molecule offers reduced oxidation due to the exchange of the methionine with noreleucine, increased stability at the N-terminal site- due to the addition of the fatty-acyl moiety and increased solubilization in lipid (the stearyl moiety). Femtomolar concentrations of SNV prevented neuronal cell death associated with the β amyloid cytotoxicity. Moreover, when delivered intranasally, SNV prevented impairments in spatial learning produced by ethyl choline aziridium-mediated cholinotoxicity in rats. These studies suggest both a novel therapeutic strategy for the treatment of Alzheimer's-related deficiencies and a means for non-invasive peptide administration to the brain (Gozes et al., 1996a).

ADNF

VIP influence on neuronal survival is mediated via factors (Brenneman et al., 1987; Brenneman et al., 1990) secreted from VIP-responsive (Gozes et al., 1991) astroglial cells (Brenneman et al., 1990), as no neuronal survival effect was observed with VIP in cultures containing neurons only (Brenneman et al., 1987). An increasing number of diverse neuronal growth factors are being discovered. Included in this group of regulatory molecules are trophic factors such as nerve growth factor (NGF) (Levi-Montalcini, 1979; Levi-Montalcini et al., 1969), ciliary neurotrophic factor (CNTF) (Lin et al., 1989), fibroblast growth factor (FGF) (Cheng et al., 1991), insulin-like growth factors 1 and 2 (IGF 1 and 2 [Ishii et al., 1994]) brain-derived neurotrophic factor (BDNF) (Leibrock, et al., 1989), neurotrophin-3 and neurotrophin-4/5 (NT3, [Cheng et al., 1994]) NT4, [Henderson et al., 1993]), and glial-derived neurotrophic factor (Lin et al., 1993). Furthermore, cytokines also have neurotrophic properties (Brenneman et al., 1992; Mehler et al., 1993). This expanding class of substances includes the various interleukins and leukemia inhibitory factor (Patterson, 1992). Although many of the classic growth factors were first recognized to play important trophic roles in neuron/target cell interactions, it is now clear that glial cells in the central nervous system (CNS) express most of these growth factors/cytokines, and that these glial cells have significant roles during development and nerve repair.

A neuroprotective, glia-derived protein (14,000 Daltons and pI 8.3+0.25), was recently isolated by sequential chromatographic methods (Brenneman and Gozes, 1996). The strategy used in isolating ADNF entailed measuring changes in neuronal survival after treatment of developing spinal cord cultures with tetrodotoxin, an agent that blocks synaptic activity. The tetrodotoxin was used to delineate neurons that were dependent on ongoing electrical activity for their survival. The end result was the isolation of ADNF, a molecule that both regulates activity-dependent neurodevelopment and elicits a wide spectrum of neuroprotection at femtomolar concentrations (Brenneman and Gozes, 1996).

Electrical blockade after treatment with tetrodotoxin has been demonstrated to inhibit the synthesis and release of trophic materials, including VIP (Brenneman et al., 1985; Agoston et al., 1991). VIP has been shown to prevent neuronal cell death associated with the envelope protein from the human immunodeficiency virus (glycoprotein 120, [Brenneman et al., 1988]), and the β amyloid peptide (putative cytotoxin in Alzheimer's disease [Gozes et al., 1996a]). We now propose that the neurotrophic activity of ADNF is mediated, at least in part, via ADNF.

During the course of studies directed to the structural characteristics of ADNF, an active peptide fragment was discovered: ADNF-14 (VLGGGSALLRSIPA). This peptide had strong homology, but not identity, to an intracellular stress protein: heat shock protein 60 (hsp60) (Brenneman and Gozes, 1996; Gozes and Brenneman, 1996b). ANDF-14, like ADNF, has been shown to exhibit neuroprotection from a wide variety of neurotoxic substances including the envelope protein from the human immunodeficiency virus, N-methyl D-aspartate (excitotoxicity), β amyloid peptide and tetrodotoxin (Brenneman and Gozes, 1996).

Classical studies on the biological effects of nerve growth factors, the foremost being NGF, relied on neutralizing antisera (Levi-Montalcini et al., 1969). Neutralizing antibodies to ADNF, now permitted the demonstration that CNS cultures contain an endogenous ADNF-like neuronal survival factor. Furthermore, these investigations have identified an active neuroprotective site and an immunogenic epitope for ADNF. Anti-ADNF serum was produced following sequential injections of purified ADNF into mice. Anti-ADNF ascites fluid (1:10,000) decreased neuronal survival by 35–50% in comparison to untreated cultures or cultures treated with control ascites. The neuronal cell killing after anti-ADNF treatment was observed in cultures derived from spinal cord, hippocampus or cerebral cortex at similar IC50's. Using a terminal deoxynucleotidyl transferase *in situ* assay to estimate apoptosis in cerebral cortical cultures, anti-ADNF was shown to produce a 70% increase in the number of labeled cells in comparison to controls. In spinal cord cultures, the anti-ADNF treatment produced a 20% decrease in choline acetyltransferase activity in comparison to controls. Neuronal cell death produced by the antiserum to ADNF was prevented in cultures co-treated with purified ADNF or ADNF-15 (VLGGGSALLRSIPAL), an active peptide derived from the parent ADNF. *In vitro* binding between the anti-ADNF and ADNF-15 was demonstrated with size exclusion chromatography. Comparative studies with other recognized growth factors (IGF-1, platelet-derived growth factor, NGF, epidermal growth factor, CNTF, and NT-3) indicated that only ADNF prevented neuronal cell death associated with electrical blockade. These investigations implied that an ADNF-like substance was present in cultures derived from multiple locations in the central nervous system and that ADNF-15 exhibited both neuroprotection and immunogenicity (Gozes et al., 1997a). ADNF appears to be both a regulator of activity-dependent neuronal survival and a neuroprotectant.

MODELS FOR ALZHEIMER'S DISEASE

Senile dementia of the Alzheimer's type afflicts 3–5 million people in the United States alone (Shapira, 1994; Brumback et al., 1994). Although the etiology of this disease remains unclear, there is increasing evidence for an involvement of several key substances. One is the β amyloid peptide, a toxic fragment of the amyloid precursor that forms deposits in the diseased brain. Another major player is acetylcholine, and a deficiency in acetylcholine is one of the most described deficiencies in Alzheimer's disease. The above described SNV and ADNF have both been shown to protect against β amyloid toxicity and cholinergic deficiencies (Gozes et al., 1996a; Brenneman and Gozes, 1996; Gozes et al., 1997a; Gozes et al., 1997b). The subject of this review is a key lipid carrier, apolipoprotein E (ApoE). ApoE is unique among the apolipoproteins in the nervous system, coordinating the mobilization and redistribution of cholesterol in repair, growth, maintenance and plasticity (Poirier, 1994). The link with Alzheimer's disease was established when one of the three common alleles of ApoE, the ApoE4 allele, was identified as a major risk factor (susceptibility gene), acting in a dose-dependent manner in late onset of sporadic and familial Alzheimer's disease (Poirier, 1994). ApoE3 may promote neuronal growth, while ApoE4 prevents it (Weisgraber et al., 1994). Furthermore, ApoE4 promotes the assembly of the β amyloid peptide into filaments (Ma et al., 1994). As indicated above, these β amyloid aggregates are deposited excessively in the brains of Alzheimer's patients, contributing to the neurodegenerative process. ApoE2 inhibits β amyloid peptide aggregation (Ma et al., 1995). In Down's syndrome patients, inheritance of the ApoE4 genotype appears to be an additional (independent) risk factor for developing higher levels of amyloid accumulation (Hyman et al., 1995). In contrast, inheritance of the ApoE2 allele protects patients with Down's syndrome from dementia (Royston et al., 1994). Additionally, a severe loss of choline acetyltransferase was found in the cortex of Alzheimer's disease patients carrying the ApoE4 allele (Poirier, 1994). Thus, ApoE plays an important role during brain development and during neurodegeneration. ApoE-deficient homozygous mice (knock-out, ApoE-deficient mice [Plump et al., 1992; Masliah et al., 1995]) may thus provide a useful *in vivo* model system for studies on the involvement of ApoE in brain development and degeneration..

SNV-MEDIATED NEUROPROTECTION IN ApoE-DEFICIENT MICE

In comparison to control animals, ApoE-deficient mice exhibited: 1) reduced amounts of VIP mRNA; 2) decreased cholinergic activity; and 3) significant retardation in the acquisition of developmental milestones: forelimb placing behavior and cliff avoidance behavior. Heterozygote animals displayed a close to median developmental pattern between control animals and ApoE-deficient homozygotes, in their acquisition of placing behavior. In contrast, heterozygote animals developed cliff avoidance behavior faster than control homozygotes, suggesting complex compensatory mechanisms. Furthermore, heterozygous animals exhibited somewhat reduced cholinergic activity. Daily injections of SNV to ApoE-deficient new-born pups resulted in increased cholinergic activity and marked improvements in the acquisition of behavioral milestones, with peptide-treated animals developing as fast as control animals. Specificity was demonstrated in that treatment with pituitary adenylate cyclase activating peptide (PACAP, a VIP-related peptide) produced only limited amelioration.

A most exciting finding was that prophylactic administration of SNV may protect against learning and memory impairments in ApoE-deficient mice. Assessments of spatial learning and memory were performed on three week-old animals in a water maze, by measurements of the time required to find a hidden platform. Two daily tests were performed. The platform location and the starting point in which the animal was placed in the water were held constant within each pair of daily trials, but both locations were changed every day. In the first test (indicative of intact reference memory) ApoE-deficient mice were significantly retarded as compared to control mice. The two groups of mice exhibited a parallel improvement over time and even after several training and testing days the ApoE-deficient mice were still retarded as compared to control animals. Similar results

Figure 1. ApoE-deficient mice exhibit a reduction in choline acetyltransferase activity that is ameliorated by SNV treatment. Incorporation of radiolabeled choline into acetylcholine (Gozes et al., 1997b; Fonnum, 1975) is depicted. Three week-old ApoE-deficient mice are designated: ApoE; 100% activity in the control animals indicated 669–758.4 pmole/ mg protein/min. Experiments were repeated ten times and results were standardized against the control calibrated at 100% per each experiment. ApoE-deficient mice daily injected with SNV=E+SNV. Statistics revealed significant differences between ApoE (E)-deficient vs control or peptide-treated animals. Het=heterozygous.

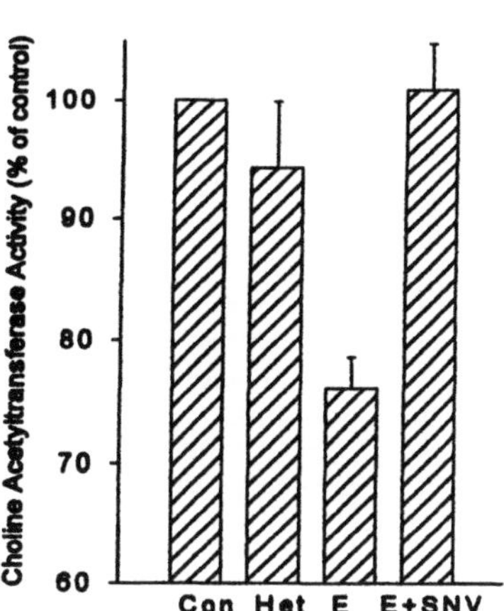

were obtained in the second daily test which is indicative of intact working memory processes. Chronic treatment of the ApoE-deficient mice with SNV for the first two weeks of life resulted in significant improvements in the performance of the animals in the water maze, in both daily tests. SNV-treated ApoE-deficient animals behaved as control animals in all test days except for day one in the first test, and exhibited only occasional minor differences from controls in the second daily test. Chronic treatment of control animals with SNV (during the first two weeks of life) also improved their performance, at 3 weeks of age, as evidenced in the first two test days in both daily trials. This study offers a new model for the evaluation of neuroprotection during development and suggests SNV as a candidate for prophylactic treatment against neurodegeneration (Gozes et al., 1997b).

FUTURE STUDIES

1. Is SNV activity mediated via ADNF *in vitro* and *in vivo?*
2. Further insight into the molecular nature of ADNF and it's active fragments.
3. Choice of the best candidate for memory enhancement in animals.
4. Potential new drugs for Alzheimer's patients?

AUTHORS COMMENTS

This short review presents the world through our own prism. As this is a part of a book summarizing a meeting, we took the liberty of describing our own work with limited background.

ACKNOWLEDGMENT

Supported in part by Fujimoto Pharmaceutical Corp., Japan; Ramot of Tel Aviv University and The US-Israel Binational Science Foundation. Prof. Illana Gozes in the incumbent of the Lily an Avraham Gildor Chair for the Investigations of Growth Factors.

REFERENCES

Agoston, D.V., Eiden, L.E., Brenneman, D.E., and I. Gozes, 1991, Spontaneous electrical activity regulates vasoactive intestinal peptide expression in dissociated spinal cord cell cultures. *Mol. Brain Res.* 10:235–240.

Brenneman, D.E., Eiden, L.E., and Siegel, R.E., 1985, Neurotrophic action of VIP on spinal cord cultures. *Peptides* 6 (suppl. 2):35–39.

Brenneman, D.E., and Eiden, L.E., 1986, Vasoactive intestinal peptide and electrical activity influence neuronal survival. *Proc. Natl. Acad. Sci. USA* 83:1159–1162.

Brenneman D.E., Neale, E.A., Foster, G.A., d'Autremont, S., and Westbrook, L.G., 1987, Nonneuronal cells mediate neurotrophic action of vasoactive intestinal peptide. *J.Cell Biology.* 104:1603–1610.

Brenneman, D.E., Westbrook, L.G., Fitzgerald, S., Ennist, L.D., Elkins, L.K., Ruff, M.R., and Pert, C.B., 1988, Neuronal cell killing by the envelope protein of HIV and its prevention by vasoactive intestinal peptide. *Nature* 335:639–642.

Brenneman, D.E., Nicol, T., Warren, D., and Bowers, L.M., 1990, Vasoactive intestinal peptide: a neurotrophic releasing agent and an astroglial mitogen. *J. Neurosci. Res.* 25:386–394.

Brenneman, D.E., Schultzberg, M., Bartfai, T., and Gozes, I., 1992, Cytokine regulation of neuronal survival. *J. Neurochem.* 58:454–460.

Brenneman, D.E., and Gozes, I. 1996. A femtomolar-acting neuroprotective peptide. *J. Clin. Invest.* 97: 2299–2307.

Brumback, R.A., and Leech, R.W., 1994, Alzheimer's disease: pathophysiology and hope for therapy. *J. Okla State Med. Assoc.* 87:103–111.

Cheng, B., and Mattson, M.P., 1991, NGF and bFGF protect rat hippocampal and human cortical neurons against hypoglycemic damage by stabilizing calcium homeostasis. *Neuron* 7:1031–1041.

Cheng, B., and Mattson, M.P., 1994, NT-3 and BDNF protect CNS neurons against metabolic/excitotoxic insults. *Brain Res.* 640:56–67.

Fonnum, F. 1975. A rapid radiochemical method for the determination of cholinacetyl transferase. *J. Neurochem.* 24:407–409.

Glowa, J.R., Panlilio, L.V., Brenneman, D.E., Gozes, I., Fridkin, M., and Hill, J.M., 1992, Learning impairment following intracerebral administration of the HIV envelope protein gp120 or a VIP antagonist. *Brain Res.* 570:49–53.

Gozes, I., Shachter, P., Shani, Y., and Giladi, E., 1988, Vasoactive intestinal peptide gene expression from embryos to aging rats. *Neuroendocrinology* 47:27–31.

Gozes, I., Meltzer, E., Rubinraut, S., Brenneman, D.E., and Fridkin, M., 1989, Vasoactive intestinal peptide potentiate sexual behavior: Inhibition by novel antagonist *Endocrinology* 125:2945–2949.

Gozes, I., McCune, S.K, Jacobson, L., Warren, D., Moody, T.W., Fridkin, M., and Brenneman, D.E., 1991, An antagonist to vasoactive intestinal peptide: effects on cellular functions in the central nervous system. *J. Pharmacol.. Exp. Ther.* 257:959–966.

Gozes, I., Glowa, J., Brenneman, D.E., McCune, S.K., Lee, E., and Westphal, H., 1993, Learning and sexual deficiencies in transgenic mice carrying a chimeric vasoactive intestinal peptide gene. *J. Mol. Neurosci.*4:185–193.

Gozes, I., Reshef, A., Salah, D., Rubinraut, S., and Fridkin, M., 1994, Stearyl-Norleucine-VIP a novel VIP analogue for noninvasive impotence treatment. *Endocrinology.* 134:2121–2125.

Gozes, I., Lilling, G., Glazer, R., Ticher, A., Ashkenazi, I.E., Davidson, A., Rubinraut, S., Fridkin, M., and Brenneman, D.E. 1995a, Superactive lipophilic peptides discriminate multiple VIP receptors. *J.Pharmacol. Exper. Therap.* 273:161–167.

Gozes, I., Fridkin, M., and Brenneman, D.E., 1995b, Stearyl-Nle-VIP: a non-invasive impotence drug and a potent agent of neuro-protection. *Drugs of the Future* 20:680–685.

Gozes, I., Bardea, A., Reshef, A., Zamostiatno, R., Zhukovsky, S., Rubinraut, S., Fridkin, M., and Brenneman, D.E., 1996a, Novel Neuroprotective strategy for Alzheimer's disease: inhalation of a fatty neuropeptide. *Proc. Natl. Acad. Sci. USA.* 93:427–432.

Gozes, I., and Brenneman D.E., 1996b, Activity-dependent neurotrophic factor (ADNF): An extracellular neuroprotective chaperonin? *J. Molec. Neurosci.* 7: 235–244.

Gozes, I., Davidson, A., Gozes, Y., Mascolo, R., Barth, R., Warren, D., Hauser, J., and Brenneman, 1997a, Antiserum to activity-dependent neurotrophic factor produces neuronal cell death in CNS cultures: immunological biological specificity. *Dev. Brain Res.* 99: 167–175.

Gozes, I., Bachar, M., Bardea, A., Davidson, A., Rubinraut, S., Fridkin, M., and Giladi, E., 1997b, Protection against developmental retardation in apolipoprotein E-deficient mice by a fatty neuropeptide: implication for early treatment of Alzheimer's disease. *J. Neurobiol.* in press.

Gressens, P., Hill, J.M., Paindaveine, B., Gozes, I., Fridkin, M., and Brenneman, D.E., 1994, Severe microcephaly induced by blockade of vasoactive intestinal peptide function in the primitive neuroepithelium of the mouse. *J. Clin. Invest.* 94:2020–2027.

Henderson, C.E., Camu, C., Mettling, Gouin, A., Poulsen, K., Karihaloo, M., Rullamas, J., Evans T., McMahon, S.B., Aramanini, M.P., Berkemeier, L., Phillips, H.S., and Rosenthal, A., 1993, Neurotrophins promote motor neuron survival and are present in embryonic limb bud. *Nature* 363:266–269.

Hill, J.M., Gozes, I., Hill, J.L., Fridkin, M., and Brenneman, D.E., 1991, Vasoactive intestinal peptide antagonist retards the development of neonatal behaviors in the rat. *Peptides.* 12:187–192.

Hill, J.M., Mervis, R.F., Politi, J., McCune, S.K., Gozes, I., Fridkin, M., and Brenneman, D.E., 1994, Blockade of VIP during neonatal development induces neuronal damage and increases VIP and VIP receptors in brain. *Ann. N.Y. Acad. Sci.* 739:211–225.

Hyman, B.T., West, H.L., Rebeck, G.W., Lai, F., and Mann, D.E., 1995, Neuropathological changes in Down's syndrome hippocampal formation. Effect of age and apolipoprotein E genotype. *Arch. Neurol.* 52:373–378.

Ishii, D.N., Glazner, G., and Pu, S.F., 1994, Role of insulin-like growth factors in peripheral nerve regeneration. *Pharmacol. Ther.* 62: 125–144.

Leibrock, J., Lottspeich, F., Hohn, A., Hofer, M., Hengerer, B., Masiakowski, P., Thoenen, H., and Barde, Y.A., 1989, Molecular cloning and expression of brain-derived neurotrophic factor. *Nature* 341: 149–152.

Levi-Montalcini, R., 1979, Recent studies on the NGF-target cells interaction, *Differentiation* 13: 51–53.

Levi-Montalcini R, Caramia, F., and Angeletti, P.U., 1969, Alteration in the fine structure of nucleoli in sympathetic neurons following NGF-antiserum treatment. *Brain Res.* 12: 54–73.

Lin, L.F., Mismer, D., Lile, J.D., Armes, L.G., Butler 3rd, E.T., Vannice, J.L., and Collins, F., 1989, Purification, cloning and expression of ciliary neurotrophic factor (CNTF). *Science* 24: 1023–1025.

Lin, L.F., Doherty, D.H., Lile, J.D., Bektesh, S., and Collins, F., 1993, GDNF: a glial cell line-derived neurotrophic factor for midbrain dopaminergic neurons. *Science* 260: 1130–1132.

Ma, J., Yee, A., Brewer Jr., H.B., Das, S., and Potter H., 1994, Amyloid-associated protein alpha 1-antichymotrypsin and apolipoprotein E promote assembly of Alzheimer beta-protein into filaments. *Nature* 372:92–94.

Ma, J., Brewer, B., and Potter, H., 1995, Promotion of the neurotoxicity of Alzheimer's A beta protein by the pathological chaperones ACT and apoE4: inhibition by A beta-related peptides and apoE2. *Soc. Neurosci. Abs.* Vol. 21:1714.

Masliah, E., Mallory, M., Ge, N., Alford, M., Veinbergs, I., and Roses, A.D., 1995, Neurodegeneration in the central nervous system of apoE-deficient mice. *Exp.Neurol.* 136:107–122.

Mehler, M.F., Rozental, R., Dougherty, M., Spray, D.C., and Kessler, J.A., 1993, Cytokine regulation of neuronal differentiation of hippocampal progenitor cells. *Nature* 362:62–65.

Patterson, P.H., 1992, The emerging neuropoietic cytokine family: first CDF/LIF, CNTF and IL6; next ONC, MGF, GCSF? *Curr Opin. Neurobiol.* 2:94–97.

Plump, A.S., Smith, J.D., Hayek, T., Aalto-Setala, K., Walsh, A., Verstuyft, J.G., Rubin, E.M., and Breslow, J.L., 1992, Severe Hypercholesterolemia and atherosclerosis in apolipoprotein E-deficient mice created by homologous recombination in ES cells. *Cell* 71:343–353.

Poirier, J., 1994, Apolipoprotein E in animal models of CNS injury and in Alzheimer's disease. *Trends Neurosci.* 17:525–530.

Royston, M.C., Mann, D., Pickering-Brown, S., Owen, F., Perry, R., Raghaven, R., Khin-Nu, C., Tyrer, S., Day, K., and Crook, R., 1994, Apolipoprotein E epsilon 2 allele promotes longevity and protects patients with Down's syndrome from dementia. *NeuroReport* 5:2583–2585.

Shapira, J., 1994, Research trends in Alzheimer's disease, *J. Gerontol. Nurs.* 20:4–9.

Weisgraber, K.H., Pitas, R.E., and Mahley, R.W., 1994, Lipoproteins, neurobiology, and Alzheimer's disease: structure and function of apolipoprotein E. *Curr. Opin. Struct. Biol.* 4:507–515.

90

CLINICAL ASPECTS OF NEUROTRANSPLANTATION OF EMBRYONAL BRAIN TISSUE

Long Term Results

Miron Šramka, Július Rattaj, and Martin Novotný

Department of Stereotactic and Functional Neurosurgery
Clinic of Neurosurgery Comenius University
Derer's Hospital Limbová str. 5
83305, Bratislava, Slovak Republic

INTRODUCTION

Experiments have shown that the transplantation of nervous brain tissue enables the regeneration of morphologic, connecting, and biochemical changes in model animals (Björklund et al., 1980). They have determined suitable anatomic sites for transplantation and also the conditions of survival are known. In 1985 Dr. Madrazzo from Mexico transplanted embryonal brain tissue from the mesencephalon of the substantia nigra area into the caudate nucleus of a parkinsonian patient (Madrazzo et al., 1985). Embryonal tissue of the mesencephalon was transplanted stereotactically (Hitchcock et al., 1989). In our department transplantations of mesencephalon embryonal brain tissue stereotactically in parkinsonian patients were performed in 1989 (Šramka et al., 1990). Transplantation of embryonal brain tissue—striatum in Huntington's chorea—via open neurosurgery and via stereotactic technique was performed in 1990 (Molina et al., 1991).

MATERIALS AND METHODS

We have operated on 6 patients-parkinsonians and two patients with Huntington's chorea to date. The patients were recommended for transplantation by their neurologists and we considered the neurotransplantation after failure of our correction with drug therapy; each patient had to sign an operation agreement. Age ranged from 44–56 years.

Progress in Alzheimer's and Parkinson's Diseases
edited by Fisher *et al.*, Plenum Press, New York, 1998.

Etiopathogenetically, there was idiopathic disease in 7 patients; in one patient the etiology was not clear at all. Duration of dopaminergic drug administration was 7–12 years. All patients were suffering from intolerance, from adverse effects, or loss of the effect of drug treatment.

The patients were examined according to a prepared scheme including history of disease, detailed physical examination of a neurologist, an internist, an immunologist, a psychiatrist and a psychologist, plus a set of screening blood examinations, and analysis of cerebrospinal fluid (CSF). Electrophysiological examinations (EMG, EEG, evoked potentials), stabilography, tremorogram and computer tomography were also conducted, so that they could be compared before and after the surgery (except for CSF and CT for radiosensitivity to the embryonal brain tissue operation). The patients were recorded on video pre- and postoperatively. We used the Hoehn-Yahr scale in our evaluation of the patients' clinical status. Our patients were tabled into the III-V stage of this scale.

The transplantation technique consisted of stereotaxy controlled by computer assisted tomography (Ružický et al., 1994). For the operation, the stereotactic Riechert-Mundinger's apparatus was used. A special canulla of our own construction enabled us to place into the brain 3–4 tissue samples on the determined trajectory by one introduction of the cannula without repeated insertion (Šramka et al., 1992).

We can obtain embryonal brain tissue by considerate vacuum-aspiration under ultrasound control. Prepared 1 cmm cubes of ventral mesencephalon were placed into the cannula by the "pick up" method and were inserted into caput nuclei caudati, in the first two patients unilaterally, in others bilaterally. We used 2–4 embryonal brains and inserted 4–5 samples into caput nuclei caudati or striatum in each operation.

Per-operative complications did not occur; postoperatively we observed elevated temperature, meningismus, hypertension, halucinations, bulimia, pylorrhea, red skin and mucosa, but only in moderate state during a duration of 3–10 days. The surgery sites were covered by the immunosupresive agent cyclosporin A. We did not observe any functional kidney disorders or adverse effects. Antiparkinsonian agents were administered as before the operation, with a gradual reduction during clinical improvement.

RESULTS

The first effects of brain grafts were observed about 8 weeks after the operation. Post-operative observation ranged between 18–30 months during which we observed changes in clinical condition of the patients as follows: 1.Rigidity decreased and kinesia improved both in extremity muscles and the axial ones; 2. Tremor was influenced least, without changes in frequency; amplitude was temporarily reduced; 3. Motility improvement was reflected in improved sociability both in the hospital and in the family, and also in the general quality of life; 4. Doses of dopaminergic agents were decreased by 40–60 %, which means a considerable economic effect regarding an increased occurence of Parkinsonism in the general population; 5. Adverse effects of dopaminergic agents (on-off effect) were diminished; and 6. Patients' condition was improved in stages 1–2 of the Hoehn-Yahr scale. We have decreased the doses of dopaminergic agents since that time.

Postoperative observation after 7–8 years: Clinical examinations performed nowadays showed similar results as two years after surgery. One female patient had generalized hypokinesia with little distinguished rigidity and almost no tremor. The clinical picture of the other two patients—males with regular dopaminergic medication—was only oscillating middle expressed rigidity. The most expressed phenomenon found in all of them was tremor on both sides, which was least influenced. Very important in all patients is the fact that the side-effect of psychic changes, especially in the area of cognitive functions, were missing. An important finding in two patients examined was progressive cachexia.

On-off effect in patients was positively expressed, decreasing with time, on phase lasted two hours on the average. We have to stress that all patients were regularly medicated with dopaminergic drugs. It is important that good therapeutic results were reached with a lower dosage. This is, in our opinion, due to the effect of neurotransplantation.

Concluding our results on behalf of classification of examined patients according to the Hoehn-Yahr scale, they are in good condition without worsening of their clinical state. According to above mentioned scale they are at the level of III-IV, which means that their state did not change significantly. The transplantation influenced mainly rigidity and akinesia, and had a lesser effect on tremor.

DISCUSSION

It is estimated that there is a 2–3% occurence of Parkinsonism in the population. The medication therapy is unsuccessful in 10% of Parkinsonians as a consequence of loss or adverse effects. Neurotransplantation is necessary to be considered as another option in these patients. In accordance with our study the application of embryonal brain tissue inserted into caput nuclei caudati and striatum seems suitable and the stereotactic technique is a considerable and acceptable method (Hitchcock et al., 1989). The application of tissue cultures with neuroendocrine effect seems to be hopeful (Ran-Ben et al., 1996). The lack of determined brain agents will be substituted by application of specific cells that will produce the absent agent. However, stereotactic destructive operations on ventral thalamus and pallidum are used to influence parkinsonian signs, mainly tremor, and neurotransplantation rigidity are decreased and kinesia is improved. Progressive cachexia is not found in the literature dealing with Parkinson disease in the picture of specific changes. The last mentioned change (cachexia)—when described—is bound with social problem of these patients. In our group of patients this social phenomenon is less important and we assume that it could be considered as a nonspecific phenomenon of Parkinson's disease. We have thus followed up the mentioned improvement for the past 6–7 years. A positive effect of the operation persists, and patients are continuing to be under our observation.

REFERENCES

Bjorklund, A., Dunnet, S.B., Stenevi, U., Lewis, M.E., Iversen, S.D., 1980, Reinnervation of the denervated striatum by substantia nigra transplants. Functional consequences as revaled by pharmacological and sensorimotor testing. *Brain Res.* 199:307–333.

Hitchcok, E.R, Kenny, B.G, Ciough, C.G, Hughes, R.C, Henderson, B.T.H, Betta, A., 1989, Stereotactic implantation of fetal Mesencephalon (STIM). In: *Abstract of X. Meeting of the World Society for Stereotact. Funct. Neurosurg.*, Maebashi, Oct. 2–5:25.

Madrazo, I., Leon, V., Torres, C., Del Carmen Aquilera Ma., Varela, G., Alvarez, F., Fraga, A., Drucker-Colin, R., Ostrovsky, F., Skurovich, M., Franco, R., 1988, Transplantation of fetal substantia nigra and adrenal medulla to the caudate nucleus in two patients with Parkinson's disease. *N. Eng. J. Med.* 318:51.

Molina, H., Šramka, M., Alvarez, L., Vojtaššák, J., Rattaj, M., Rusnák, J., Cordova, F., 1991 Neurotransplantation in Huntington's chorea . Proceedings of the Congress of the European Society for Stereotact. Funct. Neurosurg. *Acta Neurochir., suppl.* 52:68–71.

Ren-Ben, Fan Ji-Chang, Bao Yao-Dong, Liu Yie-Jian, Zhang Yi-Fan, 1990, Transplantation of foetal adrenal medullary tissue cultured to the head of caudate nucleus in 17 Parkinsonians. In: *Abstracts of 9th Congress of the European Society for Stereotactic and Functional Neurosurgery.* Marbella, Sept. 16–20:50–52.

Ružický, E., Šramka M., Jankovič, V., 1994, Mathematical methods for stereotactic neurosurgery. *Stereotact. Funct. Neurosurg.* 63(1):172.

Šramka, M., Rattaj, M., Vojtaššák, J., Rusňák, I., Belan, V., Rušický, E., 1990, Transplantation of embryonal tissue in treatment of Parkinson diseases and Huntington's chorea. In: *Summary of Int. Congress of Bioenergetical and Biological Medicine., Bratislava*:39–40.

Šramka, M., Rattaj, M., Molina, H., Vojtaššák, J., Belan, V., Rušický, E., 1992, Stereotactic technique & pathophysiological mechanisms of neurotransplantation in Huntington's chorea. *Stereotact. Funct. Neurosurg.* 58(1–4):79–83.

91

GENE THERAPY OF A RODENT MODEL OF PARKINSON'S DISEASE USING ADENO-ASSOCIATED VIRUS (AAV) VECTORS

Dong-Sheng Fan,[1,2] Matsuo Ogawa,[2] Ken-ichi Fujimoto,[2]
Kunihiko Ikeguchi,[2] Yoji Ogasawara,[1] Masashi Urabe,[1] Akihiro Kume,[1]
Masatoyo Nishizawa,[2] Imaharu Nakano,[2] Mitsuo Yoshida,[2] Hiroshi Ichinose,[3]
Toshiharu Nagatsu,[3] Gary J. Kurtzman,[4] and Keiya Ozawa[1]

[1]Department of Molecular Biology
[2]Department of Neurology
Jichi Medical School, Tochigi, Japan
[3]Institute for Comprehensive Medical Science
Fujita Health University
Aichi, Japan
[4]Avigen, Inc.
Alameda, California

INTRODUCTION

Somatic gene therapy is a logical approach to the treatment and correction of inherited disorders, and the concept that genetic manipulation might be used to treat diseases is also applied to the treatment of acquired disorders, such as cancer and AIDS. Accordingly, the types of diseases under consideration for gene therapy are diverse, and many different treatment strategies are being investigated, each with an appropriate gene transfer system. Parkinson's disease seems to be one of the appropriate target diseases for gene therapy among neurological disorders.

Parkinson's disease is a common neurodegenerative disorder which affects predominantly the elderly people. These patients display cogwheel rigidity, resting tremor, and impairment in the initiation and speed of movements. The characteristic pathological changes of Parkinson's disease are a severe loss of dopamine cell bodies in the substantia nigra and a severe decrease of dopamine in the nerve endings of the striatum (reviewed by Bemheimer et al., 1973). The severity of Parkinson's disease is proportional to the loss of local dopamine. Replacement of l-dopa, the precursor of dopamine, can restore a varying degree of motor function, since endogenous aromatic l-amino acid decarboxylase (AADC)

Progress in Alzheimer's and Parkinson's Diseases
edited by Fisher *et al.*, Plenum Press, New York, 1998.

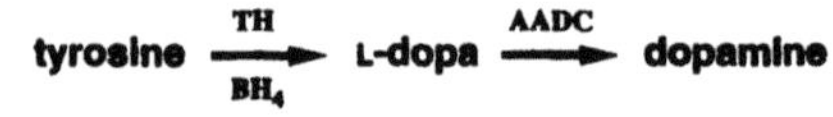

$$\text{tyrosine} \xrightarrow[\text{BH}_4]{\text{TH}} \text{L-dopa} \xrightarrow{\text{AADC}} \text{dopamine}$$

Figure 1. Dopamine biosynthetic pathway. (TH, tyrosine hydroxylase; BH$_4$, tetrahydrobiopterin, a cofactor of TH; and AADC, aromatic l-amino acid decarboxylase.)

can convert it to the neurotransmitter dopamine (Figure 1), which alleviates the symptoms of Parkinson's disease (reviewed by Nagatsu, 1992). Unfortunately, this therapy usually becomes less effective with progression of the disease and must often be discontinued due to the numerous deleterious side effects of systemic l-dopa delivery. Therefore, gene therapy has been expected as one of the novel alternative therapeutic approaches. Using model animals, most of the gene therapy strategies for amelioration of Parkinson's disease have focused on intrastriatal grafting of cells genetically modified to express tyrosine hydroxylase (TH), that catalyzes the reaction in the synthesis of l-dopa (Jiao et al., 1993); the target cells used so far include fibroblasts, muscle cells, astrocytes and even neurons (Jiao et al., 1994; reviewed by Martinez-Serrano et al., 1997). Recently, direct gene transfer into the denervated striatum of lesioned rat with the TH-expressing vector has also attracted considerable attention (During et al., 1994; Kaplitt et al., 1994).

Unlike systemic administration of l-dopa, it is believed that l-dopa produced in the local region is converted to dopamine in situ. However, the AADC activity in the striatum is considered to be very low (Tashiro et al., 1989; Kang et al., 1992). Since the source and site of decarboxylase activity have not been identified clearly, one of the basic unsolved issues in the current strategy is whether the cells genetically engineered to produce l-dopa would suffice for gene therapy of Parkinson's disease (reviewed by Jinnah et al., 1995). Therefore, expression of both TH and AADC in transduced cells may be more appropriate for gene therapy of Parkinson's disease. In vitro studies using non-neuronal cells have already shown that the co-expression of TH and AADC augmented dopamine production (Kang et al., 1993). In the present study, we co-expressed TH and AADC in primary cultures of rat striatal cells and in denervated striatum of parkinsonian rats in vivo using two separate adeno-associated virus (AAV) vectors, AAV-TH and AAV-AADC. Our objectives in this study are to examine whether two different foreign genes are able to be transferred into the same target cells using separate AAV vectors, and to determine whether co-transduction of the striatal cells with TH and AADC genes can induce better behavioral as well as biochemical changes than the TH gene alone.

VIRAL VECTORS FOR GENE THERAPY

A number of methods have been developed for introducing genes into living cells, including viral and non-viral vectors. The former is more commonly utilized for gene therapy or gene marking due to their relatively higher efficiencies of gene transfer. Several different viral vector systems are in use or under consideration for somatic gene transfer. Among them, retroviral vectors are currently most extensively investigated as gene transfer vehicles and are employed in the majority of clinical protocols. Recently, adenoviral vectors are also used in many clinical protocols, because this vector has several important properties which are different from those of retroviral vectors. AAV vector, derived from non-pathogenic virus, has potential to become an ideal vector for gene therapy. However, the difficulties in producing AAV vectors have hampered its clinical application until recently. In addition, several other types of viruses, including poxviruses, herpes viruses and a human immunodeficiency virus (HSV), are currently being developed or at least considered for this purpose.

Advantages and Disadvantages of Representative Viral Vector Systems

Retroviral vectors are widely used gene transfer vehicles, because this technique has the advantages of high-efficiency gene transfer and stable integration into the target cell genome without concomitant introduction of viral genes. Major disadvantages of retroviruses are that they infect and integrate only dividing cells and that they integrate randomly into the host genome, which may cause genetic damage (insertional mutagenesis). It was reported that infusion of replication-competent retroviruses (RCR) into non-human primates caused development of lymphoma. Another disadvantage is the variable and usually unacceptably low expression levels of transgenes after long-term observation, even if they are detectable at the DNA level. Currently, several improvements have been reported for retroviral vector system. Retroviral particles are very unstable and difficult to be concentrated by ultracentrifugation. However, the retroviral vectors containing vesicular stomatitis virus (VSV) glycoproteins allows concentration of the recombinant virus to obtain high-titer vector stocks. A novel vector system based on the human immunodeficiency virus (HIV) has been developed (Naldini et al., 1996). The ability of lentiviral vectors to deliver genes in vivo into non-dividing cells could increase the applicability of retroviral vectors in gene therapy.

Advantages of adenoviral vector system are high titers, efficient transduction of dividing and non-dividing cells. However, since adenovirus does not integrate into the host genome, defective (replication-incompetent) adenoviral vectors are not appropriate for rapidly proliferating target cells. This vector is suitable for the purposes where transient expression of transduced genes is sufficient to get therapeutic effects. Moreover, because a large part of viral genes are remained in the currently available vectors, their low-level expression causes some cytotoxic effects and induces immune reaction to transduced cells. Therefore, the best application of adenovirus vectors may be immune-mediated gene therapy for cancer. On the other hand, several groups are trying to reduce host immune responses by the removal or modification of adenoviral genes in the vector sequence.

AAV vectors possess several unique properties and are potentially useful gene transfer vehicles for gene therapy (reviewed by Muzyczka et al., 1992). Their advantages include lack of any associated disease with a wild-type virus, broad host cell range, possible integration of the gene into the host genome, and the ability to transduce non-dividing cells. Therefore, neurons, muscle cells, and hepatocytes are appropriate target cells of AAV vectors. In addition, AAV particles are remarkably stable and can be concentrated without losing infectivity. Since the AAV vectors do not contain viral genes, immune response should not occur against the transduced cells. Co-transduction with a variety of AAV vectors would also be possible. Recently, a very efficient helper-adenovirus-free system for AAV vector production has been developed by Avigen, Inc. To produce AAV vectors, 293 cells are co-transfected with the vector plasmid, which contains a therapeutic gene between the ITR (inverted terminal repeats), the helper plasmid, which supplies AAV-Rep and Cap proteins, and the plasmid containing adenovirus genes, E2A, E4, and VA (E1 genes are contained in 293 cells), in place of helper adenovirus. However, further improvement of the AAV vector production system (e.g., efficient packaging cell lines) is required for large-scale clinical trials.

Among the vector systems for neurologic gene therapy, therefore, AAV vector is one of the most attractive candidates (Kaplitt et al., 1994; Du et al., 1996). The other vectors based upon DNA viruses, such as herpes simplex virus (HSV) (During et al., 1994; Geller et al., 1995) and adenovirus vectors (Le Gal La Salle et al., 1993), are cytotoxic to the recipient cells and induce an immune response against the transduced cells, although both of them can efficiently transduce foreign genes into neurons. Retroviral vector is not appropriate, because it requires active cell division for gene transfer.

AAV VECTOR-MEDIATED GENE TRANSFER INTO NEURONS

Primary cultured neurons (rat striatal cells) were transduced with AAV vectors containing LacZ gene (AAV-LacZ). The X-gal staining showed that transduction efficiency was dose-dependent and time-dependent. Roughly 30% of cells were positive for β-galactosidase activity, and about one week was required for maximum expression.

The AAV-LacZ vector was then stereotaxically injected into the normal adult rat striatum. As a result, β-galactosidase-positive cells were detected at the injection site without any background staining for several months. Most of the positive cells were neurons, based on the morphological criteria, although it is possible that some of the positive cells were non-neuronal.

AAV VECTOR-MEDIATED TRANSFER OF TH AND AADC GENES INTO NEURONS FOR GENE THERAPY OF PARKINSONIAN RATS

Co-Transduction of Striatal Cells with AAV-TH and AAV-AADC in Vitro

Primary cultured rat striatal cells were co-transduced with AAV-TH (Kaneda et al., 1987) and AAV-AADC (Ichinose et al., 1989) vectors. Co-expression of TH and AADC in the same striatal cells was detected by dual immunofluorescent staining. Co-transduction efficiency was increased along with the increasing doses of AAV-TH/AAV-AADC vectors. The striatal cells co-transduced with AAV-TH/AAV-AADC mixture synthesized dopamine more efficiently than the cells transduced with AAV-TH alone, when the intracellular l-dopa and dopamine were measured by HPLC (high-performance liquid chromatography).

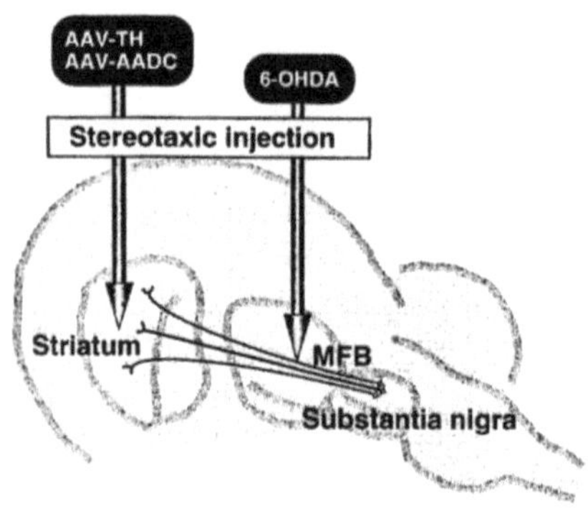

Figure 2. Gene therapy of a rodent model of Parkinson's disease using AAV vectors. (TH, tyrosine hydroxylase; AADC, aromatic l-amino acid decarboxylase; 6-OHDA, 6-hydroxydopamine; and MFB, medial forebrain bundle.)

Stereotaxic Injection of AAV-TH and AAV-AADC into Striatum of Parkinsonian Rats

A rodent model of Parkinson's disease was generated by stereotaxic injection of the catecholamine neurotoxin 6-hydroxydopamine (6-OHDA) into the left medial forebrain bundle (MFB) to destroy the nigro-striatal pathway of dopamine neurons unilaterally. This MFB lesion causes the decrease of dopamine in the striatum like Parkinson's disease. The dopamine receptors of striatal cells in the lesioned side become hypersensitive to dopamine. After the intraperitoneal administration of dopamine agonist, apomorphine, unbalance of motor function is induced, and the rats show rotational behavior. The dopamine content in the striatum can be estimated by counting the rotation after apomorphine administration.

The AAV-TH and/or AAV-AADC vectors were then stereotaxically injected into the denervated striatum of 6-OHDA-lesioned rats. A behavioral test was conducted following the injection of AAV-TH/AAV-AADC mixture, AAV-TH alone, AAV-AADC alone, AAV-LacZ, or PBS, respectively. As a result, significant decrease in rotational rate was observed in the rats injected with AAV-TH/AAV-AADC mixture and AAV-TH alone. Moreover, the decrease was more remarkable in the rats injected with AAV-TH/AAV-AADC mixture compared with the rats injected with AAV-TH alone. Co-expression of TH and AADC in the same striatal cells was confirmed with dual immunofluorescent staining.

In conclusion, this study showed that 1) AAV vectors can efficiently transfer and express foreign genes in the striatal cells in vitro and in vivo, 2) the use of two separate AAV vectors, AAV-TH and AAV-AADC, made it possible to coexpress both TH and AADC in the same striatal cells; and 3) co-transduction with these two AAV vectors resulted in more efficient dopamine production in vitro, and more remarkable behavioral recovery in 6-OHDA-lesioned rats in vivo, compared with AAV-TH alone. This study would be valuable to develop the clinically applicable protocol of gene therapy for Parkinson's disease.

ACKNOWLEDGMENTS

Supported by a Grant-in-Aid for Scientific Research on Priority Areas from the Ministry of Education, Science, Sports and Culture of Japan, grants from the Ministry of Health and Welfare of Japan, a grant from Uehara Memorial Foundation, and CREST (Core Research for Evolutional Science and Technology) of Japan Science and Technology Corporation (JST).

REFERENCES

Bemheimer, H., Birkmayer, W., Homykiewicz, O., Jellinger, K., and Seitelberger, F., 1973, Brain dopamine and the syndromes of Parkinson and Huntington: clinical, morphological and neurochemical correlations. *J. Neurol.Sci.* 20: 415–455.

Du, B., Wu, P., Boldt-Houle, D.M., and Terwilliger, E.F., 1996, Efficient transduction of human neurons with an adeno-associated virus vector. *Gene Ther.* 3: 254–261.

During, M.J., Naegele, J.R., O'Malley, K.L., Geller, and A.I., 1994, Long-term behavioral recovery in Parkinson's rats by an HSV vector expressing tyrosine hydroxylase. *Science* 266: 1399–1403.

Geller, A.I., During, M.J., Oh, Y.J., Freese, A., and O'Malley, K., 1995, An HSV-1 vector expressing tyrosine hydroxylase cause production and release of l-DOPA from cultured rat striatal cells. *J. Neurochem.* 64: 487–496.

Ichinose, H., Kurosawa, Y., Titani, K., Fujita, K., and Nagatsu, T., 1989, Isolation and characterization of a cDNA clone encoding human aromatic l-amino acid decarboxylase. *Biochem. Biophys. Res. Commun.* 164: 1024–1030.

Jiao, S., Gurevich, V., and Wolff, J.A, 1993, Long-term correction of rat model of Parkinson's disease by gene therapy. *Nature* 362: 450–453.

Jiao, S., Hogan, K., and Wolff, J.A., 1994, Gene therapy for neuromuscular disorders. *Cur. Neurol.* 14: 1–28.

Jinnah, H.A., and Friedmann, T., 1995, Gene therapy and the brain. *Bri. Med. Bull.* 51: 138- 148.

Kang, U.J., Park, D.H., Wessel, T., Baker, H., and Joh, T.H., 1992, DOPA-decarboxylation in the striata of rats with unilateral substantia nigra lesions. *Neurosci. Lett.* 147: 53–57.

Kang, U.J., Fisher, L.J., Joh, T.H., O'Malley, K.L., and Gage, F.H., 1993, Regulation of dopamine production by genetically modified primary fibroblasts. *J. Neurosci.* 13: 5203- 5211.

Kaplitt, M.G., Leone, P., Samulski, R.J., Xiao, X., Pfaff, D.W., O'Malley, K.L., and During, M.J., 1994, Long-term gene expression and phenotypic correction using adeno- associated virus vectors in the mammalian brain. *Nat. Genet.* 8: 148–154.

Kaneda, N., Kobayashi, K., Ichinose, H., Kishi, F., Nakazawa, A., Kurosawa, Y., Fujita, K., and Nagatsu, T., 1987, Isolation of a novel cDNA clone for human tyrosine hydroxylase: alternative RNA splicing produces four kinds of mRNA from a single gene. *Biochem. Biophys. Res. Commun.* 146: 971–975.

Le Gal La Salle, G,. Robert, J.J., Bernard, S., Ridoux, V., Stratford-Perricaudet, L.D., Perricaudet, M., and Mallet, J., 1993, An adenovirus vector for gene transfer into neurons and glia in the brain. *Science* 259: 988–990.

Martinez-Serrano, A., Lundberg, C., and Bjrklund, A., 1997, Use of conditionally immortalized neural progenitors for transplantation and gene transfer to the CNS. In, *Isolation, Characterization and Utilization of CNS Stem Cells.* (Gage, F. and Christen, Y., eds.), Springer-Verlag, Berlin, pp151–169.

Muzyczka, N., 1992, Use of adeno-associated virus as a general transduction vector for mammalian cells. *Curr. Top. Microbiol. Immunol.* 158: 97–129.

Nagatsu, T., 1992, Molecular biology of dopamine systems. In, *Controversies in the Treatment of Parkinson's Disease.* (Rinne, U.K. and Yanagisawa, N., eds.), PMSI, Tokyo, pp15- 26.

Naldini, L., Blmer, U., Gallay, P., Ory, D., Mulligan, R., Gage, F.H., Verma, I.M., and Trono, D., 1996, In vivo gene delivery and stable transduction of nondividing cells by a lentiviral vector. *Science* 272: 263–267.

Tashiro, T., Kaneko, T., Sugimoto, T., Nagatsu, I., Kikuchi, H., and Mizuno, N., 1989, Striatal neurons with aromatic l-amino acid decarboxylase-like immunoreactivity in the rat. *Neurosci. Lett.* 100: 29–34.

92

S 17092-1, A NEW POST-PROLINE CLEAVING ENZYME INHIBITOR: MEMORY ENHANCING EFFECTS AND SUBSTANCE P NEUROMODULATORY ACTIVITY

Pierre Lestage, Cécile Lebrun, Fabrice Iop, Anne Hugot, Nathalie Rogez, Philippe Grève, Dominique Favale, Marie-Hélène Gandon, Odile Raimbault, and Jean Lépagnol

Department of Cerebral Pathology
Institut de Recherches Servier
125, chemin de ronde
78290 Croissy sur Seine, France

INTRODUCTION

Besides acetylcholine and biogenic amines, some neuropeptides have been described for their potent biological effects and more especially for their memory enhancing properties. Among them, substance P (SP) was demonstrated as improving both learning and recall performances of rodents in a variety of memory tasks (Huston and Hasenöhrl, 1995). Other neuropeptides such as arginine-vasopressin or TRH (Dantzer et al., 1988; Giovannini et al., 1991) as well as SP (Stanfield et al., 1985; Feuerstein et al., 1996) were described as cognition enhancers with positive modulatory effects on cerebral cholinergic activity. Moreover, decreases in SP levels were reported in both cortical (Alzheimer's disease, AD) and subcortical (Parkinson's and Huntington's diseases, PD and HD) neurodegenerative diseases (Kanazawa et al., 1977; Mauborgne et al., 1983; Quigley and Kowall, 1991).

Based on these observations, the enhancement of brain neuromodulation related to certain neuropeptides could be envisaged as a promising therapeutic approach for treating the cognitive deficits associated with aging and/or neurodegenerative diseases. A common feature to the above mentioned promnesic neuropeptides is their sensitivity to a specific prolyl-targetted protease. Such an enzyme termed prolyl-endopeptidase (PEP) or post-proline cleaving enzyme (PPCE) was subsequently identified (Koida and Walter, 1976). Consequently, a PPCE inhibitor by attenuating the catabolism of neuropeptides could represent a novel therapeutical approach for the treatment of mnemocognitive deficits, associated with aging and certain neurodegenerative disorders.such as PD or HD. In this context, S 17092-1 was selected as a potent inhibitor of cerebral PPCE activity of rodents brain tissue in both *in vitro* and *in vivo* conditions (Lépagnol et al., 1996). Considering both the memory enhancing properties and cholinergic facilitatory effects of PPCE-targetted neuropeptides, notably SP, the present studies were aimed at determining whether S 17092-1 could enhance memory performances and/or prevent memory deficits. For this purpose, S 17092-1 was administered orally at PPCE inhibitory doses in the mouse (Lépagnol et al., 1996) and studied in two experimental tasks exploring different forms of memory. A spatial discrimination task was chosen in order to explore spatial reference memory in the C57bl mouse using a model based on chemically induced amnesia by scopolamine. The cognition enhancing properties of S 17092-1 were also determined with age-asociated memory deficits in the C57bl mouse by using the delayed alternation task, an expression of working memory in rodents. The present studies were also aimed at determining whether S 17092-1 could interacts with brain SP after oral administration of PPCE inhibitory doses in rodents. In this aim, neurochemical studies using radioimmunoassay (RIA) were performed in order to examine the effects of S 17092-1 on striatal SP-like immunoreactivity (SPLI) levels in the rat brain. In addition, behavioural interactions of S 17092-1 with SP were studied using a model of SP-induced grooming behaviour in NMRI mouse.This behaviour has been clearly demonstrated as specifically mediated by the striatonigral neurokininergic pathway (Katz, 1979; Van Wimersma Greidanus and Maigret, 1988; Stoessl et al., 1991).

MATERIALS AND METHODS

Animals

Procedures involving animals and their care were performed according to NIH guide for the care and the use of laboratory animals (NIH publication n° 85-23, 1985).

Young (3–5 months old) male C57bl mice (Iffa Credo) were used in the spatial discrimination test. Aged C57bl mice (21–22 months old) were used in the delayed alternation test.

Male (3 months old, 240–310g) Wistar rats (Iffa Credo) were used throughout the *in vivo* neurochemicals studies on brain SP levels.

Male NMRI mice (CER Janvier) weighing 27–33g on the day of experiments were used throughout *in vivo* behavioural studies on SP-induced grooming.

Scopolamine-Induced Amnesia in Spatial Discrimination Task in Young C57bl Mouse

The spatial discrimination test was conducted by using an elevated opened Y-maze (Imetronic, France) made of black PVC. Before experiments, mice were gradually and partially food-deprived in order to stabilize their body weight at 85% of normal values.The spatial discrimination task was conducted during 3 days. Each daily session comprised 10 trials. A learning trial was conducted as follows: after a mouse was placed on the start area of an unbaited arm, the 3 doors of the Y-maze were opened in order to allow the animals entering the goal area of one of the 2 opposite arms. The doors were closed and the mouse stayed in the chosen arm for 20s. Then, by a rotation of the maze, the animal returned to a start area for a 40 s inter-trial interval until the next trial. The entry into the baited arm followed by reward eating was noted as a correct response for the trial and the % correct choice over 10 trials per sessions was calculated for each animal. These % values were used for statistical analysis: Two-way (group x session) ANOVA with repeated measures on the session.

In order to explore the effect of oral treatment by S 17092-1 (10 mg/kg) on scopolamine-induced amnesia, the compound or vehicle (tween 80 in H_2O, 20 ml/kg) were administered during 7 days (twice daily) before the spatial memory experiment, then 60 min prior to the training sessions. A control group (n=12) was treated with the vehicle (p.o. route) and saline (i.p. route) instead of S 17092-1 and scopolamine, respectively. An amnesic group (n=14) was treated with scopolamine (0.3 mg/kg i.p. 30 min before each training session) and received the vehicle in stead of S 17092-1. A treated group (n=13) was orally treated with S 17092-1 and received scopolamine under the above mentioned conditions.

Spatial Delayed Alternation Test in Aged C57bl Mouse

All daily training sessions were conducted with a Y-shaped maze and 21–22 months old food deprived C57bl mice as described in the previous chapter. The spatial discrimination test was conducted during 4 consecutive days and 2 complementary daily session with 2 days of training interruption between the 4th and 5th session. In each daily session, the mice were submitted to 11 successivve trials. A learning session was conducted as follow: after a mouse was placed on the start area, the 3 doors of the Y-maze were opened in order to allow the animals entering the goal area of one of the 2 opposite arms and collect the food reward. The doors were closed and the mouse stayed in the chosen arm for 20 s. Then, by a rotation of the maze, the animal returned to the start area for a 20 s inter-trial interval. In each trial, except for the first, the food pellet had always to be found in the arm opposite to the one previously visited. Consequently, the animals had to alternate the arm choices in order to be rewarded. The % alternation over 10 trials (from 2th to 11th trial) per session was calculated for each animal. These % values were used for statistical analysis: Two-way (treatment x xession) ANOVA with repeated measures on the session. A group of 18 aged mice was treated orally with S 17092-1 (10 mg/kg), twice daily during 7 days before the experiments, then 60 min prior daily training sessions, included during the 2 days of training interruption. A control group (n=17) received the vehicle.

Measurement of Striatal SP-like Immunoreactivity (SPLI) in the Wistar Rat

SSPLI was measured in the Wistar rat using a standard RIA kit (Peninsula Laboratories). Each sample was incubated with 125[I]-labelled[tyr8]-SP. The bound and free peptides were separated by the addition of goat anti-rabbit iGg serum and normal rabbit serum. After 90 min at room temperature, the pellet (bound peptide) was separated by centrifugation and the radioactivity was measured. SSPLI levels were expressed as pg/mg wet tissue. For acute treatment by S 17092-1, groups of 10 rats were orally treated with S 17092-1 (1, 3, 10 or 30 mg/kg) then sacrified by decapitation 60 min later. Control group (n=10) received the vehicle. For chronic treatment by S 17092–1, groups of 10 rats were daily treated with S 17092-1 (1, 3, 10 or 30 mg/kg p.o.) during 7 days, then, sacrified by decapitation 60 min after the last administration. Control group (n=10) received the vehicle. The dose-effects of S 17092-1 on SSPLI were analysed using one way ANOVA and Dunnett's test.

SP-Induced Grooming Behaviour in NMRI Mouse

SP was injected into the right ventricle (5 µl saline/mouse) of NMRI mice (10 mice per group) at 0.5, 1, 2, 4, or 8 µg doses. Immediately after SP administration, the mice were placed individually in plexiglas boxes (10×10×10 cm) in order to observe the behaviour during 300 s. The whole duration of grooming was measured (s) and the mean values per group were calculated. S 17092–1 was orally administered at 3, 10, 30 or 100 mg/kg 60 min before the i.c.v. administration of SP (0.5 µg) and duration of grooming behaviour was measured (s). The statistical analysis was performed with one way ANOVA and Newman-Keuls test.

RESULTS

Effect of Chronic Oral Treatment by S 17092-1 on Scopolamine-Induced Amnesia in Spatial Discrimination Task in C57bl Mouse

Oral pre-treatment with S 17092-1 (10 mg/kg) during 7d (twice daily) then 60 min before each daily learning session significantly prevented the learning deficit induced by scopolamine (treatment effect, $p = 0.003$; session effect, $p = 0.001$; group x session interaction, $p = 0.646$) (Figure 1). Consequently, in the S 17092-1 treated group, learning performances were significantly greater compared to scopolamine-treated mice.

Effect of Chronic Oral Treatment by S 17092-1 on Spatial Delayed Alternation Task in Aged C57bl Mouse

Chronic oral pre-treatment with S 17092-1 (10 mg/kg) during 7d (twice daily) then 60 min before each daily training session significantly prevented the cognitive deficits associated with aging process in C57bl mouse (interaction treatment x time, $p = 0.001$) (Figure 2).

During the first 3 sessions, S 17092-1 did not modify the memory performances of treated mice compared with controls. In contrast, during the 4th session, S 17092-1 significantly increased ($p \leq 0.01$) the learning performances of aged treated mice (71.1% vs 48.2% correct responses). The cognition enhancing effect of S 17092-1 was robust as a similar value of alternation (70.0 (5.6%) was obtained in treated mice after 2 days of train-

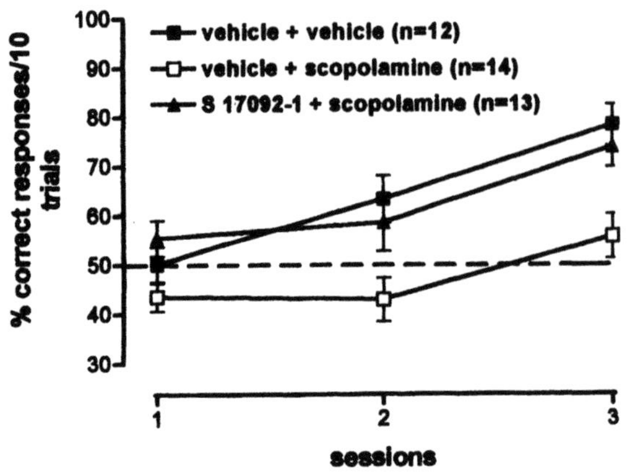

Figure 1. Effect of S 17092-1 (10 mg/kg) on scopolamine-induced amnesia in the spatial discrimination test in C57bl mouse. Values are means (±s.e.m.) % correct response over 10 trial/day session. The horizontal dotted line indicates the chance level. S 17091–1 treatment: 10 mg/kg p.o. 7 days before memory test (twice daily) then 60 min before daily training. Scopolamine treatment (0.3 mg/kg i.p.): 30 min before daily trainig. Two-way ANOVA (repeated measures on sessions): $p = 0.001$ scopolamine vs vehicle, $p = 0.03$ S 17092-1 vs scopolamine.

Figure 2. Effect of S 17092-1 (10 mg/kg p.o.) on age-associated memory deficit in a sequential reinforced alternation task in 21–22 months old C57bl mice. Animals were tested (inter-trial interval: 20s) during 4 consecutive daily session then after 72h interruption during 2 consecutive daily session. Chronic oral pre-treatment (twice daily for 7 days) with vehicle or S 17092-1 then, once daily until the end of experiment (1h before training during the memory test). Values are means (±s.e.m.) % of correct response (alternation with 20s inter-trial interval) over 10 trials/session. *: p≤0.05, **: p≤0.01 S 17092-1 vs control, two-way ANOVA with repeated measures on the session.

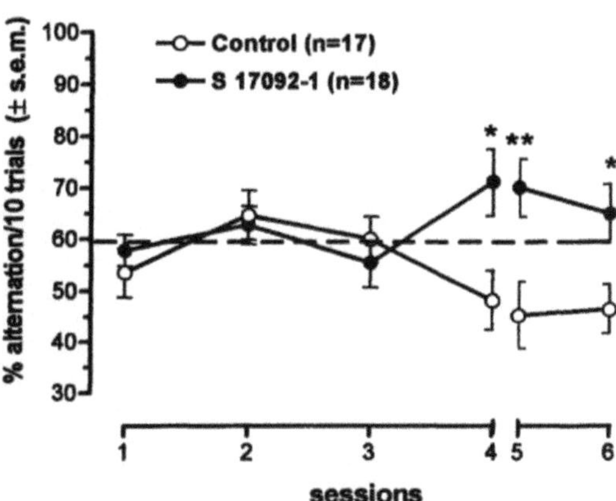

ing interruption. So, treatment with S 17092-1 maintained the memory performances at significant higher values than those of controls mice during both the 5th (p<0.001) and the 6th session (p<0.05).

Effect of Acute or Chronic Oral Treatment by S 17092-1 on Striatal SP-like Immunoreactivity Levels in the Wistar Rat

Acute oral treatment with S 17092-1 (1 to 30 mg/kg) increased, albeit non-significantly, SSPLI levels (+19%, +32% and +43% at 1, 3 and 10 mg/kg, respectively) compared with control values (Figure 3). At the highest tested dose of S 17092-1 (30 mg/kg) a significant increase of SSPLI level (+80%; p≤0.001) was observed (Figure 3).Chronic oral treatment with S 17092-1 also increased SSPLI levels. This effect was not dose-dependent, a significant effect was only observed at 10 and 30 mg/kg (+56%, p≤0.01 and +55%, p≤0.01, respectively) (Figure 3).

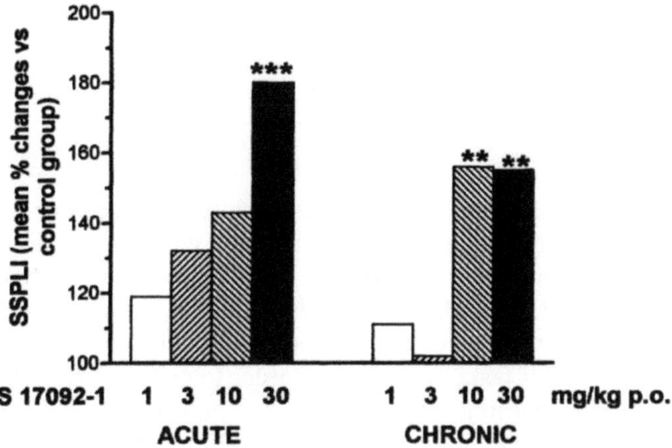

Figure 3. Effects of S 17092-1 on SSPLI levels after acute or chronic (7days) oral administration in Wistar rat. SSPLI levels were determined 60 min after the last oral administration of S 17092-1. Control groups received vehicle (tween 80 in H₂O, 20 ml/kg).Statistical analyses were performed on SSPLI values (n=10/group) with one way ANOVA and Dunnett's test. **: p<0.01, ***: p<0.001 vs. appropriate control group.

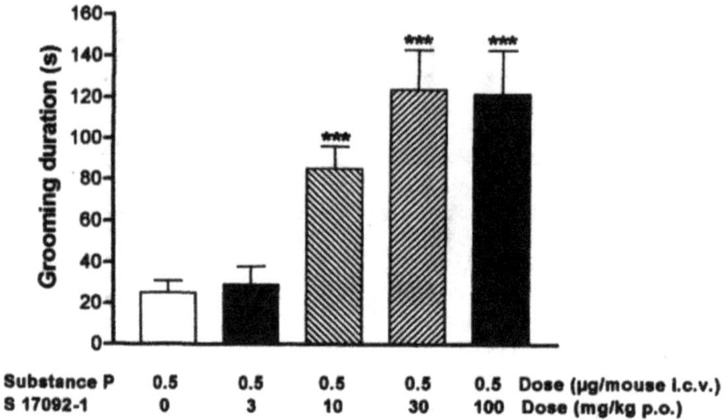

Figure 4. Potentiating effect of S 17092-1 on substance P-induced grooming behaviour after oral administration in NMRI mice. Grooming duration was measured during 5 min after i.c.v. SP injection. S 17092-1 was administered by p.o. route 60 min before SP. Values are means (s.e.m. (n=10 animals/group). ***: p<0.001, ANOVA and Newman-Keuls test.

Effect of Acute Oral Treatment by S 17092-1 on i.c.v. SP-Induced Grooming Behavior in NMRI Mouse

At 0.5 µg/mouse, SP failed to provoke a significant effect on grooming behaviour. At higher doses (1 to 8 µg/mouse) SP dose-dependently induced a significant increase of grooming duration (90 ± 17 and 167 ± 23 s for 1 and 8 µg/mouse, respectively) compared to controls.

After oral administration, S 17092-1 (3–100 mg/kg) dose-dependently potentiated the SP-induced grooming behaviour in NMRI mouse (Figure 4). At 3 mg/kg , S 17092-1 failed to modify the grooming duration induced by SP whereas at higher doses (10–100 mg/kg) S 17092-1 increased strongly and significantly (p<0.001) the duration of grooming induced by i.c.v. SP (+ 240%, + 396% and + 388 %, for 10, 30 and 100 mg/kg, respectively) (Figure 4).

DISCUSSION

Present studies demonstrated that S 17092-1 , a potent inhibitor of PPCE activity, improved learning and memory performances in both young amnesic and aged C57bl mice. In fact, the promnesic effect of S 17092-1 were observed at 10 mg/kg p.o. and this dose was clearly observed as inhibiting the brain PPCE activity by more than 50% (Lépagnol et al., 1996). Furthermore, the memory facilitating effects of S 17092-1 were evident in the 2 experimental tasks employed in order to explore different types of memory. S 17092-1 facilitated learning function related to both reference (spatial discrimination) and working (delayed alternation) memory. Taken together, these results supported the evidence that the cognition properties of S 17092-1 are intimately related to the inhibition of PPCE activity in the brain. Moreover, these results conferred to S 17092-1, a wide promnesic profile concordant with physiological clinical conditions observed in aged patients and/or in the course of neurodegenerative diseases. In fact, clinical studies have clearly demonstrated that neurodegenerative diseases are associated with marked impairment of spatial memory performances. These deficits are dramatically observed in the course of certain dementias, notably Alzheimer's or Huntington's diseases (Brown and Marsden, 1988; Adelstein et al., 1992). Experimental studies have shown that spatial memory processing could depend on cholinergic neurotransmission notably originating from basal brain nuclei (Winkler et al., 1995). Furthermore, cholinergic systems may facilitate spatial memory function by inhibiting predisposed stereotyped behaviour capable of interfering with the acquisition of spatial informations (Schallert et al., 1996). Experimental studies have demonstrated that SP positively modulate the cholinergic activity of both the basalo-cortical and septo-hippocampal pathways (Stanfield et al., 1985; Feuerstein et al., 1996). Conversely, our results (data not shown) suggest that cholinergic neurotransmission facilitated the behavioural effect of SP via nicotinic receptors since mecamylamine, a nicotinic antagonist, decreased SP-induced grooming behaviour in NMRI mice whereas scopolamine, a muscarinic receptor antagonist was devoid of any effect. In the same manner, impairment of neurokininergic pathways by specific subcortical lesions could induce memory deficits (Furtado and Mazurek, 1996) as a result of cholinergic blockade with scopolamine. All these results indicate that acetylcholine and SP are intimately associated with cognitive functions. Such a positive correlation between the two transmitters is confirmed in our studies by examination of the SP neuromodulatory activity of S 17092-1. These studies demonstrated that S 17092-1 at PPCE inhibitory doses increased the SSPLI. The increase of SPLI problably reflected an increase of SP levels in the striatum, the most enriched brain area in neurokininergic neurons. Moreover, our behavioural data on SP-induced grooming in mouse clearly indicated that S 17092-1, at PPCE inhibitory doses, could enhance the SP neuromodulation in subcortical regions such as the striatonigral pathway since SP-induced grooming in rodents have been shown to be speficically mediated by this neuronal pathway (Katz, 1979; Van Wimersma Greidanus and Maigret, 1988; Stoessl et al., 1991). In agreement, our results (data not shown) on the pharmacological characterization of SP-induced grooming behaviour in NMRI mice suggested an implication of the neurokininergic striatonigral pathway as a substrate for this behaviour. SP-induced grooming behaviour was antagonized by i.c.v injection of RP 67580, a specific NK1 receptor antagonist whereas a specific NK2 receptor antagonist (SR 48568) was devoid of any effect. Moreover , a specific D1 receptor antagonist (R(+)-SCH 23390), but not raclopride, a specific D2 antagonist, prevented, albeit partially, the grooming behaviour induced by SP. Conversely, our results suggests that the promnesic activities of S 17092-1 could be partially related to a facilitatory effect on brain SP neuromodulation via PPCE inhibition.

In conclusion, S 17092-1 could be envisaged as a potential therapeutical agent for the treatment of cognitive disorders associated with cerebral aging and for the symptomatic treatment of certain cortical (AD) or subcortical neurodegenerative diseases (PD, HD) in which pronounced changes in SP levels were recently reported.

REFERENCES

Adelstein, T.B., Kesner, R.P., and Strassberg, D.S., 1992, Spatial recognition and spatial order memory in patients with dementia of the Alzheimer's type, *Neuropsychologia* 30:59–67.

Brown, R.G., and Marsden, C.D., 1988, « Subcortical dementia »: The neuropsychological evidence, *Neuroscience* 25:363–387

Dantzer, R., Koob, G.F., Bluthe, R., and Le Moal, M., 1988, Septal vasopressin modulates social memory in male rats, *Brain Res.* 457:143–147.

Feuerstein, T.J., Gleichauf, O., and Landwehrmeyer, G.B., 1996, Modulation of cortical acetylcholine release by serotonin: the role of substance P interneurons, *Arch Pharmacol.* 354:618–626.

Furtado, J.C.S., and Mazurek, M.F., 1996, Behavioral characterization of quinolinate-induced lesions of the medial striatum: relevance for Huntington's disease, *Exp. Neurol.* 138:158–168.

Giovannini, M.G., Casamenti, F., Nistri, A., Paoli, F., and Pepeu, G., 1991, Effect of thyrotrophin releasing hormone (TRH) on acetylcholine release from different brain areas investigated by microdialysis, *Br. J. Pharmacol.* 102:363–368.

Huston, J.P., and Hasenöhrl, R.U., 1995, The role of neuropeptides in learning: focus on the neurokinin substance P, *Behav. Brain Res.* 66:117–127.

Kanazawa, I., Bird, E.D., O'Connell, R., and Powell, D., 1977, Evidence for a decrease in substance P content of substantia nigra in Huntington's chorea, *Brain Res.* 119:447–453.

Katz, R.J., 1979, Central injection of substance P elicits grooming behaviour and motor inhibition in mice, *Neurosci. Lett.* 12:133–136.

Koida, M., and Walter, R., 1976, Post-proline cleaving enzyme, *J. Biol. Chem.* 251:7593–7599.

Lépagnol, J., Lebrun, C., Morain, P., De Nanteuil, G., and Heidet, V., 1996, Cognition enhancing effects of S 17092-1, a potent and long acting inhibitor of post-proline cleaving enzyme (PPCE), *Soc. Neurosc. Abstr.* 22:142.

Mauborgne, A., Javoy-Agid, F., Legrand, J.C., Agid, Y., and Cesselin, F., 1983, Decrease of substance P-like immunoreactivity in the substantia nigra and pallidum in Parkinsonian brains, *Brain Res.* 268:167–170.

Quigley, B.J., and Kowall, N.W., 1991, Substance P-like immunoreactive neurons are depleted in Alzheimer's disease cerebral cortex, *Neuroscience* 41:41–60.

Schallert, T., Day, L.B., Weisend, M., and Sutherland, R.J., 1996, Spatial learning by hippocampal rats in the morris water task, *Soc. Neurosci. Abstr.* 22:678.

Stanfield, P.R., Nakajima, Y., and Yamaguchi, K., 1985, Substance P raises neuronal membrane excitability by reducing inward rectification, *Nature* 315:498–501.

Stoessl, A.J., Szczutkowski, C., Glenn, B., and Wtason, I., 1991, Behavioural effects of selective tachykinin agonists in midbrain dopamine regions, *Brain Res.* 565:254–262.

Van Wimersma Greidanus, T.B., and Maigret, C., 1988, Grooming behaviour induced by substance P, *Eur. J. Pharmacol.* 15:217–220.

Winkler, J., Suhr, S.T., Gage, F.H., Thal, L.J., and Fisher, L.J., 1995, Essential role of neocortical acetylcholine in spatial memory, *Nature* 375:484–487.

93

AGE DEPENDENCE OF MUSCARINIC PLASTICITY IN THE RAT HIPPOCAMPUS

J. M. Auerbach and M. Segal

Department of Neurobiology
The Weizmann Institute
Rehovot 76100, Israel

INTRODUCTION

Acetylcholine (ACh) is a member of a group of diffuse neurotransmitters which are not likely to convey precise information, but modulate reactivity of affected neurons to stimulation of other afferents. This can be achieved by changing K^+ or calcium ion channel kinetics, thereby changing excitability of the cell, by affecting release of fast neurotransmitters, or by second messenger interactions with the fast postsynaptic neurotransmitter receptors. The intuitive significance of ACh becomes evident following selective degeneration or drug treatment, resulting in severe loss of brain functions (Buresove et al., 1964, Bartus et al., 1982, Molchan et al., 1992), as is the case in Alzheimer's Disease (AD). Despite extensive research, the role of ACh at the cellular and molecular levels of cognitive functions is still unclear. In the present review, we will describe some novel actions of ACh, which may be related to the putative role of ACh in LTP, learning and memory, all of which are greatly diminished in aged brains.

The cholinergic innervation of the hippocampus arises solely from the medial septum and diagonal band of Broca (Milner et al., 1983, Lewis and Shute, 1967, Mellegren and Srebro, 1973). These are heterogeneous nuclei which also contain GABAergic neurons, also shown to innervate the hippocampus. Early stimulation and recording studies, being unaware of the complexity of the septohippocampal pathway, are likely to have obtained erroneous results due to stimulation of GABAergic fibers to the hippocampus, along with the cholinergic fibers. The cholinergic fibers, while not as precisely localized as the fast excitatory fibers arising from the entorhinal cortex and the commissural association pathway, are not at all diffuse throughout the hippocampus- a high concentration of fibers are seen in stratum oriens of CA1 as well as the dentate hilus (Milner et al., 1983, Lewis and Shute, 1967, Mellegren and Srebro, 1973).

Progress in Alzheimer's and Parkinson's Diseases
edited by Fisher *et al.*, Plenum Press, New York, 1998.

CHOLINERGIC ACTIONS IN THE HIPPOCAMPUS

There are five known subtypes of the muscarinic receptor expressed in mammalian brain, M1-M5 (Hulme et al., 1990, Levey et al. 1995, Waelbroeck et al., 1990). The main muscarinic receptor in the hippocampus, M1, is highly concentrated in stratum radiatum and oriens of CA1, whereas M2 receptor is concentrated in stratum oriens. The differential distribution of M1 receptors and the cholinergic fibers, stained for acetylcholine esterase (AChE), represents one of the classical cases of 'mismatch' of fibers/receptors, which has no simple explanation: Why is there such a high concentration of M1 receptors in an area which has few cholinergic fibers? The fact that M1 is a low affinity receptor, which may never 'see' ACh released from its terminals, due to a diffusion distance and a fast breakdown of ACh by AChE, certainly complicates interpretation of studies on the action of ACh or carbachol (CCh) applied by perfusion onto hippocampal slices, as described below.

ACh, acting on muscarinic receptors in the hippocampus causes blockade of several potassium currents including a voltage and calcium-gated potassium current which underlies the slow afterhyperpolarization (I_{AHP}), a depolarization evoked sustained K^+ current (I_M), and a resting leak K^+ current (I_L) (Cole and Nicoll, 1983, Madison et al., 1987, Dutar and Nicoll, 1988, Muller and Misgeld 1989). Blockade of these conductances results in depolarization of the cell, increase in input resistance, and enhancement of spontaneous activity and, perhaps, enhanced reactivity to afferent stimulation. Other reports suggest that ACh may actually facilitate a K^+ current (I_K (Zhang et al., 1992)). In addition, the muscarinic agonist CCh is reported to modulate a calcium dependent inward current (Fisher and Johnston, 1990, Segal, 1989). One effect of particular interest is the ACh-induced suppression of the excitatory postsynaptic potentials (EPSP) evoked by stimulation of the Schaffer collateral/commissural fibers (Segal, 1982, Segal, 1989, Sheridan and Sutar, 1990). This effect is assumed to be mediated by presynaptic muscarinic receptors. We have recently suggested that this inhibitory effect of CCh on synaptic potentials is likely to be mediated by an M3 receptor (Auerbach and Segal, 1996). These effects can be seen in most hippocampal neurons with relatively high concentrations of CCh, and are blocked by atropine. The receptor types associated with the various muscarinic effects of CCh are not entirely clear; the blockade of I_M and I_L are probably mediated by a muscarinic M1 receptor, and the blockade of I_{AHP} by an M2 receptor (Dutar and Nicoll, 1988, Muller and Misgeld 1989), but the lack of highly specific ligands for most of the muscarinic receptors hampers further progress in this field.

ACh activates second messenger systems involving phospholipases, protein kinase C, and inositol trisphosphate (IP_3) (Smith et al., 1989), as well as blockade of production of cAMP by M2, M4 receptors (McKinney et al., 1991). These, in turn, may release calcium from internal stores which can act on a number of secondary cellular processes. ACh can also cause a rise of intracellular calcium ($[Ca]i$) simply by closing potassium channels, allowing the membrane to depolarize and activate voltage-gated calcium currents (Muller and Connor, 1991). These actions will trigger several postsynaptic calcium-related, second messenger processes.

We have recently described a fast onset, selective potentiation of reactivity of hippocampal neurons to application of the glutamate agonist N-methyl D-aspartate (NMDA). This was the first demonstration of an interaction between a slow and a fast neurotransmitter, at the second messenger level in the hippocampus. The cholinergic potentiation of NMDA responses is assumed to involve activation of the IP_3 cascade (Markram and Segal,1990, 1992), and is mediated by an M2 receptor. It may function to enhance the

NMDA component of the EPSP, and allow more calcium to flow into the cell, and initiate calcium dependent plasticity. This effect is short lasting, and a recovery of NMDA responses was seen immediately following removal of the cholinergic stimulation (Markram and Segal, 1992).

ACETYLCHOLINE AND NEURONAL PLASTICITY

Insight into the role of ACh in the cellular and molecular aspects of plasticity has been gained by examining the effects of ACh on LTP. In the dentate gyrus of rat hippocampus, muscarinic activation facilitates LTP induction (Burgard and Sarvey, 1990) and physostigmine, an inhibitor of AChE, causes potentiation of population spikes resembling LTP (Ito et al., 1988, Levkovitz and Segal, 1994). The situation becomes more complex, as in area CA3-mossy fiber system, low concentrations of CCh suppress tetanus-induced LTP (Maeda et al., 1993, Williams and Johnston, 1988) via activation of a high affinity M2 receptor. In these same neurons, activation of M1 receptors facilitates LTP induction. This effect is opposite to that seen in the dentate gyrus and area CA1 (below), probably related to the fact that LTP in the mossy fiber system is mediated by different mechanisms from those in the other areas, most likely via presynaptic modulation of transmitter release.

In area CA1, CCh can enhance LTP (Blitzer et al., 1990) and the muscarinic antagonist atropine can suppress associative LTP (Sokolov and Kleschevenikov, 1995). Cholinergically induced rhythmic activity, obtained with higher concentrations of CCh, can enhance plasticity of neurons in response to afferent stimulation (Huerta and Lisman, 1993). It has also been suggested that anticholinergic drugs suppress the ability of area CA1 to express LTP (Hiratsu et al., 1989).

ACETYLCHOLINE AND LTPm

We have recently found that bath application of low concentrations (0.2–0.5µM) of CCh induces long term potentiation (LTP) of reactivity to afferent stimulation in the hippocampus (Auerbach and Segal, 1994, Fig. 1). This muscarinic LTP (LTPm) sharply contrasts

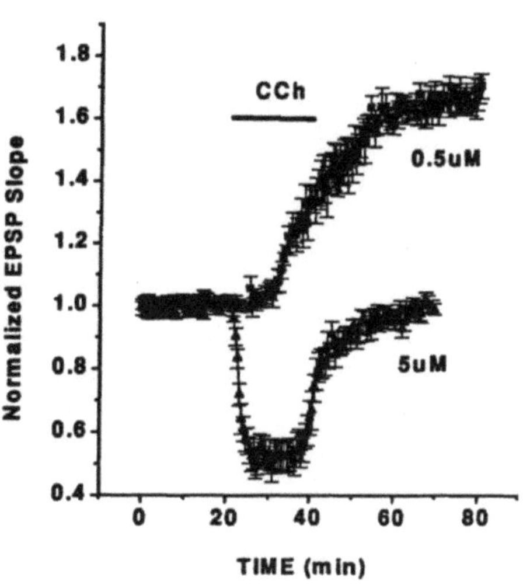

Figure 1. Dose dependent effects of CCh on reactivity of hippocampal CA1 cells to afferent stimulation. Extracellularly recorded population EPSP slopes are plotted before, during and after perfusion of the slice with either 0.5µM or 5µM CCh. The lower concentration of CCh produces a slow onset, long lasting enhancement of population EPSP slope, whereas the higher concentration of CCh produces a fast onset, fast recovery of depression of the EPSP. Ordinate EPSP slope, relative to control, predrug level. Abscissa, time. (Modified from Auerbach and Segal, 1996.)

with the response to a higher concentration of CCh, resulting in inhibition of the EPSP (Fig. 1). In fact it looks as if the two effects of CCh are mediated by totally different mechanisms. LTPm depends on cholinergic stimulation for its initiation but not for its maintenance, as it is sustained long after CCh is removed from the medium (Auerbach and Segal, 1994). LTPm is independent of activation of an NMDA receptor, as it can be produced in the presence of the NMDA antagonist 2-APV. However, it shares similarities with tetanic LTP which lie downstream of the involvement of the NMDA receptor in LTP induction e.g. application of an even lower CCh concentration (0.1 μM CCh), while having no observable effect of its own, reduces the threshold for tetanic LTP induction. Furthermore, saturation of the tetanic LTP mechanism occludes the ability of CCh to produce LTPm, and vice versa, indicating that the two types of stimulation share the same downstream mechanism.

LTPm is likely to be mediated by a genuine long term change in postsynaptic reactivity to activation of the AMPA receptor, and not by a presynaptic change in fiber excitability or release properties, as indicated by the responses to paired pulse stimulation and by the lack of change in presynaptic volley (Auerbach and Segal, 1996). Moreover, cells in the hippocampus expressed a prolonged enhancement of their reactivity to AMPA following a exposure to CCh, whereas they did enhance their reactivity to NMDA only transiently, as seen before (Auerbach and Seegal, 1996, Markram and Segal, 1992). This indicates that CCh may exert its action through some interaction with a second messenger system, which modulates the AMPA receptor. Interestingly, this second messenger interaction takes a fairly long time to develop, unlike the interaction with the NMDA receptor. In an attempt to begin deciphering this second messenger system, we first found that LTPm is dependent on a rise of intracellular calcium, but not on an influx of calcium into the cell during exposure to the drug (Auerbach and Segal, 1994). Next, we found that LTPm is likely to involve protein phophorylation as it is blocked by antagonists of both a serine/threonine kinase (H7), (ibid) and a tyrosine kinase (e.g. genestein, Auerbach and Segal, unpublished observations).

The pharmacology of LTPm was studied alongside the inhibition of EPSP produced by the higher concentration of CCh (Auerbach and Segal, 1996). The latter effect is mediated by an M3 receptor, as it was blocked by the M3 antagonist 4-DAMP (Marchi and Raiteri, 1989). LTPm was unaffected by M1 agonists or antagonists, but was blocked by methoctramine or AFDX-116, both M2 antagonists (Waelbroeck et al., 1990).

Interestingly, once the inhibition produced by higher concentration of CCh was blocked by 4-DAMP, no LTPm surfaced. If indeed LTPm is activated by an high affinity M2 receptor, why should it not be activated when the inhibitory effect, mediated by a lower affinity M3 receptor is blocked? These results indicate that there may be another player in this interaction of CCh with hippocampal neurons in the slice. One important candidate for such an interaction are the interneurons of the hippocampus, particularly those residing in stratum oriens of CA1 (Pitler and Alger, 1992). These have been shown to be innervated by cholinergic fibers of septal origin, and to possess a variety of muscarinic receptors. Blockade of GABAergic inhibition uncovered LTPm in response to high concentration of CCh (Auerbach and Segal, 1996). It appears that high CCh concentration (5 μM) may have activated interneurons which shunt the ability of the pyramidal neurons to express LTPm.

The long lasting change in efficacy of transmission in the schaffer collateral/commissural input to CA1 pyramidal neurons, produced by exposure to low concentration of CCh, is, by and large, the closest association of ACh with neuronal plasticity in the brain i.e., LTPm is long lasting, as is tetanic LTP and in fact, it shares downstream mechanisms with tetanic LTP.

LTPm AND AGING

A unique property of LTPm, which relates brain cholinergic association with learning and memory is that slices taken from aged rats totally lack LTPm (Auerbach and Segal, unpublished observations). By comparison with other reported cholinergic deficits in aged rats (Bartus et al. 1982), this effect is striking indeed, and may underly the inability of aged rats to learn spatial cognitive tasks. By contrast, the suppressive action of high CCh on synaptic responses remains intact in the aged brain. Once again, the lack of LTPm is not the only lost plastic property of aged brains. Slices taken from aged brains express a lower level of long lasting LTP, and when compared with tetanic LTP expressed in young rats, it is evident that a slow component of LTP is the one to be markedly reduced in aged rats. A major part of the slow onset tetanic LTP is an NMDA-independent component, which can be activated by repeated tetanic stimulations in the presence of an NMDA antagonist, 2-APV. We then found that aged slices are particularly deficient in non-NMDA LTP.

In searching for the cause of these differences between young and aged rats, we realized that in the aged rat brain there is a marked shift in the balance between production and breakdown of hydrogen peroxide (H_2O_2), resulting in an increase in ambient H_2O_2. Indeed, low concentrations of H_2O_2 caused a marked reduction in non-NMDA LTP, and a total suppression of LTPm. Conversely, treatment of aged slices with catalase, which shifts the balance towards a reduction in ambient H_2O_2 led to a restoration of LTPm and non-NMDA LTP in aged rats. These studies link the known oxidative stress in aged brains with specific functional deficits in these brains.

In summary, the present results bridge the gap between the cholinergic involvement in memory, and the physiological action of ACh at the single cell level. The selective loss of a specific cholinergic function in the aged rat hippocampus, and the involvement of oxidative metabolism in this function link the cholinergic innervation of the hippocampus to oxidative metabolism, know to be most sensitive to aging processes

REFERENCES

Auerbach, J. M. and Segal, M., 1994, A novel cholinergic induction of long-term potentiation in rat hippocampus. *J. Neurophys.* 72:2034–2040.

Auerbach, J. M. and Segal, M., 1996, Muscarinic Receptors Mediating Depression and Long-Term Potentiation in Rat Hippocampus. *J. Physiology* (London) 492:479–493.

Bartus, R. T., Reginald, L., Dean, R. L., Beer, B. and Lippa, A. S., 1982, The cholinergic hypothesis of geriatric memory dysfunction. *Science* 217: 08–417.

Blitzer, R. D., Gil, O. and Landau, E. M. 1990, Cholinergic stimulation enhances long-term potentiation in the CA1 region of rat hippocampus. *Neurosci. Lett.* 119:207–210.

Buresova, O., Bures, J., Bohdanecky, Z. and Weiss, T., 1964, The effect of atropine on learning, extinction, retention and retrieval in rats. *Psychopharmacologia* 5:255–263.

Burgard, E. C. and Sarvey, J. M., 1990, Muscarinic receptor activation facilitates the induction of long-term potentiation (LTP) in the rat dentate gyrus. *Neurosci. Lett.* 116:34–39.

Cole, A. E. and Nicoll, R. A., 1983, Acetylcholine mediates a slow synaptic potential in hippocampal pyramidal cells. *Science* 221:1299–1301.

Dutar, P. and Nicoll, R., 1988, Classification of Muscarinic responses in hippocampus in terms of receptor subtypes and second-messenger systems: electrophysiological studies *in vitro. J. Neurosci.* 8:4214–4224.

Fisher R. and Johnston D. 1990, Differential modulation of single voltage-gated calcium channels by cholinergic and adrenergic agonists in adult hippocampal neurons. *J. Neurophysiol.* 64:1291–1302.

Hirotsu I. Hori N. Katsuda N. and Ishihara T. 1989, Effects of anticholinergic drug on long term potentiation in rat hippocampal slices. *Brain Res.* 482:194–197.

Huerta, P. T. and Lisman, J. E. 1993, Heightened synaptic plasticity of hippocampal CA1 neurons during a cholinergically induced rhythmic state. *Nature* 364:723–725.

Hulme, E. C., Birdsall, N. J. M. and Buckley, N. J., 1990, Muscarinic receptor sybtypes. *Ann. Revi. Pharmacol. Toxicol.* 30:633–673.

Ito, T., Miura, Y., and Kadokawa, T., 1988, Physostigmine induces in rats a phenomenon resembling long-term potentiation. *Eur. J. Pharm.* 156:351–359.

Levey, A. I., Edmunds, S. M., Koliatsos, V., Wiley, R. G. and Heilman, C. G., 1995, Expression of m1-m4 muscarinic acetylcholine receptor proteins in rat hippocampus and regulation by cholinergic innervation. *J. Neurosci.* 15:4077–4092

Levkovitz, Y. and Segal, M., 1994, Acetylcholine mediates the effects of fenfluramine on dentate granule cell excitability in the rat. *Eur. J. Pharmacol.* 264:279–284.

Lewis, P. R. and Shute, C. C. D., 1967, The cholinergic limbic system: projection to hippocampal formation, medial cortex, nuclei of the ascending cholinergic reticular system and the subfornical organ and supraoptic crest. *Brain Res.* 90:521–539.

Madison, D. V., Lancaster, B. and Nicoll, R. A., 1987, Voltage clamp analysis of cholinergic action in the hippocampus. *J. Neurosci.* 7: 733–741.

Maeda T. Kaneko S. and Satoh M., 1993, Bidirectional modulation of long term potentiation by carbachol via M1 and M2 muscarinic receptors in guinea pig hippocampal mossy fiber CA3 synapses *Brain Res.* 619:324–330.

Marchi, M. and Raiteri, M., 1989, Interaction acetylcholine-glutamate in rat hippocampus: Involvement of two subtypes of M-2 muscarinic receptors. *J. Pharmacol. Exp. Ther.* 248:1255–1260.

Markram, H. and Segal, M., 1990, Long-lasting facilitation of excitatory postsynaptic potentials in the rat hippocampus by Acetylcholine. *J. Physiol.* 427:381–393.

Markram, H., and Segal, M., 1992, The inositol 1,4,5-trisphosphate pathway mediates cholinergic potentiation of rat hippocampal neuronal responses to NMDA. *J. Physiol.* 447:513–533.

McKinney, M., Miller, J. H., Gibson, V. A., Nickelson, L. and Aksoy, S., 1991, Interaction of agonists with M2 and M4 muscariniic receptor subtypes mediating cyclic AMP inhibition. *Mol. Pharmacol.* 40:014–1022.

Mellgren, S. I. and Srebo, B., 1973, Changes in acetylcholinesterase and distribution of degenerating fibers in the hippocampal region after septal lesions in the rat. *Brain Res.* 52:19–36.

Milner, T. A., Loy, R. and Amaral, D. G., 1983, An anatomical study of the development of the septo-hippocampal projection in the rat. *Dev. Brain Res.* 8:343–371.

Molchan, S. E., Martinez, R. A., Hill, J. L., Weingartner, H. J., Thompson, K., Vitiello, B. and Sunderland, T., 1992, Increased cognitive sensitivity to scopolamine with age and a perspective on the scopolamine model. *Brain Res. Rev.* 17:215–226.

Muller, W., Misgeld, U., 1989, Carbachol and pirenzepine discriminate effects mediated by two muscarinic receptor subtypes on hippocampal neurons in vitro. *Experientia* 57:114–122.

Muller W. and Connor J.A. 1991, Cholinergic input uncouples Ca+2 changes from K+ conductance activation and amplifies intradendritic Ca+2 changes in hippocampal neurons. *Neuron* 6:901–905.

Pitler, T. A. and Alger, B. E., 1992, Cholinergic excitation of GABAergic interneurons in the rat hippocampal slice. *J. Physiol.* 450:127–142.

Segal, M. 1982, Multiple actions of Acetylcholine at a muscarinic receptor studied in the rat hippocampal slice. *Brain Res.* 246:77–87.

Segal, M., 1989, Presynaptic cholinergic inhibition in hippocampal cultures. *Synapse* 4:305–312.

Smith, C. J., Court, J. A., Keith, A. B., and Perry, E. K., 1989, Increases in muscarinic stimulated hydrolysis of inositol phospholipids in rat hippocampus following cholinergic deafferentation are not paralelled by alteration in cholinergic receptor density. *Brain Res.* 485:317–324.

Sheridan, R. D. and Sutor, B., 1990, Presynaptic M_1 muscarinic cholinoceptors mediate inhibition of excitatory synaptic transmission in the hippocampus *in vitro*. *Neurosci. Lett.* 108:273–278.

Sokolov, M. V. and Kleschevnikov, A. M., 1995, Atropine suppresses associative LTP in the CA1 region of rat hippocampal slices. *Brain Res.* 672:281–284.

Waelbroeck, M., Tastenoy, M., Camus, J. and Christophe, J., 1990, Binding of selective antagonists to four muscarinic receptors (M_1 to M_4) in rat forebrain. *Mol. Pharmacol.* 38:267–273.

Zhang L. Weiner J.L. and Carlen P.L., 1992, Muscarinic potentiation of Ik in hippocampal neurons: electrophysiological characterization of the signal transduction pathway. *J. Neurosci.* 12: 4510–20.

94

MODELS OF CHOLINERGIC DEGENERATION: AF64A AND 192-IgG-SAPORIN

Thomas J. Walsh

Department of Psychology
Rutgers University
New Brunswick, New Jersey 08903

INTRODUCTION

Selective toxins have been widely used in neurobiology to unravel the molecular, cellular, anatomical, and physiological correlates of brain organization and function. They have also been used to examine the cellular events that contribute to neurodegeneration and to model neurodegenerative diseases. Cholinergic neurons in the basal forebrain are affected early in the course of Alzheimer's disease (AD) and their compromise is related to the severity of cognitive symptoms (reviewed in Walsh and Chrobak, 1991). Therefore, neurotoxins selective for cholinergic neurons should be useful tools to explore the functional biology of cholinergic systems and to model diseases of cholinergic hypofunction such as AD. The focus of this chapter is on how two specific neurotoxins, AF64A (ethylcholine mustard aziridinium) and 192-IgG-saporin, have been used to study aspects of AD. The behavioral effects of these compounds have been reviewed elsewhere (Walsh et al., 1994; 1996). Both of these compounds offer unique advantages and disadvantages to the investigator. Their careful use should provide complimentary information about: (i) the cellular and molecular mechanisms responsible for degeneration of cholinergic neurons; (ii) the functional consequences of that degeneration, and (iii) potential targets for therapeutic intervention that might retard or prevent neurodegeneration and/or promote survival of cholinergic neurons in early stages of degeneration.

ALZHEIMER'S DISEASE AND ANIMAL MODELS

AD is the most common age-related dementia. Its incidence doubles with each decade after the age of 65 and current estimates indicate that over 45% of the population over the age of 85 are affected (Cooper, 1991; Evans et al., 1989). With a limited understanding

Progress in Alzheimer's and Parkinson's Diseases
edited by Fisher *et al.*, Plenum Press, New York, 1998.

of etiology and no accepted therapies to prevent or treat the disease it is clear that AD represents a world-wide public health crisis. Research efforts focused on understanding the causes of AD and potential treatments are vital to insure the health and quality of life of the rapidly expanding 'graying' segment of our population.

CHOLINERGIC HYPOTHESIS OF ALZHEIMER'S DISEASE

The 'cholinergic hypothesis' of dementia has helped to organize a thematic research effort, test specific hypotheses, and develop new therapies. The 'cholinergic hypothesis' is based upon a wealth of evidence that links the decrease in cholinergic indices and degeneration of cholinergic neurons in the basal forebrain to the prevailing cognitive symptoms of AD (i.e., loss of episodic memory). The significance of these changes are highlighted by the significant correlation between: (i) cholinergic deficits; (ii) amyloid plaques; (iii) neurofibrillary tangles; and (iv) cognitive impairments (reviewed in Walsh and Opello, 1994). In addition, recent evidence indicates that damage to cholinergic neurons affects the expression and processing of ß-amyloid in the brain (Wallace et al., 1993). Therefore, the characteristic changes in ß-amyloid which occur in AD might be related to a primary cholinergic lesion.

Animal models promote an integrated study of the brain-behavior relationships that are affected in neurodegenerative diseases like AD. A logical strategy for developing an animal model of AD is to focus on the symptoms of episodic memory loss and changes in pre- and post-synaptic cholinergic function. Two cholinergic toxins have been used to study the role of the cholinergic system in AD; AF64A and 192-IgG-saporin (SAP).

AF64A (ETHYLCHOLINE MUSTARD AZIRIDINIUM)

AF64A targets the central events that regulate the synthesis of acetylcholine (ACh). Choline is taken into the cholinergic nerve terminal by high affinity choline transport (HAChT) and once inside it is acetylated by choline acetyltransferase (ChAT) to form ACh. AF64A is a cytotoxic analog of choline that combines a choline-like structure (ie., ethylcholine), that is recognized by the HAChT system, with a highly reactive cytotoxic aziridinium ring. Due to its structural similarity to choline, AF64A is taken into the terminal by the HAChT system and once inside the terminal the highly reactive aziridinium induces cholinergic hypofunction and the death of the cell (reviewed in Hörtnagl and Hanin, 1992; Hanin, 1996). Intraventricular (icv) injection of AF64A in rats produces a persistent cholinergic hypofunction in which all measures of presynaptic cholinergic function are decreased (ie., regional concentrations of ACh, the activity of ChAT, HAChT, K^+- and ouabain-stimulated release of ACh from hippocampal slices). The mechanisms of cell death are still under investigation but they probably involve the generation of oxidative stress and its impact on nucleic acid function (see below). The time course and specificity of AF64A are reviewed by Hanin (1996), and Walsh and Opello (1994).

AF64A appears to produce a series of toxic events in cholinergic neurons that culminate in chronic disability of the neuron or cell death. The earliest stage of toxicity involves a concentration-dependent interaction with the HAChT system located on cholinergic nerve terminals. At low concentrations (< 5 μM) AF64A competes with choline at the HAChT system for uptake into the terminal. Preventing AF64A from gaining access to the HAChT system with high levels of choline or with hemicholinium-3 averts the cholinotoxic effects of AF64A as well as the behavioral impairments that result from this compound (see Walsh and Opello, 1994). High concentrations > 22.5 µM of AF64A alkylate the proteins comprising the transport system which rapidly inhibits HAChT and prevents AF64A from gaining access to the inside of the terminal.

Once inside the cholinergic nerve terminal AF64A disrupts enzymes that use choline as a substrate such as ChAT, choline kinase, choline dehydrogenase and acetylcholinesterase, by alkylating their catalytic sites. This results in a persistent presynaptic cholinergic hypofunction in which all measures of ACh synthesis and release are affected. Enzymes that do not use choline as a substrate including alcohol dehydrogenase, lactate dehydrogenase, carboxypeptidase A, and chymotrypsinogen are not affected by AF64A even at concentrations that almost completely inhibit ChAT, choline kinase, and acetylcholinesterase activity in a cholinergic cell line (Barlow and Marchbanks, 1984; Sandberg et al., 1985).

The mechanisms that underlie AF64A-induced cell death have only recently been explored. There is now substantial evidence that AF64A produces oxidative stress which contributes to the degeneration of cholinergic neurons. Gulyaeva and colleagues (1996) reported that bilateral icv injection of AF64A increased a number of direct indices of oxidative stress measured in cerebral cortex, hippocampus and the rest of the brain, 1, 3, or 5 days after surgery. Thiobarbituric acid reactive species, a measure of free radical production, were elevated in AF64A-treated rats under basal conditions and 30 min and 60 min following the addition of $FeSO_4$ and sodium ascorbate. It was interesting to note that surgery itself, regardless of whether rats received AF64A or vehicle icv, also increased the basal levels of TBARS. However, the increase was more pronounced in the AF64A group and it appeared earlier. An increase in superoxide scavenging activity was also evident in the hippocampus of AF64A-treated rats up to 4 months following surgery. The increased superoxide scavenging activity observed in the hippocampus of AF64A-treated rats probably reflects a compensatory response to oxidative stress. Therefore, AF64A produces a long-lasting increase in oxidative stress in the hippocampus. This observation is consistent with several reports demonstrating that the anti-oxidant Vitamin E can attenuate both the cholinergic hypofunction and the memory impairments induced by AF64A (Johnson et al., 1988; Wortwein et al., 1994). There is also evidence that oxidative stress is a critical event that contributes to the neurodegenerative phenomenon observed in AD (Smith et al., 1997) and that Vitamin E might impede the progression of the disease (Sano et al., 1997).

The final phase of AF64A toxicity (ie., cell death) might relate to the effects of the compound on nucleic acid function and the transcription of genes involved in the production of ACh or in the survival of cholinergic neurons. AF64A is structurally similar to nitrogen mustard, an anti-cancer agent that produces cytotoxicity by alkylating specific sites on nuclear DNA and thereby inhibiting gene expression and cell replication. Hanin and colleagues recently demonstrated that AF64A produces concentration-dependent DNA strand breaks and premature termination of RNA transcription in cultured mouse leukemia cells (Futscher et al., 1992). It will be important to determine whether the changes in nucleic acid function represent a direct effect of AF64A or a consequence of oxidative stress. The effects of AF64A on gene expression are reviewed by Hanin (this book).

DISADVANTAGES OF AF64A

Like all biological tools AF64A is useful for addressing a restricted set of specific questions. It offers advantages and limitations. The primary limitations are that its cholinospecificity is evident over a very limited dose-response range. A corollary of this is that

AF64A can only be injected into the ventricles and not into specific neuronal sites. A very high concentration of AF64A in a restricted area will probably result in the compound being taken up into a variety of non-cholinergic cells by the ubiquitous low affinity choline transport system. The result would be a general cytotoxicity evidenced by non-specific morphological damage. In fact, icv injection of high doses of AF64A do produce non-specific tissue damage (McGurk et al., 1987). A consequence of this narrow dose-response is that low doses of AF64A (<3.0 nmoles bilateral) that guarantee cholinergic selectivity produce only a partial loss of cholinergic function; typically 30–50%. Therefore, while AF64A can produce a graded dose-related decrease in cholinergic parameters it can not produce more than a 50% loss of cholinergic function. This is problematic since a 50% decrease in a specific parameter might not represent a functional deficit due to the extent of plasticity observed in many systems. For example, the symptoms of Parkinson's disease do not emerge until more than 80% of the dopamine neurons in the substantia nigra are lost. In addition, it is impossible to use a 'partial lesion' to model the consequences of the extensive cholinergic loss observed in the late stages of AD.

An additional consideration is that icv injection of AF64A produces a select anatomical profile of toxicity. Following icv injection AF64A produces a dose-related compromise of the septohippocampal cholinergic system but a sparing of cholinergic innervation of the cortex and the cholinergic interneurons in the striatum. Therefore, AF64A cannot reproduce the widespread loss of both cortical and hippocampal cholinergic function that is observed in AD.

ADVANTAGES OF AF64A

AF64A is a useful tool to selectively compromise the cholinergic innervation of the hippocampus. This can be exploited to: (i) explore the biological and behavioral properties of this brain system; (ii) examine strategies to limit, attenuate, or reverse the functional consequences of damage to this system; (iii) determine the plasticity of this and interacting brain systems following selective insult; and finally (iv) model the functional deficits which occur following damage to this particular system in neurological disorders such as AD.

AF64A also produces a protracted time course of cholinergic degeneration which evolves over several weeks. Therefore, AF64A provides an important model of cholinergic degeneration in which the cellular events that contribute to cell death can be studied. For example, does oxidative stress produce the changes in gene expression and genotoxicity reported by Hanin and colleagues, or are these events independent? Does AF64A produce a sequential series of toxic events or parallel toxic events that lead to cell death? The time course of degeneration also offers a window of opportunity in which neuroprotective strategies can be evaluated. In this regard, anti-oxidants and neurotrophic factors have been successfully used to prevent or limit the cholinergic toxicity of AF64A (see Walsh et al., 1994). Unraveling the sequence of cellular events that produce this degeneration should cast light on the pathophysiological processes at work in AD and also it might suggest new targets for therapeutic intervention.

IMMUNOTOXINS

Immunotoxins are molecules that combine a monoclonal antibody to a specific antigen combined with a plant or bacterial toxin. The exquisite ability of the immune system to generate antibodies that target select antigen sites is combined with potent cytotoxins. The early history of immunotoxins is associated with attempts to develop selective immunotherapies for the eradication of tumor cells (see Vitetta et al., 1983). Immunotoxins using saporin or a related toxin ricin were conjugated with anti-bodies targeting selective antigens found on tumor cells. Early studies using ricin-based immunotoxins found that the it could selectively destroy tumor cells and promote survival of the host in murine leukemia models. The efficacy of immunotoxins for the treatment of human cancers is still being actively explored. It was also evident that the molecular heterogeneity of neuronal populations offered targets that might be used in the development of highly selective anti-neuronal immunotoxins. Saporin, a plant toxin derived from *Saponaria officinalis*, has been used in the production of a number of immunotoxins that target neuronal populations. Saporin is termed a ribosome-inactivating protein (RIP) since it catalytically destroys ribosomal RNA thus halting protein system and inducing cell death via apoptosis (Bergamaschi et al., 1996). An immunotoxin's antibody component recognizes and attaches to a highly specific membrane-associated antigen. The antibody and its coupled RIP is internalized by receptor-mediated endocytosis and is then transported to the cell body. Since immunotoxins recognize and destroy only antibody-targeted cells it is possible to create highly selective lesions which can mimic neurodegenerative disorders and/or address fundamental neurobiological questions. Immunotoxins have been developed that target cholinergic neurons, noradrenergic neurons, cerebellar Purkinje cells, and neuropeptidergic neurons [vasopressin, α-MSH, and neurons expressing receptors for oxytocin, LHRH, and atrial natriuretic peptide (see Wiley, 1996)].

THE ANTI-NEURONAL IMMUNOTOXIN 192 IgG-SAPORIN

Cholinergic neurons in the cholinergic basal forebrain contain p75 neurotrophin receptors which mediate the effects of NGF (Springer, 1988). SAP combines the 192 IgG monoclonal antibody to the p75 low affinity neurotrophin receptor with saporin, a potent RIP. The immunotoxin targets the p75 receptor localized on cholinergic nerve terminals in neocortex and hippocampus and on cholinergic cell bodies in the basal forebrain. Site-specific injection of SAP produces a selective loss of cholinergic neurons and neurochemical markers of ACh synthesis (Walsh et al., 1996). Since all ChAT-positive cells within the medial septum express p75 receptors, site-specific injection of SAP selectively destroys this population of cells. The brainstem cholinergic neurons do not express p75, they are not sensitive to ß-amyloid toxicity, and they do not die in AD (Woolf et al., 1989). Therefore, the expression of p75 might represent a signpost of vulnerability for degeneration of cholinergic neuronal populations in AD. 192-saporin should help to reveal the cellular and molecular properties that render cholinergic neurons susceptible or resistant to the AD disease process. We have also demonstrated that injection of SAP into the medial septum produces a dose-related decrease in high affinity choline uptake in the hippocampus, a loss of cholinergic (ChAT-immunoreactive) neurons, and delay-dependent deficits in a radial-arm maze task. These cholinergic deficits are evident without concomitant changes in regional concentrations of norepinephrine, dopamine, serotonin, or their metabolites, or a loss of GABAergic (parvalbumin-immunoreactive) neurons in the medial septum.

ADVANTAGES OF 192-IgG-SAPORIN

SAP offers several important practical advantages. It can address a number of structure-function related issues since it can be injected directly into cholinergic nuclei in the basal forebrain or into their terminal fields. This allows a precise definition of the functions of different components of the cholinergic basal forebrain. For example, the medial septum contains cholinergic neurons that project to the hippocampus, the cingulate cortex, and the entorhinal cortex. While the behavioral properties of the septohippocampal pathways have been extensively studied there has been little exploration of the functional role of the septocingulate projection. Injection of SAP into either the hippocampus or cingulate provides a way to selectively remove the cholinergic innervation of these structures and examine the behavioral results. Recent work in our laboratory indicates that the septocingulate cholinergic projection is a critical neural substrate of episodic memory (Dougherty and Walsh, in preparation). Site-specific injection of SAP also provides a way to examine the function of cholinergic innervation of different cortical target sites. Since both the septo-hippocampal and basal forebrain-cortical cholinergic pathways can be lesioned with SAP this toxin can produce a profile of cholinergic pathology that is more consistent with that observed in AD.

Another advantage of SAP is that it produces a dose-related cholinergic lesion with an acute phase of degeneration and a known mechanism of action (ie., irreversible inhibition of protein synthesis). SAP can produce either a partial or complete cholinergic lesion depending on dose.

SAP represents the advantages of immunotherapy in general; the ability to target specific cells. While SAP uses the immune system to deliver a potent cytotoxin it is also possible to use immunotherapeutic compounds to deliver drugs or trophic factors to selective populations of neurons. For example, nerve growth factor can be conjugated to an antibody for the transferrin receptor (OX-26) which actively transfers iron across the blood brain barrier. The NGF-OX-26 conjugate can be delivered peripherally and it attenuates the atrophy of cholinergic neurons and the cognitive deficits observed in aged rats (Backman et al., 1996).

DISADVANTAGES OF 192-IgG-SAPORIN

One of the few disadvantages of SAP is that it produces a rapidly evolving degeneration of cholinergic neurons. It is estimated that a single molecule of saporin is sufficient to induce cell death. Therefore, SAP produces a model of a 'completed' cholinergic lesion that will probably be resistant to neuroprotective interventions. Furthermore, due to the rapid onset of cell death it might be difficult to discern the sequence of cellular events that lead to degeneration. This limits the general utility of SAP as a model of neurodegenerative phenomena. The SAP model can be used to evaluate the efficacy of treatments that are designed to enhance cholinergic function (ie., muscarinic agonists, cholinesterase inhibitors) and promote recovery from cognitive deficits.

CONCLUSIONS

AF64A and SAP each offer distinct advantages, as well as limitations. These compounds provide complementary information about the cellular events that lead to the degeneration of cholinergic neurons and they suggest new therapeutic strategies that might prevent or slow the progression of AD or promote functional recovery following the loss of cholinergic function. AF64A models dysfunction and the degenerating neuron; SAP models the chemical, anatomical, and behavioral consequences of a completed cholinergic lesion. Both SAP and AF64A will continue to be used to address a variety of issues related to the biology of cholinergic neurons, their behavioral roles, and their involvement in degenerative diseases like AD.

ACKNOWLEDGMENT

The original work reported here was supported by NSF grant IBN9514557 and a gift in memory of Colonel Norman C. Kalmar to TJW.

REFERENCES

Backman, C., Rose, G.M., Hoffer, B.J., Henry, M.A., Bartus, R.T., Friden, P. and Granholm, A-M., 1996, Systemic administration of a nerve growth factor conjugate reverses age-related cognitive dysfunction and prevents cholinergic neuron atrophy. *J. Neurosci.* 16:5437–5442.

Barlow, P. and Marchbanks, R.M., 1984, Effect of ethylcholine mustard on choline dehydrogenase and other enzymes of choline metabolism. *J. Neurochem.* 43:1568–1573.

Bergamaschi, G, Perfetti, V., Tonon, L., Novella, A., Lucotti, C., Danova, M., Glennie, M.J., Merlini, G., and Cazzola, M., 1996, Saporin, a ribosome-inactivating protein used to prepare immunotoxins, induces cell death via apoptosis. *Brit. J. Haematol.* 93:789–794.

Cooper, B., 1991, The epidemiology of primary degenerative dementia and related neurological disorders. *Eur. Arch. Psychiat. Clin. Neurosci.* 240:223–233.

Evans, D.A., Funkenstein, H. H., Albert, M.S., Scherr, P.A., Cook, N. R., Chown, M. J., Herbert, L. E., Hennekens, C. H. and Taylor, J. O., 1989, Prevalence of Alzheimer's disease in a community population of older persons. *J. Amer. Med. Assoc.* 262:2551–2556.

Futscher, B.W., Pieper, R.O., Barnes, D.M., Hanin, I., and Erickson, L.C., 1992, DNA-damaging and transcription terminating lesions induced by AF64A in vitro. *J. Neurochem.* 58:1504–1509.

Gulyaeva, N.V., Lazareva, N.A., Libe, M.L., Mitrokhina, M.V., Yu, M. and Walsh, T.J., 1996, Oxidative stress in the brain following intraventricular administration of ethylcholine aziridinium (AF64A). *Brain Res.* 726:174–180.

Hanin, I., 1996, The AF64A model of cholinergic hypofunction: An update. *Life Sci.* 58:1955–1964.

Hörtnagl, H. and Hanin, I., 1992, Toxins affecting the cholinergic system. In: *Handbook of Experimental Pharmacology: Selective Neurotoxicity*, Herken, H. and Hucho, F., eds, Springer-Verlag, Berlin, Vol. 102, 293–331.

Johnson, G.V., M. Simanato and R.S. Jope, 1988, Dose- and time-dependent hippocampal cholinergic lesions induced by ethylcholine mustard aziridinium ion: Effects of nerve growth factor, GM1 ganglioside, and vitamin E. *Neurochem. Res.* 13:685–692.

McGurk, S.R., Hartgraves, S.L., Kelly, P.H., Gordons, M.N. and Butcher, L.L., 1987, Is ethylcholine aziridinium ion a specific cholinergic neurotoxin? *Neuroscience* 22:215–224.

Sandberg, K., Schnaar, R.L., McKinney, M., Hanin, I., Fisher, A. and Coyle, J.T., 1985, AF64A: an active site directed irreversible inhibitor of choline acetyltransferase. *J. Neurochem.* 44:439–445.

Sano, M., Ernesto, C., Thomas, R.G., Klauber, M.R., Schafer, K., Grundman, M., Woodbury, P., Growdon, J., Cotman, C.W., Pfeiffer, E., Schneider, L.S. and Thal, L.J., 1997, A controlled trial of selegiline, alpha-tocopherol, or both as treatment for Alzheimer's disease. *New Engl. J. Med.* 336:1216–1222.

Smith, M.A., Harris, P.L., Sayre, L.M., Beckman, J.S. and Perry, G., 1997, Widespread peroxynitrite- mediated damage in Alzheimer's disease. *J. Neurosci.* 17:2653–2657.

Springer, J.E., 1988, Nerve growth factor receptors in the central nervous system. *Exp. Neurol.* 102:354–365.

Vitetta, E.S., Krolick, K.A., Miyamaa-Inaba, M., Cushley, W. and Uhr, J.W., 1983. Immunotoxins: a new approach to cancer therapy. *Science* 219:644–650.

Walsh, T.J., Herzog, C., Gandhi, C., Stackman, R.W. and Wiley, R. G., 1996, Injection of IgG 192-saporin into the medial septum produces cholinergic hypofunction and dose-dependent working memory deficits. *Brain Res.* 726:69–79.

Walsh, T. J. and Opello, K. D., 1994, The use of AF64A to model Alzheimer's disease. In: *Toxin-Induced Models of Neurological Disorders*, Woodruff, M. and Nonneman, A., eds, Plenum Press, NY, 259–279.

Walsh, T.J., Kelly, R.M. and Stackman, R.W., 1994, Strategies to limit brain injury and promote recovery of function. *Neurotoxicology* 15:467–476.

Walsh, T. J. and Chrobak, J. J., 1991, Animals models of Alzheimer's disease: role of hippocampal cholinergic systems in working memory. In: *Current Topics in Animal Learning: Brain, Emotion, and Cognition.* Dachowski. L. and Flaherty, C., eds, Lawrence Erlbaum, Hillsdale, NJ, 347–379.

Wiley, R.G., 1992, Neural lesioning with ribosome-inactivating proteins: Suicide transport and immunolesioning. *Trends Neurosci.* 15:285–290.

Wiley, R.G., 1996, Targeting toxins to neural antigens and receptors. *Cancer Biol.* 7:71–77.

Woolf, N.J., Jacobs, R.W. and Butcher, L. L., 1989, The pontomesencephalotegmental cholinergic system does not degenerate in Alzheimer's disease. *Neurosci. Lett.* 96:277–282.

Wortwein, G., Stackman, R.W. and Walsh, T.J., 1994, Vitamin E prevents the place learning deficit and the cholinergic hypofunction induced by AF64A. *Exp. Neurol.* 125:15–21.

95

MOLECULAR MECHANISMS OF AF64A TOXICITY IN THE CHOLINERGIC NEURON

Israel Hanin

Department of Pharmacology
Loyola University Chicago
Stritch School of Medicine
Maywood, Illinois 60153

INTRODUCTION

When AF64A was initially developed (Fisher and Hanin, 1980; Mantione et al., 1981), it was with the goal in mind to induce a permanent cholinergic deficit in the brain, thus mimicking the neurochemical cholinergic deficiency reported in brains of patients with Alzheimer's Disease (AD) (Bowen et al., 1976; Davies and Maloney, 1976). In addition to producing this chemical deficit, rats and mice treated with AF64A were also shown to exhibit deficits in memory and learning (Chrobak et al., 1987; Walsh and Chrobak, 1991; Chrobak and Walsh, 1991). As a consequence, in the search for potential drugs for the treatment of the cognitive deficits in AD, many investigators began to use the AF64A-treated rat to test various compounds for their ability to reverse the neurochemical and cognitive deficits induced by the cholinotoxin (See review by Hanin, 1996).

More recently, molecular approaches have been employed, to explore the mechanism(s) by which AF64A may be selectively compromising the cholinergic neuron, both *in vivo* and vitro. These studies have begun to yield information about the neurotoxic events induced by AF64A in the cholinergic nerve that lead to its eventual destruction. An important and promising outcome of these studies is the realization that AF64A provides a valuable tool to model cholinergic dysfunction during the dynamic process of degeneration of the neuron, rather than presenting a state of irreversible cholinergic depletion, as seen in the 192-IgG-Saporin treated animal (Walsh, this book). AF64A can therefore be used as a tool to study dynamic changes in DNA damage, apoptosis, oxidative stress, and nerve growth factor synthesis, all of which occur as a result of AF64A treatment.

Progress in Alzheimer's and Parkinson's Diseases
edited by Fisher *et al.*, Plenum Press, New York, 1998.

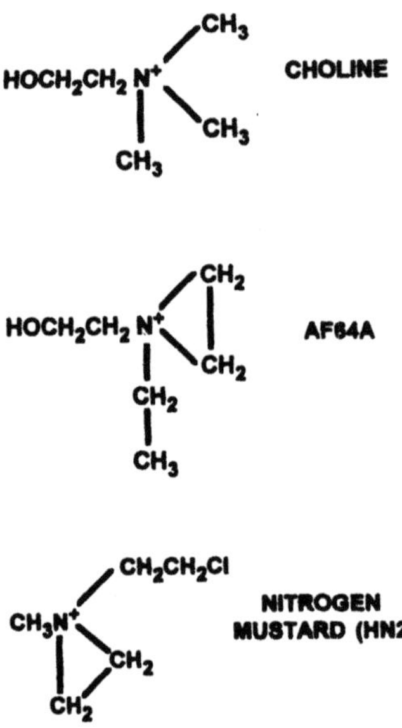

Figure 1. Choline, AF64A, and nitrogen mustard.

EFFECTS ON DNA AND RNA INTEGRITY

DNA and RNA Integrity in Cultured Cells

Santiago et al. (1997), employing Sl nuclease analysis, studied RNA isolated from LA-N-2 cells, and reported a dose- and time-dependent AF64A-induced reduction in steady state expression of N-myc. This could be averted in the presence of high concentrations of choline, or hemicholinium-3. AF64A's selectivity for the cholinergic neuron is due to its structural similarity to choline (see Figure 1). Therefore, AF64A gains access to the inside of cholinergic structures via the high affinity choline transport system (HAChT; Pittel et al., 1987; Rylett and Walters, 1990), and this effect can be competitively inhibited by agonists for the uptake system (Kelley et al., 1988; Potter et al., 1989; Gomez et al., 1993).

The effect of AF64A on the n-myc gene is explained by earlier studies from our laboratories on the human n-myc gene, using the Maxam and Gilbert DNA sequencing technique (Futscher et al. 1992). In these studies AF64A produced extensive, dose-dependent alkylations at the N-7 guanine sites on DNA, which led to termination of RNA transcription. These studies indicated that AF64A has a specific affinity for DNA, probably because of its structural similarity to the highly reactive antitumor agent nitrogen mustard (mechlorethamine) (see Figure 1).

Plasmid Cholinesterase DNA and RNA Integrity *in Vitro*

Because of the affinity of AF64A for N-7 guanine sites on DNA, we reasoned that AF64A should have a higher affinity for G, C-rich DNA (e.g. in acetylcholinesterase) than for A,T-rich DNA (e.g. in butyrylcholinesterase) (Prody et al., 1987; Soreq et al., 1990; Legay et al., 1993). Indeed, AF64A preferentially attenuated *in vitro* transcription of plasmid DNAs carrying coding sequences for the G,C-rich acetylcholinesterase (AChE) over the A,T-rich butyrylcholinesterase (BChE) genes (Hanin et al., 1995).

Cholinesterase DNA and RNA Integrity in Mammalian Brain *in Vivo*

Moreover, in several brain regions in the rat, following intracerebroventricular administration of AF64A *in vivo*, AF64A had a more pronounced inhibitory effect on AChEmRNA than on BChEmRNA, as measured using RNA polymerase chain reaction (PCR) quantification (Lev-Lehman et al., 1994). Based on these observations we concluded that AF64A exerts its effect in vivo, at least in part, by attenuating transcription of enzymes involved in regulating acetylcholine metabolism, with a higher affinity toward G,C-rich enzymes.

DNA and RNA Integrity in Mammalian Brain *in Vivo*: Choline Acetyltransferase (ChAT)

We also have conducted some studies on the *in vivo* effect of AF64A on gene expression and protein level of choline acetyltransferase (ChAT), using reverse transcription PCR analysis of ChAT mRNA in the septohippocampal pathway, and Western blot analysis, respectively. Our results demonstrated a biphasic response to AF64A administration. Initially AF64A effected a direct, inhibitory effect on the enzyme at the nerve terminal (hippocampus); this subsequently resulted in a transient, compensatory stimulatory response on ChAT gene expression in the cell body (septum). Ultimately, as the cholinergic neurons began to die, ChAT mRNA levels in the septum decreased to 42.5% of control (p<0.05) (Fan et al., unpublished).

These studies still are preliminary. They do, nevertheless, imply that AF64A may also affect gene expression of ChAT, the enzyme that synthesizes acetylcholine in the cholinergic neuron. Whether this is a direct effect of AF64A or is compensatory to damage induced at the nerve terminal, has yet to be established definitively.

APOPTOSIS AND OXIDATIVE STRESS

AF64A induces apoptosis following its *in vivo* and *in vitro* administration (Rinner et al., 1997). This effect apparently is not linked to the documented specific cholinotoxic effect of AF64A, and occurs both in neuronal and non-neuronal cells. In vivo, it expresses itself in the area surrounding the immediate locus of AF64A administration, where the concentration of the toxin initially is much higher than it is following its diffusion after its injection; it probably, therefore, is associated with the more generally localized low affinity system for the uptake of choline.

This induction of apoptosis can be prevented by zinc, implying that activation of an endonuclease may be essential in the induction of apoptosis by AF64A. Rinner and colleagues (1997) further demonstrated that initiation of apoptosis in AF64A-treated rats was strongly attenuated by Tempol, a nitroxide spin probe, which readily crosses the membrane, and acts as a free-radical scavenger.

The latter finding indicates that oxidative stress most likely is an intermediate in the development of neurodegeneration by AF64A. In concert with these findings are earlier reports in the literature showing protection from cholinotoxicity induced by AF64A, in rats pretreated with the potent antioxidant, vitamin E (Wortwein et al., 1994; Johnson et al., 1988; Maneesub et al., 1993).

NERVE GROWTH FACTOR (NGF)

Chronic NGF infusion into the lateral ventricle of rats (0.36–2.85 ug/day; 14 days) increased, in a dose-dependent manner, ChAT activity in hippocampus and septum. The effect on the septum was doubled (at the higher doses of NGF) when NGF was used in AF64A treated rats, as compared to changes measured in rats that had not been exposed to AF64A (Willson and Hanin, 1995). Thus, cholinergic neurons which are compromised exhibited an increased sensitivity to exogenously administered NGF.

This phenomenon may be linked to the observation by Hellweg and co-investigators (1997), demonstrating that mild-to-moderate lesion of the rat cholinergic septohippocampal pathway (such as is obtained by lesioning rats with low intraventricular doses of AF64A), steadily increased hippocampal NGF mRNA production over the seven-week duration of their study. Moreover, five weeks after AF64A treatment, these investigators measured an increase in septal NGF protein and a significant increase in septal ChAT activity, indicating an increase in the retrograde transport of NGF following mild-to-moderate lesion of the cholinergic septo-hippocampal system (Hellweg et al., 1997).

It is intriguing to note in this context that a partially damaged cholinergic system, such as can be generated with low doses of AF64A, appears to be necessary in order to elicit an NGF mediated repair process *in vivo*. When essentially complete cholinergic disruption was elicited in rats, following either fimbria-fornix transaction (Goedert et al., 1986; Korsching et al., 1986) or treatment with 192-IgG-saporin (Kokaia et al., 1996; Yu et al., 1996), it was not possible to measure changes in NGF MRNA levels in the septo-hippocampal system.

DISCUSSION AND SUMMARY

The presence of a highly reactive aziridinium ion in the AF64A molecule renders it toxic to many substances. AF64A has an affinity for DNA, with a higher preference for the G, C -rich variety. The cholinergic specificity of AF64A is attributable to its close similarity to choline and its vast affinity for the high affinity choline uptake system. One mechanism of AF64A-induced damage may be through the generation of reactive oxygen species. Whether, or not, AF64A-induced neuronal damage is mediated solely through its inhibitory action on DNA, or whether it also may affect axonal transport (Kasa and Hanin, 1985), and/or exert direct damage to essential components of the cholinergic neuron, has yet to be determined. As more information is gleaned about the mechanism of action of AF64A at the cellular and molecular levels, we will be able to understand more clearly processes that contribute to the degeneration of cholinergic neurons, as well as to the possible consequences of such cholinergic degeneration on other, interacting systems, in the brain.

REFERENCES

Bowen, D.M., Smith, C.B., White, P., and Davison, A.N., 1976, Neurotransmitter-related enzymes and indices of hypoxia in senile dementia and other abiotrophies. *Brain* 99:459–496.

Chrobak, J.J., Hanin, I., and Walsh, T.J., 1987, AF64A (ethylcholine aziridinium ion), a cholinergic neurotoxin, selectively impairs working memory in a multiple component T-maze task. *Brain Res.* 414:15–21.

Chrobak, J.J. and Walsh, T.J., 1991, Dose and delay dependent working/episodic memory impairments following intraventricular administration of ethylcholine aziridinium (AF64A). *Behav. Neural Biol.* 56:200–212.

Davies, P. and Maloney, A.J.F., 1976, Selective loss of cholinergic neurons in Alzheimer's disease. *Lancet* ii:403.

Fisher, A. and Hanin, I., 1980, Minireview: Choline analogs as potential tools in developing sensitive animal models of central cholinergic hypofunction. *Life Sci.* 27:1615–1634.

Futscher, B.W., Pieper, R.O., Barnes, D.M., Hanin, I., and Erickson, L.C., 1992, DNA-damaging and transcription-terminating lesions induced by AF64A *in vitro. J. Neurochem.* 58:1504–1509.

Goedert, M., Fine, A., Hunt, S.P., and Ullrich, A., 1986, Nerve growth factor MRNA in peripheral and central rat tissues and in the human central nervous system: lesion effects in the rat brain and levels in Alzheimer's disease.*Mol. Brain Res.* 1:85–92.

Gomez, C., Martin, C., Galea, E., and Estrada, C, 1993, Direct cytotoxicity of ethylcholine mustard aziridinium in cerebral microvascular endothelial cells. *J. Neurochem.* 60:1534–1539.

Hanin, I., 1996, Pharmacological Induction of Cholinergic Hypofunction as a Tool for Evaluating Cholinergic Therapies. In: *Alzheimer's Disease: From Molecular Biology to Therapy,* Becker, R. and Giacobini, E. eds., Birkhauser, Boston.

Hanin, I., Yaron, A., Ginzberg, D., and Soreq, H., 1995, The Cholinotoxin AF64A Differentially Attenuates *In Vitro* Transcription of the Human Cholinesterase Genes, In: *Alzheimer's and Parkinson's Diseases: Recent Developments,* Hanin, I., Yoshida, M. and. Fisher, A., eds., Plenum Press, New York.

Hellweg, R., Humpel, C., Lowe, A., and Hortnagl, H., 1997, Moderate lesion of the rat cholinergic septohippocampal pathway increases hippocampal nerve growth factor synthesis: evidence for long-term compensatory changes?, BRESM, in press.

Johnson, G.V., Simanato, M., and Jope, R.S., 1988, Dose- and time-dependent hippocampal cholinergic lesions induced by ethylcholine mustard aziridinium ion: Effects of nerve growth factor, GM1 ganglioside, and vitamin E. *Neurochem. Res.* 13:685–692.

Kasa, P. and Hanin, I., 1985, Ethylcholine mustard aziridinium blocks the axoplasmic transport of acetylcholinesterase in mammalian cholinergic nerve fibers of the rat. *Histochemistry* 83:343–345.

Kelley, M.C., Raizada, M.K., and Meyer, E.M., 1988, Pharmacological characterization of high affinity choline transporters in primary neuronal cultures in rat brain. *Neuropharmacology* 27:837–842.

Kokaia, M., Ferencz, I., Leanza, G., Elmer, E., Metsis, F., Kokaia, Z., Wiley, R.G., and Lindvall, O., 1996, Immunolesioning of basal forebrain cholinergic neurons facilitates hippocampal kindling and perturbs neurotrophin messenger MRNA regulation. *Neuroscience* 70:313–327.

Korsching, S., Hoemann, R., Thoenen, H., and Hefti, F., 1986, Cholinergic denervation of the rat hippocampus by fimbrial transaction leads to a transient accumulation of nerve growth factor (NGF) without a change in mRNA NGF content. *Neurosci. Lett.* 66:175–180.

Legay, C., Bon, S., Vernier, P., Coussens, F., and Massoulie, J., 1993, Cloning and expression of a rat acetylcholinesterase subunit: generation of multiple molecular forms and complementarity with a Torpedo collagenic subunit. *J. Neurochem.* 60:337–346.

Lev-Lehman, E., El-Tamer, A., Yaron, A., Grifman, M., Ginzberg, D., Hanin, I., and Soreq, H., 1994, Cholinotoxic effects on acetylcholinesterase gene expression are associated with brain-region specific alterations in G,C-rich transcripts. *Brain Res.* 661:75–82.

Maneesub, Y., Sanvarinda, Y., and Govitrapong, P., 1993, Partial restoration of choline acetyltransferase activities in aging and AF64A-lesioned rat brains by vitamin E. *Neurochem. Int.* 22:487–491.

Mantione, C.R., Fisher, A., and Hanin, I., 1981, The AF64A-treated mouse: Possible model for central cholinergic hypofunction. *Science* 213:579–580.

Pittel, Z., Fisher, A., and Heldman, E., 1987, Reversible and irreversible inhibition of high affinity choline transport caused by ethylcholine aziridinium ion. *J. Neurochem.* 49:468–474.

Potter, P. E., Tedford, C.E., Kindel, G., and Hanin, I., 1989, Inhibition of high affinity choline transport attenuates both cholinergic and noncholinergic effects of ethylcholine aziridinium (AF64A). *Brain Res.* 487:238–244.

Prody, C.A., Zevin-Sonkin, D., Gnatt, A., Goldberg, O., and Soreq, H., 1987, Isolation and characterization of full-length cDNA clones for cholinesterase from fetal human tissues. *Proc. Natl. Acad. Sci.* USA, 84:3555–3559.

Rinner, W.A., Pifl, C., Lassman, H., and Hortnagl, H., 1997, Induction of apoptosis *in vivo* by the cholinergic neurotoxin ethylcholine aziridinium. *Neuroscience*, in press.

Rylett, R.J. and Walters, S.A., 1990, Uptake and metabolism of [3H]choline mustard by cholinergic nerve terminals from rat brain. *Neuroscience* 36:483–489.

Santiago, L.R., Erickson, L.C., and Hanin, I., 1997, AF64A-induced changes in N-myc expression in the LA-N-2 human neuroblastoma cell line are modulated by choline and hemicholinium. *Neurochem. Res.* 23:747–754, 1998.

Soreq, H., Ben-Aziz, R., Prody, C., Seidman, S., Gnatt, A., Neville, L., Lieman-Hurwitz, J., Lev-Lehman, E., Ginzberg, D., Lapidot-Lifson, Y., and Zakut, H., 1990, Molecular cloning and construction of the coding region for human acetylcholinesterase reveals a G+C rich attenuating structure. *Proc. Natl. Acad. Sci. USA* 87:9688–9692.

Walsh, T.J. and Chrobak, J.J., 1991, Animal models of Alzheimer's disease: role of hippocampal cholinergic systems in working memory, In: *Current Topics in Animal learning: Brain, Emotion and Cognition,* Dachowski, L. and Flaherty, C., eds., Lawrence Erlbaum, Hillsdale, N.J.

Willson, C.A. and Hanin, I., 1995, Effect of nerve growth factor in ethylcholine mustard aziridinium (AF64A) treated rats: Sensitization of cholinergic enzyme activity in the septohippocampal pathway.*J. Neurochem.* 65:856–862.

Wortwein, G., Stackman, R.W., and Walsh, T.J., 1994, Vitamin E prevents the place learning deficit and the cholinergic hypofunction induced by AF64A. *Exp. Neurol.* 125:15–21.

Yu, J., Wiley, R.G., and Perez-Polo, J.R., 1996, Altered NGF protein levels in different brain areas after immunolesion. *J. Neurosci. Res.* 43:213–223.

96

THE AF64A MODEL OF CHOLINERGIC HYPOFUNCTION

Role of Nitric Oxide in AF64A-Mediated Neurodegeneration

M. Lautenschlager,[1] A. Arnswald,[1] D. Freyer,[2] J. R. Weber,[2] and H. Hörtnagl[1]

[1]Institute of Pharmacology and Toxicology
[2]Department of Neurology
Medical Faculty Charité
Humboldt-University at Berlin
D-10098 Berlin, Germany

INTRODUCTION

Increasing evidence indicates that nitric oxide (NO), a gaseous intra- and extracellular messenger, is involved in various neurotoxic and neurodegenerative processes. Inappropriate formation of NO is emerging as an important factor in the neurotoxicity associated with a variety of central nervous system disorders. Enhancement of NO production occurs in the central nervous system during stroke, seizures and acute and chronic inflammatory and neurodegenerative disorders (for reviews see Dawson and Dawson 1996; Scabo 1996). NO appears to be an important mediator of neuronal injury following activation of NMDA receptors (Dawson et al., 1991, 1993; Lipton et al., 1993), but also in MPTP, methamphetamine and ammonia neurotoxicity (Spencer Smith et al., 1994; Kosenko et al., 1995; Hantraye et al., 1996; Przedborski et al., 1996; Di Monte et al., 1996). NO formed by increased expression of neuronal NO synthase (NOS) may also play a role in capsaicin-induced neurotoxicity (Vizzard et al. 1995). Considerable differences in the contribution of the various isoenzymes of NOS to neuronal damage have been observed. Excessive activation of the isoform located in neurons (nNOS) appears to significantly contribute to hypoxic-ischemic brain damage (Ferriero et al., 1996) and to glutamate neurotoxicity, whereas the inducible isoform of NOS (iNOS) can be expressed under inflammatory conditions (Scabo 1996). Recent evidence in NOS mutant mice indicates that neonatal mice lacking nNOS are less vulnerable to hypoxic-ischemic injury (Ferriero et al., 1996; Panahian et al., 1996) and that malonate striatal lesions were significantly attenuated in the nNOS mutant mice but were significantly increased in the endo-

Progress in Alzheimer's and Parkinson's Diseases
edited by Fisher *et al.*, Plenum Press, New York, 1998.

thelial NOS (eNOS) mutant mice (Schulz et al., 1996). Cortical cultures from transgenic mice lacking nNOS are relatively resistant to NMDA neurotoxicity, but not to kainate neurotoxicity (Dawson et al., 1996).

However, the various roles of NO in cytotoxic events remain unclear. Neuroprotective and deleterious effects of NO on focal cerebral ischemia-induced neuronal death have been described. Enhanced NO production within the cerebral vasculature by activation of eNOS protects brain tissue during focal ischemia via hemodynamic mechanisms, whereas neuronal overproduction may mediate neurotoxicty (Dalkara et al., 1994; Verrecchia et al., 1995). Controversies also exist about the involvement of NO in neurotoxic brain injury; not any kind of neuronal damage is associated with an excessive production of NO. Inhibition of NO formation did not protect murine cortical cell cultures from NMDA neurotoxicity (Hewett et al., 1993). In quinolinic acid toxicity in the rat striatum no role of NO was observed (Mackenzie et al., 1995).

The aim of the present investigation was to define the role of NO in the pathogenesis of the neurodegeneration induced by the cholinergic neurotoxin AF64A under *in vivo* and *in vitro* conditions. *In vivo* the effect of NO was blocked by the use of various NOS inhibitors. In primary neuronal cell cultures, which have the advantage of being free from the influences of microvasulature and microglia and thus eNOS and iNOS (Dawson and Dawson 1996), the formation of NO after exposure to AF64A was measured by the accumulation of nitrite.

METHODS

In Vivo Experiments

Male Sprague Dawley rats (300–400g), anesthetized with chloral hydrate, received stereotaxic infusions (0.5 µl/min) of 1 or 2 nmol of AF64A in 3 µl or vehicle into each lateral ventricle (Hörtnagl et al., 1993). In order to block the generation of NO rats were chronically treated i.p. or s.c. with specific inhibitors of the various isoforms of NOS, starting from 12 h before the stereotaxic infusion until 2–3 days after.

The following NOS-inhibitors were applied: N-nitro-L-arginine (L-NA; 50 mg/kg i.p. twice daily) and N-nitro-L-arginine methylester (L-NAME; 100 mg/kg i.p. twice daily) for preferential inhibtion of constitutive nNOS and eNOS; 7-nitroindazole (7-NI; 30 mg/kg in 33.3% cremophor EL s.c. every 4–6 h for relatively selective inhibition of nNOS; aminoguanidine (AG; 50 mg/kg i.p. twice daily) as relatively selective inhibitor of iNOS.

Rats were decapitated 7 days after AF64A application. The rapidly removed brains were frozen at -70°C and were dissected frozen on a cold plate (-10°C). The activity of choline acetyltransferase (ChAT) was determined according to Fonnum (1969) with minor modifications (Auburger et al., 1987).

In Vitro Experiments

Primary neuronal cell cultures of septum, hippocampus and cerebral cortex were obtained from fetal rats at E15–17, dissociated using trypsin, plated in wells (15 mm diameter) in a density of 200 000 to 400 000 cells per cm^2, cultivated in serum-free neurobasal medium (Gibco) with N2 or B27-supplement, 0.5 mM glutamine and 100 U/ml penicillin/streptomycin. Half of the medium was replaced twice a week. The percentage of astroglia was less than 10%. Cultures were treated after 15 to 18 days *in vitro* with AF64A

(5–80 µM). Controls received an equivalent amount of vehicle. Condition of cells was determined morphologically by phase contrast microscopy and trypan blue staining (0.05% w/v).

MTT-assay, a live-death assay based on the cleavage of the yellow tetrazolium salt MTT to purple formazan by mitochondrial enzymes in metabolically active cells, was performed by adding 500 µg MTT/ml. After incubation at 36.5°C for 70 to 80 minutes, the reaction was stopped by 10% SDS in 0.01 M HCL, followed by 48h at 36.5°C and photometric detection at 550 nm. NO production in AF64A-treated cultures was determined by quantifying nitrite, accumulated over the period of 70–78 h after application of AF64A. For the quantitation Griess-assay was used with a detection limit of 300 nM as described previously (Freyer et al., 1996). Identification of cell-types was achieved by peroxidase-immunohistochemistry. Primary antibodies used were against GFAP for astrocytes (DAKO), NSE for neurons (DAKO), OX42 for microglia (Laboserv) and ChAT for cholinergic neurons (Chemicon).

RESULTS AND DISCUSSION

The effect of various NOS-inhibitors on the AF64A-induced decrease in ChAT activity in the rat hippocampus under *in vivo* conditions is summarized in Table 1. The pharmacological inhibition of the various isoforms of NOS did not not significantly protect the cholinergic septohippocampal pathway against the neurotoxic effect of AF64A. In contrast, a tendency towards a slight potentiation of the AF64A-induced cholinergic deficit was observed especially after unspecific inhibition of the various isoforms of NOS, including eNOS, by treatment with L-NA and L-NAME. This trend suggests rather a neuroprotective than a neurotoxic influence of NO.

Primary neuronal cell cultures reacted to AF64A with a time- and dose-dependent reduction of neuronal cell viability as seen morphologically and immunohistochemically. After 16 hours neurons showed first signs of neurite disintegration, chromatin condensation and membrane blebbing. Then they gradually underwent cytoplasmic shrinkage, nuclear fragmentation, loss of membrane integrity and neuritic processes. In the lowest dose of AF64A (5µM) this cell degeneration occured preferentially in cholinergic neurons as seen in immunohistochemical ChAT-staining (data not shown). In order to quantify the percentage of metabolic activity left after AF64A-treatment, MTT-assay was used. At the highest dosis of AF64A (80µM) MTT-metabolism was not decreased before 16 h after exposure to AF64A, but then gradually declined to levels lower than 40% after 96h. A comparable response was observed in the cell cultures of all brain regions investigated 70–78

Table 1. Effect of inhibition of NOS activity on the decrease in ChAT activity in the rat hippocampus induced by 1 or 2 nmol AF64A/ventricle

NOS-inhibitor (NOS-I)	Dose of AF64A/ventricle	ChAT activity percent of controls ± SEM			
		Vehicle/vehicle (n)	Vehicle/NOS-I (n)	AF64A/vehicle (n)	AF64A/NOS-I (n)
L-NA	2 nmol	100.0 ± 5.8 (5)	100.6 ± 4.2 (5)	54.3 ± 6.2* (5)	44.4 ± 8.2* (5)
L-NAME	2 nmol	100.0 ± 2.3 (6)	116.4 ± 4.6 (6)	63.3 ± 10.5* (5)	47.3 ± 3.6* (4)
7-NI	2 nmol	100.0 ± 1.1 (11)	103.5 ± 3.8 (10)	50.5 ± 5.2* (11)	47.7 ± 2.7* (9)
AG	1 nmol	100.0 ± 5.1 (6)	98.3 ± 4.9 (6)	75.6 ± 3.8* (6)	70.6 ± 4.0* (6)

* $p > 0.05$ versus corresponding control group (one-way ANOVA, Newman-Keuls test)

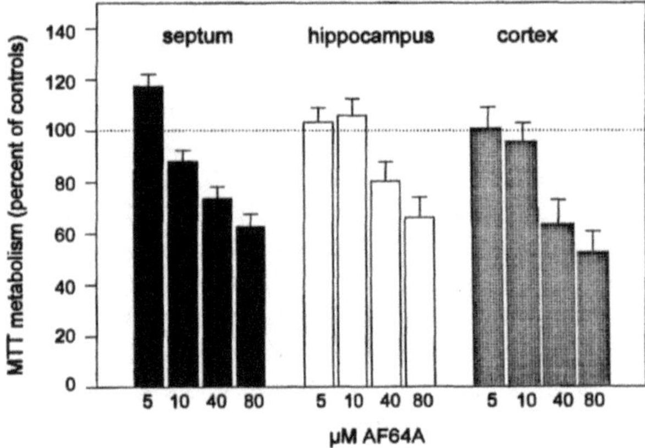

Figure 1. Dose-dependent effect of AF64A on MTT-metabolism in various primary neuronal cultures. The metabolic activity was measured by MTT-assay 70–78 h after AF64A or vehicle application (n = 4–6).

h after AF64A application (Fig.1). It was remarkable that in the lower dose ranges of AF64A even a slight increase in MTT-metabolism occurred, especially in the septal cultures, although morphological signs of neuronal cell death were evident. Preliminary immunohistochemical data indicate that in the septal cultures ChAT positive cells were preferentially damaged already at the 5µM dose of AF64A (data not shown). The increase in MTT-metabolism might reflect an metabolic activation of the less affected neuronal cells and astrocytes. At the highest dose of AF64A only astrocytes survived and showed metabolic activity in the MTT-assay (Figure 2).

Neuronal cell death, which slowly developed over several days and was extensive in the higher AF64A-dose range, was not associated with a detectable increase in NO production. Griess-assay did not reveal any detectable amounts of nitrite in the culture me-

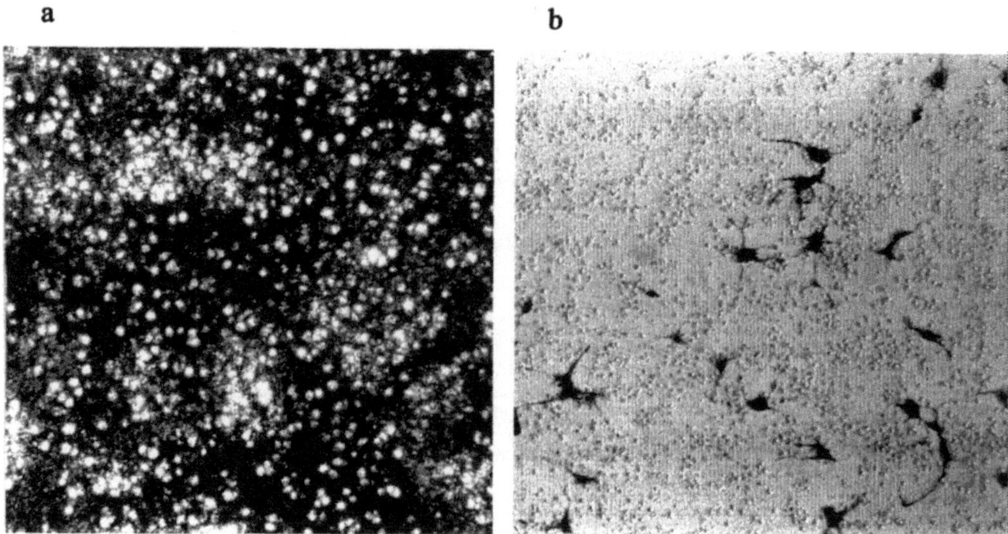

Figure 2. Changes in cell viability (MTT-assay) in primary neuronal cultures of septum 74 h after application of a high dose (80µM) of AF64A. a) In control cultures MTT is extensively metabolized to blue formazan. b) In AF64A treated cultures only astrocytes survive and show formazan staining (magnification x 125).

dium at any of the AF64A-doses studied. This finding indicates that in our primary neuronal cell cultures with a low percentage of glial cells neither neurotoxic nor neuroprotective influences of the NO-system are evident in the AF64A-mediated neurodegeneration. One possible explanation for the missing response of the NO-system to a strong neurotoxic stimulus could be the absence of microglia in our culture systems. The percentage of microglia as quantified by OX42-immunostaining was as low as 1/10 000 cells in the primary neuronal cultures from all three brain regions studied at three weeks *in vitro*. As microglia activated by various stimuli are known to show high NO-synthetizing capacity by expression of iNOS, it cannot be excluded that a detectable NO synthesis might occur in the presence of sufficient numbers of microglia. Investigation of this question requires co-culture studies with a higher percentage of microglia, which are in progress. The present *in vitro* data implicate that neither nNOS was excessively activated nor did an induction of iNOS occur in astrocytes during the various steps leading to AF64A induced neuronal cell death.

Our finding that the neurotoxic effect of AF64A on septohippocampal cholinergic neurons *in vivo* and in primary neuronal cultures *in vitro* did not substantially depend on increased NO production is in contrast to various other neurotoxins including glutamate, MPTP or methamphetamine (Dawson et al., 1991, 1993; Przedborski et al. 1996; Di Monte et al., 1996). NO has been considered as an intermediate in NMDA-receptor mediated toxicity (Dawson et al., 1991). An involvement of glutamate in the mechanism of AF64A-neurotoxicity has been excluded previously (Hörtnagl et al., 1991). It also appears that the cholinergic basal forebrain systems may respond differently, since in malonate-induced degeneration of these cholinergic neurons, which is at least partly dependent on glutamate release, only 7-NI, but not L-NA and L-NAME provided a rather modest neuroprotective effect (Connop et al., 1997).

In conclusion, the present *in vivo* and *in vitro* data do not support a prominent role of excess NO formation in the AF64A-mediated neurodegeneration. The use of AF64A thus provides a significant model for neurodegenerative mechanisms that are independent of the neurotoxic potential of NO.

ACKNOWLEDGMENTS

This study was supported by DFG (INK 21/A1-1/B8 and SFB 507/A3).

REFERENCES

Auburger, G., Heumann, R., Hellweg, R., Korsching, S. and Thoenen, H.,1987, Developmental changes of nerve growth factor and its mRNA in the hippocampus: comparison with choline acetyltransferase. *Dev. Biol.* 120:322.

Connop, B. P., Boegman, R. J., Beninger, R. J. and Ihamandas, K., 1997, Malonate-induced degeneration of basal forebrain cholinergic neurons: Attenuation by lamotridgine. *MK-801, and* 7-nitroindazole, *J. Neurochem.* 68:1191.

Dalkara, T., Yoshida, T., Trikura, K. and Moskowitz, M. A., 1994, Dual role of nitric oxide in focal cerebral ischemia. *Neuropharmacology* 33:1447.

Dawson, V. L., Dwason, T. M., London, E. D., Bredt, D. S. and Snyder, S. H., 1991, Nitric oxide mediates glutamate neurotoxicity in primary cortical cultures. *Proc. Natl. Acad. Sci.* USA 88:6368.

Dawson, V. L., Dawson, T. M., Bartley, D. A., Uhl, G. R. and Snyder, S. H., 1993, Mechanisms of nitric-oxide mediated neurotoxicity in primary brain cultures. *J. Neurosci.* 13: 2651.

Dawson, V. L. and Dawson, T. M., 1996, Nitric oxide toxicity in central nervous system cultures. *Methods Neurosci.* 30:26.

Dawson, V. L. and Dawson, T. M., 1996, Nitric oxide actions in neurochemistry. *Neurochem. Int.* 29:97.

Dawson, V. L., Kizushi, V. M., Huang, P. L., Snyder, S. H. and Dawson, T. M., 1996, Resistance to neurotoxicity in cortical cultures from neuronal nitric oxide synthase deficient mice. *J. Neurosci.* 15: 2479.

Di Monte, D. A., Royland, J.E., Jakowec, M. W. and Langston, J. W., 1996, Role of nitric oxide in methamphetamine neurotoxicity: protection by 7-nitroindazole, an inhibitor of neuronal nitric oxide synthase. *J. Neurochem.* 67:2443.

Ferriero, D. M., Holtzman, D. M., Black, S. M. and Sheldon, R. A.,1996, Neonatal mice lacking neuronal nitric oxide synthase are less vulnerable to hypoxic-ischemic injury. *Neurobiol. Dis.* 3:64.

Freyer, D., Weih, M., Weber, J.R., Bürger, W., Scholz, P., Manz, R., Ziegenhorn, A., Angstwurm, C. and Dirnagl, U.,1996, Pneumococcal cell wall components induce nitric oxide and TNF-α in astroglial-enriched cultures. *Glia* 16:1.

Hantraye, P., Brouillet, E., Ferrante, R., Palfi, S., Dolan, R., Matthews, R. T. and Beal, M.F., 1996, Inhibition of neuronal nitric oxide synthase prevents MPTP-induced parkinsonism in baboons. *Nature Medicine* 2:1071.

Hewett, S. J., Corbett, J.A., McDaniel, M. L and Choi, D. W., 1993, Inhibition of nitric oxide formation does not protect murine cortical cell cultures from N-methyl-D-aspartate neurotoxicity. *Brain Res.* 625:337.

Hörtnagl, H., Berger, M. L., Havelec, L. and Hornykiewicz, O, 1993, Role of glucocorticoids in the cholinergic degeneration in rat hippocampus induced by ethylcholine aziridinium (AF64A). *J. Neurosci.* 13:2939.

Hörtnagl, H., Berger, M. L., Reither, H. and Hornykiewicz, O., 1991, Cholinergic deficit induced by ethylcholine aziridinium (AF64A) in rat hippocampus: Effect on glutamate systems. *Naunyn-Schmiedeberg's Arch. Pharmacol.* 344:213.

Kosenko, E., Kaminsky, Y., Grau, E., Minana, M.D., Grisolia, S., Filipo, V., 1995, Nitroarginine, an inhibitor of nitric oxide synthase, attenuates ammonia toxicity and ammonia-induced alterations in brain metabolism. *Neurochem. Res.* 20:451 (1995).

Lipton, S.A., Choi, Y.B., Pan, Z. H., Lei, S. Z., Chen, H.S., Sucher, N. J., Loscalzo, J., Singel, D. J. and Stamler, J.S., 1993, A redox-based mechanism for the neuroprotective and neurodestructive effects of nitric oxide and related nitroso-compounds. *Nature* 364:636.

MacKenzie, G. M., Jenner, P. and Marsden, C. D., 1995, The effect of nitric oxide synthase inhibition on quinolinic acid toxicity in the rat striatum. *Neuroscience* 67:357.

Panahian, N., Yoshida, T., Huang, P. L, Hedley-Whyte, E. T., Dalkara, T., Fishman, M.C. and Moskowitz, M.A., 1996, Attenuated hippocampal damage after global cerebral ischemia in mice mutant in neuronal nitric oxide synthase. *Neuroscience* 72:343.

Przedborski, S., Jackson-Lewis, V., Yokoyama, R., Shibata, T., Dawson, V. L. and Dawson, T. M., 1996, Role of neuronal nitric oxide in 1-methyl-4-phenyl-1,2,3,6-tetrahydropyridine (MPTP)-induced dopaminergic neurotoxicity. *Proc. Natl. Acad. Sci.* USA 93:4565.

Scabó, C., 1996, Physiological and pathophysiological roles of nitric oxide in the central nervous system. *Brain Res. Bull.* 41:131.

Schulz, J.B., Huang, P. L., Matthews, T., Passov, D., Fishman, M.C. and Beal, M.F., 1996, Striatal malonate lesions are attenuated in neuronal nitric oxide synthase knockout mice. *J. Neurochem.* 67:430.

Smith, T. S., Swerdlow, R. H., Parker Jr., W. D. and Bennett Jr., J. P., 1994, Reduction of MPP$^+$-induced hydroxyl radical formation and nigrostriatal MPTP toxicity by inhibiting nitric oxide synthase. *NeuroReport* 5:2598.

Verrecchia, C., Boulu, R. G. and Plotkine, M., 1995, Neuroprotective and deleterious effects of nitric oxide on focal cerebral ischemia-induced neurone death. *Adv. Neuroimmunol.* 5:359.

Vizzard, M.A., Erdman, S. L. and de Groat, W. C., 1995, Increased expression of of neuronal nitric oxide synthase in dorsal root ganglion neurons after systemic capsaicin administration. *Neuroscience* 67:1.

97

EFFECT OF AF64A/NGF TREATMENT ON ChAT mRNA EXPRESSION IN THE SEPTO-HIPPOCAMPAL PATHWAY AND STRIATUM

Qing I. Fan,[1] Christopher A. Willson,[2] and Israel Hanin[1]

[1]Loyola University Chicago Stritch School of Medicine
Department of Pharmacology and Experimental Therapeutics
2160 South First Avenue
Maywood, Illinois 60153
[2]Karolinska Institutet
Medical Biochemistry and Biophysics
Laboratory of Molecular Neurobiology
Doktorsringen 12A, S171 77
Stockholm, Sweden

INTRODUCTION

In neurodegenerative diseases, such as Alzheimer's and Parkinson's disease, neurons in specific brain regions atrophy, become dysfunctional (e.g. reduced ability to produce neurotransmitters), and die. This cell death results in a loss of selective neuronal populations and the neurotransmitters that they synthesize and release. In Alzheimer's disease, the loss of basal forebrain cholinergic neurons results in a reduction of acetylcholine and its synthesizing enzyme, choline acetyltransferase (ChAT) (Nagei et al., 1983). The loss of cholinergic neurons in the basal forebrain is thought to play a role in the memory and cognitive deficits in patients with Alzheimer's disease (Hefti, 1994). Neurotrophic factors, which are known to interact with these neurons, have been proposed as a treatment for Alzheimer's disease (Hefti, 1994).

Nerve growth factor (NGF) is the classical neurotrophin protein involved in the development and maintenance of neurons in both the peripheral nervous system (PNS) and the central nervous system (CNS) (see review by Levi-Montalcini, 1987). NGF acts on sympathetic and sensory neurons of the PNS as well as on cholinergic neurons of the basal forebrain in the CNS (Longo et al., 1993). In the basal forebrain, NGF mRNA and NGF

Progress in Alzheimer's and Parkinson's Diseases
edited by Fisher *et al.*, Plenum Press, New York, 1998.

receptors have been localized in the septo-hippocampal pathway (SHP) (Lindsay et al., 1994; Senut et al., 1990; Shelton and Reichardt, 1986). In this pathway, immunoreactivity for NGF and its receptors has been co-localized with neurons expressing cholinergic phenotypic markers (Woolf, Gould and Butcher, 1989; Rylett and Williams, 1994). In addition to the SHP, NGF has been identified as having a role in the survival of cholinergic interneurons in the striatum, since NGF mRNA and receptors have been localized to the striatum (Shelton and Reichardt, 1986; Altar et al., 1991a). The localization of NGF receptors in the striatum is highly correlated with the enzyme, ChAT (Altar et al., 1991a; 1991b), indicating that cholinergic neurons in this brain region express NGF receptors. NGF-like immunoreactivity has also been identified in the striatum, although at lower levels than other brain regions (Altar, 1991b). ChAT mRNA is expressed at high levels in both the septum and striatum and at lower levels in the hippocampus, as demonstrated by reverse transcriptase (RT-PCR) (Cavicchioli et al., 1991), northern blot, and *in situ* hybridization (Ibanez et al., 1991) techniques.

In order to evaluate whether NGF could reverse cholinergic deficits in the SHP, several models of cholinergic deficits have been used. Transection of the fimbria-fornix, the major cholinergic projection from the septum to the hippocampus (Amaral and Kurz, 1985), causes a reduction in cholinergic phenotypic markers such as ChAT immunoreactivity, acetylcholinesterase staining and ChAT activity (Tuszynski et al., 1990). *In vivo* administration of NGF has been shown to reverse fimbria-fornix transection induced cholinergic deficits (Gage et al., 1988; Hagg et al., 1989; Kromer 1987; Montero and Hefti, 1988). In addition to being able to stimulate cholinergic markers in the SHP, NGF has also been shown to stimulate ChAT activity when administered into the striatum *in vivo* (Hagg et al., 1989), and it can produce recovery in ChAT activity after mechanical lesion (Altar et al., 1992).

AF64A is a neurotoxin that has been previously shown to be selective in a dose-dependent manner for cholinergic neurons in the SHP (Fisher et al., 1982). When administered into the lateral ventricle AF64A reduces ChAT and AChE activity in the hippocampus (Colhoun et al., 1986; El Tamer et al., 1992; Hanin, 1990) as well as high affinity choline transport (HAChT), acetylcholine (ACh) levels, and ChAT immunoreactivity in the SHP (El Tamer et al., 1992; Fisher et al., 1982; Leventer et al., 1985; Lorens et al., 1991). Accordingly, AF64A provides a means to produce cholinergic deficits in the SHP without the gross anatomical disruption seen when the fimbria-fornix is transected.

Although work in rats with cholinergic deficiencies indicates that NGF treatment can produce changes in cholinergic markers, studies assessing the action of NGF in normal, rats with undamaged brains, have not been as clear. Several studies have indicated that the effect of NGF on cholinergic markers in the SHP is dependent on damage or cholinergic deficiencies in this pathway (Gage et al., 1988; Hefti et al., 1984; Williams, Jodelis and Donald, 1989). Other studies indicate that NGF administration to rats with an intact SHP can increase cholinergic phenotypic markers in the medial septum and hippocampus (Fusco et al., 1989; Willson and Hanin, 1995).

The present study compared the effects of NGF administration on SHP and striatal neurons in AF64A-treated and normal, non-AF64A treated rats (Vehicle: VEH). NGF was found to increase ChAT activity in the SHP and striatum of both the AF64A treated and non-treated rats, although septal activity had a greater increase in AF64A treated rats compared with normals. In addition to evaluating changes in the level of ChAT enzyme activity, we also evaluated changes in ChAT mRNA in both these treatment groups in order to identify the possible mechanism for the stimulated ChAT activity. We demonstrate that NGF can increase ChAT mRNA in both the septum and striatum and that this increase occurs to a similar extent in both AF64A/NGF and VEH/NGF treated rats.

METHODS/RESULTS

Adult, male Sprague-Dawley rats (Zivic Miller Laboratories, Allison Park, PA.) were used for these experiments and AF64A was prepared according to standard methods (Fisher et al., 1982; El Tamer et al., 1992). Rats were anesthetized with intraperitoneal injections of equitensin (3ml/kg), and either VEH (water, pH 7.3) or AF64A (1.5 nmol/1.5 µl) were injected bilaterally into the lateral ventricles. One hour after injection, a sterile cannula-osmotic pump assembly (Alza, Palo Alto, CA), was implanted subcutaneously on the animal's back and a cannula inserted into one of the lateral ventricles. The osmotic pump contained either cytochrome C (CC; a control protein; 2.85 µg/day) or NGF (2.85 µg/day)(Harlan Bioproducts, Indianapolis, IN) dissolved in artificial cerebrospinal fluid. Therefore, this experiment had four treatment groups: VEH/CC, AF64A/CC, AF64A/NGF and VEH/NGF. The rats were infused for 14 days and then sacrificed by decapitation. The brains were dissected on ice and the tissue samples (hippocampus, septum and striatum) were immediately placed on dry ice and subsequently stored at -70°C.

For the ChAT assay, tissue samples (hippocampus, septum and striatum) were homogenized in phosphate buffer 75 mM, pH 7.4. The ChAT assay followed the Fonnum method (1975) in which 10 µl of tissue homogenate was added to 10 µl of buffer substrate containing [^{3}H]acetyl coenzyme A, 0.87 mM (20 mCi/mmol). ChAT activity was measured by subtracting the disintegrations per minute (dpm) in the blank tubes (without tissue) from the dpm in the tubes with tissue. Tissue protein levels were assessed by the method of Lowry et al. (1951). The data were calculated as nmol/mg/hr.

In order to assess ChAT mRNA levels, total mRNA was extracted from the septum and striatum according to the method of Chomczynski and Sacchi (1987). Semi-quantitative determination of ChAT mRNA levels was done by RT-PCR using 2 oligonucleotide primers for ChAT. The levels of PCR product were determined by a Betagen Betascope Analyzer and the ratio between the levels of ChAT mRNA and that of a control gene (Histone 3.3) were calculated. The data are presented as a ratio of these two gene PCR products and expressed as percentage of control (VEH/CC).

AF64A/CC treatment produced a significant decrease (25%) in hippocampal ChAT activity (Figure 1). In contrast, ChAT activity in the AF64A/NGF treatment group was reduced 19% and the VEH/NGF group had a 12% increase in activity compared to VEH/CC treated rats. NGF administration significantly increased septal ChAT activity regardless of whether it was administered after VEH or AF64A. NGF increased ChAT activity by 49% in VEH/NGF treated rats and by 113% in AF64A/NGF treated rats. This difference in the level of septal ChAT activity between these two treatment groups was significant and indicates that AF64A treated rats are more sensitive to NGF's ability to stimulate the ChAT enzyme. Striatal ChAT activity was also significantly increased by NGF administration. In the VEH/NGF treated rats, striatal ChAT activity increased 97% above control while the AF64A/NGF treated rats had an increase in ChAT activity of 116% above control. AF64A/CC treatment produced a 39% increase in striatal ChAT activity but this increase was significantly less than seen in either the VEH/NGF or AF64A/NGF treatment groups. The similar levels of striatal ChAT activity after NGF in both VEH and AF64A treated rats indicates that in this tissue, where AF64A does not produce a cholinergic deficit, AF64A treated rats are not more sensitive to NGF than VEH treated rats.

To further investigate the mechanism of the increased responsiveness of ChAT activity to NGF after AF64A administration, we investigated the effect of AF64A/NGF treatment on ChAT mRNA levels in the septum and striatum. AF64A treatment (AF64A/CC) produced a 50% reduction in the level of ChAT mRNA in the septum (Figure 2). In contrast, in

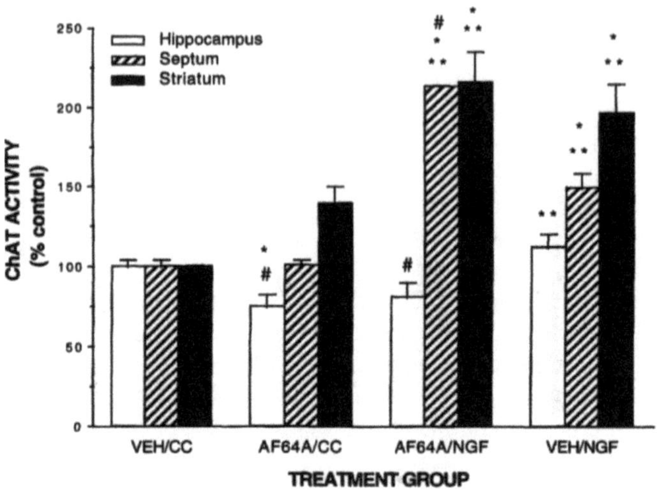

Figure 1. ChAT activity in the hippocampus, septum and striatum of rats treated with CC or NGF for 14 days after injection with either VEH or AF64A. The data are presented as the percentage of control (mean+/- SEM) for 15–20 rats per treatment group. The control rats (VEH/CC) had enzyme activities of 45 (hippocampus), 68 (septum) and 97 (striatum) nmol/mg/hr. Data were analyzed by ANOVA with LSD post-hoc analysis. * p< 0.05 vs VEH/CC, ** p<0.01 vs AF64A/CC, # p<0.01 vs VEH/NGF.

AF64A/NGF treated rats there was only an 11% reduction and the level of ChAT mRNA was 39% higher than found in AF64A/CC treated rats. The VEH/NGF treated group had a 33% increase in ChAT mRNA above control. Striatal ChAT mRNA had a robust increase when NGF was administered, regardless of whether rats were initially treated with VEH or AF64A. The AF64A/NGF treated rats showed a 106% increase above control while VEH/NGF treated rats had a 127% increase above control. Both of these increases were significant compared with mRNA levels in either VEH/CC or AF64A/CC treated rats. The levels of ChAT mRNA between the two NGF treatment groups were similar.

DISCUSSION

The present study indicates that in the SHP, animals treated with the cholinotoxin, AF64A, are more sensitive to the effects (stimulation of ChAT activity) of exogenously administered NGF when compared with non-AF64A treated rats (normals). Previous work investigating the action of NGF on cholinergic neurons in normal rats has been conflicting. NGF has been shown not to change ChAT activity in normal rats while reversing decreases in enzyme activity induced by fimbria-fornix transection (Williams, Jodelis and Donald, 1989; Hefti et al., 1984). In addition, ChAT immunoreactivity is not changed in normal rats treated with NGF (Gage et al., 1988). In contrast to these findings, several studies have shown that NGF administered to normal rats stimulates ChAT activity in both the septum and hippocampus (Vahlsing et al., 1991; Rylett and Williams 1994; Fusco et al., 1989; Williams 1991; Willson and Hanin, 1995). The results of the current study confirm the findings that normal, non-compromised cholinergic neurons of the SHP are responsive to exogenously administered NGF. In addition, our data also confirm the ability of NGF to stimulate ChAT activity in the cholinergic interneurons located in the striatum.

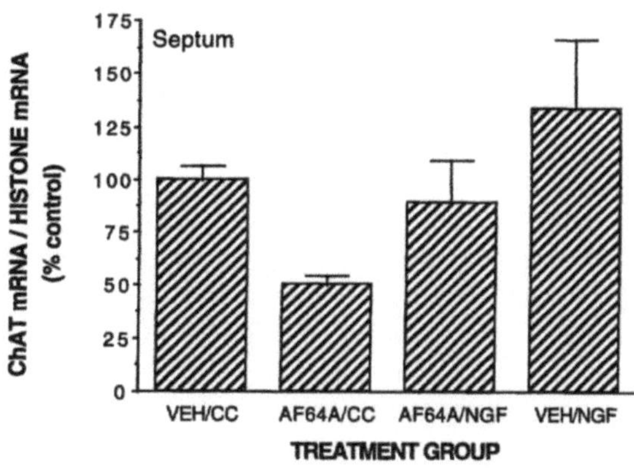

Figure 2. Measures of mRNA levels for ChAT in the septum and striatum. Levels of ChAT mRNA were determined by RT-PCR. The data are expressed as the ratio of ChAT mRNA to histone mRNA (a control gene). The data are presented as percentage of control (mean+/- SEM) for 6–7 rats per group. The mean control (VEH/CC) values for the ratios were 0.069 (+/- 0.004) in the septum and 0.067 (+/- 0.011) for striatum. Data were analyzed by ANOVA with LSD post-hoc analysis. * p< 0.05 vs VEH/CC, ** p<0.01 vs AF64A/CC.

Several groups have demonstrated that intracerebroventricular administration of NGF increases cell body size (Vahlsing et al., 1991) and ChAT activity (Altar et al., 1992) in the striatum. These data indicate that NGF administration clearly affects ChAT activity in both the SHP and striatum of normal rats and that NGF interacts with mature, uninjured cholinergic neurons.

In both the septum and striatum, NGF administration to AF64A treated rats produced a robust increase in ChAT activity. The level of increase in ChAT activity between these two brain regions was similar (113 and 116% above control for the septum and striatum respectively) indicating that both populations of neurons respond in a similar manner to exogenous NGF, even though they are comprised of different neuronal types (long projecting neurons in the septum and interneurons in the striatum). The stimulation in septal ChAT activity indicates that an interaction occurs in the SHP between the terminal and cell body of these neurons. Rats treated with AF64A/NGF demonstrated increases in septal ChAT activity to levels 113% above control. In contrast, normal rats treated with NGF had increases in their ChAT activity of 49% above control. In addition, the response of striatum of ChAT activity to exogenously administered NGF was similar in both AF64A/NGF and VEH/NGF treated rats, indicating that the increased response to NGF in the septum of AF64A/NGF treated rats is AF64A-dependent. Other studies have also found that rats with deficits in cholinergic phenotypic markers have increased sensitivity to NGF administration (Williams et al., 1989; Williams 1991; Yunshao et al., 1992; Willson and Hanin et al., 1995). Together with the current study, this indicates that when cholinergic neurons of the SHP are compromised or injured, these neurons have an increased sensitivity to the effects of exogenously administered NGF compared with neurons that are not compromised. The increased responsiveness of AF64A treated rats to NGF indicates that the action of this toxin at neuronal terminals (decrease of cholinergic enzyme activity in the hippocampus) affects the activity which occurs in the cell body (increased responsiveness to NGF in the septum). The present work therefore provides a good model of neuronal integration by demonstrating the relationship between changes that occur in the hippocampus and septum.

In order to elucidate the mechanism by which NGF increased ChAT activity in these two brain regions in the present report, we evaluated ChAT mRNA levels. NGF administration increased ChAT mRNA levels in both the septum and striatum by 33% and 127% above control, respectively. The increase in the striatum was similar between the AF64A and VEH treated rats and most likely is responsible for the increase in ChAT activity seen in this tissue. In the septum, NGF increased ChAT mRNA in both AF64A and VEH treatment groups and these increases also were similar (39% for AF64A/NGF compared with the levels in the AF64A/CC treated rats and 33% for VEH/NGF compared with the levels in the VEH/CC treated rats). It appears that NGF administration to AF64A treated rats may produce a slight recovery of septal ChAT mRNA compared to AF64A/CC treated rats (50% decrease in ChAT mRNA levels). Other studies have also shown that ChAT mRNA is increased in the septum of normal rats after exogenous NGF treatment (Cavicchioli et al., 1991). ChAT mRNA in the striatum is also increased by either intrastriatal or intracerebroventricular injection of NGF (Venero et al., 1996). The increase in ChAT mRNA in the septum (39% in AF64A/NGF compared with AF64A/CC) does not appear to be sufficient for the large increase seen in ChAT activity found in the septum of these rats. Therefore, the increase in ChAT activity found in the striatum in the present study is probably due to an increase in ChAT synthesis, while the increase in the septum may be due in part to other factors.

One possible explanation for the increased responsiveness of AF64A treated rats to NGF is that AF64A may increase the level of endogenous NGF in the SHP. Other noxious insults to the SHP such as lesions (Weskamp et al., 1986; Gall and Isackson 1989); electrical stimulation (Ernfors et al., 1991); or kainic acid administration (Gall et al., 1991), have been shown to produce an increase in NGF, its mRNA and its receptors. A recent paper by Hellweg et al., (1997) has demonstrated that NGF protein and mRNA levels in the hippocampus increase after AF64A administration. An increase in endogenous NGF would result in a higher level of NGF available to the SHP cholinergic neurons of AF64A/NGF treated rats compared with that found in rats treated with NGF alone.

Another explanation could be that AF64A inhibits axonal transport. Previous work has shown that in both the CNS and PNS, AF64A, at high doses, inhibits axonal transport (Kasa and Hanin, 1985). If axonal transport were blocked by AF64A, one would expect an accumulation of the enzyme protein in the septum and a deficit in the hippocampus. This corresponds to the data in the present study in which AF64A treated rats had a robust increase in enzyme activity in the septum and no change in the hippocampus. In normals rats, increases in enzyme activity produced by NGF were distributed evenly in the SHP, as would be expected if axonal transport was functioning properly.

In conclusion, NGF administration to both AF64A and non-AF64A treated rats produced an increase in ChAT enzyme activity. Furthermore, AF64A treated rats have an increased sensitivity to the effects of NGF on cholinergic neurons in the SHP but not in the striatum, indicating that this increased sensitivity is AF64A dependent. Septal and striatal ChAT mRNA levels were increased by NGF in both AF64A and non-AF64A treated rats. The increase in striatal levels probably accounts for the increase in ChAT activity, while the increase in the septum may only play a partial role in the increased level of enzyme activity in this tissue. These findings raise the possibility that degenerating neurons in Alzheimer's disease patients might also be more sensitive to NGF.

REFERENCES

Altar, C.A., 1991a, Nerve growth factor and the neostriatum Prog. *Neuro-Psycholpharmacol. and Biol. Psychiat.*15:157–169.

Altar, C.A., Dugich-Djordjevic, M., Armanini, M., and Bakhit, C., 1991b, Medial-to-lateral gradient of neostriatal NGF receptors: relationship to cholinergic neurons and NGF-like immunoreactivity. *J. Neurosci.* 11(3):829–836.

Altar, C.A., Armanini, M., Dugich-Djordjevic, M., Bennett, G.L., Williams, R., Feinglass, S., Anicetti, V., Sinicropi, D. and Bakhit, C., 1992, Recovery of cholinergic phenotype in the injured rat neostriatum: roles for endogenous and exogenous nerve growth factor. *J. Neurochem.*59(6):2167–2177.

Amaral, D.G., and Kurz, J., 1985, An analysis of the origins of the cholinergic and non-cholinergic septal projections to the hippocampal formation of the rat. *J. Comp. Neurol.* 240:37–59.

Cavicchioli, L., Flanigan, T.P., Dickson, J.G., Vantini, G., Dal Toso, R., Fusco, M., Walsh, F.S., and Leon, A., 1991, Choline acetyltransferase messenger RNA expression in developing and adult rat brain: regulation of nerve growth factor. *Mol. Brain Res.* 9:319–325.

Chomczynski, P., and Sacchi, N., 1987, Single-step method of RNA isolation by acid guanidinium thiocyanate-phenol-chloroform extraction. *Anal. Biochem.* 162(1):156–159.

Colhoun, E.H., Myles, L.A., and Rylett, R.J., 1986, An attempt to produce cholinergic hypofunction in rat brain using choline mustard aziridinium ion: neurochemical and histological parameters. *Can. J. Neurol. Sci.* 13:517–520.

El Tamer, A., Corey, J., Wülfert, E., and Hanin, I., 1992, Reversible cholinergic changes induced by AF64A in rat hippocampus and possible septal compensatory effects. *Neuropharmacology* 31(4):397–402.

Ernfors, P., Bengzon, J., Kokaia, Z., Persson, B., and Lindvall, O., 1991, Increased levels of messenger RNAs for neurotropic factors in the brain during kindling epileptogenesis. *Neuron* 7:165–176.

Fisher, A., Mantione, C.R., Abraham, D.J., Hanin, I., 1982, Long term central cholinergic hypofunction induced in mice by ethylcholine aziridinium ion (AF64A) *in vivo*. *J. Pharm. Exp. Ther.* 222(1):140–145.

Fonnum, F., 1975, Rapid radiochemical method for the determination of choline acetyltransferase. *J. Neurochem.* 24:407–409.

Fusco, M., Oderfeld-Nowak, B., Vantini, G., Schiavo, N., Gradkowska, M., Zaremba, M., and Leon, A., 1989, Nerve growth factor affects uninjured adult rat septohippocampal cholinergic neurons. *Neuroscience* 33(1):47–52.

Gage, F.H., Armstrong, D.M., Williams, L.R., and Varon, S., 1988, Morphological response of axotomized septal neurons to nerve growth factor. *J. Comp. Neurol.* 269:147–155.

Gall, C.M., Isackson, P.J., 1989, Limbic seizures increase neuronal production of messenger RNA for nerve growth factor. *Science* 245:758–761.

Gall, C., Murray, K., and Isackson, P.J., 1991, Kainic acid-induced seizures stimulate increased expression of nerve growth factor mRNA in rat hippocampus. *Mol. Brain Res.* 9:113–123.

Hagg, T., Fass-Holmes, B., Vahlsing, H.L., Manthorpe, M., Conner, J.M., and Varon, S., 1989, Nerve growth factor (NGF) reverses axotomy induced decreases in choline acetyltransferase, NGF receptor and size of medial septum cholinergic neurons. *Brain Res.* 505:29–38.

Hanin, I., 1990, AF64A-induced cholinergic hypofunction. In: *Progress in Brain Research*, Aquilonius, S.M. and Gillberg, P.G., eds. Elsevier Science, Amsterdam, 84:289–299.

Hefti, F., Dravid, A., and Hartikka, J., 1984, Chronic intraventricular injections of nerve growth factor elevate hippocampal choline acetyltransferase activity in adult rats with partial septo-hippocampal lesions. *Brain Res.* 293:305–311.

Hefti, F., 1994, Neurotrophic factor therapy for nervous system degenerative diseases. *J. Neurobiol.* 25(11):1418–1435.

Hellweg, R., Humpel, C., Löwe, A., and Hörtnagl, H., 1997, Moderate lesion of the rat cholinergic septohippocampal pathway increases hippocampus nerve growth factor synthesis: evidence for long-term compensatory changes? *Mol. Brain Res.* 45:177–181.

Ibanez, C.F., Ernfors, P., and Persson, H., 1991, Development and regional expression of choline acetyltransferase mRNA in the rat central nervous system. *J. Neurosci. Res.* 29:163–171.

Kása, P., and Hanin, I., 1985, Ethylcholine mustard aziridinium blocks the axoplasmic transport of acetylcholinesterase in cholinergic nerve fibers of the rat. *Histochemistry* 83:343–345.

Kromer, L.F., 1987, Nerve growth factor treatment after brain injury prevents neuronal death. *Science* 235:214–216.

Leventer, S., McKeag, D., Clancy, M., Wülfert, E., and Hanin, I., 1985, Intracerebroventricular administration of ethylcholine mustard azirdinium ion (AF64A) reduces release of acetylcholine from rat hippocampal slices. *Neuropharmacology* 24(5):453–459.

Levi-Montalcini, R., 1987, The nerve growth factor 35 years later. *Science* 237:1154–1162.

Lindsay, R.M., Wiegand, S.J., Altar, C.A., and DiStefano, P.S., 1994, Neurotrophic factors: from molecule to man. *Trends Neurosci.* 17(5):182–190.

Longo, F.M., Holtzman, D.M., Grimes, M.L., and Mobley, W.C., 1993, Nerve growth factor in the peripheral and central nervous system. In: *Neurotrophic Factors*, Loughlin, S.E., and Fallon, J.H., eds., Academic Press, CA, 209–256.

Lorens, S.A., Kindel, G., Dong, X.W., Lee, J.M., and Hanin, I., 1991, Septal choline acetyltransferase immunoreactive neurons: dose-dependent effects of AF64A. *Brain Res. Bull.* 26:965–971.

Lowry, O.H., Rosebrough, N.J., Farr, A.L., and Randall, R.J., 1951, Protein measurement with the folin phenol reagent. *J. Biol. Chem.* 195:265–267.

Montero, C.N., and Hefti, F., 1988, Rescue of lesioned septal cholinergic neurons by nerve growth factor: specificity and requirement for chronic treatment. *J. Neurosci.* 8:2986–2999.

Nagei, T., McGeer, P.L., Peng, J.H., McGeer, E.G., and Dolman, C.E., 1983, Choline acetyltransferase immunohistochemistry in brains of Alzheimer's patients and controls. *Neurosci. Lett.* 36:195–199.

Rylett, R.J., and Williams, L.R., 1994, Role of neurotrophins in cholinergic-neurone function in the adult and aged CNS. *Trends Neurosci.* 17(11):486–490.

Senut, M.C., Lamour, Y., Lee, J., Brachet, P., and Dicou, E., 1990, Neuronal localization of the nerve growth factor precursor-like immunoreactivity in the rat brain. *Int. J. Dev. Neurosci.* 8:65–80.

Shelton, D.L., and Reichard, L.F., 1986, Studies on the expression of the â nerve growth factor (NGF) gene in the central nervous system: level and regional distribution of NGF mRNA suggest that NGF functions as a trophic factor for several distinct populations of neurons. *Proc. Natl. Acad. Sci.* 83:2714–2718.

Tuszynski, M.H., Armstrong, D.M., and Gage, F.H., 1990, Basal forebrain cell loss following fimbria/fornix transection. *Brain Res.* 508:241–248.

Vahlsing H.L., Hagg, T., Spencer, M., Conner, J.M., Manthorpe, M., and Varon, S., 1991, Dose-dependent responses to nerve growth factor by adult rat cholinergic medial septum and neostriatum neurons. *Brain Res.* 552:320–329.

Venero, J.L., Hefti, F., and Knusel, B., 1996, Trophic effect of exogenous nerve growth factor on rat striatal cholinergic neurons: comparison between intraparenchymal and intraventricular administration. *Mol. Pharm.* 49(2):303–310.

Weskamp G., Gasser, U.E., Dravid, A.R., and Otten, U., 1986, Fimbria-fornix lesion increases nerve growth factor content in adult rat septum and hippocampus. *Neurosci. Lett.* 70:121–126.

Williams, L.R., Jodelis, K.S., and Donald, M.R., 1989, Axotomy-dependent stimulation of choline acetyltransferase activity by exogenous mouse nerve growth factor in adult rat. *Brain Res.* 498:243–256.

Williams, L.R., 1991, Exogenous nerve growth factor stimulates choline acetyltransferase activity in aging Fischer 344 male rats. *Neurobiol. Aging* 12:39–46.

Willson, C.A., and Hanin, I., 1995, Effect of nerve growth factor in ethylcholine mustard aziridinium (AF64A)-treated rats: sensitization of cholinergic enzyme activity in the septohippocampal pathway. *J. Neurochem.* 65(2):856–862.

Woolf, N.J., Gould, E., and Butcher, L.L., 1989, Nerve growth factor receptor is associated with cholinergic neurons of the basal forebrain but not the pontomesencephalon. *Neuroscience* 30(1):143–152.

Yunshao, H., Zhibin, Y., Yaoming, G., Guobi, K., and Yici, C., 1992, Nerve growth factor promotes collateral sprouting of cholinergic fibers in the septohippocampal cholinergic system of aged rats with fimbria transection. *Brain Res.* 586:27–35.

98

INDUCTION, SECRETION, AND PHARMACOLOGICAL REGULATION OF β-APP IN ANIMAL MODEL SYSTEMS

V. Haroutunian,[1] S. A. Ahlers,[2] N. Greig,[3] and W. C. Wallace[3]

[1]Department of Psychiatry
The Mount Sinai School of Medicine and Bronx VA Medical Center
New York, New York
[2]Naval Medical Research Institute
Bethesda, Maryland
[3]Laboratory of Cellular and Molecular Biology
National Institutes on Aging
Bethesda, Maryland

The deposition of Alzheimer's amyloid β-protein (Aβ) in neuritic plaques and the degeneration of cholinergic neurons originating in the basal forebrain are among the hallmarks of Alzheimer's disease (Selkoe et al., 1986; Selkoe, 1994; Masters et al., 1985; Bierer et al., 1995; Perry et al., 1978; DeKosky et al., 1992; Citron et al., 1992; Goate et al., 1991). That these neuropathological and neurochemical abnormalities may be related to each other or may interact with each other has been explored only recently. *In vitro* and *in vivo* studies have shown that the synthesis, processing and secretion of β-amyloid precursor protein (β-APP) can be regulated by the neurotransmitter systems affected in Alzheimer's disease.

A link between the forebrain cholinergic system and β-APP has been established by *in vivo* studies. The infusion of neurotoxins into the region of the nucleus basalis of Meynert (nbM), the nucleus of origin of the cholinergic innervation of the cerebral cortex, causes not only the expected loss of cholinergic marker activity in the cerebral cortex, but also an increase in the synthesis of β-APP (Wallace et al., 1991) and an increase in the cerebrocortical levels of β-APP mRNA (Wallace et al., 1993). The induction of β-APP is rapid, occurring within 1–2 hours of lesioning, and persistent. The levels of β-APP mRNA remain elevated in the cortices of 20 month old rats that were lesioned when they were 2 months old. More detailed studies have shown that the induction of β-APP mRNA is coupled to the loss of cholinergic activity in the cortex and not to the physical loss of the cholinergic neurons or surgical trauma. When the spontaneous release of acetylcholine

(ACh) in the cortex is temporarily blocked by the infusion of lidocaine into the nbM, the levels of β-APP mRNA in the cortex increase. β-APP mRNA levels in the cortex return to baseline levels as the local anesthetic effects of lidocaine diminishes and cortical acetylcholine release is restored to baseline levels. The neurotransmitter dependent induction of β-APP is not restricted to the forebrain cholinergic system. Lesions of the forebrain projecting noradrenergic and serotonergic systems also induce β-APP in the cortices of the lesioned rats. When 6-hydroxydopamine was infused into the dorsal bundle, or when 5-7-dihydroxytryptamine was injected into the dorsal raphe nucleus, the levels of noradrenaline and serotonin, respectively, were significantly reduced in the cerebral cortex. Both types of lesions caused a nearly two fold increase in the levels of β-APP mRNA in the cortices of the same animals.

The induction of cortical β-APP (APPs) following lesions of forebrain projecting neurotransmitter systems is accompanied by a concomitant rise in the levels of secreted β-APP (APPs) measured in the cerebro-spinal fluid (CSF) (Wallace et al., 1995). In these experiments different groups of rats received lesions of forebrain cholinergic, noradrenergic, or serotonergic systems using axon-sparing neurotoxic lesioning procedures. The rats were then anesthetized at different times after the lesioning or sham-lesioning procedure and clear CSF was collected by cisternal puncture. Initially, during the 24–72 hours post-lesioning (time course dependent upon the neurotransmitter system lesioned) the levels of APPs in the CSF were found to be reduced relative to sham operated rats, but the levels of APPs rose above baseline within 7 days of the lesioning procedure. The increased levels of APPs in the CSF of nbM lesioned rats were found to persist for at least 18 months after lesioning. This forebrain cholinergic lesion-induced increase in the levels of APPs in the CSF was found to be significantly exaggerated when the lesions were made in aged rats relative to forebrain cholinergically lesioned young adult rats. The increase in the levels of APPs in the CSF of nbM lesioned rats was accompanied by a similar increase in the levels of c-terminal fragments of β-APP in the cerebral cortex(Wallace et al., 1995). Similar increases in the levels of c-terminal fragments have been observed in the hippocampi of rats sustaining lesions of the septo-hippocampal pathway(Beeson et al., 1994).

The regulation of β-APP by pharmacological agents that affect the cholinergic system has been demonstrated by *in vitro* and *in vivo* experiments. Tissue culture and cortical and hippocampal slice preparation studies have shown that the metabolism and secretion of β-APP and its various fragments can be altered by pharmacological agents that affect the cholinergic system by the inhibition of cholinesterases (Lahiri et al., 1994; Lahiri, 1994) or by stimulation of muscarinic receptors and the M1 subtype of the muscarinic receptors (Lahiri et al., 1992; Buxbaum et al., 1992; Farber et al., 1995; Nitsch et al., 1992; Pittel et al., 1996). *In vivo* studies have also shown that the levels of APPs in the CSF can be regulated by the pharmacological manipulation of the cholinergic system. In one series of studies we administered various cholinomimetic agents acutely to naive rats. The cholinesterase inhibitor physostigmine (0.3 mg/kg), a relatively specific acetylcholinesterase inhibitor phenserine (Brzostowska et al., 1992; Greig et al., 1995) (3.0 mg/kg), a butyrylcholinesterase specific analogue of phenserine(2.5 mg/kg), and the M1 receptor subtype specific agonist AF102B (1 mg/kg) were administered. Cerebrospinal fluid was then collected 1–1.5 hours after treatment and the CSF levels of APPs determined by immunoblot analysis using the 22C11 antibody. Relative to vehicle treated controls, these cholinomimetic agents all reduced the levels of APPs in the CSF (Haroutunian et al., 1997a). In a similar series of studies, the acetylcholinesterase inhibitor phenserine and the organophosphate cholinesterase inhibitor DFP were administered to nbM lesioned rats for 7 days following lesioning. The reversible acetylcholinesterase specific inhibitor phenserine normalized the lesion-induced increase in CSF-APPs, but the non-specific cholinesterase inhibitor, DFP had no significant effect on APPs (Haroutunian et al., 1997b). The muscarinic receptor antagonist scopolamine can also influence the induction and secretion of β-APP. The chronic (7-days) treatment of rats with scopolamine (0.5 mg/kg/hour) administered subcutaneously led to increases in the CSF levels of APPs that were comparable in magnitude to that observed by neurotoxic lesions of the nbM (Haroutunian et al., 1997b). β-APP mRNAs were also increased in the cortices of scopolamine treated rats (Acevedo et al., 1997). Interestingly, the administration of scopolamine to nbM lesioned rats failed to raise the CSF levels of APPs beyond that observed in nbM lesioned rats receiving saline infusions (Haroutunian et al., 1997b).

These results taken as a whole show an intimate relationship between central neurotransmission and the synthesis and secretion of β-APP. Experimentally induced deficits in some of the neurotransmitter systems involved in Alzheimer's disease lead to the induction of β-APP and increased secretion of its fragments. Pharmacological agents which enhance cholinergic neurotransmission reduce the levels of secreted fragments of β-APP and normalize their levels in the CSF of rats with forebrain cholinergic lesions. At a more speculative level, these findings suggest that the therapeutic effects of cholinomimetics may extend beyond the palliative treatment of cognitive deficits in AD and influence amyloidogenic processes.

REFERENCES

Acevedo, L. D., Haroutunian, V., Sherman-Baust, C. A., Norton, D. D., and Wallace, W. C., 1997, Increased APP induction following muscarinic receptor blockade *in vivo. Soc.Neurosci. Abstract.*

Beeson, J., Shelton, E., Chan, H., and Gage, F., 1994, Age and Damage Induced Changes in Amyloid Protein Precursor Immunohistochemistry in the Rat Brain. *J. Comp. Neurol.* 342: 69–77.

Bierer, L., Haroutunian, V., Gabriel, S., Knott, P., Carlin, L., Dushyant, P., Perl, D., Schmeidler, J., Kanof, P., and Davis, K., 1995, Neurochemical Correlates of Dementia Severity in Alzheimer's Disease: Relative Importance of the Cholinergic Deficits. *J. Neurochem.* 64:749–760.

Brzostowska, M., He, X. S., Greig, N. H., Rapaport, S., and Brossi, A., 1992, Selective inhibition of acetyl-and butyrylcholinesterases by phenylcarbamates of (-)-eseroline, (-)-(N1)-noreseroline and physovenol. *Med. Chem. Res.* 2: 238–246.

Buxbaum, J., Oishi, M., Chen, H., Pinkas-Kramarski, R., Jaffe, E., Gandy, S., and Greengard, P., 1992, Cholinergic agonists and interleukin 1 regulate processing and secretion of the Alzheimer B/A4 amyloid protein precursor. *Proc. Natl. Acad. Sci.* U S A 89:10075–10078.

Citron, M., Oltersdorf, T., Haass, C., McConlogue, L., Hung, A. Y., Seubert, P., Vigo-Pelfrey, C., Lieberburg, I., and Selkoe, D. J., 1992 Mutation of the β-amyloid precursor protein in familial Alzheimer's disease increases B-protein production. *Nature* 360:672–674.

DeKosky, S. T., Harbaugh, R. E., Schmitt, F. A., Bakay, R. A., Chui, H. C., Knopman, D. S., Reeder, T. M., Shetter, A. G., Senter, H. J., and Markesbery, W. R., 1992, Cortical biopsy in Alzheimer's disease: diagnostic accuracy and neurochemical, neuropathological, and cognitive correlations. Intraventricular Bethanecol Study Group. *Ann. Neurol.* 32:625–632.

Farber, S. A., Nitsch, R. M., Schulz, J. G., and Wurtman, R. J., 1995, Regulated Secretion of β-Amyloid Precursor Protein in Rat Brain. *J. Neurosci.* 15:7442–7451.

Goate, A., Chartier-Harlin, M., Mullan, M., Brown, J., Crawford, F., Fidani, L., Giuffra, L., Haynes, A., Irving, N., James, L., Mant, R., Newton, P., Rook, K., Roques, P., Talbot, C., Pericak-Vance, M., Roses, A., Williamson, R., Rossor, M., Owen, M., and Hardy, J., 1991, Segregation of a missense mutation in the amyloid precursor protein gene with familial Alzheimer's disease. *Nature* 349:704–706.

Greig, N. H., Pei, X. F., Soncrant, T. T., Ingram, D. K., and Brossi, A., 1995, Phenserine and ring C hetero-analogues: drug candidates for the treatment of Alzheimer's disease. *Med. Res. Rev.* 15:3–31.

Haroutunian, V., Ahlers, S. T., Acevedo, L. D., Utsuki, T., Gluck, R., Davis, K. L., and Wallace, W. C., 1997a,. Cholinergic pharmacology of secreted Alzheimer's β-amyloid precursor protein levels in the CSF of rats. *Soc. Neurosci. Abstract.*

Haroutunian, V., Greig, N., Pei, X.-F., Utsuki,, T., Gluck, R., Acevedo, D.L., Davis, K. L., and Wallace, W. C., 1997b, Pharmacological modulation of Alzheimer's β-amyloid precursor protein levels in the CSF of rats with forebrain cholinergic lesions. *Brain Res. Mol. Brain Res.* 46:161–168.

Lahiri, D., 1994, Reversibility of the effect of tacrine on the secretion of the β-amyloid precursor protein in cultured cells. *Neurosci. Lett.* 181:149–142.

Lahiri, D., Lewis, S., and Farlow, M., 1994, Tacrine alters the secretion of the beta-amyloid precursor protein in cell lines. *J. Neurosci. Res.* 37:777–787.

Lahiri, D. K., Nall, C., and Farlow, M. R., 1992, The cholinergic agonist carbachol reduces intracellular beta-amyloid precursor protein in PC 12 and C6 cells. *Biochem. Int.* 28:853–860.

Masters, C. L., Simms, G., Weinman, N. A., Multraup, G., McDonald, B. L., and Beyreuther, K., 1985, Amyloid plaque core protein in Alzheimer's disease and Downs syndrome. *Proc. Natl. Acad. Sci.* U S A 82:4245–4249.

Nitsch, R. M., Slack, B. E., Wurtman, R. J., and Growdon, J. H., 1992, Release of Alzheimer amyloid precursor derivatives stimulated by activation of muscarinic acetylcholine receptors. *Science* 258:304–307.

Perry, E. K., Tomlinson, B. E., Blessed, G., Bergmann, K., Gibson, P. H., and Perry, R. H., 1978, Correlation of cholinergic abnormalities with senile plaques and mental test scores in senile dementia. *Br. Med. J.* 2:1457–1459.

Pittel, Z., Heldman, E., Barg, J., Haring, R., and Fisher, A., 1996, Muscarinic control of amyloid precursor protein secretion in rat cerebral cortex and cerebellum. *Brain Res.* 742:299–304.

Selkoe, D. J., Abraham, C. R., Podlisny, M. B., and Duffy, L. K., 1986, Isolation of low-molecular-weight proteins from amyloid plaque fibers in Alzheimer's disease. *J. Neurochem.* 146:1820–1834.

Selkoe, D. J., 1994, Normal and abnormal biology of the β-amyloid precursor protein. *Annl. Rev. Neurosci.* 17:489–517.

Wallace, W., Ahlers, S. T., Gotlib, J., Bragin, V., Sugar, J., Gluck, R., Shea, P. A., Davis, K. L., and Haroutunian, V., 1993, Amyloid precursor protein in the cerebral cortex is rapidly and persistently induced by loss of subcortical innervation. *Proc. Natl. Acad. Sci.* U S A,.90:8712–8716.

Wallace, W., Lieberburg, I., Schenk, D., Vigo-Pelfrey, C., Davis, K., and Haroutunian, V., 1995, Chronic elevation of secreted amyloid precursor protein in subcortically lesioned rats, and its exacerbation in aged rats. *J. Neurosci.* 15:4896–4905.

Wallace, W. C., Bragin, V., Robakis, N. K., Sambamurti, K., Vanderputten, D., Merril, C. R., Davis, K. L., Santucci, A. C., and Haroutunian, V., 1991, Increased biosynthesis of Alzheimer amyloid precursor protein in the cerebral cortex of rats with lesions of the nucleus basalis of Meynert. *Brain Res. Mol. Brain Res.* 10:173–178.

99

ANAPSOS IMPROVES LEARNING AND MEMORY IN RATS WITH ßA(1-28) DEPOSITS INTO THE HIPPOCAMPUS

Antón Alvarez,[1] José Javier Miguel-Hidalgo,[1] Lucía Fernández-Novoa,[1] Joaquín Díaz,[2] José Miguel Sempere,[2] and Ramón Cacabelos[1]

[1]EuroEspes Biomedical Research Center
A Coruña, Spain
[2]ASAC Pharmaceutical International
Alicante, Spain

INTRODUCTION

Anapsos is a vegetal extract obtained from dried rhizhomes of the fern Polypodium leucotomos growing in Central America. This extract is devoid of toxic effects in animals and humans at therapeutic doses and is commercially available in Spain. An antitumoral effect of anapsos was found in early studies (Horwath et al., 1967), and this effect was confirmed by other authors suggesting an interaction of anapsos with cytoplasm receptors (Vargas et al., 1981). These studies show that anapsos has anabolic effects in normal tissues *in vivo* oppossite to the catabolic action exerted by cytostatics. Furthermore, Anapsos exerts immunoregulatory effects in control subjects (Sempere et al., 1997; Vargas et al., 1983) and in patients with atopic dermatitis (Jiménez et al., 1987), psoriasis (Padilla et al., 1974) or vitiligo (Mohamed, 1989), and increases the allograft survival in rats and mice with skin transplants (Pérez de las Casas et al., 1987; Tuominen et al., 1991). In healthy subjects anapsos increases the lymphoblast response to mitogens, serum immunoglobulin levels and the proportion of $CD8^+$ cells in a dose-dependent manner (Vargas et al., 1983). Anapsos also stimulates cell proliferation, reduces LPS-stimulated IL-1ß levels and delays the peak response of IL-1ß to LPS+PHA in human PBMC cultures (Sempere et al., 1997). Recently, we have found that anapsos improves learning and reduces brain IL-1ß levels in normal rats; reverses learning impairment and brain IL-1ß overexpression in rats with lesions in the nucleus basalis of Meynert; improves motor functioning and influences the production of brain immune factors as histamine and IL-1ß in aged mice; and reduces behavioral deficits and neuronal degeneration induced by ß-amyloid implants into the hippo-

Progress in Alzheimer's and Parkinson's Diseases
edited by Fisher *et al.*, Plenum Press, New York, 1998.

campus, modulating IL-1ß and superoxide dismutase (SOD) activity levels in the brain of ßA-injected rats (Alvarez et al., 1992, 1995, 1996c, 1997; Fernández-Novoa et al., 1997).

Recent data showing that neuroimmune mechanisms are involved in Alzheimer's disease (AD) pathology suggest that the intense immunoreactive-inflammatory process observed in AD brains may contribute to neurodegeneration (Alvarez et al., 1996a; Cacabelos et al., 1994a,b; Dickson and Rogers, 1992; Eikelenboom et al., 1994; McGeer et al., 1994). Thus, the neurotoxic effect of the immune activation, together with a failure of neurotrophic factors to stimulate degenerating neurons, can lead to accelerated cell death. Consequently, we propose that a therapeutic intervention in this cascade of neuroimmune-neurotrophic events in the CNS would be of some help in limiting neurodegeneration and cell death and in alleviating cognitive decline in AD (Cacabelos et al., 1994b). Furthermore, preventive strategies with neuroimmunotrophic drugs given chronically to people with genetic risk for developing AD might be implemented by given drugs for years prior to the onset of the disease. In this regard, anapsos has a good pharmacological profile to be used with a preventive purpose in neurodegenerative and age-related disorders.

In this study we have investigated the effects of anapsos (0, 20, 40, and 100 mg/kg/day; 7 days; i.p.) on learning and memory performance in a step-down passive avoidance paradigm in rats with hippocampal injections of the ß-amyloid fragment 1–28 (ßA). The stabilized anapsos powder contains 40% anapsos and 60% maize starch. The dose of anapsos used in the present experiments is based on the content (40%) of active compound in the purified extract.

MATERIAL AND METHODS

Animals

We have used female Sprague Dawley rats (N=16 rats/group), weighing 250–300 g (Santiago University, Santiago de Compostela, Spain). Animals were housed in groups of five in transparent macrolon cages containing sawdust with free access to food and tap water one week before learning testing. Rats were kept in a constant temperature room (21±1°C) with lights on from 08.00 to 20.00 hours.

Neurosurgery

Rats were anesthesized with sodium thiopental (50–60 mg/kg; i.p.) and injected unilaterally (half of the animals) or bilaterally (the other half of the animals) with the fragment 1–28 of the ß-amyloid protein (3 nmoles/2 µl water) into the hippocampus. Stereotaxic coordinates according to the atlas of Paxinos and Watson (1982) were: 3.8 mm posterior to bregma, 2 mm lateral to the midline, and 3.5 mm ventral to the dorsal surface of the skull, respectively. Control rats were not operated.

Drugs and Chemicals

Amyloid ß-protein fragment 1–28 (Sigma Chemical Co, St Louis, MO, U.S.A) was dissolved in ultrapure water at a final concentration of 1.5 nmol/µl, the solution was placed for 48 h at room temperature to facilitate its aggregation. Commercial sodium thiopental was dissolved in ultrapure water. Anapsos (A.S.A.C. Pharmaceutical International) was dispersed in a 0.9% saline solution.

Treatment

Anapsos (0, 20, 40 or 100 mg/kg/day; i.p.) was injected since 2 days before and until 5 days after ßA implants.

Passive Avoidance Learning (PAL)

PAL was tested in a step-down paradigm in which rats had to learn to stay 30 s. on a neutral platform (18×18 cm) in order to avoid a 0.25 mA continuous electric foot-shock in the surrounding area. Learning acquisition (10 trials) and retention (5 trials) sessions were done 24 hours apart on days 4 and 5 after surgery, respectively. Intertrial interval was 30 s. The number of complete (30 s) avoidances and mean time spent on the platform per trial (latency) were measured. The increase in mean scape latency per trial from the acquisition (first 5 trials) to the retention session was also evaluated as an index of memory.

Statistics

Data were analyzed by using the Mann-Whitney U test.

RESULTS AND DISCUSSION

Anapsos improved learning acquisition in rats with ßA implants into the hippocampus, inducing a significant increase in the number of avoidances (ßA0=3.1±0.4 av; ßA40=4.8±0.3 av; p<0.05) and in mean trial latency at the 40 mg/kg dose (ßA0=17.3±0.9 s; ßA40=21.6±0.8; p<0.01) (Table 1). In the retention session, anapsos, at doses of 20 mg/kg and 40 mg/kg, increased mean latency per trial (ßA0=19.4±1.7 s; ßA20=25.0±1.3* s, ßA40=25.6±0.8** s; *p<0.05 and **p<0.01 vs ßA0) and the number of avoidances (ßA0=2.1±0.4 av; ßA20=3.3±0.4* av; ßA40=3.5±0.3* av; *p<0.05 vs ßA0) (Table 1). Finally, the increase in mean trial latency from the acquisition (firs five trials) to the retention session, an index of the task recall, was also enhanced by 20 mg/kg of anapsos (ßA0=7.7±1.8 s; ßA20=13.3±1.7; p<0.05) (Table 1, Figure 1).

These results demonstrate that injections of the amyloid ß-protein fragment 1–28 into the hippocampus produce learning and memory deficits and that anapsos is able to reverse this cognitive impairment in rats with ßA1–28 implants. In previous studies it has been re-

Table 1. Effects of anapsos on learning and memory in rats with ßA(1–28) deposits into the hippocampus

Group	N	Learning acquisition (10 trials)		Memory Retention (5 trials)		Retention-acquisition
		Avoidances (n°)	Latency (s)	Avoidances (n°)	Latency (s)	Latency increase (s)
Control	16	5.1±0.3**	21.0±0.6**	3.7±0.3*	26.8±0.7**	13.6±1.0*
ßA0	16	3.1±0.4	17.3±0.9	2.2±0.4	19.3±1.8	8.7±1.6
ßA20	16	4.5±0.4	18.9±1.1	3.3±0.4*	25.0±1.3*	13.3±1.7*
ßA40	16	4.8±0.3*	21.6±0.8**	3.5±0.3*	25.6±0.8**	10.7±0.8
ßA100	16	4.2±0.6	19.7±1.3	3.0±0.4	23.2±1.5	9.6±1.4

Results: mean±SEM. *p<0.05 & **p<0.01 vs ßA0

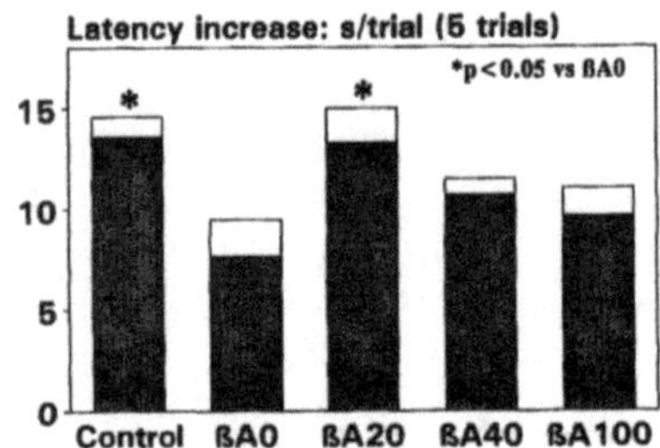

Figure 1. Effect of anapsos on learning improvement from the acquisition to the retention session in a PAL paradigm. The increase in mean latency per trial (first five trials of each session) is represented as an index of the task recall (memory). Anapsos (0, 20, 40 and 100 mg/kg/day; i.p.) was injected since 2 days before and until 5 days after ßA implants (ßA0, ßA20, ßA40, ßA100). Control rats were not operated. X±SEM.

ported that ßA1–28 impairs learning acquisition in the same passive avoidance task both 1 and 4 weeks after surgery (Alvarez et al., 1996b), reduces retention in mice tested in a T-maze paradigm after intrahippocampal or intracerebroventricular injections (Flood et al, 1991), and impairs performance in water maze and passive avoidance tasks in rats when infused into the cerebral ventricles for two weeks (Nabeshima and Nitta, 1994). Thus, animals with brain deposits of exogenous ßA have memory and learning deficits and seem to constitute a reliable model for testing drugs with potential neuroprotective activity. The improvement in learning and memory induced by anapsos in this animal model of neurodegeneration is consistent with the promnesic and antiamnesic effects exerted by this extract in intact rats and in animals with neurotoxic lesions in the nucleus basalis of Meynert (Alvarez et al., 1992, 1995, 1996c, 1997), and might be mediated by a neuroprotective action of the compound involving neuroimmune and/or antioxidative mechanisms. In this regard, we have found that anapsos reduces neuronal loss in the hippocampus of ßA-injected rats at the 20 mg/kg dose (Alvarez et al., 1996c), modulates brain interleukin-1ß and superoxide dismutase (SOD) activity levels (Alvarez et al., 1996c; Fernández-Novoa et al., 1997) and reduces glial activation (J.J. Miguel-Hidalgo, unpublished results) in these animals in a dose-dependent manner. Therefore, anapsos may reverse cognitive deficits in ßA rats by preserving the integrity and the functional capacity of hippocampal neurons, specifically in CA1-CA3 areas, as a consequence of its effects on neuroimmune and oxidative processes.

According to the present results showing that anapsos improves learning and memory performance in rats with hippocampal neurodegeneration at doses similar to those reducing neuronal death in the same animal model, we conclude that anapsos has procognitive and neuroprotective effects and might be useful in treating neurodegenerative diseases.

REFERENCES

Alvarez, X.A., Franco, A., Fernández-Novoa, L., and Cacabelos, R., 1992, Effects of anapsos on behavior and brain cytokines in rats. *Ann. Psychiat.* 3:329–341.

Alvarez, X.A., Zas, R., Lagares, R., Franco, A., Maneiro, E., Miguel-Hidalgo, J.J., Lao, J.I., Fernández-Novoa, L., Díaz, J., and Cacabelos, R., 1995, Neuroimmunomodulatory and neurotrophic activity of anapsos: studies with laboratory animals. *Ann. Psychiat.* 5:267–280.

Alvarez, X.A., Franco, A., Fernández-Novoa, L., and Cacabelos, R., 1996a, Blood levels of histamine, IL-1ß and TNF-α in patients with mild to moderate Alzheimer's disease. *Mol. Chem. Neuropathol.* 29:237–252.

Alvarez, X.A., Miguel-Hidalgo, J.J., Fernández-Novoa, L., Beyer, K., Lao, J.I., Vecino, B., and Cacabelos, R., 1996b, Behavioral deficits in rats with hippocampal neurodegeneration induced by ß-amyloid implants. *Ann. Psychiat.* 6:159–171.

Alvarez, X.A., Zas, R., Lagares, R., Fernández-Novoa, L., Franco, A., Miguel-Hidalgo, J.J., Cacabelos, R., Díaz, J., and Sempere, J.M., 1996c, Anapsos: new therapeutic strategies for neurodegeneration and brain aging with neuroimmunotrophic factors. In: *Alzheimer Disease: From Molecular Biology to Therapy*, Becker, R., and Giacobini, E., eds., Birkhäuser, Boston, pp. 367–372.

Alvarez, X.A., Franco-Maside, A., Zas, R., and Cacabelos, R., 1997, Anapsos reverses interleukin-1ß overexpression and behavioral deficits in nbm-lesioned rats. *Meth. Find. Exp. Clin. Pharmacol.*, in press

Cacabelos, R., Alvarez, X.A., Fernández-Novoa, L., Franco, A., Mangues, R., Pellicer, A., and Nishimura, T., 1994a, Brain interleukin-1beta in Alzheimer's disease and vascular dementia. *Meth. Find. Exp. Clin. Pharmacol.* 16:141–151.

Cacabelos, R., Nordberg, A., Caamaño, J., Franco-Maside, A., Fernández-Novoa, L., Gómez, M.J., Alvarez, X.A., Takeda, M., Prous, J.Jr., Nishimura, T., and Winblad, B., 1994b, Molecular strategies for the first generation of antidementia drugs (I). Tacrine and related compounds. *Drugs Today* 30: 295–337.

Dickson, D.W., and Rogers, J., 1992, Neuroimmunology of Alzheimer's disease: A conference report. *Neurobiol. Aging* 13:793–798.

Eikelenboom, P., Zhan, S-S., van Gool, W.A., and Allsop, D., 1994, Inflammatory mechanism in Alzheimers's disease. *TIPS* 15:447–450.

Fernández-Novoa, L., Alvarez, X.A., Sempere, J.M., Miguel-Hidalgo, J.J., Díaz, J., Franco-Maside, A., and Cacabelos, R., 1997, Effects of anapsos on the activity of the Cu-Zn-superoxide dismutase in an animal model of neuronal degeneration. *Meth. Find. Exp. Clin. Pharmacol.* 19:99–106.

Flood, J.F., Morley, J.E., and Roberts, E., 1991, Amnestic effects in mice of four synthetic peptides homologous to amyloid ß protein from patients with Alzheimer disease. *Proc. Natl. Acad. Sci. USA.* 88:3363–3366.

Horvath, A., Alvarado, F., Szöcs, J., De Alvarado, Z.N., and Padilla, G., 1967, Metabolic effects of Calagualine, an antitumoral saponine of Polypodium Leucotomos. *Nature* 214:1256–1258.

Jiménez, D., Naranjo, R., Doblaré, E., Muñoz, C., and Vargas, J.F., 1987, Anapsos, an antipsoriatic drug, in atopic dermatitis. *Allergol. Immunopathol.* 15:185–189.

McGeer, P.L., Rogers, J., and McGeer, E.G., 1994, Neuroimmune mechanisms in Alzheimer disease pathogenesis. In: *Alzheimer's Disease and Associated Disorders*, Giacobini, E., and Becker, R., eds., Raven Press, New York, pp. 149–158.

Mohamed, A., 1989, Vitiligo repigmentation with anapsos, polypodium leucotomos. *Int. J. Dermatol.* 28:479.

Nabeshima, T., and Nitta, A., 1994, Memory impairment and neuronal dysfunction induced by beta-amyloid protein in rats. *Tohoku J. Exp. Med.* 174:241–249.

Padilla, H.C., Laínez, H., Pacheco, J.A., 1974, A new agent (hydrophilic fraction of Polypodium leucotomos) for management of psoriasis. *Int. J. Dermatol.* 13:276–282.

Paxinos, G., and Watson, C., 1982, The Rat Brain in Sereotaxic Cordinates. *Academic Press*, Sydney.

Pérez de las Casas, O., Rodríguez, E., González, P., Diaz-Flores, L., González, F., Alarcó, A., 1987, Aloinjertos cutáneos tras la administración de extractos de polipodium leucotomos (estudio experimental). *Rev. Barcelona Quirurg.* 6:303–311.

Sempere, J.M., Rodrigo, C., Campos, A., Villalba, J.F., and Díaz, J., 1997, Effect of anapsos (polypodium leucotomos extract) on in vitro production of cytokines. *British J. Clin. Pharmacol.* 43:85–89.

Tuominen, M., Bohlin, L., Lindbom, L-O., and Rolfsen, W., 1991, Enhancing effect of Calaguala on the prevention of rejection on skin transplants in mice. *Phytotherapy Res.* 5:234–236.

Vargas, J., García, E., Gutiérrez, F., and Osorio, C., 1981, Síntesis de ácidos nucleicos y niveles de AMP cíclico en tumores murinos después del tratamiento in vitro con Anapsos. *Arch. Fac. Med. Madrid* 40:39–46.

Vargas, J., Muñoz, C., Osorio, C., García-Olivares, E., 1983, Anapsos, an antipsoriatic drug which increases the proportion of suppressor cells in human peripheral blood. *Ann. Immunol.* (Inst. Pasteur) 134:393–400.

100

IN VIVO NEUROTOXICITY OF ß-AMYLOID 1-40 IN THE RAT HIPPOCAMPUS

José Javier Miguel-Hidalgo, Antón Álvarez, and Ramón Cacabelos

Department of Basic Neuroscience
EuroEspes Biomedical Research Center, 15166
Bergondo, La Coruña, Spain

INTRODUCTION

The hippocampus is a privileged brain center for the study of neuronal plasticity and the responses of neurons to various types of injury. Specific degeneration of different neuronal populations occurs in the hippocampus after particular aggressions (Miguel-Hidalgo and Cacabelos, 1997). A classical example is the degeneration of CA1 neurons following a short period of ischemia (Pulsinelli, 1988). In this instance it is already known that excess extracellular glutamate caused by prolonged depolarization of hypoxic neurons contributes greatly to neuronal degeneration. In the dentate gyrus, granule cells are specifically sensitive to corticosteroid deprivation specially in rodents, although in this case the mechanisms of cell death are not yet well understood (Sloviter et al. 1993). Specific neuronal depletion is found also in the dentate gyrus as a consequence of small injections of fluids into the hippocampus (Vietje and Wells, 1989), but the mechanisms involved are unknown. Neuronal degeneration in the hippocampus, among other structures, is a characteristic of the Alzheimer's disease (AD) that very likely contributes to the overhelming memory deficits observed in AD patients (Hyman et al., 1984; Hyman and Van Hoesen, 1989). Accordingly, models of degeneration involving hippocampal neurons are relevant to AD therapy whenever it is possible to show that particular pharmacological molecules are capable of protecting the neurons that degenerate in those models. With this consideration in mind, we have been studying the effects of injecting small volumes of ß-amyloid peptide fragments dissolved with water or water alone into the rat hippocampus in order to assess the degenerative effects on hippocampal neurons at the morphological and behavioral levels.

Progress in Alzheimer's and Parkinson's Diseases
edited by Fisher *et al.*, Plenum Press, New York, 1998.

MATERIAL AND METHODS

We employed 35 female Sprague-Dawley rats (250–275 g). The animals were anesthetized with pentothal (60 mg/kg) and located in a stereotaxic apparatus. Then, either 2 µl of water alone (vehicle), ß-amyloid protein fragment 1–28 (Aß 1–28) in vehicle or ß-amyloid protein fragment 1–40 (Aß 1–40) were injected into the hippocampus with a Hamilton syringe. The injections were aimed to the hippocampal fisure and made at 3.8 mm from the bregma point in the caudal direction and 2 mm laterally from the rostrocaudal midline. ßAP fragments were dissolved in water (1.5 nmol/µl) and kept in solution for 48 hours before being injected. Five or seven days after the implants the animals were anesthetized with a lethal dose of pentothal and perfused with fixative solution (4% formaldehyde in phosphate buffer, pH 7.4). The brains were extracted out and sections were obtained on a paraffin microtome. The sections were stained with haematoxylin or cresyl violet, or processed for immunohistochemistry of microtubule-associated protein 2 (MAP2) in order to assess morphological changes occurred after the treatments given and confirm the complete degeneration of neurons in the CA1 subfield and the gyrus dentatus, respectively. In haematoxylin- and cresyl violet-stained sections we estimated the degree of neuronal degeneration in the CA1 subfield and the gyrus dentatus by measuring the maximum lateromedial extent of those layers that was deprived of neurons or that contained only small dense nuclei with loss of staining of Nissl substance in cell bodies and MAP2 immunoreactivity in dendrites. Measurements were made with an image analysis computer program on images captured with a video camera attached to the microscope. Alternate sections were deparaffinated and processed for *in situ* detection of fragmented DNA by means of terminal deoxynucleotide transferase-mediated dUTP-biotin nick end labeling (TUNEL) using the Apoptag kit from Oncor and following the maker's instructions.

RESULTS

Our experiments have taken advantage of previous studies by other researchers about the effects of injections of small amounts of fluids into the hippocampus. The common finding in these studies has been that injections directed to the dentate gyrus cause massive and, in many cases, complete neuronal loss in the lateral blade of the dentate gyrus (LBGD). Neurons in the CA1 and CA3 subfields do not degenerate in most of those experiments. Only larger amounts of fluid or injections with potent excitotoxins (for example, ibotenic or kainic acid) cause major degeneration in areas other than the gyrus dentatus. We have performed experiments in our laboratory with small injections of ultrapure water (1–2 µl) aimed to the dentate gyrus, just beyond the hippocampal fissure. In this experiments we have found, in confirmation with results of other investigators (Vietje and Wells, 1989; Games et al., 1992), that there is specific degeneration of LBGD neurons while the lesion in the CA1 area is very small, only at the site of penetration of the injection needle. Furthermore, we have injected in the same location equal amounts of a solution containing fragment 1–28 of the ß-amyloid peptide (Aß1–28) or ß-amyloid fragment 1–40 (Aß1–40). In principle, these solutions should be expected to cause non-specific degeneration of LBGD neurons and we actually found that this is the case in 60–70 % of animals per experiment. When the ß-amyloid solutions were injected immediately after reconstituting the lyophilized ß-amyloid peptides (Sigma) in water, no specific degeneration was found in other areas of the hippocampus except for the small discontinuity in the CA1 subfield caused by the penetration of the injection needle. However, when the Aß1–40 solution was left incubating for 48–72 hours and then deposited into the hippocampus, extensive degeneration was observed in the CA1 subfield just along the place where Aß1–40 was deposited, and, consequently, all further experiments were carried out with the long incubation period. The importance of neuronal degeneration in the gyrus dentatus and the CA1 subfield was easily quantified as the longitudinal maximal extension in the mediolateral plane of any of the layers that is deprived of neurons or only contains dramatically shrunken neuronal nuclei with complete loss of Nissl staining in their somata. We confirmed this criterion of degeneration by the absence of immunostaining for MAP2 in the place where the dendrites of the degenerating neurons are normally situated. When we compared the extension of neuronal degeneration in animals with deposits of either water alone (vehicle), Aß1–28 in vehicle or Aß1–40 in vehicle we found that all of them produced extensive degeneration of the LBGD of some animals without significant differences among groups, although a clear tendency for larger lesions in the group with Aß1–40 was found. However, only the deposits of Aß1–40 caused dramatic neuronal degeneration in the CA1 subfield while in animals with water or Aß1–28 there were only the remains of the site where the injection needle had penetrated (Fig. 1). These effects were found as early as 5 days after the injection of Aß1–40 into the hippocampus. Microscopic examination of sections from animals with Aß1–40 and stained with haematoxylin or after *in situ* detection of fragmented DNA by means of terminal deoxynucleotide transferase-mediated dUTP-biotin nick end labeling (TUNEL) technique revealed conspicuous signals of apoptotic neurodegeneration such as dramatic cell nucleus shrinkage, perinuclear condensed chromatin or picnotic nuclei. These findings are relevant for the sudy of AD etiopathogenesis since some authors have reported significant presence of apoptotic profiles in the autopsied brains of AD patients (Su et al., 1994; Lassman et al., 1995; Smale et al., 1995).

DISCUSSION

Earlier reports attributed to cores of senile plaques injected into the hippocampus the degeneration of cells in the denatate gyrus (Frautschy et al., 1991). Other researchers

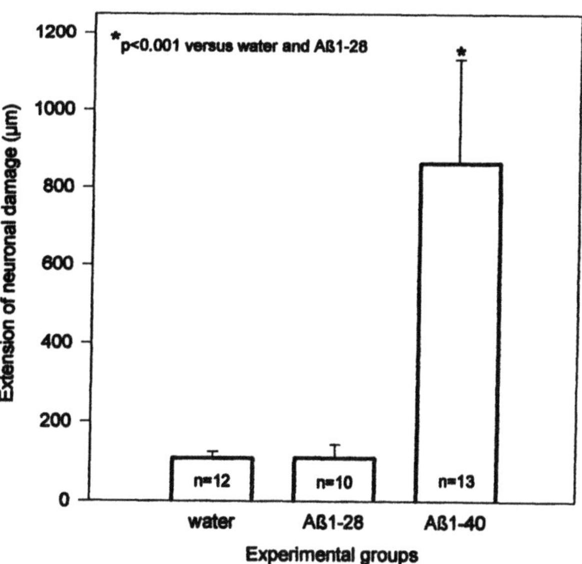

Figure 1. Graph representing the extension of neuronal damage in the CA1 subfield as measured in coronal sections through the hippocampus of rats that received intrahippocampal deposits of 2µl of either water (vehicle), Aß1–28 in vehicle or Aß1–40 in vehicle. Note the highly significant difference (Mann-Whitney U test) of the average region of neuronal damage in the animals injected with Aß1–40 as compared to that in either of the other two groups.

found that the degeneration in the dentate gyrus was actually undistinguishable from the effects of injecting water or other fluids into the hippocampus (Vietje and Wells, 1989; Games et al. 1992; Rush et al., 1992). In addition, some of these latter authors injected Aß fragments into the hippocampus, but found no extensive neuronal degeneration in areas other than the dentate gyrus and consequently ruled out any specific degenerative effects of Aß1–40 when injected in small volumes (Games et al., 1992; Stein-Behrens et al. 1992). By using a different protocol we have found that Aß1–40 causes neurodegeneration in the CA1 subfield while the fragment Aß1–28 does not. Our findings are in agreement with what is known of the neurodegenerative effects of fibrils or aggregates of Aß1–40 in cell culture where they are neurotoxic, cause abnormal growth of dendritic processes, or induce apoptosis (Forloni et al., 1993; Loo et al., 1993; Watt et al., 1994; Copani et al., 1995). In some animal models deposition of Aß actually is associated with abundant signs of apoptosis (LaFerla et al., 1995), increases in Aß1–40 and Aß1–42, plaque formation, and memory deficits (Hsiao et al., 1996).

REFERENCES

Copani, A., Bruno, V., Battaglia, G., Leanza, G., Pellitteri, R., Russo, A., Stanzani, S., and Nicoletti, F., 1995, Activation of metabotropic glutamate receptors protects cultured neurons against apoptosis induced by ß-amyloid peptide. *Mol. Pharmacol.* 47:890–897.

Forloni, G., Chiesa, R., Smiroldo, S., Verga, L., Salmona, M., Tagliavini, F., and Angeretti, N., 1993, Apoptosis mediated neurotoxicity induced by chronic application of ß-amyloid fragment 25–35. *Neuroreport* 4:523–526.

Frautschy, S.A., Baird, A., and Cole, G.M., 1991, Effects of injected Alzheimer ß-amyloid cores in rat brain. *Proc. Natl. Acad. Sci. USA* 88:8362–8366.

Games, D., Khan, K.M., Soriano, F.G., Keim, P.S., Davis, D.L., Bryant, K., and Lieberburg, I., 1992, Lack of Alzheimer pathology after ß-amyloid protein injections in rat brain. *Neurobiol. Aging* 13:569–576.

Hsiao, K., Chapman, P., Nilsen, S., Eckman, C., Harigaya, Y., Younkin, S., Yang, F., and Cole, G., 1996, Correlative memory deficits, Aβ elevation, and amyloid plaques in transgenic mice. *Science* 274:99–102.

Hyman, B. T., and . Van Hoesen, G. W., 1989, Hippocampal and entorhinal cortex cellular pathology in Alzheimer's disease. In: *The Hippocampus: New Vistas.* Chan-Palay, V. and Köhler, C. eds., Alan R. Liss, NY. 449–512.

Hyman, B.T., Van Hoesen, G.W., Damasio, A.R., and Barnes, C.L., 1984, Alzheimer's disease: cell specific pathology isolates the hippocampal formation. *Science* 225:1168–1170.

LaFerla, F.M., Tinkle, B.T., Bieberich, C.J., Haudenschild, C.C., and Jay, G., 1995, The Alzheimer's Aß peptide induces neurodegeneration and apoptotic cell death in transgenic mice. *Nature Genet.* 9:21–30.

Lassmann, H., Bancher, C., Breitschopf, H., Wegiel, J., Bobinski, M., Jellinger, K., and Wisniewski, H.M., 1995, Cell death in Alzheimer's disease evaluated by DNA fragmentation in situ. *Acta. Neuropathol. (Berl)* 89:35–41.

Loo, D.T., Copani, A., Pike, C.J., Whittemore, E.R., Walencewicz, A.J., and Cotman, C.W., 1993, Apoptosis is induced by ß-amyloid in cultured central nervous system neurons. *Proc. Natl. Acad. Sci. U. S. A.* 90:7951–7955.

Miguel-Hidalgo, J.J. and Cacabelos, R., 1997, Modeling neuronal degeneration in the rodent hippocampus: an approach for studying degenerative neuropathology in dementia. *Meth. Find. Exp. Clin. Pharmacol.* 19:133–142.

Pulsinelli, W.A., 1988, Selective neuronal vulnerability: morphological and molecular characteristics. *Prog. Brain Res.* 63:29–37.

Rush, D.K., Aschmies, S., and Merriman, M.C., 1992, Intracerebral ß-amyloid(25–35) produces tissue damage: is it neurotoxic? *Neurobiol. Aging* 13:591–594.

Sloviter, R.S., Sollas, A.L., Dean, E., and Neubort, S., 1993, Adrenalectomy-induced granule cell degeneration in the hippocampal dentate gyrus: characterization of an *in vivo* model of controlled neuronal death. *J. Comp. Neurol.* 330:324–336.

Smale, G., Nichols, N.R., Brady, D.R., Finch, C.E., and Horton, W.E., Jr., 1995, Evidence for apoptotic cell death in Alzheimer's disease. *Exp. Neurol.* 133:225–230.

Stein-Behrens, D.A., Adams, K., Yeh, M., and Sapolsky, R., 1992, Failure of beta-amyloid protein fragment 25–35 to cause hippocampal damage in the rat. *Neurobiol. Aging* 13:577–579.

Su, J.H., Anderson, A.J., Cummings, B.J., and Cotman, C.W., 1994, Immunohistochemical evidence for apoptosis in Alzheimer's disease. *Neuroreport* 1994:2529–2533.

Vietje, B.P. and Wells, J., 1989, Selective lesions of granule cells by fluid injections into the dentate gyrus. *Exp. Neurol.* 106:275–282.

Watt, J.A., Pike, C.J., Walencewicz, A.J., and Cotman, C.W., 1994, Ultrastructural analysis of ß-amyloid-induced apoptosis in cultured hippocampal neurons. *Brain Res.* 661:147–156.

101

IMPAIRMENTS OF CHOLINERGIC BUT NOT OF NIGROSTRIATAL DOPAMINERGIC PROJECTIONS IN APOLIPOPROTEIN E DEFICIENT MICE

Shira Chapman and Daniel M. Michaelson

Department of Neurobiochemistry
The George S. Wise Faculty of Life Sciences
Tel-Aviv University, Israel

INTRODUCTION

The ε4 allele of apolipoprotein E (apoE) has been implicated as a major risk factor for the development of late onset Alzheimer's disease (AD) (Roses, 1994). Recent studies have shown that the degree of cholinergic deficiency in AD brains, as monitored by the extent of reduction in cortical and hippocampal ChAT levels, correlates positively with the ε4 alelle copy number (Poirier et al., 1995). Similar attempts to link the apoE genotype with additional neurodegenerative disorders such as Parkinson's disease (PD) or multiple sclerosis revealed no specific association between the apoE genotype and these disorders (Rubinsztein et al., 1994). Since degeneration of nigrostriatal dopaminergic neurons is a major neuropathological hallmark of PD, this raises the possibility that, the neurobiology of the nigrostriatal dopaminergic neurons, unlike that of basal forebrain cholinergic neurons, is less dependent on apoE for its' normal function and maintenance.

Previous findings from our laboratory reveal that apoE deficient mice have distinct cognitive and cholinergic deficiencies (Gordon et al., 1995), suggesting that this is a good model for studying the role of apoE in neuronal function. Further studies indicated that cholinergic neurons projecting from the basal ganglia, but not cholinergic interneurons in the striatum, are particularly vulnerable in apoE deficient mice (Fisher et al., 1997). In the present study we examined whether the neuronal derangements in apoE deficient mice are specific to basal forebrain cholinergic neurons, and whether nigrostriatal dopaminergic projections are also affected in these mice. This was pursued by histochemical measurments of the levels of dopaminergic striatal nerve terminals and of cortical and hippocampal cholinergic synapses in brains of apoE deficient mice and comparing them to those of control mice.

Progress in Alzheimer's and Parkinson's Diseases
edited by Fisher *et al.*, Plenum Press, New York, 1998.

METHODS

Control and apoE deficient mice derived from the same parent line (C57BL/CJ) were kindly provided by Dr. J. L. Breslow (Plump et al., 1992). Fourteen weeks old male mice (10 in each group) were subjected to a Morris-water maze test as previously described (Gordon et al., 1995), with the minor modifications that the maximal trial length and inter trial interval were reduced to 60 seconds. Following the behavioral test, the animals were sacrificed, and their brains excised and rapidly frozen in a mixture of hexane and dry ice. Frozen coronal sections (20 µ) were then cut, mounted on gelatin coated glass slides and stored at −80°C until used. The synaptic density of cholinergic neurons was determined by evaluation of AChE activity and ChAT immunoreactivity, while the dopaminergic synapses were monitored autoradiografically, utilizing [^{3}H]GBR 12,935 which binds specifically to the presynaptic DA transporters (Mennicken et al., 1992). AChE activity was measured histochemically according to Karnovsky et al (1964). In brief, frozen sections were incubated for 30 minutes at 37°C in 0.1 M acetic-citric buffer which contained 0.03 M cupric sulfate, 0.005 M potassium ferricyanide and 5 µM of acetylthiocholine-Iodide as substrate. The stained sections were then washed and fixed in 4% buffered paraformaldehide. ChAT immunohistochemistry was pursued utilizing rabbit anti ChAT antiserum Ab143 (Chemicon Int.), diluted 1/100 in PBS containing 10% normal rabbit serum and alkaline phosphatase conjugated second antibodies (AP-RED 95-6142, Zymed Ltd.). The dopaminergic presynaptic transporters were visualized autoradiographically using the tritiated ligand: [^{3}H]GBR 12,935 as described by Mennicken et al (1992). In breif, sections were incubated for 20 hours at 4°C in 50 mM Tris-HCl buffer (pH = 7.5) containing 300 mM NaCl, 0.2% BSA and 2 nM [^{3}H]GBR 12,935 (30 Ci/mmol) (NEN). Non-specific binding was measured by performing the binding experiment in the presence of mazindol (50 µM). The incubation was terminated by rinsing the slides (4 × 5 minutes) in cold buffer, afterwhich they were dried and placed apposite to tritium-sensitive film (Amersham) for two weeks. Quantitation of the intensity of staining was performed utilizing the Cue-2 Image Analysis System (Galai Corp.) and the NIH image software (NIH). Three consecutive sections for each brain area of both the cholinergically and dopaminergically stained sections were measured and averaged. The intensity of staining of control and apoE deficient mice was analyzed by one-way ANOVA.

RESULTS

Behavioral Studies

The cognitive performance of apoE deficient and control mice was compared by Morris water maze utilizing a learning and short term memory paradigm. This paradigm is based on the difference in performance of the mice between two daily trials, over a period of ten days. While the first daily trial monitors the learning curve or reference memory of the mice during the 10 day duration of the experiment, the ratio between the second daily trial, (performed 1 minute following the termination of the first trial), and the first daily trial is considered a measurement of short term or working memory. The results thus obtained of the ratios of path lengths between the two daily trials of the two groups are depicted in Figure 1. As can be seen, while control mice improved in performance from the first to the second daily trial (ratio < 1), the apoE deficient mice did not improve but rather performed worse on their second daily trial (ratio > 1; p < 0.05). This finding is in accord-

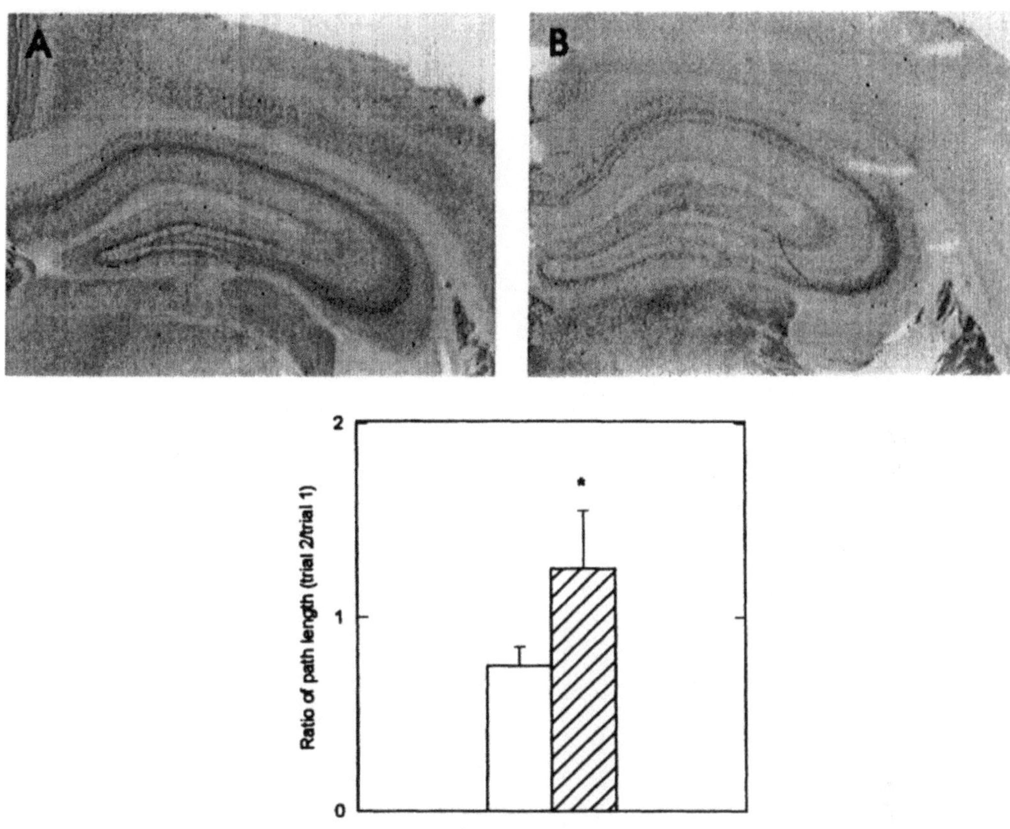

Figure 1. Ratios of path lengths in Morris water swim test of apoE deficient (striped) and control (empty) mice. Results presented correspond to the ratio of trial 2/trial 1, and are the mean ± SEM of 10 mice in each group for 10 days. *p < 0.05.

ance with previous findings (Gordon et al., 1995), and suggests that apoE deficient mice have working memory deficits.

Cholinergic Histochemistry

The synaptic density of basal forbrain cholinergic neurons of apoE deficient and control mice was monitored histochemically by measurments of the level of AChE activity and of ChAT immunohistochemistry in the brain areas to which they project. Representative stained sections thus obtained are depicted in the upper panels of Figures 2 and 3. As can be seen, AChE and ChAT staining in the hippocampus and parietal cortex of apoE deficient mice was markedly lower than those of the controls. Quantitation of the AChE results by computed densitometry revealed that AChE levels in the hippocampus and parietal cortex of apoE deficient mice decreased by respectively 33.8 ± 5.7% and 29.6 ± 7.4% as compared to control mice, and that AChE levels in other brain areas such as the striatum, were unaffected (Fig. 2, lower panel).

Quantitation of the ChAT immunohistochemical results which is depicted in the lower panel of Figure 3, revealed decreases in the hippocampus and cortex of apoE defi-

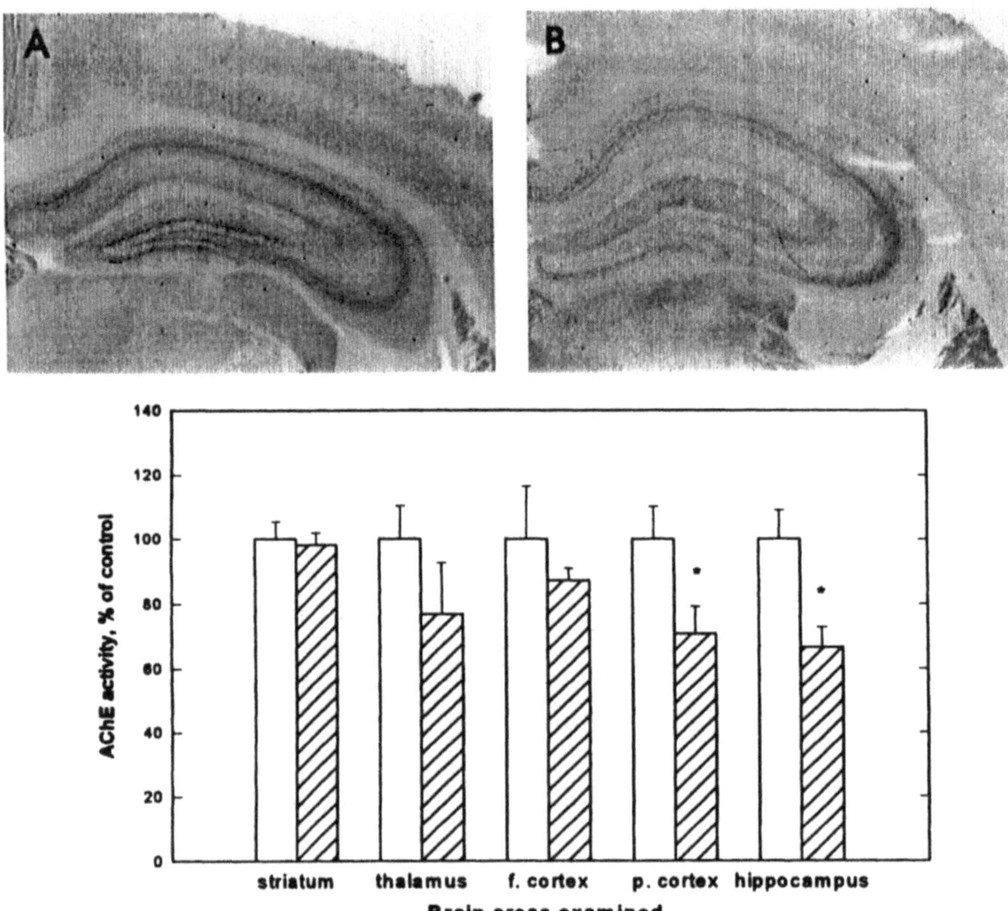

Figure 2. Comparison of the brain levels of AChE staining of brains of apoE deficient and control mice. Upper panel: representative brain coronal sections, at the level of the hippocampus, of a control (A) and an apoE deficient (B) mouse. Lower panel: comparison of the histologically measured levels of AChE activities of the indicated brain areas of apoE deficient (striped) and control (empty) mice. Results presented are the mean ± SEM of the data obtained from 5 mice in each group. *p < 0.01.

cient mice very similar to those which were obtained in the AChE experiments (respectively 27.6 ± 3.7 and 27.8 ± 3.9 percent of control). These results are consistent with previous findings in which ChAT activity was measured, and which showed that cortical and hippocampal levels of apoE deficient mice are decreased but that their striatal ChAT activity levels do not change (Gordon et al., 1995).

Dopaminergic Autoradiography

The densities of dopaminergic nerve terminals of apoE deficient and control mice were measured at the level of the striatum utilizing [^{3}H]GBR 12,935 which binds specifically to presynaptic dopaminergic transporters. The results thus obtained are depicted in Figure 4. As can be seen, unlike with the cholinergic neurons, the levels of striatal dopaminergic nerve terminals of apoE deficient was not lower than those of control mice.

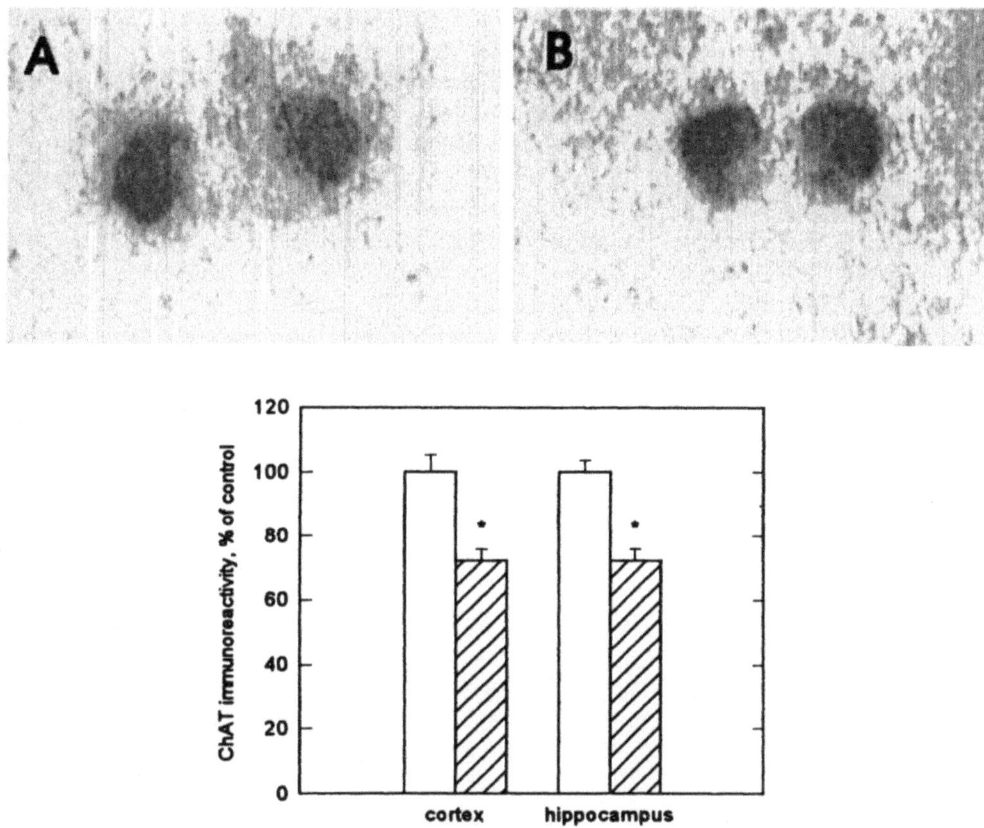

Figure 3. Comparison of the brain levels of ChAT immunoreactivities of apoE deficient and control mice. Upper panel: representative brain coronal sections, at the level of the hippocampus, of a control (A) and an apoE deficient (B) mouse. Lower panel: comparison of the intensities of the ChAT immunohistochemical staining in the cortex and hippocampus of apoE deficient (striped) and control (empty) mice. Results presented are the mean ± SEM of the data thus obtained from 5 mice in each group. *p < 0.05.

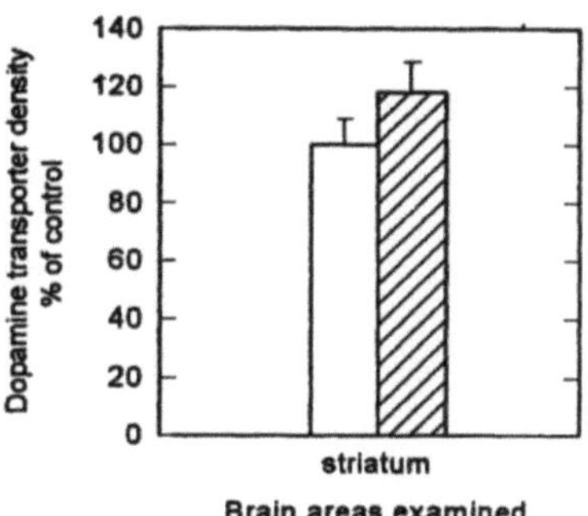

Figure 4. Comparison of the density of striatal dopaminergic nerve terminals of apoE deficient and control mice. Upper panel: representative brain coronal section at the level of the striatum of control (A) and apoE deficient (B) mouse following autoradiographic exposure to [³H]GBR 12,935. Lower panel: quantitation of the intensities of dopaminergic staining at the level of the striatum of apoE deficient (stripped) and control (empty) mice.. Results represented are the mean ± SEM of the data thus obtained of 5 mice in each group.

DISCUSSION

The present study employed apoE deficient and control mice for studying the effects of apoE deficiency on cognitive function and on the integrity of the synaptic terminals of distinct neuronal pathways. The loss of memory demonstrated in this work confirms previous results with apoE deficient mice (Gordon et al., 1995, Fisher et al., 1997). Taken together with the observed cholinergic deficits, in cognitively relevant brain areas such as the hippocampus and parietal cortex, this suggests that at least part of the memory deficits of apoE deficient mice might be related to cholinergic dysfunction.

The finding that cholinergic nerve terminals but not nigrostriatal dopaminergic nerve terminals are affected in apoE deficient mice, is novel and suggests that these pathways differ in their dependence on apoE for their normal function. Since apoE, the major lipoprotein in the brain, is presumed to play an important role in intracellular lipid transport (Mahley, 1988), it is possible that dopaminergic neurons are better able to synthesize cholesterol and other lipids internally than do the cholinergic neurons. Further studies of the relative abilities of these neurons to synthesize lipids and to interact with apoE will contribute to our understanding of this issue. Parkinson's disease whose neuropathological hallmark is degeneration of dopaminergic neurons is, unlike AD, not associated with apoE genetics (Rubinztein et al., 1994). It is therefore possible that unraveling the mechanisms underlying the differential susceptibilies of the dopaminergic and cholinergic neurons to apoE deficiency, will contribute to the understanding of the neuron specific mechanisms which play a role in neurodegeneration in these diseases.

ACKNOWLEDGMENTS

This work was supported in part by grants to DMM from the United States-Israel Binational Science Foundation (grant no. 95116), from the fund for Basic Research of the Israel Academy of Sciences and Humanaties (grant no. 670/96), from Revah-Kabelli Fund and from the Jo and Inez Eichenbaum Foundation.

REFERENCES

Fisher, A., Brandeis, R., Chapman, S., Pittel, Z. and Michaelson, D.M., 1997, M1 muscarinic agonist treatment reverses cognitive and cholinergic deficiencies of apolipoprotein E-deficient mice, submitted for publication.

Gordon, I., Grauer, E., Genis, I., Sehayek, E., and Michaelson, D.M., 1995, Memory deficits and cholinergic impairments in apolipoprotein E-deficient mice. *Neurosci. Lett.* 199;1–4.

Karnovsky, M.J. and Roots, L., 1964, A "direct coloring" thiocholine method for cholinesterases. *J. Histochem. Cytochem.* 12:219.

Mahley, R.W., 1988, Apolipoprotein E:cholesterol transport protein with expanding role in cell biology. Science 240:622–630.

Mennicken, F., Savasta,M., Peretti-Renucci, R., and Feuerstein, C., 1992, Autoradiographic localization of dopamine uptake sites in the rat brain with 3H-GBR 12935. *J. Neural Transm* [GenSect] 87:1–14.

Plump, A.S., Smith, J.D., Hayek, T., Aalto-Setala, K., Walsh, A., Verstuyft, J.G., Rubin, E.M. and Breslaw, J.L., 1992, Severe hypercholestrolemia and atherosclerosis in apolipoprotein E-deficient mice created by homologous recombination in ES cells. *Cell* 16:343–353.

Poirier, J., Delisle, M.C., Quirion, R., Aubert, I., Farlow, M., Lahiri, D., Hui, S., Bertrand, P., Nalbantoglu, J., Gilfix, B.M., *et al.,* 1995, Apolipoprotein E4 allele as a predictor of cholinergic deficits and treatment outcome in Alzheimer disease. *Proc. Natl. Acad. Sci.* 92:12260–12264.

Roses, A.D., 1994, Apolipoprotein E affects the rate of Alzheimer disease expression: beta-amyloid burden is of secondary consequence dependent on APOE genotype and duration of disease. *J. Neuropathol. Exp. Neurol.* 53(5):429–437.

Rubinztein, D.C., Hanlon, C.S., Irving, R.M., Goodburn, S., Evans, D.G.R., Kellar-Wood, H., Xuereb, J.H., Bandmann, O. and Harding, A.E., 1994, Apo E Genotype in multiple sclerosis, Parkinson's disease, schwannomas and late-onset Alzheimer's disease. *Mol Cell. Probes* 8:519–525.

102

INTERVAL HYPOXIC TRAINING PREVENTS OXIDATIVE STRESS IN STRIATUM AND LOCOMOTOR DISTURBANCES IN A RAT MODEL OF PARKINSONISM

Natalia V. Gulyaeva,[1] Mikhail Yu. Stepanichev,[1] Mikhail V. Onufriev,[1] Ilya V. Sergeev,[1] Olga S. Mitrokhina,[1] Yulia V. Moiseeva,[1] and Elena N. Tkatchouk[2]

[1]Institute of Higher Nervous Activity and Neurophysiology RAS
5A Butlerov Street Moscow 117865, Russia
[2]Hypoxia Medical Clinical Research Laboratory
Moscow, Russia

INTRODUCTION

In Parkinson's disease, a progressive degeneration of nigro-striatal dopaminergic neurons results in akinesia, muscular rigidity and tremor. MPTP (1-methyl-4-phenyl-1,2,3,6-tetrahydropyridine) is a neurotoxin that is responsible for the Parkinson-like symptoms seen in humans using illicit synthetic opiate analogs of meperidine containing MPTP as a contaminant (Langston et al., 1983). Rodents are highly susceptible to the neurotoxic effects of MPTP and may be useful animal models for Parkinson's disease (Hallmann et al., 1985; Takada et al., 1987). Administration of MPTP to rodents results in a significant loss of nervous cells in the substantia nigra (Takada et al., 1987) and a marked reduction in neostriatal content of dopamine and its metabolites (Heikkila et al., 1984; Fuller and Hemrick-Luecke, 1984).

Oxidative stress inducing nigro-striatal degeneration of dopamine neurons is believed to be one of the mechanisms of Parkinson's disease development, as well as of other neurodegenerative diseases (Halliwell, 1992; Gulyaeva and Erin, 1995; Fisher and Gage, 1995). Continued research aimed at developing therapies for Parkinson's disease that could restore dopamine, its metabolites and precursors level, and/or prevent oxidative stress is being carried out. Reactive oxygen species, including hydroxyl radical, have been implicated in dopaminergic toxicity caused by MPTP (Chiueh et al., 1993) indicating that MPTP model of parkinsonism is sutable for studying therapeutic interventions for this diseases targeted for the protection from oxidative stress.

Progress in Alzheimer's and Parkinson's Diseases
edited by Fisher *et al.*, Plenum Press, New York, 1998.

Hypoxic training, a method of so called adaptive medicine (Meerson, 1993) has been shown to increase the adaptive capacity of the organism raising its resistance against different external factors. Interval hypoxic training (IHT) is the most promising method of adaptation to hypoxia (Tkatchouk et al., 1993). Enhancement of antioxidant defense systems is one of the most important adaptive effects resulting from IHT (Sazontova et al., 1994, 1995). This "antioxidative" effect caused by IHT makes it possible to limit, or even to prevent the oxidative stress, the main damaging factor mediating effects of various unfavorable factors. The beneficial effects of IHT has been demonstrated in treatment of different diseases and in health promotion (Tkatchouk et al., 1993), however, the potential of IHT application in treatment of cerebral pathologies remains obscure.

The aim of this study was to investigate effects of IHT on brain free radical-mediated processes and locomotor activity in rat model of Parkinsonism induced by 1-methyl-4-phenyl-tetrahydropyridine (MPTP).

METHODS

Animals

Male Wistar rats (n=40), weighing 300–350 g at the beginning of the experiment, were housed five per cage and maintained on a natural light/dark cycle. Food and water were provided ad libitum. Rats were randomly divided into four groups (n=10 each): control, MPTP-treated, IHT, and IHT+MPTP.

Interval Hypoxic Training

Normobaric hypoxic training was performed in a special device designed in the "Hypoxia Medical" Laboratory. Atmosphere with low oxygen content (10%) was developed in the chamber connected to the device creating and pumping hypoxic gas mixture. Gas analyzer was used to control oxygen content in the chamber and in the gas mixture. 20 daily training sessions were performed. The training started with total 35 min of hypoxia once a day. Each session included 7 hypoxic periods 5 min each with the intervals of breathing atmospheric air (3 min). By the 10 session total time of hypoxic exposure was increased to 60 min (6 hypoxic periods 10 min each with breaks of 3 min). In order to prevent carbon dioxide accumulation in the chamber during hypoxic session, CO_2 control was performed along with the additional pumping of hypoxic mixture. The animals from the control and MPTP groups were placed into the similar chamber, with atmospheric air pumped at the same mode as the hypoxic mixture for experimental animals.

Bilateral MPTP Lesions

Parkinsonian syndrome was modeled by bilateral intranigral administration of MPTP, (Takada et al., 1987). Animals under ketamine anesthesia (150 mg/kg) (Calipsol, Gedeon Richter, Hungary) were positioned in a stereotaxic instrument. Then a midline sagittal incision was made in the scalp and the skull was drilled at the place of injection. The drug was administered with the microsyringe according to the following coordinates: A -5.3; DV -8.1; L± 2.0 . Each animal received 40 mg of MPTP diluted with 2 ml of isotonic NaCl solution (administration time 2 min). The needle stayed at the place of injection for 3 min. Animals of the control group received similar injections of NaCl solution.

Intranigral MPTP injection to experimental animals and NaCl injections to the control group was performed in 3 days after the IHT termination.

"Open Field" Test

The "open field" test (Kelley, 1993) was carried out on the 2nd and 4th days after MPTP injection. The following parameters were evaluated during 5 min: latency of movement start, horizontal and vertical locomotor activity, number of entries to the center of the lighted area, grooming, defecation number, freezing time.

Preparation of Brain Samples and Analysis of Free Radical-Mediated Processes

The animals were decapitated on the 2nd or 4th days after the surgery, brain was immediately taken out and washed in isotonic NaCl solution. Striatum and cerebral cortex were isolated (cortex was used as less sensitive area in comparison to striatum in the situation of MPTP-induced nigro-striatal dopaminergic degeneration). Brain tissue samples were kept frozen in liquid nitrogen before analysis. Then the tissue was homogenized in Potter's homogenizer with 2 volumes of buffer containing 50 mM N-2-hydroxy-ethylpiperasin-N'-2- ethanesulphonic acid (HEPES), pH 7,4. Homogenate aliquots were centrifuged at 3000xg for 10 min, and supernatants were used to analyze free radical-mediated oxidative processes.

The method of chemiluminescence can be used for detection of active oxygen species. The analysis of H_2O_2-induced luminol-dependent chemiluminescence makes it possible to assess free radical generation (FRG) in tissues (Betts, 1987). Chemiluminescence (maximal light emission) was evaluated using chemiluminometer CHLM-3m (Russia) at $20°$ C as described earlier (Gulyaeva et al., 1994). FRG was calculated as the ratio of total light emission of the sample containing biological material to the control without biological material.

2-Thiobarbituric acid reactive products (TBARP), both basal and induced in Fe^{2+}/ascorbate system were detected using spectrophotometric method (Kagan et al., 1979). Protein concentration was determined by using the method of Bradford

Materials

All chemicals were from Sigma, unless otherwise stated.

Statistical Analysis

Statistical analysis of the data was performed using Kruskal-Wallis ANOVA and Mann-Whitney criterion. The data are presented as means±S.E.M.

RESULTS

Effects of IHT and MPTP on Free Radical-Mediated Processes

IHT had no statistically significant effect on free radical-mediated processes in brain of the sham operated animals: FRG values and TBARP levels remained unchanged in striatum and brain cortex on 2nd and 4th days after the surgery (Figure 1).

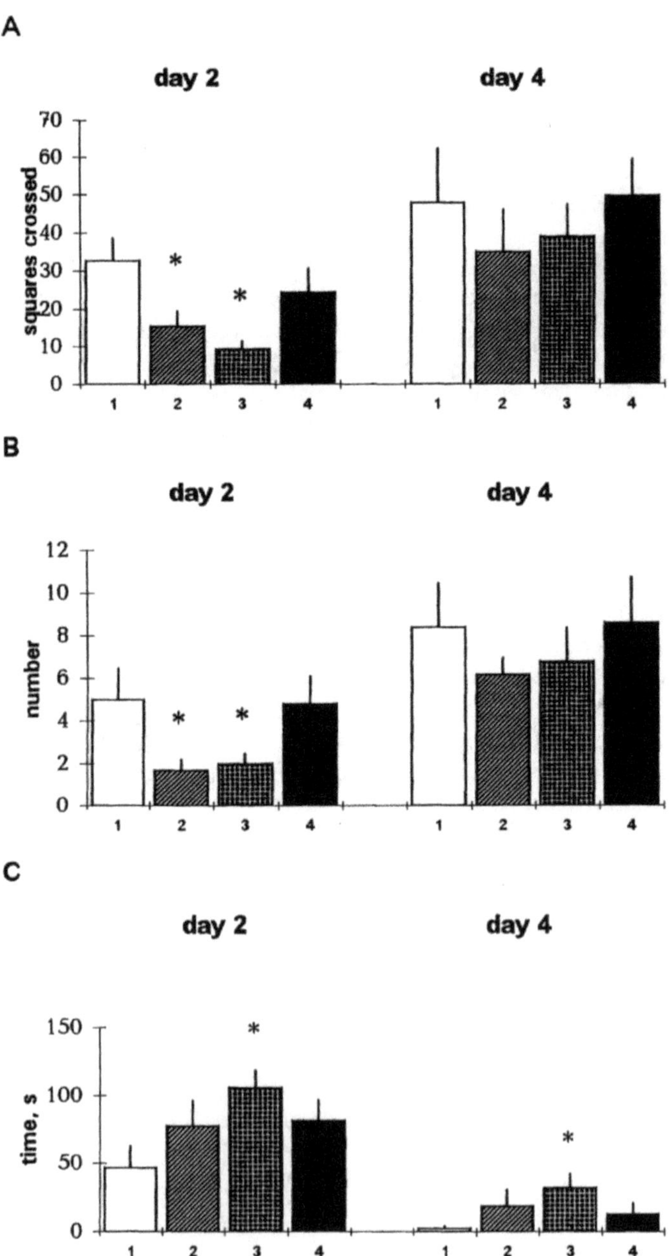

Figure 1. Effects of MPTP and IHT on free radical generation (A), basal TBARP (B) and Fe/ascorbate induced TBARP (C) in rat striatum. 1 - sham operated controls, 2 - IHT, 3 - MPTP, 4 - IHT+MPTP. *P<0.05 indicates difference from sham operated group.

Kruskal-Wallis analysis revealed a significant effect of MPTP on both FRG and Fe2+/ascorbate induced TBARP (P<0.05). MPTP induced oxidative stress in striatum of rats. FRG intensity in striatum of MPTP-treated animals increased by 30% on the 2nd day after the surgery. Though basal TBARP level remained unchanged, Fe/ascorbate induced TBARP doubled both on the 2nd and on the 4th days (Fig. 1). As a rule, MPTP effects were observed only in striatum, and were not found in cerebral cortex (data not shown).

IHT prevented both Fe2+/ascorbate-induced TBARP accumulation and FRG activation in striatum (Fig.1).

Behavioral Effects of MPTP and IHT

Kruskal-Wallis analysis revealed effects of both MPTP and IHT on locomotor activity of rats (p<0.05). Intranigral MPTP administration resulted in behavioral disturbances specific for Parkinsonian syndrome modeled in rodents: lower locomotor activities, both horizontal and vertical (on the 2nd day after the surgery), as well as striking increase in freezing time.

Preliminary IHT, as a rule, prevented locomotor disorders induced by MPTP administration (Figure 2), though effects of IHT itself were similar to that of MPTP.

DISCUSSION

Dopaminergic system (striatal one, in particular) is among primary targets when brain is exposed to hypoxia (Brooderic, 1989). Proceeding with the investigation of IHT effect on free radical-mediated processes in rat brain under administration of dopaminergic neurotoxin, we considered its specific effect on dopaminergic neurons and its ability to induce oxidative stress (Chiueh et al.,1993). It could be supposed that training of the dopaminergic system as a result of adaptation to interval hypoxia would provide the protection from the neurotoxin effects. Moreover, a protective effect of IHT by enhanced capacity of antioxidative systems could be expected.

In this study, we showed the protective effect IHT against MPTP-induced disturbances in striatal free radical mediated processes and in locomotor activity. Considering damage to nigro-striatal brain dopaminergic system induced by intranigral MPTP administration and irreversible neurodegeneration, it may be supposed that IHT provides a stable physiological adaptation of dopaminergic system and of other brain systems, as well, as of the organism as a whole. Basing only on the results obtained in this study and without any morphological investigation it cannot be suggested whether the preliminary IHT contributes to lower nigro-striatal dopaminergic neuro -degeneration, however, it can be suggested that some adaptive and compensatory mechanisms slowing oxidative processes are more expressed in brain after IHT. The results of the present study provide the basis for further investigation of IHT effect on the adaptive brain capacity and its resistance to the extreme factors.

Though IHT itself did not influence FRG and TBARP level in the brain, it clearly affected locomotor activity. The possible reason for the depression of locomotor activity by IHT may be the effect of adaptation to hypoxia on the catecholamine metabolism in brain, including inhibition of dopamine synthesis (Brooderic, 1989). In fact, dopaminergic system is the target of both hypoxia and MPTP effects. It should be also remembered that along with specific IHT and MPTP effects on the 2nd and 4th day after the surgery the effect of the surgery itself is to be considered as well (pain syndrome, anesthesia, etc.). The

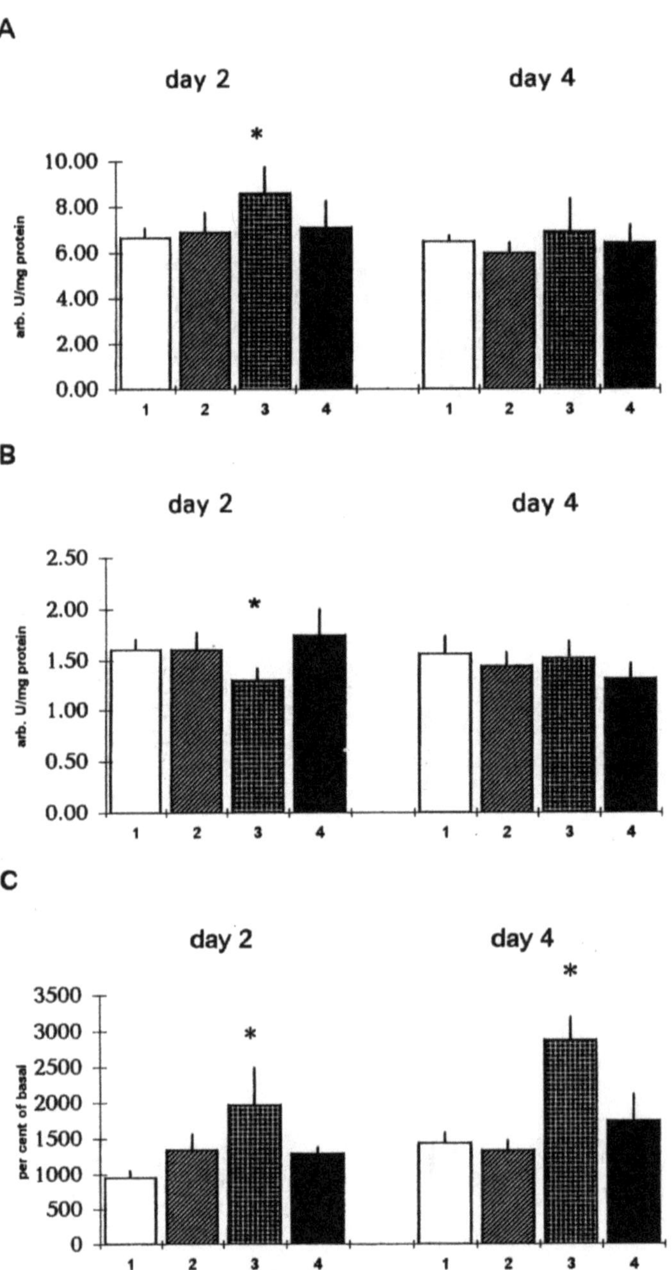

Figure 2. Effects of MPTP and IHT on locomotor activity in the "open field" test: horizontal activity (A), vertical activity (B) and freezing time (C). 1 - sham operated controls, 2 - IHT, 3 - MPTP, 4 - IHT+MPTP. * P<0.05 indicates difference from sham operated group.

control group of sham operated animals is used to consider the surgery effect to much extent, however, it cannot entirely accommodate all the possibile different factors interaction.

The present study was the first attempt to investigate the IHT effects in a model of cerebral pathology. The results of the study demonstrated that IHT prevented oxidative stress and locomotor disturbances induced by dopaminergic neurotoxin. Continued research aimed at studying effects of IHT in neurodegenerative diseases may very well lead to important insights as well as discovery of prophylactic treatments that protect against neurodegeneration.

REFERENCES

Betts, W.H., 1987. Detection of radicals by chemiluminescence, In: *CRC Handbook of Methods for Oxygen Radical Research*, Greenwald, R.A., ed., CRC Press, Boca Raton., pp. 197–201.

Bradford, M.M., 1976, A rapid and sensitive method for the quantitation of microgram quantities of protein using the principle of protein-dye binding, *Anal. Biochem.* 72:248–254.

Brooderic, P.A., 1989, Dopamine and serotonin in rat striatum during in vivo hypoxic hypoxia, *Metab. Brain. Dis.* 4:143–153.

Chiueh, C.C., Miyake, H., and Peng, M.T. Role of dopamine autoxidation, hydroxyl radical generation, and calcium overload in underlying mechanisms involved in MPTP-induced parkinsonism, *Adv. Neurol.* 60:251–259.

Fuller, R.W., and Hemrick-Luecke, S.K., 1984, Deprenyl protection against striatal dopamine depletion by 1-methyl-4-phenyl-1,2,3,6-tetrahydropyridine in mice, *Res. Commun. Substance Abuse.* 5:241–247.

Gulyaeva, N.V., Onufriev, M.V., and Stepanichev, M.Yu., 1994, NO synthase and free radical generation in old rats: Correlations with individual behavior, *NeuroReport* 6:94–96.

Gulyaeva, N.V., and Erin, A.H., 1995, The role of free radical-mediated processes in the development of neurodegenerative diseases, *Neurochemistry (Neurok- himija, Rus).* 12:3–15.

Halliwell, B. 1992, Reactive oxygen species and the central nervous system., *J. Neurochem.* 59:1609–1623.

Hallman H., Lange, J ., Olson, L., Stromberg, I., and Jonsson, G., 1985, Neurochemical and histochemical characterization of neurotoxic effects of 1-methyl-4-phenyl-1,2,3,6-tetrahydropyridine on brain catecholamine neurons in the mouse, *J. Neurochem.* 44:117–122.

Heikkila, R.E., Hess, A., and Duvoisin, R.C., 1984, Dopaminergic neurotoxicity of 1-methyl-4-phenyl-1,2,3,6-tetrahydropyridine in mice, *Science (Wash. D.C.).* 224:1451–1453.

Kagan, V.E., Prilipko, L.L., Savov, V.M., Pisarev, V.A., Eluashvili, I.A., Kozlov Yu.P., 1979, Participation of free active forms of oxygen in enzymatic peroxidation of lipids in biomembranes, *Biochemistry (Biokhimija)* 44:379–385.

Kelley, A.E., 1993, Locomotor activity and exploration, In: *Behavioral Neuroscience. V. 2. A Practical Approach*, Sahgal A., ed., IRL Press. Oxford et al., pp. 1–21.

Langston, J.W.P,. Ballard, P., Tetrud, J.W., and Irwin I., 1983, Chronic parkinsonism in humans due to product of meperidine-analog synthesis, *Science (Wash. D.C.).* 219:979–981.

Meerson F.Z., 1993, Adaptation to hypoxia: Mechanisms and protective effects, in: *Essentials of Adaptive Medicine: Protective Effects of Adaptation (A Manual)*, Meerson F.Z., ed., Moscow. Hypoxia Medical LTD, pp. 142–199.

Sazontova, T.G., Tkatchouk, E.N., Kolmykova, S.N., Ehrenburg, I.V., Meerson, F.Z., Arkhipenko, Yu.V., 1994, Comparative analysis of of peroxidation and antioxidant enzyme activities in rats adapted to different regimens of normobaric hypoxia, *Hyp. Med. J.* 2:4–7.

Sazontova, T.G., Tkatchouk, E.N., Golantsova, N.E., Ehrenburg, I.V., Meerson, F.Z., Arkhipenko, Yu.V., 1995, The state of sarcoplasmatic reticulum Ca-pump and the activity of myocardial antioxidant defense in adaptation to normobaric hypoxia, *Hyp. Med. J.* 3:5–8.

Takada, M., Li, Z.K., and Hattori, T., 1987, Intracerebral MPTP injections in the rat cause cell loss the substantia nigra, ventral segmental area and dorsal raph, *Neurosci. Lett.* 78:145–150.

Tkatchouk, E.N., Gorbatchenkov, A.A., Kolchinskaya,A.Z., Ehrenburg, I.V., Kondrykinskaya, I.I., 1993, Adaptation to interval hypoxia for the purpose of prophylaxis and treatment, In: *Essentials of Adaptive Medicine:Protective Effects of Adaptation (A Manual)*, Meerson F.Z., ed., Moscow. Hypoxia Medical LTD, pp. 200–224.

AN α_2-ADRENOCEPTOR AGONIST, CLONIDINE, DISRUPTS ATTENTIONAL PERFORMANCE

Pekka Jäkälä,[1,2] Kosti Kejonen,[2] Matti Vanhanen,[2] Esa Koivisto,[1] and Paavo Riekkinen, Jr.[1,2]

[1]Department of Neuroscience and Neurology
University of Kuopio and
[2]University Hospital of Kuopio
P.O. Box 1627 - FIN-70211
Kuopio, Finland

INTRODUCTION

Noradrenaline-containing neurons of the locus coeruleus (LC), arising from the brainstem, form one of the ascending modulatory systems innervating the forebrain (Foote and Morrison, 1987). Based on electrophysiological and behavioral studies, noradrenaline and its α_2-adrenoceptors play an important role in behavioral activation, responses to novel/salient stimuli, arousal, vigilance, selective attention, as well as effortful processing of information (Foote and Morrison, 1987; Harley, 1987; Aston-Jones et al., 1990; Buzsáki et al., 1990; Riekkinen Jr. et al., 1990; Berridge and Foote, 1991; Cole and Robbins, 1992; Jäkälä et al., 1992; Robbins and Everitt, 1994; Sirviö et al., 1994).

Three subtypes of α_2-adrenoceptors (α_{2A}, α_{2B} and α_{2C}) have been cloned in humans (Scheinin et al., 1994). The subtypes have a different distribution in brain areas involved in separate functional systems, suggesting that drugs that would selectively modulate these subtypes might possess qualitatively different behavioral actions. Unfortunately, no such subtype selective ligands are available. However, the various actions of unselective α_2-agonists can be dissociated based on their relative affinities for each receptor subtype. For example, the adverse effects (sedation, hypotension) of α_2-agonists may be dissociable from their beneficial (cognition-enhancing) effects (Arnsten et al., 1996).

The approach of using comparable psychopharmacological manipulations with analogous tests in animals and humans is a valuable tool to reveal the neurochemical basis of different cognitive functions. A single test of attentional performance (*i.e.* the 5-choice serial reaction time task which is considered to assess sustained attention and vigilance) with a variety of different neurochemical manipulations, has been used to probe the neurochemical

Progress in Alzheimer's and Parkinson's Diseases
edited by Fisher *et al.*, Plenum Press, New York, 1998.

basis of attention in rats (Cole and Robbins, 1992; Jäkälä et al., 1992; Robbins and Everitt, 1994; Sirviö et al., 1994). The Cambridge Neuropsychological Test Automated Battery (CANTAB) is a computerized test for humans which is based on those tests of animal psychology that have proved useful in establishing the neural substrates and neuropharmacology of certain types of cognitive functions, such as attention (Sahakian and Owen, 1992).

The aim of the present study was to elucidate the role of α_2-adrenoceptors in the modulation of attention in humans. Therefore, we studied the effects of α_2-agonists on the performance of normal healthy young volunteers in the CANTAB attention battery. To elucidate the relative contribution of different α_2-adrenoceptor subtypes in the modulation of attention in humans we compared the effects of an unselective α_2-agonist, clonidine, to those of a more selective α_{2A}-agonist, guanfacine (Uhlen and Wikbeg, 1991). The tasks were given as a part of our larger-scale project investigating the role of α_2-adrenoceptors in attentional, executive and memory functions, aimed at revealing novel therapeutic strategies to alleviate cognitive deficits associated with Alzheimer's and Parkinson's diseases.

METHODS

Subjects

Normal healthy young (23–35 years of age, n=43) volunteers free of concurrent medication or illnesses and medical conditions that could interfere with central nervous system functions took part in the study. The studies were approved by the local ethics committee and national drug regulatory authority. All the subjects provided a written informed consent, and were covered by insurance.

Pharmacological Manipulations and Experimental Design

Groups 1 (n=6), 2 (n=8) and 3 (n=8) received 0.5, 2.0 and 5.0 µg/kg, respectively, of clonidine hydrochloride (Catapressan®, Boehringer Ingelheim) p.o. in tablet form, or appropriate oral placebo. Groups 4 (n=9) and 5 (n=12) received 7 and 29 µg/kg, respectively, of guanfacine hydrochloride (Estulic®, Sandoz Oy) p.o. in tablet form, or appropriate oral placebo. Subjects attended on two occasions with at least seven days between sessions. A placebo-controlled double-blind cross over design was used. The testing began 90 min post-ingestion of tablets. The test session lasted for 60–90 min.

Neuropsychological Tests

The tasks were part of the CANTAB attention battery (Sahakian and Owen, 1992), and were run on an IBM PS/2 Model 30 486 personal computer, with a high resolution Taxan 770+ colour monitor fitted with an Intasolve touch-sensitive screen.

Motor Screening Test

A series of crosses was shown in different locations on the screen. The subjects had to point to crosses as they appeared on the screen as quickly and accurately as possible. Measures of speed and accuracy were taken to provide an index of the subjects' motor performance. Mean of ten trials for both the latency to point accurately to a cross after it appeared, and accuracy ("error") *i.e.* the distance between the first point touched by the subject and the actual cross, were recorded.

Following a Simple Rule and Its Reversal Test

Subjects were presented with a large and a small dot and required to point as quickly as possible at first the smaller dot for 20 trials and then to the larger dot for the following 20 trials. The number and the latency to correct responses were recorded.

Simple and Choice Reaction Time Test

At the first stage, subjects had to touch the screen when a yellow dot appeared in the centre, neither being too early nor too late. At the second stage, the dot appeared in one of five locations. At the third stage the subjects were required to release their hand from a touch pad as quickly as possible after a dot appeared in a single location on the screen. At the fourth stage the subjects were required to hold down a touch pad until a single dot appeared in the centre of the screen and then to touch the position of the dot as quickly as possible (Simple Reaction Time Test). At the fifth stage, a Choice Reaction Time Test, the subjects were required to hold down the touch pad until the dot appeared at one of five locations on the screen, and then point to the position on the screen where the dot was presented. At this stage, the subjects were presented with a maximum of 40 trials to reach a criterion of 7/8 correct. Both accuracy (the proportion of correct) and speed of response were recorded.

Visual Analogue Scale

After completion of the test, the subjects were asked to rate themselves for subjective feelings of "sedation/tiredness" by asking them to place a mark on a 10 cm line numbered from 1 to 10, 1 representing "not at all" and 10 representing "very much".

Monitoring of Blood Pressure

Blood pressure was measured before the subjects received the study drug or matching placebo tablet, just before beginning and after completion of the test session.

Statistics

To reveal possible practice effects, which may confound the validity of statistical interactions in the repeated measures cross-over design, we had beforehand tested a separate group (n=12) of normal young healthy subjects without any drug treatment with the same test battery on two occasions with no less than 1 week between sessions. No significant practice effects on the parameters analyzed in the present study were found. Therefore, paired samples T-test was used in statistical analysis.

RESULTS

Motor Screening Test

Neither clonidine nor guanfacine affected latency or accuracy to point to a cross (data not shown) (p > 0.05).

Table 1. The effects of clonidine and guanfacine on the performance in an attentional test (Choice Reaction Time Test)

	Correct responses	Reaction latency	Total moves
C 0.5	8.0±0	411±58	8.0±0
	(7.8±0.2)	(403±66)	(8.0±0)
C 2	7.6±0.4	423±98	8.0±0
	(7.8±0.2)	(403±43)	(8.0±0)
C 5	6.7±0.4[a]	439±56[a]	8.0±0
	(7.8±0.2)	(398±60)	(8.0±0)
G 7	7.8±0.3	404±66	8.0±0
	(8.0±0)	(402±63)	(8.0±0)
G 29	8.0±0	429±43	8.0±0
	(8.0±0)	(433±76)	(8.0±0)

Drug values are given first, with corresponding placebo values in brackets below them. Abbreviations: C=clonidine; G=guanfacine. Doses are expressed as µg/kg. Results are expressed as means ± S.D. Clonidine 5.0 µg/kg decreased the number of correct responses, and increased reaction latency (expressed in milliseconds). The number of total moves was not affected by either of the drugs. [a] $p < 0.05$, paired samples two-tailed t-test.

Following a Simple Rule and Its Reversal Test

Neither clonidine nor guanfacine affected the number of correct responses or the latency to correct responses (data not shown) ($p > 0.1$).

Simple and Choice Reaction Time Test

Clonidine 5.0 µg/kg decreased the number of correct responses ($p < 0.05$), and increased reaction latency ($p < 0.05$) in the Choice reaction Time Test (stage 5). The number of total moves in Choice Reaction Time Test was not affected by clonidine or guanfacine ($p > 0.1$). In lower stages of this test, no drug treatment effects on accuracy or speed of response were found (data not shown; $p > 0.1$) (Table 1).

Table 2. The effects of clonidine and guanfacine on subjective ratings for sedation on Visual Analogue Scale

	Placebo	Drug
C 0.5	3.3±1.1	3.0±1.7
C 2	3.2±1.4	3.3±1.3
C 5	3.1±1.5	5.0±1.3[a]
G 7	3.0±1.3	3.3±1.4
G 29	3.2±1.4	4.5±1.3[a]

Values (range 0-10; 1 representing not at all tired/sedated, and 10 representing extremely tired/sedated) represent ratings after completion of the test session (about 180 min after taking the study drug or matching placebo). Abbreviations: C=clonidine; G=guanfacine. Doses are expressed as µg/kg. Results are expressed as means ± S.D. [a] $p < 0.05$, paired samples two-tailed t-test,

Table 3. The effects of clonidine and guanfacine on blood pressure

	Placebo			Drug		
	0 min	+ 90 min	+ 180 min	0 min	+ 90 min	+ 180 min
C 0.5	128/79	126/78	128/78	126/78	125/78	127/79
C 2	126/78	126/78	126/78	126/78	123/78	122/75
C 5	127/78	125/77	128/79	127/78	120/74[a]	114/70[a]
G 7	125/78	124/78	125/78	124/79	126/78	128/80
G 29	127/77	129/78	126/78	129/77	122/78[a]	117/75[a]

Abbreviations: +90 min=90 min after taking the study drug or matching placebo, *i.e.* just before starting the test session; +180 min=180 min after taking the study drug or matching placebo, *i.e.* after completion of the test session; C=clonidine; G=guanfacine. Doses are expressed as µg/kg and blood pressure values (means of systolic/diastolic pressures) as mmHg. [a] p < 0.05, paired samples two-tailed t-test.

Visual Analogue Scale

Clonidine 5 and guanfacine 29 µg/kg increased subjective feelings of sedation (p < 0.05) (Table 2).

Blood Pressure

Clonidine 5 and guanfacine 29 µg/kg reduced both systolic and diastolic blood pressures (p < 0.05) (Table 3).

DISCUSSION

A non-subtype selective α_2-agonist, clonidine, at 5.0 µg/kg disrupted performance at the Choice Reaction Time Test, which is analogous to the rat 5-choice serial reaction time task, considered to assess sustained attention (Sahakian and Owen, 1992). Performance at easier levels of the test, requiring less effortful information processing capacity, was unaffected by clonidine. Furthermore, simple motor performance or the ability to follow a simple rule and its reversal were not disrupted by clonidine. Thus, the deficits in the Choice Reaction Time Test were not secondary to slowing or inaccuracy of motor performance. The lack of deficits by clonidine on the performance of easier tasks can be interpreted in terms of clonidine having had no effect on more automatic forms of information processing.

Another α_2-agonist, guanfacine, had no impairing effects on attentional performance. Furthermore, simple motor performance and the ability to follow a simple rule and its reversal were not affected by guanfacine. These findings are in line with previous animal data. In both aged, and young hyperactive and inattentive monkeys, guanfacine improved prefrontal cortical functions (delayed-response performance) without the sedative or hypotensive effects which accompanied clonidine administration (Arnsten et al., 1996). This was suggested to be related to the relative selectivity for the α_{2A} binding site for guanfacine over clonidine, and is consistent with the presence of the most dense immunocytochemistry of α_{2A} subtype in monkey prefrontal cortex Aoki et al., 1994).

Clonidine 5 and guanfacine 29 µg/kg lowered systolic and diastolic blood pressures. In mutant mice lacking α_{2A}-adrenoceptor subtype, the hypotensive response to α_2-agonists was lost, demonstrating that α_{2A}-adrenoceptors play a major role in this response

(MacMillan et al., 1996). Thus, clonidine 5 and guanfacine 29 µg/kg may have equally effectively stimulated brainstem α_{2A}-adrenoceptors.

In the Choice Reaction Time Test, clonidine 5 µg/kg both increased reaction latencies and reduced the number of correct responses. This suggests that when treated with clonidine 5 µg/kg, the study subjects may have adopted a speed/accuracy trade-off strategy (Cole and Robbins, 1992), *i.e.* by responding more slowly they may have tried to maintain the tendency to respond deliberately at a lower level to reduce the possibility of responding inaccurately or too soon and so maintain a high level of response accuracy. The slowed reaction latencies after clonidine 5 µg/kg could not be simply due to sedation, as an equally sedating dose of guanfacine (29 µg/kg), had no effect on reaction latencies or the number of correct responses. Thus, the effects of clonidine and guanfacine on attentional performance vs. sedation could be dissociated from each other.

The deficit in attentional performance by clonidine 5 µg/kg could relate to stronger α_{2B} (and/or α_{2C})-adrenoceptor stimulation by this dose of clonidine. α_{2B} mRNA labelling in the rat brain is found exclusively in the thalamus (Scheinin et al., 1994), and clonidine can modulate arousal through actions at postsynaptic α_2-adrenoceptors in the rat thalamus (Buzsáki et al., 1990). The α_{2C}-adrenoceptors are located at the hippocampus, cortex and striatum (Scheinin et al., 1994). Interestingly, the sedative action of an α_2-agonist, dexmedetomidine, on cortical EEG arousal in mice lacking α_{2C}-adrenoceptors was enhanced compared with that of the control mice (Puoliväli et al., 1997), and overexpression of α_{2C}-adrenoceptors did not enhance the EEG arousal sedating effects of dexmedetomidine (Björklund et al., 1996), suggesting that α_{2C}- and $\alpha_{2A/B}$-adrenoceptors may have antagonistic effects on cortical EEG arousal and that α_{2C}-adrenoceptors are not essential for the sedative actions of α_2-agonists. These data suggest thalamic α_{2B}-related mechanisms as being involved in the attention defect induced by clonidine.

In conclusion, clonidine 5 µg/kg disrupted sustained attention under conditions requiring effortful processing of information, while leaving performance in more automatic tasks intact. An equally sedating dose of a more selective α_{2A}-agonist, guanfacine (29 µg/kg), had no effect on attentional performance, indicating that the effects of clonidine on attention could be dissociated from its sedative effects. Based on previous results, we suggest that activation of α_{2B}-adrenoceptors by clonidine may account for its ability to disrupt sustained attention in young healthy volunteers. Further studies with Alzheimer's and Parkinson's disease patients with clonidine and guanfacine are underway in our laboratory.

ACKNOWLEDGMENTS

This study was supported by the Finnish Academy of Sciences.

REFERENCES

Aoki, C., Go, C.-G., Venkatesan, C., and Kurose, H., 1994, Perikaryal and synaptic localization of α-2A-adrenergic receptor-like immunoreactivity. *Brain Res.* 650: 81–204.

Arnsten, A.F.T., Steere, J.C., and Hunt, R.D., 1996, The contribution of α_2-noradrenergic mechanisms to prefrontal cortical cognitive function. *Arch. Gen. Psychiatry* 53:448–455.

Aston-Jones, G., Shipley, M. T., Ennis, M., Williams, J. T., and Pieribone, V. A., 1990, Resticted afferent control of locus coeruleus neurones revealed by anatomical, physiological, and pharmacological studies. *In: The Pharmacology of Noradrenaline in the Central Nervous System*, D. J. Heal and C. A. Marsden, eds., New York: Oxford University Press, pp.187–247.

Berridge, C. W., and Foote, S. L., 1991, Effects of locus coeruleus activation on electroencephalographic activity in neocortex and hippocampus. *J.Neurosci.* 11: 3135- 3145.

Björklund, M.G., Riekkinen, M., Puoliväli, J., Santtila, P., Sirviö, J., Sallinen, J., Scheinin, M., Haapalinna, A., and Riekkinen, P. Jr., 1996, Alpha2c-adrenoceptor overexpression impairs development of normal water maze search strategy in mice. *Soc. Neurosci. Abstract* 26th Annual Meeting, Washington D.C., p. 682.

Buzsáki, G., Kennedy, B., Solt, V. B., and Ziegler, M., 1990, Noradrenergic control of thalamic oscillation: The role of α-2 receptors. *Eur. J. Neurosci.*3:222–229.

Cole, B. J., and Robbins, T. W., 1992, Forebrain norepinephrine: Role in controlled information processing in the rat. *Neuropsychopharmacology* 7: 29–142.

Foote, S. L., and Morrison, J. H., 1987, Extrathalamic modulation of cortical function. *Ann. Rev. Neurosci.* 10:67–95.

Harley, C. W, 1987, A role for norepinephrine in arousal, emotion, and learning? Limbic modulation by norepinephrine and the key hypothesis. *Prog. Neuropsychopharmacol. Biol. Psychiatry* 11:419–458.

Jäkälä, P., Sirviö, J., Riekkinen, P.Jr., Haapalinna, A. and Riekkinen, P.J., 1992, Effects of atipamezole, an α_2-adrenoceptor antagonist, on the performance of rats in a five-choice serial reaction time task. *Pharmacol. Biochem. Behav.* 42:903–907.

MacMillan, L.B., Hein, L., Smith, M.S., Piascik, M.T., and Limbird, L.E., 1996, Central hypotensive effects of the α_{2a}-adrenergic receptor subtype. *Science* 273:801–803.

Puoliväli, J.T., Björklund, M., Riekkinen, M., Sallinen J., Scheinin, M., Haapalinna, A., Kobilka, B., and Riekkinen, P. Jr., 1997, Alpha2c-adrenoceptor knock out increases the sedative effect of alpha-agonist. *2nd European Meeting: Cognitive Dysfunction. Pharmacol. Biochem. Behav., Abstracts.*

Riekkinen, P. Jr., Sirviö, J., Jäkälä, P., Lammintausta, R., and Riekkinen, P., 1990, Effect of alpha$_2$ antagonists and an agonist on EEG slowing induced by scopolamine and lesion of the nucleus basalis. *Neuropharmacology* 29:993–272.

Robbins, T.W., and Everitt, B. J., 1994, Arousal systems and attention. *In: The Cognitive Neurosciences,* M.S. Gazzaniga , ed., Cambridge, Mass. MIT Press, pp. 703–720.

Sahakian, B.J., and Owen, A.M., 1992, Computerized assessment in neuropsychiatry using CANTAB: discussion paper. *J. Royal Soc. Med.* 85:399–402.

Scheinin, M., Lomasney, J.W., Hayden-Hixson, D.M., Schambra, U.B., Caron, M.G., Lefkowitz, R.J., and Fremeau, R.T., 1994, Distribution of α-2-adrenergic receptor subtype gene expression in rat brain. *Mol. Brain Res.* 21:133–149.

Sirviö, J., Mazurkiewicz, M., Haapalinna, A., Riekkinen, P. Jr., Lahtinen, H., and Riekkinen, P. J. Sr., 1994, The effects of selective alpha-2 adrenergic agents on the performance of rats in a 5-choice serial reaction time task. *Brain Res. Bull.* 35:451–455.

Uhlen, S, and Wikberg, J.E.S., 1991, Delineation of rat kidney α-2A and α-2B-adrenoceptors with [3H]RX821002 radioligand binding: computer modeling reveals that guanfacine is an α-2A-selective compound. *Eur. J. Pharmacol.* 202:235–243.

FUNCTIONAL NEUROIMAGING REVEALS DECLINE FROM PREMORBID FUNCTIONING IN AD

Isak Prohovnik

Department of Diagnostic Radiology
Yale University School of Medicine
New Haven, Connecticut 06510

INTRODUCTION

Correct and early diagnosis of Alzheimer's disease (AD) is critical to exclude other, treatable, conditions, and is now achieving greater importance with the growing availability of specific treatments. Some of the new dementia treatments are associated with significant toxicity, requiring caution in their widespread use. There is also growing recognition of a wide spectrum of geriatric degenerative diseases that may be pathophysiologically and biochemically distinct. This may, in the near future, require a fundamental rethinking of diagnostic and therapeutic strategies.

Clinical Diagnosis

The accuracy of clinical diagnosis of AD is variable; experts in specialized centers sometimes approach 90% accuracy against neuropathological criteria, but a general practice would be expected to be significantly less accurate (Gearing et al., 1995; Ashford et al., 1996). In a recent large series, Galasko et al. (1994) reviewed the clinicopathological correlations in a selected population that had extensive clinical evaluations at a tertiary AD Center. In this sample, of 111 clinical diagnoses of probable AD 60% had neuropathological diagnoses of pure AD, and 93% had neuropathological findings including AD and other pathologies, mainly Lewy Bodies and cerebrovascular disease (CVD). Of 26 possible AD diagnoses, the neuropathological rates were 50% and 77%, respectively. Sensitivity of the combined probable and possible diagnoses against pure AD pathological findings was 93%, and against all AD findings was 84%. Growdon (1995) reported a similar series where about 84% of clinical AD diagnoses were confirmed by autopsy, whereas 2–5% (each) were found to have Lewy Body Disease, Pick's disease or

CVD. It has recently been estimated that the likelihood ratio of current clinical AD criteria results in 25% error rate (Jobst, 1995) with false positives rising to as much as 50% for maximum sensitivity.

The actual situation is likely to be even worse. Accuracy of clinical diagnosis is a function of skill and experience, and it is probably the experienced researchers that tend to publish their achievements, rather than the poor performers, thus biasing the literature. Second, many published reports assess the accuracy of final clinical diagnosis, based on long-term follow-up, rather than the initial diagnosis. Finally, several screening instruments, most notably the MMS, and probably the clinical diagnosis itself, are affected by cultural and educational factors (Ashford et al., 1996). In fact, most clinicians diagnose this disease by assuming a certain premorbid level of functioning, and assessing the decline from that level; that theoretical premorbid functioning is culturally determined.

It seems clear, therefore, that the clinical diagnosis of AD will benefit from a valid and reliable laboratory marker of the disease. Such a marker would, ideally, be independent of cultural and educational bias. This is the focus of the current report.

Neuroimaging in AD

Traditional, anatomical brain imaging has not proved useful for the diagnosis of AD (Growdon, 1995). Structural brain imaging by means of CT has been used to exclude other conditions associated with cerebral lesions. Attempts to achieve specificity for AD by quantifying atrophy have been unsuccessful (Smith, 1987). The introduction of MRI added high sensitivity to white-matter lesions, recently found useful as a major correlate of Vascular Dementia (VaD), but still no specificity with respect to AD. Both methods are effective at finding generalized atrophy, but such atrophy cannot discriminate degenerative disease from normal aging. One of the most ambitious attempts was performed by the CERAD consortium (Davis et al., 1992), and resulted in low reliability among neuroradiologists in the visual interpretation of MRI scans.

In contrast, functional brain imaging is a successful adjunct to the diagnosis of Alzheimer's disease. The sensitivity of these methods is not yet fully established, especially for mild disease, although a recent paper (Rieman et al., 1996) suggests that the typical metabolic deficits are clearly detectable in brains of healthy individuals homozygous for the ApoE4 allele, and therefore at high risk for developing the disease. Specificity is already known to be satisfactory, and a positive result is of diagnostic value (Prohovnik et al., 1988; Holman et al., 1992; Claus et al., 1994). Since the late 1980s, the bulk of the literature suggests that AD is characterized by a focal reduction of blood flow and metabolism in parietotemporal cortex (Jagust et al., 1987; Prohovnik et al., 1988). This finding is sensitive even to mild disease stages, and highly specific against the major psychogeriatric conditions that may be misdiagnosed as AD, including major depression (Sackeim et al., 1993), VaD (Prohovnik et al., 1991; Prohovnik & Wu, 1996) and Frontal Lobe Dementia (FLD, Risberg et al., 1993; Alexander et al., 1995). Thus, it has been proposed as a highly accurate diagnostic marker, with good predictive validity (Holman et al., 1992). The only possible false positive involves demented patients with Parkinson's disease, who may also reveal an AD-like parietotemporal perfusion deficit (Liu et al., 1992; Tachibana et al., 1993), but they also share neuropathological findings (Gearing et al., 1995).

This description is true at the time of writing, but may soon need revision, because recent findings suggest a possible diagnostic role even for structural imaging. It has long been known that the mesial temporal lobe is among the sites earliest affected neuropathologically in AD, but imaging technology was inadequate to the task. Recently, CT and MRI studies suggested that focal atrophy of mesial temporal cortex may be a sensitive indicator of early AD (Growdon, 1995). In the only prospective study of both CT and SPECT, mesial temporal atrophy on CT had a specificity of 80%, compared to 84% of the parietotemporal SPECT deficit; both measures combined had a specificity of 94% (Jobst et al., 1994, 1995). Of course, SPECT itself may also show the mesial temporal deficit (e.g., Prohovnik & Wu, 1996), and MRI may be more accurate than CT. The success of these methods depends partly on enhanced spatial and temporal resolution, and partly on the development of more intelligent quantification and analysis algorithms.

These data suggest that neuroimaging is a useful adjunct to clinical diagnosis: the studies below will additionally emphasize that functional neuroimaging may also overcome the problem of variable premorbid status.

OVERCOMING DIAGNOSTIC BIASES

Based partly on Katzman (1993), consider the following hypotheses:

1. The critical characteristic of AD patients, for both diagnosis and severity staging, is their speed of deterioration from premorbid functional level, rather than their current deficits.
2. It is not possible to accurately infer the rate of deterioration from current level of functioning, because the rate is variable, and premorbid functioning heterogeneous. Yet, this is usually the major basis for clinical evaluation.
3. It is very difficult to accurately quantify this rate of deterioration from the patient's or caregiver's reports.
4. This is particularly problematic at early stages of the disease, and in populations with low premorbid functioning.

The general problem can be stated as follows: given that clinical diagnosis will tend to be biased by the unknown deterioration from premorbid functional level, can a laboratory marker be found to quantify this deterioration. Evidence will be reviewed below to suggest that functional neuroimaging can provide such a marker. The three studies have utilized the ^{133}Xe rCBF technique to quantify cortical perfusion. The parietotemporal deficit was quantified by a standard index and used for all numerical comparisons. Actual images were presented in the original publications.

Review of Findings

Since actual premorbid intellectual ability is rarely known, indirect indices need to be used. The most obvious of those is educational achievement. It is plausible that higher educational achievements are proportional to intellectual ability, either as a result (the smarter you are, the higher your educational attainments) or as a cause (the more education you receive, the more developed your intellect). This association is known from epidemiological studies that report a higher prevalence of Alzheimer's disease (AD) in individuals with fewer years of education (Zhang et al., 1990; Moritz & Petitti, 1993). This may represent an artifact: individuals with lower educational levels perform more poorly on screening tests for dementia, which results in a higher rate of detection. This in turn introduces high false positive rates in individuals with low education and high false negative rates in those with more education. Alternatively, the prevalence of AD in the higher education ranges may actually be lower, indicating protection. The first hypothesis, involving bias, would be supported if we could show that the extent of their disease is mild, despite poor performance.

In the first experiment of this series (Stern et al., 1992), 58 AD patients were divided into three education groups: <12 years of education (range 3 to 11 years), high school graduate (12 years), and greater than high school (13 to 24 years). The three groups were otherwise matched on clinical and demographic characteristics, including age, duration of disease, and current severity of disease quantified by the mMMS and BDRS.

Parietotemporal perfusion was found to be reduced in the AD patients, as expected, and the deficits were inversely proportional to education: greater flow reduction in the highest education group relative to the other groups. In contrast, within 34 aged normal controls there was no association between any perfusion measure and education. Although range of education is truncated in the controls, it does include education levels whose flow differed significantly in the AD patients. This suggests that the relation between education and flow is specific to the demented group.

If education is the result of cognitive abilities, rather than their precursor, it is possible that lifetime occupational experience may offer an equally good index of intellect. Further, educational experience occurs over a relatively brief period, whereas occupational experiences last longer. Finally, those individuals denied proper education for social reasons may still show their abilities by occupational achievements. For example, gifted children from very low socio-economic status may not receive the education they deserve. Similarly, elderly women who grew up in the beginning of the 20th century may also have been denied proper education in some societies.

For these reasons, we designed the second experiment (Stern et al., 1995). We classified primary lifetime occupations of 51 AD patients using the Dictionary of Occupational Titles of the US Department of Labor and derived 6 factor scores describing intellectual, interpersonal and physical job demands. After controlling for age and clinical dementia severity, relative perfusion in the parietotemporal region showed significant inverse correlations with job complexity and interpersonal skills factor scores. These results are complicated by the strong correlations of education with occupational attainments, and their interpretation was not simple, but they further strengthen the association between life experiences and the extent of brain damage, as reflected by parietotemporal cortex perfusion in AD: patients with higher achievements, and presumably higher premorbid functioning, show greater brain damage with equal clinical disease severity.

Both education and occupations are indirect indices, of course, of premorbid functioning. The optimal test of the hypothesis that functional neuroimaging reveals deterioration in AD would consist of rigorous follow-up of elderly subjects from normal functioning to eventual onset of the disease, and such a study would be prohibitively expensive. However, the excellent norms developed over the years for the standard intelligence test, the WAIS-R, allowed us to approach this situation. Previous work has established that it is possible to generate an accurate IQ estimate (in the US) from the demographic factors of age, sex, race, education, occupation, region of residence, and urban vs. rural residence. We (Keilp & Prohovnik, 1996) used these equations to estimate premorbid IQ in 27 patients with early AD. Following estimation of premorbid IQ's, the estimate of IQ decline associated with the diagnosis of AD was computed. This estimate was generated by subtracting estimated from currently assessed IQ.

The results were as follows. Over the estimated disease duration of 3.8 ± 2.2 years, Full-Scale IQ declined by an estimated 28.0 ± 15.5 points. Current parietotemporal perfusion was well correlated with the individual IQ decline (r=.66, p<.001). This association was linear, and stronger than those with any measure of current disease severity. A multiple stepwise regression analysis suggested that IQ decline alone accounted for the variance in parietotemporal perfusion related to clinical deterioration. Actual images showed a mild blood flow deficit in patients with the smallest estimated IQ declines, but deep and extensive lesions in patients with large declines. These results suggest that the decline from premorbid baseline, rather than current level of functioning, best predicts the extent of brain damage reflected in rCBF abnormality.

COMMENT

These results confirm that the parietotemporal deficit of perfusion and metabolism is a useful index of disease severity in AD. However, disease severity in this context appears to reflect each individual patient's decline from premorbid functioning, not just their deviation from population norms.

These data are limited by the fairly homogenous nature of the samples, derived from a tertiary care center in a large American city. They need to be replicated in other populations. The data are also limited in being derived from a single imaging technique, which reveals only cortical perfusion and at low spatial resolution. The final major limitation involves the known weakness of clinical diagnosis in AD. It is possible that some of our patients suffered from diseases other than AD, but the proportion of such errors is likely to be low and would not affect the overall findings. Nevertheless, it would be highly interesting to repeat such studies with neuropathological diagnostic confirmation, which could also directly validate the concept of metabolic or perfusion deficits reflecting "brain damage".

For the time being, these data suggest that functional neuroimaging should not be expected to reveal major cerebral deficiencies in patients with mild decline from premorbid levels. This is not a problem of low sensitivity, but a true biological reflection of neurophysiological processes. Further, the data suggest that the results of therapeutic trials may need to be evaluated in a new light. Currently, patients' baseline status is characterized by measures of current severity, such as the MMS. Some of the resulting heterogeneity in response to therapeutic compounds may be related to variable premorbid functioning, and the inability of standard instruments to reveal such variability.

ACKNOWLEDGMENTS

This work was partially supported by grants from the National Psychobiology Institute, Israel, and NIH grant NIA RO1 05433.

REFERENCES

Alexander, G.E., Prohovnik, I., Sackeim, H.A., Stern, Y., and Mayeux, R., 1995, Cortical Perfusion and Gray-Matter Weight in Frontal Lobe Dementia. *J. Neuropsychiatry Clin.* Neurosci. 7:315–322.
Ashford, J.W., Schmitt, F.A. and Kumar,V., 1996, Diagnosis of Alzheimer's Disease. *Psychiatric Ann.* 26:262–268.
Davis, P.C., Gray, L., Albert, M., et al., 1992, The Consortium to Establish a Registry for Alzheimer's Disease (CERAD) Part III: Reliability of a Standardized MRI Evaluation of Alzheimer's Disease. *Neurology* 42:676–1680.

Galasko, D., Hansen, L.A., Katzman, R., Wiederholt, W., Masliah, E., Terry, R., Hill, R., Lessin, P. and Thal, L.J., 1994, Clinical-Neuropathological Correlations in Alzheimer's Disease and Related Dementias. *Arch. Neurol.* 51:888–895.

Gearing, M., Mirra, S.S., and Hedreen, J.C., et al., 1995, The Consortium to Establish a Registry for Alzheimer's Disease (CERAD) Part X: Neuropathology Confirmation of the Clinical Diagnosis of Alzheimer's Disease. *Neurology* 45:461–466.

Growdon, J.H., 1995, Advances in the Diagnosis of Alzheimer's Disease. In: *Research Advances in Alzheimer's Disease and Related Disorders*, K. Iqbal et al.,eds., John Wiley & Sons, pp. 139–153.

Jagust, W.J., Budinger, T.F., and Reed, B.R., 1987, The Diagnosis of Dementia with Single Photon Emission Computed Tomography. *Arch. Neurol.* 44:258–262.

Jobst, K.A., Hindley, N.J., King, E. and Smith, A.D., 1994, The Diagnosis of Alzheimer's Disease: A Question of Image ? *J. Clin. Psychiatry;*55(Suppl):22–31.

Jobst, K.A. SPECT in the Diagnosis of Dementia, In: *The Clinical Use of SPECT*, M.A. Schuckit, ed., pp 539–542

Katzman R., 1993; Education and the prevalence of dementia and Alzheimer's disease. *Neurology* 43:13–20.

Keilp, J.G., and Prohovnik, I., 1995, Intellectual Decline Predicts the Parietal Perfusion Deficit in Alzheimer's Disease. *J. Nucl. Med.* 36:1347–1354.

Moritz, D,J, and Petitti, D.B., 1993, Association of education with reported age of onset and severity of Alzheimer's Disease at presentation: Implications for the use of clinical samples. *Am. J. Epidemiol.* 137(4): 456–462.

Prohovnik, I., Alexander, G., Tatemichi, T.K., et al., 1991, Cortical Perfusion in Vascular and Alzheimer's Dementia. *Neurology* 41(Suppl. 1):358.

Prohovnik, I., Mayeux, R., Sackeim, H.A., Smith, G., Stern, Y. and Alderson, P.O., 1988, Cerebral Perfusion as a Diagnostic Marker in Early Alzheimer's Disease. *Neurology,* 38:931–937.

Prohovnik, I., Wade, J., Knezevic, , S., Tatemichi, T. K. and Erkinjuntti, T., 1996, Vascular Dementia , John Wiley & Sons, Ltd., in press.

Reiman EM, Casselli RJ, Yun LS, et al.: Preclinical Evidence of Alzheimer's Disease in Persons Homozygous for the e4 Allele for Apolipoprotein E. *NEJM* 1996;334:752–758.

Sackeim, H.A., Prohovnik, I., and Moeller, J.R., et al., 1993, Regional Cerebral Blood Flow in Mood Disorders, II: Comparison of Major Depression and Alzheimer's Disease. *J. Nucl. Med.* 34:1090–1101.

Stern, Y., Alexander, G.E., Prohovnik, I., and Mayeux, R., 1992, Inverse Relationship between Education and Parietotemporal Perfusion Deficit in Alzheimer's Disease. *Ann. Neurol.* 32:371–375.

Stern, Y., Alexander, G.E., Prohovnik, I., Stricks, L., Link, B., Lennon, M.C and Mayeux, R., 1995, Relationship between Lifetime Occupation and Parietal Flow: Implications for a Reserve against Alzheimer's Disease Pathology. *Neurology* 45:55–60.

Tatemichi T.K., Desmond D.W., Prohovnik I., Cross, D.T., Gropen, T.I., Mohr, J.P., and Stern, Y., 1992, Confusion and Memory Loss from Capsular Genu Infarction: A Thalamocortical Disconnection Syndrome. *Neurology* 42:1966–1979.

Tatemichi, T.K., Desmond, D.W., Prohovnik, I., and Eidelberg, D., 1995, Dementia Associated with Bilateral Carotid Occlusions: Neuropsychological and Hemodynamic Course Following EC-IC Bypass Surgery. *J. Neurol. Neurosurg. Psychiatry* 58:633–636.

Zhang, M.Y., Katzman, R., Salmon, D., et al., 1990, The prevalence of dementia and Alzheimer's disease in Shanghai, China: Impact of age, gender, and education. *Ann. Neurol.*27:428–437.

105

NOVEL PHENYLTROPANES: AFFINITY TO MONOAMINE TRANSPORTERS IN RAT FOREBRAIN

John L. Neumeyer,[1] Ross J. Baldessarini,[2,3] Nora S. Kula,[2,3] and Gilles Tamagnan[4]

[1]Alcohol and Drug Abuse Research Center and
[2]Mailman Research Center
McLean Division of Massachusetts General Hospital
115 Mill Street
Belmont, Massachusetts 02178
[3]Consolidated Department of Psychiatry and Neuroscience Program
Harvard Medical School
Boston, Massachusetts
[4]Department of Psychiatry
Yale University and VAMC
West Haven, Connecticut 06516

INTRODUCTION

The active, natural (–)-isomer of cocaine (compound 1; Figure 1) preferentially binds to dopamine transporter (DA_T) proteins in the cell membranes of DA neurons, with lesser interactions at transporters for norepinephrine (NE_T) and serotonin (5-hydroxytryptamine, $5-HT_T$) (Harris and Baldessarini, 1973; Reith et al., 1980; Kennedy and Hanbauer, 1983; Calligaro and Elderfrawi, 1987, 1988; Madras et al., 1989). The DA_T is essential to the major physiological process for inactivating DA released extracellularly at synapses by neuronal reuptake, Its inhibition by cocaine or other psychostimulant drugs enhances dopaminergic neurotransmission in the forebrain (Reith et al., 1986; Ritz et al., 1987; Bergman et al., 1989). Saturable binding sites for (–)-cocaine at the DA_T associated specifically with DA-containing nerve terminals have been identified in caudate-putamen (neostriatum) tissue in the forebrain of rodents (Calligaro and Elderfrawi, 1988), nonhuman primates (Madras et al., 1989), and man (Schoemaker et al., 1985).

Progress in Alzheimer's and Parkinson's Diseases
edited by Fisher *et al.*, Plenum Press, New York, 1998.

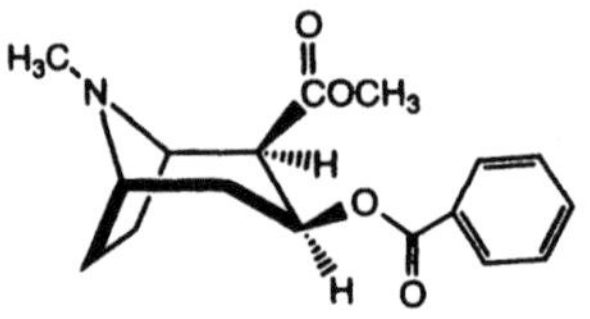

(−)-Cocaine (1) 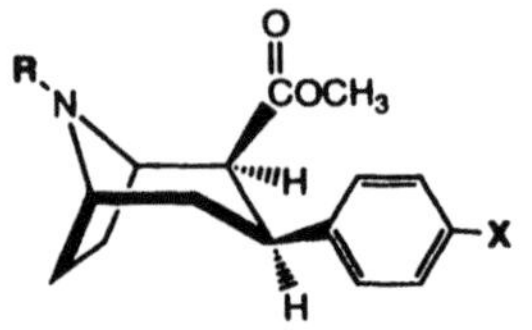   (−)-Phenyltropanes (2–5)

2 (nor-β-CIT) R = H, X = I
3 (β-CIT) R = CH₃, X = I
4 (β-CFT) R = CH₃, X = F
5 (FE-CIT) R = CH₂CH₂F, X = I
6 (FP-CIT) R = CH₂CH₂CH₂F, X = I

Figure 1. Cocaine and phenyltropane analogs.

Synthetic halophenyltropane analogs of cocaine (Fig. 1), including 2β-carbomethoxy-3β-(4'-iodophenyl)tropane (β-CIT or RTI-55; 3) has very high affinity at DA_T, and its 4'-fluorophenyl congener (β-CFT; WIN-35,428; 4) has somewhat less affinity at DA_T, but considerably greater selectivity for DA_T over $5\text{-}HT_T$ (Table 1). In contrast to readily hydrolyzed cocaine, a 3β-benzoyltropane ester, the phenyltropanes are much longer-acting (Neumeyer et al., 1991). Although both β-CIT and β-CFT bind to the DA_T, they also interact avidly with the $5\text{-}HT_T$ (Innis et al., 1991; Neumeyer et al., 1991; Carroll et al., 1992; Shaya et al., 1992; Baldwin et al., 1993; Laruelle et al., 1993; Wong et al., 1993; Table 1). Nevertheless, they appear to label DA_T selectively in the basal ganglia in vivo, evidently reflecting the higher natural abundance of DAt in that DA-rich brain region compared to 5-HT and its transporter (Kennedy and Hanbauer, 1983; Schoemaker et al., 1985; Calligaro and Elderfrawi, 1988; Madras et al., 1989).

Radiolabeled [¹²³I]β -CIT (Neumeyer et al., 1991; Shaya et al., 1992; Carroll et al., 1992; Baldwin et al., 1993; Brüke et al., 1993; Laruelle et al., 1993; Kuikka et al., 1995) and [¹¹C]β-CFT (Frost et al., 1993; Wong et al., 1993) are useful brain imaging agents for computed single photon emission tomography (SPECT) and positron emission tomography (PET), respectively. Such radioligands have particularly important potential for clinical applications in the neuroradiological diagnosis of Parkinson's disease and for monitoring progressive losses of DA neurons in this common idiopathic neurodegenerative disorder, and its potential modification by treatment (Innis et al., 1993).

Cocaine and its phenyltropane analogs have a tertiary amino nitrogen in the tropane ring system which is sufficiently basic to be protonated at physiological pH. Since interactions between cocaine and amine transporters may involve electrostatic or hydrogen bonding, N-substitution that changes electron density at the tropane nitrogen atom or lipophilicity may alter the affinity of phenyltropanes for amine transporter proteins. For example, we found previously that N-fluoroalkyl phenyltropanes including N-(3-fluoropropyl)-2β-carbomethoxy-3β-(4'-iodophenyl) nortropane (FP-CIT; 5), N-(2-fluoroethyl)-2β-carbomethoxy-3β-(4'-iodophenyl)nortropane (FE-CIT; 6), and their isopropyl ester congeners retained high affinity for the DA_T in rat caudate-putamen tissue, as well as even higher affinity for $5\text{-}HT_T$ (Neumeyer et al., 1994; Table 1).

These compounds have also been developed as neuroradiological tracers, including the PET radio-ligand [¹⁸F]FP-CIT (Chaly et al., 1996; Ishikawa et al., 1996) and SPECT radioligand [¹²³I]FP-CIT (Neumeyer et al., 1994; Baldwin et al., 1995; Chaly et al., 1996, Ishikawa et al., 1996; Booij et al., 1997a, 1997b) derived from FP-CIT (5; Fig. 1, Table 1).

Table 1. Affinities of phenyltropanes at monoamine transporters in rat forebrain tissue

Compound number	R^1	R^2	X	Y	Z	Ki (nM)			Selectivity	
						DA_T	$5\text{-}HT_T$	NE_T	$5\text{-}HT_T$	DA_T vs. NE_T
1 ([–]-Cocaine)	–	–	–	–	–	350	>10,000	>30,000	28.6	85.7
2 (nor-CIT)	H	$COOCH_3$	I	H	H	0.42	0.062	1.85	0.15	4.40
7*	CH_3	$COOCH_3$	I	NO_2	H	0.85	1.19	3.53	1.40	4.15
8*	CH_3	$COOCH_3$	I	I	H	0.89	0.26	24.4	0.29	27.4
3 (β-CIT)	CH_3	$COOCH_3$	I	H	H	0.96	0.46	2.80	0.48	6.09
9*	$CH_3OC_6H_4CH_2S(CH_2)_3$	$COOCH_3$	Cl	H	H	1.15	0.35	95.7	0.30	83.2
10	$F(CH_2)_3$	$COOCH(CH_3)_2$	I	H	H	1.20	48.7	≥10,000	40.6	8,300
11*	$O_2NPh(CH_2)_2$	$COOCH_3$	Cl	H	H	1.32	0.25	3.04	0.19	2.30
12*	CH_3	CH_2OH	Cl	H	H	1.61	25.9	40.8	16.1	25.3
13*	CH_3	$CH_2O(CH_2)_3I$	I	H	H	1.66	1.04	60.5	0.63	36.4
14*	CH_3	$COOCH_3$	I	NH_2	H	1.69	1.37	83.1	0.81	49.2
15*	CH_3	CH_2OH	I	H	H	1.80	3.03	106	1.68	68.9
16	Phthalimido$(CH_2)_4$	$COOCH_3$	I	H	H	2.38	0.21	192	0.09	80.7
17	Phthalimido$(CH_2)_5$	$COOCH_3$	I	H	H	2.40	0.34	55.9	0.14	23.3
18	Br$(CH_2)_3$	$COOCH_3$	I	H	H	2.56	0.35	164	0.14	64.1
19	Phthalimido$(CH_2)_8$	$COOCH_3$	I	H	H	2.98	0.20	74.5	0.07	372
20*	Phthalimido$(CH_2)_8$	$COOCH_3$	Cl	H	H	3.04	1.78	17.6	0.59	5.79
21	Cl$(CH_2)_3$	$COOCH_3$	I	H	H	3.10	0.32	96.0	0.10	31.0
5 (FP-CIT)	$F(CH_2)_3$	$COOCH_3$	I	H	H	3.53	0.11	63.0	0.032	17.8
6 (FE-CIT)	$F(CH_2)_2$	$COOCH_3$	I	H	H	3.67	0.86	93.0	0.23	25.3
22	Phthalimido$(CH_2)_2$	$COOCH_3$	I	H	H	4.23	0.84	441	0.20	104
23	Cyclopropyl-CH_2	$COOCH_3$	I	H	H	4.34	1.30	198	0.30	45.6
24	$F(CH_2)_2$	$COOCH(CH_3)_2$	H	H	H	4.40	21.7	>10,000	4.93	2,300
25*	$F(CH_2)_3$	$COOCH_3$	I	NH_2	H	4.92	7.33	441	1.49	89.6
26*	$F(CH_2)_3$	$COOCH_3$	I	NO_2	H	5.35	7.88	6.29	1.47	1.18
27	OH$(CH_2)_3$	$COOCH_3$	I	H	H	5.39	2.50	217	0.46	40.3
28	$(CH_3O)_2CHCH_2$	$COOCH_3$	I	H	H	6.80	1.69	110	0.25	16.2
29	Phthalimido$(CH_2)_3$	$COOCH_3$	I	H	H	9.10	0.59	73.7	0.06	8.10
30	$(CH_3)_2NCOCH_2$	$COOCH_3$	I	H	H	12.2	6.4	522	0.14	42.8
4 (β-CFT)	CH_3	$COOCH_3$	F	H	H	14.7	181	635	12.3	43.2

(*) Novel compounds not previously reported. The SE of all reported Ki values averaged ±12.1% (not shown).

These radio-pharmaceuticals have been used successfully to label DA neurons in brain tissue of normal human subjects and patients with Parkinson's disease (Neumeyer et al., 1994; Innis et al., 1993; Baldwin et al., 1995; Chaly et al., 1996; Ishikawa et al., 1996; Booij et al., 1997a, 1997b).

In an ongoing program to develop additional probes of monoamine transporters and to better define the sites of action of cocaine, we have synthesized and evaluated the binding affinity of a growing series of phenyltropane analogs substituted at the tropane nitrogen atom, the 2β position, and on the phenyl ring. Selected examples of recent findings are summarized in this report.

EXPERIMENTAL METHODS

Experimental tropanes were synthesized and evaluated with membrane preparations of forebrain tissue of young adult male Sprague-Dawley rats for their affinity (K_i, nM) to DA_T, $5\text{-}HT_T$, and NE_T. Test agents were stored at $-5°C$ in dimethylsulfoxide in ethanol (1:1, vols) until used for transporter affinity assays with dilution in a large excess of each assay buffer. Agents were tested in duplicate in at least six concentrations with membrane fractions of forebrain homogenates. Assays of DA_T used rat caudate-putamen tissue in 50 mM Tris-citrate buffer (50 mM; pH 7.4) containing NaCl (120 mM) and $MgCl_2$ (4 mM), with [^{3}H]GBR-12935 (13 Ci/mmol; Kd = 1.0 nM) as the radioligand at a concentration (L) of 0.4 nM, incubated for 45 min at 4°C, with or without excess (30 µM) (±)-methylphenidate included as a "blank" to define nonspecific binding.

For assays of affinity to $5\text{-}HT_T$ and NE_T, frontoparietal cerebral cortex tissue was similarly prepared in Tris-HCl buffer (50 mM; pH 7.4), containing NaCl at either 120 mM ($5\text{-}HT_T$) or 300 mM (NE_T) and KCl (5 mM). The $5\text{-}HT_T$ assay used [^{3}H]paroxetine (20 Ci/mmol; Kd = 0.15 nM) at L = 0.2 nM, incubated for 60 min at 20°C, using excess (1 µM) (±)-fluoxetine (donated by Eli Lilly Labs.; Indianapolis, IN) as the blank agent. For the NE_T assay, we used [^{3}H]nisoxetine (50 Ci/mmol; Kd = 0.8 nM) at L = 0.3 nM, with 2 µM desipramine (donated by Marion Merrell Dow; Kansas City, MO) as the blank, and incubating for 180 min at 4°C. Radioligands were from NEN (Boston, MA). Concentration-inhibition curves were analyzed by microcomputer with the ALLFIT program (provided by the National Institutes of Health; Bethesda, MD) to determine $IC_{50} \pm SE$, which was converted to K_i by the relationship: $K_i = IC_{50}/(1 + [L/K_d])$. These methods have been described in detail previously (Habert et al., 1985; Andersen 1987; Kula and Baldessarini, 1991; Tejani-Butt, 1992; Neumeyer et al., 1994).

RESULTS AND DISCUSSION

Selected findings are summarized in Table 1, with test agents listed in descending order by affinity ($1/K_i$) to the DA_T. Most of the phenyltropanes tested showed higher affinities (K_i) to DA_T and $5\text{-}HT_T$ than to NE_T, and all showed much greater DA_T affinity than that of (−)-cocaine (**1**). The highest DA_T affinity among compounds reported in Table 1 was found with previously reported (Neumeyer et al., 1991) nor-β-CIT (**2**; Ki = 420 pM), and this agent had even greater affinity (6.8-fold) for the $5\text{-}HT_T$ (K_i = 62 pM). Phenyltropanes that were doubly substituted on the phenyl ring at the 3' and 4' positions produced a slight gain of affinity for DA_T (850–890 vs. 960 pM) compared to the mono-iodinated, N-methyl congener β-CIT (**3**), but 3'-nitro-4'-iodo (**7**) substitution yielded even greater reduction of affinity to the $5\text{-}HT_T$ and improved DA_T-over-$5\text{-}HT_T$ selectivity, whereas the 3',4'-di-iodo (**8**) substituted congener showed a striking reduction of affinity for NE_T sites and a substantial gain in DA_T-over-NE_T selectivity.

Substitution at the tropane amino nitrogen atom produced highly variable changes in the affinity and selectivity of phenyltropanes for the DA_T. For example, the N-fluoroethyl (**6**), N-fluoropropyl (**5**), and N-bromopropyl (**18**) derivatives of nor-β-CIT retained similarly high affinity for the DA_T (2.56–3.67 nM), with somewhat lower affinity for the $5\text{-}HT_T$ found with the N-fluoropropyl compound (**5**; Ki = 1.68 nM) compared to the other two congeners (**6,18**; Ki = 0.35–0.86 nM). Such N-fluoroalkyl iodophenyltropanes have been successful in recent clinical applications as radioligands for imaging the DA_T, as was reviewed above.

Other bulkier N-substituents also changed the affinity and selectivity for specific amine transporters. Among several N-phthalimidoalkyl derivatives (**16,17,19,20,22,29**), there was some loss of affinity to DA_T, compared to β-CIT (**3**; 2.40–4.23 nM vs. 0.96 nM), but those with long alkyl chains showed a gain in affinity to the $5\text{-}HT_T$ over the DA_T, particularly in compound **19** with an 8-carbon spacer between the tropane and phthalimido rings ($5\text{-}HT_T$ K_i = 0.20 nM and selectivity = 15-fold over DA_T and 370-fold over NE_T). Such agents, with potent interactions with $5\text{-}HT_T$ as well as DA_T might be of interest as leads to novel mood-elevating agents for clinical use in the treatment of major depression, attention disorder, early dementia, or other disorders in which antidepressants or stimulants have useful effects (Baldessarini, 1996).

With regard to potential pharmaceutical development of novel phenyltropanes, it is noteworthy that the molar affinity of the standard selective serotonin-reuptake inhibitor antidepressant (±)-fluoxetine (Prozac®) for the $5\text{-}HT_T$ (Ki = 3.55 nM) was 18-times lower than that of compound **19** (and well below those of analogous compounds; **16,17,19,20,22,29**), and 57-times lower than that of nor-β-CIT (**2**) under the same assay conditions (not shown). Moreover, many of the experimental phenyltropanes have much higher DA_T affinity and much longer duration of behavioral action than (−)-cocaine (800-times lower DA_T affinity than nor-β-CIT) or other standard, clinically employed psychostimulants including (+)-amphetamine (2,000-times) and (±)-methylphenidate (350-times), or the dopaminergic antidepressants nomifensine (recalled due to toxicity; 100-times) and bupropion (475-times).

A general conclusion from the present observations is that the inclusion of more polar, larger, or more electronegative substituents at the tropane nitrogen of phenyltropanes, or the placement of electronegative 3' or 4' substituents in the phenyl ring did not produce marked losses of affinity to the DA_T (Table 1). Such tolerance for major molecular modifications indicates a good deal of leeway for producing potentially useful derivatives bearing radioactive or other substituents that might serve as markers for monoamine transporters, particularly of the DA_T and $5\text{-}HT_T$ types.

ACKNOWLEDGMENT

Supported in part by NIMH grants MH-34006, MH-47370, an award from the Bruce J. Anderson Foundation, and awards from the Mailman Research Center Private Donors Fund for Neuropharmacology Research (to RJB).

REFERENCES

Andersen, P.H., 1987, Biochemical and pharmacological characterization of [³H]GBR-12935 binding in vitro to rat striatal membranes: Labeling of the dopamine uptake complex, *J. Neurochem.* 48:1887–1896.

Baldessarini, R.J., 1996, Drugs and the treatment of psychiatric disorders. In: *Goodman and Gilman's The Pharmacological Basis of Therapeutics*, Hardman, J.G., Limbird, L.E., Molinoff, P.B., Ruddon, R.W., and Gilman, A.G., eds., McGraw-Hill Press, New York, ninth edition Chapters 18 and 19 pp 399–459.

Baldwin, R.M., Zea-Ponce, Y., Zoghbi, S.S., Laruelle, M., Al-Tikriti, M., Sybirska, E., Malison, R.T., Zoghbi, S.S., Neumeyer, J.L., Milius, R.A., Wang, S., Stabin, M., Smith, E.O., Charney, D.S., Hoffer, P.B., and Innis, R.B., 1993, Evaluation of the monoamine uptake site ligand [¹²³I]methyl-3β-(4-iodophenyl)tropane-2β-carbomethoxylate ([¹²³I]β -CIT in nonhuman primates: Pharmacokinetics, biodistribution and SPECT brain imaging coregistered with MRI, *Nucl. Med. Biol.* 20:597–606.

Baldwin, R.M., Zea-Ponce, Y., Al-Tikriti, M.S., Zoghbi, S.S., Seibyl, J.B., Charney, D.S., Hoffer, P.B., Wang, S., Milius, R.A., Neumeyer, J.L., and Innis, R.B., 1995, Regional brain uptake and pharmacokinetics of

[^{123}I]N-β-fluoroalkyl-2β-carboxy-3β-(4-iodophenyl)nortropane esters in baboons, *Nucl. Med. Biol.* 22:2311–219.

Brüke, T. Kornhuber, J., Angelberger, P., Asenbaum, S.A., Frassine, H., and Podrecka, I., 1993, SPECT imaging of dopamine and serotonin transporters with [^{123}I]β --CIT: Binding kinetics in the human brain, *J. Neural Transmission* 94:137–146.

Booij, J., Tissingh, G., Boer, G.J., Speelman, J.D., Stoof, J.C., Janssen, H.G.M., Wolters, E.C., and Van Royen, E.A., 1997a, [^{123}I]FP-CIT SPET shows a pronounced decline of striatal dopamine transporters labeled in early and advanced Parkinson's disease, *J. Neurol. Neurosurg. Psychiatry* 62:133–140.

Booij, J., Tissingh, G., Winogradzka, A., Boer, G.J., Stoof, J.C., Wolters, E.C., and Van Royer, E.A., 1997b, Practical benefit of [^{123}I]FP-CIT SPET in the demonstration of the dopaminergic deficit in Parkinson's disease, *Eur. J. Nucl. Med.* 24:68–71.

Bergman, J., Madras, B.K., and Spealman, R.D., 1989, Effects of cocaine and related drugs in nonhuman primates: Self-administration by squirrel monkeys, *J. Pharmacol. Exp. Ther.* 251:150–155.

Calligaro, D.O., and Elderfrawi, M.E., 1987, Central and peripheral cocaine receptors, *J. Pharmacol. Exp. Ther.* 243:61–67.

Calligaro, D.O., and Elderfrawi, M.E., 1988, High-affinity stereospecific binding of [^{3}H]cocaine in striatum and its relationship to the dopamine transporter, *Membrane Biochem.* 7:87–106.

Carroll, F.I., Gao, Y., Rahman, M.A., Abraham, P., Lewin, A.H., Parham, K.A., Boja, J.W., and Kuhar, M.J., 1992, Synthesis, ligand binding, QSAR, and coMFA study of 3β-(p-substituted phenyl)-tropane-2β-carboxylic acid methyl ester, *J. Med. Chem.* 35:2719–2725.

Chaly, T., Dhawan, V., Kazumata, K., Antonini, A., Margouleff, C., Dahl, J.R., Belakhlef, A., Margouleff, D., Yee, A., Wang, S., Tamagnan, G., Neumeyer, J.L., and Eidelberg, D., 1996, Radiosynthesis of [^{18}F]N-3-fluoro-propyl-2β-carbomethoxy-3β-(4-iodophenyl)tropane and the first human study with positron emission tomography, *Nucl. Med. Biol.* 23:999–1004.

Frost, J.J., Rosier, A.J., Reich, S.G., Smith, J.S., Ehlers, M.D., Snyder, S.H., Savert, H.T., and Dannals, R.F., 1993, Positron emission topographic imaging of the dopamine transporter with [^{11}C]WIN-35,428 reveals marked declines in mild Parkinson's disease, *Ann. Neurology* 34:423–431.

Habert, E., Graham, D., Aahraoui, L., Claustre, Y., and Langer, S.Z., 1985, Characterization of [^{3}H]paroxetine binding to rat cortical membranes, *Eur. J. Pharmacol.* 118:107–114.

Harris, J.E., and Baldessarini, R.J., 1973, Uptake of [^{3}H]-catecholamines by homogenates of rat corpus striatum and cerebral cortex: Effects of amphetamine analogues. *Neuropharmacology* 12:669–679.

Innis, R.B., Baldwin, R.M., Sybirska, E., Zea-Ponce, Y., Laruelle, M., Al-Tikriti, M., Charney, D.S., Zoghbi, S.S., Smith, E.O., Wisniewski, G., Hoffer, P.B., Wang, S., Milius, R.A., and Neumeyer, J.L., 1991, Single photon emission computed tomography imaging of monoamine reuptake sites in primate brain with [^{123}I]β - CIT, *Eur. J. Pharmacol.* 200:369–370.

Innis, R.B., Seibyl, J.B., Scanley, B.E., Laruelle, M., Abi-Dargham, A., Wallace, E., Baldwin, R.M., Zea-Ponce, Y., Zoghbi, S., Wang, S., Gao, Y., Neumeyer, J.L., Charney, D.S., Hoffer, P., and Marek, K.L., 1993, SPECT imaging demonstrates loss of striatal monoamine transporters in Parkinson's disease, *Proc. Natl. Acad. Sci. U.S.A.* 90:11965–11969.

Ishikawa, T. Dhawan, V., Kazumata, K., Chaly, T., Mandel, F., Neumeyer, J.L., Margouleff, C., Babchyck, B., Zanzi, I., and Eidelberg, D., 1996, Comparison of nigrostriatal dopaminergic imaging with [^{123}I]β -CIT-FP/SPECT and [^{18}F]DOPA/PET, *J. Nucl. Med.* 37:1760–1765.

Kennedy, L.T., and Hanbauer, I.. 1983, Sodium-sensitive cocaine binding to rat striatum membrane: Possible relationship to dopamine uptake sites, *J. Neurochem.* 41:172–178.

Kuikka, J.T., Bergstrom, K.A., Ahonen, A., Hiltunen, H.J., Haukka, J. β-carbomethoxy-3β-(4-iodophenyl)tropane and 2β-carbomethoxy-3β-(4-iodophenyl)-N-(3-fluorophenyl)nortropane for imaging of the dopamine transporter in the living human brain, *Eur. J. Nucl. Med.* 22:356–360.

Kula, N.S., and Baldessarini, R.J., 1991, Lack of increase in dopamine transporter binding or function in rat brain tissue after treatment with blockers of neuronal uptake of dopamine, *Neuropharmacology* 30:89–92.

Laruelle, M., Baldwin, R.M., Malison, R.T., Zea-Ponce, Y., Zoghbi, S.S., Al-Tikriti, M., Sybirska, E., Malison, R.T., Zoghbi, S., Neumeyer, J.L., Milius, R.A., Wang, S., Stabin, M., Smith, E.O., Roth, R.H., Charney, D.S., Hoffer, P.B., and Innis, R.B., 1993, SPECT imaging of dopamine and serotonin transporters with [^{123}I]β -CIT: Pharmacological characterization of brain uptake in nonhuman primates, *Synapse* 13:295–309.

Madras, B.K., Fahey, M.A., Bergman, J., Canfield, D.R., and Spealman, R.D., 1989, Effects of cocaine and related drugs in nonhuman primates: [^{3}H]Cocaine binding sites in caudate-putamen, *J. Pharmacol. Exp. Ther.* 251:131–141.

Neumeyer, J.L., Wang, S., Milius, R.A., Baldwin, R.M., Zea-Ponce, Y., Hoffer, P.B., Sybirska, E., Al-Tikriti, M. Charney, D.S., Malison, R.T., Laruelle, M., and Innis, R.B., 1991, [^{123}I]2β-carbomethoxy-3β-(4-iodophenyl)tropane: High-affinity SPECT radiotracer of monoamine reuptake sites in brain, *J. Med. Chem.* 34:3144–3146.

Neumeyer, J.L., Wang, S., Gao, Y., Milius, R.A., Kula, N.S., Campbell, A, Baldessarini, R.J., Zea-Ponce, Y., Baldwin, R.M., and Innis, R.B., 1994, N-ù-fluoroalkyl analogs of (1R)-2β-carbomethoxy-3β-(4-iodophenyl)tropane (β-CIT): Radiotracers for PET and SPECT imaging of dopamine transporters. *J. Med. Chem.* 37:1558–1561.

Reith, M.E.A., Sershen, H., and Lajtha, A., 1980, Saturable [³H]cocaine binding in central nervous system of mouse, *Life Sci.* 27:1055–1062.

Reith, M.E., Meisler, B.E., Sershen, H., and Lajtha, A., 1986, Structure requirements for cocaine congeners to interact with dopamine and serotonin uptake sites in mouse brain and to include stereotyped behavior, *Biochem. Pharmacol.* 35:11233–1129.

Ritz, M.C., Lamb, R.J., Goldberg, S.R., and Kuhar, M.J., 1987, Cocaine receptors on dopamine transporters are related to self-administration of cocaine, *Science* 237:1219–1223.

Schoemaker, H., Pimoule, C., Arbilla, S., Scatton, B., Javoy-Agid, F., and Langer, S.Z., 1985, Sodium-dependent [³H]cocaine binding associated with dopamine uptake sites in rat striatum and human putamen decrease after dopaminergic denervation and in Parkinson's disease, *Naunyn-Schmiedeberg's Arch. Pharmacol.* 329:227–235.

Shaya, E.K., Schettel, U., Dannals, R.F., Ricaurte, G.A., Carroll, F.I., Wagner, H.N., Kuhar, M.J., 1992, In vivo imaging of dopamine reuptake sites in the primate brain using single photon emission computed tomography (SPECT) and iodine-123 labeled RTI-55, *Synapse* 10:1169–1172.

Tejani-Butt, S.M., 1992, [³H]Nisoxetine: A radioligand for quantitation of norepinephrine uptake sites by autoradiography or by homogenate binding, *J. Pharmacol. Exp. Ther.* 260:4237–436.

Wong, D.F., Yong, V., Dannals, R.F., Shaya, E.K., Ravert, H.T., Chen, C.A., Chan, B., Folio, T., Scheffel, U., Ricaurte, G.A., Neumeyer, J.L., Wagner, H.N., and Kuhar, M.J., 1993, In vivo imaging of baboon and human dopamine transporters by positron emission tomography using [¹¹C]CFT, *Synapse* 15:130–142.

106

APP ISOFORMS IN PLATELETS

A Peripheral Marker of Alzheimer's Disease

M. Di Luca,[4] A. Padovani,[1] L. Pastorino,[4] A. Bianchetti,[2] J. Perez,[4]
S. Govoni,[2] L. A. Vignolo,[1] G. L. Lenzi,[3] M. Trabucchi,[2] and F. Cattabeni[4]

[1]Institute of Neurology, University of Brescia
p.za Ospedale 1, 25124 Brescia
[2]Institute Sacro Cuore-Centro Alzheimer
via dei Pilastroni 4, 25123 Brescia
[3]Department of Neurological Sciences
University of Rome La Sapienza
V.le dell'Universita' 30, 00185 Rome, Italy
[4]Institute of Pharmacological Sciences
University of Milan
via Balzaretti, 9, 20133 Milan

INTRODUCTION

Alzheimer disease is a neurodegenerative disorder characterized by progressive intellectual decline associated with senile plaques, neurofibrillary tangles and amyloid angiopathy as main pathological hallmarks.

Similar lesions are present in brains of Down's syndrome patients and to a lesser extent in normal aging (Glenner and Wong 1984). The amyloid β protein (Aβ) is derived from a larger precursor: the Amyloid Precursor Protein (APP) (Weidemann et al., 1989). This integral transmembrane cell-surface protein is present as numerous alternatively spliced isoforms derived from a single gene localized on human chromosome 21, in both neuronal as well as non neuronal tissues (Golde et al., 1990). Indeed much evidence supports the hypothesis that the presence of APP in peripheral cells, i.e. endothelial and blood cells, may contribute to Aβ deposition (Ghilardi et al., 1996; Shayo et al., 1997). If this is the case, Aβ of circulating origin might have important implications both in the diagnosis and in the pathogenesis of the disease.

Platelets represent an important peripheral source of APP, containing a large fraction of the vascular pool of this protein (Gardella et al., 1990; Schlossmacher et al., 1992). In fact it has been reported that the three major APP isoforms with apparent MW in the range

Progress in Alzheimer's and Parkinson's Diseases
edited by Fisher *et al.*, Plenum Press, New York, 1998.

of 100–130 kDa are present in membranes of resting platelets (Bush et al., 1990). In addition, it has been shown that activated platelets release membrane fragments containing the full length 130 kDa APP 770–751 (Cole et al., 1990). Stimulated platelets release amyloid β-protein precursor. When stimulated with thrombin, calcium ionophore or collagen, platelets are also able to release the soluble, carboxyl-truncated form of APP (protease nexin 11, PN2) (Van Nostrand et al., 1990). Moreover Smith et al. (Smith et al., 1990) reported that, upon stimulation, platelets release a protein functionally identical to the platelet coagulation factor Xla inhibitor, that has been shown to be a truncated form of APP containing the Kunitz domain. The large amount of APP found in platelets suggests that this protein, in addition to its role in the regulation of blood coagulation, may also serve to deliver a conspicuous amount of APP to the circulation. Nevertheless, the question whether the levels of APP in platelets of AD patients are affected has not yet found experimental support.

The aim of the present work was, therefore, to investigate if a correlation between levels of platelet APP isoforms and Alzheimer disease could be detected. The population studied comprised 37 Alzheimer patients and 35 age-matched control subjects. AD patients (mean age ± SD; 71.8 ± 7.1, range 45–86) fulfilled both DSM IIIR and NINCDS-ADRDA diagnostic criteria for probable AD (McKhann et al., 1984). Control subjects (67.6 years ± 13.5, range 40–86) were drawn from a series of either healthy subjects or non-demented hospitalized neurological patients. Exclusion criteria for all the subjects to be included in the study, were the following: head trauma, metabolic dysfunction, haematologic diseases, alcohol abuse, delirium, mood disorders, and actual treatment with acetylcholinesterase inhibitors or with medications affecting platelet functions. Neither control cases nor patients had family history of Alzheimer's disease. Informed consent was obtained from all subjects.

A blood sample was collected from all subjects included in the study and platelets separated by centrifugation at room temperature as previously described (Di Luca et al., 1996). Whole platelet homogenates from each subject were then processed for Western Blot analysis using monoclonal 22C11 antibody raised against the N-terminal domain of APP and therefore recognizing all APP isoforms. The staining of the upper band (130 kDa), corresponding to the full length mature APP was markedly reduced in AD patients when compared to control subjects. On the other hand immunostaining for the two lower forms showed similar intensity, both in control cases and in AD patients. After measuring the intensity of the bands at 130 kDa and 106–110 kDa by image analysis, a highly statistically significant difference was found in the ratio of these isoforms between AD patients and control subjects (mean ± SD): control subjects 0.84 ± 0.2; AD group 0.31 ± 0.12; AD vs control group: p< 0.001 (Figure 1).

The mechanism by which the ratio in levels of platelet APP isoforms is decreased in AD patients is at present only a matter of speculation. One possible explanation could reside in a decreased expression of a specific APP isoform in platelets of AD patients. To address this point, RT-PCR experiments were performed by using primers that flank the alternative splice site, following the method described by Golde et al (Golde et al., 1990). RT-PCR products from platelet MRNA of control subjects and AD patients were revealed by agarose gel and ethidium bromide. The pattern of gene expression was similar among groups (data not shown), thus suggesting that the differential level of APP isoforms observed in AD cannot be ascribed to a decreased/absent level of MRNA encoding either for APP770 or for APP 751.

There is evidence indicating that modifications in the concentration/processing of APP in platelets are expressed in advanced stages of AD and it has been reported that plate-

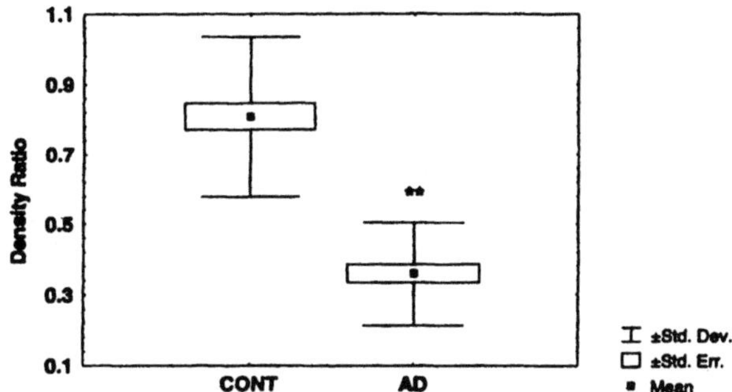

Figure 1. Optical density ratio of the bands corresponding to the high molecular weight (130 kDa) APP isoform and the low molecular weight (106–110 kDa) isoforms in platelets of aged-matched control subjects and AD patients. **p<0.001.

lets from individuals with AD show alterations in membrane fluidity. Our data showing a differential level of platelet APP isoforms in AD patients in absence of any modifications of the transcripts encoding for the three isoforms present in platelets, strongly support the hypothesis of an alteration in processing/secretion of the mature APP isoforms in AD.

These findings have several implications. First, APP processing abnormalities believed to be an early change in AD, do occur in extraneuronal tissues, lending support to the view that AD is a systemic disorder.

Secondly our data suggest that APP751/770 may be oversecreted in platelets from AD and that APP of circulating origin and Aβ deposits are often found in specific structures which are not readily accessible to tissue-derived peptides. This could have implications for novel therapeutic approaches to prevent the progressive deposition of Aβ. Finally, our data strongly indicate that a differential level of platelet APP isoforms can be considered as a potential peripheral marker of AD.

REFERENCES

Bush, A.I., Martins, R.N., Rumble, B., Moir, R., Fuller, S., Milward, E., Currie, J., Ames, D., Weidemann, A., Fisher, P., Multhaup, G., Beyreuther, K., and Masters, C.L., 1990, The Amyloid precursor protein of Alzheimer's disease is released by human platelets. *J. Biol. Chem.* 265:15977–15983.

Cole, G.M., Galasko, D., Shapiro, I.P., and Saitoh, T., 1990, Stimulated platelets release amyloid β protein precursor. *Biochem. Biophys. Res. Comm.* 170:288–295

Di Luca, M., Pastorino, L., Cattabeni, F., Zanardi, R., Scarone, S., Racagni, G., Smeraidi, E., and Perez, J., 1996. Abnormal pattern of platelet APP isoforms in Alzheimer disease and Down syndrome. *Arch. Neurol.* 53:1162–1166.

Gardella, J.E., Ghiso, J., Gorgone, G.A., Marratta, D., Kaplan, A.P., Frangione, B., and Gorevic, P.D., 1990, Intact Alzheimer amyloid precursor protein (APP) is present in platelet membrane and is encoded by platelet MRNA. *Biochem. Biophys. Res. Commun.* 173:1292–1298.

Ghilardi, J.R., Catton, M., Stimson, E.R., Rogers, S., Walker, L.C., Maggio, J.E., and Mantyh, P.W., 1996, Intra-arterial infusion of [1–125]A beta-1–40 labels amyloid deposits in the aged primate brain *in vivo. Neuroreport* 7:2607–2611.

Glenner, G.G., and Wong C.W., 1984, Alzheimer's disease and Down's syndrome: sharing of a unique cerebrovascular amyloid fibril protein. *Biochem. Biophys. Res. Commun.* 122:1131–1135.

Golde, T., Estes, S., Usiak, M., Yankin, L., and Yankin, S., 1990, Expression of β amyloid protein precursor mRNAs: recognition of a novel alternatively spliced form and quantitation in AD using PCR. *Neuron* 4:253–267.

McKhann, G., Drachman, D., Folstein, M., Katzman, R., Price, D., and Stadlan, E.M., 1984, Clinical Diagnosis of Alzheimer's disease: report of the NINCDS-ADRDA Work group under the auspices of department of Health and the human services task force on Alzheimer's disease. *Neurology* 34:939–944.

Schlossmacher, M.G., Ostaszewski, B.L., Hecker, L.I., Celi, A., Haas, C., Chin, D., Lieberburg, I., Furie, B.C., Furie, B., and Selkoe D.J., 1992, Detection of distinct isoform patterns of the β-amyloid precursor protein in human platelets and lymphocytes. *Neurobiol. Aging* 13:421–434.

Shayo, M., Mclay, R.N., Kastin, A.J., and Banks, W.A., 1997, The putative blood-brain barrier transporter for the beta-amyloid binding protein apolipoprotein J is saturated at physiological concentrations. *Life Sci.* 60:115–118.

Smith, R.P., Higuchi, D.A., and Broze, G.J.Jr., 1990, Platelet coagulation factor Xla-inhibitor, a form of Alzheimer amyloid precursor protein. *Science* 248:1126–1128.

Van Nostrand, W.E., Schmaier, A.H., and Farrow, J. S. Cunningham, D.D., 1990, Protease Nexin II (Amyloid β-Protein Precursor): A platelet α-granule protein. *Science* 248:745–748.

Weidemann, A., Konig, G., Bunke, D., Fisher, P., Salbaum, J.M., Masters, C.L., and Beyreuther, K., 1989, Identification, biogenesis and localization of precursors of Alzheimer's disease A4 Amyloid protein. *Cell* 57:115–126.

107

NEUROPSYCHOLOGICAL AND POSITRON EMISSION TOMOGRAPHIC COMPARISONS OF ALZHEIMER'S, MULTI-INFARCT, AND PARKINSON'S DISEASE DEMENTIAS

Daphne Alroy Harris,[1] Rowena Gomez,[2] Gerardo Bedolla,[3] Edward Lee,[3] Ingrid Ochoa,[3] Bond Ren,[3] Susan Vasquez,[3] and Joseph Harris[4,5,6]

[1]Memory Clinic
Chaim Sheba Medical Center
Tel-Hashomer, Israel
[2]Department of Psychology
Washington University
St. Louis, Missouri
[3]Neuropsychology Program
University of California
Berkeley, California
[4]Psychology Program
Institute of Technology, Arts and Sciences
Holon, Israel
[5]Neuropsychology Unit for Treatment and Rehabilitation
Tel-Aviv, Israel
[6]Herczeg Institute on Aging
Tel-Aviv University
Ramat Aviv, Israel

INTRODUCTION

In the study of dementia, diagnostic criteria as well as differential diagnosis remain issues to be resolved, hindering both effective research and developing effective treatments. Further, there has been a need to combine brain metabolism studies with specific forms of cognitive analysis. Dementia is characterized by chronic and substantial decline in two or more areas of cognitive function. The cognitive deficits should include a memory impairment and at least one other cognitive disturbance, such as aphasia, agnosia or a disturbance in executive functioning. The impairments must be severe enough to cause oc-

Progress in Alzheimer's and Parkinson's Diseases
edited by Fisher *et al.*, Plenum Press, New York, 1998.

cupational and /or social impairment and must represent a significant decline from previous functioning (American Psychiatric Association, 1994).

Alzheimer's disease (AD) is a human neurodegenerative disorder of insidious onset and progressive course, and is the most common cause of dementia. Neuroanatomically, the most pronounced atrophy in AD is found in the temporoparietal and anterior frontal regions (Cummings & Benson, 1992). Neuropsychological changes—particularly the memory deficits—are most obvious in the early stage of this disease. Attention, verbal functions, visuospatial competence as well as reasoning and abstraction functions have been reported to be impaired (Thompson, 1988; Kolb and Whishaw, 1995).

Studies of brain metabolism in Alzheimer patients most consistently indicate reduced metabolic activity in both anterior and posterior association areas, occurring most severely in posterior temporal, parietal, and occipital regions (Chase at al., 1984; Cutler et al., 1985; Foster, Van Hoesen and Damasio, 1987). In a review of AD and Positron Emission Tomography research literature, Harris (1993) describes metabolic reductions throughout the neocortex in AD groups of equivalent dementia severity. In each level of dementia, frontal, parietal, and temporal association cortices appeared more severely affected than the subcortical, and primary sensorimotor regions.

Multi infarct dementia (MID), the second most common cause of dementia, clinically reflects typical characteristics of cerebral vascular events: rapid and abrupt onset, focal neurological signs and symptoms, stepwise progression with a fluctuating course, the presence of other vascular disease, and hypertension. This dementia has been characterized as being "subcortical" in contrast to the "cortical" dementia of AD (Cummings & Benson, 1983).

There is surprisingly little agreement about the pathological basis of vascular dementia. It appears that dementia can be produced by multiple small but well-placed infarcts, particularly those involving the thalamus or cortical association areas or pathways (e.g. Ladurner et al., 1982). It has been suggested that MID patients with multiple subcortical lacunes present deficits in set shifting, impaired executive functions, and decreased verbal fluency (Wolfe et al., 1990). Compared to AD patients, MID patients are marked with relatively better memory test performance, and reduced output on verbal description and unstructured construction tasks (Mendez and Asha-Mendez, 1991). PET imaging of MID presents a random constellation of metabolic deficits (Benson et al., 1982). MID patients may have focal metabolic deficiencies scattered throughout the cortex, white matter, thalamus, caudate, and cerebellum (Kuhl et al., 1985).

Another degenerative disorder is Parkinson's disease (PD). PD produces a complex motor system disturbance including bradykinesia, cogwheel rigidity, tremor, masked faces, loss of associated movements, and disturbances of gait, posture, and equilibrium. PD is primarily a condition of progressive basal ganglia dysfunction usually resulting from degeneration of the substantia nigra (Agid, et al., 1987; Freedman, 1990; Strange, 1992) and consequently may result in frontal disconnections (Sullivan et al., 1989).

The principle neuropsychological features of Parkinson's disease dementia (PDD) include failure to initiate activities spontaneously, inability to develop a successful approach to problem solving, impaired and slowed memory, impaired visuospatial perception, impaired concept formation, poor word list generation, impaired set shifting, and reduced rate of information processing (Talland and Schwab, 1964; Loranger et al., 1972b; Bowen et al., 1975; Albert, 1978; Wilson et al., 1980; Mayeux et al., 1981b; Matison et al., 1982; Pirozzolo et al., 1982; Levin et al., 1989). PET shows diffused reductions in cerebral glucose metabolism (Kuhl et al., 1984). Some demented Parkinsonian patients exhibit diminished parietal glucose metabolism bilaterally, resembling the characteristic AD cerebral hyopometablic pattern.

Table 1

Score	(N)	Age		Education		Hamilton	
		Mean	SD	Mean	SD	Mean	SD
Alzheimer's disease	(56)	68.4	8.38	12.6	3.49	7.9	8.07
Parkinson's disease dementia	(20)	69.4	5.84	12.4	2.26	10.7	4.38
Multi-infarct dementia	(18)	67.3	7.24	11.5	1.47	7.8	3.17

This study will examine AD, MID, and PDD; their neuropsychological and cerebral glucose metabolism in an attempt to elucidate unique profiles and differences.

METHODS

Subjects

Ninety-four outpatients diagnosed with either Alzheimer's, Multi-infarct or Parkinson's disease dementia participated in this study. The demographics of the subject groups are summarized in Table 1.

Subject groups are age and education level matched and gender-balanced. All subjects were screened for health status, which consisted of a thorough history, physical, neurological, and neuropsychological exams, as well as laboratory diagnostics to rule out other causes of dementia. All testing was performed at least one month after discontinuance of medications.

Neuropsychological Testing

Measures used include the Mini-Mental State Examination, (MMSE: Folstein et al., 1975), Hamilton Depression Scale. (Hamilton, 1967), Wechsler Memory Scale-Revised, Memory Quotient (WMS-R MQ:Wechsler, 1987), Boston Naming Test (BNT: Kaplan et al, 1978),Wechsler Adult Intelligence Scale-Revised, (FSIQ: Wechsler, 1981) Subtests: Digit span, Picture completion, Similarities,Blessed Dementia Rating Scale (BDRS: Blessed et al, 1968) and the Clinical Dementia Rating (CDR: Hughes et al., 1982). These neuropsychological measurements were administered along with a battery of other neuropsychological measures during individual sessions with each subject.

Positron Emission Tomography

Positron emission tomography scans were performed within 30 days of psychological testing using a Siemens 921-08/12, whole body, multi-slice positron emission tomography tomograph with an in-plane resolution of 4 mm FWHM and a Z-axis resolution-9.5 mm separated by 5.75 mm. Five horizontal slices were used, the cantho-meatal line and the two adjacent slices above and below the line. This was an ^{18}F-2-fluoro-deoxy-D-glucose (^{18}FDG) resting-state study. Regions of interest were defined by an automated program dividing the cortex into 16 equal sections. The average of two adjacent regions were then computed to provide eight cortical regions (left and right: frontal, parietal, temporal, occipital) for the present analysis. Eight subcortical regions (left and right: caudate, putamen, thalamus, cerebellum) were manually defined and drawn from visually identifiable anatomical landmarks. These structures were co-identified by the third author and two independent observers. The formula used to determine rCMRglc is described elsewhere (cf. Sokoloff, 1977).

RESULTS

The data analysis consisted of multiple one-way ANOVAs. Subsequent analyses using the Scheffe procedure confirmed significance. For all analyses, results were considered statistically significant with a $p < .01$. No differences were found in analyses of age $F= (2, 91)\ 0.37$; education level $F= (2, 91)\ 0.92$; Hamilton Score: $F= (2, 91)\ 1.41$; MMSE: $F= (2, 91)\ 1.75$; WMS-MQ: $F= (2, 91)\ 1.23$; or BNT: $F= (2, 91)\ 0.36$.

Performance differences were found on WAIS-R Subtests: Digit Span: $F= (2, 91)\ 4.96$, $p < 0.01$; Picture Completion: $F= (2, 91)\ 6.55$, $p < 0.01$; Similarities: $F= (2, 91)\ 8.10$, $p < 0.001$ and the FSIQ: $F= (2, 91)\ 6.77$, $p < 0.01$. Significant differences were also found with the CDR: $F= (2, 91)\ 5.93$, $p < 0.01$ and the BDRS: $F= (2, 91)\ 9.29$, $p < 0.01$. Of particular interest were differences found on composite scores: VIQ - PIQ: $F= (2, 91)\ 6.66$. $p < 0.01$; and FSIQ - MQ: $F= (2, 91)\ 4.85$. $p < 0.01$. Main effect differences were found on all PET regions [except for the parietal region: $F= (2, 91)\ 0.78$]: caudate: $F= (2, 91)\ 6.95$, $p < 0.01$; putamen: $F= (2, 91)\ 16.75$, $p < 0.0001$; thalamus: $F= (2, 91)14.11$, $p < 0.0001$; cerebellum: $F= (2, 91)\ 15.32$, $p < 0.0001$; frontal: $F= (2, 91)\ 8.90$, $p < 0.001$; temporal: $F= (2, 91)\ 14.47$, $p < 0.01$; and occipital $F= (2, 91)\ 10.18$, $p < 0.01$.

Pair-wise comparisons within the ANOVAs yielded some results that may better assist in understanding the differences between the dementia groups. As a group MID subjects performed significantly worse than AD subjects on Picture Completion: $p < 0.005$; Similarities: $p < 0.0006$, FSIQ: $p < 0.002$; CDR: $p < 0.004$; BDRS: $p < 0.0003$; and VIQ - PIQ: $p < 0.001$. PDD subjects scores were significantly different than AD subjects on VIQ - PIQ composite score $p < 0.0001$. AD subjects scores were significantly lower on the FSIQ - MQ composite score than MID $p < 0.0001$ and PDD subjects on $p < 0.0001$.

When we examine comparisons within the ANOVAs for rCMRglc differences we find that in the caudate: MID < AD and PDD; putamen: MID < AD and PDD; thalamus: MID < AD and PDD, cerebellum: MID and PDD < AD; frontal: MID and PDD < AD; temporal: PDD < AD and MID; parietal: AD_MID_PDD; occipital: MID < AD and PDD. All of these pair-wise comparisons are significant to $p < 0.01$.

DISCUSSION

A relatively endless number of studies have been performed, examining and noting the difficult task of differential diagnosis in dementia. The results of this study suggest that the task of distinguishing among three forms of dementia can indeed seem like a guessing game. Even though the three groups' neuropsychological performance and cerebral glucose metabolic patterns appear generally similar, there are nevertheless some unique characteristics to AD, MID and PDD that may make the task of differential diagnosis more reliable.

It is common knowledge that one of the most distinguishing features of AD is memory loss. While all three groups, matched for dementia severity level, appeared to have similar levels of memory impairment as demonstrated by their WMS-R Memory Quotient, when a composite score was used, subtracting memory quotient (overall memory abilities) from FSIQ (overall cognitive abilities), only the AD patients had a significant disparity between these two scores. Further, while all three groups had a significant decline in overall abilities, the AD patients stood alone as a group in having an additional memory decrease on top of the compromised overall cognitive ability. When PET results were examined, aside from finding the typical AD temporoparietal and frontal hypo-metabolic pattern, AD patients had higher rCMRglc rates in the cerebellar and frontal regions than did the PDD and MID groups. The relatively preserved metabolism in the AD group cerebellum is supported by previous research, and in turn supports the use of this brain region in future AD studies as a reference point for relative PET measures. AD patients' performance on the abstract thinking task (WAIS-R Similarities subtest) may be attributed to their higher rCMRglc frontal rates.

The MID group's neuropsychological performance was consistently the lowest among the three patient groups, across most measures and areas of cognitive functions tested. When looking at the PET results, the MID group's rCMRglc rates were significantly lower than those of the other groups, with the exception of the temporal and parietal region decreases, which were similar to those found in AD patients. It has been previously reported that the manifestations of MID may sufficiently resemble those of AD to misdiagnose one with the other (e.g., Scheinberg, 1978; Walton, 1994).

The most notable finding in this study related to the neuropsychological functioning of PDD subjects is the difference between their verbal and performance abilities. This is evident when we examined the composite score of WAIS-R PIQ subtracted from VIQ. While all groups exhibited a significant decline in Verbal as well as Performance IQ, the PDD group were unique in that they exhibited a further significant decline in their Performance IQ, compared to the AD and MID groups. This finding may be attributed to Parkinsonian bradykinesia. In analyses of rCMRglc, the PDD group had a significantly lower metabolic rate in the temporal region, compared to the MID and AD group rates.

A final consideration in the evaluation and diagnosis of dementias pertains to the perceptions of clinicians and caregivers of the dementia patient. Although the three groups were matched for age, education level, dementia severity, and overall did not present with obviously contrasting neuropsychological and metabolic profiles, both clinicians and caregivers rated the groups at significantly different levels of dementia severity. Both clinicians and caregivers consistently rated MID patients as suffering from significantly more cognitive deficits than PDD patients. They also rated PDD patients as being more cognitively impaired than AD patients. It is possible that this incongruity stems from over-rating the MID patient personality changes and the physical demands of the PDD patient, thus overshadowing the more diagnostically relevant cognitive symptoms.

ACKNOWLEDGMENT

Research was supported in part by the Ford Foundation, American Psychological Association, NIA Grant #1RO3AG12780-01, NIA Grant #P50AG0867, NIH Grant #2R01NS24896 and the Howard Hughes Center for Academic Excellence, University of California, Irvine.

REFERENCES

Agid, Y., Ruberg, M., DuBois, B., and Pillon, B., 1987, Anatomoclinical and biochemical concepts of subcortical dementia, In: *Cognitive Neurochemistry*, Stahl, S.M., Iversen, S.D. and Goodman E.C., eds., Oxford: Oxford University Press.

Albert, M.L., 1978, Subcortical dementia, In: *Alzheimer's Disease: Senile Dementia and Related Disorders*, Katzman, R., Terry, R.D., and Bick, K.L., eds., New York: Raven Press, pp. 173–196.

American Psychiatric Association, 1994, *Diagnostic and Statistical Manual of Mental Disorders*, 4th ed., Washington, D.C.: American Psychiatric Association.

Benson, D.F., Cummings, J.L., and Tsai, S.Y., 1982, Angular gyrus syndrome simulating Alzheimer Disease, *Arch Neurol.* 39:616–620.

Bowen, F.P., Kamienny, R.S., Burns, M.M., and Yahr, M.D., 1975, Parkinsonism: Effects of levodopa treatment on concept formation, *Neurology* 25:701–704.

Cummings, J.L., and Benson, D.F., 1983, *Dementia: A Clinical Approach*, Boston: Butterworth's.

Cummings, J.L., and Benson, D.F., 1992, *Dementia: A Clinical Approach*, Boston: Butterworth's.

Cutler, N.R., Haxby, J.V., Duara, R., et al., 1985, Clinical history, brain metabolism, and neuropsychological function in Alzheimer's disease, *An. Neurol.* 18:298–309.

Folstein, M.F., Folstein, S.E., and McHugh, P.R., 1975, "Mini-Mental State" a practical method for grading the cognitive state of patients for the clinician, *J. Psychiatric Res.* 12:189–198.

Foster, N.L., Chases, T.N., Mansi, L., Brooks, R., Fedio, P., Patronas, N.J., and DiChiro, G., 1984, Cortical abnormalities in Alzheimer's disease, *An. Neurol.* 16:649–654.

Freedman, M., 1990, Parkinson's disease. In: *Subcortical Dementia*, Cummings, J.L. ed., New York: Oxford University Press.

Hamilton, M., 1967, Development of a rating scale for primary depressive illness. *Br. J. Soc Clin. Psychology* 6:278–296.

Harris, J., 1993, *Assessing Dementia in Alzheimer's Disease*, Berkeley, CA: University of California Press.

Kaplan, E., Goodglass, H., and Weintraub, S., 1978, *The Boston Naming Test*, Boston: E. Kaplan & H. Goodglass.

Kolb, B. and Whishaw, I.Q., 1995, *Fundamentals of Human Neuropsychology*, 4th ed., Boston: W.H. Freeman and Company.

Kuhl, D.E., Metter, E.J., and Riege, W.H., 1985, Patterns of cerebral glucose utilization in depression, multiple infarct dementia, and Alzheimer's disease, In: *Brain Imaging and Brain Function*, Sokologg, L., ed., New York: Raven Press.

Ladurner, G., Lliff, L.D., and Lechner, H., 1982, Clinical factors associated with dementia in ischemic stroke, *J. Neurol. Neurosurg. Psychiatry* 45:97–101.

Levin, B.E., Llabre, M.M., and Weiner, W.J., 1989, Cognitive impairments associated with early Parkinson's disease, *Neurology* 39:557–561.

Loranger, A.W., Goodell, H., McDowell, F.H., Lee, J.H., and Sweet, R.D., 1972, Intellectual impairment in Parkinson's syndrome, *Brain* 95:405–412.

Matison, R., Mayeux, R., Rosen, J., and Fahn, S., 1982, "Tip-of-the-tongue" phenomenon in Parkinson's disease, *Neurology* 32:567–570.

Mayeux, R., Stern, Y., Rosen, J., and Leventhal, J., 1981, Depression, intellectual impairment, and Parkinson disease, *Neurology* 31:645–650.

Mendez, M.F. and Ashla-Mendez, M., 1991, Differences between multi-infarct dementia and Alzheimer's disease on unstructured neuropsychological tasks, *J. Clin. Exp. Neuropsychol.* 13:923–932.

Pirozzolo, F.J., Hansch, E.C., Mortimer, J.A., Webster, D.D., and Kuskowski, M.A., 1982, Dementia in Parkinson's disease: a neuropsychological analysis, *Brain and Cogn.* 1:71–83.

Scheinberg, P., 1978, Multi-infarct dementia. In : *Alzhiemer's Disease: Senile Dementia and Related Disorders*, Katzman, R., Terry, R.D. and Bick K.L.,eds, New York: Raven Press.

Strange, P.G., 1992, *Brain Biochemistry and Brain Disorders*, Oxford: Oxford University Press.

Sullivan, E.V., Sagar, H.J., Gabrieli, J.D.E., et al., 1989, Different cognitive profiles on standard behavioral tests in Parkinson's disease and Àlzheimer's disease, *J. Clin. Exp, Neuropsychol.* 11:799–820.

Talland, G.A., and Schwab, R.S., 1964, Performance with multiple sets in Parkinson's disease, *Neuropsychologia* 2:45–53.

Thompson, R.F., 1988, Brain substrates of learning and memory, In: *Clinical Neuropsychology and Brain Function: Research, Measurement, and Practice*, Boll T. and. Bryant B.K eds.,Washington, D.C.: American Psychological Association.

Van Hoesen, G.W., and Damasio, A.R., 1987, Neural correlates of cognitive impairment in Alzheimer's disease, In: *Handbook of Physiology, Vol. 5: The Nervous System*, Plum F., ed., New York: Oxford University Press.

Walton, J.N., 1994, *Brains, Diseases of the Nervous System*, 10th ed., Oxford: Oxfrod Univeristy Press.

Wechsler, D., 1981, *Wechsler Adult Intelligence Scale-Revised*, New York: Psychological Corporation.

Wechsler, D., 1987, *Wechsler Memory Scale-Revised*, New York: Psychological Corporation.

Wilson, R.S., Kaszniak, A.W., Klawans, H.L., Jr., and Garron, D.C., 1980, High speed memory scanning in Parkinsonism, *Cortex* 16:67–72.

Wolfe, N., Linn, R., Babikian, V.L., Knoefel, J.E., and Albert, M.L., 1990, Frontal systems impairment following multiple lacunar infarcts, *Arch. Neurol.* 47:129–132.

α1-ANTICHYMOTRYPSIN AND APOLIPOPROTEIN E POLYMORPHISM IN ALZHEIMER'S DISEASE

Akira Ueki,[1] Mieko Otsuka,[1] Yoshio Namba,[2] Takeshi Ishii,[2] and Kazuhiko Ikeda[2]

[1]Department of Neurology, Jichi Medical School
Omiya Medical Center, Amanuma 1-847
Omiya City 330, Japan
[2]Department of Ultrastructure
Tokyo Institute of Psychiatry
Kamikitazawa, Tokyo 156, Japan

INTRODUCTION

The apolipoprotein E-ε4 allele (apoE-ε4) is a major risk factor for late onset, familial and sporadic Alzheimer's disease (AD). The frequency of ε4 in patients with AD is about three times higher than yhat in controls, and approximately 60% of AD patients have at least one copy of the ε4 allele (Strittmatter et al., 1993; Poirier et al., 1993; Saunders et al., 1993a; Saunders et al., 1993b; Rebeck et al., 1993; Ueki et al., 1993; Dai et al., 1994). ApoE-ε4 reduces the onset age of dementia in a gene dosage manner (Corder et al., 1993). However, ε4 is not a sufficient factor for developing AD, and some individuals carrying ε4 remain cognitively intact past age 90 (Lehtovirta et al., 1995; Asada et al., 1996). Furthermore, the prevalence of AD in various ethnic groups does not correlate simply with variations of ε4 frequencies in general populations (Hendrie et al., 1995). These facts suggest additional genetic or environmental factors must be involved in the manifestation of the disease. Family history of dementia (Duara et al., 1996), VLDL-receptor gene polymorphism (Okuizumi et al., 1995; Mui et al., 1996), low density lipoprotein-like receptor (LRP) gene polymorphism (Mui et al., 1996), C/G polymorphism in the apoE intron 1 enhancer element (Lendon et al., 1997), α1-antichymotrypsin (ACT) signal peptide gene polymorphism (Kamboh et al., 1995), and past history of head trauma (Mayeux et al., 1995) are the candidates factors.

Among these factors, ACT polymorphism is of interest. ACT has been shown to deposit in senile plaques of AD brains (Abraham et al., 1988) and it appears to promote fibril formation of β-amyloid peptideformatio (Ma et al., 1994; Eriksson et al., 1995). Furthermore, plasma concentration of ACT is elevated in AD patients (Matsubara et al., 1990; Hinds et al., 1994). ACT The gene of ACT is located on the chromosome 14 q31-q32.3 (Rabin et al., 1986). Recently, Kamboh et al. (Kamboh et al., 1995) have shown that the apoE-ε4 dosage effect associated with AD risk is significantly modulated by ACT signal peptide gene polymorphism. The ACT signal peptide gene has biallelic polymorphism, namely ACT/A and ACT/T, with Ala to Thr substitution at codon 15. They found that among three ACT genotypes (ACT/AA, ACT/AT, and ACT/TT), the frequency of ACT/AA was significantly higher in AD patients compared with controls and concluded that AA acts as an additional risk factor of ε4 for developing AD.

To test their results, we examined ACT genotypes in Japanese patients with AD and age-matched controls. We also measured plasma levels of ACT and compared them with the apoE and ACT genotypes.

METHODS

Patients and Controls

The 66 sporadic AD patients (29 men and 37 women) meeting the standard clinical criteria for AD (DSM-IV) (American Psychiatric Association, 1994) were recruited in this study. The average onset age of dementia was 72.9 (±5.9) years. Onset age of dementia was defined as when the first cognitive changes were noticed by family members or by a review of the medical records. Controls were 129 persons (69 men and 60 women) with no memory complaints and with a negative family history of AD and other mental disorders. The averge age of controls was 74.4 (±7.8) years. Both patients and controls were largely unrelated Japanese who resided in the same geographical area. Informed consent was obtained from all participants before obtaining blood samples.

Genotyping ApoE and ACT

DNA was extracted from peripheral lymphocytes according to standard prosedures. The ACT polymorphism was determined by the PCR-based methods described by Kamboh et al (Kamboh et al., 1995). The 124-bp fragment encompassing the signal peptide polymorphism of was amplified during 40 cycles of denaturation (1 min at 94°C), annealing (1.75 min at 55°C), and extension (2 min at 72°C). Amplification was preceded by a prerun of 3 min at 95°C and followed by a final extension for 5 min at 72°C. The amplification product was digested with MvaI (Toyobo Ltd, Japan) and separated on a 10% polyacrylamide gel. The apoE was genotyped acording to the conventional method described by Wenham et al (Wenham et al., 1991).

Determination of Serum ACT Level

The serum concentration of ACT was measured using the immunoturbidity method.

Statistics

Allelic and genotypic frequencies of ACT and apoE in different subgroups were compared using χ^2 test. Correlations between ACT genotypic frequencies and apoE-ε4 gene dose was tested using Cochran-Armitage trend test. Onset age of dementia and serum ACT levels between subgroups were compared using Student's *t*-test.

Table 1. ApoE genotypes and allele frequencies

	AD patients (n=66)		Controls (n=129)	
	n	(%)	n	(%)
apoE genotypes				
E4/4	6	(9.1)	0	(0.0)
E4/3	32	(48.5)	26	(20.2)
E4/2	2	(3.0)	0	(0.0)
E3/3	26	(39.4)	98	(76.0)
E3/2	0	(0.0)	4	(3.0)
E2/2	0	(0.0)	1	(0.8)
apoE alleles				
ε4*	0.349		0.101	
ε3	0.636		0.876	
ε2	0.015		0.023	

*apoE-ε4 allele frequency was significantly increased in AD patients (χ^2 = 35.6, p<0.0001).

RESULTS

ApoE Genotypes and Allele Frequencies

As expected, the frequency of ε4 in AD patients was significantly higher than in controls (p < 0.0001) (Table 1). Odds of developing AD for those with ε4 homozygotes was 10.3 (95% CI 1.17–90.00, p= 0.010), and the odds for those with ε4 heterozygotes was 4.5 (95% CI 2.30–8.87 , p = 0.0001). AD aptients and controls were divided into subgroups according to ε4 status. Forty AD patients were ε4 carriers and 26 were not. Twenty-six controls carried ε4 and the remaining 91 controls did not.

ACT Genotypes and Allele Frequencies Differed between AD Patients and Controls

Distribution of ACT genotypes did not differ significantly when the entire AD patient group and entire control group were compared (p = 0.148), though there was a tendency for AA genotype to be slightly higher (18.0% vs. 10.3%) and the TT genotype inversely lower (32.8% vs. 44.0%) in AD patients compared to controls (Table 2). The frequency of ACT/A or ACT/T did not differ significantlly between AD pateints and controls (p = 0.079).

Table 2. ACT genotypes and frequencies in AD patients and controls

	AD patients (n=66)		Controls (n=129)	
	n	(%)	n	(%)
ACT genotypes				
AA	11	(16.7)	16	(12.4)
AT	32	(48.5)	51	(39.5)
TT	23	(34.8)	62	(48.1)
ACT alleles				
A	0.409		0.322	
T	0.591		0.678	

Table 3. ACT genotypes and frequencies among AD patients and controls with or without apoE-ε4 allele

	ε4 carriers				Non-ε4 carriers			
	AD patients (n=40)		Controls (n=26)		AD patients (n=26)		Controls (n=103)	
	n	(%)	n	(%)	n	(%)	n	(%)
ACT gneotypes								
AA	7	(17.5)	2	(7.7)	4	(15.4)	14	(13.6)
AT	22	(55.0)	9	(34.6)	10	(38.4)	42	(40.8)
TT*	11	(27.5)	15	(57.7)	12	(46.2)	47	(45.6)
ACT alleles								
A**	0.450		0.250		0.346		0.340	
T**	0.550		0.750		0.654		0.660	

*The TT genotype differed significantly between ε4 carriers of AD patients and controls (P=0.014).
**The frequencies of allele A and allele T differed significantly between ε4 carriers of AD patients and controls (P=0.020).

The ACT/TT Genotype Was Overexpressed in Controls and Underexpressed in AD Patients Carrying ε4

When AD patients and controls were divided into subgroups of ε4 carriers and non-ε4 carriers, the differences between AD patients and controls became clearer (Table 3). In ε4 carriers, the TT genotype was significantly lower in AD patients compared to controls (26.3% vs. 56.0%; p = 0.017). The odds ratio for developing AD by individuals with the TT genotype compared to those with the AA or AT genotype was 0.281 (95% CI,0.096–0.818; p = 0.017), suggesting a protective effect of the TT genotype for ε4 carriers. The AA genotype was higher in AD patients, but the difference was not significant (18.4% vs. 8.0%; p = 0.248). The frequency of ACT/A allele was significantly higher (0.461 vs. 0.260), and that of ACT/T allele was significantly lower (0.539 vs. 0.740) in AD patients compared to controls (p = 0.023). In contrast, the distribution of ACT genotypes and allele frequencies were almost identical in non-ε4 carriers in both the AD patient and control groups (p = 0.403).

ACT Genotypes among Three AD Groups with Zero, One, and Two Copies of ε4 Alleles

The frequencies of AA were almost identical in three AD subgroups with zero, one, and two copies of ε4 (Table 4). In contrast, there was a trend that the frequency of ACT/TT became lower with increasing number of ε4 . The frequency of TT genotype was highest in AD patients with no copy of ε4 (43.5%) followed by the patients with one copy of ε4 (27.3%), and those with two copies of ε4 (20.0%). However, this trend did not reach statistical significance because of the small number of AD patients with ε4 homozygotes.

The Effects of ACT Genotypes on Onset Age of AD

Mean onset age of dementia for patients with the AA, AT, and TT genotypes were 68.7±7.8, 73.5±5.0, and 72.1±5.0 years respectively. All groups had a wide range of 20 years from 60 to 80 years (Figure 1). Six out of seven patients with the AA genotype exhibited dementia before the age of 72 and seemed to become demented earlier. However,

Table 4. Distribution of ACT genotypes based upon the presence of one copy and two copies of apoE-ε4

| | AD patients (n=66) | | | | | | Controls (n=129) | | | | | |
| | 0 | | 1 | | 2 | | 0 | | 1 | | 2 | |
Number of ε4	n	(%)	n	(%)	n	(%)	n	(%)	n	(%)	n	(%)
Genotypes												
AA	4	(15.4)	6	(17.7)	1	(16.7)	14	(13.6)	2	(7.7)	0	(0.0)
AT	10	(38.4)	18	(52.9)	4	(66.6)	42	(40.8)	9	(34.6)	0	(0.0)
TT§	12	(46.2)	10	(29.4)*	1	(16.7)	47	(45.6)	15	(57.7)*	0	(0.0)

§Significant difference between AD patients and controls have one copy of ε4 and the TT genotype. *(p=0.028).

the difference between AD patients with the AA genotype and with the AT genotype was only marginally sign ificant (Student's *t* test, p = 0.066). Differences between patients with the AA or TT genotype, or between patients with the AT or TT genotype were not significant.

Plasma Concentrations of ACT

Plasma levels of ACT in total AD patients were significantly higher than that in total controls (p=0.0004), though there were many overlaps between patients and controls (Fig. 2a). ACT levels did not differ in ε4 carriers and non-ε4 carriers of AD and controls (Fig. 2b). Plasma ACT concentrations did not also correlate with any of ACT genotypes (figure not shown).

DISCUSSION

There are ethnic variations of ACT/A and ACT/T allele frequencies. In our Japanese study, the frequency of the ACT/A allele was 0.322 which is much lower than those in caucasians ranging from 0.439 to 0.510 (Kamboh et al., 1995; Nacmias et al., 1996; Müller et al., 1996; Haines et al., 1996). Inversely, the frequency of the ACT/T allele in Japanese is higher than those of caucasians.

In contrast to the original report by Kamboh et al. (Kamboh et al., 1995), we failed to find any hazardous effects of the ACT/AA genotype, independently or combined with ε4, for the developement of AD. In the original report by Kamboh et al. (Kamboh et al., 1995), they concluded that the AA genotype carried a risk for AD based on the findings that in the presence of the AA genotype, an individual's risk increased to almost twofold with one ε4 copy and to threefold with two ε4 copies. However, in the present result, the

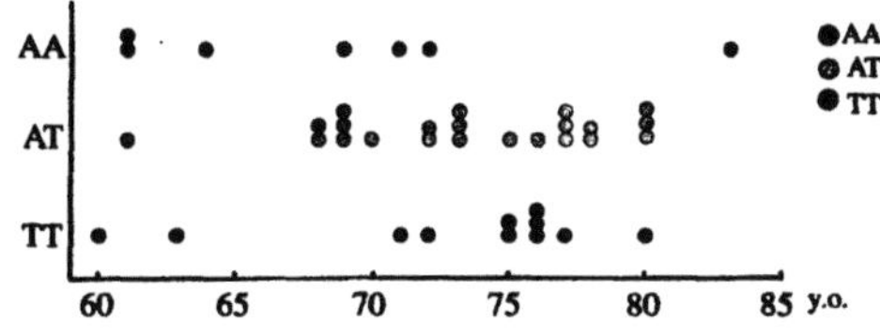

Figure 1. Onset age of dementia in AD patients with different ACT genotypes.

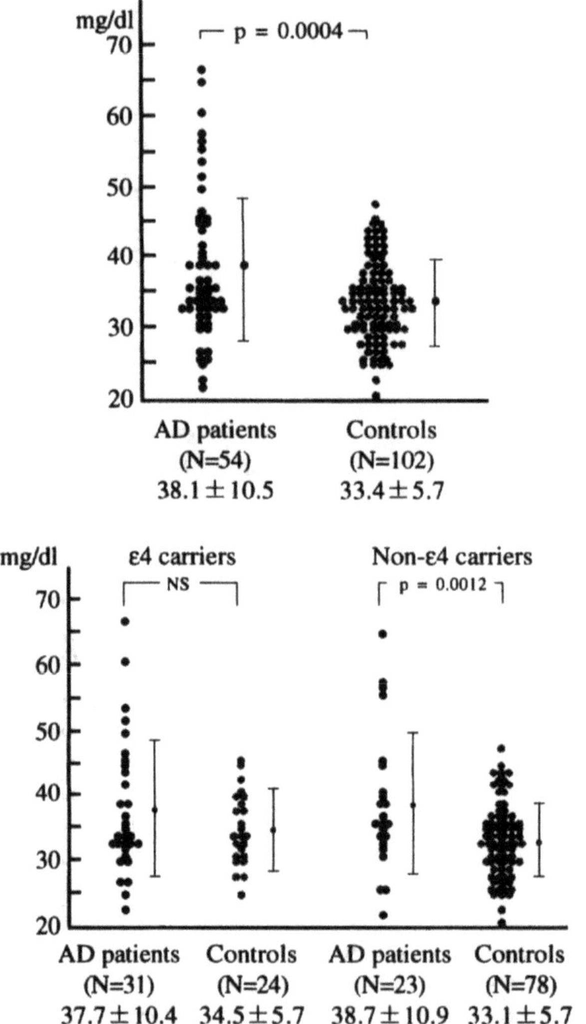

Figure 2. a) Plasma ACT levels in AD patients and controls. b) Plasma ACT levels in ε4-carriers (left) and non ε4-carriers (right) of AD patients and controls.

frequency of AA genotype did not increase significantly among any subgroups of AD, and no correlation with ε4 gene dose was found. Several studies (Nacmias et al., 1996; Müller et al., 1996; Haines et al., 1996) following Kamboh et al. also do not support the hazardous effects of the ACT/AA genotype, independently or combined with ε4, for the developement of AD. Possibly the synergistic effects of the AA genotype to ε4 apply only to certain ethnic groups.

Instead, we found an apparent protection against AD by the TT genotype for ε4 carrying individuals. This protective effect of the TT genotype was also mentioned by Kamboh et al. (Kamboh et al., 1995) in their findings that the TT genotype had the same risk with either one or two copies of the ε4 allele. However, this possible protective effect of the TT genotype is not confirmed also in other previous studies (Haines et al., 1996). We could not find any good explanation for this difference. Since our study might be possible as a chance positive result, studies in a more large size and in various ethnic background are necessary before we can reach substantial conclusions that the TT genotype has the protective effect for the developement of AD.

Plasma concentration of ACT is increased significantly as previously reported (Matsubara et al., 1990; Hinds et al., 1994) However, there are many overlaps between AD patients and controls, limiting the clinical use of ACT levels as a diagnostic marker of AD. Present results fail to explain the wide range of ACT concentrations by the difference of apoE or ACT polymorphism.

In conclusion, the clinical usefulness of ACT, both genotypic polymorphism and plasma concentrations, as a biological marker for AD, is limited despite its close association with the pathological process of β-amyloid deposition. Though the apoE-ε4 is a major risk factor of AD, search for other factors either independent or associated with ε4 is necessary since AD is a disease of complex etiology.

ACKNOWLEDGMENTS

We wish to thank to Dr. Origasa H, Department of Biostatistics, Toyama Medical-Pharmacological University, for his advice on statistical analysis. This research was supported in part by a Grant-in Aid for Scientific Research from the Ministry of Education, Science, and Culture of Japan.

REFERENCES

Abraham, C.R., Selkoe, D.J., and Potter, H., 1988, Immunohistochemical identification of the serine protease inhibitor alpha 1-antichymotrypsin in the brain amyloid deposits of Alzheimer's disease, *Cell* 52:487–501.

American Psychiatric Association, 1994, "Diagnostic and Statistical Manual of Mental Disorders" 3rd ed. revised (DSM-IV), American Psychiatric Association, Washington D.C.

Asada, T., Yamagata, Z., Kinoshita, T., Kinoshita, A., Kariya, T., Asaka, A., and Kakuma, T., 1996, Prevalence of dementia and distribution of apoE alleles in Japanese centenarians: an almost-complete survey in Yamanashi Prefecture, Japan, *J. Am. Geriatr. Soc.* 44:151–155.

Corder, E.H., Saunders, A.M., Strittmatter, W.J., Schmechel, D.E., Gaskell, P.C., Small, G.W., Roses, A.D, Haines, J.L., and Pericak-Vance, M.A., 1993, Gene dose of apolipoprotein E type 4 allele and the risk of Alzheimer's disease in late onset families, *Science* 261:921–923.

Dai, X.Y., Nanko, S., Hattori, M., Fukada, R., Nagata, K., Isse, K.,Ueki, A., and Kazamatsuri, H., 1994, Association of apolipoprotein ε4 with sporadic Alzheimer's disease is more pronounced in early onset type, *Neurosci Lett.* 175:74–76.

Duara, R., Barker, W.W., Lopez-Alberola, R., Loewenstein, D.A., Grau, L.B., Gilchrist, D., Sevush, S., and St. George-Hyslop, P.H., 1996, Alzheimer's disease: interaction of apolipoprotein E genotype, family history of dementia, gender, education, ethnicity, and age of onset, *Neurology* 46:1575–1579.

Eriksson, S., Janciauskiene, S., and Lannfelt, L., 1995, α1-Antichymotrypsin regulates Alzheimer β-amyloid peptide fibril formation, *Proc. Natl. Acad. Sci. U.S.A.* 92:2313–2317.

Haines, J.L., Pritchard, M.L., Saunders, A.M., Schildkraut, J.M., Grwodon, J.H., Gaskell, P.C., Farrer, L.A., Auerbach, S.A., Gusella, J. F., Locke, P.A., Rosi, B. L., Yamaoka, L., Small, G.W., Conneally, P.M., Rose, A. D., and Pericak-Vance, M.A., 1996, No genetic effect of α1-antichymotrypsin in Alzheimer Disease. *Genomics* 33:53–56.

Hendrie, H.C., Hall, K.S., Hui, S., Unverzagt, F.W., Yu, C.E., Lahiri, D.K., Sahota, A., Farlow, M., Musick, B., Class, C.A., Brashear, A., Burdine, V.E., Osuntokun, B.O., Ogunniyi, A.O., Guereje, O., Baiyewu, O., and Schellenberg, G.D., 1995, Apolipoprotein E genotype and Alzheimer's disease in a community styudy of elderly African Americans, *Ann Neurol.* 37:118–120.

Hinds, T.R., Kukull, W.A., Van Belle, G., Schellenberg, G.D., Villacres, E.C., and Larson, E. B., 1994, Relatioship between serum α1-antichymotrypsin and Alzheimer's disease, *Neurobiol. Aging* 15:21–27.

Kamboh, M.I., Sanghera, D.K., Ferrell, R.E., and DeKosky, S.T., 1995, APOE*4 associated Alzheimer's disease risk is modified by α1-antichymotrypsin polymorphism, *Nature Genet.* 10:486–488.

Lehtovirta, M., Helisalmi, S., Mannermaa, A., Soininen, H., Koivisto, K., Ryynan, M., and Riekkinen Sr, P., 1995, Apolipoprotein E polymorphism and Alzheimer's disease in Eastern Finland, *Neurosci. Lett.* 185:13–15.

Lendon, C.L., Talbot, C.J., Craddock, N.K., Han, S.W., Wragg, M., Morris, J. C., and Goate, A.M., 1997, Genetic association studies, between dementia of the Alzheimer's type and three receptors for apolipoprotein E in a Caucasian population, *Neurosci. Lett.* 222:187–190.

Ma, J., Yee, A., Brewer, H.B.Jr., Das, S., and Potter, H., 1994, Amyloid-associated proteins α1-antichymotrypsin and apolipoprotein E promote assembly of Alzheimer b-protein into filaments, *Nature* 372:92–94.

Matsubara, E., Hirai, S., Amari, M., Shoji, M., Yamaguchi, H., Okamoto, K., Ishiguro, K., Harigaya, Y., and Wakabayashi, K., 1990, α1-antichymotrypsin as a possible biochemical marker for Alzheimer-type dementia, *Ann. Neurol.* 28:561–567.

Mayeux, R., Ottman, R., Maestre, G., Nagai, C., Tang, M.-X., Ginsberg, H., Chun, M., Tycko, B., and Shelanski, M., 1995, Synergistic effects of traumatic head injury and apolipoprotein-ε4 in patients with Alzheimer's disease, *Neurology* 45:555–557.

Mui, S., Briggs, M., Chung, H., Wallance, R.B., Gomez-Isla, T., Rebeck, G.W., and Hyman, B.T., 1996, A newly identified polymorphism in the apolipoprotein E enhancer gene region is associated with Alzheimer's disease and strongly with the ε4 allele, *Neurology* 47:196–201.

Müller, U., Bödeker, R.-H., Gerundt, I., and Kurz, A., 1996, Lack of association between α1-antichymotrypsin polymorphism, Alzheimer's disease, and allele ε4 of apolipoprotein E. *Neurology* 47:1575–1577.

Nacmias, B., Tedde, A., Latorraca, S., Piacentini, S., Bracco, L., Amaducci, L., Guarnieri, B.M., Petruzzi, C., ortenzi, L., and S. Sorbi, 1996, Apolipoprotein E and α1-antichymotrypsin polymorphism in Alzheimer's disease. *Ann. Neurol.* 40:678–680.

Okuizumi, K., Onodera, O., Namba, Y., Ikeda, K., Yamamoto, T., Seki, K., Ueki, A., Nanko, S., Tanaka, H., Takahashi, H., Oyanagi, K., Mizusawa, H., Kanazawa, I., and Tsuji, S., 1995, Genetic association of very low density lipoprotein (VLDL) receptor gene with sporadic Alzheimer's disease. *Nature Genet.* 11:207–209.

Poirier, J., Davignon, J., Bouthillier, D., Kogan, S., Bertrand, P., and Gauthier, S., 1993, Apolipoprotein E polymorphism and Alzheimer's disease, *Lancet* 342:697–699.

Rabin, M., Watson, M., Kidd, V., Woo, S.L.C., Berg, W.R., and Ruddle, F.H., 1986, Regional location of α1-antichymotrypsin and α1-antitrypsin genes on human chromosome 14, *Somat. Cell Mol. Genetics* 12:209–214.

Rebeck, G.W., Reite, J.S., Strickland, D.K., and Hyman, B.T., 1993, Apolipoprotein E in sporadic Alzheimer's disease: allelic variation and receptor interactions, *Neuron* 11:575–580.

Saunders, A.M., Strittmatter, W.J., Schmechel, D., St. George-Hyslop, P.H., Pericak-Vance, M.A., Joo, S.H., Rosi, B.L., Gusella, J.F.,Crapper-MacLachlan, D.R., Alberts, M.J., Hulette, C., Crain, B., Goldgraber, D., and Roses, A.D., 1993a, Association of apolipoprotein E allele ε4 with late-onset familial and sporadic Alzheimer's disease, *Neurology* 43:1467–1472.

Saunders, A.M., Schmader, K., Breitner, J.C.S., Benson, M.D., Brown, W.T., Goldfarb, L., Goldgaber, D., Manwaring, M.G., Szymanski, M.H., McCown, N., Dole, K., Schmechel, D.E., Strittmatter, W.J., Pericak-Vance, M.A., and Roses, A.D., 1993b, Apolipoprotein E ε4 allele distributions in late-onset Alzheimer's disease and in other amyloid-forming diseases, *Lancet* 342:710–711.

Strittmatter, W.J., Saunders, A.M., Schmechel, D., Pericak-Vance, M., Enghild, J., Salvesen, G.S., and Roses, A.D., 1993, Apolipoprotein E:high-avidity binding to β-amyloid and increased frequency of type 4 allele in late-onset familial Alzheimer disease, *Proc. Natl. Acad.Sci. U.S.A.* 90:1977–1981.

Ueki, A., Kawano, M., Namba, Y., Kawakami, M., and Ikeda, K., 1993, A high frequency of apolipoprotein E4 isoprotein in Japanese patients with late-onset nonfamilial Alzheimer's disease, *Neurosci. Lett.* 163:166–168.

Wenham, P.R., Price, W.H., and Blundell, G., 1991, Apolipoprotein E genotyping by one-stage PCR, Lancet 337:1158–1159.

109

INFLUENCE OF THE APOE GENOPTYPE ON SERUM ApoE LEVELS IN ALZHEIMER'S DISEASE PATIENTS

L. Corzo, L. Fernández-Novoa, R. Zas, K. Beyer, J. I. Lao, X. A. Alvarez, and R. Cacabelos

EuroEspes Biomedical Research Center
Santa Marta de Babío 15166 Bergondo
La Coruña, Spain

INTRODUCTION

Alzheimer's disease (AD) is a devastating neurologic disorder that affects more than 20 million individuals of all races and ethnic backgrounds. The incidence of AD in the general population is about 1%, with a prevalence of 5–15% in people older than 65 years of age. AD is an etiologically and genetically heterogeneous disorder. So far, 4 chromosomes have been implicated in the etiopathogenesis of AD. Several missense mutations in the amyloid precursor protein gene (APP) on chromosome 21 have been found in about 3% of familial early-onset AD. This familial pattern is consistent with an autosomal dominant inheritance (St. George-Hyslop et al., 1987). In 1992, two different groups discovered genetic linkage to a major familial AD gene defect on chromosome 14 in the region14q24.3 (St.George-Hyslop et al., 1992; Schellenberg et al., 1992). In that region, several candidate genes have been postulated, including c-fos and presenilin 1 (Van Broeckhoven et al., 1992; Mullan et al., 1992; Sherrington et al., 1995). An intronic polimorphism located at 3′ to exon 8 of the presenilin 1 (PS1) gene was described (Wragg et al., 1996). The most common allele has an adenine at nucleotide position 16 (allele 1) in the intron, while the variant allele has a cytosine at the same position (allele 2). Neither the 1/2 genotype nor the 2/2 genotype were associated with increased risk for AD, whereas the 1/1 genotype was associated with an approximately 2-fold risk.The STM2 gene maps on chromosome 1 and was also found to have two point mutations segregating in early-onset AD families (Levy-Lahad et al., 1995). In the nineties several groups showed evidence for an AD susceptibility gene on chromosome 19 (Pericak-Vance et al., 1991; Farrer et al., 1992; Stritmatter et al., 1993). The responsible gene was the APOE gene located at 19q13.2, which encodes apolipoprotein E (ApoE), a 34 kD glycosilated protein associated with plasma lipoproteins (Weisgraber, 1994; Hallmann et al., 1991). Three common APOE variants are encoded by three APOE alleles: ε2, ε3 and ε4. Several groups have reported an association between late-onset AD or sporadic AD and the APOε4 allele (Saunders et al., 1993; Beyer et al., 1996). The risk of suffering AD-type dementia increases with the number of associated genetic factors identified in an individual. Consistent with the APOE ε4-late onset AD association, the presence of ApoE4 in the characteristic AD brain lesions, such as senile plaques, and neurofibrillary tangles has been demonstrated (Namba et al., 1991). It is known that *in vitro* Apo ε4 binds more avidly to β-amyloid peptide (βA) than ApoE3 in order to form stable ApoE-βA complexes that would result in βA deposition (Strittmatter et al., 1993; Sanan et al., 1994). In contrast, another major protein implicated in AD, tau protein, binds strongly *in vitro* to ApoE3 but not to ApoE4. One hypothesis proposes that Apo E3-tau interactions serve as a protective mechanism against tau phosphorilation (Strittmatter et al., 1994). It is well known the function of ApoE in peripheral lipid metabolism and in the homeostasis of cholesterol. The role of ApoE in the brain is not well understood although it seems to be related to the redistribution of cholesterol within neuronal tissues undergoing repair or remodeling (Boyles et al., 1989). Poitier et al (1991) demonstrated that ApoE is important in the transport and redistribution of cholesterol during membrane remodelling in the central nervous system of the rat. Serum ApoE levels were measured by different groups in healthy and disease states. ApoE concentrations vary as a function of different biological factors as age, decreasing ApoE levels after the age of 60 (Siest et al., 1995). Several other groups also studied the levels of ApoE in AD patients. Lehtimäki et al. in 1995 found that ApoE concentrations in cerebrospinal fluid were lower in AD patients than in healthy subjects, but they did not find differences among ApoE phenotypes. Serum ApoE levels in AD patients could also be different from healthy subjects due to the implication of ApoE in the etiopathogenesis of AD. In this study, we measured serum ApoE, total-cholesterol, triglycerides and lipoproteins-cholesterol levels in AD patients and control subjects in order to know the influence of the APOE genotype on the serum levels of these biochemical parameters, and to assess if AD patients have a different lipid and lipoprotein profile than controls.

MATERIAL AND METHODS

Subjects

This study was carried out on a group of thirty-nine subjects, 10 healthy age-matched controls (APOE genotype 3/3) with no personal record or known family history of AD and twenty-nine patients who met DSM-IV and NINCDS-ADRDA criteria for the diagnosis of probable AD (Diagnostic and Statistical Manual of Mental Disorders, 1994; McKhann et al., 1984). AD patients were classified according to APOE genotype (3/3, 3/4 and 4/4). Patients and controls were of the same age and body weight and none was taking drugs known to affect lipid metabolism.

Genetic Analysis

Genomic DNA was extracted from peripheral blood by a conventional method without phenol-chloroform. The APOE and PS1 genotypes were carried out under blind conditions by procedures reported previously (Beyer et al., 1997; Wragg et al., 1996).

Measurement of ApoE

Levels of apolipoprotein E were measured in serum using a commercial enzyme-linked immunosorbent monoclonal/polyclonal sandwich assay Apo-Tek Apo E™ (PerImmune, Inc.) for the quantitative determination of apolipoprotein E in human serum or plasma.

Measurement of Total-Cholesterol, Triglycerides, HDL-C, LDL-C

Total-cholesterol in serum was measured spectrophotometrically by a conventional cholesterol oxidase/peroxidase (CHOD-PAP) enzymatic method. Triglycerides were measured by the enzymatic Trinder method. The precipitation method with phosphotungstic acid and $MgCl_2$ was used for measuring HDL-C levels. LDL-C was calculated by the Friedewald formula.

Statistical Methods

Data were statistically analyzed by using the non parametric Mann-Whitney U test. Results are expressed as mean ± S.D. in tables and figures.

RESULTS

Results of the present study show that AD patients have significant lower serum ApoE levels than age-matched healthy individuals (AD=0.271±0.071 g/l; C=0.188±0.053 g/l; p<0.05).

When we compare the concentration of ApoE observed in AD patients and controls with an APOE genotype 3/3, no significant differences were found (Table 1, Figure 1). In the group of AD patients, ApoE levels were significantly lower in those with an APOE 4/4 than in APOE 3/3 subjects (Table 1, Figure 1). AD patients with APOE genotype 3/4 also have significantly lower ApoE levels than control subjects. Circulating levels of total-cholesterol, triglycerides, HDL-C and LDL-C levels were similar in AD patients and controls, and did not show variations as a function of APOE genotype in AD (Table 2).

The percentage of AD patients that present (positive) or not (negative) the 1/1 genotype of the presenilin 1 is presented in Table 2. PS1 genotype 1/1 was most frequent in

Table 1. Serum levels of ApoE, total-cholesterol (T-Cho), triglycerides (TG), HDL-cholesterol (HDL-C), and LDL-cholesterol (LDL-C) in Alzheimer's disease (AD) patients and control subjects according to APOE genotype

Subjects	ApoE (g/l)	T-Cho (mmol/l)	TG (mmol/l)	HDL-C (mmol/l)	LDL-C (mmol/l)
Control					
APOE genotype 3/3	0.271 ± 0.071	5.579 ± 0.722	1.426 ± 0.464	1.070 ± 0.181	3.857 ± 0.613
AD					
APOE genotype 3/3	0.215 ± 0.057**	5.297 ± 0.939	1.207 ± 0.323	1.095 ± 0.162	3.645 ± 0.950
APOE genotype 3/4	0.188 ± 0.033*	5.952 ± 0.810	1.376 ± 0.984	1.204 ± 0.273	4.113 ± 0.799
APOE genotype 4/4	0.158 ± 0.056*	5.989 ± 0.576	1.517 ± 0.505	1.053 ± 0.243	4.239 ± 0.651

Results are expressed as mean ± S.D. * p<0.01 vs Control ** p<0.05 vs APOE genotype 4/4

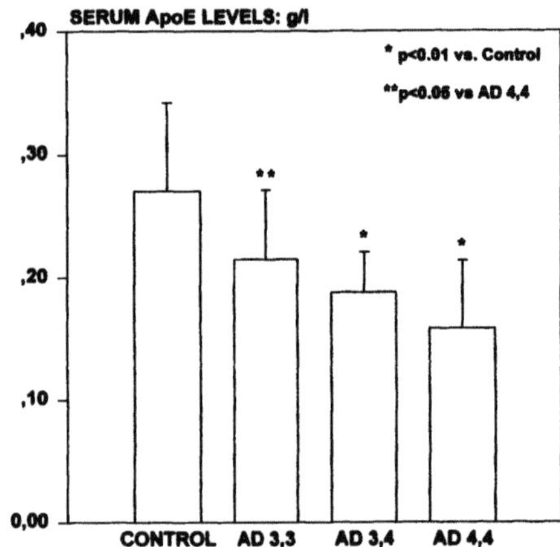

Figure 1. Serum ApoE levels in Alzheimer's disease (AD 3/3, 3/4 and 4/4) and control subjects (APOE genotype 3/3) according to the APOE genotype. Results are expressed as mean ± S.D.

APOE 3/3 patients than in those with an APOE genotype 4/4. Serum ApoE concentrations were not significantly different (p=0.0706) in patients bearing (positive; n=10, ApoE=0.210 ± 0.047g/l) or not the PS1 genotype 1/1 (negative; n=17, ApoE=0.176 ± 0.051 g/l).

DISCUSSION

The present results clearly show an association between low serum ApoE levels and AD. In agreement with our data, other authors have found decreased ApoE levels in the cerebrospinal fluid of AD patients (Lehtimäki et al., 1995). These data might indicate that this biochemical parameter is intimately related to AD development. In fact, it has been demonstrated that ApoE is present in AD brain lesions, as senile plaques and neurofibrillary tangles (Strittmatter et al., 1993; Sanan et al., 1994), and some studies have also found the presence of its receptor, low density lipoprotein receptor-related protein (LRP), in AD amyloid plaques (Rebeck et al., 1993). We postulate that the observed decrease in serum ApoE levels in AD patients could be due to the deposition of ApoE in amyloid plaques, through the interaction of ApoE with LRP or directly by its binding to β-amyloid peptide. When we studied serum ApoE concentrations in AD patients with different APOE genotype, we observed a clear reduction in ApoE values as a function of the ε4 allele dose, these data clearly showed that there is an association between low serum ApoE levels and the presence of the ε4 allele. Our results might be explained taking into account that ApoE ε4 has more affinity for β-amyloid peptide than ApoE3 (Sanan et al., 1994). In this regard, patients with an

Table 2. Percentage of the presence (positive) or absence (negative) of the 1/1 genotype of presenilin 1 in Alzheimer's disease patients with different APOE genotypes

Presenilin 1 genotype 1/1	APOE 3/3 (n=9)	APOE 3/4 (n=10)	APOE 4/4 (n=8)	Total (n=27)
Positive (%)	556	400	125	37
Negative (%)	444	600	875	63

APOE genotype 4/4 would have lower serum ApoE levels owing to its greater deposition to form amyloid plaques. In this study we have also measured the levels of total-cholesterol, tryglicerides, HDL-C and LDL-C in AD patients and controls, and in patients as a function of the APOE genotype, and no significant variations in the levels of these parameters were observed. Some groups reported a different lipid pattern in AD patients with respect to controls (Giubilei et al., 1990), mainly in HDL-cholesterol (Muckle et al., 1985), and significantly higher plasma cholesterol levels in AD patients homozygotic for ApoE4 (Czech et al., 1994). However, other authors, like us, did not find any significant difference in lipid profile between AD and healthy subjects (Wieringa et al., 1997). According to our results, it seems unlikely that the role of ApoE in the etiopathogenesis of AD may be mediated by changes in serum lipid levels. These data support the hypothesis of the involvement of ApoE in AD etiology through a protein-association mechanism.

Another risk factor described for AD is the 1/1 genotype of the PS1 gene, which is associated with a 2-fold increased AD prevalence. We compared serum ApoE levels as a function of the presence or absence of the 1/1 genotype, and no significant differences among genotypes were observed. The percentage of AD patients that present or not the 1/1 genotype of the PS1 gene was also calculated for the different APOE genotypes. Apparently, there is not an association between the APOE 4/4 and the PS1 genotype 1/1. However, the concurrence of these two genetic variants in the same individual may have an important implication on the disease progression.

Finally, we conclude that low serum ApoE levels are observed in AD patients and may have pathogenic implications in this disease. If the present results are confirmed in a more extensive sample, measurement of serum ApoE levels might be of utility for the diagnosis and follow-up of AD patients.

ACKNOWLEDGMENTS

We gratefully acknowledge the assistance of the Nursery Department and we also thank Drs. Miguel-Hidalgo and E. Maneiro for their valuable comments. This study was supported by the EuroEspes Foundation.

REFERENCES

Beyer K., Lao J.I., Alvarez X.A., Cacabelos R., 1997, A general method for DNA polymorphism identification in genetic assessment and molecular diagnosis. *Meth. Find. Exp. Clin. Pharmacol. 19: 87–91.*

Beyer K., Lao J.I, Alvarez X.A., Cacabelos R., 1996, Different implications of APO ε4 in Alzheimer's disease and vascular dementia in the Spanish population. *Alzheimer's Res.* 2: 215–220.

Boyles J.K., Zoellner C.D., Anderson L.J., Kosik L.M., Pitas R.E., Weisgraber K.H., 1989, A role for apolipoprotein E, apolipoprotein A-I and low density lipoprotein receptor in cholesterol transport during regeneration and remyelination of the rat sciatic nerve. *J. Clin. Invest.* 83:1015–1031.

Czech H., Förstl F., Hentschel F., Mönning U., Besthorn C., Geiger-Kabish C., Sattel H., Masters C., Beyreuther K., 1994, Apolipoprotein E-4 gene dose in clinically diagnosed Alzheimer's disease: prevalence, plasma cholesterol levels and cerebrovascular change. *Psychiatry Clin. Neurosci.* 243:291–292.

Diagnostic and Statistical Manual of Mental Disorders (4th ed). Washington, DC: *Am. Psychiatric Assoc.* 1994:133–55.

Farrer L.A., Stice L., 1992, Susceptibility genes for familial Alzheimer's disease on chromosome 19 and 21: A reality check. *Genet. Epidemiol.* 9:123–127.

Giubilei F., d'Antona R., Antonini R., Lenzi GL., Ricci G., Fieschi C., 1990, Serum lipoprotein pattern variations in dementia and ischemic stroke. *Acta Neurol. Scand.* 81:84–6.

Hallmann D.M., Boerwinkle E., Saha N., Sandholzer C., Menzel H.J., Czazar A., Utermann G., 1991, The apolipoprotein E polymorphism: a comparison of alelle frequencies and effects in nine populations. *Am. J. Hum. Genet.* 45:793–802.

Lehtimäki T., Pirttilä T., Mehta P.D., Wisniewski H.M., Frey H., Nikkari T., 1995, Apolipoprotein E (apoE) polymorphism and its influence on ApoE concentrations in the cerebrospinal fluid in Finnish patients with Alzheimer's disease. *Hum. Genet.* 95:39–42.

Levy-Lahad E., Wasco W., Pookaj P., Romano D.M.,Oshima J., Pettingell W.H., Yu Ch., Jondro P.D., Schmidt D., Wang K., Crowley A.C., Fu Y.-H., Guenette S.Y., Galas D., Nemens E., Wijsman E.M., Bird T.D., Schellenberg G.D., Tanzi R.E., 1995, Candidate gene for the chromosome 1 familial Alzheimer's disease locus. *Science* 269:973–977.

McKhann G., Drachman D., Folstein M., Katzman R., Price D., Stadlan E.M., 1984, Clinical diagnosis of Alzheimer's disease: Report of NINCDS-ADRDA Work Group. *Neurology* 34:939–944.

Muckle TJ., Roy JR., 1985, High-density lipoprotein cholesterol in differential diagnosis of senile dementia. *Lancet* i:1191–3.

Mullan M., Houlden H., Windelspecht M., Fidani L., Lombardi C., Diaz P., Rossor M., Crook, R., Hardy J., Duff K., Crawford F., 1992, A locus for familial early onset Alzheimer's disease on the long arm of chromosome 14, proximal to the alpha$_1$-antichymotrypsin gene. *Nat. Genet.* 2:340–342.

Namba Y., Tomonoga M., Kawasaki H., Otomo E., Ikeda K., 1991, Apolipoprotein E immunoreactivity in cerebral amyloid deposits and neurofibrillary tangles in Alzheimer's disease and kuru plaqueamyloid in Creutzfeldt-Jakob disease. *Brain Res.* 541:163–166.

Pericak-Vance M.A., Bebout J.L., Gaskell Jr. P.C., Yamaoka L.H., Hung W.Y., Alberts M.J., Walker A.P., Bartlett R.J., Haynes C.A., Welsn C.A., Earl N.L., Heyman C.A., Clark C.M., Roses A.D., 1991, Linkage studies in familial Alzheimer disease: evidence for chromosome 19 linkage. *Am J Hum. Gen.* 48:1034–1050.

Poitier J., Hess M., May P.C., Finch C.E., 1991, Astrocytic apolipoprotein E mRNA and GFAP mRNA in hippocampus after entorhinal cortex lesioning. *Mol. Brain Res.* 11:97–106.

Rebeck GW., Reiter JS., Strickland DK., Hyman BT., 1993, Apolipoprotein E in sporadic Alzheimer's disease: allelic variation and receptor interactions. *Neuron* 11:575–580.

Sanan D.A. Weisgraber K.H., Russell S.J., Mahley R.W., Huang D., Saunders D.A., Schmechel D., Wisniewski T., Frangione B., Roses B., Strittmatter W.J., 1994, Apolipoprotein E associates with beta amyloid peptide of Alzheimer's disease to form novel monofibrils. Isoform apoE4 associates more efficiently than apo E3. *J. Clin. Invest.* 94:860–869.

Saunders A.M., Strittmatter W.J., Schmechel D., St George-Hyslop P.H., Pericak-Vance M.A., Joo S.H., Rosi B.L., Gusella J.F., Crapper-MacLachlan D.R., Alberts M.J., Hulette C., Crain B., Goldgaber D., Roses A.D., 1993, Association of apolipoprotein E allele ε4 with late-onset familial or sporadic Alzheimer's disease. *Neurology* 43:1467–1472.

Schellenberg G.D., Bird T.D., Wijsman E.M., Orr H.T., Anderson L., Nemens E., White J.A., Bonnycastle L., Weber J.L., Alonso M.E., Potter H., Heston L.L., Martin G.M., 1992, Genetic linkage evidence for a familial Alzheimer's disease locus on chromosome 14. *Science* 258:668–671.

Sherrington R., Rogaev E.I., Liang Y., Rogaeva E.A., Levesque G., Ikeda M., Chi H., Lin C., Li G., Holman K., Tsuda T., Mar L., Foncin J.-F., Bruni A.C., Montesi M.P., Sorbi S., Rainero I., Pinessi L., Nee L., Chumakov I., Polien D., Brookes A., Sanseau P., Polinsky R.J., Wasco W., Da Silva H.A.R., Haines J.L., Pericak-Vance M.A., Tanzi R.E., Roses A.D., Fraser P.E., Rommens J.M., St George-Hyslop P.H., 1995, Cloning of a gene bearing missense mutations in early-onset familial Alzheimer's disease. *Nature* 375:754–760.

Siest G., Pillot T., Régis-Bailly A., Leininger-Muller B., Steinmetz J., Galteau M.-M., Visvikis S., 1995, Apolipoprotein E: an important gene and protein to follow in laboratory medicine. *Clin. Chem.* 41:1068–1086.

St. George-Hyslop P.H., Tanzi R.E., Polinski R.J., Haines J.L., Nee L., Watkins P.C., Meyers R.H., Feldman R.G., Pollen D., Drachman D., Growdonn J., Bruni A., Foncin J.F., Salmon G., Fromheld P., Amaducci L., Sorgi S., Placentini S., Steward G.D., Hobbs W., Conneally P.M., Gusella J.F., 1987, The genetic defect causing familial Alzheimer's disease maps on chromosome 21. *Science* 235:885–890.

St. George-Hyslop P.H., Haines J.L., Rogaev E., Mortilla M., Vaula G., Pericak-Vance M., Foncin J.F., Montesi M., Bruni A., Sorbi S., Rainero I., Pinessi L., Pollen D., Polinsky R., Nee L., Kennedy J., Macciardi F., Rogaeva E., Liang Y., Alexandrova N., Lukiw W., Schlumpf K., Tanzi R., Tsuda T., Farrer L., Cantu J.M., Duara R., Amaducci L., Bergamini W., Gusella J., Roses A., Crapper McLachlan D., 1992, Genetic evidence for a novel familial Alzheimer's disease locus on chromosome 14. *Nat. Genet.* 2:330–334.

Stritmatter W.J., Saunders A.M., Schmechel D., Pericak-Vance M.A., Enghild J., Salvesen G.S., Roses A.D., 1993, Apolipoprotein E high avidity binding to β-amyloid and increased frecuency of type 4 allele in late-onset familial Alzheimer's disease. *Proc. Natl. Acad. Sci.*USA 90:1977–1981.

Strittmatter W.J., Weisgraber K.H., Huang D.Y., Dong L.M., Salveser G.S., Pericak-Vance M., Schmechel D., Saunders A.M., Goldgaber D., Roses A.D., 1993, Binding of human apolipoprotein E to synthetic amyloid ß-peptide: isoform specific effects and implications for late-onset Alzheimer disease. *Proc. Natl. Acad. Sci. USA* 90:8098–8102.

Strittmatter W.J., Weisgraber K.H., Goedert M., Saunders A.M., Huang D., Corder E.H., Dong L.M., Jakes R., Alberts M.J., Gilbert J.R., Han S.-H., Hulette Ch., Einstein G., Schmechel D.E., Pericak-Vance M., Roses A.D., 1994, Hypothesis: microtubule instability and paired helical filament formation in the Alzheimer disease brain are related to apolipoprotein E genotype. *Exp. Neurol.* 125:163–171.

Van Broeckhoven C., Backhovens H., Crusts M., Winter G., de Bruyland M., Cras P., Martin J.J., 1992, Mapping of a gene predisposing to early-onset Alzheimer's disease to chromosome 14q24.3. Nat. Genet. 2:335–339.

Weisgraber K.H., 1994, Apolipoprotein E: Structure-function relationship. Adv. Prot. Chem. 45:249–320.

Wieringa G.E., Burlinson S., Rafferty JA., Gowland E., Burns A., 1997, Apolipoprotein E genotypes and serum lipid levels in Alzheimer's disease and multi-infarct dementia. Int. J. Geriat. Psychiatry 12: 359–362.

Wragg M., Hutton M., Talbot C., 1996, Alzheimer's Disease Collaborative Group. Genetic association betweeen intronic polymorphism in presenilin-1 gene and late-onset Alzheimer's disease. Lancet 347:509–512.

110

DEVELOPMENT OF A SPECIFIC DIAGNOSTIC TEST FOR MEASUREMENT OF β-AMYLOID (1-42) [βA₄(1-42)] IN CSF

H. Vanderstichele,[1] K. Blennow,[2] N. D'Heuvaert,[1] M.-A. Buyse,[1] A. Wallin,[2] N. Andreasen,[3] P. Seubert,[4] A. Van de Voorde,[1] and E. Vanmechelen[1]

[1]Innogenetics NV
Industriepark Zwijnaarde 7
B-9052, Ghent, Belgium
[2]Department of Clinical Neuroscience
University of Göteborg
Sahlgrenska University Hospital
S-431 80 Mölndal, Sweden
[3]Department of Rehabilitation
Piteå RiverValley Hospital
Piteå, Sweden
[4]Athena Neurosciences
800 Gateway Boulevard
South San Francisco, California 94080

INTRODUCTION

Alzheimer's disease (AD) is considered as the most important of all neurodegenerative diseases, due to its frequent occurrence and devastating consequences. AD appears to be a very heterogeneous group of disorders sharing clinical characteristics and pathological hallmarks. Neuropathologically, the brains of AD patients are characterized by the presence of intracellular accumulations of neurofibrillary tangles (primarily composed of a hyperphosphorylated form of the microtubule associated protein tau) in the hippocampus and temporal lobe of the cerebral cortex, the extracellular deposition of amyloid fibrils in the senile plaques, and the degeneration of neurons and their synapses. Neither plaques or tangles are restricted to AD (Selkoe, 1991).

Since AD is a disease which is clinically restricted to the brain, it is reasonable to examine whether the most pronounced changes will occur also in the cerebrospinal fluid (CSF). Since some causes of dementia are treatable or even potentially reversible, prompt recogni-

Progress in Alzheimer's and Parkinson's Diseases
edited by Fisher *et al.*, Plenum Press, New York, 1998.

tion of AD is of major importance. For both routine clinical evaluation and basic research studies, there is a pressing need for biochemical diagnostic markers of AD, especially to help in the early diagnosis of the disease. Today, several acetylcholinesterase inhibitors have been, or are in the processes of being registered for the treatment of AD patients; while drugs with potential effects on the disease process, such as neuroprotective compounds affecting aggregation of β-amyloid (Aβ), are being tested or under development. Therapeutic compounds have the greatest potential of being effective when they can be used in the early phase of the disease, before the degenerative process has gone too far. However, in the early phase, the symptoms are often vague and diffuse, and the clinical diagnosis is especially difficult to make. In addition, biochemical markers may also be useful to monitor the effect of therapeutic compounds, and to select patients that will respond to these compounds.

Evidence is now accumulating that both tau and Aβ, the main components of tangles and plaques respectively, are useful tools for AD diagnosis. The presence of elevated levels of tau in CSF from AD patients was confirmed in 14 studies worldwide, involving over a thousand subjects (Vanmechelen et al., 1997).

While total amyloid levels in the CSF were not different between control, Parkinson's or AD patients, analysis of Aβ (1-42) was found to be an important tool in the confirmation of the diagnosis (Motter et al., 1995). Aβ (1-42) has been identified in senile plaques from AD patients; Aβ(1-42) is more amyloidogenic than Aβ (1–40); Aβ (1-42) deposition is one of earliest pathological signs in Down's syndrome patients (Selkoe, 1996); increased Aβ (1-42) levels were found in plasma from early-onset familial AD genes (PS1, PS2, βAPP717) (Scheuner et al. 1996), in skin fibroblasts cultured from PS1, PS2, or APP 670/671 mutation carriers (Citron et al., 1994; Johnston et al., 1994; Scheuner et al. 1996), in human 293 embryonic kidney cells, double transfected with APP695 carrying the Swedish APP mutation and PS1, PS2 mutations or in PS1 transgenic mice (Citron et al., 1997). Surprisingly, Aβ (1-42) concentrations in the CSF were found to be lower in AD patients, compared to age-matched controls, presumably due to increased deposition into plaques or otherwise failing to be cleared into the CSF (Motter et al., 1995, Tamaoko et al. 1997).

The present study describes the optimization and evaluation of a sandwich-type ELISA for specific measurement of β-Amyloid (1-42) in CSF using two epitope-specific mouse monoclonal antibodies.

MATERIALS AND METHODS

Monoclonals

21F12 and 3D6 monoclonal antibodies, were generated against the carboxy- or amino-terminus of β-amyloid (1-42), respectively. The characteristics of the monoclonals are described in Citron et al. (1997). The affinity of the antibodies for binding different amyloid peptides was verified by ELISA and BIAcore.

Peptides

Synthetic peptides were obtained from Sigma or Bachem.

ELISA

β-amyloid (1-42) was measured by a sandwich-type ELISA using two epitope-specific monoclonal antibodies, 21F12 and 3D6. 21F12 was used as coating antibody; biotinylated 3D6 as capturing antibody. The amount of bound antibody was quantified by HRP-streptavidin (Jackson Laboratories). Total tau was measured with the tau antigen test, using AT120 as coating antibody and biotinylated HT7-BT2 as capturing antibody (IN-NOTEST hTau antigen, Innogenetics, Ghent, Belgium).

Patients and Controls

The diagnosis of "probable AD" was made by way of exclusion, according to NINCDS-ADRDA criteria (McKhann et al., 1984). The control group consisted of individuals without history, symptoms or signs of psychiatric or neurological diseases, malignant diseases, or systemic disorders. CSF samples were obtained by lumbar puncture in the L3/L4 or L4/L5 interspace. CSF samples with more than 500 erythrocytes per μl were excluded. Several tube types (glass, polypropylene, polystyrene) were evaluated for storage of the CSF or β-amyloid peptides. Samples were stored at -80°C until assay.

RESULTS AND DISCUSSION

Characteristics of the ELISA

The intra-assay variability was less than 3%; the inter-assay variability was below 10%. In its present configuration, the sensitivity of the test for detection of Aβ (1-42) in CSF was 38 pg/ml. The 21F12/3D6 ELISA was highly specific for amyloid peptides starting at amino acid 1 and ending at the carboxy-terminus at amino acid 42 or 43. Comparison of (1-42) and (1-43) synthetic peptides revealed that the highest sensitivity was obtained with the (1-42) peptide, as confirmed by ELISA (Figure 1) and BIAcore.

During the optimization phase of the test, we observed that overall levels of Aβ(1-42) were influenced by the composition or material of the test tubes. When solutions of β-amyloid (1-42) were aliquoted in glass vials, and stored one day at 4°C, more than 25% of the reactivity was lost. The impact of the test tube on the measurable amount of Aβ (1-42) was even more pronounced for CSF samples. Seven frozen samples of CSF were thawed and aliquoted again in several vial types. Approximately 7.2%, 30.2% or 27.4% of the Aβ (1-42) was lost after storage for three hrs at 4°C in polypropylene, polystyrene or glass vials, respectively (Figure 2). No differences were measured for tau with respect to the tube

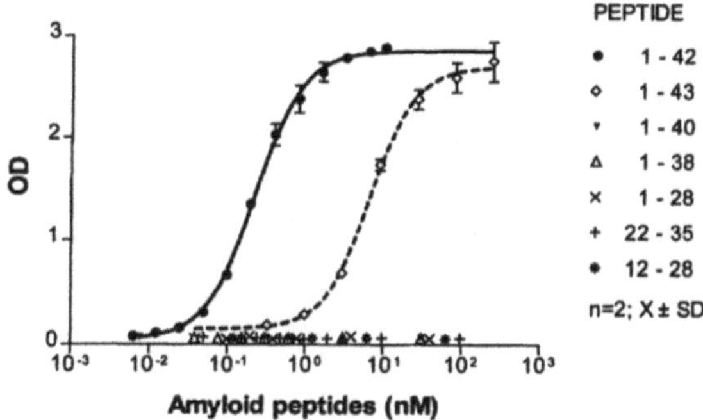

Figure 1. 21F12/3D6 ELISA: peptide specificity.

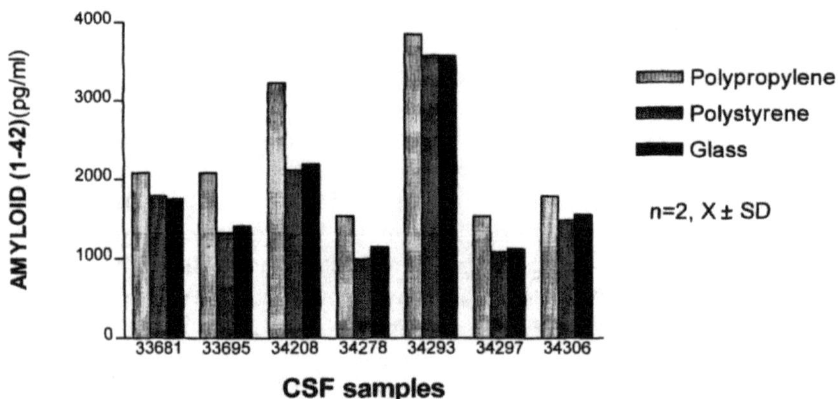

type. These reductions are probably caused by hydrophobic interactions with the test tubes, indicating that methodological differences might, at least partially, account for different absolute values of the amyloid peptides found between different research groups (Motter et al., 1995; Tamaoka et al. 1997, present study).

Clinical Validation of the Test

Paired CSF and serum samples were obtained from 26 patients with variable blood-brain barrier dysfunctions (CSF/serum albumin ratios ranging from 0.0037 to 0.0899) to study the extent of serum participation in the observed changes in the CSF. The highest concentration of Aβ (1-42) was found in the CSF. No correlation was found between blood-brain-barrier defects and tau or amyloid concentrations, suggesting that both tau and Aβ (1-42) are produced within the central nervous system. While concentration gradients were found along the spinal cord for some proteins such as albumins, IgG, and transthyretin (Blennow et al., 1993), no major concentration gradients were found in the lumbar CSF from demented patients for Aβ (1-42) or tau, indicating that the volume of CSF collected is not critical.

In another series of experiments, CSF from 15 control patients, 4 FLD and 81 probable AD patients were collected (C: control; AD: Alzheimer's Disease; FLD: Frontal Lobe Dementia). Individual values are shown in Figure 3B, mean values of patient groups in Table 1.

Table 1. CSF determination of tau and β-amyloid (1-42) in control and AD patients

	Control	AD
N° of samples	15	81
Age (years)	70.9 ± 6.6	73.8 ± 6.7
CSF		
Total Tau (pg/ml)	274 ± 133.0	487 ± 230.6 **
Aβ (1-42) (pg/ml)	2145 ± 407.7	1600 ± 366.2 **

Mean ± SD; ** p (0.01

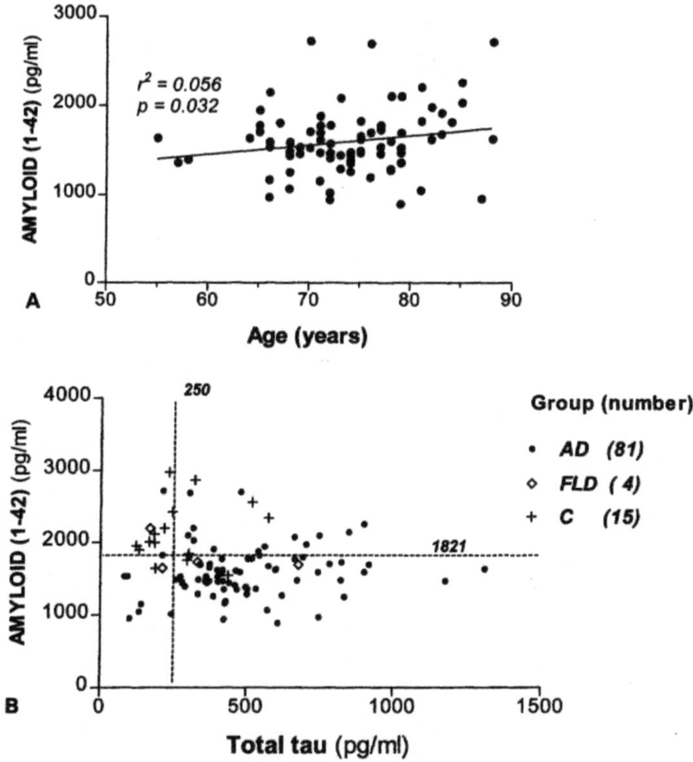

Figure 3. A) Influence of age on amyloid(1-42) levels in CSF from AD patients. B) Detection of tau and amyloid (1-42) in CSF.

Within the AD group, a fully factorial multiple ANOVA, with CSF-tau or Aβ (1-42) as dependent variables, gender as factor, and age, duration, and Mini Mental State Examination score as co-variates, showed that neither of the parameters covaried with CSF-tau or Aβ (1-42) (p ⟨ 0.01) (Figure 3A).

These results confirmed the significantly higher levels of tau in CSF from AD patients. In addition, CSF Aβ (1-42) was significantly decreased in the AD group as compared with the control group (Figure 3B). A cut-off level of 1821 pg/ml for Aβ (1-42) or 250 pg/ml for tau gave the best separation of AD patients and controls. The specificity of the test, defined as [(true negative)/(true negative+false positive)] x 100%, as calculated in the control group was 67%, 80% and 93% for CSF-tau, CSF Aβ (1-42) or CSF-tau+Aβ (1-42), respectively. The sensitivity of the test, based on AD samples, and defined as [(true positive)/(true positive + false negative)] x 100% was 90%, 81% or 74% for CSF-tau, CSF Aβ (1-42) or CSF-tau+Aβ (1-42), respectively.

CONCLUSION

The Research Version of the β-amyloid (1-42) test is able to reproducibly measure the amount of Aβ (1-42/43) in patient CSF for use as a diagnostic marker for AD. CSF amyloid (1-42) is intrathecally produced, and thus reflects changes in the central nervous system. Potential confounding factors, such as blood-brain barrier function, or concentration gradients do not affect the results. However, care must be taken to use non-absorbing test tubes. The specificity of the determination of amyloid (1-42) levels in the CSF from AD patients versus other dementia disorders must be further studied.

REFERENCES

Blennow, K., Fredman, P., Wallin, A., Gottfries, C.-G., Längström, L., Svennerholm, L., 1993, Protein analyses in cerebrospinal fluid: I. Influence of concentration gradients for proteins on cerebrospinal fluid/serum albumin ratio. *Eur. Neurol.* 33:126.

Citron, M., Vigo-Pelfrey, C., Teplow, D. B., Miller, C., Schenk, D., Johnston, J., Winblad, B., Venizelos, N., Lannfelt, L., Selkoe, D. J., 1994, Excessive production of amyloid β-protein by peripheral cells of symptomatic and presymptomatic patients carrying the Swedish familial Alzheimer disease mutation. *Proc. Natl. Acad. Sci.* 91:11993.

Citron, M., Westaway, D., Xia, W., Carlson, G., Diehl, T., Levesque,G., Johnson-Wood, K., Lee, M., Seubert, P., Davis, A., Kholodenko, D., Motter, R., Sherrington, R., Perry, B., Yao, H., Strome, R., Lieberburg, I., Rommens, J., Kim ,S., Schenk, D., Fraser, P., St George Hyslop, P., Selkoe, D.J., 1997, Mutant presenilins of Alzheimer's Disease increase production of 42-residue amyloid β-protein in both transfected cells and transgenic mice. *Nature Med.* 3:67.

Johnston, J. A., Cowburn, R. F., Norgren, S., Wiehager, B., Venizelos, N., Winblad, B., Vigo-Pelfrey, C., Schenk, D., Lannfelt, L., O'Neill, C., 1994, Increased β-amyloid release and levels of amyloid precursor protein (APP) in fibroblast cell lines from family members with the Swedish Alzheimer's disease APP670/671 mutation. *FEBS Lett.* 354:274.

McKhann, G., Drachman, D., Folstein, M., Katzman, R., Price, D., Stadlan, E.M., 1984, Clinical diagnosis of Alzheimer's disease: Report of the NINCDS-ADRDA work group under the auspices of department of health and human services task force on Alzheimer's disease. *Neurology* 34:939.

Motter, R., Vigo-Pelfrey, C., Kholodenko, D., Barbour, R., Johnson-Wood, K., Galasko, D., Chang, L., Miller, B., Clark, C., Green, R., Olson, D., Southwick, P., Wolfert, R., Munroe, B., Lieberburg, I., Seubert, P., Schenk, D.,1995, Reduction of β-amyloid peptide $_{42}$ in the cerebrospinal fluid of patients with Alzheimer's Disease. *Ann. Neurol.* 38:643.

Scheuner, D., Eckman, C., Jensen, M., Song, X., Citron, M., Suzuki, N., Bird, T.D., Hardy, J., Hutton, M., Kukull, W., Larson, E., Levy-Lahad, E., Viitanen, M., Peskind, E., Poorkaj, P., Schellenberg, G., Tanzi, R., Wasco, W., Lannfelt, L., Selkoe, D., Younkin, S., 1996, Secreted amyloid β-protein similar to that in the senile plaques of Alzheimer's disease is increased *in vivo* by the presenilin 1 and 2 and APP mutations linked to familial Alzheimer's disease. *Nature Med.* 2:864.

Selkoe, D.J., 1996, Amyloid β-protein and the genetics of Alzheimer's disease. *J. Biol. Chem.* 217:18295.

Tamaoka, A., Sawamura, N., Fukushima, T., Shoji, S., Matsubara, E., Shoji, M., Hirai, S., Furiya, Y., Endoh, R., Mori, H., 1997, Amyloid β protein 42(43) in cerebrospinal fluid of patients with Alzheimer's disease. *J. Neurol. Sci.* 148:41.

Vanmechelen, E., Blennow, K., Davidsson, P., Cras, P., Van De Voorde, A., 1997, Combination of tau/phospho-tau with other biochemical markers for Alzheimer cerebrospinal fluid diagnosis and tau in cerebrospinal fluid as marker for neurodegeneration, In: *Alzheimer's disease: Biology, Diagnosis and Therapeutics,* Iqbal, K., Winblad, B., Nishimura, T., Takeda, M., Wisniewski, H.M., eds., John Wiley and Sons, Chichester:197.

111

INDICES OF OXIDATIVE STRESS IN THE PERIPHERAL BLOOD OF *DE NOVO* PATIENTS WITH PARKINSON'S DISEASE

Tihomir V. Ilic,[1] Marina Jovanovic,[2] Aco Jovicic,[1] and Mirjana Tomovic[1]

[1]Department of Neurology
[2]Institute for Medical Research
Military Medical Academy
Belgrade, Yugoslavia

INTRODUCTION

Parkinson's disease (PD) represents a clearly defined neurodegenerative disorder with unique clinical features. In spite of enormous efforts directed toward understanding the etiology and pathogenesis of PD, the cause of this disorder is still unknown. Among numerous causative agents, various hypotheses presume that the illness may be due to hereditary factors (Markopoulou et al., 1995; Ward et al., 1983), intrauterine events (Mattock et al., 1988), viral infection (Poskanzer et al., 1963), or environmental factors such as exogenous toxins, including 1-methyl-4-phenyl-1,2,3,6-tetrahydropyridine (MPTP) (Snyder et al., 1986; Jovanovic et al., 1994). Intensive research over the last decade has generated several lines of evidence from both human and experimental studies, which support the possibility that free radical mechanisms may initiate cell damage (Jovicic et al., 1995).

There is an increasing amount of findings related to oxidative stress as a possible pathogenic mechanism of the neuronal degeneration of neurons in the *pars compacta* of the *substantia nigra* (SN) in patients with PD (Olanow, 1992). The actual physiopathological concept is based on a selective increase in levels of malondialdehyde (a stable intermediate formed during lipid peroxidation) (Dexter et al., 1989), decreased levels of reduced and total glutathione (Riederer et al., 1989; Perry et al., 1986), decreased glutathione peroxidase (GPx) activity (Kish et al., 1985), and an increase in superoxide dismutase (SOD) activity in the parkinsonian SN (Saggu et al., 1989). Also mitochondrial abnormalities have been found, in the form of a selective reduction of NADH-CoQ reductase activity in SN and platelets in those patients (Schapira et al., 1990; Parker et al., 1989). The latter findings focused attention on a possible undefined genetic pattern of PD and possibilities of widespread oxidative stress damage of extracerebral tissues. In the present study we have investigated the content of reactive oxidative species and the activity of enzymatic antioxidative defense systems in peripheral blood of *de novo* patients with PD, with the aim to determine the above mentioned speculations.

PATIENTS AND METHODS

Twenty patients with PD according to clinical criteria were included in study (Hughes et al., 1992). These patients were diagnosed as having late onset PD. They were evaluated with the Hoehn & Yahr staging (Hoehn et al., 1967) (Table 1).

The following exclusion criteria were applied to these patients:

1. therapy with antiparkinsonian drugs, including vitamin E;
2. previous history of severe chronic systemic disease;
3. infectious diseases or parasitosis.

Patients with PD were all slightly to moderately affected, and had a shortstanding history of disease which did not require levodopa therapy.

The control group comprised 15 age-matched patients, otherwise free of neurologic, psychiatric or other organic disease.

Venous blood samples (5 ml) were taken from each fasted patient or control between 8.00 and 9.00 a.m. The blood samples were collected in vials prepared with sodium heparin and 5mM EDTA, and centrifuged for 15 minutes at 6000 g. The plasma specimens were frozen at -70°C until analysis, while the precipitates were used for preparation of erythrocyte haemolysate. Samples were always evaluated blind.

Lipid peroxidation was determined as the content of thiobarbituric acid reactive substances (TBARs) formed during *in vitro* stimulation by Fe^{2+} salts, while n-butanol was used for extraction (Andreeva et al., 1988).

Nitroblue tetrazolium (NBT) reduction in the alkaline nitrogen saturated medium was used as a probe for superoxide anion generation at 515 nm (Auclair et al., 1985).

Glutathione reductase activity was measured in Tris-HEPES buffer (100 mM, pH-7.2) containing NADPH (1mM), EGTA (1mM) and oxidized glutathione (3mM). Reaction was started by the sample addition and stopped after 15 min with HCl (1M), that destroys NADPH. Fluorescence of $NADPH^+$ formed was measured after treatment with NaOH (6 M) at 340/460 nm) (Lowry et al., 1974).

Superoxide dismutase activity was measured as an inhibition of epinephrine autoxidation at 480 nm. Kinetics were followed in sodium carbonate buffer (50mM, pH-10.2) containing EDTA (0.1 mM) after addition of epinephrine (10 mM) (Sun et al., 1978).

Table 1. Clinical data of PD patients and control group

	PD-Patients	Controls
No. of subjects	20	15
Age (years)	55.67 ± 13.38	60.5 ± 9.31
Female	14	7
Male	6	8
Duration of PD (years)	1.93 ± 1.67	
Hoehn & Yahr stage	1.83 ± 0.65	

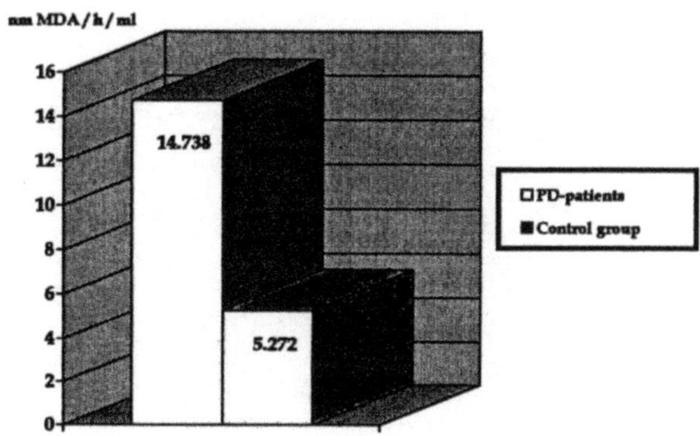

Figure 1. Plasma levels of malondialdehyde in patients with PD and control group.

The results are expressed as means ± SD. The statistical analysis used the SPSS for Windows version 5.1, and included the two-tailed student's t-test, and calculations of Pearson's and Spearman's correlation coefficient when appropriate (SPSS, 1992).

RESULTS

Mean plasma levels of malondialdehyde differed significantly between PD patients and the control group (Figure 1). Namely, the content of MDA was increased two-fold compared to control. These results are summarized in Table 2 which includes other measured quantitative variables.

The amount of superoxide anion radical in erythrocyte haemolysate was significantly higher in PD patients when compared to controls (Figure 2).

Furthermore, we found significantly increased activities of both SOD (Figure 3) and GSH-R (Figure 4) enzymes in the erythrocyte haemolysate of PD patients, when compared to the other study group.

Levels of all of the above-mentioned quantitative variables were not influenced significantly by age, gender, duration of illness or Hoehn & Yahr staging. MDA content and GSH-R activity were positively correlated.

Table 2. Levels of malondialdehyde, superoxide anion radical,
SOD, and GSH-R in peripheral blood of patients
with PD, and in control subjects

	PD-patients	Controls
Malondialdehyde	14.738 ± 7.411*	5.27 ± 1.48
Superoxide anion radical	0.082 ± 0.024*	0.047 ± 0.011
SOD	2089 ± 938**	382 ± 194
GSH-R	13.62 ± 3.43*	4.62 ± 1.61

Biochemical parameters are expressed as: nM MDA/h/ml for MDA content; μM NADP$^+$/mg Hb, as activity of GSH-R; U/mg Hb , as activity of SOD; μM NBT/ mg Hb/min for superoxide anion radical content.
*p < 0.05
**p < 0.001

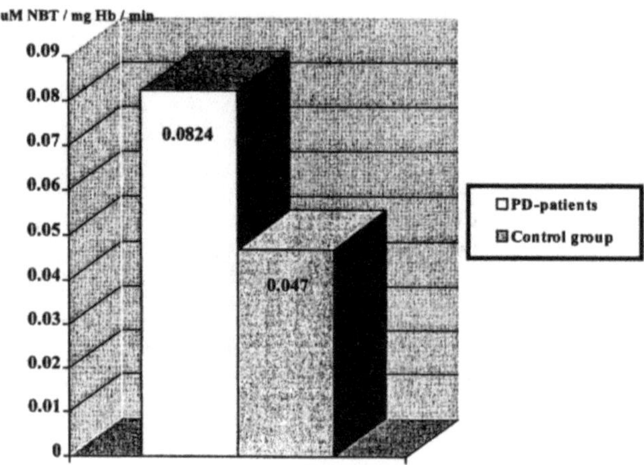

Figure 2. Superoxide anion radical in erythrocyte haemolysate in patients with PD and control group.

DISCUSSION

Oxidative stress hypothesis has been evoked in Parkinson's disease because of the coalition of several biochemical features, particularly around the major site of neuronal damage—dopaminergic cells in the *substantia nigra* (Fahn et al., 1992). Evidence which has been collected relates to enzymatic and autooxidative processes of metabolic degradation of dopamine (Graham, 1978), increased content of iron in the *pars reticulata* SN (Dexter et al, 1991), presence of neuromelanin (Ben-Schachar et al., 1991), and particularly *postmortem* pathological biochemical studies. Further support is provided *via* findings of a selective reduction of activity in the mitochondrial enzyme specific to complex I - NADH-CoQ reductase, and a reduced efficacy of antioxidant defense mechanism, possibly based on a genetic or environmental basis (Swerdlow et al., 1996). The latter possibil-

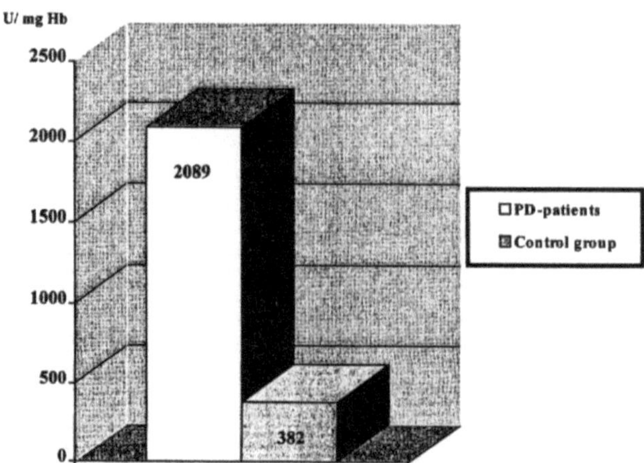

Figure 3. Activity of SOD in erythrocyte haemolysate in patients with PD and control group.

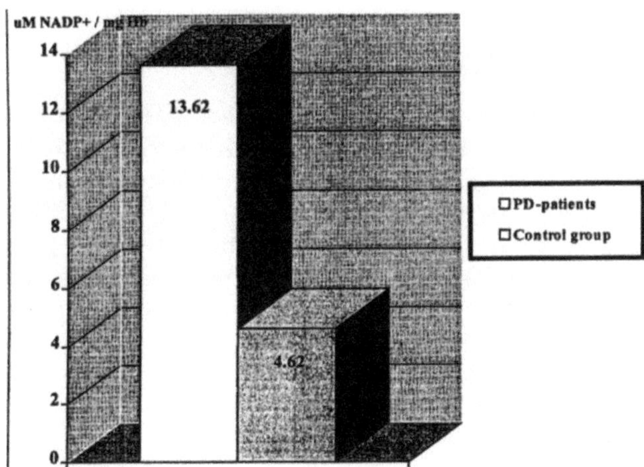

Figure 4. Activity of GSH-R in erythrocyte haemolysate in patients with PD and control group.

ity provides a rational basis for investigations of indices of oxidative stress in peripheral blood of patients with PD.

In our investigation we found a two-fold increase in lipid peroxidation, measured as malondialdehyde content in peripheral blood, which suggests an adequate environment for initiation and further perpetuation of those chain reactions. Namely, it is known that during lipid peroxidation hydroxyl radicals can react with polyunsatured fatty acids incorporated in cellular membranes, with the consequent formation of peroxyl radicals as intermediates, which would continue further free radicals reactions (Olanow, 1992). The final result is damage of the structural integrity of membranes and cell degeneration.

The primary source of superoxide anion radical (O_2^-) generation is the mitochondrial electron transport chain. Electrons and oxidative species formed in these reactions are tightly bound to the active sites of enzyme, although some leakage of superoxide can occur. In such cases high levels of protective enzymes SOD and GPx help to remove reactive oxidative species (Jesberger et al., 1991; Jovicic et al., 1994). Therefore, findings of increased formation of superoxide radical implicate inefficacy of antioxidant defense enzymes.

On the other hand, we measured activities of the protective enzymes—SOD and GSH-R. The role of the latter enzyme is regeneration of oxidized glutathione (GSSG) into a reduced form (GSH) (Jenner et al., 1991). Namely, the glutathione pathway has a key role in the detoxification of hydrogen peroxide, related to redox properties of glutathione, so altered activity of GSH-R could suggest changes of this detoxifying mechanism.

As our results showed, we found a highly statistical significant increase of activity in those enzymes. This can be paradoxical at first sight, because we also found evidence of increased formation of reactive oxidative species. Furthermore, there have been findings of decreased activity of SOD in peripheral blood of patients with PD (Gatto et al., 1996). In spite of that, our results do not contradict previous reported changes, because we examined exclusively newly diagnosed patients with short duration of disease, while the other groups of investigators had a different population sample; patients who were in late stages of PD, with significant longer duration of the disease.

Therefore, the observed changes could represent a continuum of the same biological process, registered at opposite time points—the early and late stages of the disease. If we accept this explanation, the increased activity of antioxidant defense enzymes, which was found in our study, could suggest a compensatory defense reaction, in order to overcome an increased formation of reactive oxidative species.

The absence of a correlation between our clinical data and the measured biochemical parameters, except for MDA content and GSH-R activity, could be explained by the relative short duration of PD and homogenous distribution of clinical variables in our study population. However, the mutual dependence of MDA and GSH-R could suggest a compensatory reaction of antioxidative defense enzymes in the early stage of the illness.

In conclusion, our findings provide further evidence for the oxidative stress hypothesis of PD pathogenesis.

REFERENCES

Andreeva, J.L., Kozemjakin, A.L, and Kiskun, A.A., 1988, Modifikacija metoda opredelenija perekisej lipidov v teste s tiobarbiturovoj kislotoi. *Lab. Delo.* 11:41–43.

Auclair, C., and Voisin, E., 1985, Nitroblue tetrazolium reduction. In: *Handbook of Methods for Oxygen Radical Rresearch.*, Greenwald, R.A., ed., CRC Press Inc., Boca Raton. pp 123–132.

Ben-Schachar, D., Riederer, P., and Youdim , M.B., 1991, Iron-melanin interaction and lipid peroxidation: Implication for Parkinson's disease. J. Neurochem. 57:1609–1614.

Dexter, D.T., Carayon, A., Javoy-Agid, F., and Agid, Y., 1991, Alterations in the levels of iron, ferritin, and other trace metals in Parkinson s disease and other neurodegenerative diseases affecting the basal ganglia. *Brain* 114:953–75.

Dexter, D.T., Carter, C.J., Wells, F.R. et al., 1989, Basal lipid peroxidation in substantia nigra is increased in Parkinson's disease. J.Neurochem. 52:381–89.

Fahn, S., and Cohen, G., 1992, The Oxidant Stress Hypothesis in Parkinson's Disease: Evidence Supporting It. *Ann. Neurol.* 32:804–812.

Gatto, E.M., Carreras, M.C., Pargament, G.A., Riobo, N.A., Reides, C., Repetto, M., Fernandez, Pardal, M.M., Llesuy, S., Poderoso, J.J., 1996, Neutrophil Function, Nitric Oxide, and Blood Oxidative Stress in Parkinson's Disease. *Mov. Disord.* 11:261–267.

Graham, D.G., 1978, Oxidative pathways for catecholamines in the genesis of neuromelanin and cytotoxic quinones. *Mol. Pharmacol.* 14:633–643.

Hoehn, M.M., and Yahr, M.D., 1967, Parkinsonism: onset, progression and mortality. *Neurology* 17:427–442.

Hughes, A.J., Daniel, S.E., Kilford, L., Lees, A.J., 1992, Accuracy of clinical diagnosis of idiopathic Parkinson's disease: a clinico-pathological study of 100 cases. *J. Neurol. Neurosurg. Psychiatry* 55:181–184.

Jenner, P., Dexter, D.T., Sian, J., Schapira, A.V.,and Marsden, C.D., 1992,. Oxidative Stress as a Cause of Nigral Cell Death in Parkinson's Disease and Incidental Body Disease. *Ann. Neurol.* 32:S82-S87.

Jesberger, J.A., and Richardson, J.S., 1991, Oxygen free radicals and brain dysfunction. *Int. J. Neurosci.* 57:1–17.

Jovanovic, M., Jovicic, A., Ivanovic, L., Cernak, I., Mrsulja, B.B., 1994, Free radicals in MPTP-induced parkinsonism. *Iugoslav. Physiol. Pharmacol. Acta* 30:197–203.

Jovicic, A., Djordjevic, D., Raicevic, R., Maric, D., and Jovanovic, M., 1995, Racionalne osnove za formiranje programa lecenja Parkinsonove bolesti. *Vojnosanit. Pregl.* 52:253–260.

Jovicic, A., Ivanisevic, V., Markovic, M., and Simovic, M., 1994, Uloga azotnog oksida u fizioloskim funkcijama i patoloskim stanjima. *Vojnosanit. Pregl.* 51:126–131

Kish, S.J., Morito, C., and Hornykiewicz, O., 1985, Glutathione peroxidase activity in Parkinson's disease. *Neurosci. Lett.* 58:343–346.

Lowry, O.H., Passonneau, J.V., 1974, In: *A Flexible System of Enzymatic Analysis.* Academic Press, New York , pp. 231–256.

Markopoulou, K., Wszolek, Z.K., and Pfeiffer, R.F., 1995; A Greek-American kindred with autosomal dominant, levodopa-responsive parkinsonism and anticipation. *Ann. Neurol.* 38: 373–78.

Mattock, C., Marmot, M., and Stern, G., 1988, Could Parkinson's disease follow intra-uterine influenza?: A speculative hypothesis. *J. Neurol. Neurosurg. Psychiatry* 51:753–756.

Olanow, C.W., 1992. An Introduction to the Free Radical Hypothesis in Parkinson's disease. *Ann.* Neurol. 32:S2-S9.

Parker, W.D., Boyson, S.J., and Parks, J.K., 1989, Abnormalities of the electron transport chain in idiopathic Parkinson's disease. *Ann. Neurol.* 26:719–23.

Perry, T.L. , and Yong, V.W., 1986, Idiopathic Parkinson's disease, progressive supranuclear palsy and glutathione metabolism in the substantia nigra of patients. *Neurosci. Lett.* 67:269–274.

Poskanzer, D.C., and Schwab, R.S., 1963,. Cohort analysis of Parkinson's syndrome. Evidence for a single etiology related to subclinical infection about 1920. *J. Chronic Dis.* 16:961–973.

Riederer, P., Sofic, E., and Rausch, W., 1989, Transition metals, ferritin, glutahione and ascorbic acid in parkinsonian brains. *J. Neurochem.* 52:515–520.

Saggu, H., Cooksey, J., and Dexter, D.T. 1989,. A selective increase in particulate superoxide dismutase activity in parkinsonian substantia nigra. *J. Neurochem.* 53:692–697.

Schapira, A.H.V., Mann, V.M., and Cooper, J.M., 1990, Anatomic and disease specificity of NADH CoQ1 reductase (complex I) deficiency in Parkinson's disease. *J. Neurochem.* 55:2142–2145.

Snyder, S.H., and D'Amato, R., 1986, MPTP: A neurotoxin relevant to the pathophysiology of Parkinson's disease. *Neurology* 36:250–258.

SPSS., 1992, Statistical Package for the Social Sciences. Windows version, release 5.0. Chicago, III: SPSS Inc.

Sun, M., and Zigman, S., 1978, An improved spectrophotometric assay for superoxide dismutase based on epinephrine autooxidation. *Anal. Biochem.* 90:81–89.

Swerdlow, R.H., Parks, J.K., Miller, S.W., Tuttle, J.B., Trimmer, P.A., and Sheehan, J.P., 1983, Origin and Functional Consequences of the Complex I Defect in Parkinson's Disease. *Ann. Neurol.* 40:663–671.

Ward, C.D., Duoisin, R.C., and Ince, S.E., 1983, Parkinson's disease in 65 pairs of twins and in a set of quadriplets. *Neurology* 33:815–824.

112

ACYLPHOSPHATASE LEVELS IN ALZHEIMER'S DISEASE CULTURED SKIN FIBROBLASTS

S. Latorraca,[1] C. Cecchi,[2] A. Pieri,[2] G. Liguri,[2] L. Amaducci,[1] and S. Sorbi[1]

[1]Department of Neurological and Psychiatric Sciences
[2]Department of Biochemical Sciences
University of Florence, Italy

INTRODUCTION

Alzheimer's disease (AD) is a degenerative disorder of the central nervous system which causes progressive cognitive decline during mid to late adult life. The primary causes of AD have not yet been identified. Mutated genes have been located on chromosomes 21,14, and 1, leading to the early onset familial form of the disease (EOFAD) (Shellenberg, 1995; Sorbi, 1993). The first presenile AD gene encoding for β-amyloid precursor protein (APP) was identified in 1991 (Goate et al., 1991). The most frequent pathogenic mutation in exon 17, a Val-Ile substitution at codon 717, has been described in more than 10 families (Levy-Lahad et al., 1996). The largest portion of early onset FAD cases have been associated with mutations in Presenilin 1 (PS1) gene and Presenilin 2 (PS2) gene (Van Broeckhoven, 1995; Rogaev et al., 1995; Levy-Lahad et al., 1995). Fibroblasts from patients and pre-symptomatic carriers of mutations in PS1 and PS2 contain increased amounts of Aβ1-42 peptide (Scheuner et al., 1996). Moreover, the allele E4 of APOE gene has been associated with increased risk for late-onset familial form of AD (Saunders et al., 1993). Apolipoprotein E is the first identified genetic susceptibility factor for sporadic AD. The familial AD form account for 10% of all AD cases (Van Broeckhoven, 1995).

AD leads to alteration of several metabolic properties in cultured skin fibroblasts, and other peripheral tissues indicating both impairment of energy metabolism and alteration of calcium homeostasis (Kumar et al,. 1994; Parker et al., 1994; Sheu et al., 1994; Sims et al., 1987; Sorbi et al., 1995; Peterson et al., 1986). Furthermore, recent studies have highlighted the role that altered calcium homeostasis could play in the physiopathology of AD, such as the described alternative proteolytic processing of β-amyloid precursor protein (Mattson et al., 1993; Querfurth et al., 1994), the hyperphosphorylation of tau-mi-

Progress in Alzheimer's and Parkinson's Diseases
edited by Fisher *et al.*, Plenum Press, New York, 1998.

crotubule-associated protein (Grundke-Iqbal et al., 1986), and the altered protein tyrosine phosphorylation (Shimohama et al., 1993).

Acylphosphatase (AcPase) is a cytoplasmic enzyme able to hydrolyze very efficiently the phosphointermediate formed during the catalytic cycle of Ca^{2+}-ATPase, the main regulatory protein of calcium homeostasis (Nediani et al., 1996). Although the regulatory effect of this interaction with respect to cellular free calcium levels has not been fully elucidated, in vitro experiments demonstrated a marked calcium membrane transport decrease when AcPase in physiological amounts was added to reversed plasmalemmal vesicles (Nassi et al., 1991; Stefani et al., 1995). The hydrolytic activity of AcPase toward the phosphointermediate that is formed during the catalytic mechanism of both Na^+,K^+-ATPase and Ca^{2+}-ATPase may also affect the energy metabolism increasing the rate of ATP hydrolysis (Nediani et al., 1996).

In a previous study we investigated AcPase levels in cultured skin fibroblasts from patients affected by EOFAD linked to presenilin mutations (Liguri et al., 1996). AcPase content was increased by about 100% in EOFAD fibroblasts compared to age-matched control (AC) fibroblasts.

In order to clarify if this alteration only pertains to patients with presenilin mutations, we investigated the AcPase levels in cultured skin fibroblasts from patients affected by sporadic or familial form of Alzheimer's disease bearing the APP Val717Ile missense mutation. Moreover, with the aim to elucidate if AcPase alterations occur early during pathogenesis we analyzed the AcPase content even in a pre-symptomatic carrier of PS1 mutation.

MATERIALS AND METHODS

The following subjects have been studied: 4 subjects belonging to two different Italian families bearing the APP Val717Ile mutation on chromosome 21; 4 subjects affected by the sporadic form of Alzheimer's disease; 2 unaffected young subjects belonging to a family (FAD4) carrying the PS1 Met146Leu missense mutations on chromosome 14, one of them bearing the mutation. Clinical diagnosis of AD was assigned as described by Bracco et al. (1992), fulfilled the NIH-NINCDS criteria, and was confirmed in each family at autopsy. We also studied six age-matched apparently normal controls (Table 1).

Skin biopsies of 3 mm punch were obtained from the volar side of the upper arm of FAD patients and controls. Two explants were performed from each biopsy and plated in 25-cm^2 flasks. Cells were grown in Dulbecco modified Eagle's medium, supplemented with 10% foetal bovine serum, and harvested at confluence in T-25 flasks, 7 days after previous subculture. All fibroblast lines were subjected to an equal number of passages (ranging from 10 to 15) and analyzed twice before confluence in two different weeks together with an age-matched fibroblast line. Cells were washed one time in PBS, than twice in 50 mM Tris-HCl, pH 7.2 containing 0.1 mM PMSF. They were scraped and homogenized with 30 strokes in a glass-glass homogenizer and soluble fractions were separated from the membrane fraction by centrifugation at 24,000 g for 60 min. AcPase activity was determined on the cytosols using 2-methoxybenzoylphosphate as substrate by a continuous fluorimetric test (Paoli et al., 1995). The cytosolic fractions were also subjected to 15% SDS-PAGE and then electrotransferred to nitrocellulose membranes. These membranes were incubated with antibodies against the two isoforms of AcPase, the muscle and the erythrocyte isoenzymes, and detection was performed using HRP conjugated anti-rabbit antibody by enhanced chemiluminescence (ECL). Erythrocyte isoenzyme con-

Table 1. Main parameters of the fibroblast lines analyzed

Fibroblasts	Family	Age (years)	Sex	Mutation
Sporadic AD	AD 1	75	F	
	AD 2	64	M	
	AD 3	51	F	
	AD 4	65	M	
FAD	APP 1	52	F	APPVal717Ile
	APP 2	57	F	APPVal717Ile
	APP 3	60	M	APPVal717Ile
	APP 4	50	F	APPVal717Ile
Young PS 1 mutated subjects	Y 1	18	M	
	Y 2	19	F	PS1Met146Leu
Controls*	C 1	52	M	
	C 2	52	M	
	C 3	50	F	
	C 4	55	M	
	C 5	49	F	
	C 6	40	F	

*All subjects were tested and none of them carried the FAD mutations

tent was carried out by a non-competitive enzyme linked immunosorbant assay (ELISA) performed using affinity-purified anti-human AcPase antibodies. Results obtained were evaluated using Student's t-test for significance.

RESULTS AND DISCUSSION

AcPase enzymatic activity showed comparable value in APP Val717Ile mutated fibroblasts and sporadic AD fibroblasts with respect to age-matched control lines (Figure 1).

In order to exclude the possible contribution of other non-specific phosphatases present in the cytosols and to discriminate between the two isoforms of the enzyme, we carried out, as a first semiquantitative approach, a Western blotting against the two AcPase isoforms. Neither the muscle or the erythrocyte isoenzyme showed a consistent variation between APPVal717Ile and sporadic AD fibroblasts with respect to age-matched fibroblasts (Figure 2).

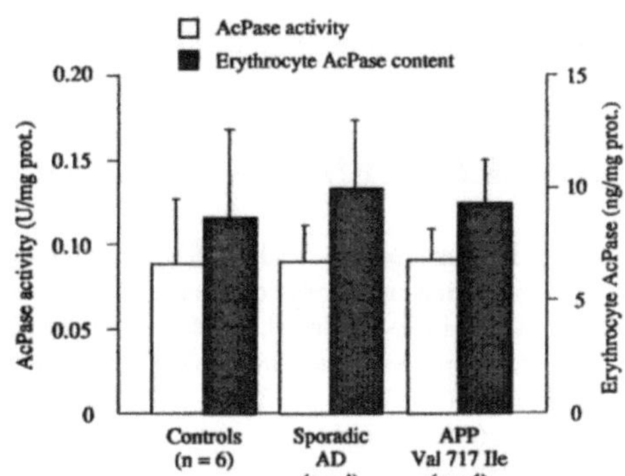

Figure 1. Total AcPase activity and levels of erythrocyte AcPase in controls, sporadic AD and APP Val717Ile mutated FAD fibroblasts. Values are means ± SD of two independent experiments, each performed in triplicate.

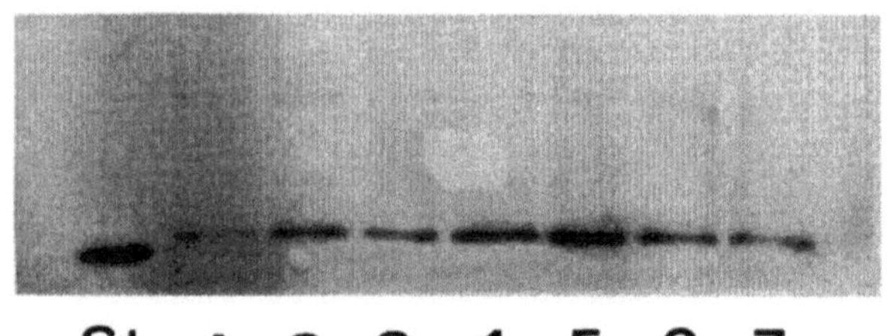

Figure 2. Western blots of AD (lanes 1, 3, 5, 7) and controls (lanes 2, 4, 6). Cytosols recognized with anti-erythrocyte acylphosphatase antibodies. St, erythrocyte acylphosphatase standard.

The non-competitive ELISA against the erythrocyte isoenzyme confirmed the previous data, showing no statistical difference (Figure 1). ELISA performed on the two isoenzymes of confluence fibroblast lines subjected to a number of passages ranging from 10 to 15 remained stable (about 10 ng/mg of cytosolic protein) during one week growth in T-25 flasks. The trend of the two isoenzymes levels was confirmed by Western blotting.

In order to investigate if the alteration of the AcPase levels found in affected subjects bearing one of the Presenilin mutations (Liguri et al., 1996) was strictly related to the mutation rather then to the disease, we tested the two FAD4 young subjects. No differences were found in the AcPase activity and content.

Previous results provided strong evidence that an alteration of erythrocyte AcPase expression or turnover occurs in some EOFAD pedigrees (Liguri et al. 1996). Both isoenzymes of AcPase are able to modulate the efficiency of calcium transport by hydrolyzing very efficiently the phosphointermediate formed during the catalytic cycle of Ca^{2+}-ATPase from several tissues (Nassi et al., 1991). It can therefore be hypothesized that in fibroblasts carring the genetic presenilin lesions, altered AcPase levels could lead to aberrant free calcium homeostasis, a common feature of AD (Peterson et al., 1986).

Preliminary results reported in this paper suggest that the AcPase alteration seems to occur only in the fibroblasts from patients with the familial form of AD linked to mutations of the presenilin genes. Thus it is possible that a pathway exists whereby dysfunctional presenilin proteins lead to increased amyloid β-protein (β1–42) production and that AcPase could function in this pathway through a disruption of calcium homeostasis or an impairment of energy metabolism.

ACKNOWLEDGMENT

This work was supported by grants from MURST, ex quota 60%, Telethon, n. 686 and Targeted Project on Aging N. (CNR - Italy).

REFERENCES

Bracco, L., Amaducci, L. and the SMID group. Italian multicenter study on dementia, 1992, A protocol for data collection and clinical diagnosis of Alzheimer's disease. *Neuroepidemiology* 11:39.

Goate, A., Chartier-Harlin, M.C., Mullan, M., et al., 1991, Segregation of a missense mutation in the amyloid precursor protein gene with familial Alzheimer's disease. *Nature* 349:704.

Grundke-Iqbal, I., Iqbal, K., Tung, Y-C., Quinlan, M., Wisniewski, H.M. and Binder, L., 1986, Abnormal phosphorilation of the microtubule-associated protein tau in Alzheimer cytoskeletal pathology. *Proc. Natl. Acad. Sci.* 83:4913.

Kumar, U., Dunlop, D.M. and Richardson, J.S., 1994, Mithocondria from Alzheimer's fibroblasts show decreased uptake of calcium and increased sensitivity to free radicals. *Life Sci.* 54:1855.

Levy-Lahad, E., Wasco, W., Poorkaj, P., Romano, D.M., et al., 1995, Candidate gene for the chromosome 1 familial Alzheimer's Disease locus. *Science* 269:973.

Levy-Lahad, E. and Bird, T.D., 1996, Genetic factors in Alzheimer's Disease: a review of recent advanced. *Ann. Neurol.* 40:829.

Liguri, G., Cecchi, C., Latorraca, S., Pieri, A., Sorbi, S., Degl'Innocenti, D. and Ramponi, G., 1996, Alteration of acylphosphatase levels in familial Alzheimer's disease fibroblasts with presenilin gene mutations. *Neurosci. Lett.* 210:153.

Mattson, M.P., Barger, S.W., Cheng, B., Lieberburg, I., Smith-Swintosky, V.L. and Rydel, R.E., 1993, β-amyloid precursor protein metabolites and loss of neuronal Ca^{2+} homeostasis in Alzheimer's disease. *TINS* 16:409.

Nassi, P., Nediani, C., Liguri, G., Taddei, N., Ramponi, G., 1991, Effects of acylphosphatase on the activity of erythrocyte membrane Ca^{2+} pump. *J. Biol. Chem.* 266:10867.

Nediani, C., Fiorillo, C., Marchetti, E., Pacini, A., Liguri, G. and Nassi, P., 1996, Stimulation of cardiac sarcoplasmic reticulum calcium pump by acylphosphatase. *J. Biol. Chem.* 271:19066.

Paoli, P., Camici, G., Manao, G. and Ramponi, G., 1995, 2-Methoxybenzoyl phosphate: a new substrate for continuous fluorimetric acyl phosphate assays. *Experientia* 51:57.

Parker, W.D., Mahr, M.S., Filley, C.M., Parks, J., Hughes, M.A., Young, D.A. and Cullum, C.M., 1994, Electron platelet cytochrome c oxidase activity in Alzheimer's disease. *Neurology* 44:1086.

Peterson, C. and Goldman, J.E., 1986, Alterations in calcium content and biochemical processes in cultured skin fibroblasts from aged and Alzheimer donors. *Proc. Natl. Acad. Sci.* 83:2758.

Querfurth, H.W., and Selkoe, D.J., 1994, Calcium ionophore increases amyloid β peptide production by cultured cells. *Biochemistry* 33:4550.

Rogaev, E.I., Sherrington, R., Rogaeva, E.A. et al., 1995, Familial Alzheimer's disease in kindreds with missense mutations in a gene on chromosome 1 related to the Alzheimer's disease type 3 gene. *Nature* 376:775.

Saunders, A.M., Strittmatter, W.J., Schmechel, D., George-Hyslop, P.H., et al., 1993, Association of Apolipoprotein E allele e4 with late-onset familial and sporadic Alzheimer's disease. *Neurology* 43:1467.

Schellemberg, G.D., 1995, Genetic dissection of Alzheimer Disease, a heterogeneous disorder. *Proc. Natl. Acad. Sci.* 92:8552.

Scheuner, D., Eckman, C., Jensen, M., Song, X. et al., 1996, Secreted amyloid β-protein similar to that in the senile plaques of Alzheimer's disease is increased in vivo by the presenilin 1 and 2 and APP mutations linked to familial Alzheimer's disease. *Nat. Med.* 2:864.

Sheu, K.F.R., Cooper, A.J.L., Koike, M., Lindsay, J.G. and Blass, J. P., 1994, Abnormality of the α-ketoglutarate dehydrogenase complex in fibroblasts from familial Alzheimer's disease. *Ann. Neurol.* 35:312.

Shimohama, S., Fujimoto, S., Taniguchi, T., Kameyama, M., Kimura, J., 1993, Reduction of low-molecular-weight acid phosphatase activity in Alzheimer brains. *Ann. Neurol.* 33:616.

Sims, N.R., Finegan, J.M. and Blass, J.P., 1987, Alterated metabolic properties of cultured skin fibroblasts in Alzheimer's disease. *Ann. Neurol.* 21:451.

Sorbi, S., 1993, Molecular genetics of Alzheimer's disease, *Aging Clin. Exp. Res.* 5:417.

Sorbi, S., Piacentini, S., Latorraca, S., Piersanti, P. and Amaducci, L., 1995, Alterations in metabolic properties in fibroblasts in Alzheimer's disease. *Alzheimer. Dis. Assoc. Disord.* 9:73.

Stefani, M., Ramponi, G., 1995, Acylphosphate phosphohydrolases. *Life Chem. Rep.* 12:271.

Van Broeckhoven, C., 1995, Presenilins and Alzheimer disease. *Nat. Genet.* 11:230.

113

CENTROMERIC DISTURBANCES AFFECTING ALL CHROMOSOMES OF CULTURED LYMPHOCYTES OBTAINED FROM ALZHEIMER'S DISEASE PATIENTS

José Ignacio Lao Villadóniga,[1] Katrin Beyer,[1] and Ramón Cacabelos[2]

[1]EuroEspes Biomedical Research Center
Department of Molecular and Clinical Genetics
[2]Department of Neurogeriatry
Santa Marta de Babío, s/n
15166 Bergondo, A Coruña, Spain

INTRODUCTION

In Familial Alzheimer's disease (FAD), a devastating neurodegenerative process mainly characterized by loss of learning and memory, the genetic contributions are been clarified day by day. Mutations on chromosome 21 and 19 AD-related have been described and well documented in some patients and their relatives (St. George-Hyslop et al., 1987; Murrell et al., 1991; Chartier-Harlin et al., 1991; Pericak-Vance et al., 1991). Further studies have shown mutations on chromosome 14, the locus FAD-3 placed in 14q24.3, as responsible of about 70% of the early-onset FAD (Schellenberg, et al., 1992; Bonnycastle et al., 1993). In this locus, the S182 gene (presenilin 1 gene) has been recently mapped and postulated as a possible FAD gene (Selkoe et al., 1995). Another gene, the STM2 on chromosome 1 (presenilin 2 gene), has also been related with some pedigrees of AD; and, curiously, this gene is very close related in its function with the S182 (Levy-Lahad et al., 1995) . At the cytogenetic level, some authors have reported certain chromosomal abnormalities associated with this disorder. In two sisters with late-onset AD, an unusual elongated short arm of chromosome 22 has been described, and this marker was also demonstrated in other 24 biological relatives of these patients (Percy et al., 1991). Other reports postulate that a nondisjunction, mainly affecting chromosome 21, may lead to AD through the same mechanism by which Down syndrome patients develop the disease (having an extra copy of chromosome 21) (Potter, 1991). An increase of chromosome breaks, acentric chromosomes, chromatid exchanges and high sensitivity to damage induced by chemical o physical agents reveal the fragility of the chromosomes in these patients (Nakanishi et al., 1979; Noderson et al., 1980; Ettinger et al.,

1994). Another age-related cytogenetic event more recently described was the formation of micronuclei and a significant increase in the loss of chromosomes in both males and females with age, especially involving chromosome X in females and chromosome Y in males (Hando et al., 1994). In this paper, we present some cytogenetic findings observed in metaphases of AD lymphocytes in comparison with an age-matched healthy eldery controls.

SUBJECTS AND METHOD

We selected 18 patients (age: 65.7±5.1 years) from the Department of Neurogeriatrics of the EuroEspes Biomedical Center in Coruña, Spain, with probable diagnosis of AD, and 18 age-matched control subjects (age: 68±5 years). AD diagnosis was obtained according to DSM-IV and NINCDS-ADRDA criteria and using our own clinical protocol EuroEspes-Eudenet (Cacabelos, 1991). We inoculated 400 µl of whoole venous blood from each person under study into the culture tubes, containing 4 ml of a medium composed by RPMI 1640, 10% of fetal calf serum, 1% of penicillin (5000 IU/ml), 1% of streptomycin (5000 µg/ml) and, 1% of L-Glutamine (200 mM). Previously, we had added PHA^L at 1% into the tubes to stimulate lymphocyte division. After 72 hours of incubation at 37°C, we added colchicine, as a metaphase arresting agent, at a final concentration of 0.1 µg/ml. We left the culture in the incubation chamber at 37°C for 2 aditional hours, and then, we provoked an hypotonic shock using 0.075 M KCl. The following step was the fixation with a mixture of 3 parts of methanol and 1 part of glacial acetic acid. Then, we extended the metaphases into clean microscope slides and allowed them to dry overnight. Finally, we developed the trypsin-giemsa G-banding, and the C-banding pattern using conventional techniques (Benn et al., 1979). Metaphase analyses were carried out by cytogenetists in a microscope Olympus C35AD/4.

This process was developed each time for patients and their respective controls at the same time, in order to minimize possible influences inherent to the manipulation and to the growth cell environment.

RESULTS

In 16 out of 18 patients we found a 30–40% of cells with premature centromere division (PCD) (Figure 1) as a more remarkable sign of AD lymphocyte metaphases (Figure 2). This phenomenon was observed in only 3 normal controls (Figure 2). We found a high frequency of acentric chromosomes (AC) in the AD group (8 out of 18). This cytogenetic sign was not present in the controls. Another alteration involving centromeres was a dicentric chromosome formation (DIC) which was found in 5 patients but not in controls (Figure 2).

Some of the AD analised metaphases (8 out of 18) also showed several chromatid breaks and gaps signs (CBS) forming acentric fragments the loss parts. Other chromosomes appear in a ring-shape conformation (R), and there also are minute chromosomes (MC) surrounding normal chromosomes (Figure 3).

DISCUSSION

The present results demonstrate clear differences between AD patients and their respective age-matched controls regarding chromosomic abnormalities in lymphocyte cell cultures.

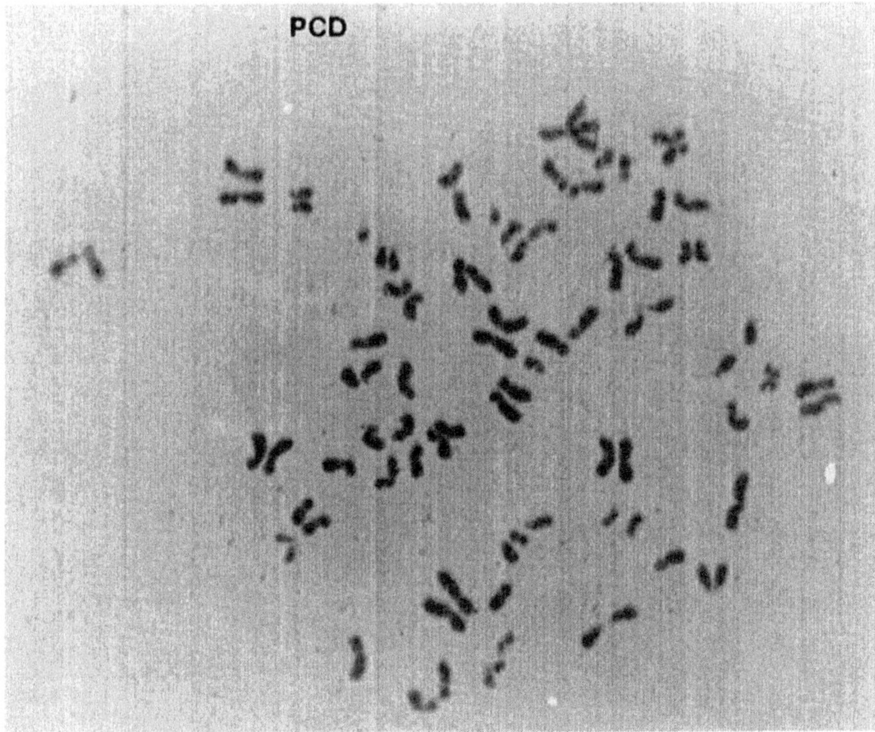

Figure 1. Premature rupture of centromeres in the early metaphase.

AD patients showed an increased frequency of premature rupture of centromeres and signs of chromosome breakages. These changes were shown at a higher frequency than in age-matched healthy eldery controls.

An elevated incidence of numeric aberrations, consistent with the previously reported by other researchers (Potter et al., 1991; Ward et al., 1979), and an enhaced prevalence of premature centromere division observed in AD lymphocyte cultures might

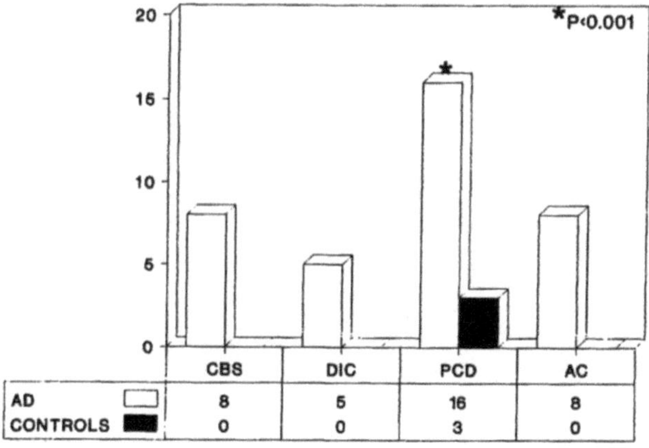

		CBS	DIC	PCD	AC
AD	☐	8	5	16	8
CONTROLS	■	0	0	3	0

Figure 2. Total of patients by cytogenetic signs observed in the AD group in comparison with the control group.

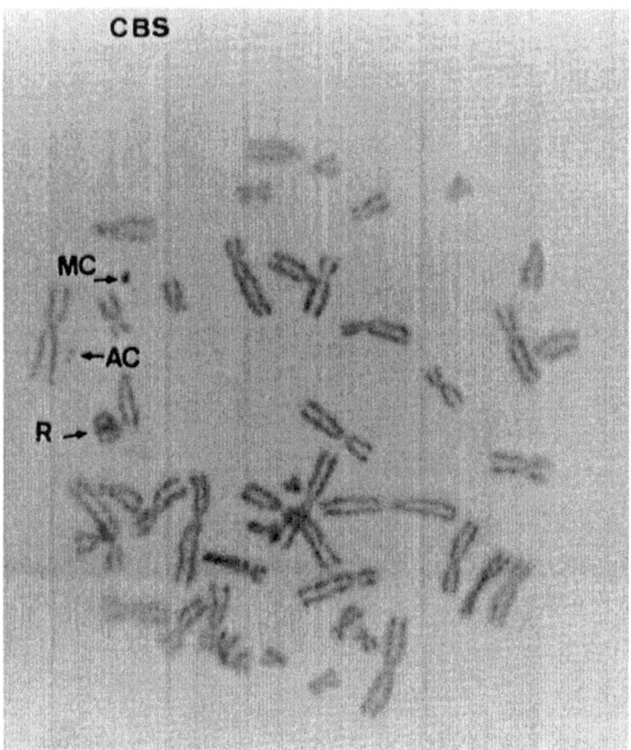

Figure 3. Centromere disturbances found in some AD metaphases.

suggest the possibility of the existence of an aberrant mitotic process affecting AD patients. However, this mechanism associated with other cytogenetic abnormalities (acentric fragments, gaps, micronuclei formations), also reported by other authors (Benn et al., 1979; Cook et al., 1979; Hughel et al., 1994), demonstrate a loss of genetic information that seems to take place in AD. The chromosome breakage signs found in AD patients are similar to those observed in syndromes of chromosomal instability (Ataxia-Telangiectasia or Progeria, Cockayne, and Werner syndrome) also associated with premature senescence (Mattevi et al., 1975) or in subjects exposed to strong mutagenic influences (Tawn et al., 1992). These finding would be consistent with a possible replication defect which could be taken place in AD and it would be related with a high rate of spontaneous sister chromatid exchange. Some of these cytogenetic figures observed in the premature senescence syndromes are also demonstrated in neoplasias and they are related to the catastrophic genetic imbalance inherent to these entities (Mandahl et al., 1992). However, none of the mentioned syndromes nor demonstrable malignant illness were present in any of the patients included in this study. Signs of fragmented DNA and the apparent incapacity of AD lymphocytes to preserve the DNA stability seems to reflect a possible failure in the DNA preservative systems inherent to the AD cells in general.

Principal signs we show in this paper are mainly involving centromeres (Figure 2). It may suggests that there is an abnormal mitotic process due to some centromere disturbances affecting AD cells. Furthermore, premature centromere division as a potential cause of improper chromosome segregation, which is one of the principal finding in the AD patients analysed in the present study, has been also found to be positively correlated with age by other authors (Nakagome et al., 1984). From all the evidence it is highly probable that a predisposition to abnormal mitosis could be inheritable (due to mutations in some yet uknown gene or genes which regulate the chromosome segregation), or it also could be environmentally determined (due to influences of some agents which may cause centromere disturbances). In this sense, both genetic and sporadic forms of AD can be explained.

Further analysis have to determine chromosomes or chromosome regions mainly implicated in the AD origin in which could be placed a gene or genes with a major effect in the AD pathogenesis. In fact, it has been described some families with a potential AD mutation on chromosome 21 different from the beta-protein gene and closer to the centromere. In this sense, there is reason to believe that the main AD gene is mainly implicated in a yet uknown mechanism designed to preserve the genetic information.

CONCLUSIONS

Cytogenetic signs demonstrated in the AD group are consistent with a marked genomic instability resulting in a failure of the normal cell division process that might suggest new hypotheses to explain AD as a result of disturbances in the cellular mechanisms available to preserve the genomic integrity. An inherited or environmentally adquired defect in these mechanisms might provoke an important depletion of genetic information that could be essential for the normal cell replacement process, leading to degeneration and cell death.

ACKNOWLEDGMENT

This study was supported in grant in aid by EuroEspes Foundation.

REFERENCES

Benn, P.A., Perle, M.A., 1992, Chromosome staining and banding techniques. Human Cytogenetics.A Practical Approach I., 2nd ed., Oxford: Rooney & Czepulkowski.

Bonnycastle, L.L.C., Yu, C.-E., Wijsman, E.M., Orr, H.T., Patterson, D., Clancy, K.P., Goddard, K.A.B., Alonso, M.E., Nemens, E., White, J.A., Heston, L.L., Martin, G.M., Bird, T.D., Schellenberg, G.D., 1993, The c-fos gene and early-onset Alzheimer's disease. *Neurosci. Lett.* 160:33–36.

Cacabelos, R., 1991, Enfermedad de Alzheimer. JR Prous International Publishers, Barcelona.

Chartier-Harlin, M.-C., Crawford, F., Houlden, H., 1991, Early-onset Alzheimer's disease caused by mutations on codon 717 of the ß-amyloid precursor protein gene. *Nature* 353:844–846.

Cook, B.E, Ward, B.E, Austin, J.H., 1979, Studies in ageing of the brain: IV Familial AD: relation to transmissible dementia, aneuploidy, and microtubular defects. *Neurology* 29:1402–1412.

Ettinger S, Weksler ME, Zhou X, Blass, J., Szabo P., 1994, Chromosomal fragility associated with familial Alzheimer's disease. *Ann. Neurol.* 36:190.

Hando, J.C, Nath, J., Tucker, J.D., 1994, Sex chromosomes, micronuclei and ageing in women. *Chromosoma* 103:186–192.

Hughel, A., Mielke, R., 1994, Cytogenetic Investigations from Lymphocyte Cultures of Patients with Probable Alzheimer's Disease. *Dementia* 5:310–313.

Levy-Lahad, E., Wasco, W., Poorkaj, P., Romano, D.M., Oshima, J., Pettingell, W.H., Yu, C., Jondro, P.D., Schmidt, S.D., Wang, K., Crowley, A.C., Fu, Y.-H., Guenette, S.Y., Galas, D., Nemens, E., Wijsman, E.M., Bird, T.D., Schellenberg, G.D., Tanzi, R.E., 1995, Candidate Gene for the Chromosome 1 Familial Alzheimer's disease locus. *Science* 269:973–976.

Mandahl, N., 1992, Methods in solid tumor. Human cytogenetics. A practical Approach I., 2nd ed., Oxford: Rooney & Czepulkowski.

Mattevi, M.S., Salzano, F.M., 1975, Senescence and human chromosome changes. Humangenetik 27:1–8.

Murrell, J., Farlow, M., Ghetti, B., Benson, M.D., 1991, A mutation in the amyloid precursor protein associated with hereditary Alzheimer's disease. *Science* 254:97–99.

Nakagome, Y., Abe, T., Misawa, S., Takeshita, T., Iinuma, K., 1984, The loss of centromeres from chromosomes of aged women. *Am. J. Hum. Genet.* 36:398–404.

Nakanishi, Y., Kram, D., Schneider, E.L., 1979, Aging and sister chromatid exchange. *Cytogenet Cell Genet* 24:61–67.

Noderson, I., Adolfsson, R., Beckman, G., Bucht, G., Winblad, B., 1980, Chromosomal abnormality in dementia of Alzheimer type. *Lancet* 1:481–482.

Percy, M.E, Markovic, V.D, Crapper McLachlan, D.R., Berg, J.M., Hummel, J.T., Laing, M.E., Dearie, T.G., Andrews, D.F., 1991, Family with 22-derived marker chromosome and late-onset dementia of the Alzheimer type I. Application of a new model for stimation of the risk of disease associated with the marker. *Am. J. Med. Genet.* 39:307–313.

Pericak-Vance, M.A., Bebout, J.L., Gaskell, P.C., Jr., Yamaoka, L.H., Hung, W.-Y., Albert, M.J., Walker, A.P., Bartlett, R.J., Haynes, C.A., Welsch, K.A., Earl, N.L., Heyman, A., Clark, C.M., Roses, A.D., 1991, Linkage studies in familial Alzheimer's disease: evidence for chromosome 19 linkage. *Am. J. Hum. Genet.*48:1034–1050.

Potter, H., 1991, Review and hypothesis: Alzheimer Disease and Down Syndrome-Chromosome 21 Nondisjunction may underlie both disorders. *Am. J. Hum. Genet.* 48:1192–1200.

Schellenberg, G.D., Bird, T.D., Wijsman, E.M., Orr, H.T., Anderson, L., Nemens, E., White, J.A., Bonnycastle, L., Weber,J.L., Alonso, M.E., Potter, H., Heston, L.L., Martin, G.M.,1992, Genetic linkage evidence for a familial Alzheimer's disease locus on chromosome 14. *Science* 258:668–671.

Selkoe, D.J., 1995, Missense on the membrane. *Nature* 375:734–735.

St.George-Hyslop, P.H., Tanzi, R.E., Polinsky, R.J., Haines, J.L., Nee, L., Watkins, P.C., Meyers, R.H., Feldman, R.G., Pollen, D., Drachman, D., Growdonn, J., Bruni, A., Foncin, J.F., Salmon, G., Fromheld, P., Amaducci, L., Sorgi, S., Placentini, S., Steward, G.D., Hobbs, W., Conneally, P.M., Gusella, J.F., 1987, The genetic defect causing familial Alzheimer's disease maps on chromosome 21. *Science* 235:885–890.

Tawn, E.J., Holdsworth, D., 1992, Mutagen-induced chromosome damage in human lymphocytes. Human Cytogenetics. A Practical Approach I. 2nd ed. Oxford: Rooney & Czepulkowski.

Ward, B.E., Cook, R.H., Robinson, A., Austin, J.H., 1979 Increased aneuploidy in Alzheimer's disease. *Am. J. Med. Gen.* 3:137–142.

114

APOE GENOTYPE-RELATED BLOOD PRESSURE IN SENILE DEMENTIA

Ricardo Mouzo, X. Antón Alvarez , V. Manuel Pichel, Angeles Sellers,
Jose M. Caamaño, Marta Laredo, Katrin Beyer, Jose I. Lao, Paula Perez,
Margarita Alcaraz, M. Carmen Rúa, Lola Corzo, Lucía Fernández-Novoa,
René Fernández, and Ramón Cacabelos

Department of Neurogeriatry
Santa Marta de Babio
15166 Bergando, A Coruña, Spain

INTRODUCTION

Both senile dementia (SD) and hypertension (HBP) are pathologies with a high prevalence (Applegate, 1989; Cacabelos, 1995). SD is the third health problem in developed countries after cardiovascular disease and cancer (with a prevalence of 5–15 % after the age of 65 (Cacabelos, 1995). Hypertension is a risk factor classically associated with SD of the vascular type (Sokoog, 1994, 1996, Strandgaard, 1994). Genetic factors, and particularly Apolipoprotein E (APOE), have been associated with SD (Saunders, 1993; Basun, 1995; Cacabelos, 1996; Beyer, 1996) although no specific factors correlating SD and HBP have yet been identified.

The association between the APOE polymorphism, atherosclerosis and cardiovascular disease has been widely studied (Uterman, 1975; Davignon, 1988; Uusitupa, 1994). Differences in ε4 allele frequency between populations explain the different prevalence rates of cardiovascular disease. Recently, we have published a study about the different implications of APOE ε4 in Alzheimer's disease (AD) and Vascular Dementia (VD) in the Spanish population (Beyer, 1996). Our results suggest that APOE ε4 plays a different role in AD and VD. In AD, APOE ε4 may act as a precipitating factor that could modify the clinical course of the disease when there are additional familial AD-genes segregating in an affected family. In VD, APOE ε4 represents a vulnerability factor which might enhance its pathogenic effects in an age and dose-dependent manner under negative endogenous and/or exogenous influences.

In 1994 contradictory data concerning the relationship between the APOE phenotype and blood pressure were reported. Uusitupa et al. (1994) showed that in a selected

Progress in Alzheimer's and Parkinson's Diseases
edited by Fisher *et al.*, Plenum Press, New York, 1998.

Finnish population sample, APOE 4/4 and 4/3 phenotypes appear most frequently associated with high systolic blood pressure than phenotypes 3/3, 2/3, or 2/4, suggesting a relationship between APOE, serum cholesterol and blood pressure. However, Knijff et al. (1994) could not find any consistent influence of the APOE on blood pressure in an unselected sample.

The relationship between blood pressure and the APOE genotype in senile dementia patients has not been yet documented. In the present study we evaluated blood pressure according to the presence or not of the allele ε4, the most prevalent APOE genotype (4/4, 3/4, 3/3, 2/3), and the global deterioration scale (GDS) staging in patients with senile dementia and in age-matched control subjects.

MATERIALS AND METHODS

Sixteen elderly subjects were used as controls (C) (age 68.5 ± 8 years, range: 60–85); and 87 patients with clinical diagnosis of SD (74 ± 7.9 years, range: 57–89) were included: a) Alzheimer disease (AD) (n = 23; age 70.65 ± 7.9 years, range: 57–86); b) vascular dementia (VD) (n = 26; age 77.6 ± 5 years, range: 64–85); c) mixed dementia (MD) (n = 38; age 75.9 ± 7.5 years, range: 57–89). Disease staging according to the Global Deterioration Scale[21] was 3–6 in SD patients and 1–2 in controls subjects. Anthropometric measures (height, weight and body mass index) were similar among the four groups evaluated. The patients were diagnosed according to ICD-10, DSM-IV (American Psychiatric Association, 1994), and NINCDS-ADRDA criteria (Mc Khann, 1984). The diagnostic criteria for high blood pressure was established according to the World Health Organization) Expert Committee Report (WHO, 1978), reassesment for Working Group in 1985; and the JNC-4 Criteria (Fourth Joint National Committee, 1988). Blood pressure measurements were obtained at rest in a supine position for at least five minutes, with a validated semi-automatic sphygmomanometer (Boso-medicus. BOSCH + SOHN. GMBH. U. Co. Germany™).

APOE genotyping was carried out in a blind condition for the clinicians following the procedure previously reported. The allellic frequencies were stimated for controls, AD, VD and MD groups by counting alleles and calculating sample proportions. ANOVA and Student's *t* Test and Mann Whitney *u* Test were used for parametric and non parametric analysis. The frequency of high, normal or low blood pressure levels in dementia patients with different aetiology were compared by the chi-square test.

RESULTS

Systolic blood pressure (SBP) values were higher in VD (147.7 ± 26 mmHg; $p < 0.05$) and MD (144.9 ± 24.9 mmHg; $p < 0.05$) than in AD (129.7 ± 19.6 mmHg) (Table 1). The allelic frequencies for ε4 were 12.5%, 34.4%, 13.4% and 43.4% for C, EA, VD and MD respectively. No significant differences were found when BP scores were analyzed as a function of the presence or absence of the ε4 allele, the APOE genotype (Figure 1) or the GDS stage (Table 2).

HBP, systolic, diastolic and systo-diastolic, was more frequent in VD (n = 14; 53.84%; $p < 0.05$) and MD (n = 16; 42.1%; ns) than in AD (n = 13; 13.04%).

In HBP subjects, SBP and DBP levels did not vary according to the presence of the ε4 allele, the APOE genotype or the GDS stage.

Table 1. Blood pressure and anthropometric parameters

Dementia type	Age years (range)	Sex (M/F)	Weight (kg)	Height (cm)	BMI	SBP mmHg (range)	DBP mmHg (range)
Alzheimer (n = 23)	70.6 ± 7.9 (57–86)	4/19	66 ± 15	159 ± 7	26.1	129.7 ± 19.6 (98–172)	77 ± 9 (60–101)
Vascular (n = 26)	77.6 ±5.4 (64–85)	12/14	64 ± 9	158 ± 7	25.2	147.7 ± 26* (102–210)	81 ± 15 (57–123)
Mixed (n = 38)	75.9 ± 7.5 (57–89)	10/28	62 ± 9	154 ± 9	26	144.9 ± 24.9* (107–220)	80 ± 12 (56–109)
No dementia (n = 16)	68.5 ± 8 (60–85)	6/10	70 ± 12	161 ± 11	26.9	141 ± 20 (110–185)	82 ± 7 (72–95)

M/F: Male/Female; BMI: Body Mass Index; SBP: Systolic Blood Pressure; DBP: Diastolic Blood Pressure.
*p < 0.05 vs AD.

DISCUSSION

The prevalence of high blood pressure in caucasian elderly people is about 33–50%. In our study 38% of SD patients had high blood pressure, 42.5% showed normal values and 19.5% of the subjects had low BP. No significant differences in BP were obtained when all SD patients were compared with controls. Conversely, SBP in VD and MD was higher than in AD and controls.Any relationship between HBP and APOE genotyping coul not be proved.

Although no significant differences were found in BP according to the GDS staging, we observed the highest DBP levels in advanced stages of the disease.

In our sample, AD patients had lower BP than the other dementia types, BP being normal or low in 62% of the SD patients. In this regard, Guo et al. (1996) observed that the relatively low blood pressure is probably a complication of the dementia process, paticularly in Azheimer's disease. They showed that people with SBP below 140 mmHg or DBP below 75 mmHg were more often diagnosed as demented. Both systolic and diastolic blood pressures were inversely proportional to the prevalence of dementia in elderly people.

We found that patients with VD and MD had higher SBP than those with AD. The relationship between hypertension and VD has already been described (Strandgaard, 1997). The diagnosis of VD is ussually supported by Computed Tomography (CT) and/or Magnetic Resonance Imaging (MRI). However Soppe et al. (1995), recently reported that the diagnosis of VD based on CT or MRI should not be made, because the occurrence of cerebral white matter lesions is a non- specific finding which is observed in up to 50% of the elderly subjects. This is an important conclusion because it could be necesary to obtain complementary information about cerebral blood flow for the evaluation of VD and MD.

Table 2. APOE 4-related blood pressure levels in senile dementia

ε4	Alzheimer		Vascular		Mixed		No-Dementia	
	Yes	No	Yes	No	Yes	No	Yes	No
SBP (mmHg)	130 ± 19 (n = 11)	130 ± 20 (n = 12)	146 ± 31 (n = 7)	143 ± 25 (n = 19)	140 ± 24 (n = 22)	151 ± 26 (n = 16)	125 ± 15 n = 2	144 ± 19 n = 14
DBP (mmHg)	76 ± 8 (n = 11)	77 ± 12 (n = 12)	78 ± 16 (n = 7)	82 ± 15 (n = 19)	78 ± 10 (n = 22)	82 ± 14 (n = 16)	86 ± 2 n = 2	82 ± 7 n = 14

ε4: Allele ε4; SBP: Systolic Blood Pressure; DBP: Diastolic BloodPressure

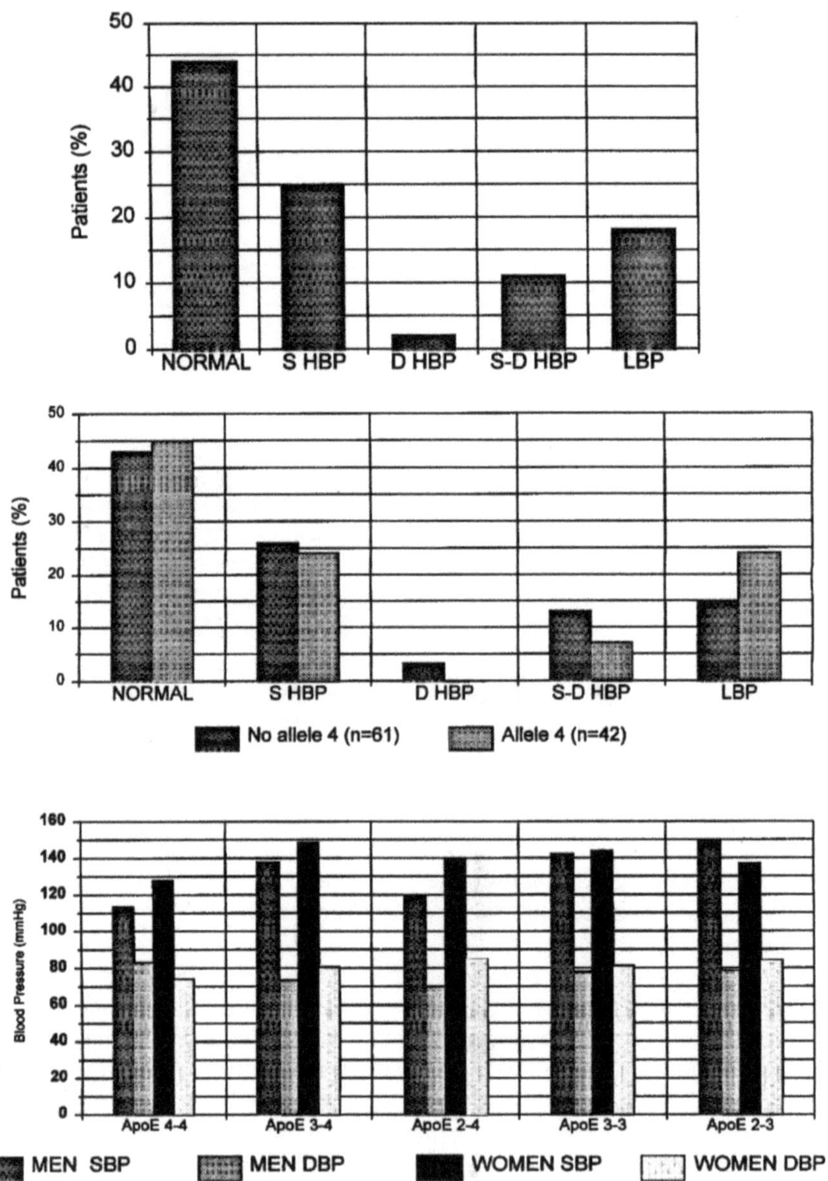

Figure 1. a) Distribution of patients according to the BP levels and the presence or not the APOE ε4 allele. b) BP levels according to sex and APOE genotype. c) Distribution of SD patients according to BP levels. (**S HBP:** Systolic High Blood Pressure; **D HBP:** Diastolic High Blood Pressure; **S-D HBP:** Systolic-Diastolic High Blood Pressure; **LBP:** Low Blood Pressure).

In transcranial doppler studies (Caamaño, 1994; Pichel, 1997), our group demostrated that in SD there is a general brain hypoperfusion from the beginning of the disease, independent of the dementia type and the APOE genotype, and that this hemodynamic pattern is more evident in advanced stages of the disease.

The lack of association between the APOE genotype and BP levels in SD reported in this paper is in agreement with the results obtained by de Knijff et al. (1994) when evaluating the influence of the APOE phenotype and BP in an unselected population.

The absence of any relationship between the presence or absence of the allele ε4 and any APOE genotype and BP levels in SD observed suggest that the HBP present is not determined by apolipoprotein-E in these patients. As it was reported in nondemented patients, our results support the idea that other different genetic factors might be associated with HBP in senile dementia.

REFERENCES

Applegate, W.O., 1989, Preface, Hypertension. *Clin. Geriatr. Med* 5:xi

American Psychiatric Association, 1994, Diagnostic and Statistical Manual of Mental Disorders. *4th ed.*, Washington, D.C.

Beyer, K., Lao, J.I., Alvarez ,X.A., Cacabelos, R., 1996, Different implications of APOE E4 in Alzheimer's disease and vascular dementia in the Spanish population. *Alzheimer's Res.* 2:215–220.

Basun, H., Grut, M., Winblad, B., Lannfelt, L, 1995, Apolipoprotein E4 allele and disease progression in patients with late-onset Alzheimer's disease. *Neurosci. Lett.* 183:32–34.

Caamaño J., Gómez, M.J., Vinagre, D., Franco-Maside, A., Cacabelos, R., 1994, Trancranial doppler ultrasonography in senile dementia. *Drugs of Today* 30:283–293.

Cacabelos, R., 1995, Alzheimer's disease: Etiopathogenic factors. *Neurogerontol. Neuorgeriat.* 1:299–328.

Davignon, J., Gregg, R.E., Sing, C.F., 1988, Apolipoprotein E polymorphism and atherosclerosis. *Arteriosclerosis* 8:1–21.

de Knijff, P., Boomsma, D.I., Feskens, E.J.M, Jespersen, J., Johansen, L.G., Kluft, C., Kromhout, D., Haevekes, L.,1994, Apolipoprotein E phenotype and blood pressure. *Lancet* 343:1234–5.

Guo, Z., Viitanen, M., Fatiglioni, L., Winblad, B., 1996, Low blood pressure and dementia in elderly people: the Kungsholmen project. *B.M.J.* 312:805–8.

Joint National Committee on Detection, Evaluation, and Treatment of High Blood Pressure, 1988. *Arch. Intern.Med.* 148:1023.

Mc Khann, G., Drachman, D., Folstein, M., Katzman, R., Price, D., Stadlan, E.M., 1984, Clinical diagnosis of Alzheimer's disease: Report of the NINCDS-ADRDA work group under the auspices of departament of health and human services task force on Alzheimer's disease. *Neurology* 34:939–44.

Pichel, V.M., Caamaño, J.M., Sellers, A., Mouzo, R., Alvarez, X.A., Perez, P., Laredo, M., Alcaraz, M., Lao, J.I., Beyer, K., Cacabelos, R., 1997, Changes in cerebral blood flow associated with disease staging and APOE genotyping in patients with senile dementia. In: *Progress in Alzheimer's and Parkinson's Diseases.* NewYork, in press

Saunders, A.M., Strittmatter, W.J., Schmeche,l D., 1993, Association of apolipoprotein E allele E4 with late onset familial and sporadic Alzheimer's disease. *Neurology* 43:1467–1472.

Sokoog, I., 1994, Risk factors for vascular dementia: A review. *Dementia.* 5:137–144.

Sokoog, I., Lernfelt, B., Landahl, S., Palmertz, B., Andreasson, L., Nilsson, L., Persson, G., Odén, A., Svanborg, A., 1996, 15-year longitudinal study of bood pressure and dementia. *Lancet* 347:1141- 1145.

Stoppe, G., Staed, J., Bruhn, H., 1995, Patchty changes in white matter in cranial computerized and magnetic resonance tomography-significance for diferential diagnosis of dementia of the Alzheimer type and vascular dementia. *Fortschr. Neurol. Psyciatr.* (11) 63:425–40.

Strandgaard, S., Paulson, O.B., 1997, Cererobrascular consequences of hypertension. *Lancet* 344:519–21.

Uterman, G., Jaeschke, M., Menzel, J., 1975, Familial hyperlipoproteinemia type III. Deficiency of a specific apoliporpotein (apo EIII) in the very low density lipoproteins. *FEBS Lett.* 56:352–5.

Uusitupa, M., Sarkkinen, E., Kervinen, K., Kesaniemi, Y., 1994, Apolipoprotein E phenotype and blood pressure. *Lancet* 343:57.

WHO Expert Committee Report, 1980, Arterial Hypertension, *Technical Report Series 628. World Health Organization.*

Working Group on Risk and High Blood Pressure. 1985, *Hypertension* 7:641.

115

APOLIPOPROTEIN E (ApoE) PHENOTYPE IN ALZHEIMER'S DISEASE, VASCULAR DEMENTIA AND PARKINSON'S DISEASE WITH AND WITHOUT DEMENTIA IN NORTHERN IRELAND

Cathal J. Foy,[1] Anthony P. Passmore,[1] Djamil M. Vahidassr,[1] Ian S. Young,[2] Michael Smye,[2] and John T. Lawson[3]

[1]Department of Geriatric Medicine
The Queen's University of Belfast
Whitla Medical Building
97 Lisburn Road
Belfast BT9 7BL
[2]Department of Clinical Chemistry
Royal Victoria Hospital
Grosvenor Road
Belfast BT12 6BA
[3]Department of Radiology
Belfast City Hospital
Lisburn Road
Belfast BT9 7AB

INTRODUCTION

Apolipoprotein E (Apo E) is important in the transport of lipid to and from the liver and peripheral tissues. The three Apo E phenotypes have been shown to have different lipid transporting characteristics, E2 being the most efficient and E4 being the least efficient. E3 is the ancestral isoform and has transporting characteristics intermediate to E2 and E4 (reviewed by Mahley, 1988). Apo E also has important roles in the repair and re-modelling of central neurones by facilitating the transport of lipid to damaged and repairing cells. Lipid is closely related to neurological tissue; myelin is mainly composed of lipid, and phospholipid and cholesterol are major components of neuronal membranes.

Progress in Alzheimer's and Parkinson's Diseases
edited by Fisher *et al.*, Plenum Press, New York, 1998.

It has been hypothesised that E4 causes inefficient lipid transport to and from central cells analogous to its transport characteristics in the peripheral circulation. Thus the ability of neurones to repair and remodel cell membranes and myelin sheaths may be compromised in those individuals with one or more copies of E4 (the neuronal repair hypothesis). The generation of neuronal synapses also requires an adequate supply of lipid and therefore may also be restricted in those with the Apo E4 phenotype. It has been shown in post mortem studies that cognitively intact elderly people, despite age related neurone loss, have synaptic densities similar to young deceased. Alzheimer's brains show neuronal loss and decreased synaptic density (for reviews see Poirier, 1994 and Ignatius, 1994).

A clear association of Apo E4 with Alzheimer's Disease (AD) has been established in a number of populations (Saunders et al., 1993a; Van Duijin et al., 1994; Dai et al., 1994) Less clear associations with other dementias and neurological diseases have been reported (Frisoni et al., 1994; Arai et al., 1994; Benjamin et al., 1994; Pickering Brown et al., 1994). However no association with the closely related disorder PD without dementia has been observed.

We wished to test the association of Apo E4 with AD in a Northern Ireland population and establish if an association exists with Vascular dementia (VaD) and Parkinson's Disease with dementia (P Dem) and Parkinson's Disease without dementia (PD). Such an relationship would increase evidence for the neuronal repair hypothesis and demonstrates that this phenotype has important implications in other central nervous system diseases.

METHODS

All subjects were recruited and screened by the same physician. Subjects were resident in Northern Ireland and belonged to the ethnic population. Written informed consent was obtained from subjects and carers prior to inclusion in the study and the study had gained approval from the local ethics committee prior to recruitment. Dementia patients were assessed using a structured interview and examination that included the Folstein Mini Mental State Examination (MMSE) (Folstein et al., 1975), Geriatric Depression Scale, (Yesavage, 1988) Barthel index of activities of daily living (Mahoney 1965) and the Hachinski Ischaemic Scale (Hachinski et al., 1974). A blood screen for systemic causes of dementia, analysed and CT scan of brain performed. Data collected conformed to the recommended minimum required for research studies on AD (Wilcock et al., 1989). Diagnoses were made as probable AD and probable VaD according to the DSM IV and NINCDS ADRDA (McKhann et al., 1984), and AIREN (Roman et al., 1993) criteria respectively. Patients with mixed and other forms of dementia, except P Dem were excluded.

PD patients were classified as PD with and without dementia. Those with concomitant disease and or atypical features were excluded. A diagnosis of PD was made in accordance with the UKPDSBB criteria (Gibb and Lees, 1988) and dementia was established by MMSE and DSM III R criteria. A second younger control group was used to age and sex match the PD without dementia group as these subjects were significantly younger than those with dementia.

Blood samples were collected and serum separated and stored at -70°C for subsequent analyses. Apo E phenotyping was determined by agarose gel electrofocusing combined with immunoblotting as described by McDowell et al. (1989).

The resulting Apo E phenotype distributions within subject groups were described as phenotype frequencies. A chi squared test was used to test statistical significance in both studies. Significance was accepted at the 5% level.

Table 1. Summary descriptions of dementia and control populations

	n	Male	Female	Median age	Age quartile	Minimum age	Maximum age
Controls	59	26	33	74	69-80	58	92
AD	78	29	49	79	72-83	55	90
VaD	37	18	19	79	69-85	55	90
P Dem	18	8	10	72	67-84	55	90

RESULTS

Dementia, Parkinson's and control populations are described in Tables 1 and 3. Numbers of resulting phenotypes varied slightly from these as small numbers of samples deteriorated during laboratory processing. There were no significant differences with respect to age between dementia and control groups and PD and controls groups. Apo E phenotype distributions are described in Tables 2 and 4, and in Figures 1 and 2. Significant differences in phenotype distribution were observed between dementia and control groups $p<0.05$ (Table 2 and Figure 1). There were no significant differences between PD and controls $p=0.886$ (Table 4 and Figure 2). The most marked difference in Apo E distribution, was an increase in E4 frequency in AD. E4 frequency was more than double that of the control population (124% increase). E4 was also over represented, but to a lesser degree, in VaD and P Dem, approximately 60% increased in each group compared to controls. E2 was equally reduced in all dementia groups and was half of the control frequency. Apo E phenotype distribution in PD was similar to that of the control population.

DISCUSSION

Previous studies have demonstrated a strong association of E4 with AD in different populations (Saunders et al, 1993a; Van Duijin et al., 1994; Poirer et al., 1993; Dai et al., 1994). A possible association of E4 with VaD has been reported by Frisoni *et al*, (1994) and a less strong associations with Lewy body dementia and PD with dementia have been reported by Arai et al., (1994), Benjamin *et al.*, (1994) and Pickering Brown et al., (1994). E2 has also been reported to have a possible protective effect against the development of AD (Talbot et al., 1994, Hardy et al., 1995).

The association of E4 with AD and other dementia syndromes has not been investigated in a Northern Irish population prior to the present study. Apo E phenotype or geno-

Table 2. Apo E phenotype frequencies dementias
and controls

	n	E2	E3	E4
Controls	55	.06	.76	.17
AD	73	.03	.59	.38
VaD	35	.03	.70	.27
P Dem	18	.03	.69	.28

$\chi^2 = 14.140$, Degrees of Freedom = 6, P= 0.029.
(As 3 cells have expected counts less than 5.0, chi-squared test
should be interpreted with discretion)

Table 3. Summary descriptions of PD without dementia and control populations

	n	Male	Female	Median age	Age quartile	Minimum age	Maximum age
Controls	40	25	16	67	59-74	29	88
PD	40	25	16	67	61-74	32	88

Table 4. Apo E phenotype frequencies PD and controls

	n	E2	E3	E4
Controls	40	.06	.75	.19
PD	40	.08	.76	.16

$\chi^2 = 0.242$, Degrees of Freedom = 2, P = 0.886

type distribution in Northern Ireland is of particular interest as few immigrants have settled in this area over the last century. Therefore this population represents an opportunity to study Apo E polymorphism in an almost pure European Caucasian race. Findings may be contrasted with other European studies and with other races.

The strong association with AD was demonstrated in our population and less strong associations with the other 2 dementia syndromes were also observed. E2 was noted to be equally reduced in all dementia groups and this may indicate that the presence of E2 confers the same degree of protection from each of the three dementias studied.

The observed associations of E4 with VaD and P Dem provides increased evidence for associations with other neurological disease and also suggests a role for the E4 in the common pathogenesis of dementia. It may be that E4 acts in synergism with central neuronal injury from a variety of pathologies to potentiate their injurious effects on cognitive function. Frisoni et al., (1994) hypothesised that different insults, whether vascular or degenerative, may result in greater damage when E4 is present. Alberts et al., (1995) observed that after haemorrhagic stroke, the functional and neurological outcome in subjects

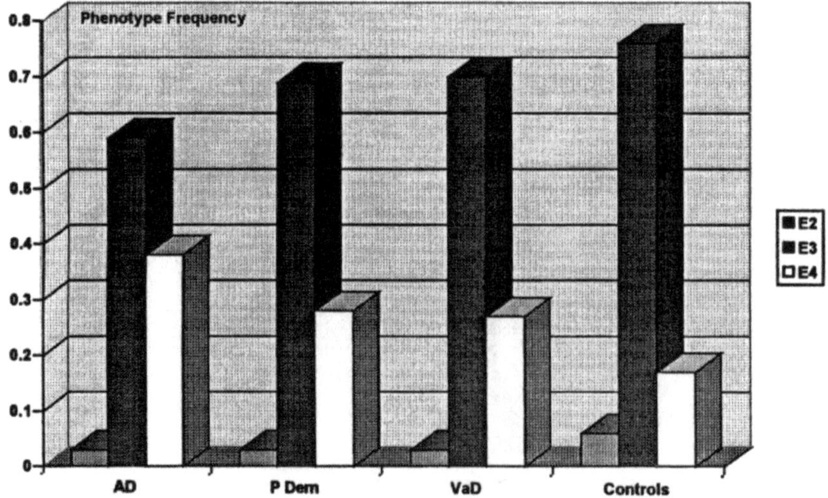

Figure 1. Frequency distribution of Apo E phenotypes in dementias and age matched controls.

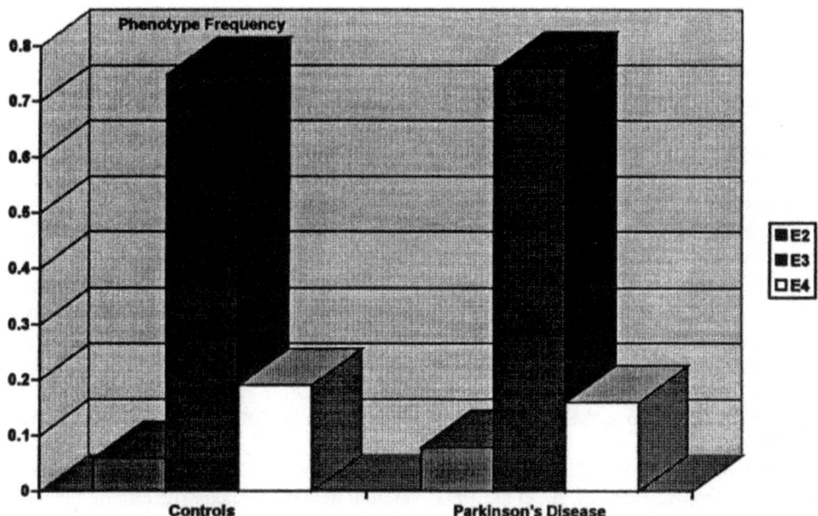

Figure 2. Frequency distribution of Apo E phenotypes in Parkinson's Disease and age matched controls.

with the Apo E4 allele (ε4) was worse and survival reduced compared to with subjects without the ε4 and suggested that stroke is more harmful in carriers of this gene. E4 may cause inefficient central lipid transport necessary to repair neurones and is analogous to the defect in peripheral lipid transport associated with this phenotype (Poirier, 1994). Evidence against the neuronal repair hypothesis is provided by those studies where there was no association of E4 with other neurological disease. In the present study no association with PD without dementia was found. The neuronal repair hypothesis would suggest that E4 should potentiate most central neurological diseases through a generalised central lipid transport inefficiency to all parts of the brain. However it appears that those neuronal diseases associated with dementia syndromes are specifically potentiated and there may be a further factor or factors, as yet undiscovered, responsible for this relationship.

REFERENCES

Alberts, M. J., Graffagnino, C., Delong, D., Strittmatter, W., Saunders, A. M, Roses, A. D., 1995, Apo E genotype and survival from intracerebral haemorrage. *Lancet.* 346:575.

Arai, H., Muramatsu, T., Higuchi, S., Sasaki, H., Trojanowski, J. Q., 1994, Apolipoprotein E gene in Parkinson's disease with or without dementia. *Lancet* 344:889.

Benjamin, R., Leake, A., Edwardson, J. A., McKeith, I. G., Ince, P. G., Perry, R. H., Morris, C. M., 1994, Apolipoprotein E genes in Lewy body and Parkinson's disease. *Lancet* 18 343:1565.

Dai, X. Y., Nanko, S., Hattori, M., Fukuda, R., Nagata, K., Isse, K., Ueki, A., Kazamatsuri, H, 1994, Association of apolipoprotein E4 with sporadic Alzheimer's disease is more pronounced in early onset type. *Neurosci. Lett.* 175:74–6.

Gibb, W. R., Lees, A. J., 1988, The relevance of the Lewy body to the pathogenesis of idiopathic Parkinson's disease. *J. Neurol. Neurosurg. Psychiat.* 51:745–52.

Folstein, M. F., Folstein, S. E., McHugh, P. R., 1975, "Mini-mental state". A practical method for grading the cognitive state of patients for the clinician. *J. Psychiat. Res.* 12:189–98.

Frisoni, G. B., Calabresi, L., Geroldi, C., Bianchetti, A., D'Acquarica, A. L., Govoni, S., Sirtori, C. R., Trabucchi, M., Franceschini, G., 1994, Apolipoprotein E epsilon 4 allele in Alzheimer's disease and vascular dementia. *Dementia* 5:240–2.

Hachinski, V. C., Lassen, N. A., Marshall, J., 1974, Multi-infarct dementia. A cause of mental deterioration in the elderly. *Lancet* 27(874):207–10.

Hardy, J., 1995, Apolipoprotein E in the genetics and epidemiology of Alzheimer's disease. *Amer. J. Med. Genetics* 60:456–60.

Ignatius, M. J., Gebicke-Haerter, P. J., Pitas, R. E., Shooter, E. M., 1987, Apolipoprotein E in nerve injury and repair. *Prog. Brain Res.* 71:177–84.

Mahley, R. W., 1988, Apolipoprotein E: cholesterol transport protein with expanding role in cell biology. *Science* 29:622–30.

Mahoney, F. I., Barthel, D. W., 1965, Functional evaluation: Barthel Index, *Maryland State Med..J.* 14:61–5.

McDowell, I. F., Wisdom, G. B., Trimble, E. R., 1989, Apolipoprotein E phenotype determined by agarose gel electrofocusing and immunoblotting. *Clin. Chem.* 35:2070–3.

McKhann, G., Drachman, D., Folstein, M., Katzman, R., Price, D., Stadlan, E. M., 1984, Clinical diagnosis of Alzheimer's disease: report of the NINCDS-ADRDA Work Group under the auspices of Department of Health and Human Services Task Force on Alzheimer's Disease. *Neurol.* 34:939–44.

Poirier, J., 1994, Apolipoprotein E in animal models of CNS injury and in Alzheimer's disease. *Trends in Neurosci.* 17:525–30.

Rea, I. M., McDowell, I. F., Smye, M., et al., 1995, Apolipoprotein E alleles in nonagenarian subjects. Abstract, *Atherosclerosis* 112:261.

Roman, G. C., Tatemichi, T. K., Erkinjuntti, T., Cummings, J. L., Masdeu, J. C., Garcia, J. H., Amaducci, L., Orgogozo, J. M., Brun, A., Hofman, A., et al., 1993, Vascular dementia: diagnostic criteria for research studies. Report of the NINDS-AIREN International Workshop. *Neurolology* 43:250–60.

Saunders, A. M., Strittmatter, W. J., Schmechel, D., George-Hyslop, P. H., Pericak-Vance, M. A., Joo. S. H., Rosi, B. L., Gusella, J. F., Crapper-MacLachlan, D. R., Alberts, M. J., et al., 1993a, Association of apolipoprotein E allele epsilon 4 with late-onset familial and sporadic Alzheimer's disease. *Neurology* 43:1467–72.

Saunders, A. M., Schmader, K., Breitner, J. C., Benson, M. D., Brown, W. T., Goldfarb, L., Goldgaber, D., Manwaring, M. G., Szymanski, M. H., McCown, N., et al., 1993b, Apolipoprotein E epsilon 4 allele distributions in late-onset Alzheimer's disease and in other amyloid-forming diseases. *Lancet* 342:710–1.

Schachter, F., Faure-Delanef, L., Guenot, F., Rouger, H., Froguel, P., Lesueur-Ginot, L., Cohen, D., 1994, Genetic associations with human longevity at the APOE and ACE loci. *Nature Genetics* 6:29–32.

Talbot, C., Lendon, C., Craddock, N., Shears, S., Morris, J. C., Goate, A., 1994, Protection against Alzheimer's disease with apoE epsilon 2. *Lancet* 343:1432–1433.

Van Duijn, C. M., de Knijff, P., Cruts, M., Wehnert, A., Havekes, L. M., Hofman, A., Van Broeckhoven, C., 1994, Apolipoprotein E4 allele in a population-based study of early-onset Alzheimer's disease. *Nature Genetics* 7:74–8.

Wilcock, G. K., Hope, R. A., Brooks, D. N., Lantos, P. L., Oppenheimer, C., Reynolds, G. P., Rossor. M. N., Davies, M. B., 1989, Recommended minimum data to be collected in research studies on Alzheimer's disease. The MRC(UK) Alzheimer's Disease Workshop Steering Committee. *J. Neurol. Neurosur. Psychiat.* 52:693–700.

Yesavage, J. A., 1988, Geriatric Depression Scale. *Psychopharmacol. Bull.* 24:709–11.

116

CHANGES IN CEREBRAL BLOOD FLOW ASSOCIATED WITH DISEASE STAGING AND APOE GENOTYPING IN PATIENTS WITH SENILE DEMENTIA

V. M. Pichel, J. M. Caamaño, A. Sellers, R. Mouzo, X. A. Alvarez, P. Pérez, M. Laredo, and R. Cacabelos

EuroEspes Biomedical Research Center
15166 Bergondo
A Coruña, Spain

INTRODUCTION

Senile Dementia (SD) represents a problem of growing interest because of its increased prevalence in occidental countries. At present the prevalence of SD is about ten times higher than that detected at the beginning of this century (Cacabelos, 1991), and it is expected that the number of people with severe dementia will increase aproximately 60% in the next decade (Mortimer et al., 1985).

Cerebral vascular blood flow dysfunctions have been reported in patients with Alzheimer's disease (AD) and vascular dementia (VD) (Ries et al., 1993; Caamaño et al., 1993, Sattel et al., 1996). Decreased blood flow velocities in the middle cerebral arteries (MCA) were found in both types of dementia, whereas peripheral vascular resistances are significantly higher in VD than in AD. Recent studies also showed an association between late-onset and sporadic AD cases and the presence of the allele e4 of the Apolipoprotein E gene (APOE), and we have documented an increased prevalence of the of the APOE4 in VD patients as well (Beyer et al., 1996). On the other hand, the involvement of APOE on atherosclerosis and cardiovascular disease is well established (Uusitupa et al., 1994; de Knijff et al., 1994). Relevant factors involved in the ethiopathogenesis of cerebrovascular disease include: 1) high blood pressure; 2) cardiac dysfunctions; 3) occlusive extracranial carotid diseases; 4) intracranial carotid disorders; and 5) vascular risk factors such as hypercholesterolemia, hyperglycemia and hemorheological disorders (Forete et al., 1991; Philips et al., 1992; Mendel et al., 1992). So, since cardiovascular alterations play a very important role in the development of the different types of dementia, especially in vascu-

Table 1. Brain hemodynamic parameters in SD according to disease staging

Parameters	Side	Controls	SD	GDS 3	GDS 4	GDS 5	GDS 6
Mv cm/sec.	Right	51.3±16.1	39.49±11.66**	40.1±9.6**	39.1±11.3	39.4±13.6	37.4±14.0
	Left	51.8±13.8	40.17±12.38**	41.0±11.1*#	42.8±14.4#	41.4±13.6#	32.3±5.9
Sv cm/sec.	Right	73.4±22.7	62.95±17.70	64.3±14.6	64.2±19.8	61.4±19.3	58.4±19.4
	Left	75.2±19.7	64.76±18.72	66.2±18.2#	71.4±21.9#	65.3±18.2#	51.8±8.3
Dv cm/sec.	Right	35.7±12.6	24.35±8.08**	24.5±7.0**	23.4±7.4	25.3±10.1	22.9±8.0
	Left	35.5±10.0	25.16±9.11**	24.9±7.5**	27.2±11.2#	26.6±10.1	20.2±5.0
EPR	Right	13.7±7.8	0.89±8.51**	0.3±7.8**	−1.6±9.0	3.3±9.8	1.9±6.3
	Left	12.2±7.7	1.03±8.20**	0.2±7.9**	0.7±8.9	2.6±9.3	0.8±5.4
Age		62.3±9			73.5±8.2		
N		13	93	30	22	19	12

*p<0.05 vs Controls
**p<0.01 vs Controls
#p<0.05 vs GDS 6

lar dementia (Cacabelos, 1991), it is expected that some APOE genotypes might be associated with cerebrovascular deficits in SD. To date, however, there are no studies evaluating the possible influence of the APOE genotype in the cerebrovascular dysfunction observed in senile dementia. In this work we investigated changes in cerebral blood flow parameters (Mv, Sv, Dv, and EPR), according to the disease stage and the APOE genotype in senile dementia patients.

PATIENTS AND METHODS

Ninety three patients affected with Senile Dementia (SD; age=73.5±8.2) and thirteen control subjects (C; age=62.3±9.3) were included in the study (Table 1). The diagnosis of SD was carried out according to the NINCDS-ADRDA (Mac Kann et al., 1984) and DSM-IV criteria (American Psychiatric Association, 1994) . All subjects were submitted to the same research protocol: physical examination, EEG and/or brain mapping, EKG, laboratory tests, monitorization of biological parameters, neuroimaging (CT-Scan) and TCD study.

Transcraneal Doppler Ultrasonography (TCD) is a non-invasive technique used for measuring blood flow parameters (Mv, Sv, Dv,and EPR) in the Circle of Willis, which allows for the follow-up of several cerebrovascular risk factors (Aaslid et al.,1982; Arnolds et al., 1986). TCD examination was undertaken by a multifrequency Transcraneal Doppler Ultrasound TC-2000S (Eden Medical Electronics, Uberlinguen, Germany) with automatic data processing. This machine uses pulsatile ultrasound waves at a 2MHz frequency with a cylindrical probe and a beam aperture of 15mm.

TCD recordings were obtained with the patient laying in a supine position and in somatosensory rest, approaching the artery thru the temporal window. The vessel identification criteria we use are: 1) blood flow velocities; 2) depth of insonation; 3) physiological direction of the blood flow; 4) wave form; 5) insonation angle; and 6) window used (Hennerici et al., 1987; Russo et al., 1986). To identify the MCA a 2MHz probe was positioned over both temporal regions with an insonation depth between 46 and 58 mm, and the blood flow direction towards the probe. To obtain the hemodynamic parameters in the extracraneal carotid territory we used a 4MHz probe. No carotid compressions were performed to avoid any possible cerebrovascular risks. Mv, Sv, Dv, and EPR were the brain hemodynamic parameters studied (Gosling et al., 1974; Pourcelot, 1974).

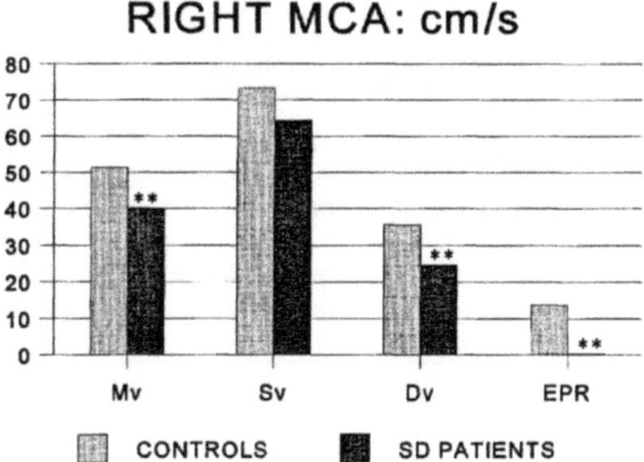

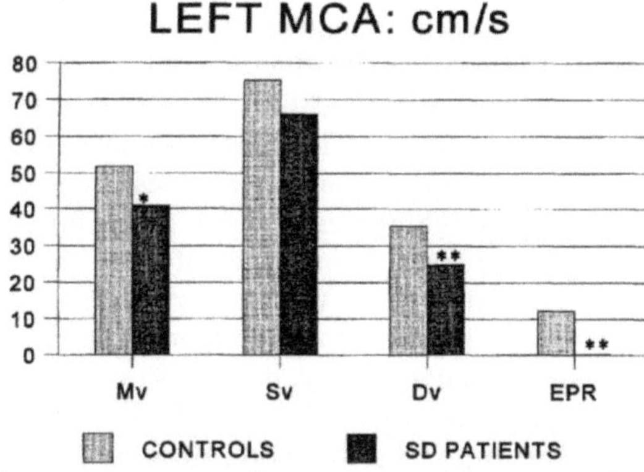

Figure 1. Brain Hemodynamic parameters in the right and left MCA in control subjects and in patients with mild SD (GDS 3). *P<0.05 vs controls; **P<0.01 vs controls.

RESULTS

Scores in brain hemodynamic parameters were lower in patients with SD than in control subjects in the right [Mv (cm/s): SD=39.49±11.66**, C=51.3±16.1; Sv (cm/s): SD=62.95±17.70; C=73.4±22.7, Dv(cm/s): SD=24.35±8.08**, C=35.7±12.6; EPR (cm/s): SD=0.89±8.51**; C=13.7±7.8;**p<0.01 vs C] and left [Mv (cm/s): SD=40.17±12.38**, C=51.8±13.8; Sv(cm/s): DS=64.7±18.72, C=75.2+19.7; Dv (cm/s): SD=25.16±9.11**, C=35.5+10.0; EPR(cm/s): SD=1.03±8.20**, C=12.2±7.7; **p<0.01 vs C] MCA (Table 1). These differences between SD patients and controls were observed from the initial disease stage (GDS=3) in both right [Mv=40.1±9.6**; Sv=64.3±14.6; Dv=24.5±7.0**; EPR=0.3±7.8**;**p<0.01 vs C] and left [Mv=41.0±11.1*; Sv=66.2±18.2; Dv=24.9±7.5**; EPR=0.2±7.9**; *p<0.05 & **p<0.01 vs C] MCA (Figure 1). Decreased blood flow velocities were also observed in the left MCA of patients with severe dementia (GDS=6) as compared with mild to moderate SD cases (GDS=3–5) (Table 1). Although no significant differences were found in cerebrovascular parameters when analyzed as a function of the ApoE genotype, a clear trend to a worse cerebral perfusion was observed in patients with APOE3/4 in comparison with APOE 3/3 carriers (Table 2).

Table 2. Brain hemodynamic parameters in SD according to APOE Genotype

APOE	N	Mv	Sv	Dv	EPR
Right middle cerebral artery					
4-4	15	42.48 ± 8.94	65.04 ± 11.0	26.90 ± 6.15	4.34 ± 7.39
3-4	25	39.20 ± 13.47	63.56 ± 19.18	24.13 ± 9.91	−0.23 ± 9.15
3-3	28	45.63 ± 14.50	70.43 ± 21.74	29.17 ± 10.89	4.37 ± 11.33
Left middle cerebral artery					
4-4	15	40.02 ± 7.72	62.38 ± 10.01	25.36 ± 6.73	2.99 ± 8.17
3-4	25	42.24 ± 15.39	68.29 ± 24.00	26.42 ± 11.98	0.37 ± 8.31
3-3	28	45.10 ± 14.98	71.64 ± 20.22	29.40 ± 10.42	4.28 ± 10.73

CONCLUSIONS

The present results showing that hemodynamic parameters are similar in patients with distinct APOE genotypes seem to indicate that cerebrovascular dysfunction observed in senile dementia patients is not associated with ApoE variants. However, a tendency for lower cerebral blood flow velocities and EPR values is observed in patients with the APOE Genotype 3/4. These results are concordant with increased prevalence of the APOE genotype 3/4 in subjects with carotid atheroma plaques (Venarucci et al., 1996), and suggest that this APOE genotype might represent a risk factor for cerebrovascular alterations. Finally, we cannot exclude the possible influence of other genetic factors on brain perfusion deficits in SD. In agrement with previous reports (Ries et al., 1993; Caamaño et al., 1993), we found that there is a general brain hypoperfusion in SD patients as compared to age-matched control subjects. Interestingly, deficits in cerebral blood flow are observed from the early stages of the disease (GDS = 3), which indicates that TCD examination might be of diagnostic value in SD. Furthermore, since blood flow values in the left MCA are significantly lower in advanced disease stages (GDS = 6) than in the early ones (GDS = 3–5), TCD appears to be also useful in evaluating the progession in SD patients. In summary, our results show that there is a general brain hypoperfusion pattern in SD patients from the beginning of the disease not significantly related to the APOE genotype, this pattern being more pronounced in advanced disease stages. Therefore, we conclude that TCD is a useful tool for the monitoring of cerebrovascular functioning in SD, constituting a valuable help in the diagnosis and follow-up of the disease.

REFERENCES

Aaslid, R., Markwalder, T., and Normes, H., 1982, Non-Invasive Transcranial Doppler Ultrasound recording of flow velocity in basal cerebral arteries. *J. Neurosurg.* 57:769–774.

American Psychiatric Association, 1994, Diagnostic and Statistical Manual of Mental Disorders. 4th edition. DSM IV. Am. Psychiatric Assoc., Washington, DC.

Arnolds, B.J., and Von Rautenberg, W., 1986, Trancranial Doppler Ultrasonography. Examination Technique and normal reference values. *Ultrasound Med. Biol.* 12 :115–123.

Beyer, K., Lao, J.I., Álvarez, X.A., and Cacabelos, R., 1996, Different implications of ApoE, ε4 in Alzheimer's disease and vascular dementia in the Spanish population. *Alzheimer's Res. 2.*

Caamaño, J., Gómez, M.J., and Cacabelos, R., 1993, Transcranial Doppler Ultrasonography in senile dementia: Neuropsychological correlations. *Meth. Find. Exp. Clin. Pharmacol.* 15 (3):93–199.

Cacabelos, R., ed, 1991, Alzheimer's disease. Prous Science Publishers, Barcelona.

de Knijff, P., Boomsma, D.I., Feskens, E.J.M., Jespersen, J, Johansen, L.G., Kluft, C., Kromhout, D., and Haevekes, L., 1994, Apolipoprotein E and blood pressure. *Lancet* 343:1234–5.

Forete, F., and Boller, F., 1991, Hypertension and the risk of dementia in the elderly. *Am.. J. Med.* 90:145–195.

Hennerici, M., Rautenberg, W., Sitzer, G., and Schwartz, A., 1987, Transcranial Doppler Ultrasound for the assessment of intracranial arterial flow velocity part 1. Examination technique and normal values. *Surg. Neurol.* 27:439–448.

Mac Kann, G., Drachman, D., Folstein, M., Cathman, R., Price, D., and Stadland, E.M., 1984, Clinical diagnosis of Alzheimer's disease: Report of NINCDS-ADRDA work group. *Neurology* 34:939–944.

Mendel, T., Jura, E., Mizgalska, J., and Zambrowska, A., 1992, Demostration of cardiac arrhythmias in multi-infarct dementia and ischemic stroke using Holter monitoring. *Neurol. Neurochir. Pol.* 26:605–611.

Mortimer, J.A., and Hutton, J.T., 1985, Epidemiology and ethiology of Alzheimer's disease. Senile dementia of the Alzheimer type. Hutton, J.T., Kenny, A.D., eds,. Alan R. Liss, New York.

Philips, S.J., and Whisnant, J.P., 1992, Hypertension and the brain. The National High Blood Pressure Education Program. *Arch. Intern. Med.* 152:938–945.

Poucelot, L., 1974, Applications cliniques de L'Examen Doppler Transcrânien. Les colloques de L'institut National de la Santé et de la Recherché Médicale. *INSERM* 21.

Ries, F., Horn, R., Hillecamp, J., Honisch, C., König, M., and Solimosi, L., 1993, Differentiation of multi-infarct and Alzheimer's dementia by intracranial hemodynamic parameters. *Stroke* 24:28–235.

Russo, G., Profeta, G., Acampora, S., and Troisi, F., 1974, Transcranial Doppler Sonography. Examination Gosling RG, King DH. In: Cardiovascular aplications of ultrasound, Reneman, R.E., ed, North Holland, Amsterdam, pp. 266–282.

Sattel, H., Fâorstl, H., Biedert, S., 1996, Senile dementia of Alzheimer's type and multi-infarct dementia investigated by transcraneal doppler sonography. *Dementia* 7:41–46.

Uusitupa, M., Sarkkinen, E., Kervinen, K., and AnteroKesaniemi, Y., 1994, Apolipoprotein E phenotype and blood pressure. *Lancet* 343:357.

Venarucci, B., Venarucci, V., Casado, A., and De la Torre, R., 1996, Atheroma plaque and APOE alleles. *Minerva Cardioangiol.* 44:1–2, 15–18.

APOLIPOPROTEIN E ε4 ALLELE DOES NOT INFLUENCE THE DEVELOPMENT OF DEMENTIA IN PARKINSONIAN PATIENTS

D. Paleacu,[1] R. Inzelberg,[2] J. Chapman,[1] E. Orlov,[1] A. Asherov,[1] and A. D. Korczyn[1]

[1]Department of Neurology
Tel Aviv Medical Center
Sackler Faculty of Medicine
Tel Aviv University
Ramat-Aviv, Israel
[2]Department of Neurology
Hillel Yaffe Medical Center
Hadera, Israel

INTRODUCTION

James Parkinson in 1817 in his famous Essay on the Shaking Palsy described the "involuntary tremulous motion, with lessened muscular power, in parts not in action and even when supported; with a propensity to bend the trunk forwards, and to pass from a walking to a running pace: the senses and intellects being uninjured" (Parkinson, 1817). Indeed the possibility that PD is associated with dementia has been negated by neurologists for several decades. It should be mentioned that antedating levodopa therapy patients could not be formally cognitively tested because of their motor disability, bradyphrenia and speech impairment. There was also a tendency to attribute dementia in old age (and the great majority of PD patients are aged) to concurrent "senility" or "cerebral aterosclerosis". Once levodopa and dopa-agonist therapy was instituted this situation, surprisingly, did not change and the impression emerged that dementia is common in PD, more so in patients with advanced PD (Korczyn et al., 1986). Since then, overwhelming proof has accumulated that PD is accompanied by dementia in at least 20% of the cases. The debate over the issue of coincidental AD in demented PD patients is still not entirely resolved since some of the clinical and pathological features of the two dementias are similar.

The apolipoprotein E (APO E) ε4 allele has been associated with increased prevalence of AD in the general population (Corder et al., 1993; Saunders et al., 1993; Roses et

Progress in Alzheimer's and Parkinson's Diseases
edited by Fisher *et al.*, Plenum Press, New York, 1998.

al., 1996). A number of previous studies (Koller et al., 1995; Marder et al., 1994) including our own (Inzelberg et al., 1997) have not found an association of APO E ε4 alleles with the dementia of PD. Since all these studies were retrospective there is still a possibility that selection biases, such as the diagnosis of parkinsonian dementia as being dementia with extrapyramidal signs, obscured an effect of APO E ε4. We therefore addressed this issue by a prospective study which examined the effect of APO E ε4 alleles on the incidence of dementia in PD patients.

SUBJECTS AND METHODS

Among 125 consecutive PD patients examined at the Parkinson's Disease Outpatient Clinic of the Tel Aviv Medical Center in 1994, 78 patients who were not demented at the time of their first visit were followed up for a period of 21 months (December 1994-August 1996). An interview was conducted with the patient and a family member at each visit, at intervals 3 to 6 months apart. Besides the neurological examination a detailed inquiry about changes in the mental status and activities of daily living (ADL) and a Short Mental Test (SMT; Treves et al., 1990) of the patients was carried out during these visits. Subjects were classified as demented if they matched the DSM-IV criteria (American Psychiatric Association, 1994) for dementia.

All subjects had venous blood drawn in EDTA, and DNA was obtained from blood leukocytes by standard procedures. The relevant portion of the APO E gene was amplified by PCR using the method of Wenham et al., 1991. In order to identify ε4 alleles, PCR fragments were digested with the restriction enzyme Afl III (New England Biolabs). Cleavage of the PCR fragments from ε2 or ε3 alleles result in two fragments of 170 and 57 bp, in contrast to the (4 allele in which this site is absent and from which undigested 227 bp fragments were obtained. This method enables the identification of subjects who are heterozygous or homozygous for the (4 allele, as well as those not carrying one (Asherov et al., 1995).

Comparison of the proportion of patients carrying the ε4 allele in different groups was performed utilizing the chi-square test.

RESULTS

The average age of the patients who developed dementia (71.8±7.4 years) was not different from those who remained cognitively intact (71.6±8.2 years).

Of the 78 non demented patients, 33 patients were lost to follow up and 2 died during the observation period. Of the remaining 43, 16 (37.2%) became demented; of these, 4 (33.3%) had one ε4 allele (no individual was homozygous for ε4). Of the 27 patients with no ε4 allele a similar proportion of 12 (38.7%) developed dementia. There was no significant difference in the proportion of patients carrying the ε4 allele in the demented PD patients as compared to the non demented PD patients (χ^2 =0.45, p=0.5).

The PD patient allelic distribution is detailed in Figure 1.

DISCUSSION

Many similarities are shared between the dementia of PD and that of AD (Jellinger et al, 1986; Korczyn et al., 1986). For this latter it has been widely shown that the pres-

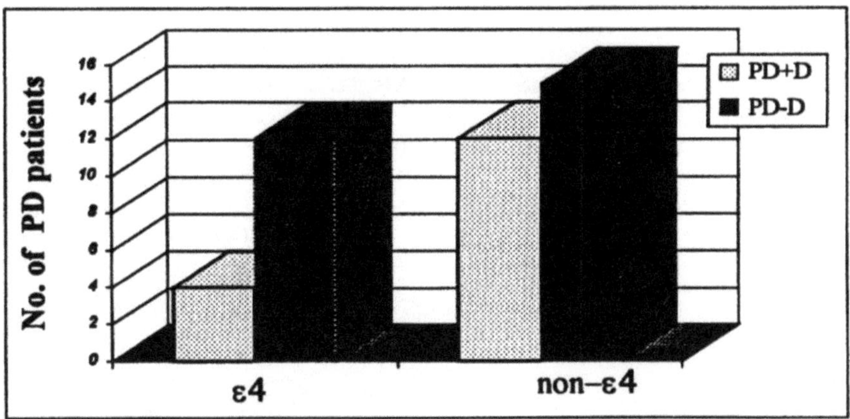

Figure 1. Allelic distribution of parkinsonian patients (PD+D = demented parkinsonian patients, PD-D = non-demented parkinsonian patients, ε4 = patients with one APOE ε4 allele, non-ε4 = patients with no ε4 allele).

ence of the ε4 allele represents a risk factor (Corder et al., 1993; Saunders et al., 1993; Roses et al., 1996). The ε4 allele of APO E has been associated with greater accumulation of β amyloid in the elderly with and without dementia (Povlikovsky et al., 1995). The age of onset of mental deterioration is influenced by the presence of APO E allele, but APO E genotype does not influence the rate of cognitive decline in AD (Growdon et al., 1996; Kurz et al., 1996; Plassman et al., 1996). Virtually all patients with Down syndrome have the neuropathological characteristics of AD by the age of 40. It has been shown that the age of onset of dementia in patients with Down syndrome too is influenced by the presence of the ε4 allele of APO E (Schupf et al., 1996). In PD dementia however, previous studies (Marder et al., 1994; Koller et al., 1995) including ours (Inzelberg et al., 1997) have shown that the frequency of the ε4 allele was not higher among demented PD patients. A meta-analysis of all previous studies raising the issue of APO E in PD has demonstrated that the presence of dementia was not correlated with the ε4 allele suggesting that these two occur independently from each other (Inzelberg et al., 1997). Indeed, the frequency of ε4 allele in our cohort was 10%, a figure which is similar to that found in epidemiological studies in Israel (Treves et al., 1996). The frequency of the ε4 allele was 16% among PD patients as a whole, while it was 17% among those without and 14 % among those with dementia (Rubinsztein et al., 1994).

Despite the fact that in a given PD population the ε4 allele does not occur more frequently among demented patients it is still possible that its presence influences the clinical course of dementia reflected by the age of onset and the rate of decline of cognitive functions upon time. This latter effect would then be reflected in a prospective study that aims at following periodically these patients. The present study verified this hypothesis and. our results indicate that APO E ε4 alleles do not influence the incidence of dementia in PD. The age of parkinsonian demented patients was not younger among the patients who carried the ε4 allele. These findings strongly suggest that the APO E allele is not correlated with the presence and time of occurrence of dementia in PD or its rate of progression. An observation that stands out in our cohort is the lack of homozygous patients among PD patients, as observed also by others (Rubinsztein et al., 1994; Growdon et al, 1996). This finding could possibly suggest that ε4 homozygosity being a risk factor for AD, leads to mental decline before the appearance of the extrapyramidal signs (Korczyn, 1995). The ε4 allele frquency has been studied in amyloid forming diseases other than AD and higher frequencies have been found in the Lewy body variant of AD and lower in diffuse Lewy body disease expressed as parkinsonism and mental deterioration (Benjamin et al., 1994; Galasco et al., 1994; Pickering-Brown et al., 1994). One can then observe that the highest correlation with APO E alleles occur in AD, followed by its Lewy body variant, while this latter expressed by parkinsonism and PD itself are not correlated with APO E. These observations suggest different pathogenetic mechanisms underlying AD and the dementia of PD.

REFERENCES

American Psychiatric Association, 1994, Diagnostic and Statistical Manual of Mental Disorders, 4th ed., Washigton D.C.

Asherov, A., Chapman, J., Kipperwasser, S., Inzelberg, R., and Korczyn, A.D., 1995, Apo E haplotype in Parkinson's disease and its relation to dementia. *Neurology* 45:(suppl 4):A340.

Benjamin, R., Leake, A., Edwardson, J.A., McKeith, I.G., Ince, P.G., Perry, R.H., and Morris, C.M., 1994, Apolipoprotein E genes in Lewy body and Parkinson's diseases. *Lancet* 343:1565.

Corder, E.H., Saunders, A.M., Strittmatter, W.J., Schmechel, D.E., Gaskell, P.C., Small, G.W., Roses, A.D., Haines, J.L., and Pericak, Vance M.A., 1993, Gene dose of apolipoprotein E type 4 allele and risk of Alzheimer's disease in late onset families. *Science* 261:921–923.

Galasko, D., Saitoh, T., Xia, Y., Thal, L.J., Katzman, R., Hill, L., and Hansen, L., 1994, The apolipoprotein E allele e4 is overrepresented in patients with the Lewy body variant of Alzheimer's disease. *Neurology* 44:1950–1951.

Growdon, J.H., Locascio, J.J., Corkin, S., Gomez-Isla, T., and Hyman, B.T., 1996, Apolipoprotein E genotype does not influence rates of cognitive decline in Alzheimer's disease. *Neurology* 47:444–448.

Inzelberg, R., Chapman, J., Treves, T.A., Kipperwasser, S., Orlov, E., Klimovitzky, S, Verchovsky, R., and Korczyn, A.D., 1997, Apolipoprotein E4 in Parkinson's disease and dementia: New data and meta-analysis of published studies. *Alz. Dis Assoc Disord* (in press).

Jellinger, K, 1986, Overwiev of morphological changes in Parkinson's disease. In: *Advances in Neurology*, vol 45, Yahr, M.D. and Bergman, K.J., ed., Raven Press, New York, pp 1–18

Koller, W.C., Glatt, S.L., Hubble, J.P., Paolo, A., Troster, A.I., Handler, M.S., Horvat, R.T., Martin, C., Schmidt, K., and Konst, A., 1995, Apolipoprotein E genotypes in Parkinson's disease with and without dementia. *Ann Neurol* 37:242–245.

Korczyn, A.D., Inzelberg, R., Treves, T.A., Neufeld, M.Y., Reider, I., and Rabey, M.J., 1986, Dementia of Parkinson's Disease. In: *Advances in Neurology*, vol 45, Yahr, M.D. and Bergman, K.J., Raven Press, New York pp 399–403.

Korczyn, A.D., 1995, The apolipoprotein e4 allele in Parkinson's disease with and without dementia.. (letter) *Neurology* 45:1025.

Kurz, A., Egensperger, R., Haupt, M., Lautenschlager, N., Romero, B., Graeber, M.B., and Muller, U., 1996, Apolipoprotein E e4 allele, cognitive decline and deterioration of everyday performance in Alzheimer's disease. *Neurology* 47:440–443.

Marder, K., Maestre, G., Cote, L., Mejia, H., Alfaro, B., Halim, A., Tang, M., Tycko, B., and Mayeux, R., 1994, The apolipoprotein e4 allele in Parkinson's disease with and without dementia. *Neurology* 44:1330–1331.

Parkinson, J., 1817, An Essay on the Shaking Palsy. London. Sherwood, Neely and Jones.

Pickering-Brown, S.M., Mann, D.M.A., Bourke, J.P., Roberts, D.A., Balderson, D., Burns, A., Byrne, J., and Owen, F., 1994, Apolipoprotein e4 and Alzheimer's disease pathology in Lewy body disease and in other (-amyloid forming diseases. *Lancet* 343:1155–1158.

Plassman, B.L., and Breitner, J.C.S., 1996, Apolipoprotein E and cognitive decline in Alzheimer's disease. *Neurology* 47:317–320.

Polvikoski, T., Sulkava, R., Haltia, Kainulainen, K, Vuorio, A., Verkkoniemi, A., Niinisto, L., Halonen, R., and Kontula K, 1995, Apolipoprotein E, dementia and cortical deposition of β-amyloid protein. *N. Engl. J. Med.* 333:1242–1247.

Roses, A.D., 1996, Apolipoprotein E alleles as risk factors in Alzheimer's disease. *Ann. Rev. Med.* 47:387–400.

Rubinszstein, D.C., Hanlon, C.S., Irving, R.M., Goodburn, S., Evans, D.G., Kellan-Wood, H., Huereb, J.H., Bandmann, O., and Harding, A.E., 1994, Apo E genotypes in multiple sclerosis, Parkinson's disease, Schwanomas and late onset Alzheimer's disease. *Mol. Cell Probes* 8:519–525.

Saunders, A.M., Strittmatter, W.J., Schmechel, D., St. George Hyslop, P.H., Pericak, Vance M.A., Rosi, B.C., Gusella, J.F., Crapper, Mac Lachlan, D.R., Alberts, M.J., Hullette, C., Crain, B., Goldgaber, D., Roses, A.D., 1993, Association of apolipoprotein E allele e4 with late onset familial and sporadic Alzheimer's disease. *Neurology* 43:1467–1472.

Schupf, N., Kapell, D., Lee, J.H., Zigman, W., Canto, B., Tycko, B., and Mayeux, R., 1996, Onset of dementia associated with apolipoprotein E ε4 in Down syndrome. *Ann. Neurol.* 40:799–801.

Treves, T.A., Ragolsky, M., Gelernter, I., and Korczyn, A.D., 1990, Evaluation of a short mental test for the diagnosis of dementia. *Dementia* 1:102–108.

Treves, T.A., Bornstein, N.M., Chapman, J., Klimovitzky, S., Verchovsky, R., Asherov, A., Veshchev, I.O., and Korczyn AD, 1996, APOE epsilon 4 in patients with Alzheimer's disease and vascular dementia. *Alz. Dis. Assoc. Disord.* 10:189–191.

Wenham, P.R., Price, W.H., and Blundel, G., 1991, Apolipoprotein E genotyping by one-stage PCR. *Lancet* 337:1158–1159.

118

A SIMPLE PROCEDURE OF IMMUNOCHEMICAL DETECTION OF AMYLOID β PROTEINS USING MILLIGRAM AMOUNTS OF BRAIN TISSUES OF PATIENTS WITH ALZHEIMER'S DISEASE

B. Kaplan,[1] B. Martin,[2] S. Yakar,[1] M. Pras,[1] T. Wisniewski,[3,4] J. Ghiso,[3] B. Frangione,[3] and G. Gallo[3]

[1]Heller Institute of Medical Research
Sheba Medical Center, Israel
[2]Clinical Neuroscience Branch, NIH
[3]Department of Pathology
[4]Department of Neurology
NYU Medical Center
New York, New York

INTRODUCTION

Formation of neurofibrillary tangles and extracellular accumulation of fibrillar β-amyloid (Aβ) in the brain are major neuropathological hallmarks of Alzheimer's disease (AD). In AD patients, Aβ is found within senile plaques and in the walls of leptomeningeal and intracortical vessels. In addition to the fibrillar Aβ deposits, the brain gray matter accumulates a diffuse nonfibrillar form of amyloid. Recent evidence suggests that deposition of this diffuse form of amyloid plaques may be an early event in the pathology of AD (Frangione et al., 1993).

The immunochemical techniques are important analytical tools providing precise detection and identification of Aβ proteins in AD tissues. These techniques are widely applied in different studies aimed to understand the formation of Aβ deposits and AD pathogenesis. However, the common protocols used for the extraction and partial purification of Aβ are complex and time consuming. They require relatively large amounts of starting tissue material and can be applied for analysis of only autopsy, not biopsy specimens (Sipe et al., 1990; Frucht et al., 1993; Harigaya et al., 1995; Permanne et al., 1995).

Progress in Alzheimer's and Parkinson's Diseases
edited by Fisher *et al.*, Plenum Press, New York, 1998.

The aim of our study was to develop a simple procedure for immunochemical detection of Aβ proteins by using milligram amounts of brain tissue from AD patients.

EXPERIMENTAL

Brain Tissues

Brain tissues were obtained at autopsy from two control individuals and five patients with AD, confirmed neuropathologically. Cortical tissue specimens of the AD patients were taken from four brain areas: hippocampal and temporal cortex (rich in neuritic plaques) and insular and cingulate cortex (containing predominantly diffuse plaques).

Extraction of Amyloid β Proteins

The cerebral gray matter was separated from leptomeninges and white matter and homogenized with several volumes of cold saline. In some experiments the tissue homogenates were sieved through a series of nylon mesh of 350, 150, 170 and 30 μm in order to remove small vessels. Tissue homogenates were centrifuged in an Eppendorf microfuge for 10 min at 14,000 rpm. The resulting pellett was washed with saline, dispersed in 20% acetonitrile containing 0.1% trifluoroacetic acid (Ac-TFA) for 1 h and centrifuged (10 min, 14,000 rpm). The supernatant was collected and the extraction with Ac-TFA was repeated twice (Kaplan et al., 1993). The Ac-TFA soluble material was pooled and lyophilized, and the insoluble residue was dispersed in formic acid (FA) for 30 min at room temperature. The mixture was centrifuged with a Beckman L7 ultracentrifuge for 40 min at 100,000 g at 4°C and the obtained supernatant was collected and lyophilized.

High Performance Liquid Chromatography (HPLC)

The HPLC equipment consisted of a Spectra-Physics 8700 solvent delivery system, a 8500 dynamic mixer and 8750 organizer, coupled to a Jasco Uvidec 100IV spectrophotometer with an 8μl cassette type cell, and a Hewlett-Packard 3390 A integrator. The lyophilized samples of Ac-TFA tissue extract were redissolved in 20% acetonitrile / 0.1% TFA (20 mg/ml) and applied to a Vydac 214TP54 (Alltech, Deerfield, IL, USA) column (250 × 4.6mm, I.D.). A linear gradient from 20 to 75% acetonitrile in 0.1% TFA over 30 min was used. The elution of proteins was monitored by UV absorbance at 220 nm. The fractions of interest were collected and lyophilized. Synthetic Aβ 1–40 peptide was run as a standard under the same conditions.

Sodium Dodecyl Sulphate Polyacrylamide Gel Electrophoresis (SDS-PAGE) and Western Blot Analysis

The specimens of tissue extracts and HPLC fractions were solubilized in Laemmli sample buffer (125 mM Tris, 6% SDS, 2%β-mercaptoethanol, 6M urea, 4 mM Na₂EDTA, and 0.2 M sucrose) pH 6.8, resolved in a 17% SDS-PAGE (Laemmli, 1970) and electrotransferred to nitrocellulose membranes (Schleicher and Schuell, Dassel, Germany) using Towbin's buffer (Towbin et al., 1979). Unbound sites were blocked with 6% skimmilk in PBS. Monoclonal 6E10 (Kim et al., 1998) (recognizing residues 1–17 of Aβ was used as a

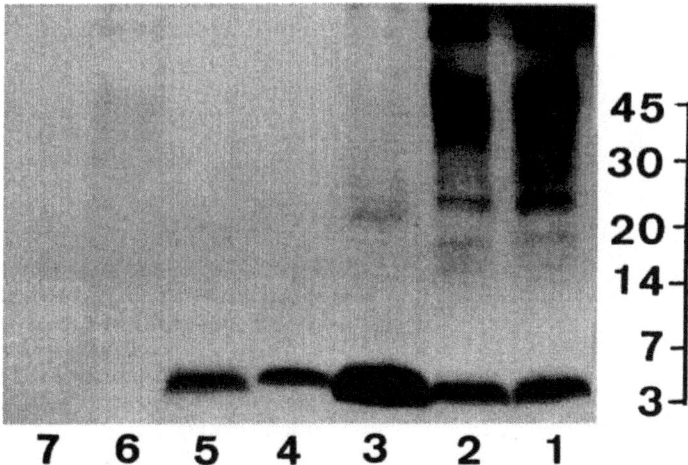

Figure 1. Western blot of brain tissue extracts obtained from the AD patient (lanes 1–3,5) and control individual (6, 7). 1, 2, 6 - Ac-TFA soluble tissue extracts; 3, 5, 7 - FA soluble tissue extracts; 1, 3, 6, 7 - tissue preparations containing microvessels; 2, 5 - tissue preparation free from microvessels; 4 - synthetic Aβ1–40 peptide.

primary antibody (1:300). Anti-mouse IgG horseradish peroxidase linked F(ab')2 fragment (from sheep) (Amersham, Arlington, IL, USA) was used as a secondary antibody (1:3000). Proteins were visualized via ECL Western Blotting detection system (Amersham).

RESULTS

The brain tissue extracts (1g of the initial cortical tissue material) were prepared by using consecutively Ac-TFA and FA as described above. The samples were run on SDS-PAGE and immunoblotted (Fig. 1). The 4 kDa protein bands immunoreactive with 6E10 antibody were detected in the Ac-TFA and FA extracts from AD tissues (Fig. 1, lanes 1–3, 5); their mobilities were equal to the standard, Aβ1–40 (lane 4). This immunoreactivity was absent in the specimens from control individuals (Fig. 1, lanes 6, 7). The immunoreactive 4kDa bands were revealed in the AD tissue specimens containing microvessels (Fig. 1, lanes 1, 3), as well as after their removal (Fig. 1, lanes 2, 5).

The Ac-TFA extracts from AD tissues were fractionated by reverse phase HPLC (Fig. 2A). The HPLC fraction with the elution time corresponding to that of synthetic Ab1–40 peptide (Fig. 2B) was collected and lyophilized. Western blotting showed that this HPLC fraction contained the 4kDa proteins immunoreactive with 6E10 antibodies (Fig. 3).

Scheme 1 (Fig. 4) illustrates the small-scale extraction procedure applied for the immunochemical detection of Aβ species using milligram amounts of the AD brain tissue. Tissue specimens of three different brain regions from one AD patient and of two brain regions from each of four other AD patients were used. The Ac-TFA soluble Aβ proteins were found in all cortical AD preparations tested (n=11). Fig. 5 shows that 5–10 mg of cortical tissue is sufficient to obtain a clearly visible immunochemical signal.

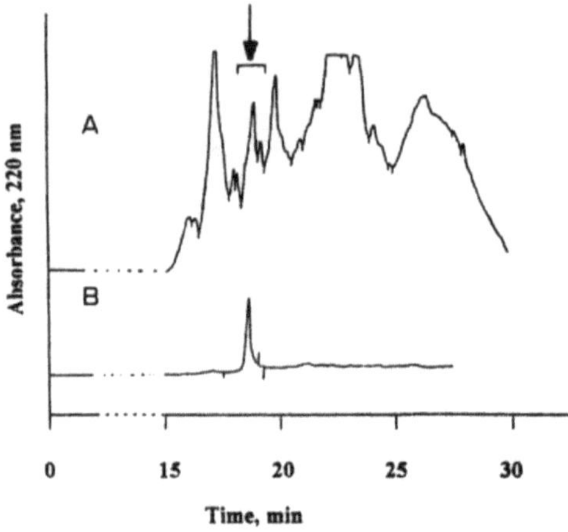

Figure 2. HPLC of the Ac-TFA soluble brain tissue extract from AD patient (A) and synthetic Aβ1–40 peptide (B). The samples were run on Vydac 214TP54 column as described in Experimental. The effluent was monitored by UV absorbance at 220 nm. Arrow indicates to Ac-TFA fraction (k'= 4.7) collected for further analysis (see Fig. 3).

DISCUSSION

Several species of Aβ peptides were found to accumulate in AD brains. Cerebrovascular amyloid contains mostly Aβ1–39/40, while senile plaque Aβ starts with heterogeneous N-termini at positions 1, 2, 4, 15 and ends with C-termini 42/43 (Glenner et al., 1984; Masters et al., 1985; Selkoe et al., 1986; Miller et al., 1993; Roher et al., 1993). The major component of diffuse plaques is Aβ17 - 42 (Gowing et al., 1994; Lalowski et al., 1996; Wisniewski et al., 1996). Aβ proteins are also different in respect to their solubility. AD brains accumulate the TBS soluble Aβ proteins (Harigaya et al., 1995), as well as the more insoluble Aβ forms, which could be extracted by using guanidinium salts, 10% SDS and formic acid[5,11] (Masters et al., 1985; Harigaya et al., 1995). We found that substantial amounts of the insoluble Aβ (accumulating in brain regions rich in senile, as well as diffuse plaques) could be solubilized and easily extracted with 20% acetonitrile / 0.1% TFA solvent. Based on these findings, a new simple procedure for immunochemical Aβ detection was developed. The procedure is rapid and does not require any special equipment. It

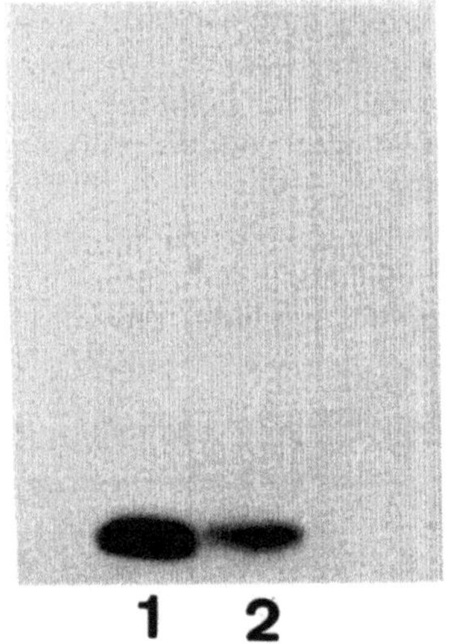

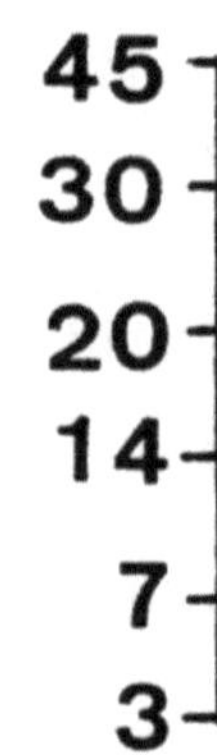

Figure 3. Western blot of the HPLC fraction of Ac-TFA soluble AD tissue material with the elution time identical of that of standard Aβ1–40. 1: HPLC fraction, 2: synthetic Aβ1–40 peptide.

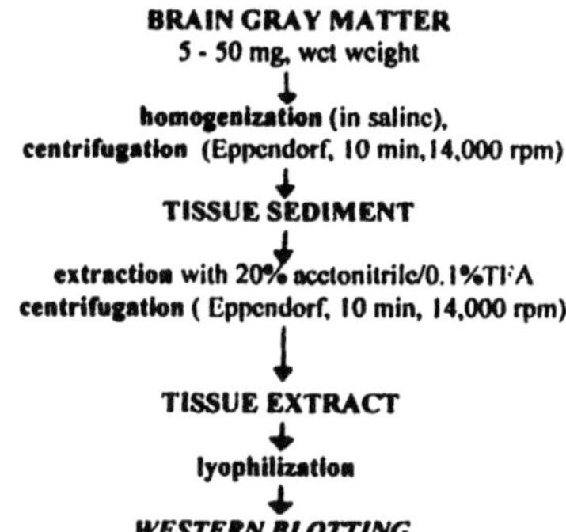

Figure 4. (Scheme 1) A procedure for extraction and immunochemical detection of Aβ in milligram amounts of brain tissue.

can be performed by using only a few milligrams of tissue, that is comparable with the tissue amount obtained by stereotactic brain biopsy. This is in contrast to the common protocols based on the solubility of Aβ in formic acid (Frucht et al., 1993; Harigaya et al., 1995; Permanne et al., 1995), which utilize a larger amount of tissue, employ extensive washings of tissue homogenates with SDS and protease inhibitors prior to their treatment with formic acid and require several prolonged ultracentrifugation steps. The developed

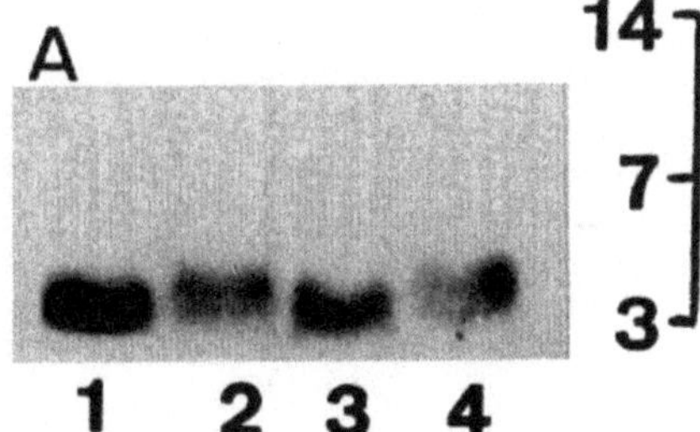

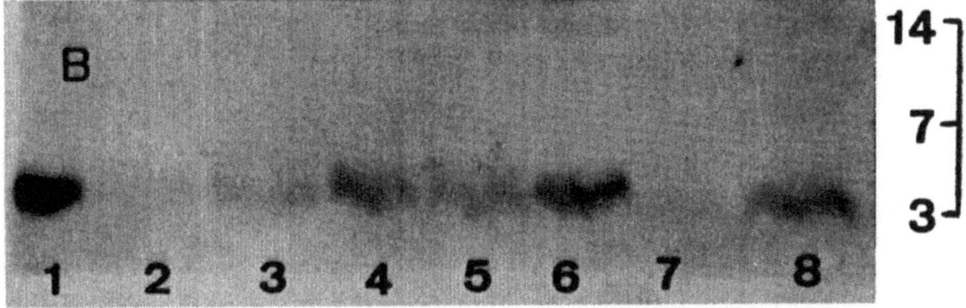

Figure 5. Western blots of the Ac-TFA soluble brain tissue material obtained from AD patients: A: 1: MP-94 temporal, 25mg; 2: MP-94 cingulate, 25mg; 3: OC-493 hippocampal, 25mg; 4:OC-493 insular, 25mg. B: 1: OC-515 insular, 5mg; 5 - OC-493 insular, 4mg; 2: OC-514 cingulate, 4mg; 6 - OC 493 hippocampal, 11mg; 3: OC-517 temporal, 4mg; 7 - MP-94 cingulate, 2mg; 4: OC-491 hippocampal, 8mg; 8 - MP-94 temporal, 7mg.

procedure allows detection of Aβ not only in the brain regions rich in senile plaques, but also in the areas containing predominantly diffuse plaques. The feasibility of the developed technique for early detection of AD is under study.

ACKNOWLEDGMENT

This work was supported by a grant from the Chief Scientist's Office, Ministry of Health, Israel.

REFERENCES

Frangione, B., Wisniewski, T., and Ghiso, J., 1993, Alzheimer's disease and amyloid β, *In: Amyloid and Amyloidosis.* R.Kisilevsky, M.D.Benson, B.Frangione et al., eds., New York:Pantheon Publishing 310–315.

Frucht, S.J., Koo, E.H., 1993, β-Amyloid protein is higher in Alzheimer's diseaserains; description of a quantitative biochemical assay, *J. Neuropathol. Exp. Neurol.* 52:640–647.

Glenner, G.G., and Wong, C.W., 1984, Alzheimer's disease: initial report of the purification and characterization of a novel cerebrovascular amyloid protein, *Biochem. Biophys. Res. Commun.* 120:885–890.

Gowing, E., Roher, A.E., Woods, A.S., Cotter, R.J., Chaney, M., Little, S.P., and Ball, M.J., 1994, Chemical characterization of Aβ17–42 peptide, a component of diffuse amyloid deposits of Alzheimer's disease, *J. Biol. Chem.* 269:10987–10990.

Harigaya, Y., Shoji, M., Kawarabayashi, T., Kanai, M., Nakamura, T., Iizuka, T., Igeta, Y., Saido, T.C., Sahara, N., Mori, H., and Hirai, S., 1995, Modified amyloid b protein ending at 42 or 40 with different solubility accumulates in the brain of Alzheimer's disease, *Biochem. Biophys. Res. Commun.* 211:1015–1022.

Kaplan, B., German, G., and Pras, M., 1993, Isolation and characterization of amyloid proteins from milligram amounts of amyloid-containing tissue, *J. Liq. Chromatogr.* 16:2249–2268.

Kim, K.S., Miller, D.L., Sapienza, V.J., Chen, C.M.J., Bai, C., Grungke-Iqbal, I., Currie, J., Wisniewski, H.M., 1988, Production and characterization of monoclonal antibodies reactive to synthetic cerebrovascular peptide, *Neurosci. Res. Commun.* 2:121–130.

Laemmli, U.K., 1970, Cleavage of structural proteins during assembly of the head of the bacteriophage T4, *Nature* 227:680–682.

Lalowski, M., Golabek, A.A., Lemere, C.A., Selkoe, D.J., Wisniewski, H.M., Beavis, R.C., Frangione, B., and Wisniewski, T, 1996, *J. Biol. Chem.* 271:33623–33631.

Masters, C.L., Simms, G., Weinman, N.A., .Muthaup, G., .McDonald, B.L., and Beyreuther, K., 1985, Amyloid plaque core protein in Alzheimer's disease and Down syndrome, *Proc.Natl. Acad. Sci.* 82:4245–4249.

Miller, D.L., Papayannopoulos, I.A., Styles, J., Bobin, S.A., Lin, Y.Y., Biemann, K., and Iqbal, K, 1993, Peptide composition of cerebrovascular and senile plaque core amyloid deposits in Alzheimer's disease, *Arch. Biochem. Biophys.* 301:41–52.

Permanne, B., Buee, L., David, J.P., Fallet-Bianko, C., Di Menza, C., and Delacourte, A., 1995, Quantitation of Alzheimer's amyloid peptide and identification of related amyloid proteins by dot-blot immunoassay, *Brain Res.* 685:154–162.

Roher, A.E., Lowenson, J.D., Clarke, S., Wolkow, C., Wang, R., Cotter, R.J., Rearson, I.M., Zurcher-Neely, H.A., Heinrikson, R.L., Ball, M.J., and Greenburg, B.D., 1993, Structural alterations in the peptide backbone of b-amyloid core may account for its deposition and stability in Alzheimer's disease, *J. Biol. Chem.* 268:3072–3083.

Selkoe, D.J., Abraham, C.R., Podlisny, M.B., and Duffy, L.K., 1986, Isolation of low molecular weight proteins from amyloid plaque deposits in Alzheimer's disease, *J. Neurochem.* 46:1820–1834.

Sipe, J.D., De Beer, F.C., Pepys M., et al., 1990, Report on special session on bioassays and standartization of amyloid proteins and precursors, *In: Amyloid and Amyloidosis.*Natvig, J.B,.Forre, Q,.Husby G et al., eds London: Kluwer Academic Publishers 203–206.

Towbin, J., Stachelin, T., and Gordon, J., 1979, Electrophoretic transfer of proteins from polyacrylamide gels to nitrocellulose sheets, *Proc. Natl. Acad. Sci. USA* 76:4350–4354.

Wisniewski, T., Lalowski, M., Bobik, M., Russel, M., Strosznajder, J., and Frangione, B., 1996, Amyloid Ab 1–42 deposits do not lead to Alzheimer's neuritic plaques in aged dogs, *Biochem. J.* 313:575–580.

119

BRIDGING STUDIES IN ALZHEIMER'S DISEASE

Finding the Optimal Dose for Efficacy Studies

Neal R. Cutler and John J. Sramek

California Clinical Trials Medical Group
8500 Wilshire Boulevard
Beverly Hills, California 90211

INTRODUCTION TO BRIDGING STUDIES

Phase I studies in healthy normal volunteers have traditionally provided the only preliminary clinical safety data prior to efficacy studies in patients. However, drug effects can vary widely between the target population and healthy volunteers (Cutler et al., 1991, 1992, 1993). Bridging studies, designed to determine the maximum tolerated dose (MTD) in the target population, provide an intermediate step and optimize selection of a dose range for Phase II efficacy studies.

In order to determine the MTD of an investigational compound, the minimum intolerated dose (MID) is ascertained. The MID is the dose at which a majority (50% or more) of the subjects receiving active drug experience severe or multiple moderate adverse events, or the dose at which a serious adverse event occurs in one patient. The dose which falls just below the MID is considered the MTD.

We have often based the dosing regimen in bridging studies on the MTD in healthy volunteers. (Cutler and Sramek, 1995a, 1995b). Patients are enrolled in one of approximately five fixed-dose panel (n=6 in each panel, 4 active, 2 placebo). Patients in panel number one would receive a dose 50% below the MTD of healthy normals. Subsequent panels would receive doses at 25% below, MTD, 25% above, 50% above, and so on, until the MID for the target population is reached. Once again, the dose just below the MID would be considered the MTD; another panel of new patients at this dose is recommended to verify safety at this level.

Progress in Alzheimer's and Parkinson's Diseases
edited by Fisher *et al.*, Plenum Press, New York, 1998.

Table 1. MTD values for healthy normals vs. probable AD patients

	Healthy young	Healthy elderly	Probable AD	% Change from healthy MTD to AD MTD
Velnacrine	not determined	100 mg tid	75 mg tid	–25%
Eptastigmine	32 mg tid	32 mg qd	48 mg tid	+50%, +350%
CI-979	1 mg q6h	not determined	2 mg q6h	+100%
Xanomeline	not determined	50 mg bid	100 mg bid	+100%
Besipirdine	not determined	100 mg bid	50 mg bid	–50%
Lu 25-109	not determined	130 qid	150 mg tid	–13%

BRIDGING STUDIES IN THE TREATMENT OF ALZHEIMER'S DISEASE

Research indicates that a loss of cholinergic neurons and choline acetyltransferase is associated with Alzheimer's Disease (AD). As a means of counteracting these deficits, many experimental therapeutics for the treatment of AD involve compounds which enhance cholinergic function. Unfortunately, the efficacy of cholinergic compounds appears to be limited, and significant adverse events often occur with their use. Furthermore, our review of multiple studies in cholinergic treatments for AD reveal a possible impact of cholinergic deficits on the pharmacodynamic profiles of these compounds. These circumstances have rendered the clinical investigations of cholinergic agents as model studies for the application of bridging (Cutler et al., 1992b). Table 1 summarizes the differences in MTD's between healthy and probable AD volunteers.

VELNACRINE

In Phase I studies of velnacrine, an acetylcholinesterase inhibitor, no MTD was reached, but 200 mg qd was well tolerated in young, healthy normal subjects. In healthy, normal elderly subjects, 300 mg qd was well tolerated and the MTD was found to be 100 mg tid. However, in a bridging study involving AD patients, the MTD was reached at 75 mg tid—twenty five percent *below* the MTD in the control group due to the appearance of a serious adverse event (seizure) at higher doses (Puri et al., 1988, 1989, 1990; Cutler et al., 1990).

EPTASTIGMINE

The compound eptastigmine, also an acetylcholinesterase inhibitor, was similarly studied in young, healthy normal subjects. Twenty mg qd was tested (not to MTD) and found to be well tolerated. The MTD for this population was 32 mg tid. Likewise, the MTD among the healthy elderly population was 32 mg qd (no multiple dose studies were conducted). In a bridging study of AD patients, the MTD was *higher*: 48 mg tid. (Goldberg et al., 1991; Sramek et al., 1994).

CI-979

The muscarinic agonist, CI-979, was studied in multiple doses only, and produced an MTD in young healthy control subjects of 1 mg q6h. Similar tolerance was observed in the elderly control population. In contrast, AD patients in a bridging study demonstrated a substantially greater MTD of 2 mg q6h. (Reece et al., 1992; Sramek et al., 1995a).

XANOMELINE

Xanomeline was well tolerated at a single dose of 150 mg in a young, healthy population. An MTD was not reached, but it was shown that 75 mg bid was also well tolerated. An MTD of 50 mg bid was established in the elderly control group. Once again, a significantly higher MTD was found in the AD bridging population: 100 mg tid. (Sramek et al., 1995b).

BESIPIRDINE

The MTD was not reached in a panel of healthy young volunteers in Phase I studies of besipirdine, but a 30 mg qd dose was well tolerated. No multiple dose studies were conducted in this population, nor was a single dose study conducted in an elderly, healthy control group. However, this latter population reached an MTD at 100 mg bid. The MTD in the target population was discovered in bridging studies to be 50 mg bid—half of the control group MTD. (Sramek et al., 1995c)

LU 25-109

The most recent bridging study conducted at our unit involved the partial M_1 agonist, (with M_2/M_3 antagonistic properties) Lu 25-109. An elderly control group previously demonstrated tolerance at 130 mg qid. The MTD among probable AD patients was found at 150 mg tid, which was not improved in a titration scheme. (Cutler, 1997).

CONCLUSION

Bridging studies have provided tremendous benefit to the drug development process. In this review we have addressed specific applications of bridging in AD.

Though not thoroughly understood, it has been observed that similar doses of cholinergic compounds can invoke sometimes radically different tolerance in healthy normals than those with probable AD. A possible explanation appears to be differences in pharmacodynamics between patients and normals, since pharmacokinetics are typically not altered appreciably. Unquestionably, intensive studies into these issues are needed. But in the interim period, compounds such as cholinergics which have shown relative safety and promising efficacy can be more rapidly brought to market by adding the short, efficient step of bridging. Performing bridging studies in cholinergic drugs eliminates doses which may be well below the effective dose in cases where AD patients have greater tolerance than healthy patients. Bridging also eliminates potentially toxic doses in cases where AD patients experience lesser tolerance. Preliminary data on adverse events in patients also prepare investigators with an expected profile of the compound in patients. As a result of these factors, Phase II efficacy studies can be performed in less time with greater confidence, endangering the fewest possible patients.

As bridging is embraced by clinical researchers, similar advantages in a number of other therapeutic areas are possible. Many other indications share the characteristic of AD that patients show significantly different response in safety studies than their healthy counterparts. These indications include psychiatric disorders such as schizophrenia, depression, and anxiety. Even non-neurological medical conditions, such as hypertension, demonstrate features which make early safety/tolerance studies ideal candidates for bridging.

REFERENCES

Cutler, N.R., Murphy, M.J, Nash, R.J., and Prior PL., 1990, Clinical safety, tolerance, and plasma levels of HP 029 in Alzheimer's disease. *J. Clin. Pharmacol.* 30:556–561.

Cutler, N.R., Sramek, J.J., and Narang, P.K. 1991, Geriatrics: clinical trials in an aging population. *J. Clin. Pharmacoepidem.* 5:241–53.

Cutler, N.R., Sramek, J.J., Murphy, M.F., and Nash, R.J., 1992a, Commentary: Alzheimer's patients should be included in Phase I clinical trials to evaluate compounds for Alzhemier's disease. *J. Geriatr. Psychiatry Neurol.* 5:192–194.

Cutler, N.R., Sramek, J.J., Murphy, M.F., and N ash, R.J.. 1992b, Implications of the study population in the early evaluation of anticholinesterase inhibitors for Alzheimer's disease. *Ann. Pharmacother.* 26:1118–1122.

Cutler, N.R., Sramek, J.J., Seifert, R.D., and Sawin, S.F., 1993, *Alzheimer's Disease: Advances in Clinical and Basic Research*, Corain, B., ed, John Wiley & Sons, Ltd., Sussex, England, pp. 559–562.

Cutler, N.R., and Sramek, J.J., 1995a, Clinical safety, tolerance, and plasma levels of HP 029 in Alzheimer's disease. *J. Clin. Pharmacol.* 30:556–561.

Cutler, N.R., and Sramek, J.J., 1995b, The target population in phase I clinical trials of cholinergic compounds in Alzheimer's disease: the role of the "bridging study". *Alzheimer Dis. Assoc. Disord.* 9:139–145.

Culter, N.R., Forrest, M., Mengel, H., and Sramek, J.J., 1997, A bridging study of the muscarinic compound LU 25–109 in patients with probable Alzheimer's disease. Accepted for Presentation at the Fourth International Conference on Progress in Alzheimer's and Parkinson's Disease, May.

Goldberg, M.R., Barchowsky, A., McCrea, J., et al. 1991,Heptylphysostigmine (L-693, 487). Safety and cholinesterase inhibition in a placebo-controlled rising-dose healthy volunteer study. Presented at: Second International Springfield Symposium on Advances in Alzheimer Therapy.

Puri, S.K., Hsu, R., Ho, I., and Lassman, H.B., 1988, Single-dose safety, tolerance and pharmacokinetics of HP029 in elderly men: a potential Alzheimer agent. *Curr. Ther. Res.* 44:766–780.

Puri, S.K., Hsu, R.S., Ho, I., and Lassman, H.B., 1989, Singel dose safety, tolerance and pharmacokinetics of HP029 in healthy young men: A potential Alzheimer agent. *J. Clin. Pharmacol.* 29:278–284.

Puri, S.K., Ho, I., Hsu, R., and Lassman, H.B., 1990, Multiple dose pharmacokinetics, safety and tolerance of velnacrine (HP029) in healthy elderly subjects: a potential therapeutic agent for Alzheimer's disease. *J. Clin. Pharmacol.* 30:948–955.

Reece, P.A., Bockbrader, H., and Sedman, A.J., 1992, Safety, pharmacodynamics, and pharmacokinetics of a new muscarinic agonist, CI-979. *Clin. Exp. Pharmacol. Physiol.* 21 (Suppl): 8.

Sramek, J.J., Block, G.A., Reines, S.A., Sawin, S.F., Barchowsky, A., and Cutler, N.R. 1994, A multiple-dose safety trial of eptastigmine in Alzheimer's disease, with pharmacodynamic observations of red blood cell cholinesterase. *Life Sci.* 56:19–326.

Sramek, J.J., Sedman, A.J., Reece, P.A., Underwood, B., Seifert, R.D., Bockbrader, H., and Cutler, N.R. 1995a, Safety and tolerability of CI-979 in patients with Alzheimer's disease. *Life Sci.* 57:503–510.

Sramek, J.J., Hurley, D.J., Wardle, T.S., Satterwhite, J.H., Hourani, J., Dies, F., and Cutler, N.R.. 1995b, The safety and tolerance of xanomeline tartrate in patients with Alzheimer's disease. *J. Clin. Pharmacol.* 35:800–806.

Sramek, J.J., Viereck, C., Huff, F.J., Wardle, T., Hourani, J., Steward, J.A., and Cutler, N.R., 1995c, A "bridging" (Safety/Tolerance) study of besipirdine hydrochloride in patients with Alzheimer's disease. *Life Sci.* 57:1241–1248.

120

HOW CAN WE IMPROVE THE DRUG DEVELOPMENT PROCESS IN ALZHEIMER'S DISEASE?

C. Brazell and T. H. Corn

CNS Clinical Research
Glaxo Wellcome Research and Development
Greenford Road, Greenford, Middlesex
UB6 0HE, United Kingdom

INTRODUCTION

The drug development process and clinical evaluation of a potential drug for Alzheimer's disease (AD) is strongly influenced by the guidelines issued by regulatory authorities world-wide.Since the early 1990s these have been primarily those issued by the Food and Drug Administration (FDA) in the United States and by the Committee for Proprietary Medicinal Products (CPMP) in Europe. Such guidelines reflect both regulatory policy and the prevailing consensus of expert scientific and medical opinion. They cover the theoretical and practical issues affecting the validity and reliability of clinical investigations carried out in dementia. The guidelines are not regulations as such, but they do summarize the advice that agency staff give to those seeking direction on how to obtain an antidementia drug claim. It is therefore understandable that drug developers adhere closely to the guidelines and dementia trials to date have had a common format. This is clearly demonstrated by the similarity in the design of the trials supporting the approval of Cognex™ and Aricept™ for AD.

The guidelines however, do not prevent researchers from investigating methodologies that may improve the drug development process and allow an efficacious and safe medication to reach the patient more quickly. Some of the strategies that address this issue and are currently being explored are discussed in this chapter.

Progress in Alzheimer's and Parkinson's Diseases
edited by Fisher *et al.*, Plenum Press, New York, 1998.

CURRENT PHASE II CLINICAL STUDIES

Patients

As with any phase II study the goal of a trial in AD is to document efficacy and identify the parameters of the treatment regime, e.g., dose, dose interval, that are likely to maximize the product's therapeutic ratio. Accordingly phase II studies commonly enroll patients who have a well characterised dementia, meeting DSM-IV and NINCDS-ADRDA AD diagnostic criteria, have a mild to moderate disease classification and suffer fewer medical illnesses than typical patients with dementia.

Clinical Efficacy Variables

To gain an antidementia indication for a product, both the CPMP and the FDA require the drug to demonstrate action on the core manifestations of dementia, e.g. memory, praxis, language, judgement and orientation, and for this to be shown to translate into a clinically meaningful effect. The guidelines require results from:

1. a performance based objective test instrument which provides a comprehensive assessment of cognitive functions and
2. a global assessment performed by a skilled clinician.

The drug must show superiority to an appropriate control treatment on both of these measures. In addition, improvement in behaviors closely connected to activities of daily living is of importance.

The two scales most widely used to satisfy the dual assessment requirement have been the cognitive subsection of the Alzheimer's Disease Assessment Scale (ADAS-Cog) (Rosen et al, 1984) and the Clinician's Interview Based Impression of Change (CIBIC) (Leber, 1990). On occasions the CIBIC Plus, which allows information from a caregiver to be incorporated, has also been used.

Trial Duration

The number of patients enrolled in phase II studies is a balance between concern over needlessly exposing patients to a pharmacologically active, yet potentially harmful, substance and achieving the exposure required to demonstrate therapeutic efficacy. When using the ADAS-Cog as the primary efficacy variable, statistical power calculations dictate that it is necessary to randomise approximately 100 patients per treatment arm in order to detect a minimally clinically meaningful difference of 3 points over a 3–6 month study period. Phase II studies are usually of parallel group, double-blind, placebo-controlled design employing three well separated dose groups. So far, an active control has not been required.

The total duration of a phase II programme is approximately 19 months, usually comprised of:

Study set up time	3 months
Treatment duration	3–6 months
Recruitment period	9 months
Finalization of database	1 month

Duration of the study will naturally be increased if Phase I data indicates that more doses should be tested. Whilst this may be unwelcome news for the developer, a clear dose response will be critical for Phase III design.

STRATEGIES FOR ACCELERATED DRUG DEVELOPMENT

Whilst the drug treatment period may be sometimes judged as outside the control of the developer (safety data requirements may be paramount), all four components of development time may be subject to reduction over the program as a whole. For example, any system which allows a seamless interface between the research scientist and the clinical department will allow reductions in study set-up time. The use of advertising agencies and press relations organizations appealing to patients directly may assist recruitment, and a good relationship between drug developer and the investigators is vital to ensure rapid recruitment of patients. Finally, database completion may be greatly facilitated by computerized remote data entry systems.

Within the trial itself, acceleration will be achieved by:

1. reducing the number of patients required to demonstrate efficacy and select dose, and
2. reducing the duration of treatment required to document efficacy.

Strategies for achieving these objectives may be:

1. to refine further the current diagnostic criteria to eliminate patient heterogeneity, and possible variation in drug response, and
2. to employ outcome measures of greater sensitivity than the conventional clinical instruments.

REFINEMENT OF THE DIAGNOSIS OF ALZHEIMER'S DISEASE

Several potential candidates for improving diagnostic criteria have been proposed including biological markers, cerebral imaging techniques and genotyping. Of these, genotyping seems to have the greatest potential.

Potential of Genetic Markers for AD

Genetic factors predisposing to AD are given in Table 1 (adapted from Selkoe, 1997).

The three early-onset genes APP, PS_1 and PS_2 are autosomal dominant genes, associated with early onset AD, usually seen in patients younger than 60 and thus responsible for only a small fraction of AD cases.

The fourth gene implicated in AD, apolipoprotein E (apoE), is a susceptibility gene. Inheritance of one or two apoE ε4 alleles increases the likelihood and decreases the age of onset of AD (Corder et al., 1993), but does not predict rate of cognitive decline of patients with AD. Until recently, the ε4 allele was thought to play a role in about 50 % of cases of late-onset AD. Currently apoE ε4 testing is reported to have a positive predictive value of 97% and a negative predictive value of 42%. This means that 97% of patients diagnosed clinically as having AD and carrying two apoE ε4 alleles, will have the diagnosis confirmed at autopsy, whereas 42% of AD patients, who are non-ε4 carriers will also have their diag-

Table 1. Genetic classification of Alzheimer's disease

AD type	Chromosome	Gene defect	Age of onset
Early-onset familial, autosomal dominant	21	Amyloid Precursor Protein (APP)	50s
Early-onset familial, autosomal dominant	14	Presenilin-1 (PS_1)	40s and 50s
Variable-onset familial, autosomal dominant	1	Presenilin-2 (PS_2)	50s
Late-onset familial and sporadic susceptibility gene	19	ApoE polymorphism	60-70s
Late-onset susceptibility genes	12, 3, ?	?	70+

nosis confirmed after death. However, evidence from a recent study indicates that apoE ε4 is a risk factor only among patients who develop the disease before age 70 (Skoog et al., 1997) whilst more than 90% of AD cases occur in individuals older than 70 years. Unlike the ε4 allele, the apoE ε2 allele appears to decrease the risk of developing AD.

ApoE testing is therefore not appropriate for predicting whether someone will develop AD, but could be a useful diagnostic adjunct in selected patients suspected of having AD. The argument for the use of apoE genotyping in combination with standard phenotypic measures in the differential diagnosis of patients with dementia is based on evidence that for patients presenting with dementia at a certain stage, the likelihood that other diagnostic evaluations would show a reversible cause of dementia is less for carriers of the ε4 genotype (Roses, 1995). In view of the genetic heterogeneity of the AD population, it is probably not suprising that recent evidence suggests this may influence drug response. Analysis of the clinical response to tacrine, an acetylcholinesterase inhibitor, has suggested a reduced efficacy among patients with the ε4 allele, compared to those lacking the ε4 allele (Poirier, 1995).

Currently therefore, there appears that little is to be gained from employing genotype as an inclusion criterion for phase II clinical trials as we cannot know *a priori* which genotype group will be responsive to a novel therapy. However stratifying the general AD population by genotype in the analysis of a clinical trial may pick out treatment responsive subgroups for further study. Moreover, it should be remembered that whilst using genotype as a diagnostic criterion may suggest that fewer patients need to be randomized, the same number of patients will still need to be screened to select a specific population. Furthermore, regulatory authorities may take the view that findings in a specific genotype group cannot be generalized to the AD population as a whole.

REFINING OUTCOME MEASURES

Clinical Efficacy Markers

Whilst the outcome variables that are currently used for determining drug efficacy are highly valid as assessments of AD, the resultant scores show a high level of variability, even within a very select clinical trial population. For example, the population cited in the tacrine (Cognex ™) product label has an ADAS-Cog score which ranges from 7–62 at entry. This scatter is considerable when one considers that the scale ranges from 0 (no impairment) – 70 (maximum impairment). This issue of variability is compounded by the fact that the ADAS-Cog changes on average 9.6 points (standard deviation 8.2) over a 12 month time period (Stern et al., 1994) whilst the trial duration was only 6 months.

In theory though, it may be possible to select an Alzheimer's disease population who are undergoing a high rate of change in cognitive test scores and thereby reduce both the variability in scores and the time in which such a population would show a drug–placebo difference. Stern et al., 1994, have shown that patients presenting with an ADAS-Cog score in the range 35–40 show an annual change of nearly 13 points, whereas those patients having a score of either under 20 or over 60 have a change closer to 5 points per annum. In addition the authors clearly demonstrate that reliability of the measured change increases with longer follow-up.

More recently, researchers have started to develop predictive algorithms which use clinical features to estimate the length of time likely to elapse before a patient requires nursing home care or dies (Stern et al., 1997). It may prove possible, by combining clinical scores in several domains in this way to produce a composite measure of clinical status which shows less variability and greater sensitivity to change than its component parts.

Indices of Disease Severity

The identification of a severity index or prognostic marker which is clearly correlated with AD progression and severity of neurodegeneration could greatly enhance our ability to accelerate the drug development process. In order to achieve this, such a marker would need to be readily accessible to the investigator and would need to show less variability than conventional clinical testing so that trials could be conducted in smaller numbers of patients over shorter periods of time. Refinements of cognitive testing have thus far failed to provide such tools but candidate surrogate markers are emerging in the fields of biology and imaging.

Potential Biological Markers

Many potential biological markers have been reported, and because of conflicting results continue to be investigated. For example, the iron binding protein p97 has been reported to be expressed on reactive microglial cells associated with amyloid plaques in post-mortem brain tissue and to be elevated in the serum of AD patients (Kennard et al., 1996). CSF apoE levels have likewise been reported elevated in AD (Merched et al., 1997). However, whether such changes are specific to AD and not evident in patients suffering from other neurological and related diseases has yet to be determined. For example higher levels of CSF apoE were also present in a sub-set of patients with meningioencephalitis, motor neurone disease and lower back pain, thus underlying the importance and the difficulty of selecting a control population and raising the possibility that levels may be a reflection of neuronal damage and/or an inflammatory action that may be common to neurological diseases. Thus far none of these markers has been shown to be clearly correlated with disease progression rather than simply with disease presence and there is as yet no evidence that changes can be observed in individuals over time courses shorter than those currently employed in phase II clinical trials.

Potential Imaging Markers

Positron emission tomography (PET), computer-assisted tomography (CT), single photon emission computed tomography (SPECT) and magnetic resonance imaging (MRI) have all been employed in the investigation of AD. Indeed in the clinic these techniques have become standard in the diagnostic work-up of dementia patients to eliminate reversible causes of dementia and to refine the diagnosis of AD.

Both MRI and PET offer techniques which chart the progression of AD in ways that are linked to neurodegeneration. The exquisite anatomical accuracy of MRI allows more precise measurement of cerebral atrophy in life while PET allows measurement of the metabolic consequences of that atrophy. Both MRI and PET therefore hold the promise of providing surrogate markers for AD progression. Using MRI, Fox et al. (1996) have shown rates of cerebral atrophy to be up to 70 times higher in AD patients than in controls, although the time course over which this was observed (12 months) was no shorter than that required to detect deterioration with a standard clinical assessment scale. Similarly Jagust et al. (1996) have used PET to demonstrate changes in glucose metabolism in posterior temporal and visual cortex which are correlated with changes in the MMSE score. Once again however, this was over an extended study period of 2.5 years. It seems unlikely therefore that either of these techniques could currently allow a significant reduction in the duration of treatment trials and, given the restrictions on repeat PET scanning and the inherent resolution problems of PET it seems unlikely that PET will ever provide such a technique. MRI perhaps holds more promise for the future. Image resolution continues to improve and there are no safety restrictions on repeat scanning, but further work must be undertaken to validate MR as an outcome measure over periods of time of 6 months or less.

Interestingly Reiman et al. (1996) have shown that cognitively normal individuals carrying the ApoE ε4 allele show reductions of glucose metabolism on PET scanning which are very similar to those shown by AD patients. If it can be demonstrated that these observed reductions progress PET could, in the future, offer a way to test treatments designed to prevent the development of AD in susceptible populations.

Treatment Specific Surrogate Markers

Whilst it may not yet be possible to employ surrogate markers for the disease process itself it may be possible in the case of a drug with a clearly defined mechanism of action to employ a surrogate marker which is specific to that mechanism. For example levels of erythrocyte cholinesterase activity and salivary amylase activity may have the potential to provide information, albeit indirectly, about cholinesterase inhibition and muscarinic agonist activity in the brain (Cutler et al., 1994).

When employing a peripheral marker it is clearly vital to know that the potential therapeutic agent penetrates the CNS. To answer this question PET and CSF sampling can be included in the development process. However, these techniques are either expensive or invasive or both and so it will often be necessary to rely on peripheral markers for early dose finding work without the reassurance of knowing the relationship between plasma and brain levels of the novel agent.

PHASE III

With the exception of fewer dose groups, possibly longer treatment duration and recruitment of more heterogeneous populations, the basic design of the Phase III trial is similar to that employed in Phase II. Outcome measures and treatment duration will be decided primarily on the basis of regulatory requirements. Given the inflexibility of this design it is vital that the general strategies employed in Phase II should be employed in Phase III.

With the current uncertain status of surrogate end-points, it is highly unlikely that any such alternative measure will become acceptable to regulatory authorities in the foreseeable future. This however, does not preclude the use of phase III trials for the investigation and validation of surrogate markers which may then be available for use with novel agents.

CONCLUSION

Despite the rapid rate of progress in understanding the molecular and neuropathological basis of AD much work has yet to be done to translate this to the clinical environment. The need to continue development of diagnostic and outcome measurements, both those that are clinical and biological/ technology based is evident. This issue becomes crucial if we are to identify patients in the early stages of the disease, or have an early efficacy marker for drugs that alter the underlying etiology of the disease without causing an improvement in symptomatology. The controlled environment of the clinical trial may provide an ideal setting for such research.

REFERENCES

Corder, E.H, Saunders, A.M, Strittmatter, W.J, Schemechel, D.E, Gaskell , P.C. et al, 1993, Gene dose of apolipoprotein E type 4 allele and the risk of Alzheimer's disease in late onset families. *Science.* 261:921.

Cutler, N. R., Sramek, J. J., and Veroff, A. E., 1994, Peripheral end-organ responses: Red blood cell cholinesterase and salivary amylase. *Alzheimer's Dis. Optim. Drug Develop. Strat.* ISBN 0471951455:73:88.

Fox, N. C., Freeborough, P. A., and Rossor, M. N., 1996, Visualization and quantification of rates of atrophy in Alzheimer's disease. *The Lancet.* 348:94:97.

Jagust, W. J., Haan, M. N., Eberling, J. L., Wolfe, N., and Reed B. R., 1996, Functional imaging predicts cognitive decline in Alzheimer's disease. *J. Neuroimaging,* 6, 156:160.

Kennard, M. L., Feldman, H., Yamada, T., and Jefferies, W. A., 1996, Serum levels of the iron binding protein p97 are elevated in Alzheimer's disease. *Nat. Med.* 2(N11):1230:1235.

Leber, P., 1990, Guidelines for the clinical evaluation of antidementia drugs. Rockville, *MD: US Food and Drug Admin.*

Merched, A., Blain, H., Visvikis, S., Herbeth, B., Jeandel, C., and Siest G., 1997, Cerebrospinal fluid apolipoprotein E level is increased in late-onset Alzheimer's disease. *J. Neurol. Sci.* 145(N1):33:39.

Poirier, J., Delisle, M., Quirion, R., Aubert, I., Farlow, M., Laiiri, D., Hui , S., Bertrand, P., Nalbantoglu, J., Gilfix, B. M., and Gauthier S., 1995, Apolipoprotein E4 allele as a predictor of cholinergic deficits and treatment outcome in Alzheimer disease. *Neurobiology.* 92:12260:12264.

Reiman, E. M., Caselli, R. J., Yun Lang, S., Chen, K., Bandy, D., Minoshima,, S., Thibodeau, S. N., and Osborne D., 1996, Preclinical evidence of Alzheimer's disease in persons homozygous for the E4 allele for apolipoprotein E. *N. Engl. J. Med.* 334(N12):752:758.

Rosen, W.G., Mohs, R.C., and Davis, K.L., 1984, A new rating scale for Alzheimer's disease, *Am. J. Psychiatry.* 141:1356:1364.

Roses, A. D., 1995, Apolipoprotein E genotyping in the differential diagnosis, not prediction, of Alzheimer's disease. *Ann. Neurol.* 38:6:14.

Selkoe, D.J, 1997, Alzheimer's Disease: Genotypes, Phenotype, and Treatments, *Science.* 275:630:631.

Skoog, I., Hesser, C., Fredman, P., Andreasson, L.A., Palmertz, B., and Blennow, K., 1997, Apolipoprotein E in cerebrospinal fluid in 85-year-old subjects - relation to dementia, apolipoprotein E polymorphism, cerebral atrophy and white matter lesions. *Arch. Neurol.* 54(N3):267:272.

Stern, R.G., Mohs, R.C., Davidson, M., Schmeidler, J., Silverman, J. M., Kramer-Ginzberg, E., Searcey, T., Bierer, L. M., and Davis, K. L., 1994, A longitudinal study of Alzheimer's disease: measurement, rate and predictors of cognitive deterioration. *Am. J. Psychiatry.* 151:390:396.

Stern, Y., Tang, N., Albert, M. S., Brandt, J., Jacobs, D. M., Bell, K., Marder, K., Sano, M., Devanand, D., Albert, S. M., Bylsma, F., and Tsai, W., 1997, Predicting Time to Nursing Home Care and Death in Individuals with Alzheimer Disease. *JAMA.* 277(N10):806:812.

121

TRIAL TO PREVENT NEURODEGENERATION IN PERSONS GENETICALLY PREDISPOSED TO ALZHEIMER'S DISEASE

Natalia Ponomareva, Vitaly Fokin, and Natalia Selesneva

Brain Research Institute
Obucha-by-Street, 5
103064, Moscow, Russia

INTRODUCTION

Genetic factors are of great importance in the development of Alzheimer's disease (AD)—a common progressive dementia of late age. The risk of AD is higher in first order relatives of the AD patients, than in other groups of the population (Amaducci et al., 1992). Genetic studies have shown that patients with AD can have mutations in one of three genes: β–amyloid precursor protein (βAPP) gene located in chromosome 21, presenilin 1 gene (PS-1) located in chromosome 14 and presenilin -2 gene (PS-2) located in chromosome 1 (St. George-Hyslop et al., 1987). A polymorphism of the Apolipoprotein E gene (ApoE) located in chromosome 19 is well established as accounting for much of the genetic risk in senile AD (Mullan, Crawford, 1993). At the present time there are no biochemical or genetic markers which could be used as predictors of AD development in relatives of AD patients before the clinical manifestation of the disease.

It has been shown that relatives of AD patients, predisposed to the AD development, can have some peculiarities of brain function organization before the beginning of the disease, which are not manifested clinically, due to compensatory mechanisms, but which can be revealed by neurophysiological methods (Ponomareva et al., 1995). Neurophysiological alterations in relatives of AD patients may increase the risk of further AD development.

We suggest that for the prevention of AD in persons genetically predisposed to the disease the normalization of brain functional activity can be helpful. To normalize brain activity we applied pykamilon—a medicine which stimulates GABA receptors and combines nootropic and tranquillizing properties.

The following study was aimed at determining neurophysiological alterations in AD patients' relatives, and at examining the effect of pykamilon on these alterations. We used visual evoked potentials to a flash to characterize the relatives' brain functions because that method is very effective for revealing brain function disturbances in patients with AD and their relatives (Harding et al., 1985; Ponomareva et al., 1995).

EXPERIMENTAL PROCEDURES

5 groups of people were examined:

1. 14 first-order AD patients' relatives (mean age 43.5 ± 2.9 years).
2. The same AD patients' relatives after one-month therapy with pycamilon (20 mg twice a day).
3. 15 middle aged healthy subjects, age-matched with the relatives (mean age 41.6 ± 2.6 years).
4. 20 patients with AD (the mean age 61.9 ± 1.4 years).
5. 20 healthy elderly subjects, age-matched with the AD patients years (mean age 60.8 ± 1.2).

All patients corresponded NINCDS-ADRDA criteria for probable Alzheimer's disease (McKhann et al., 1984). They were suffering from progressive mental impairment. None had a history of cerebral vascular disease and none had a focal brain abnormality in the CT scan. In all cases, folic acid deficiency, hypothyroidism, tertiary neurosyphilis, pernicious anaemia and alcohol abuse were ruled out.

The healthy volunteers and the AD patients relatives were normal on neurological examination; also, they had no history of cerebral vascular or psychiatric disease.

VEP to the flash were registered using evoked response recorder "Neuropack 11" (Nihon Kohden) at standard conditions (Harding et al., 1985). Subjects were awake and seated comfortably in the chairs with eyes closed. The impedance was maintained at below 5 kOm. Active electrodes were applied to the scalp over the occipital areas, points O1, O2. Reference electrodes were placed on the central areas, points C3, C4; a grounding electrode was positioned on the forehead (Fpz) (10–20 International System). Subjects were tested at a distance of 30 cm. The intensity of the flash was 0.3 Dg, and duration -0.1 ms. Stimuli were presented in random order. The sweep time was 500 ms. For each trial 128 sweeps were averaged. Latencies and amplitudes were measured at the highest peak of each wave component.

Data from each group were tested for normal distribution by the Wilk-Shapiro test, and in no cases were the data skewed. A statistical evaluation included the calculation of the means, standard deviations and standard error of each VEP component's latencies and amplitudes. The significance of the differences between the VEP parameters in the groups was estimated using One-Way ANOVA analysis (F-values). The differences were estimated as significant at the $p < 0.05$ level.

RESULTS

Table 1 presents the mean latencies of the VEP components in the middle aged and elderly healthy subjects, the patients with AD and their relatives. The same table gives the significance of differences between the groups as the result of ANOVA (F criteria).

The comparison of the parameters of healthy subjects of middle and old age indicated that the latencies of VEP components tended to be longer with aging, but the shifts of the la-

Table 1. Latencies of different components of visual evoked potentials in healthy subjects of middle and old age (H1, H2 respectively), in AD patients (AD) and their relatives before treatment (R) and under pykamilon (RP). Significance of differences between the groups of the VEP latencies according to results of ANOVA (F-value)

	P1		N1		P2		N2		P3		N3	
	d	S	d	s	D	s	d	s	d	s	d	s
H1												
X	56.3	57.6	81.6	81.5	115.3	116.7	142.4	142.8	173.5	173.9	222.5	219.7
SE	1.4	1.2.	2.2	1.5	4.8	4.1	7.6	7.7	10.1	9.8	10.8	10.9
H2												
X	60.7	59.6	88.0	85.7	121.3	120.1	153.5	154.5	181.9	181.7	229.2	228.7
SE	1.3	1.3	2.5	2.1	3.6	3.5	7.5	7.3	8.9	8.9	9.6	10.0
F-value N2/N1	–	–	–	–	–	–	–	–	–	–	–	–
R												
X	60.0	60.0	85.9	85.9	129.4	129.1	191.1*	190.9*	230.0*	231.5*	273.5*	271.5*
SE	1.9	1.9	1.6	1.6	5.5	6.3	9.4	9.3	8.5	7.9	11.2	11.7
F-value R/N1	–	–	–	–	–	–	15.112	14.735	13.854	15.404	9.022	9.070
RP												
X	59.5	59.3	82.5	82.5	117.0	115.8	174.3*	173.0*	209.3	209.3	247.8	253.8
SE	1.9	2.0	2.6	2.6	5.2	4.8	13.7	13.7	16.3	16.3	19.5	19.8
F-value RP/N1 Fvalue	–	–	–	–	–	–	4.872	4.377	–	–	–	–
RP/R	–	–	–	–	–	–	–	–	–	–	–	–
AD												
X	57.3	57.4	91.1	93.9	136.8*	139.3*	194.3*	198.4*	251.7*	246.3*	302.1*	296.6*
SE	2.8	2.9	5.9	5.9	6.5	6.6	12.5	13.3	18.9	20.0	19.7	20.1
F-value AD/N2	–	–	–	–	4.311	6.734	7.839	8.351	12.324	10.003	19.7	11.397

*P<0.05 (AD patients' relatives versus age-matched normal controls; AD patients versus age-matched normal controls).
X - mean
SE- standard error
Only significant (p<0.05) F-values are given in the table

tencies were not significant. Compared with the age-matched normal controls all VEP late component latencies (P2, N2, P3, N3) were considerably increased in AD patients.

In the AD patients' relatives the latencies of the N2, P3 and N3 late components were significantly longer than in age-matched normal controls.

Table 2 gives the mean VEP component amplitudes in the different groups. The statistical significance of differences between groups as the result of ANOVA (F criteria) is presented in the same table.

There was no significant difference in amplitude parameters between healthy subjects of different age. In AD patients compared with the age-matched controls the amplitudes of the P1 component in the left hemisphere and the N1 in the right hemisphere were increased and the amplitude of N3 component in both hemispheres was decreased. In the AD patients relatives, in comparison with the age-matched normal controls, a significant increase in the amplitude of P2 (in the right hemisphere) and N2 components was observed.

Under pykamilon the neurophysiological abnormalities were reduced in the AD patients' relatives. The VEP late components latencies tended to decrease (Table 1). After the treatment only the latencies of N2 components in the AD patients' relatives were significantly longer than in the age-matched normal controls. The shift of the latencies of P3 and N3 components in the group of relatives after the treatment was not significant.

Table 2. Amplitudes of different components of visual evoked potentials in healthy subjects of middle and old age (H1,H2 respectively), in AD patients (AD) and their relatives before treatment (R) and under pykamilon (RP). Significance of differences between the groups of the VEP latencies according to results of ANOVA (F-value)

	P1		N1		P2		N2		P3		N3	
	d	S	d	s	D	s	d	s	d	s	d	s
H1												
X	3.6	3.8	8.0	7.9	9.3	9.8	5.9	5.8	7.7	7.2	11.5	11.7
SE	0.4	0.5	0.7	0.8	1.3	1.4	1.3	1.1	1.3	1.0	1.5	1.3
H2												
X	3.3	3.4	7.0	7.1	10.0	10.1	7.7	7.4	6.5	6.2	9.9	10.3
SE	0.5	0.5	0.7	0.7	1.2	0.8	1.4	1.3	0.8	0.8	1.3	1.20
F-value N2/N1	–	–	–	–	–	–	–	–	–	–	–	–
R												
X	4.6	4.8	9.1	9.6	14.8*	13.4	15.6*	14.7*	7.2	6.8	7.1	7.4
SE	0.9	0.6	1.3	1.3	2.0	1.7	1.5	1.3	1.5	1.3	1.1	1.3
F-value R/N1	–	–	–	–	5.820	–	20.758	25.905	–	–	–	–
RP												
X	3.3	3.5	8.0	7.3	12.9	12.2	11.1*+	11.2*	7.5	7.5	7.2	8.6
SE	0.3	0.3	1.4	1.2	1.9	1.6	1.4	1.5	0.9	0.7	1.5-	1.1
F-value RP/N1	–	–	–	–	–	–	6.360	8.635	–	–	–	–
F-value RP/R	–	–	–	–	–	–	4.485	–	–	–	–	–
AD												
X	4.7	5.2*	9.9*	9.3	11.4	12.0	10.6	11.0	6.6	6.2	5.6*	4.8*
SE	0.5	0.5	0.9	1.2	1.3	1.4	1.3	1.4	1.2	1.1	1.1	0.9
F-value AD/N2	–	6.036	6.223	–	–	–	–	–	–	–	6.269	13.366

*P<0.05 (AD patients' relatives versus age-matched normal controls; AD patients versus age-matched normal controls)
+P<0.05 (AD patients' relatives versus AD patients' relatives under pykamilon)
X - mean
SE - standard error
Only significant F-values (p<0.05) are given in the table

The significant decrease of the amplitude of the N2 component in the right hemisphere was observed in the group of relatives under pykamilon compared with the same parameter before treatment (Table 2). The differences in the amplitude of the P2 component between the relatives and age-matched normal controls were not significant after the treatment.

DISCUSSION

VEP is widely used in neurophysiology and in clinical practice for the analysis of brain alterations with normal and pathological aging (Harding et al., 1985). Our previous studies showed that VEP parameters were also useful for investigating neurophysiological changes in AD patients' relatives (Ponomareva et al., 1995).

Analysis of the VEP component latencies in AD patients agrees with the results of the preceding studies, which showed a considerable delay of late components latencies with AD. A more pronounced shift of the late component latencies may be due to the atrophic alterations of the limbico-reticulo-cortical pathways, especially cholinergic ones, and associative visual areas with AD (Moore et al., 1992).

Our results show that in the middle aged AD patients' relatives there is the delay of the VEP N2, P3 and N3 late component latencies . These findings may be considered as signs of neurodegeneration in limbico-reticulo-cortical pathways, lesser than in the patients with AD. These data may reflect the early subclinical stages of the disease process. Obviously the neurodegeneration touches only certain brain systems, especially the cholinergic one, because the generation of the shifted components is connected with the rich cholinergic visual association areas 18 & 20.

The other neurophysiological peculiarity of the AD patients' relatives is the increase of the amplitude of the P2, N2 VEP late components. Such an increase reflects high reaction to afferent stimulation, connected with the hyperactivity of brain structures. It was observed in stress situations, under the effect of drugs, provoking the excitation of the brain (Zenkov and Melnitchuk, 1985).

The pathological hyperactivity in AD patients' relatives may be due to the presence of a small amount of β–amyloid peptide. β–amyloid has an excitotoxic effect on brain cells and often provokes epileptiform discharges of neurones (LaFerla, 1995). Besides, the presence of β–amyloid increases the neurotoxic effect of excitatory mediators. Its surplus leads to the activation of proteolytic enzymes, causing the proteolysis of the nervous cells (Seubert et al., 1988). Neuronal damage is also caused by oxidative stress (Fokin et al., 1989).

All these data allow us to suggest that the probable cause of the premature neurodegeneration in AD patients' relatives is the pathological hyperactivity of limbico-reticulo-cortical structures. A continuous increase in the degenerative alterations caused by pathological hyperactivity may be one of the factors of the manifestation of AD.

After one-month treatment with pycamilon, which combines nootropic and tranquillizing properties, the features of pathological hyperactivity of limbico-reticulo-cortical structures were reduced in AD patients' relatives: the amplitude of VEP late components was decreased. The shift of the latencies of the VEP late components tended to decrease. It is therefore suggested that pharmacological correction of neurophysiological disturbances in persons genetically predisposed to the disease can promote the prevention of AD.

REFERENCES

Amaducci, L., Falcini, M., Lippi, A., 1992, Descriptive epidemiology and risk factors for Alzheimer's disease. *Acta Neurol, Scand.* Suppl. 139:21–25.

Fokin, V. F., Ponomareva, N. V., Orlov, O. N., et al., 1989, Relations between electricity reactions of the brain and lipid peroxidation in patients with pathological ageing. *Bull. Exp. Biol. Med.* 54: 682–684 (rus).

Harding, G. F., Wright, C. E., Orwin, A, 1985, Primary presenile dementia. The use of visual evoked potential as a diagnostic indicator. Br. *J. Psychiatry* 147:532–539.

LaFerla, F.M., 1995, The Alzheimer's beta-amyloid peptide induces neurodegeneration and apoptotic cell death in transgenic mice. *Behav. Pharmacol.* Suppl. 6:55–56.

McKhann, G., Drachman, D., Folstein, M., Katzman, R., et al., 1984, Clinical diagnosis of Alzheimer's disease: Report of the NINCDS-ADRDA Work Group under the auspices of Department of Health and Human Services Task Forces on Alzheimer's Disease. *Neurology.* 34:933–944.

Moore, N. C., Tucker, K. A., Jann, M. W. et al., 1992, Flash P2 delay is a probable biological marker of primary degenerative dementia of the Alzheimer type. *Clinical Neuropharmacology. Proceeding of the 18 Collegium International Neuropharmacologicum Congress.* 15:291 B.

Mullan, M., Crawford, F., 1993, Genetic and molecular advances in Alzheimer's disease. *Trends Neurosci.* 16:398–403.

Ponomareva, N.V., Fokin, V.F., Selesneva, N.D., et al., 1995, Neurophysiological alterations and emotional disturbances in persons genetically predisposed to Alzheimer's disease. *Behav. Pharmacol.* Suppl. 6:57–58.

Seubert, P., Larson, J., Oliver, M. et al., 1988, Stimulation of MMDA receptors induces proteolysis of spectrin in hippocampus. *Brain Res.* 460:189–194.

St. George-Hyslop, P.H., Tanzi, R.E., Polinsky, R.J et al., 1987, The genetic defect causing familial Alzheimer's disease maps on chromosome 21. *Science* 235:885–890.

Zenkov L. R., Melnitchuc P. V., 1985, Central mechanism of afferentation in human brain. Medicina: Moscow. (rus).

122

DELAYING ENDPOINTS IN ALZHEIMER'S DISEASE AND MILD COGNITIVE IMPAIRMENT

Leon J. Thal

Department of Neurosciences
University of California San Diego
School of Medicine
La Jolla, California

INTRODUCTION

Alzheimer's disease (AD) is the nation's third most costly disease after cancer and heart disease (Ernst et al., 1994). In the United States in 1991, direct medical and social service costs averaged $48,000 per case per year while the total of direct and indirect costs were approximately $174,000 per annum. Total U.S. health care costs including direct and indirect were estimated at $67.3 billion in 1991 and are projected to exceed $80 billion by 1997 (Ernst et al., 1994). This enormous financial burden argues for approaches designed to slow the rate of decline or delay the onset of appearance of the disease.

Numerous studies have indicated that AD is infrequent below the age of 65. However, prevalence rises rapidly and approximately doubles with every five year epoch after the age of 65. These figures indicate that delaying the onset of AD by five years would halve the prevalence of this disorder in one generation. Similarly, if the age of onset could be delayed by 10 years, the prevalence would be decreased by 75% within one generation (Khachaturian, 1992).

Several classes of agents are available which might slow the decline or delay the onset of appearance of AD. These include:

- anti-inflammatory agents
- hormones, especially estrogens
- anti-oxidants
- growth factors
- agents that modify apolipoprotein E status
- drugs that alter the metabolism of amyloid

Progress in Alzheimer's and Parkinson's Diseases
edited by Fisher *et al.*, Plenum Press, New York, 1998.

Recently, a controlled clinical trial of selegiline, α-tocopherol or both was reported as treatment for AD (Sano et al., 1997). Selegiline is a monoamine oxidase inhibitor which acts as an anti-oxidant, increases lifespan in animals (Knoll, 1983), and increases levels of catecholamines. In short term trials in patients with AD, small but significant improvements in cognition (Piccinin et al., 1990), and overall rating of function (Mangoni et al., 1991) were reported. α-tocopherol is a lipid soluble vitamin which traps free radicals (Halliwell et al., 1991). It has also been reported to reduce cell death associated with β-amyloid neurotoxicity (Behl et al., 1992).

In this trial, 341 moderately demented AD patients from 23 participating Alzheimer's Disease Cooperative Study (ADCS) sites were enrolled in a two year placebo-controlled study. The primary endpoint for the study was the time to occurrence of any of the following: death, institutionalization, loss of the ability to perform basic activities of daily living, or severe dementia defined as a Clinical Dementia Rating of three (Morris, 1993). Subjects entered the trial with a Clinical Dementia Rating of two and were randomized to one of four groups: placebo, selegiline 5 mg bid, α-tocopherol 1000 IU twice daily, and the combination of selegiline and α-tocopherol. A series of secondary outcome measures were collected including measures of cognition (Alzheimer Disease Assessment Scale–Cognitive [ADAS-Cog] and Mini Mental State Examination [MMSE]), functional measures (Blessed Dementia Rating Scale and Dependency Scale), psychiatric assessment (CERAD Behavioral Scale), and the development of extrapyramidal findings as measured by the Unified Parkinson's Disease Rating Scale.

At baseline, patients were well-matched on age, education and duration of illness. The MMSE score was approximately two points higher in the placebo group than in the α-tocopherol group and mean MMSE scores for all four groups ranged from 11.3 to 13.3. A Cox Proportional Hazards Model that included the baseline score on the MMSE as a covariant was carried out and demonstrated significant delays in the time to the primary outcome for the patients treated with selegiline (medium time, 215 days), α-tocopherol (medium time, 230 days), or combination therapy (medium time, 145 days) as compared with the placebo group. In an analysis examining the percentage of subjects reaching each individual endpoint, there was a significantly lower rate of institutionalization for patients treated with α-tocopherol when compared to placebo. On secondary outcome measures, there was no difference in the rate of decline on the MMSE or the ADAS-Cog. Patients treated with any of the treatment regimens showed less decline on the Blessed Dementia Scale, a measure of loss of function. Both drugs were well-tolerated although there was a slightly increased rate of falls and syncope in subjects on combined selegiline and α-tocopherol therapy. We conclude that in patients with moderately severe AD, treatment with selegiline, α-tocopherol or both delays the time to important functional endpoints.

In attempting to delay the onset of AD, a potential strategy to pursue would include primary prevention trials. Unfortunately, because of the low incidence of AD, primary prevention trials require the enrollment of large numbers of subjects. Sample sizes to carry out a primary prevention trial are in the range of 6–8,000 with a follow up period of approximately 5 years. At present, the only primary prevention trial in AD is an add-on trial to the woman's Health Initiative (WHI), known as the WHI Memory Study (Shumaker et al., 1996). In this trial, approximately 8000 non-demented women over the age of 65 who are being randomized to hormone replacement therapy (estrogen alone or estrogen plus progesterone) will be cognitively evaluated over 5–8 years to determine if therapy with these agents can reduce incident cases of dementia. Because of the high cost and long duration of such studies, more efficient trial designs are needed.

An alternate strategy is to use a population "at risk". At Alzheimer's Disease Research Centers, individuals with mild cognitive impairment convert to AD at a rate of about 15% per annum or 45% after 3 years (Grundman et al., 1996). Thus, with three years of follow up, sufficient subjects will develop diagnosable AD to allow for the detection of a 30% decrease "at risk" subjects in a sample of 500 patients or fewer. Endpoints in such a trial would be the development of clinically diagnosable AD. This design would be considerably more efficient than conducting an incidence study in a healthy population.

ACKNOWLEDGMENT

Supported by NIH AGO 10483.

REFERENCES

Behl, C., Davis, J., Cole, G.M., and Schubert, D., 1992, Vitamin E protects nerve cells from amyloid-beta protein toxicity. *Biochem. Biophys Res. Commun.* 186:944–950.

Ernst, R.L., and Hay, J.W., 1994, The U.S. economic and social costs of Alzheimer's disease revisited. *Am. J. Public Health* 84:1261–1264.

Grundman, M., Petersen, R.C., Morris, J.C., Ferris, S., Sano, M., Farlow, M.R., Doody, R.S., Galasko, D., Ernesto, C., Thomas, R.G., Thal, L.J., and the ADCS Cooperative Study, 1996, Rate of dementia of the Alzheimer type (DAT) in subjects with mild cognitive impairment. *Neurology* 46:A403.

Halliwell, B., and Gutteridge, J.M.C., 1985, Oxygen radicals in the nervous system. *Trends Neurosci.* 8:22–26.

Khachaturian, Z., 1992, The five-five, ten-ten plan for Alzheimer's disease (editorial). *Neurobiol. Aging* 13:197–198.

Knoll, J., 1983, Deprenyl (selegiline): The history of its development and pharmacological action *Acta Neurol. Scand. Suppl.* 95:57–80.

Mangoni, A., Grassi, M.P., Frattola, L., Piolti, R., Bassi, S., Motta, A., Marcone, A., and Smirne, S., 1991, Effects of a MAO-B inhibitor in the treatment of Alzheimer's disease. *Eur. Neurol.* 31:100–107.

Morris, J.C., 1993, The Clinical Dementia Rating (CDR): Current version and scoring rules. *Neurology* 43:2412–2414.

Piccinin, G.L., Finali, G., and Piccirilli, M., 1990, Neuropsychological effects of L-deprenyl in Alzheimer's type dementia. *Clin. Neuropharmacol.* 13:147–163.

Sano, M., Ernesto, C., Thomas, R.G., Klauber, M.R., Schafer, K., Grundman, M., Woodbury, P., Growdon, J., Cotman, C.W., Pfeiffer, E., Schneider, L., and Thal, L.J., 1997, A controlled trial of selegiline, alpha-tocopherol, or both as treatment for Alzheimer's disease. *N. Engl.J. Med.* 336:1216- 1222.

Shumaker, S., and Rapp, S., 1996, Hormone therapy in dementia prevention: The Women's health initiative memory study. *Neurobiol. Aging* S17:S9.

CURRENT NEUROTRANSMITTER STRATEGIES IN AD DRUG DEVELOPMENT

Paul T. Francis, J. Tracy Alder, Kate L. Cole, Kirsten E. Heslop, Stephen L. Minger, and Maria J. Ramirez

Dementia Research Laboratory
Division of Biochemistry and Molecular Biology
United Medical and Dental Schools of Guy's and St. Thomas' Hospitals
London, United Kingdom

INTRODUCTION

Detection of very substantial deficits in the enzyme responsible for the synthesis of acetylcholine, choline acetyltransferase (ChAT), in the neocortex (Bowen et al., 1976; Davies and Maloney, 1976; Perry et al., 1977) and correlation with dementia rating (Francis et al., 1985) provided the first rational therapeutic target for the treatment of Alzheimer's disease (AD). Current drug therapies in use and under development for the treatment of AD have, therefore, tended to concentrate on restoring the cholinergic deficits associated with the disease. Continuing research is beginning to identify other possible therapeutic approaches to treating AD. Cholinoceptive glutamatergic pyramidal neurones have been proposed to play a central role in both the pathogenesis and cognitive impairment associated with AD. Enhancing the activity of these cells may provide a further target for therapeutic strategies to combat the progression of the disease (Francis, 1996). The development of new drugs for the treatment of affective disorders in general could also be applied to the specific area of AD drug development to enable treatment of behavioural changes associated with AD, including depression, anxiety, psychosis and overactivity (Hope and Fairburn, 1992). These abnormal behaviours are often identified by carers as the most difficult aspect of the disease to cope with and usually determine admission to long-stay residential care with the associated costs. The neurochemical basis of such symptoms in AD patients has only recently received significant attention (Esiri, 1996). These alternative neurotransmitter-based strategies for the treatment of AD, in addition to the current use of cholinomimetics with their limited success in clinical trials, forms the basis of this review on AD drug development.

Progress in Alzheimer's and Parkinson's Diseases
edited by Fisher *et al.*, Plenum Press, New York, 1998.

Neurotransmitter Biochemistry of AD

Analysis of AD brains has revealed extensive but selective neuronal loss with associated changes in neurotransmitter levels. In the cortex of AD brains, glutamatergic pyramidal neurones are primarily affected, with relative sparing of GABAergic interneurones. Subcortical neurones from ascending pathways are also lost resulting in reduced cortical cholinergic and serotonergic markers, however, dopamine and noradrenaline levels are relatively unaffected. The strongest correlates of dementia in AD patients are cholinergic dysfunction and chemical and histopathological markers of glutamatergic cortical pyramidal neurones. Cortical pyramidal neurone (DeKosky and Scheff, 1990) and synapse loss (DeKosky and Scheff, 1990), tangle counts (Wilcock and Esiri, 1982) and glutamate concentration (Francis et al., 1993) have all been shown to correlate with dementia rating. No markers of other transmitters have been demonstrated to correlate with dementia rating in more than a small number of studies. These findings clearly indicate that pyramidal neurones and their transmitter glutamate play a major role in the cognitive symptoms of the disease. They may, therefore, represent a therapeutic target in addition to the current use of cholinomimetics. Candidate drugs should, therefore, be selected for their ability to modify the activity of such neurones.

A severe loss of serotonergic dorsal raphe neurones which innervate the neocortex has been reported (Halliday et al., 1992) with several studies reporting reduced serotonin (5-HT) levels in the neocortex of postmortem AD brain (e.g. Palmer et al., 1987). Recent PM evidence indicates an altered balance between 5-HT_{1A} and 5-HT_{2A} receptors in the presence of preserved 5-HT concentrations (Chen et al., 1996). These changes could be proposed to further compound the glutamatergic hypoactivity as electrophysiological studies indicate that 5-HT inhibits pyramidal cells via 5-HT_{1A} receptors (McCormick and Williamson, 1989) while 5-HT_{2A} receptors are excitatory (Araneda and Andrade, 1991).

Neurotransmission and AD Pathology

The hyperphosphorylation of the microtubule-associated protein tau is believed to be the key event that changes normal adult brain tau to paired helical filament-tau and hence neurofibrillary lesions. Experimental data suggest that treatment of cells with glutamate or muscarinic agonists can lead to increases in dephosphorylated tau compared to control (Davis et al., 1995; Sadot et al., 1996). Similarly, glutamatergic and/or cholinergic agonists increase the production of APP and reduce β-amyloid formation (Nitsch, 1996). Thus, in addition to restoring a degree of cholinergic neurotransmission, treatment with cholinomimetics may increase secretion of APP with its associated neuroprotective properties, decrease the production of ß-amyloid and decrease the phosphorylation status of tau. Therefore, cholinomimetics may serendipitously affect the spread of AD pathology.

TREATMENT STRATEGIES FOR COGNITIVE IMPAIRMENT IN AD

Current Treatment

It is now well established that the strongest correlates of dementia in AD patients are cholinergic dysfunction and neurochemical and histopathological markers of glutamatergic cortical pyramidal neurones (Francis et al., 1993). In the cortex, the main target for cholinergic neurotransmission is glutamatergic pyramidal neurones, therefore in AD the loss of glutamatergic neurones is compounded by the cholinergic deficit. This is supported by experimental data. The activity of pyramidal neurones can be investigated in rat using glutamate release from the cortico-striatal pathway as a marker. In such studies both the acetylcholinesterase (AChE) inhibitor physostigmine (im) or the muscarinic M_1 agonist PD142505–0028 (applied topically to the cortex) increased striatal glutamate release measured by in vivo microdialysis (Dijk et al., 1995a). Trials with the AChE inhibitor tacrine have shown that while this drug does produce some improvement and slowing of cognitive decline, the benefit is modest (Byrne and Arie, 1994). A so called second generation of AChE inhibitors are in the final stages of development, however, a number of other approaches could be exploited to enhance the neuronal excitability of remaining pyramidal neurones in an attempt to overcome cognitive deficits.

Serotonergic Modulation of Glutamatergic Activity

Studies indicating the role of 5-HT in cognition indicate that decreased availability of 5-HT can enhance learning and memory while increased 5-HT impairs learning and memory tasks (McEntee and Crook, 1991). It is possible that the substrate for this action is modulation of either cholinergic or glutamatergic neurotransmission (Dijk et al., 1995b). In support of this, the effect of the muscarinic agonist PD142505-0028 on glutamate release was potentiated by co-application of WAY100-135 (Dijk et al., 1995a). The development of specific 5-HT_{1A} antagonists has allowed studies of the behavioural and biochemical effects of blockade of 5-HT_{1A} receptors. In marmosets WAY100-135 has been shown to ameliorate cognitive impairment following a fornix-fimbria transection (Harder et al., 1996). Another 5-HT_{1A} antagonist NAN-190 has been shown to compensate for septohippocampal cholinergic deficiency (caused by intra-hippocampal scopolamine) in the working memory of rats (Ohno and Watanabe, 1997).

Dialysis and behavioural studies indicate that 5-HT_{1A} antagonists may provide a useful treatment for the cognitive impairment in combination with either an AChE inhibitor or an M_1 agonists. Such polypharmacy may have additional benefits for AD patients with noncognitive behavioural problems (see below). For example, clinical trials using the β-blocker pindolol which has 5-HT antagonist action has shown that this combination treatment is effective in both overcoming the initial delay in the onset of antidepressant action and in producing an antidepressant effect in previously resistant patients (Artigas, 1995).

Serotonergic Modulation of ACh Release

The relationship between the serotonergic system and ACh release has been extensively studied in recent years. Drugs acting at different 5-HT receptor subtypes have been tested for their ability to modify ACh release in several brain regions. For example, 5-HT_3 receptors have been shown to inhibit ACh release from rat entorhinal cortex slices and from synaptosomes of human cerebral cortex (Maura et al., 1992). 5-HT_3 receptor antagonists, such as ondansetron and granisetron, produce a concentration-dependent increase in both spontaneous and K^+-evoked ACh release in rat striatal and entorhinal cortex slices, and it has been suggested that 5-HT_3 receptors could exert a tonic inhibitory control of ACh release. 5-HT_3 receptor antagonists may suppress this inhibition and promote augmented ACh release. In the entorhinal cortex it has been suggested that 5-HT_3 receptor antagonists are able to block a hypothetical excitatory influence of 5-HT on 5-HT_3 receptors located on GABA neurones, which inhibit the cholinergic system. A concomitant blockade of 5-HT_3 and $GABA_A$ receptors would thus contribute to restore a diminished cholinergic function (Ramirez et al., 1996).

The effects of ondansetron and other 5-HT$_3$ receptor antagonists on ACh release may provide a basis for the use of 5-HT$_3$ receptor antagonists in the treatment of cognitive disorders. This is supported by the observations that these drugs are able to improve performance in a behavioural test to evaluate cognitive function and to antagonize memory impairment induced by the muscarinic antagonist scopolamine or by cholinergic lesions (Cassel and Jeltsch, 1995).

Serotonin and GABAergic Action

The effects of 5-HT$_3$ receptor antagonists on cognition have also been related with the ability of these class of drugs to antagonize the inhibitory effect of 5-HT on the induction of the long-term potentiation in the hippocampus (Staubli and Xu, 1995). In the CA1 region of the rat hippocampus it has been shown that 5-HT can enhance the GABA-mediated inhibitory postsynaptic potentials. The increase in the activity of GABAergic interneurones produced by 5-HT would be related to the involvement of 5-HT$_3$ receptors in the blockade of LTP induced by primed burst stimulation in the CA1 region. It has also been suggested that the induction of the LTP in the mossy fibre-CA3 system is inhibited by an activation of 5-HT$_3$ receptors through the facilitation of GABAergic neurones and also through the inhibition of cholinergic neurones.

Nerve Growth Factor Treatment

Cholinergic neurones of the basal forebrain are the major neuronal population in the CNS which express receptors for nerve growth factor (NGF) (Mufson et al., 1989). Numerous studies have shown that procedures which result in the deafferentation of basal forebrain neurones from their target projection fields results in the atrophy and/or degeneration of cholinergic neurones and corresponding impairments in tests designed to assess learning and memory (see for example, Nilsson et al., 1987). Moreover, intracerebral administration of exogenous NGF can significantly ameliorate cholinergic neuronal degeneration and reverse lesion-induced behavioural deficits (Gage et al., 1986) suggesting that basal forebrain cholinergic neurones remain dependent on target-derived neurotrophic support for both long-term survival and integrative functioning within the brain.

There are, however, significant difficulties in delivering exogenous NGF to the brain as it does not readily cross the blood-brain barrier. Therefore, alternative means of administering NGF to circumvent this problem have been proposed, including the conjugation of NGF to antibodies specific for the transferrin receptor (Frieden et al., 1993) and intracerebral implantation of cells genetically modified to synthesize and release NGF (for review, see Suhr and Gage, 1993). Both approaches have resulted in enhanced cholinergic neuronal survival and attenuation of cognitive deficits comparable to that observed with direct intracerebral NGF administration.

The results of animal lesioning studies, therefore, suggest that the administration of neurotrophic factors (especially NGF) might be beneficial in supporting the survival of residual vulnerable neurones in human neurodegenerative conditions, in particular cholinergic neurones in the AD brain. There are, however, fundamental objections to the central role of NGF in cholinergic neuronal survival. Several experimental studies have shown that cholinergic neurones are capable of long-term survival despite the widespread loss of their target neurones and neurotrophic factor support (Sofroniew et al., 1993; Minger and Davies, 1992b; Minger and Davies, 1992a). More importantly, no consistent reductions in neurotrophic factors protein/mRNA nor alterations in neurotrophic receptor functioning have been reported in AD brain that might function as aetiological factors for cholinergic neuronal degeneration (see for example, Allen et al., 1991; Scott et al., 1995). Therefore, it is not surprising that to date, only a single case report of one patient treated with intraventricular NGF has appeared. Although cerebral blood flow and nicotinic receptor binding were transiently increased by NGF treatment, no significant cognitive improvement was observed (Olson et al., 1992).

Cholinergic Neuronal Replacement Therapy

Another potential therapeutic option for the treatment of AD is the repopulation of lost cholinergic neurones with replacement cells from developing brain. Numerous rodent and primate studies have shown that the implantation of cholinergic-rich foetal basal forebrain tissue into the target regions of cholinergic neuronal projections is capable of long-term survival and host-brain integration following implantation (for review, see Fisher and Gage, 1993). Moreover, these grafts have been shown to release acetylcholine under appropriate physiological conditions and to reverse many of the behavioural deficits normally observed in cognitively impaired aged animals or those subjected to surgical or excitotoxic lesions of the cholinergic system. This approach is attractive given the reports of long-term survival of grafted foetal dopaminergic neurones with corresponding clinical improvement in Parkinson's disease patients. However, the routine implantation of human foetal brain tissue is subject to a number of practical issues including significant difficulty in obtaining the necessary quantity of foetal tissue of the appropriate age as well as ethical concerns regarding the source of such tissue. Recent progress in extending *in vitro* neuronal proliferation and subsequent long-term survival following engraftment (see for example, Minger et al., 1996) offer hope that similar techniques may be applicable to human foetal tissue.

Despite the consistent findings of pronounced cholinergic hypo-/dysfunction in AD, modest progress has been made in regards to pharmacological therapies which attempt to increase the availability of acetylcholine at target synapses in the AD brain. Attempts to simulate production of ACh directly or to prolong its action at the synaptic cleft with inhibitors of AChE have met with modest clinical success. One novel approach, however, suggests that even diffuse local release of acetylcholine in the cortex may significantly influence cognition. Fisher and colleagues have demonstrated that fibroblasts genetically modified to synthesize ACh and implanted into the cerebral cortex significantly attenuated lesion-induced cognitive deficits in comparison to similarly deafferentated lesioned animals implanted with unmodifed fibroblasts (Winkler et al., 1995). Whether such local and tonic release of ACh will prove beneficial in primate and/or human studies remains to be determined, but these studies convincingly demonstrate that nonpharmacological methods of increasing acetylcholine concentrations at target synapses may be another route to cognitive enhancement in AD.

TREATMENT STRATEGIES FOR NONCOGNITIVE BEHAVIOURAL IMPAIRMENT IN AD

The cognitive decline associated with AD is often accompanied by behavioural disturbances such as, depression, anxiety, psychosis and overactivity (Hope and Fairburn, 1992). Knowledge of the neurochemical correlates of these behaviours may indicate rational therapeutic regimes. Previous studies have correlated serotonergic dysfunction in

AD with retrospectively assessed behavioural problems. These studies and the observation that several psychotropic drugs are believed to exert their action through modification of serotonergic transmission (Esiri, 1996), has prompted an investigation into the relationship between prospectively assessed behavioural problems and markers of the serotonergic system in AD.

Pathologically confirmed postmortem AD brains from a unique longitudinal study of prospectively assessed behaviour and cognition in community recruited patients (Hope and Fairburn, 1992) have been studied. Histochemical examination of these cases revealed a 40% reduction of ascending serotonergic neurones in the raphe nuclei which was not related to the behavioural disturbances observed. Somewhat surprisingly, the magnitude of loss was not uniformly reflected by the presynaptic neocortical markers examined in the same AD cases (Chen et al., 1996). 5-HT concentration was found to be unaltered in the two neocortical areas studied, while, the turnover of 5-HT (5-HIAA/5-HT ratio) was significantly increased in both the frontal and the temporal cortex. The maintained 5-HT concentrations and the increase in the turnover of 5-HT suggest a compensatory change in the remaining presynaptic terminals. Examination of the drug history of the cases revealed that those patients receiving neuroleptic medication had reduced cortical 5-HT concentrations which correlated with dorsal raphe neurone loss . This is in keeping with previous studies that reported reduced cortical 5-HT in predominantly institutionalised patients who were probably receiving chronic neuroleptic treatment (Esiri, 1996). This suggests that neuroleptic medication may inhibit potentially useful compensatory increases in serotonergic turnover. In light of this and due to the reported limited effectiveness of neuroleptic medication in the treatment of the behavioural disorders of dementia (for review, see Herrmann et al., 1996), neuroleptics should be used with caution in AD.

Paroxetine binding to the serotonin reuptake site, which has been used as a marker for serotonergic terminals, was reduced in both the frontal and temporal cortex in AD compared with controls; however, this reduction was significantly correlated with depression in these AD cases (12 out of 20 AD cases were depressed). Nondepressed AD cases had paroxetine binding densities similar to controls. The lack of correlation between dorsal raphe cell loss and paroxetine binding in nondepressed AD may be due to collateral sprouting of the remaining serotonergic innervation. The association between reduced serotonergic terminals and depression in AD suggests a theoretical benefit of selective serotonin reuptake inhibitors and indeed they have been used clinically with some success (Nyth and Gottfries, 1990).

Postsynaptic serotonergic receptors were differentially altered in this study of AD. 5-HT_{1A} receptor binding density was unchanged, whereas, the 5-HT_{2A} receptor was reduced in both regions compared with controls. However, anxious AD patients had preserved 5-HT_{2A} receptor levels which were not significantly different from controls, which suggests that anxiolytics such as the 5-HT_2 antagonist ritanserin (Pangalila-Ratu Langi and Jansen, 1988) may be useful for the treatment of anxiety in AD. It is important to note that the behavioural syndromes reported in Alzheimer's disease are not always distinct pathologies, indeed seven of the eight anxious cases in this study were also depressed, therefore, the overlap in symptoms must be considered.

CONCLUSIONS

In summary, the main focus for the amelioration of the cognitive deficit in AD is the enhancement of glutamatergic pyramidal neurone activity. This could be achieved in a number of ways including enhancement of excitatory input through cholinomimetics—muscarinic and nicotinic agonists, AChE inhibitors, nonpharmacological cholinergic approaches, $5HT_{1A}$ and $5HT_3$ antagonists. The treatment of noncognitive behavioural impairment has to date been largely overlooked. Postmortem data support the more widespread use of (serotonergic) drugs currently prescribed for similar symptoms in nondemented elderly patients. Through continuing research and drug development, the prospect of a symptomatic treatment of AD with a combination of therapies can now be envisaged, allowing for improvement in both cognitive and noncognitive deficits. These may also have the additional benefit of slowing the progression of the disease with consequent socioeconomic benefits.

REFERENCES

Allen, S. J., MacGowan, S. H., Treanor, J. J. S., Feeney, R., Wilcock, G. K., and Dawbarn, D., 1991, Normal β-NGF content in Alzheimer's disease cerebral cortex and hippocampus. *Neurosci. Lett.* 131:135–139.

Araneda, R. and Andrade, R., 1991, 5-Hydroxytryptamine2 and 5-hydroxytryptamine1A receptors mediate opposing responses on membrane excitability in rat association cortex. *Neuroscience* 40:399–412.

Artigas, F., 1995, Pindolol, 5-hydroxytryptamine and antidepressant augmentation. *Arch. Gen. Psychiat.* 52:969–971.

Bowen, D. M., Smith, C. B., White, P., and Davison, A. N., 1976, Neurotransmitter-related enzymes and indices of hypoxia in senile dementia and other abiotrophies. *Brain* 99:459–496.

Byrne, E. and Arie, T., 1994, Tetrahydroaminoacridine and Alzheimer's disease. *Br. Med. J.* 308:868–869.

Cassel, J.-C. and Jeltsch, H., 1995, Serotonergic modulation of cholinergic function in the central nervous system: cognitive implications. *Neuroscience* 67:1–41.

Chen, C. P. LH., Alder, J. T., Bowen, D. M., Esiri, M. M., McDonald, B., Hope, T., Jobst, K. A., and Francis, P. T., 1996, Presynaptic serotonergic markers in community-aquired cases of Alzheim's disease: correlation with depression and neuroleptic medication. *J. Neurochem.* 66:1592–1598.

Davies, P. and Maloney, A. J. F., 1976, Selective loss of central cholinergic neurones in Alzheimer's disease. *Lancet* ii:1403.

Davis, D. R., Brion, J., Gallo, J., Hanger, D. P., Ladhani, K., Lewis, C., Miller, C. C. J., Rupniak, T., Smith, C., and Anderton, B. H., 1995, The phosphorylation state of the microtubule-associated protein tau as affected by glutamate, colchicine and β-amyloid in primary rat cortical neuronal cultures. *Biochem. J.* 309:941–949.

DeKosky, S. T. and Scheff, S. W., 1990, Synapse loss in frontal cortex biopsies in Alzheimer's disease: correlation with cognitive severity. *Ann. Neurol.* 27:457–464.

Dijk, S. N., Francis, P. T., Stratmann, G. C., and Bowen, D. M., 1995a, Cholinomimetics increase glutamate outflow by an action on the corticostriatal pathway: Implications for Alzheimer's disease. *J. Neurochem.* 65:2165–2169.

Dijk, S. N., Francis, P. T., Stratmann, G. C., and Bowen, D. M., 1995b, NMDA-induced glutamate and aspartate release from rat cortical pyramidal neurones: evidence for modulation by a $5-HT_{1A}$ antagonist. *Br. J. Pharmacol.* 115:1169–1174.

Esiri, M. M., 1996, The basis for behavioural disturbances in dementia. *J. Neurol. Neurosurg. Psychiatry* 61:127–130.

Fisher, L. J. and Gage, F. H., 1993, Grafting in the mammalian central nervous system. *Physiol. Rev.* 73:583–616.

Francis, P. T., Palmer, A. M., Sims, N. R., Bowen, D. M., Davison, A. N., Esiri, M. M., Neary, D., Snowden, J. S., and Wilcock, G. K., 1985, Neurochemical studies of early-onset Alzheimer's disease. Possible influence on treatment. *N. Engl. J. Med.* 313:7–11.

Francis, P. T., Sims, N. R., Procter, A. W., and Bowen, D. M., 1993, Cortical pyramidal neurone loss may cause glutamatergic hypoactivity and cognitive impairment in Alzheimer's disease: investigative and therapeutic perspectives. *J. Neurochem.* 60:1589–1604.

Francis, P. T., 1996, Pyramidal neurone modulation: a therapeutic target for Alzheimer's disease. *Neurodegeneration* 5:461–465.

Frieden, P. M., Walus, L. R., Watson, P., Doctrow, S. R., Kozarich, J. W., Bergman, H., Hoffer, B., Bloom, F., and Granholm, A.-C., 1993, Blood brain barrier penetration and *in vivo* activity of an NGF conjugate. *Science* 259:373–377.

Gage, F. H., Wictorin, K., Fischer, W., Williams, L. R., Varon, S., and Bjorklund, A., 1986, Retrograde cell changes in medial septum and diagonal band following fimbria-fornix transection: quantitative temporal analysis. *Neuroscience* 19:241–255.

Halliday, G. M., McCann, H. L., Pamphlett, R., Brooks, W. S., Creasey, H., McCusker, E., Cotton, R. G. H., Broe, G. A., and Harper, C. G., 1992, Brain stem serotonin-synthesising neurons in Alzheimer's disease: a clinicopathological correlation. *Acta Neuropathol.* 84:638–650.

Harder, J. A., Maclean, C. J., Alder, J. T., Francis, P. T., and Ridley, R. M., 1996, The 5-HT$_{1A}$ antagonist WAY 100635, ameliorates the cognitive impairment induced by fornix transection in the marmoset. *Psychopharmacology* 127:245–254.

Herrmann, N., Lanctot, K. L., and Naranjo, C. A., 1996, Behavioural disorders in demented elderly patients. *CNS Drugs* 6:280–300.

Hope, T. and Fairburn, C. G., 1992, The present behavioral examination (PBE)—the development of an interview to measure current behavioral abnormalities. *Psychol. Med.* 22:223–230.

Maura, G., Andrioli, G. C., Cavazzani, P., and Raiteri, M., 1992, 5-HT3 receptors sited on cholinergic axon terminals of human cerebral cortex mediate inhibition of acetylcholine release. *J. Neurochem.* 58:2334–2337.

McCormick, D. A. and Williamson, A., 1989, Convergence and divergence of neurotransmitter action in human cerebral cortex. *Proc. Natl. Acad. Sci. USA.* 86:8098–8102.

McEntee, W. J. and Crook, T. H., 1991, Serotonin, memory, and the aging brain. *Psychopharmacology* 103:143–149.

Minger, S. L. and Davies, P., 1992a, Persistent innervation of the rat neocortex by basal forebrain cholinergic neurons despite the massive reduction of cortical target neurons. II. Neurochemical analysis. *Exp. Neurol.* 117:139–150.

Minger, S. L. and Davies, P., 1992b, Persistent innervation of the rat neocortex by basal forebrain cholinergic neurons despite the massive reduction of cortical neurons. I. Morphometric analysis. *Exp. Neurol.* 117:124–138.

Minger, S. L., Fisher, L. J., Ray, J., and Gage, F. H., 1996, Long-term survival of transplanted basal forebrain cells following in-vitro propagation with fibroblast growth factor-2. *Exp. Neurol.* 141:12–24.

Mufson, E. J., Bothwell, M., Hersh, L. B., and Kordower, J. H., 1989, Nerve growth factor receptor immunoreactive profiles in the normal, aged human basal forebrain: colocalization with cholinergic neurons. *J. Comp. Neurol.* 285:196–217.

Nilsson, O. G., Shapiro, M. L., Gage, F. H., Olton, D. S., and Bjorklund, A., 1987, Spatial learning and memory following fimbria-fornix transection and grafting of fetal septal neurons to the hippocampus. *Exp. Brain Res.* 67:195–215.

Nitsch, R. M., 1996, From acetylcholine to amyloid: neurotransmitters and the pathology of Alzheimer's disease. *Neurodegeneration* 5:477–482.

Nyth, A. L. and Gottfries, C. G., 1990, The clinical efficacy of citalopram in treatment of emotional disturbances in dementia disorders. *Br. J. Psychiat.* 157:894–901.

Ohno, M. and Watanabe, S., 1997, Blockade of 5-HT$_{1A}$ receptors compensates for loss of hippocampal cholinergic neurotransmission involved in working memory of rats. *Brain Res.* 736:180–188.

Olson, L., Nordberg, A., Von Holst, H., Backman, L., Ebendal, T., Alafuzoff, I., Amberla, K., Hartving, A., Herlitz, A., Lilja, A., Lundqvist, H., Langstrom, B., Meyerson, B., Persson, A., Vitanen, M., Winblad, B., and Seiger, A., 1992, Nerve growth factor affects $_{11}$C-nicotine binding, blood flow, EEG, and verbal episodic memory in an Alzheimer patient (Case Report). *J. Neural Transm.* 4:79–95.

Palmer, A. M., Francis, P. T., Benton, J. S., Sims, N. R., Mann, D. M., Neary, D., Snowden, J. S., and Bowen, D. M., 1987, Presynaptic serotonergic dysfunction in patients with Alzheimer's disease. *J. Neurochem.* 48:8–15.

Pangalila-Ratu Langi, E. A. and Jansen, A. A., 1988, Ritanserin in the treatment of generalized anxiety disorders: a placebo-controlled trial. *Hum. Psychopharm.* 3:207–212.

Perry, E. K., Gibson, P. H., Blessed, G., Perry, R. H., and Tomlinson, B. E., 1977, Neurotransmitter enzyme abnormalities in senile dementia. Choline acetyltransferase and glutamic acid decarboxlyase activities in necropsy brain tissue. *J. Neurol. Sci.* 34:247–265.

Ramirez, M. J., Cenarruzabeitia, E., Lasheras, B., and Delrio, J., 1996, Involvement of GABA systems in acetylcholine-release induced by 5-HT3 receptor blockade in slices from rat entorhinal cortex. *Brain Res.* 712:274–280.

Sadot, E., Gurwitz, D., Barg, J., Behar, L., Ginzburg, I., and Fisher, A., 1996, Activation of M$_1$ muscarinic acetylcholine receptor regulates ô phosphorylation in transfected PC12 cells. *J. Neurochem.* 66:877–880.

Scott, S. A., Mufson, E. J., Weingartner, J. A., Skau, K. A., and Crutcher, K. A., 1995, Nerve growth factor in Alzheimer's disease: increased levels throughout the brain coupled with declines in nucleus basalis. *J. Neurosci.* 15:6213–6221.

Sofroniew, M. V., Cooper, J. D., Svendsen, C. N., Crossman, P., Lindsay, R. M., Zafra, F., and Lindholm, D., 1993, Atrophy but not death of adult septal cholinergic neurons after ablation of target capacity to produce mRNAs for NGF, BDNF and NT-3. *J. Neurosci.* 13:5263–5276.

Staubli, U. and Xu, F. B., 1995, Effects of 5-HT$_3$ receptor antagonism on hippocampal theta rhythm, memory and LTP induction in the freely moving rat. *J. Neurosci.* 15:2445–2452.

Suhr, S. T. and Gage, F. H., 1993, Gene therapy for neurologic disease. *Arch. Neurol.* 50:1252–1268.

Wilcock, G. K. and Esiri, M. M., 1982, Plaques, tangles and dementia. *J. Neurol. Sci.* 56:343–356.

Winkler, J., Suhr, S. T., Gage, F. H., Thal, L. J., and Fisher, L. J., 1995, Essential role of neocortical acetylcholine in spatial memory. *Nature* 375:484–487.

HARMONIZATION OF DRUG APPROVAL GUIDELINES IN ALZHEIMER'S AND PARKINSON'S DISEASES

Rachelle Smith Doody,[1] Michael Davidson,[2] Ira Shoulson,[3] and Peter Whitehouse[4]

[1]Baylor College of Medicine
Houston, Texas
[2]Sackler School of Medicine
Hashomer, Israel
[3]University of Rochester Medical Center
Rochester, New York
[4]University Hospitals of Cleveland
Cleveland, Ohio

INTRODUCTION

The world's population is aging at an accelerated rate. In the United States, Western Europe and Japan where individuals over the age of 60 represent more than 20% of the population, the most rapidly growing population segment is people age 85 and over. Countries in South America and Asia, such as China and India, are aging at an even more rapid rate. Current projections suggest that more older people will be living in the developing world than in the developed world. It is therefore expected that most countries of the world will experience a rapid rise in diseases of aging, such as Alzheimer's disease and Parkinson's disease.

Recent academic advances have lead to new understanding of the pathophysiologies of these conditions and new approaches to treatment. The pharmaceutical industry, academia and governments are concerned about the cost of research and technology transfer. Governments have recognized that unnecessary impediments to drug development should be modified and eliminated if possible in order to improve the efficiency of the process (D'Arcy and Harron, 1991, 1993). In Europe there was recognition of the need to consolidate European drug regulatory practices as part of the development of the European Union. Thus, the European Medicines Evaluation Agency (EMEA) was formed in London in January 1995. It is now possible for pharmaceutical companies to submit applications for

Progress in Alzheimer's and Parkinson's Diseases
edited by Fisher *et al.*, Plenum Press, New York, 1998.

approval either to particular European countries individually or to all of Europe at once. For many disease states, governmental regulatory agencies have attempted to provide guidelines for drug approval.

By the 1990s, draft or unofficial guidelines for approval of dementia drugs either exist or are under development in the United States, Europe, Canada, Japan, and China. Through a consensus process, the U. S. Food and Drug Administration (FDA) created drug development guidelines in draft form at the time Tacrine was approved in 1993. These guidelines, which remain in draft form in 1997, consider various aspects of trial design focusing on drugs to improve cognition. Perhaps most important was the requirement for outcome measures which include objective psychometric testing as well as some measure of clinical meaningfulness (either a clinical global impression of change or an Activity of Daily Living scale). In Europe, the EMEA along with the Committee for Proprietary Medicinal Products (CPMP) has also developed multiple drafts of guidelines for dementia drug approval. In Japan, the Ministry and Health and Welfare have recently begun the process of modifying previous guidelines aimed at the approval of cerebral metabolic enhancers and vasoactive drugs, and the process of drafting guidelines is at an early stage in China. Current efforts will likely provide separate guidelines for the approval of drugs for vascular dementia and for Alzheimer's disease. Guidelines for the approval of other drugs, such as those to treat Parkinson's disease, would also benefit from a coordinated, global approach.

There emerged out of this environment a sense that drug studies in dementia could be conducted more efficiently if there were greater agreement among the academic, regulatory and pharmaceutical industry communities around the world. The International Working Group on the Harmonization of Dementia Drug Guidelines (IWG) was officially formed in July 1994 in Minneapolis at the International Alzheimer's Disease Conference. Approximately 50 invited opinion leaders discussed the feasibility of forming a group to examine how global drug development could be conducted more efficiently. Dr. Paul Leber from the U. S. Food and Drug Administration attended. Because there was active debate and discussion about regulatory guidelines at that time, the group decided to make harmonization of those guidelines its initial goal. The group also decided to address how academics, regulators and pharmaceutical industry representatives can cooperate to improve the efficacy of drug development internationally. A steering committee selected the word "harmonization" and a logo incorporating the Asian symbol for balance and harmony (yin-yang) to convey that this group will not try to standardize regulatory practices (it does not have that authority anyway), but rather that it will work for greater understanding of the process of efficient drug development, built on firm foundations of trust and careful intellectual inquiry.

Following the decision to form a group, leading academics, regulators, and industry scientists were surveyed about their interest in participating and their opinions on which topics would be most important to the harmonization process. Based on the results, committees were formed which focused on topics such as trial design and outcome measurement, as well as broader issues such as culture and ethics. Committees on pharmacoeconomics and quality of life were also established, to acknowledge the need for broad measures of the impact of drugs on patients and caregivers and the costs to society as a whole. With their membership spread across the world, the committees used modern communication technologies such as e-mail and facsimile to initiate development of the position papers that appear in this supplement.

Contacts were also made with organizations that might endorse the process, including Alzheimer's Disease International (ADI), the International Psychogeriatrics Association, the

World Federation of Neurology, the World Health Organization, and the International Federation of Pharmaceutical Manufacturer's Association. The latter is the secretariat for the International Conference on Harmonization, a group that is considering issues of standardization in global regulatory mechanisms for drugs. There was already FDA representation in the process, and regulators in Japan and Europe were also invited to participate.

Financial support was obtained principally from industry. A request was made for block grants from a number of companies, which allowed a meeting to be held in London in September 1995. This meeting was divided between plenary sessions and committee work sessions. Topics discussed in plenary sessions included the status of regulatory guidelines in different countries, practical problems for the pharmaceutical industry in drug development across national boundaries, and issues confronting developing countries that are not part of the major pharmaceutical markets or the International Conference on Harmonization. The committees met in working sessions and then presented their draft papers to the group as a whole.

After the London meeting, the committees continued to develop their papers, and revisions were presented to the overall group at the 1996 International Alzheimer's Disease Conference in Osaka. To facilitate comment and revision, a World Wide Web site was developed where the drafts of the committee papers were posted, and an information systems committee was formed to support the Web site. At the London meeting Dr. Eric Abadie of the EMEA discussed the evolution of the European guidelines, and their state of harmonization with the Japanese guidelines were reviewed. In addition, pharmaceutical companies made presentations about drugs that were in the late stages of clinical development and indicated some of the difficulties they were having with their global development programs.

In addition to the meetings in Minneapolis, London, and Osaka, several satellite meetings have been held in conjunction with other organizations. Canadian investigators met in April 1996 to discuss seeking official recognition of the Canadian guidelines. Japanese regulators, pharmaceutical company scientists and investigators discussed world guidelines and outcomes assessment in Tokyo, after the Osaka meeting. As the harmonization process became better known, members were invited to present at different meetings, including the International Geneva/Springfield Symposium on Advances in Alzheimer Therapy in Nice.

The IWG is now composed of 250 individuals from industry, academia and regulatory agencies. In general, there is significant agreement on many issues concerning trials for improving cognition. Some differences remain to be resolved concerning efficacy measurement, the nature of trial design, and the standardization of safety assessments. The FDA guidelines remain relatively static, although they have become a standard for comparison with other regulations. The EMEA guidelines are in their seventh version and continue to be revised, with debate about outcomes measures, responder analyses, and the length of studies. The Japanese Ministry is also working to revise its guidelines. Its drafts have been submitted to working committees. The Chinese Ministry of Health is working with investigators in that country to draft guidelines.

Internationally agreed upon approval criteria for anti-dementia drugs will serve both humanistic and commercial purposes. Although AD occurs in all populations which have been studied to date, the disease goes undiagnosed and unrecognized in many countries of the world. In other countries, it is thought of as an untreatable psychiatric disorder, often with social stigma attached to the diagnosis. Within most countries currently active in developing AD drugs, AD is a recognized illness known to have a biological and sometimes genetic basis, although practitioners vary widely in their understanding of its diagnosis and treatment.

This cultural background clearly affects regulations for the approval of AD drugs. The regulations vary as a reflection of local bureaucratic and research practices and as a function of how AD is viewed in the local society. Attitudes toward AD (within and between countries) include: it is disgraceful; it is embarrassing; it is part of normal aging; it is a mental illness; it is a brain disease; and it is abnormal, but inevitable. The predominant attitudes often shape local practices regarding the care of AD patient. For example, in sub-populations which regard AD as part of normal aging, there are often high levels of family involvement in providing care. Attempts to harmonize dementia drug guidelines must take cultural attitudes into account, must recognize that subcultures exist within every culture, and must acknowledge the impact that the harmonization process may have upon such cultural attitudes and practices.

Cultural differences also affect the process of actually carrying out clinical trials in diverse locales. Normative scores cannot be applied across diverse groups; assessment measures have to be translated for cultural equivalence (rather than simply linguistic equivalence); researchers have their own preferred clinical measures which may not be known internationally; diagnostic criteria and their application vary; standards of efficacy and safety vary; and clinical researchers play differing roles in relation to the regulatory agencies in their countries.

Industrial sponsors and others engaged in global AD drug development often remark that Alzheimer's disease seems to manifest and progress differently in different countries (reflected, for example, in divergent performance of placebo groups); that uniform procedures are difficult to achieve as personnel with radically different backgrounds may assume the same roles in clinical trials; and that the regulatory climate and hurdles for approval seem arbitrary across national boundaries.

The IWG aims to acknowledge these cultural factors in the process of helping to shape the development of approval guidelines. The ultimate goals are to: make it possible for multiple countries to simultaneously participate in a scientifically sound approval study; make studies conducted in diverse locales more relevant to local regulators with or without local participation when deciding whether or not to approve; make more agents available to more AD patients worldwide as quickly as possible; and reduce costs involved in global drug development.

Some of the questions to be addressed by future studies or by consensus groups within the IWG are:

1. How to design trials which test drugs to prevent AD or delay emergence of symptoms, and how to identify populations at risk which would facilitate such trials.

2. How to design ethical trials of novel compounds when mildly to moderately effective drugs are already marketed.

3. Do cholinomimetic show specificity for enhancing memory in AD patients or are they nonspecific drugs which improve cognitive functions regardless of specific etiology.?

4. Is the exclusion of patients with signs and symptoms of central vascular lesions from AD drug trials justified?

5. Do cost/benefit analysis discriminate against drugs for the treatment of AD in comparison with drugs used by younger non-demented patients?

6. What is the role of regulators and advocacy groups in influencing reimbursement policies for the currently available drugs for the treatment of AD?

Research and development of new treatments for Parkinson's disease in North America has been enhanced by the activities of the Parkinson Study Group (PSG). The PSG is a consortium of academic investigators who are committed to the cooperative planning, implementation, analysis, and reporting of controlled therapeutic trials for Parkinson's disease. The PSG now includes more than 150 investigators, coordinators and scientists from 56 participating academic sites in the United States and Canada.

The PSG is committed to the principles of open scientific communication, peer-review, full disclosure of potential conflicts-of-interest, and democratic governance of its organization and activities. Founded in 1986, the PSG is governed by a constitution and bylaws and an elected executive committee which is primarily responsible for the direction and oversight of its research projects and activities.

Since 1986, the PSG has completed and reported ten major multi-center trials under government and industry sponsorships. All PSG trials have been carried out under appropriate regulatory scrutiny (US Food and Drug Administration, Canadian Health Protection Board) and in keeping with efforts to harmonize standards of research and clinical practices.

In 1994–95, the PSG and the NORDIC Study Group carried out similar phase III multi-center trials examining the efficacy of the catechol-O-methaltransferase-(COMT)-inhibitor, entacapone. Despite predetermined differences in design, the results of the two 24-week independent trials were remarkably similar (Kieburtz, Rinne, et al., 1996). Additional efforts are underway to harmonize therapeutic trials in Parkinson's disease and related neurodegenerative disorders.

The development and operation of independent academic consortia have provided the means for ensuring high standards of research in the increasingly active but complicated environment of experimental therapeutics.

In conclusion, diseases like Alzheimer's disease and Parkinson's disease already pose a major financial burden to the world's governments, and this burden will clearly increase over the next decade or more. The International Working Group on the Harmonization of Dementia Drug Guidelines has been established to aid regulatory agencies, academic researchers, and pharmaceutical industry representatives in the process of efficiently testing promising anti-dementia drugs on a global basis and expediting their approval if they are found to be meritorious. The Parkinson's Study Group in the United States provides one model for rapid and scientifically sound assessments of putative anti-parkinsonian agents. It remains to be seen whether this model could be adapted effectively in other cultural settings. Clearly, an organized and global approach to evaluating therapies for Alzheimer's and Parkinson's diseases will make it possible for multiple countries to simultaneously participate in scientifically sound approval studies, will make such studies relevant to local regulators in countries not participating in trials, will make more agents available to more patients worldwide, and will reduce the cost involved in global drug development.

REFERENCES

D'Arcy, P.F., Harron, D.W.G., eds., 1991, International Conference on Harmonisation of Technical Requirements for Registration of Pharmaceuticals for Human Use. *Proc. First Int. Conf. Harmonisation*, Orlando, Florida.

D'Arcy, P.F., Harron, D.W.G., eds., 1993, International Conference on Harmonisation of Technical Requirements for Registration of Pharmaceuticals for Human Use. *Proc. Second Int. Conf. Harmonisation*, Orlando, Florida.

Kieburtz, K., Rinne, U.K., et al., 1996, The COMT Inhibitor Entacapone Increases "On" Time in Levodopa-Treated PD Patients with Motor Fluctuations; Report of Two Randomized, Placebo-Controlled Trials. *Mov. Dis. Abstract,.* 11(5): 595–596.

INDEX

A23187 calcium ionophore, 137–138
ABT-418, 466
Acetylcholine
  β-amyloid precursor protein-mediating activity of,
    137, 509
  brain membrane lipid phase effects of, 185–186
  dopamine interaction, in Parkinson's disease,
    484–485
  long-term potentiation effects, 663–665
  muscarinic receptor effects, 509, 662
  synthesis of, 668
    acetylCoA source, 587
    choline source for, 301, 305
    cholinesterase inhibitor-enhanced, 855
Acetylcholinesterase, 531, 541
  acetylcholine hydrolysis by, 523
  AF64A-induced disruption of, 669
  β-amyloid aggregation-mediating activity of, 542,
    553
  antisense oligonucleotides-induced inhibition of,
    553–554
  apolipoprotein E e4 allele-related activity increase,
    14
  brain membrane lipid phase, effect of antioxidants
    on, 183–186
  cerebral blood flow effects, 446
  cholinesterase inhibitor complexes, 523–530, 532
  crystallographic structural analysis, 531, 532
  G1/G4 forms of, 448–449
  Hu mutants, complexes with cholinesterase inhibi-
    tors, 531–539
    active center acidic residues in, 532–536
    edrophonium, 532, 533, 535–536
    huperzine A, 532, 533, 534–535
    tacrine, 532, 533, 534, 535–537
  membrane-bound, effect of antioxidants on, 177–181
  neuronal growth-regulating function of, 552
  precursor replacements for, 446
  retinospheroid effects, 544, 545–547
  mRNA, antisense oligodeoxynucleotide-dependent
    suppression of, 557–562

Acetylcholinesterase (*cont.*)
  tacrine-related inhibition, 568
  Torpedo
    cholinesterase inhibitor complexes, 523–530
    structure, 523
Acetylcholinesterase inhibitors: *see* Cholinesterase in-
    hibitors
N-Acetylcysteine, effect on dopaminergic cell apop-
    tosis, 110
Acetyl salicyclic acid, neuroprotective activity of, mo-
    lecular characterization of, 99–104
Actin gene
  developmental regulation of, 242
  up-regulation of, in β-amyloid precursor protein-ex-
    pressing cells, 3
Activities of daily living impairments (ADLIs), of
    Parkinson's disease patients, 373–374
Activity-dependent neurotrophic factor, 636, 637–638,
    640
Acylphosphatase, fibroblast content, in early-onset fa-
    milial Alzheimer's disease, 787–791
Adenosine triphosphate, effect on β-amyloid precursor
    protein processing, 137
S-Adenosylmethioine decarboxylase, 160
Adenoviral vector systems, in Parkinson's disease
    gene therapy, 647–652
Adenylate cyclase, muscarinic acetylcholine receptor-
    mediated increase of, 503
α₂ Adrenoceptors, in attentional performance, 725
Advanced glycation end products (AGE), 78, 79
AF64A, 667, 688–693
  advantages of, 670
  disadvantages of, 669–670
  gene expression of, 669
  neurotoxicity
    in cholinergic neurons, 511–512, 675–680
    hippocampal cholinergic pathway lesions,
      511–512
    nitric oxide in, 681–686
    mechanisms of, 668–669
  nucleic acid function effects of, 669

AF102B
  β-amyloid precursor protein processing and secretion effects of, 506, 510, 517, 518, 696
  clinical trials of, 519
  neurotrophic-like effects of, 517
  signal transduction effects of, 516
AF150, signal transduction effects of, 516
AF150(S)
  neurotrophic-like effects of, 517
  signal transduction effects of, 516
AF151, signal transduction effects of, 516
AF151(S), signal transduction effects of, 516
African Americans, Parkinson's disease prevalence in, 371
Agitation
  Alzheimer's disease-related, 317
  senile dementia-related, 318, 319, 320, 321
  as sleep disorder cause, 325
Agmatine, 160–161
Agnosia, senile dementia-related, 318, 319, 320, 321, 751
Akinesia, Parkinson's disease-related, 330, 437
Alcohol dehydrogenase, 669
Aluminum, cerebral content, in Alzheimer's disease, 293–300
  energy dispersive X-ray spectroscopic analysis of, 294, 296, 297, 298, 299
  in isolated nuclei, 294, 295, 296, 297–298
  secondary ion mass spectrometric analysis of, 294, 295–296, 298
Alzheimer's disease
  age-related factors in, 113–114
    Na,K-ATPase as mRNA expression as, 113–119
  β-amyloid cascade hypothesis of, 187–190
  β-amyloid precursor protein platelet isoform markers, 747–750
  apolipoproteins associated with: see specific apolipoproteins
  autosomal dominant inheritance of, 59
  cerebral blood flow in, 811
    acetylcholinesterase inhibitor-related increase, 446
    as diagnostic marker, 734–737
    focal reduction of, 734
    relationship to apolipoprotein genotype, 811–815
    relationship to premorbid functioning decline, 734–737
  cholinergic hypothesis of: see Cholinergic deficits, Alzheimer's disease-related
  cognitive impairments of, 317, 752
    cholinergic deficits associated with, 445–446
    drug therapy for, 478–479, 526, 587–593, 847–849
    generalized impairment subtypes, 272–273
    prevalent language impairment subtype, 272, 273–274
    prevalent visuo-spatial impairment subtype, 272, 273–274
    relationship to glucose metabolism, 587–593
    relationship to synapse concentration, 3
    severity, 445–446
    subtypes, 271–275

Alzheimer's disease (cont.)
  dementia of: see Dementia, Alzheimer's disease-related
  drug development process for, 833–839
    accelerated drug development, 835
    bridging studies, 829–832
    Phase II studies, 834–838
    Phase III studies, 838–839
    refining outcome measures, 838–838
  genetic markers, 835–836, 838
    with extrapyramidal features, 347
  health care costs of, 847
  incidence, 667, 765
  intraneuronal inclusions in, insolubility of, 77–78
  memory impairment associated with, 318, 319, 320, 321
    "amnesia pattern" of, 268, 269
    β-amyloid in, 563–564
    animal models of, 553, 563–564, 711–716
    antipsychotic drug-related, 319–320
    apolipoprotein E e4 allele and, 13–16
    cholinergic neuron impairment in, 711–716
    ENA 713 therapy for, 587–593
    episodic, 265–270
    excess acetylcholinesterase-related, 553
    huperzine A therapy for, 526
    muscarinic agonist therapy for, 518
    quaternary-lipophilic carbamate therapy for, 595–600
    release from "proactive inhibition" effect in, 309–315
  neuropsychological subtypes, relationship to disease progression rate, 271–275
  neurotrophic hypothesis of, 615, 616
  onset age, see also Alzheimer's disease, early-onset
    relationship to 1-antichymotrypin genotypes, 760–761
  paired helical filament assembly in, 231
  pathogenesis, 1–5; see also β-Amyloid; β-Amyloid precursor protein; Amyloidosis; Cholinergic deficits; Neurofibrillary tangles; Senile plaques
  predictors of, 15
  prevalence, 667, 765, 847
    projected increase, 861
  progression rate, 588
    relationship to β-amyloid formation rate, 188
  relationship to dementia with Lewy bodies, 456–457, 459–460
  sleep disorders associated with, 323–237
  stages of, relationship to neurofibrillary deposits distribution, 223
  survival time in, 319
Alzheimer's disease, early-onset
  β-amyloid precursor protein mutations associated with, 25
  familial
    β-amyloid precursor protein gene mutations associated with, 187
    chromosome mutations associated with, 187, 787
    fibroblast acylphosphatase levels in, 787–791

Alzheimer's disease, early-onset (*cont.*)
  presenilin gene mutations associated with, 25, 141,
    187
  tau protein abnormalities in, 7–11
Alzheimer's disease, familial, *see also* Alzheimer's
    disease, early-onset, familial
  centromere disturbances in, 793–798
  chromosomal mutations associated with, 187, 188,
    793
Alzheimer's disease, late-onset, apolipoprotein E e4
    allele associated with, 187, 811
Alzheimer's disease, sporadic
  a1-antichymotrypsin gene polymorphism in,
    757–764
  apolipoprotein E e4 allele associated with, 811
  environmental insult-related, 187
  fibroblast acyltransferase levels in, 788–790
  head trauma-related, 187
  reduced cerebral glucose metabolism in, 587
  risk factors for, 587
Alzheimer's Disease Assessment Scale, 834, 836–837,
    848
Alzheimer's Disease Cooperative Study, 848
Alzheimer's Disease International, 862–863
Alzheimer's disease patients, relatives of
  as caregivers, 371–376
  visual evoked potentials in, 841–845
Alzheimer's Disease Research Center, 849
γ-Aminobutyric acid, cerebral hemispheric localiza-
    tion, 280
γ-Aminobutyric acidergic neurons, effect of serotonin
    on, 854
Ammonia, nitric oxide-mediated neurotoxicity, 681
Amnesia
  β-amyloid (25–35)-induced, 92, 94, 97
  scopolamine-induced, effect of S12024–2 on,
    470–471, 472, 474–475
"Amnesia pattern," of Alzheimer's disese, 268, 269
Amylase, saliva content, 838
Amylin, as amyloid precursor protein, 214, 217
Amyloid A, 4'-iodo-4'-deoxydoxorubicin binding of,
    199
β-Amyloid, 121
  as Alzheimer's disease marker, 2
  in Alzheimer's disease pathogenesis, 1–3
  apolipoprotein E2-related inhibition of, 638
  apolipoprotein E e4 allele-related accumulation of,
    13
  apoptosis-inducing activity
    antioxidants and, 45
    oxidative stress in, 47–48, 50
  cerebral expression of, effect of cholinergic injury
    on, 668
  cerebrospinal fluid content
    ELISA detection of, 773–778
    immunochemical detection of, 823–828
  classification, 214
  in cystic fibrosis, 214
  definition of, 213–214

β-Amyloid (*cont.*)
  in diabetes, 213, 215, 217
  in dialysis patients, 213
  in Down's syndrome, 121
  excitotoxicity, 845
  fibril structure, 191–192
  formation of, 488
    in cell-free system, 492
    endocytic pathway in, 488–489, 490
    rate of, 188
    tacrine-related decrease, 563–569
  forms of, 121
  heparin binding growth associated molecule associ-
    ated with, 121–131
  hereditary cerebral hemorrhage with amyloidosis-re-
    lated, 121
  inflammatory response to, 188
  in leprosy, 214
  localization, 823
  neurotoxicity, 2, 188, 495
    of β-amyloid (25–35), 89–99
    antioxidants' lack of efficacy against, 48–49
    cholinesterase-mediated protection against, 466
    estrogen-mediated protection against, 466
    mechanisms of, 495
    nicotine-mediated protection against, 466
    in RN46A cell cultures, 495–502
    vasoactive intestinal peptide-mediated protection
      against, 637
  non-Alzheimer's disease associations of, 1, 213,
    214, 215, 217
  N-terminal of, solubilty epitope of, 205–211
  in osteomyelitis, 214
  polymerization of, peptidoorganic inhibitors of,
    191–195
  solubility-related epitopes of, monoclonal antibody
    binding to, 205–211
    aggregation-inhibiting effects, 207–210
    binding profiles, 206
  effect on tetrazolium salts reduction, 496–500
  in tuberculosis, 214
β-Amyloid cascade hypothesis, of Alzheimer's dis-
    ease, 187–190
β-Amyloid metabolism-altering drugs, as Alzheimer's
    disease prophylaxis, 847
Amyloidosis
  amyloid associated proteins of, 121
  animal models of, 214–219
  British type, heparin binding growth associated
    molecule in, 122, 126, 128
  definition of, 197
  meningocerebrovascular Hungarian-type, 122, 127
β-Amyloid plaques: *see* Senile plaques
β-Amyloid precursor protein, 133–134
  astrocytic expression of, 588
  cleavage, 488, 509
    enzymes involved in, 188, 488, 509, 517, 563
    muscarinic receptor-induced, 517
  immunochemical detection of, 823–828

β-Amyloid precursor protein (*cont.*)
  isoforms, in platelets, as Alzheimer's disease
    marker, 747–750
  muscarcinic agonist-induced inhibition of, 517–518,
    520–521
  neuronal localization and trafficking of, 487–494
    anterograde transport, 489
    characterization of APP-containing organelles in,
      490–493
    cytoplasmic proteins' role in, 492–493
    endocytic pathway of, 488–489, 490
    insertion in nerve-terminal plasma membrane,
      489–490
    localization, 489
    retrograde transport, 490
  presenilin complex formation, 141, 144–145
  processing of, 133–139
    as β-amyloid source, 197
    calcineurin (protein phosphatase 2B) in, 136
    calcium in, 137–139
    muscarinic acetylcholine receptors in, 509–513
    non-amyloidogenic, 503, 506–507
    protein kinase C in, 133–136, 137, 138
    protein kinase C/phospholipase C-linked first
      messenger in, 137
    protein phosphatase 1 line, 136
  relationship to forebrain cholinergic system,
    695–697
  secretion
    cholinomimetics-related increase, 852
    muscarinic acetylcholine receptor-mediated,
      510–511
    tacrine-related reduction of, 563–569
  synthesis, 2
β-Amyloid precursor proteins
  proteolysis, 492
  release into extracellular space, 488
β-Amyloid precursor protein-expressing cells, actin
  gene up-regulation in, 3
β-Amyloid precursor protein gene mutations, 2, 487
  as familial Alzheimer's disease marker, 198, 765,
    835, 836
  gene locus, 841
  effect on β-amyloid precursor protein processing,
    188
  Swedish mutations, 133, 139
Anapsos, 699–703
Anesthesia, 458
Animal models, of Alzheimer's disease, 668
  AF64A neurotoxicity in, 668–670
  β-amyloid (25–35) neurotoxicity in, 90–97
  of amyloidosis, 214–219
  β-amyloid precursor protein induction, secretion,
    and pharmacological regulation in, 695–698
  β-amyloid precursor protein mutations in, 25–30
  apolipoprotein E-deficient
    cholinergic neuronal impairments in, 711–716
    dopaminergic neuronal impairments in, 711 712,
      714–715, 716

Animal models, of Alzheimer's disease (*cont.*)
  of cognitive impairment, S12024–2 therapy for,
    471–476
  192-Ig-saporin neurotoxicity in, 668, 670–672
  of memory deficits
    anapsos-related improvement, 699–703
    neuropeptide-related improvement, 653–660
  of tau hyperphosphorylation, 251–256
Animal models, of Parkinson's disease
  glial cell line-derived neurotrophic factor effects in,
    607–614
  interval hypoxic training of, 717–723
Anthracyclines
  amyloidosis-inhibiting activity of, 198–203
    in experimental scrapie, 201–203
  structure, 198
Anticholinergic drugs: *see* Cholinesterase inhibitors
Anticholinesterase inhibitors: *see* Cholinesterase in-
    hibitors
1-Antichymotrypsin gene polymorphism, in Alzhe-
    imer's disease
  Alzheimer's disease onset age and, 760–761
  antichymotrypsin plasma levels and, 758, 761, 762,
    763
  apolipoprotein E genotype and, 758, 759–763
  ethnic group-related variations in, 761
Anticonvulsive therapy, for Parkinson's disease-re-
    lated seizures, 361
Antidepressant therapy, for Alzheimer's disease pa-
    tients, 317
Anti-inflammatory agents, as Alzheimer's disease pro-
    phylaxis, 847
Antioxidants, *see also specific antioxidants*
  as Alzheimer's disease prophylaxis, 847
  effect on membrane-bound acetylcholinesterase,
    177–181
  in oxidative stress, 79
  ultra-low doses of, effect on brain membrane, lipid
    phase acetylcholinesterase, 183–186
Antipsychotic drugs, adverse effects of, 319–320, 321
Antisense oligodeoxynucleotides, acetylcholinesterase-
    suppressing activity, 553–554, 557–562
Anxiety
  Alzheimer's disease drug therapy-related, 851,
    855–856
  Alzheimer's disease-related, 317
  senile dementia-related, 318, 319, 320, 321
Apathy, Alzheimer's disease-related, 317
Aphasia, senile dementia-related, 318, 319, 320, 321,
    751
Apolipoprotein A gene, 397
Apolipoprotein A-I, 122
Apolipoprotein A-II, 214, 215
Apolipoprotein B, as oxidation target, 31
Apolipoprotein E
  β-amyloid-like fibril promotion/inhibition by, 130
  in atherosclerosis, 811
  in cardiovascular disease, 811
  cholesterol transport function, 31

Apolipoprotein E (*cont.*)
  as familial Alzheimer's disease risk factor, 787
  functions of, 31, 638
  intron 1 enhancer element C/G polymorphism, 757
  isoforms, cysteine and methionine content, 36
  as ligand, 17
  oxidation, 31
    C-terminal lipoprotein fragments in, 36–37
  phospholipid redistribution function, 31
  polymorphism of, Alzheimer's disease-associated, 509
  as senile plaque component, 495
  serum levels, effect of apolipoprotein E genotype on, 765–771
Apolipoprotein E2, 638
  lipid transport properties, 805
  oxidation, differential susceptibility of, 31–37
Apolipoprotein E2 allele, 31, 836
Apolipoprotein E3
  amino acid substitution, 17
  cellular accumulation, comparison with apolipoprotein E4, 17–23
  interaction with tau protein, 252
  lipid transport properties, 805
  neuronal growth-promoting activity of, 638
  oxidation, differential susceptibility of, 31–37
Apolipoprotein E3/3
  relationship to serum apolipoprotein E levels, 767–768
  in senile dementia, relationship to cerebrovascular function, 813, 814
Apolipoprotein E3/4
  relationship to serum apolipoprotein E levels, 767, 768
  in senile dementia, relationship to cerebrovascular function, 813, 814
Apolipoprotein E4
  Alzheimer's disease association, 806–809
  amino acid substitutions, 17
  cellular accumulation, comparison with apolipoprotein E 3, 17–23
  lipid transport properties, 805, 806, 808
  neuronal growth-inhibiting activity of, 638
  neuronal repair hypothesis of, 806, 809
  oxidation, differential susceptibility of, 31–37
  relationship to Parkinson's disease, 806–809
    with dementia, 390, 391–392
  vascular dementia association, 806–809
Apolipoprotein E4/4
  relationship to serum apolipoprotein E levels, 767–769
  in senile dementia, relationship to cerebrovascular function, 814
Apolipoprotein E-deficient mice
  cholinergic neuronal impairments in, 711–716
  peptide-mediated neuroprotection in, 635–636, 639–640
  tau protein hyperphosphorylation in, 251–256

Apolipoprotein E e4 allele, 3, 39–43, 766, 799, 836, 841
  β-amyloid deposition associated with, 133–134
  in dementia with Lewy bodies, 454
  depression associated with, 39–43
  Down's syndrome relationship, 819
  frequency of, 757
    ethnic group-related variations in, 757
  in hemorrhagic stroke patients, 808–809
  impaired antioxidant activity of, 252
  lack of relationship to cognitive impairment, 757
  as late-onset familial Alzheimer's disease risk factor, 17–18, 638, 835–368
  membrane repair and biosynthesis defects associated with, 251–252
  memory impairment and, 13–16
  Parkinson's disease dementia relationship, 817–821
  S12024–2 activity and, 470, 475
  vascular dementia relationship , 799
Apolipoprotein E-modifying drugs, as Alzheimer's disease prophylaxis, 847
Apolipoprotein J, 126
Apomorphine
  antioxidant and cytoprotective properties of, 421–427
  as Parkinson's disease therapy, 421, 423
    effect on motor status, 435, 436–438
  as parkinsonism freezing phenomenon treatment, 332
Apoptosis, 3–4, 45–52
  AF64A-induced, 668, 669, 670, 677
  as alternative effector pathway, 81
  β-amyloid-induced, 46
    β-amyloid (25–35)-induced, 89–90
    antioxidants' lack of neuroprotective against, 45, 48
    in hippocampal neurons, 705–709
    lipid peroxidation in, 49–50
    neuroprotection against, 45, 46, 47–48
    oxidative stress-induced, 46, 50
    in PC12 cells, 257–263
    relationship to tau phosphorylation, 257, 259–262
    in tau-transfected CHO cells, 257–263
  as β-amyloid secretion cause, 3
  calcium homeostasis and, 89–90
  definition of, 105
  DNA mismatch repair system in, 83–84, 85
  excitotoxicity-induced, 84
  glucose metabolism reduction-induced, 47
  in hippocampal CA1 neurons, β-amyloid-induced, 705–709
  mitochondrial dysfunction-related, 60–61
  neurotrophin-mediated, 615, 616
  1-methyl-4-phenylpyridinium ion-induced, 109
  N-methyl(R)salsolinol-induced, 105–111
    effect of antioxidants on, 106, 107, 110
    effect of cycloheximide on, 107, 109
  oxidative stress-induced, 46, 50, 414
  p53-related promotion of, 81, 82–83

Apoptosis (*cont.*)
   presenilin-enhanced, 144–145
   protein kinase A-mediated pathway of, 89–90
   in tau-transfected CHO cells, 257–263
   transcriptional cascade in, 84–85
APP: *see* β-Amyloid precursor protein
Apraxia, senile dementia-related, 318, 319, 320, 321
Arachidonic acid, muscarinic acetylcholine receptor-
      mediated release, 503
Arginine-vasopressin, memory-enhancing activity, 653
Aricept: *see* E2020
Aromatic 1-amino acid decarboxylase gene, adeno-asso-
      ciated virus vector-mediated transfer, 650–651
Aromatic 1-amino acid decarboxylase, in dopamine
      conversion, 647–648
Ascorbic acid: *see* Vitamin C
Aspirin, neuroprotective activity of, molecular charac-
      terization of, 99, 100, 102
Assistive devices, for Parkinson's disease patients,
      373–374
Astrocytes
   antioxidant vitamin and enzyme content, 166–167
   matrix metalloproteinases of, cytokines-related
      modulation, 149–157
Astrogliosis
   Alzheimer's disease-related, 197
   β-amyloid precursor protein gene mutation-related,
      198
Atherosclerosis, apolipoprotein E in, 811
Attention, tacrine-related improvement of, 478–479
Autism, alterations in consciousness associated with,
      452
Axonal injury, effect on tau protein mRNA expres-
      sion, 244, 247–248
   cytoskeletal protein gene expression and, 242, 243
Axons, terminal, loss of, 3
Axoplasmic flow, in Alzheimer's disease, 3

Basal forebrain, cholinergic neurons of, nerve growth
      factor receptors, 854
Basal ganglia, in dementia with Lewy bodies, 456
bcl-2, 411
Behavioral disorders
   Alzheimer's disease-related, 851, 855–856
   senile dementia-related, 319–0321
1-Benzyl-1,2,3,4-tetrahydroisoquinoline, 431
Besipirdine, maximum tolerated dose, 830, 831
BH4, partial deficiency, hereditary progressive
      dystonia-associated, 365, 368
Biological markers, of Alzheimer's disease, 837
Blood flow, cerebral, in Alzheimer's disease, 811
   acetylcholinesterase inhibition-related increase, 446
   as diagnostic marker, 734–737
   focal reduction of, 734
   relationship to apolipoprotein E genotypes, 811–815
   relationship to glucose metabolism abnormalities,
      588, 589, 591
   relationship to premorbid functioning decline,
      734–737

Blood pressure
   clonidine-related decrease, 729–730
   guanfacine-related decrease, 729–730
   relationship to apolipoprotein E genotype, 799–803
Boston Naming test scores, of Alzheimer's disease,
      Parkinson's disease, and Huntington's cho-
      rea patients, 378, 379, 381
Bradykinesia, Parkinson's disease-related, 437, 752
Bradykinin, effect on β-amyloid precursor protein
      processing, 137
Bradyphrenia, 348
Brain
   in Alzheimer's disease, *see also* Neurofibrillary tan-
      gles; Senile plaques; specific areas of the
      brain
      aluminum content, 293–300
      apoptosis-inducing agents' effects on, 46–47
      atrophy, 278, 279
      comparison with non-demented brains, 278
      c-peptide content, 287–292
      insulin-like growth factor I receptor density, 288,
         290–291
      insulin receptor density, 287–292
      lipid composition, 301–307
      neuroimaging of, 734–737
   β-amyloid protein content
      effect of cholinergic injury on, 668
      immunochemical detection of, 823–828
   neuronal membrane permeability, β-amyloid
      (25–35)-related increase, 90
   in Pick's disease, 279
Brain banking, of Alzheimer's disease brains, 277–285
   brain specimens
      fixation, freezing, and storage of, 282–284
      hemispheric asymmetry of, 280, 282
      nucleus basalis of Meynert of, 279–280, 281
   postmortem factors in, 277–279
Brain derived neurotrophic factor, 496, 627
Brain derived neurotrophic factor gene, 627–633
Brain injury
   as Alzheimer's disease risk factor, 588–589
   polyamine treatment of, 160–161
Brainstem, thalamic inputs to, 457
Bridging studies, in Alzheimer's disease drug therapy,
      829–823
   maximum tolerated dose, 829, 830, 831
   minimum intolerated dose, 829
Brown Peterson task scores, of Alzheimer's disease,
      Parkinson's disease, and Huntington's
      chorea patients, 382
bul-2, 54
Butyrycholinesterase, in Alzheimer's disease, 541
   cross-reactivity with anticholinesterase inhibitors,
      552
   tacrine-related inhibition, 568
Butyrycholinesterase gene, mutations of, 552

Calbindin-28K, mRNA, cerebral expression, in Alzhe-
      imer's disease brains, 114

Calcineurin, effect on β-amyloid precursor protein processing, 136

Calcium, effect on β-amyloid precursor protein processing, 137–139

Calcium homeostasis, in Alzheimer's disease pathology, 3
  relationship to acylphosphatase levels, 787–788, 790

Carbachol
  effect on β-amyloid precursor protein secretion, 510
  effect on long-term potentiation, 662, 663–665

Carbamates, quaternary-lipophilic, 595–600

Carbonyls, 78

Carboxypeptidase A, resistance to AF64A, 669

Cardiovascular disease, apolipoprotein E in, 811

Caregivers, of Parkinson's disease patients, 371–376

β-Carotene, in haloperidol-induced neurotoxicity, 165, 166, 16

Carotid sinus syndrome, 456

Catalase, antioxidant activity of, 54, 415
  in dopaminergic cell apoptosis, 107, 110

Catecholamines, neurotoxicity of, 422–423

Catechol-*O*-methyltransferase gene, mutant alleles of, in Parkinson's disease, 396–397

Catechol-*O*-methyltransferase inhibitors, 865

CDR(R) molecule, 622, 615

CDTF, effect on β-amyloid neurotoxicity, 496

Centromeres, Alzheimer's disease-related disturbances of, 793–798

Cerebellum
  β-amyloid (25–35) neurotoxicity in, 93, 94
  β-amyloid precursor protein secretion from, 510
  phospholipid content, in Alzheimer's disease, 302, 303, 305

Cerebral cortex
  β-amyloid (25–35) neurotoxicty in, 93, 94
  β-amyloid precursor protein secretion from, 510
  cholinesterase inhibiting activity in, 448
  phospholipid content, in Alzheimer's disease, 302, 303, 305

Cerebrospinal fluid
  β-amyloid content, ELISA detection of, 773–779
  β-amyloid precursor protein content, 509
    effect of cholinesterase inhibitors on, 696–697
    effect of forebrain neurotransmitter system lesions on, 696
    effect of muscarinic acetylcholine receptors in, 511
  apolipoprotein E levels in, 768, 837
  in Parkinson's disease
    1-benzyl-1,2,3,4-tetrahydroisoquinoline content, 431
    cytokine content, 407–412
  pH of, in Alzheimer's disease autopsy specimens, 277, 280
  pyruvate content, in Alzheimer's disease, 587

Cerebrospinal fluid sampling, use in drug development process, 838

Cerebrovascular disease, Alzheimer's disease misdiagnosed as, 733–734

c-fos gene, 765

Charles Bonnet syndrome, 455

China, senile dementia incidence and prevalence in, 389–392

Chloramine, apolipoprotein E isoforms' differential response to, 32–37

Chlorpromazine, extrapyramidal effects of, 163

Cholesterol, in Alzheimer's disease
  influence of apolipoprotein E genotype on, 766–769
  apolipoprotein E-related transport of, 31
  brain membrane content, effect of antioxidants on, 183–186
  membrane remodelling function of, effect of apolipoproteins on, 766
  oxidative stress sensitivity effects of, 56

Choline
  as acetylcholinesterase precursor, 446
  high affinity transport of, 668–669

Choline acetlytransferase
  AF64A-related disruption of, 669, 677
  Alzheimer's disease-related deficits of, 531, 687, 851
    apolipoprotein E allele and, 14
    correlation with cognitive impairment severity, 445–446
  choline acetylation by, 668
  dementia with Lewy bodies-related deficits of, 457
  gene expression of, effect of AF64A on, 677
  nerve growth factor-related increase, 678

Choline kinase
  AF64A-related disruption of, 669
  brain content, in Alzheimer's disease, 305

Cholinergic agonists, effect on β-amyloid precursor protein processing, 137

Cholinergic deficits
  Alzheimer's disease-related, 445, 515, 531, 668, 851
    apolipoprotein E e4 allele and, 13
  as cognitive deficit cause, 445–446, 553
    drug therapy for, 851–855
    peptide-mediated neuroprotection against, 638–640
  nerve growth factor-mediated reversal of, 688–694
  Parkinson's disease-related, 481

Cholinergic inhibitors: *see* Cholinesterase inhibitors

Cholinergic neuronal replacement therapy, 855; *see also* Embryonal brain tissue transplants

Cholinergic neurons
  AF64A neurotoxicity in, 511–512, 675–680
  in apolipoprotein E-deficient mice, 711–716
  nerve growth factor neuroprotection in, 854–855
  neurotoxins specific for, 667
    192-IgG-saporin, 667, 671–673
    AF64A, 667, 668–670, 672–673
  Parkinson's disease-related loss, in cognitive impairment without dementia, 348
  during REM sleep, 458–459

Cholinesterase(s), *see also* Acetylcholinesterase
  brain selectivity of, 447–448
  metabolism of, 447–448
  molecular forms of, 448–449
  in neurodegeneration, 541–549

Cholinesterase inhibitors, 531, 551–555, 595; *see also names of specific cholinesterase inhibitors*
  acetylcholesterase-promoting activity of, 553
  adverse response to, genetic predisposition to, 552
  clinical trials of, 571–573
  cognitive effects of
    comparative study of, 571–576
    long-term, 574
    relationship to percentage of acetylcholinesterase inhibition, 573–575
  combined with β-amyloid precursor protein releasers, 575–576
  combined with β-amyloid precursors, 575–576
  combined with estrogens, 575–576
  combined with muscarinic agonists, 575–576
  combined with nicotonic agonists, 575–576
  crystallographic structural analysis of, 532–538
  dosage, 552
  efficacy of, comparative studies of, 571–575
  Food and Drug Administration-licensed, 523
  effect on glutaminergic neurons, 446
  high-dose formulations, 552
  mode of inhibitory action of, 447
  effect on neurotransmission, 445, 446, 447–448
  as Parkinson's disease therapy, 607
  peripheral cholinergic stimulation by, 447–448
  preclinical studies of, 447–448
  quaternary-lipophilic carbamates as, 595–600
  side effects, 574
  slow-release formulations, 574–575
Cholinomimetics, as Alzheimer's disease therapy, 851, 852–857; *see also* Cholinesterase inhibitors
Chromosome 1
  as Alzheimer's disease gene locus, 371, 765
  mutations of, early-onset familial Alzheimer's disease-related, 787
  as presenilin gene locus, 3
Chromosome 4, as Parkinson's disease gene locus, 348, 371
Chromosome 4q-q23, as Parkinson's disease gene locus, 394–395
Chromosome 6q25.2–27, as Parkinson's disease gene locus, 401–406
Chromosome 14
  as Alzheimer's disease gene locus, 371, 765
  mutations, 2
    early-onset familial Alzheimer's disease-related, 787, 793
    presenilin Met146Leu missense, 788, 789, 790
  as presenilin gene locus, 3, 141
Chromosome 19
  as Alzheimer's disease gene locus, 765–766
  mutations of, familial Alzheimer's disease-related, 793
Chromosome 21
  as Alzheimer's disease gene locus, 371
  as β-amyloid precursor protein gene locus, 747
  mutations, 2
    β-amyloid precursor protein, Val717Ile mutation, 788, 789
    familial Alzheimer's disease-related, 787, 793, 797

Chromosome 22, elongated short arm, in familial Alzheimer's disease, 793
Chromosome X, age-related loss of, 794
Chromosome Y, age-related loss of, 794
Chymotrypsinogen, resistance to AF64A, 669
CI-979, maximum tolerated dose, 83–831
Ciliary nerve growth factor, in electrical blockade-related neuronal apoptosis, 638
Ciliary neurotrophic factor, 637
4-CIN, effect on lactate-supported synaptic function, 172, 173–175
Cingulate cortex, β-amyloid (25–35) neurotoxicity in, 93
Cingulate gyrus, Lewy bodies in, 353, 355
Circadian rhythm changes
  Alzheimer's disease-related, 323, 324–326
  senile dementia-related, 319, 320, 321, 324, 325
Clinical Dementia Rating, 848
Clinical trials
  of Alzheimer's disease drugs, 829–832
  cultural differences affecting, 864
  of Parkinson's disease drugs, 865
  Phase II
    clinical efficacy variables, 834
    optimal dose determination for, 829–832
    outcome measures, 836–838
    trial duration, 834–835
  Phase III, 838–839
Clinician's Interview Based Impression of Change, 834
Clonidine, attentional performance effects of, 725–731
Clozapine
  extrapyramidal effects, 163
  seizure-inducing activity of, 361
Cocaine, phenyltropane analogs of, 739–745
Cognex, 833
  efficacy determination, 836–837
Cognitive deficits, Alzheimer's disease-related, 317; *see also* Memory deficits; Alzheimer's disease-related
  comparison with Parkinson's disease-related and Huntington's chorea-related deficits, 377–383
  effect of drug therapy on, 478–479, 526, 847–849
    comparative study of, 571–576
    long-term effects of, 574
  glucose metabolism in, 587–588
    effect of ENA713 on, 587–593
  relationship to synapse concentration, 3
  severity of, correlation with cholinergic deficits, 445–446
Cognitive deficits, Parkinson's disease-related, 337–341
Committee for Proprietary Medicinal Products, 833, 834, 862
Computed tomography (CT), 734, 837–838
Consciousness
  alterations in, dementia with Lewy bodies-related, 454, 456–460
  conditions affecting, 451–452
  definition, 451

Convulsions, senile dementia-related, 319, 320, 321
Cox Proportional Hazards Model, 848
C-peptide, cerebral, in Alzheimer's disease, 287–292
Creutzfeld Jakob disease, 197
    meningocerebrovascular Hungarian-type, 122
    nucleus basalis of Meynert in, 279
Crystallographic studies, of acetylcholinesterase-choli-
        nesterase inhibitor complexes, 523–530
Cybrid models, of mitochondrial dysfunction
    in Alzheimer's disease, 61–66
    in Parkinson's disease, 69–73
Cycloheximide, effect on apoptosis, 107, 109
    in N-methyl(R)salsolinol-induced apoptosis, 107,
        109
Cyclosporin A, 136
CYP1A1, mutant alleles, Parkinson's disease-associ-
        ated, 396
CYP2D6, mutant alleles, Parkinson's disease-associ-
        ated, 396
Cysteine, 36
Cystic fibrosis, β-amyloid in, 214
Cytochrome c oxidase, Alzheimer's disease-related de-
        fects of, 60, 61
    in cybrid models, 61–64
Cytochrome oxidase 1 gene mutations, familial Alzhe-
        imer's disease-associated, 187
Cytochrome oxidase 2 gene mutations, familial Alzhe-
        imer's disease-associated, 187
Cytokines
    matrix metalloproteinases modulation by, in astro-
        glial cells, 149–157
    neurotrophic properties of, 637, 638
Cytoplasmic proteins, in β-amyloid precursor protein
        processing, 492–493
Cytoskeletal changes, Alzheimer's disease-related, 197
Cytoskeletal proteins, mRNA expression, 242–248
    following axonal injury, 242, 243
Cytoskeleton, neuronal, 3

D 1 agonists, seizure-inducing activity of, 361
D2–4 dopamine receptor genes, Parkinson's disease-
        associated, 397
Decamethonium, 524
Delusions, 452
    Alzheimer's disease-related, 317, 459
    dementia with Lewy bodies-related, 454
Dementia, senile
    Alzheimer's disease-related
        apoptosis and, 3
        cerebral c-peptide in, 287–292
        cerebral glucose metabolism in, 587–588, 751–756
        cerebral insulin in, 287–292
        cerebral insulin-like growth factor in, 287–292
        in China, incidence and prevalence of, 389, 390
        comparison with Parkinson's disease and Hunt-
            ington's chorea, 377–383
        cortical pathology of, 752
        drug therapy for, 848
        neuropathology of, 752
        effect on recall of Rabin's assassination, 385–387

Dementia, senile (cont.)
    apolipoprotein E genotype-related blood pressure
        in, 799–803
    cerebral blood flow in, 811–815
    cognitive impairment associated with, 317–322,
        751–752
    cortical, memory performance in, 265
    depression relationship of, 39
    diagnostic criteria for, 751
    differential diagnosis of, use of glucose metabolism
        for, 751–756
    fronto-temporal lobe, 452
    fronto-temporal with parkinsonism, 347
    huperzine therapy for, 526
    Lewy body, 451–462
        apolipoprotein E e4 allele frequency in, 819–820
        clinical criteria for, 351
        hallucinations associated with, 452, 453, 454,
            455–456, 460
        effect of tacrine on, 485
    mixed
        cognitive symptoms of, 320
        noncognitive symptoms of, 318, 320
        sleep disorders associated with, 324, 325, 326
    multi-infarct: see Dementia, senile, vascular
    noncognitive symptoms of, 317–322
    Parkinson's disease-related
        age-related prevalence of, 343
        apolipoprotein E associated with, 390, 391–392,
            806–809, 817–821
        cerebral glucose metabolism in, 752–755
        with coincidental Alzheimer's disease, 817
        cortical pathology of, 344
        incidence of, 343
        effect on interpersonal relations with family mem-
            bers, 373
        neuropsychological features of, 752
        prevalence of, 343–350, 481, 817
        relationship to disease severity, 347
        tacrine treatment for, 481–486
        without dementia, 806–809
    prevalence, 343–350, 391, 481, 799, 811, 817
    sleep disorders associated with, 323–327
    subcortical, memory performance in, 265, 269
    transcranial Doppler ultrasound monitoring of, 812–814
    vascular
        apolipoprotein E genotype-blood pressure rela-
            tionship in, 799, 800, 801
        apolipoprotein E phenotypes associated with,
            806–809
        brain phospholipid content, 302–305
        cerebral glucose metabolism in, 752–755
        cognitive symptoms of, 320
        relationship to hypertension, 391, 392
        incidence and prevalence in China, 389, 390, 391,
            392
        neuropathology of, 752
        noncognitive symptoms of, 318, 320
        relationship to cerebrovascular disease, 391, 392
        sleep disorders associated with, 324, 325, 326

Dementia-Associated Sleep Disorders Scale, 324
Dementia Differential Diagnostic Schedule, 389
Dentate gyrus
β-amyloid (1–40)-induced degeneration in, 705–709
granule cells of, NMDA-mediated damage to, 101
Deprenyl
antioxidant activity of, 415
effect on dopaminergic cell apoptosis, 107
Depression
alterations of consciousness associated with, 452
Alzheimer's disease drug therapy-related, 851, 855–856
Alzheimer's disease-related, 317
as sleep disorder cause, 323, 325
apolipoprotein E e4 allele and, 39–43
in Parkinson's disease patients, 374
in Parkinson's disease patients' caregivers, 372, 373, 374
relationship to senile dementia, 39, 318, 319, 320, 321
Desferrioxamine, neuroprotective properties of, 423, 424
lack of, in haloperidol-induced neurotoxicity, 165, 166, 168
DFP, effect on cerebrospinal fluid amyloid precursor protein levels, 697
Diabetes, β-amyloid in, 213, 215, 217
Diagnosis, of Alzheimer's disease, accuracy of, 733–734
Diagnostic and Statistical Manual-III, dementia diagnostic criteria of, 389
Dialysis patients, amyloid in, 213
Diffuse Lewy body disease, 347
Dimethyl dichlorovinyl phosphate, as metrifonate metabolite, 580, 581, 582–583
1,2-Dimethyl-6,7-dihydroxyisoquinolinium ion, 106, 109–110, 417, 418, 419
1(R),2(N)-Dimethyl-6,7-dihydroxy-1,2,3,4-tetrahydroisoquinoline, neurotoxicity of, in Parkinson's disease, 413–420
3-(4,5-Dimethylthiazol-2yl)-2,5-diphenyltetrazolium, 496, 497, 498–500
0,0-Dimethyl-2,2,2-trichloroethyl phosphonate: *see* Metrifonate
Dipalmitoyl phosphatidylcholine, interaction with apolipoprotein E, 32–37
Disorientation, senile dementia-related, 318, 319, 320, 321
DMSO, neuroprotective activity, in haloperidol-induced neurotoxicity, 165, 167, 168
DNA, AF64A affinity for, 676–677, 678
DNA damage, AF64A-induced, 669
Domperidone, 423
Donepezil, 447
efficacy of, comparative studies of, 572, 573, 574
inhibitory action mode of, 447
side effects of, 572
DOPA: *see* Levodopa

Dopamine
antioxidant properties of, 423, 424, 425–426
effect on 1-benzyl-1,2,3,4-tetrahydroisoquinoline-induced toxicity, 430–432
biosynthetic pathway of, 648
as endogenous 6-OHDA source, 422–423
haloperidol neurotoxicity-potentiating effect of, 165, 167
nicotinic acetylcholine receptor-mediated secretion, 463
in Parkinson's disease
deficiency of, 647–648
interaction with acetylcholine, 484–485
Dopamine neurons
in apolipoprotein E-deficient mice, 711, 712, 714–715, 716
effect of brain derived neurotrophic factor on, 631–633
cholinergic mediation of, 484
effect of interval hypoxic training on, 717–723
N-methyl (R) salsolinol-induced apoptosis in, 105–111
in Parkinson's disease
in cognitive impairment without dementia, 348
effect of glial cell line-derived neurotrophic factor on, 607–614
Dopamine transporter gene, 397
Dopamine transporter proteins, phenyltropanes' affinity for, 739–743
Down's syndrome
Alzheimer's disease neuropathology associated with, 198
Alzheimer's disease progression in, 191
β-amyloid accumulation in, 2, 638, 774
β-amyloid precursor protein gene associated with, 198
apolipoproptein E2 allele in, 638
apolipoprotein E e4 allele in, 819
apolipoprotein E4 genotype in, 638
chromosome 21 gene locus in, 371, 793
dementia of, 819
Drug therapy, *see also specific drugs*
for Alzheimer's disease, drug approval guidelines for, 861–865
as sleep disorder cause, 324, 325
Dyscrasia, plasma-cell, amyloidosis reversal in, 198–199
Dystonia, hereditary progressive, with marked diurnal fluctuation, 363–370

E2020, 373, 833
action mechanism of, 552
dosage, acetylcholinesterase specificity of, 552
Food and Drug Administration approval of, 523, 595
Edema, cerebral, as cognitive and memory impairment cause, 589
in animal models, 590–591
treatment of, 590–591
Edrophonium, 524
complexes with HuAChE mutants, 532, 533, 535–536

Educational level, of Alzheimer's disease patients, 733–735
Elderly population, increase of, 390, 861
Electroconvulsive therapy, 353, 357
Embryonal brain tissue transplants, 855
  acetylcholinesterase-containing, 447
  complications of, 644
  as Huntington's chorea treatment, 643–646
  long-term results of, 644–645
  as Parkinson's disease treatment, 643–646
ENA-713, 595
  brain selectivity of, 448, 449
  effect on acetylcholinesterase G1/G4 forms, 448–449
  effect on cognitive impairment, 587–593
  efficacy of, comparative study of, 572, 574
  inhibitory action mode of, 447, 449
  lipophilicity of, 448
  metabolism of, 447
  side effects of, 572
Encephalopathy, spongiform, 198, 216
Endoglycosidase F/N glycosidase F, 236
Entacapone, 865
Entorhinal cortex
  β-amyloid-containing plaques, 1
  β-amyloid (25–35) neurotoxicity in, 93, 95
  neurofibrillary pathology in, 7, 9
  tau protein abnormalities in, 7
Enzyme-linked immunoassay (ELISA), for β-amyloid cerebrospinal content detection, 773–778
Enzymes, see also specific enzymes
  antioxidant activity, 54
Epidermal growth factor, in electrical blockade-related neuronal apoptosis, 638
Epilepsy, Parkinson's disease-related, case history of, 359–361
Eptastigmne
  efficacy of, comparative study of, 572, 573, 574
  maximum tolerated dose, 830
  side effects of, 572
Erythrocytes
  cholinesterase content, 838
  membrane-bound acetylcholinesterase content, effect of antioxidants on, 177–181
Estrogens, neuroprotective properties of, 466, 847
  combined with cholinesterase inhibitors, 575–576
Ethnic factors
  in 1-antichymotrypsin plasma concentration, 761
  in apolipoprotein E e4 allele frequency, 757
Ethylcholine mustard aziridinium: see AF64A
European Medicines Evaluation Agency (EMEA), 861–862, 863
Executive functions deficits, dementia-related, 751
Extrapyramidal symptoms, dementia-related, 319

Farnesyl thiosalicilate, 506, 507
Fas antigen/APO-1, 410
Fasciculin-acetylcholinesterase complex, 524–525

Fatty acids, brain content, in Alzheimer's disease, 302, 303, 304, 305, 306
Fe65 protein, 493
Fenton reaction, 90, 422, 423
Fetal tissue grafts: see Embryonal brain tissue transplants
Fibroblast(s), acylphosphatase content, in familial Alzheimer's disease, 787–791
Fibroblast cultures, apolipoprotein E3/apolipoprotein E4 differential accumulation in, 19–21
Fibroblast growth factor, 637
  basic, 506
Fibroblast implants, as acetylcholine source, 855
Food and Drug Administration (FDA)
  Alzheimer's disease drug development guidelines of, 833, 834
  drug approval guidelines of, 862, 863
Free radicals
  apolipoprotein E isoforms' differential response to, 32–37
  catecholamine-derived, 422–423
  sources of, 53–54
Frontal cortex
  Lewy bodies of, 354
  phospholipid content, in Alzheimer's disease, 301, 303, 305
Frontal-striatal loops, Parkinson's disease-related disruption of, 348
Fronto-parietal cortex, β-amyloid (25–35) neurotoxicity in, 93, 95, 96
Fronto-temporal lobe dementia, 452

Gait disorders, Parkinson's disease-related, 752
  as freezing phenomenon, 329–335
Galanthamine, inhibitory action mode of, 447
Gallamine, effect on hippocampal β-amyloid precursor protein levels, 511
GAP43, 2
Gender differences, in Parkinson's disease prevalence, 371
Gene therapy, for Parkinson's disease, with adeno-associated virus vectors, 647–652
Geriatric Mental State Examination, 389
Gertsman-Sträussler-Scheinker disease, 121
  meningocerebrovascular Hungarian-type, 122, 124
Glial cell line-derived neurotrophic factor, neuroprotective properties, 164
  in Parkinson's disease, 607–614
Glial cells, haloperidol-induced neurotoxicity inhibition in, 165, 166–167
Glial derived neurotrophic factor, 637, 638
Glial fibrillary acidic protein, mRNA, expression in Alzheimer's disease brains, 114
Glial S-100, mRNA, expression in Alzheimer's disease brains, 114
Global Deterioration Scale scores, of Alzheimer's disease and Parkinson's disease patients, 266
Glucose, as neuronal posthypoxia energy substrate, 171, 173–175

Glucose metabolism, cerebral
  Alzheimer's disease-related impairment of, 587–588
    as cognitive impairment cause, 589–591
    differential diagnosis of dementia and, 751–756
  Parkinson's disease-related impairment of, 752
  positron emission tomographic assessment of, 838
  reduction of, neurodegenerative effects of, 47
GLUT 1 transporter, 588
GLUT 4 transporter, 588
Glutamate
  excitotoxicity of, effect of salicylates on, 100–101,
      102
  locus coeruleus immunoreactivity of, 90
  neurotoxicity, 84–85
    in AF64A neurotoxicity, 685
    apoptosis-inducing activity, 84–85
    astrocytes in, 90
  nicotinic acetylcholine receptor-mediated secretion,
      463
Glutamatergic pyramidal neurons, cholinoreceptive,
      drug-enhanced activity, 851, 852–853, 855,
      856–857
Glutamic acid decarboxylase, cerebral hemispheric lo-
      calization, 280
Glutamine, neuroprotection against, 466
Glutaminergic neurons, effect of cholinesterase inhibi-
      tors on, 446
Glutathione
  antioxidant activity of, 54, 415
  reduced
      in dopaminergic cell apoptosis, 106, 107, 110
      in haloperidol-induced neurotoxicity, 166–167, 168
      oxidized/total ratio, age-related changes in, 54
Glutathione reductase, Parkinson's disease-related de-
      crease, 779, 780, 781, 783, 784
Glutathione S-transferase, 397
Glycation, 78, 79
Glycerol-3-phosphorycholine, brain content in, in
      Alzheimer's disease, 301
Glycerol-3-phosphorycholine phosphodiesterase, brain
      content, in Alzheimer's disease, 305
Glycerophosphocholine, brain content, in Alzheimer's
      disease, 301
Glycerophosphorylcholine, brain content, in Alzhe-
      imer's disease, 305
Glycerophosphorylethanolamine, brain content, in
      Alzheimer's disease, 305
Golgi apparatus
  dispersion of, 3
  size of, in Alzheimer's disease, 279–280, 281, 282
G-proteins, muscarinic agonist coupling by, 516, 519,
      520–521
Grooming behavior, substance-induced, effect of post-
      proline cleaving enzyme inhibitor on, 654,
      656, 658, 659
GTS21, 475
Guanfacine, effect on attentional performance, 725–731
Guanosine triphosphate cyclohydrolase I gene, het-
      erozygotic donor of, 363–364, 365, 368

H-7, β-amyloid precursor protein-inhibiting activity
      of, 134
Hallucinations
  Alzheimer's disease-related, 317, 452
  dementia with Lewy bodies-related, 353, 356, 452,
      453, 454, 455–456, 460, 457
    cholinesterase inhibitor control of, 460
  Parkinson's disease-related, 452, 460
  schizophrenia-related, 452
Haloperidol
  extrapyramidal effects of, 163
  neurotoxicity
    antioxidant-related neuroprotection against, 164,
      165–168
    in mouse embryo brain tissue, 163–170
H antagonists, 455
HB-GAM protein: see Heparin binding growth associ-
      ated molecule (HB-GMA)
Head injury, see also Brain injury
  as Alzheimer's disease risk factor, 757
Heme oxygenase-1, in oxidative stress response, 79
Hemispheric lateralization, neurotransmitter distribu-
      tion and, 280, 282
Heparin binding growth associated molecule (HB-
      GAM), in cerebral amyloidoses, 121–131
  β-amyloid binding activity, 122, 123, 126, 128, 129,
      130
  immunohistochemistry of, 122–123, 124–126, 127
Heparin sulfate proteoglycan
  interaction with amyloid A, 218
  as senile plaque component, 495
Heptylphysostigmine, effect on acetylcholinesterase
      G1/G4 forms, 448
Hereditary cerebral hemorrhage with amyloidosis-
      Dutch type, heparin binding growth associ-
      ated molecule in, 122, 124, 125, 128
High performance liquid chromatography, for cerebral
      β-amyloid protein detection, 824, 826
Hippocampus, see also Entorhinal cortex
  β-amyloid in vivo neurotoxicity in, 705–709
  β-amyloid (25–35) neurotoxicity in, 90, 93, 94, 95
  β-amyloid precursor protein levels in, effect of mus-
      carinic receptors on, 511
  anti-inflammatory drug-related neuroprotection in,
      100–101
  atrophy of, 13
  CA1 neurons
    age-dependent muscarinic plasticity of, 661–
      666
    β-amyloid-induced degeneration, 705–709
    β-amyloid (25–35) neurotoxicity in, 93
    DNA mismatch repair system in, 84
    immunocytology of, 9–10
    ischemia-induced degeneration of, 705
    lactate-mediated posthypoxia synaptic recovery
      of, 171–176
    N-methyl-D-asparate-mediated injury to, 101
    serotonin receptor-enhanced GABAergic action
      of, 854

Hippocampus (*cont.*)
CA3 neurons
β-amyloid (25–35) neurotoxicity in, 93, 95
anapsos-mediated neurodegeneration in, 699–703
N-methyl-D-aspartate-mediated injury to, 101
serotonin receptor-related long-term potentiation inhibition of, 854
cholineacetyltransferase activity in, effect of nitric oxide on, 682–685
cholinesterase inhibiting activity in, 448
phospholipid content, 302, 303, 305
tau protein abnormalities in, 7
volume decrease, relationship to memory impairment, 13, 14
Human immunodeficency virus (HIV), envelope protein, neurotoxicity of, 637
Human immunodeficiency virus (HIV) vector system, 649
Huntington's chorea
embryonal brain tissue transplant treatment for, 643–646
memory impairment associated with, 265
Mini Mental State Examination scores in, 377, 378, 381–382
Huperzine A, 601–605
acetylcholinesterase complexes, 525–528
HuAChE mutants, 532, 533, 534–535, 536–537
C-substituted analogues, 602–605
molecular modeling of, 603–605
Hydrogen peroxide
apoptosis-induced activity, 45
in long-term potentiation, 665
in oxidative stress, 425–426
pro-oxidant activity, 54
as reactive hydroxyl radicals source, 422
Hydroperoxyl radicals, 54
6-Hydroxydopamine, endogenous, 421
antioxidant protection against, 425–426
interaction with mitochondrial enzymes, 423
in Parkinson's disease, 422–423
sources of, 422–423
6-Hydroxydopamine-lesioned rats, as Parkinson's disease model, gene therapy in, 651
Hydroxyl radicals, pro-oxidant activity of, 54
Hydroxynoneal, 78
Hypertension, dementia associated with, 389, 390, 391, 392, 799–803
Hypokinesia, Parkinson's disease-related, dopaminergic responsiveness of, 435–438
Hypoxia, lactate-mediated neuronal recovery following, 171–176
Hypoxic-ischemic injury, nitric oxide in, 681–682
Hypoxic training, interval, 717–723

Imaging studies, of Alzheimer's disease, 837–838
Immune function, anapsos-related enhancement of, 699
192-Immunoglobulin G-saporin, 667–674

Immunoglobulin light chain
as β-amyloid precursor protein, 214, 215–216
4'-iodo-4'-deoxydoxorubicin binding of, 199
Immunotoxins, 670–671
Incontinence, senile dementia-related, 319, 320, 321
Indomethacin, neuroprotective properties of, 99, 100, 102
Inflammation-associated protein, 218–219
Inflammatory processes, in Alzheimer's disease, 588
salicylate therapy for, 99–104
Insulin
as β-amyloid precursor protein, 214, 215
cerebral activity of, in Alzheimer's disease, 287–292, 588
Insulin-like growth factor, cerebral, 287–292
Insulin-like growth factor-1, 164, 637
in electrical blockade-related neuronal apoptosis, 638
Insulin-like growth factor 1 receptors, 288, 290–291
Insulin-like growth factor-2, 637
Insulin receptors, cerebral, 287–292
Intelligence quotient, of Alzheimer's disease patients, correlation with parietotemporal blood flow decrease, 736–737
Interferon-β and γ, matrix metalloproteinease-modulating activity of, 150, 152, 153
Interleukin(s), neurotrophic properties of, 637, 638
Interleukin-1, in Alzheimer's disease
effect on β-amyloid precursor protein processing, 137
brain and cerebrospinal fluid content, 137
Interleukin-1β
cerebral content, anapsos-related decrease, 699–700
in Parkinson's disease, 409–410
Interleukin-2
in Alzheimer's disease, hippocampal content, 410
in Parkinson's disease, cerebrospinal fluid content, 409–410
Interleukin-3, in Alzheimer's disease, hippocampal content, 410
Interleukin-4
in Alzheimer's disease, hippocampal content, 410
in Parkinson's disease, cerebrospinal fluid content, 409–410
Interleukin-6
in Alzheimer's disease, hippocampal content, 410
matrix metalloproteinase-modulating activity, 149–151, 152, 153, 154, 155
in Parkinson's disease, cerebrospinal fluid content, 409–410
International Alzheimer's Disease Conference, 862, 863
International Federation of Pharmaceutical Manufacturers' Association, 862–863
International Geneva/Springfield Symposium on Advances in Alzheimer's Therapy, 863
International Psychogenic Association, 862–863
International Working Group on the Harmonization of Dementia Drug Guidelines, 862–865

Interval hypoxic training, 717–723
4'-Iodo-4'-deoxydoxorubicin
    amyloidosis-inhibiting activity of, 198–203
        in experimental scrapie, 201–203
    structure, 198
Iron
    in Alzheimer's disease, 422
    antioxidant protection against, 47–48, 50
    apoptosis-inducing activity, 45
    brain accumulation, 422
    dopamine-induced chelation of, 424
    free radical potentiating activity, 79, 90, 422
    in Huntington's disease, 422
    as hydroxyl radical catalyst, 79
    in multisystem atrophy, 422
    in neurofibrillary tangles, 79
    in Parkinson's disease, 422
    as reactive hydroxyl radical source, 422
    in supranuclear palsy, 422
Irritability, Alzheimer's disease-related, 317
Ischemia, cerebral, nitric oxide in, 681–682

K252a, 506–507
Kinesin, in β-amyloid precursor protein transport, 489
Korsakoff's disease, 279

Lactate, as posthypoxia neuronal energy substrate,
        171–76, 171–176
Lactate dehydrogenase
    effect on 1-benzyl-1,2,3,4-tetrahydroisoquinoline-in-
        duced toxicity, 430–432
    as membrane activity indicator, 564, 565, 566–567
    resistance to AF64A, 669
    secretion, effect of tacrine on, 564, 565, 566–567
Language impairment, Alzheimer's disease-related,
        272, 273–274
L-dopa: see Levodopa
Learning
    anapsos-related enhancement of, 699–703
    effect of excess acetylcholinesterase on, 553
    metrifonate-related enhancement of, 584
Leber, Paul, 862
Lecithin, as choline and acetylcholine precursor, 446
Leprosy, β-amyloid in, 214
Leukemia inhibitory factor, 637, 638
Levodopa
    as hallucination cause, 455
    as Parkinson's disease therapy, 421, 647–648
        motor fluctuation effects of, 439–444
    as parkinsonism freezing phenomenon treatment, 332
Lewy bodies
    in autosomal dominant parkinsonism, 401–402
    familial Parkinson's disease-related degeneration,
        401–402
    influence on response to tacrine, 477–480
    insolubility of, 78
Lewy body dementia: see Dementia, Lewy body
Lewy body-positive autosomal dominant Parkinson's
        disease, 393–394, 395

Lewy body-positive autosomal recessive Parkinson's
        disease, 394–395
Lipid peroxidation
    β-amyloid-induced, 49–50
    antioxidant-related inhibition of, at ultra-low doses,
        183–186
    end products of, 78, 79
    iron-induced, 49–50
    as oxidative damage index, 78
    in Parkinson's disease, 780, 783
    vitamin E-related prevention of, 168
Lipid transport, by apolipoprotein E phenotypes, 805,
        806, 808–809
Lipofuscin, in membrane lipid peroxidation, 54
Lipoproteins
    serum levels of, influence of apolipoprotein E geno-
        types on, 766–769
Lobeline, 475
Locomotor disturbances, in Parkinson's disease, effect
        of interval hypoxic training on, 717–723
Locus coeruleus, noradrenaline-containing neurons of,
        725
Low density lipoprotein-like receptor gene, polymor-
        phism of, 757
Low density lipoprotein receptor, 17, 21
Low density lipoprotein receptor gene family, 17
Low density lipoprotein receptor-related protein, 768
    apolipoprotein E ligand, 17, 18, 20, 21
L-threo-DOPS, as parkinsonism freezing phenomenon
        treatment, 332–33
Lu 25–109, 519
    maximum tolerated dose, 830, 831
Lymphocyte cultures, Alzheimer's disease, cen-
        tromeric disturbances in, 793–798
Lymphocytes, nicotinic receptor expression on, 465
Lysosomal enzymes, effect on β-amyloid formation,
        489

Magnetic resonance imaging, 734, 837–838
Malondialdehyde
    in Alzheimer's disease, 78
    in Parkinson's disease, 779, 781, 783, 784
Manganese superoxide dismutase gene, polymorphism
        segregation of, 402–404
    in autosomal recessive juvenile Parkinson's disease,
        402–405
Mania, alterations in consciousness associated with,
        452
Mannitol, effect on dopaminergic cell apoptosis, 110
Matrix metalloproteinases, in astroglial cells, cytokine-
        related modulation of, 149–157
MCI antibody, 8, 9–10
Mecamylamine, 466
Medullary cell cultures, β-amyloid neurotoxicity in,
        495–502
Membrane lipids, oxidative stress sensitivity and,
        55–57
Membrane permeability, β-amyloid (25–35)-related in-
        crease of, 90

Memory deficits
Alzheimer's disease-related, 318, 319, 320, 231
β-amyloid in, 90–97, 563–564
"amnesia" pattern of, 268, 269
anapsos therapy for, 699–703
animal models of, 553, 563–564, 711–716
antipsychotic drug-related, 319–320
apolipoprotein E e4 allele and, 13–16
cholinergic neuron impairment in, 711–716
ENA713 therapy for, 587–593
episodic, 265–270
excess acetylcholinesterase-related, 553
huperzine therapy for, 526
muscarinic agonist treatment for, 518–518
post-proline cleaving enzyme therapy for, 653–660
effect of quaternary-lipophilic carbamates on, 595–600
release from "proactive inhibition" effect in, 309–315
Parkinson's disease-related, 265–270
Mesencephalic slice culture, 1-benzyl-1,2,3,4-tetrahy-droisoquinoline toxicity in, 429–433
dopamine-induced decrease of, 431, 432–433
lactate dehydrogenase-induced decrease in, 430–432
Methamphetamine, nitric oxide-mediated neurotoxic-ity, 681
Methionine residues, apolipoproptein E isoform con-tent, 36
N-Methyl-D-aspartate
hallucinations and, 455
salicylate-mediated neurotoxicity, 101
4-Methyl-2,6-ditertiary butylphenol, 178–179
RS-Methyl-1(morpholinyl-2 methoxy)-8 tetrahydro-1,2,3,4-quinoline, in nicotinic neurotransmis-sion, 469–476
1-Methyl-4-phenylpyridinium ion, 67, 413
1-Methyl-4-phenyl-1,2,3,6-tetrahydropyridine, neuro-toxicity of, 105
antioxidant-mediated, 167
nitric oxide-mediated, 681
parkinsonism-inducing activity of, 67, 607–614
1-Methyl-4-phenyl-1,2,3,6-tetrahydropyridine-lesioned rats, interval hypoxic training of, 717–723
1-Methyl(R)salsolinol, apoptosis-inducing activity, 105–111
effect of antioxidants on, 106, 107, 110
1-Methyl-1,2,3,4-tetrahydroisoquinoline
as Parkinson's disease-inducing and prophylactic agent, 429
structure, 430
1-Methyl-1,2,3,6-tetrahydropyridine, 779
N-Methyltransferases, in Parkinson's disease, 413, 414
cerebral levels, 417–418
cerebrospinal fluid levels, 419
lymphocytic activity, 418
Metrifonate, as Alzheimer's disease therapy, 447, 579–585
cholinesterase inhibiting activity, 581–582
cognitive enhancing activity, 583–584
efficacy of, comparative study of, 572, 573, 574
prodrug activity, 580
Metrifonate, as Alzheimer's disease therapy (cont.)
safety and tolerability, 582–583
side effects of, 572
Microglia, synaptic degeneration-related activation, 3–4
Microgliosis, Alzheimer's disease-related, 197, 198
β-Microglobulin
4'-iodo-4'-deoxydoxorubicin binding by, 199
in Parkinson's disease, striatal content, 410–411
Microsomal membranes, as free radical source, 54
Microtubules
absence from neurofibrillary tangle neurons, 235–236
cortical neuronal, deficiency of, 3
tau protein-related assembly of, 236
Midbrain reticular formation, 457
Millard reaction (glycation), 78
Mini-Mental State Examination scores, 389, 848
of Alzheimer's disease patients, 266, 338
comparison with Parkinson's disease and Hunt-ington's chorea patients, 377, 378, 381–382
effect of tacrine on, 478, 479
cultural and educational factors affecting, 734
of parkinsonism patients, 338, 339, 340
of Parkinson's disease patients, 266, 344, 345, 377, 378, 381–382
effect of tacrine on, 482, 483
Minnesota Multiphasic Personality Inventory, use with Parkinson's disease patients' caregivers, 372, 377
Misidentifications, Alzheimer's disease-related, 317
Mitochondrial dysfunction
Alzheimer's disease-associated, 59–66
cybrid models of, 61–64
cytochrome c oxidase defects in, 61–64
pseudogene DNA/mtDNA ratio in, 62–63
Parkinson's disease-associated, 68–70
complex I in, 67–75
cybrid models of, 69–73
Monoamine oxidase gene, Parkinson's disease-associ-ated, 397
Monoclonal antibodies
β-amyloid epitope binding, 205–211
aggregation-inhibiting effects, 207–210
binding profiles, 206
for tau protein, 7, 8–10
Motor dysfunction
Parkinson's disease-related, effect of tacrine on, 481, 483, 484, 485
senile dementia-related, 318, 319, 320, 321
Motor memory, of Alzheimer's disease patients, 309–315
MSH2, effect on apoptosis, 81, 83–84, 85
Multiple sclerosis, memory impairment associated with, 265
Muscarinic acetylcholine receptors, in Alzheimer's dis-ease, 445
in β-amyloid precursor protein processing, 509–513
decrease of, 515

Muscarinic acetylcholine receptors, in Alzheimer's disease (*cont.*)
   hippocampal, age-dependent plasticity of, 661–666
   as muscarinic agonist target, 503
   subtypes
      as Alzheimer's disease treatment target, 516
      in oxidative stress vunerability, 57
Muscarinic agonists, 459, 460
   effect on β-amyloid precursor protein processing,
      517–518, 520–521
   effect on β-amyloid production, 137
   combined with cholinesterase inhibitors, 575–576
   G-protein coupling, 516, 519, 520–521
   hallucinations and, 455
   memory-enhancing properties of, 518–519
   muscarinic receptor selectivity of, 516
   neurotrophic-like effects of, 516–517, 520
   non-selective, 446
   selective, 446–447
   signal transduction effects of, 503–508, 516–519,
      520–521
Muscarinic antagonists, selective, 446–447
Music therapy, for Parkinson's disease patients,
   373–374
Myoclonus, senile dementia-related, 319, 320, 321

Na,K-ATPase, isoform mRNA, expression in brains of
   Alzheimer's disease patients, 113–119
NAC (non-β-amyloid component), 166, 168, 495
NADH-CoQ reductase, Parkinson's disease-related reduction of, 779, 782
NADH:ubiquinone oxidoreductase (complex 1) dysfunction, in Parkinson's disease, 67–75
   cybrid models of, 69–73
NAN-190, 853
Neocortex, β-amyloid (25–35) neurotoxicity in, 93
Nerve cell death, *see also* Apoptosis
   effect of polyamines on, 159–162
Nerve growth factor, 637
   as Alzheimer's disease treatment, 854–855
   in electrical blockade-related neuronal apoptosis,
      638
   effect on non-amyloidogenic β-amyloid precursor
      protein processing, 506
   as p75 ligand, 615–616, 617
   receptors, cholinergic neuronal expression, 688
   mRNA, in AF64A-lesioned rats, 678
   septo-hippocampal pathway localization, 687–688
   transferrin receptor conjugate, 672
   as tyrosine kinase receptor ligand, 615–616
      agonistic polyclonal antibodies for, 619–622
      artificial Trka ligand development and, 617–616
      binding domains, 616–619
      diagnostic and therapeutic applications, 622–616
      nerve growth factor analog development and,
         617–616
Netherlands Brain Bank, 277–285
Neurite outgrowth, acetylcholinesterase in, 557–
   562

Neurofibrillary tangles, 1–2, 773
   apolipoprotein E e4 allele-related accumulation of, 13
   in dementia with Lewy bodies, 453
   formation of, 7, 235–236
   immunocytochemistry of, 9–10
   insolubility of, 77–78
   paired helical filaments' dissociation from, 238
   relationship to Alzheimer's disease progression, 235
   RNA content, 231
   solubility of, 78
   tau protein incorporation into, 77–78
Neurofilament proteins, gene expression, developmental regulation of, 242
Neurogenesis, cholinesterases in, 541–549
Neuroimmunotrophic drugs, as Alzheimer's disease
   prophylaxis, 700, 702
Neuroleptic malignant syndrome, dementia with Lewy
   bodies-associated, 351–357
Neuroleptics, *see also* Chlorpromazine; Clozapine;
   Haloperidol
   effect on serotonergic neuronal turnover, 856
   as unconsciousness cause, in dementia with Lewy
      bodies, 456
Neuromelanin, 422, 782
Neuronal degeneration, Alzheimer's disease-related,
   773
   anapsos-mediated neuroprotection against, 699–703
   tau phosphatase-mediated prevention of, 238
Neurons
   Alzheimer's disease-related loss of, 806
   β-amyloid precursor protein trafficking and processing in, 488–493
      anterograde transport, 489
      characterization of APP-containing organelles,
         490–493
      cytoplasmic proteins' role in, 492–493
      endocytic pathway, 488–489, 490
      insertion in nerve-terminal plasma membrane,
         489–490
      localization, 489
      retrograde transport, 490
Neurotransmitters, in Alzheimer's disease drug development, 851–859
Neurotrophic factors, as Alzheimer's disease treatment, 687
Neurotrophin(s), 615, 616
Neurotrophin 3, 637, 638
Neurotrophin 4/5, 637, 638
NF-KB transcription factor, 84–85
   salicylate-related inhibition of, 101–102
Nicotine, neuroprotective activity of, 466
Nicotinic acetylcholine receptors
   Alzheimer's disease-related decrease of, 445
   as Alzheimer's disease target, 463–468
   effect of cholinesterase inhibitors on, 465–466
   interaction with anesthetic agents, 458
   interaction with S 12024–2, 469–476
   effect of nicotinic agonists on, 465, 466, 467
   neurotransmitter modulating function of, 463, 464

Nicotinic agonists, 460, 466
    as Alzheimer's disease therapy, 446–447
    combined with cholinesterase inhibitors, 575–576
    effect on nicotinic acetylcholine receptors
Nitric oxide, lack of effect on AF64A neurotoxicity,
        681–686
Nitric oxide synthase, 397, 681
n-myc gene, effect of AF64A on, 676
Non-β-amyloid component (NAC), 166, 168, 495
Noradrenaline neurons, Parkinson's disease-related
        loss of, 348
Noradrenergic system, neurotoxin-induced β-amyloid
        precursor protein secretion in, 696
NORDIC Study Group, 865
Norepinephrine transporter proteins, phenyltropanes'
        affinity for, 739–743
Northern Ireland population, apolipoprotein E-Alzhe-
        imer's disease association in, 806–809
Notch receptor signaling pathway, 188
Nuclear membranes, as free radical source, 54
Nucleus basalis of Meynert
    in Alzheimer's disease, 541
        Golgi apparatus size in, 279–280, 281, 282
    effect of neurotoxins on, 695–696
Nutritional therapy, for Parkinson's disease, 373–374

Occupational therapy, for Parkinson's disease, 373–374
Okadaic acid, 136
Olfactory cortex, β-amyloid (25–35) neurotoxicity in,
        93, 95
Oligodendrocytes, antioxidant vitamin and enzyme
        content, 166–167
Ondansetron, 854
Opioid antagonists, 455
Ornithine decarboxylase, stress-related activity in-
        crease, 160
Osteomyelitis, β-amyloid in, 214
Overactivity, Alzheimer's disease drug therapy-re-
        lated, 851, 855–856
Oxidation
    apolipoprotein E isoforms' susceptibility to, 31–38
    effect on apolipoprotein E-mediated phospholipid
        redistribtion, 32–37
Oxidative stress
    AF64A-induced, 677
    aging-related sensitivity to, 55–57
        tests for, 54–57
    β-amyloid (25–35) neurotoxicity-related, 89–99
    as Alzheimer's disease cause, 3, 60–61, 77–80
        antioxidant neuroprotection against, 79
    definition of, 53
    interval hypoxic training-related prevention of,
        717–723
    in iron-mediated neurotoxicity, 47–48, 50
    as Parkinson's disease cause, peripheral blood indi-
        ces of, 779–785
    sources of, 53–54
    as tardive dyskinesia cause, 167
Oxotremorine, 511, 516–517

p3 peptide, formation of, 488
    protein kinase C-enhanced, 134–135
    p97 protein, 837
Paired helical filaments, 235; see also Neurofibrillary
        tangles
    dephosphorylation of, 237–238
    microtubule-associated protein content, 235–236
Pallidotomy, 333, 607
Palsy, progressive supranuclear, 279, 330, 331
Paralysis agitans, 337
    of early-onset with marked diurnal fluctuation of
        symptoms, 402, 405
Parietal cortex, phospholipid content, in Alzheimer's
        disease, 301–305
Parkinson, James, 337, 817
Parkinson's disease
    Alzheimer's disease-like parietotemporal perfusion
        deficits associated with, 734
    animal models of
        glial cell line-derived neurotrophic factor effects
            in, 607–614
        interval hypoxic training in, 717–723
    apolipoprotein E associated with, in Northern Ire-
        land population, 806–809
    apoptosis associated with, 105, 413
    autosomal recessive juvenile, manganese superox-
        ide dismutase gene polymorphism in,
        402–405
    cerebrospinal fluid in
        1-benzyl-1,2,3,4-tetrahydroisoquinoline content, 431
        cytokine content, 407–412
    coexistence with Alzheimer's disese, 371
    cognitive impairment without dementia
        neuropathology of, 348
        prevalence of, 343–350
        relationship to disease severity, 347
    in Contursi kindred, 348
    definition of, 407
    dementia of: see Dementia, Parkinson's disease-re-
        lated
    diagnostic criteria for, 347
    dopaminergic degeneration associated with, 413
        chromosome 6q25.2–27 gene locus of, 401–406
    embryonal brain tissue transplant treatment for,
        643–646
    epilepsy associated with, case history of, 359–361
    extrapyramidal symptoms, effect of cholinergic
        drugs on, 481, 483, 484
    familial
        autosomal dominant Lewy body-positive,
            393–394, 395
        autosomal recessive Lewy-body negative,
            394–395
        clinical phenotypes, 395
    freezing phenomenon of, 329–335
        clinical features of, 331–332
        pathophysiology of, 331
        treatment for, 332–333
    genetic factors-related, 779

Parkinson's disease (*cont.*)
hallucinations associated with, 452
idiopathic
cognitive impairment of, 337–340
prevalence, 371
intraneuronal inclusions in, insolubility of, 77–78
intrauterine events-related, 779
iron in, 423
levodopa-responsive, autosomal recessive form,
401–402
levodopa therapy, 421, 647–648
relationship to motor fluctuations and dyskineisa,
435–438
Lewy bodies associated with, 347, 348
memory impairment associated with, 265–270
mitochondrial dysfunction in, cybrid models of, 69–73
neuropathology of, 421, 752
cytokines associated with, 407–412
neurotoxin-induced, 105
nucleus basalis of Meynert in, 279, 279
peripheral blood oxidative stress indices of, 779–785
pharmacological therapy, 373, 607; *see also* Parkinson's disease, levodopa therapy
post-encephalitic, 344
prevalence, 371
projected increase of, 861
relationship to dementia with Lewy bodies,
452–453, 454, 455, 460
sporadic, genetic predisposition in, 396–396
surgical treatment, 373, 607
symptoms of, 393, 607, 752
relationship to severity of dopamine neuron destruction, 670
tacrine treatment for, effect on motor function, 481,
483, 484, 485
viral infection-related, 779
Parkinson's disease patients, interpersonal relations
with family members, 371–376
Parkinsonism
autosomal-recessive early onset, diurnal fluctuation
in, 367, 368
dementia associated with, 319
dystonic juvenile, 367, 368
MPTP-induced, 105
vascular, freezing phenomenon of, 330, 331
Parkinson Study Group, 865
Parkinson syndrome, atypical, cognitive impairment
of, 337–340
Paroxetine, as serotonergic terminals marker, in depression, 856 257–263
PD142505–0028, 853
Pentosidine, 78
Peptidoorrganic inhibitors, 191–195
Peroxidase, antioxidant activity, 54
Phenosan, ultra-low dose, 183–186
effect on membrane-bound acetylcholinesterase ac-
tivity, 178–791
Phenserine, effect on cerebrospinal fluid β-amyloid
precursor protein levels, 696–697

Phenyltropane analogs, affinity for forebrain
monoamine transporters, 739–645
Phosphatidylcholine
brain content, in Alzheimer's disease, 302, 303,
304, 305, 306
membrane, 301
Phosphatidylethanolamine, brain content, in Alzheimer's disease, 302, 304, 305
Phosphatidylinositol, brain content, in Alzheimer's disease, 302, 304
Phosphatidylserine, brain content, in Alzheimer's disease, 302, 304
Phosphoaminoacids, 9
Phosphoepitopes, of tau protein, antibody recognition
of, 9
Phosphoinositide, hydrolysis of, effect of muscarinic
agonists on, 503, 504–505
Phospholipase A, β-amyloid (25–35)-related stimulation, 90
Phospholipase C
β-amyloid (25–35)-related stimulation, 90
muscarinic agonist binding by, 517
effect on tau protein phosphorylation, 446
Phospholipase D, β-amyloid (25–35)-related stimulation, 90
Phospholipids
apolipoprotein E interaction, 31, 32–37
brain content, in Alzheimer's disease, 301–307
Phosphoprotein phosphorylases, in tau protein dephosphorylation, 237–238
Physical therapy, for Parkinson's disease, 373–374
Physostigmine, 595
effect on acetylcholinesterase G1/G4 forms, 448
effect on cerebral blood flow, 446
effect on cerebrospinal fluid β-amyloid precursor
protein levels, 511, 696
efficacy, comparative study of, 573
effect on glutamate release, 853
effect on hippocampal β-amyloid precursor protein
levels, 511
half-life of, 595
inhibitory action mode of, 447
lack of effect on amyloid precursor protein secretion, 568
as Parkinson's disease treatment, 373
toxicity of, 595
Pick's disease
Alzheimer's disease misdiagnosed as, 733–734
cerebral atrophy in, 279
nucleus basalis of Meynert in, 279
Plasma membranes, β-amyloid precursor protein localization in, 489–490
Platelet-derived growth factor, 638
Platelets, β-amyloid precursor protein isoforms in, as
Alzheimer's disease marker, 747–750
Polyamine-stress-response, 159–162
Polyneuropathy, familial amyloid, 214, 216
Polypodium leucotomos, 699
Positron emission tomography, 751–756, 837–838

Post-proline cleaving enzyme inhibitor, as cognitive
    deficit therapy, 653–660
PPI-368 (Cholyl-L-leucyl-L-valyl-L-phenylalanyl-L-
    phenylalanyl-L-alanine), 194
Presenilin
    apoptosis-related, 144–145
    effect on Golgi apparatus, 3
Presenilin 1
    localization, 141
    peptide binding by, random peptide display library-
        assisted detection of, 141–147
Presenilin 1 gene
    as Alzheimer's disease gene locus, 765
    as early-onset familial Alzheimer's disease marker,
        835, 836
    genotype 1/1, influence on serum apolipoprotein E
        content, 767–769
    mutations of, 28–29, 509, 841
        β-amyloid accumulation associated with, 198, 487
        as autosomal dominant trait, 187
        early-onset familial Alzheimer's disease-related,
            787
        intronic, 187
        Leu286-Val, 144, 146
    S182, as familial Alzheimer's disease gene, 793
Presenilin 2, peptide binding to, 141, 142, 144–145
Presenilin 2 gene, Alzheimer's disease-associated mu-
        tations of, 835, 836, 841
    β-amyloid accumulation associated with, 198, 487
    as autosomal dominant trait, 187
    as early-onset familial Alzheimer's disease marker,
        787, 835, 836
Presenilin gene mutations, early-onset familial Alzhe-
        imer's disease-related, fibroblast acylphos-
        phatase levels in, 787–791
Presenilin proteins, interaction with Notch receptor
        signaling pathway, 188
Prion protein
    as β-amyloid precursor protein, 214, 216
    protease-resistant (PrP^{res}), β-amyloid fibril aggregat-
        ing activity of, 198
        anthracycline-related inhibition of, 198–203
Prion protein amyloid plaques, 121
Prion-related disorders, 198
    anthracyclin-related protease resistant prion protein
        inhibition in, 201–203
    heparin binding growth associated molecule in, 121–131
Probucol, neuroprotective activity of
    against β-amyloid-induced apoptosis, 49, 50
    lipid peroxidation-inhibiting activity, 49–50
    against oxidative damage, 47, 48
Proinsulin, 291
Propyl gallate, neuroprotective activity, 47–48, 110
Prostaglandin endoperoxide H synthase enzyme, 101
Proteases, antioxidant activity, 54
Protein kinase C
    β-amyloid-induced inhibition of, 492
    in β-amyloid precursor protein processing,
        133–136, 137, 138, 506–507

Protein kinase C/phospholipase C-linked first messen-
        gers, 137
Protein phosphatase 1, 136
Protein phosphatase 2B, 136
β-Protein precursor, as β-amyloid precursor protein,
        214, 217–218
Pseudogene DNA/mtDNA ratio, 62–63
Psychiatric disorders, Alzheimer's disease-related, 317
Psychosis
    Alzheimer's disease drug therapy-related, 851,
        855–856
    senile dementia-related, 319, 320, 321
Psychotherapy, for Parkinson's disease patients,
        373–374
Pykamilon, effect on visual evoked potentials,
        841–845
Pyridostigmine
    derivatives of, as Alzheimer's disease inhibitors,
        595–600
    as myasthenia gravis therapy, 595
    as poisoning prophylactic, 595
Pyrraline, 78
Pyruvate dehydrogenase, as acetylCoA source, 587

Rabin, Ytzak, assassination of, 385–387
Racial differences, in Parkinson's disease prevalence,
        371
Random peptide display libraries, 141–147
Raphe neurons, serotonergic dorsal, in Alzheimer's
        disease, 852
ras protein, in β-amyloid precursor protein processing,
        506–075
Reactive hydroxyl radicals, iron-generated, 422
Reactive oxygen species
    in neurodegenerative diseases, 422
    as protein carbonyl source, 424
Respiratory therapy, for Parkinson's disease patients,
        373–374
Retinoic acid, effect on dopaminergic cell apoptosis,
        107, 110
Retinospheroids
    acetylcholinesterase effects on, 544, 545–547
    butyrylcholinesterase effects on, 544–545
    as retinogenesis *in vitro* assay system, 542–544
Retroviral vectors, 649
Rey Auditory Verbal Learning Test scores, of Alzhe-
        imer's disease, Parkinson's disease, and
        Huntington's chorea patients, 378, 379–380,
        381
Rey-Osterieth Complex Figure test scores
    of Alzheimer's disease, Parkinson's disease, and
        Huntington's chorea patients, 378, 380
Ribose-inactivating proteins, 671
Ricin, 671
Rigidity, Parkinson's disease-related, dopaminergic re-
        sponsiveness of, 435–438
Ritanserin, 856
RN46A cell cultures, β-amyloid neurotoxicity in,
        495–502

RNA, effect on paired helical filament assembly, 230–231
RNA transcription, AF64A-induced premature termination, 669
mRNA
    acetylcholinesterase, antisense oligodeoxynucleotide-dependent suppression of, 553–554, 557–562
    β-amyloid precursor protein, 695–696
    glial fibrillary acidic protein, 114
    Na,K-ATPase, expression in brains of Alzheimer's disease patients, 113–119

S 12024–2, interaction with nicotonic neurotranmission, 469–476
S 17092–1, memory-enhancing effects, 653–660
Salicylates, neuroprotective activity, molecular characterization of, 99–104
SB-202026, 519
Schistosomiasis, metrifonate therapy for, 579
Schizophrenia, 452
Scopolamine, 458
    effect on cerebrospinal fluid β-amyloid precursor protein levels, 511, 697
Scrapie, protease-resistant prion protein accummulation in, 198
    anthracyclines-related inhibition of, 201–203
Secretase, 563
Secretase-a, 188, 488, 509, 517
Secretase-b, 488, 509
Secretase-y, 188, 509
Selective serotonin reuptake inhibitors, 856
Selegiline, 332, 848
Selenium, in haloperidol-induced neurotoxicity, 165, 166, 168
Semicarbazide, antioxidant activity of, 415
    in dopaminergic cell apoptosis, 107, 110
Senile plaques, 197
    C-terminal lipoprotein fragment content, 36–37
    dystrophic neurites of, 198
    structure of, 495
    in transgenic mice, 198
Septo-hippocampal pathway, cholinergic deficits of, nerve growth factor reversal of, 688–694
Serotonergic system
    acetylcholinesterase release modulation by, 853–854
    glutamatergic activity modulation by, 853
    effect of neuroleptic drugs on, 856
    neurotoxin-induced β-amyloid precursor protein secretion by, 696
Serotonin
    delusions and, 459
    pyramidal cell-inhibiting activity, 852
Serotonin receptors
    effect on acetyltransferase release, 853–854
    altered balance with $5HT_{2A}$ receptors, 852
    in anxiety, 856
Serotonin receptor antagonists, 853–854, 856
Serotonin transporter proteins, phenyltropanes' affinity for, 739–743

Severity index, of Alzheimer's disease, 837
Signal transduction, effect of muscarinic agonists on, 503–508, 516, 519, 520–521
Single photon emission computed tomography, 837–383
Sleep, REM
    acetylcholine levels during, 457
    dreaming during, 458–459
Sleep disorders
    Alzheimer's disease-related, 317–318
    senile dementia-related, 319, 320, 321, 323–327
Social memory, effect of S12024–2 on, 471, 473, 475
Social withdrawal, by Alzheimer's disease patients, 317
Sodium chloride, as hypertension risk factor, 391, 392
Sodium dodecyl sulfate polyacrylamide gel electrophoresis, 824–825, 827–828
Sodium valproate, as Parkinson's disease-related seizure therapy, 361
Speech therapy, for Parkinson's disease patients, 373–374
Sphingomyelin
    brain content, in Alzheimer's disease, 302, 304
    effect on oxidative stress sensitivity, 56–57
Stearyl-Nle^{17}-VIP, 635–637, 639–640
Stereotactic surgery, 333, 643, 644, 645
Stratospheroids, 543
Stress, polyamine-stress-response, 159–162
Stress proteins, 159
Striatum
    acetylcholine-stimulated dopamine release from, 484–485
    cholinergic deficits of, nerve growth factor-related reversal, 688–694
    in Parkinson's disease
        cytokine content, 407–412
        iron content, 423
    substance P-like immunoreactivity in, effect of post-proline cleaving enzyme inhibitor on, 654–655, 657–658, 659
Substance P, memory-enhancing activity, 653
Substance P-like immunoreactivity, effect of post-proline cleaving enzyme inhibitor on, 564–655, 657–658, 659
Substantia nigra
    apoptosis in, 105, 107
    iron content of, in Parkinson's disease, 422
    Lewy bodies in, 354
    in Parkinson's disease, 422, 442, 779
Subthalamic nucleus, deep brain stimulation of, 333
Superoxide dismutase
    antioxidant activity, 54
    Parkinson's disease-related increase, 779, 780, 781, 782, 783
Superoxide scavenging/generating activity, β-amyloid (25–35)-related, 91, 92, 93
Surrogate markers, for Alzheimer's disease, 838
Synapses
    Alzheimer's disease-related loss of, 3, 197, 198
    β-amyloid precursor protein localization in, 489, 491, 492, 493

Synaptic density, in Alzheimer's disease, 806
Synaptogenesis, in Alzheimer's disease, 15
Synaptosomes, membrane-bound acetylcholinesterase
      of, effect of antioxidants on, 177–181
α-Synuclein, 348, 394

Tacrine, 14
  acetylcholinesterase G1/G4 forms and, 448
  as acetylcholinesterase ligand, 524
  β-amyloid neurotoxicity inhibition by, 466
  clinical response to, effect of apolipoprotein E e4 al-
      lele on, 836
  cognitive effects, 853
  complexes with HuAChE mutants, 532, 533, 534,
      535–537
  efficacy of, 551–552, 595
    comparative study of, 572, 573, 574
    minimal, 373
  Food and Drug Administration approval of, 523, 595
  gastrointestinal side effects, 595
  hepatotoxicity of, 595
  effect on hippocampal β-amyloid precursor protein
      levels, 511
  interaction with nicotinic acetylcholine receptors,
      465
  Lewy body influenec on efficacy of, 477–480
  lysosomotropic action of, 568
  metabolism of, 447
  as Parkinson's disease-related dementia treatment,
      481–486
  pKa of, 568
  side effects of, 572
  effect on soluble β-amyloid secretion, 563–569
Tardive dyskinesia, vitamin E therapy for, 164, 167
Tau protein
  advanced glycation end products-induced, 79
  apolipoprotein E binding by, 13, 766
  cerebrospinal fluid content, enzyme-linked immu-
      noassay for, 775–776, 777
  as cytoskeletal protein, 241
  dephosphorylation of
    muscarinic acetylcholine receptor-mediated, 503
    muscarinic agonist-mediated, 518, 520
    site-specific, 237
  developmental regulation of, 242
  diagnostic applications of, 223
  in early Alzheimer's disease, 7–11
  expression during development, 241
  hyperphosphorylation, 3, 77, 235–236
    age dependency of, 252–255
    apolipoprotein E3-related prevention of, 252
    in apolipoprotein E-deficient mice, 251–256
    brain area specificity of, 252–255
    effect of cholimimetics on, 852
    ERK-1/ERK-2 expression in, 260–261, 262
    glycogen synthase kinase-3β expression in, 257,
      261–263
    microtubule-associated protein binding and, 236
    mitogen activated protein kinase expression in, 257

Tau protein (*cont.*)
  hyperphosphorylation (*cont.*)
    in PC12 and CHO cells, 257–263
    phosphatase inhibitors in, 260, 262
    protein phosphatases in, 236–237
    relationship to neurofibrillary tangles formation,
      77–78
  monoclonal antibodies, 7, 8–10
  mRNA isoforms
    in Alzheimer's disease, 247–248
    developmental expression of, 243–248
    following neuronal injury, 244, 247–248
  number of moles of phosphate in, 236
  in paired helical filament assembly, 224, 227–231
  phosphorylation, 224
    abnormal: *see* Tau protein, hyperphosphorylation
    developmental regulation, 242
    normal, 257
    phospholipase C-related reduction of, 446
  structure and conformation
    antibody reactivity and, 8
    microtubule binding domain-associated, 8
    relationship to paired helical filaments, 224–231
Tau-PHF protein, 7
Temporal cortex
  Lewy bodies in, 353, 355
  phospholipid content, in Alzheimer's disease, 303,
    305
Temporal lobe, apolipoprotein E e4 allele vulnerabil-
    ity of, 15
Tert-butylhydroperoxide, oxidative stress-induced ac-
    tivity, 47
Tertiary butyl hydroperoxide, 45
1,2,3,4-Tetrahydroisoquinoline (TIQ)
  as Parksinson's disease-inducing and prophylactic
    agent, 429
  structure, 430
Tetrazolium salts, metabolism of, effect of β-amyloid
    on, 497–500
TG3 antibody, 9–10
Thalamus, conscious awareness role of, 457, 460
Thiobarbituric acid reactive substances, 49, 50, 168
  β-amyloid (25–35)-related, 91–92, 93, 97
  apomorphine inhibition of, 423–424
  effect of interval hypoxic training on, 719, 720, 721
Thioflavin T, 123–124
Thranthyretin, 4'-iodo-4'-deoxydoxorubicin binding
    of, 199
Thrombin, 137
Thyroid-releasing hormone, 280
Tissue inhibitors of metalloproteinases (TIMPS),
    149–150, 153, 156
α-Tocopherol, as Alzheimer's disease treatment, 848
Trail Making Test scores, of Alzheimer's disease,
    Parkinson's disease, and Huntington's cho-
    rea patients, 378, 380
Transcranial Doppler ultrasonography, 812–814
Transentorhinal cortex, neurofibrillary pathology in, 7
Transferrin receptor, nerve growth factor conjugate, 672

Transgenic animal models
  of Alzheimer's disease, 217–218
  of β-amyloidosis, 215, 216–217
  of β-amyloid polymerization, 191
  of β-amyloid precursor protein mutations, 25–30
  anti-acetylcholinesterase antisense therapy in, 554
  of apolipoprotein E expression, 25, 28
Transthyretin, as β-amyloid precursor protein, 214, 216–217
Tremor, Parkinson's disease-related, 752
  dopaminergic responsiveness of, 435–438
Triglycerides, serum levels of, influence of apolipoprotein E genotype on, 766–769
Tris, effect on dopaminergic cell apoptosis, 110
Trolox, neuroprotective activity, 47–48
Tuberculosis, amyloid in, 214
Tubulin, gene expression, developmental regulation of, 242
Tubulin-α, fetal isoform, in Alzheimer's disease, 247
Tumor growth factor-α
  in Parkinson's disease, cerebrospinal fluid levels, 409–410
Tumor necrosis factor-α
  in Alzheimer's disease, 410
  matrix metalloproteinase-modulating activity, 149–151, 152, 153, 155, 156
  in Parkinson's disease, 409, 410
Tumor necrosis factor-β, matrix metalloproteinease-modulating activity, 150–151, 152, 154, 156
Tyrosine hydroxylase
  in hereditary progressive dystonia, 365, 366–368
  locus coeruleus immunoreactivity, 90
  memory-enhancing activity, 653
  as Parkinson's disease therapy, 648
Tyrosine hydroxylase gene
  adeno-associated virus vector-mediated transfer, 650, 651
  mutant, alleles, Parkinson's disease-associated, 397
Tyrosine kinase, in β-amyloid precursor protein processing, 506
Tyrosine kinase receptor, nerve growth factor ligands, 615–616
  agonistic polyclonal antibodies for, 619–622
  artificial Trka ligand development and, 617–616
  binding domains, 616–619
  diagnostic and therapeutic applications, 622–616
  nerve growth factor analogs and, 617–616

U-83836E, 90

Vasoactive intestinal peptide, neuroprotective activity of, 636
Vasoactive intestinal peptide agonist, 635–637
Velnacrine, maximum tolerated dose, 830
Very low density lipoprotein, apolipoprotein-enriched, 17–23
Very low density lipoprotein gene, polymorphism of, 757
Visual evoked potentials, in relatives of Alzheimer's disease patients, 841–845
Visuo-spatial impairment, Alzheimer's disease-related, 272, 273–274
Vitamin C
  antioxidant activity, 54
  lack of neuroprotective activity, in haloperidol-induced neurotoxicity, 165, 166, 168
Vitamin E
  neuroprotective activity, 51, 54, 90
    against AF64A-induced cholinotoxicity, 677
    in apoptosis, 45
    in haloperidol-induced neurotoxicity, 165, 166–167, 168
    in lipid peroxidation, 168
  as tardive dyskinesia therapy, 164, 167

WAL2014, effect on β-amyloid precursor protein secretion, 510, 517
WAL2014 YM-796, 519
WAY100–135, 853
Wechlser Adult Intelligence Scale scores, of Alzheimer's disease patients, Parkinson's disease, and Huntington's chorea patients, 344, 345, 346, 378, 379, 380
Western blot analysis, for cerebral β-amyloid protein detection, 824–825, 826, 827
Wisconsin Card Sorting Test scores, of Alzheimer's disease patients, Parkinson's disease, and Huntington's chorea patients, 344, 345, 346, 378
Women's Health Initiative Memory Study, 848
World Health Organization, 214, 862–863

Xanomeline, 517, 519, 517

Y337, 601–602

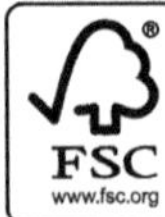